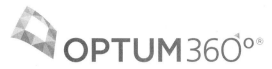

OB/GYN

A comprehensive illustrated guide to coding and reimbursement

2021

optum360coding.com

Publisher's Notice

Coding Companion for OB/GYN is designed to be an authoritative source of information about coding and reimbursement issues affecting obstetrics and gynecological procedures. Every effort has been made to verify accuracy and all information is believed reliable at the time of publication. Absolute accuracy cannot be guaranteed, however. This publication is made available with the understanding that the publisher is not engaged in rendering legal or other services that require a professional license.

American Medical Association Notice

CPT © 2020 American Medical Association. All rights reserved.

Fee schedules, relative value units, conversion factors and/or related components are not assigned by the AMA, are not part of CPT, and the AMA is not recommending their use. The AMA does not directly or indirectly practice medicine or dispense medical services. The AMA assumes no liability for data contained or not contained herein.

CPT is a registered trademark of the American Medical Association.

The responsibility for the content of any "National Correct Coding Policy" included in this product is with the Centers for Medicare and Medicaid Services and no endorsement by the AMA is intended or should be implied. The AMA disclaims responsibility for any consequences or liability attributable to or related to any use, nonuse or interpretation of information contained in this product.

Our Commitment to Accuracy

Optum360 is committed to producing accurate and reliable materials.

To report corrections, please email accuracy@optum.com. You can also reach customer service by calling 1.800.464.3649, option 1.

Copyright

Property of Optum360, LLC. Optum360 and the Optum360 logo are trademarks of Optum360, LLC. All other brand or product names are trademarks or registered trademarks of their respective owner.

© 2020 Optum360, LLC. All rights reserved.

Made in the USA

ISBN 978-1-62254-605-3

Acknowledgments

Marianne Randall, CPC, *Product Manager*

Stacy Perry, *Manager, Desktop Publishing*

Karen Krawzik, RHIT, CCS, AHIMA-approved ICD-10-CM/PCS Trainer, *Subject Matter Expert*

Anita Schmidt, BS, RHIA, AHIMA-approved ICD-10-CM/PCS Trainer, *Subject Matter Expert*

Tracy Betzler, *Senior Desktop Publishing Specialist*

Hope M. Dunn, *Senior Desktop Publishing Specialist*

Katie Russell, *Desktop Publishing Specialist*

Kimberli Turner, *Editor*

Subject Matter Experts

Karen Krawzik, RHIT, CCS, AHIMA-approved ICD-10-CM/PCS Trainer

Ms. Krawzik has expertise in ICD-10-CM, ICD-9-CM, CPT/HCPCS, DRG, and data quality and analytics, with more than 30 years' experience coding in multiple settings, including inpatient, observation, ambulatory surgery, ancillary, and emergency room. She has served as a DRG analyst and auditor of commercial and government payer claims, as a contract administrator, and worked on a team providing enterprise-wide conversion of the ICD-9-CM code set to ICD-10. More recently, she has been developing print and electronic content related to ICD-10-CM and ICD-10-PCS coding systems, MS-DRGs, and HCCs. Ms. Krawzik is credentialed by the American Health Information Management Association (AHIMA) as a Registered Health Information Technician (RHIT) and a Certified Coding Specialist (CCS) and is an AHIMA-approved ICD-10-CM/PCS trainer. She is an active member of AHIMA and the Missouri Health Information Management Association.

Anita Schmidt, BS, RHIA, AHIMA-approved ICD-10-CM/PCS Trainer

Ms. Schmidt has expertise in ICD-10-CM/PCS, DRG, and CPT with more than 15 years' experience in coding in multiple settings, including inpatient, observation, and same-day surgery. Her experience includes analysis of medical record documentation, assignment of ICD-10-CM and PCS codes, and DRG validation. She has conducted training for ICD-10-CM/PCS and electronic health record. She has also collaborated with clinical documentation specialists to identify documentation needs and potential areas for physician education. Most recently she has been developing content for resource and educational products related to ICD-10-CM, ICD-10-PCS, DRG, and CPT. Ms. Schmidt is an AHIMA-approved ICD-10-CM/PCS trainer and is an active member of the American Health Information Management Association (AHIMA) and the Minnesota Health Information Management Association (MHIMA).

Contents

Getting Started with Coding Companion

Coding Companion for OB/GYN is designed to be a guide to the specialty procedures classified in the CPT® book. It is structured to help coders understand procedures and translate physician narrative into correct CPT codes by combining many clinical resources into one, easy-to-use source book.

The book also allows coders to validate the intended code selection by providing an easy-to-understand explanation of the procedure and associated conditions or indications for performing the various procedures. As a result, data quality and reimbursement will be improved by providing code-specific clinical information and helpful tips regarding the coding of procedures.

CPT Codes

For ease of use, evaluation and management codes related to OB/GYN are listed first in the *Coding Companion*. All other CPT codes in *Coding Companion* are listed in ascending numeric order. Included in the code set are all surgery, radiology, laboratory, and medicine codes pertinent to the specialty. Each CPT code is followed by its official CPT code description.

Resequencing of CPT Codes

The American Medical Association (AMA) employs a resequenced numbering methodology. According to the AMA, there are instances where a new code is needed within an existing grouping of codes, but an unused code number is not available to keep the range sequential. In the instance where the existing codes were not changed or had only minimal changes, the AMA assigned a code out of numeric sequence with the other related codes being grouped together. The resequenced codes and their descriptions have been placed with their related codes, out of numeric sequence.

CPT codes within the Optum360 *Coding Companion* series display in their resequenced order. Resequenced codes are enclosed in brackets for easy identification.

ICD-10-CM

Overall, the 10th revision goes into greater clinical detail than did ICD-9-CM and addresses information about previously classified diseases, as well as those diseases discovered since the last revision. Conditions are grouped with general epidemiological purposes and the evaluation of health care in mind. New features have been added, and conditions have been reorganized, although the format and conventions of the classification remain unchanged for the most part.

Detailed Code Information

One or more columns are dedicated to each procedure or service or to a series of similar procedures/services. Following the specific CPT code and its narrative, is a combination of features. A sample is shown on page ii. The black boxes with numbers in them correspond to the information on the pages following the sample.

Appendix Codes and Descriptions

Some CPT codes are presented in a less comprehensive format in the appendix. The CPT codes appropriate to the specialty are included in the appendix with the official CPT code description. The codes are presented in numeric order, and each code is followed by an easy-to-understand lay description of the procedure.

The codes in the appendix are presented in the following order:

- HCPCS
- Surgery
- Radiology
- Pathology and Laboratory
- Medicine Services
- Category III

Category II codes are not published in this book. Refer to the CPT book for code descriptions.

CCI Edit Updates

The *Coding Companion* series includes the list of codes from the official Centers for Medicare and Medicaid Services' National Correct Coding Policy Manual for Part B Medicare Contractors that are considered to be an integral part of the comprehensive code or mutually exclusive of it and should not be reported separately. The codes in the Correct Coding Initiative (CCI) section are from version 26.3, the most current version available at press time. The CCI edits are located in a section at the back of the book. Optum360 maintains a website to accompany the Coding Companions series and posts updated CCI edits on this website so that current information is available before the next edition. The website address is http://www.optum360coding.com/ProductUpdates/. The 2021 edition password is: **SPECIALTY21**. Log in each quarter to ensure you receive the most current updates. An email reminder will also be sent to you to let you know when the updates are available.

Index

A comprehensive index is provided for easy access to the codes. The index entries have several axes. A code can be looked up by its procedural name or by the diagnoses commonly associated with it. Codes are also indexed anatomically. For example:

69501   Transmastoid antrotomy (simple mastoidectomy)

could be found in the index under the following main terms:

Antrotomy
    Transmastoid, 69501

OR

Excision
    Mastoid
        Simple, 69501

General Guidelines

Providers

The AMA advises coders that while a particular service or procedure may be assigned to a specific section, it is not limited to use only by that specialty group (see paragraphs two and three under "Instructions for Use of the CPT Codebook" on page xiv of the CPT Book). Additionally, the procedures and services listed throughout the book are for use by any qualified physician or other qualified health care professional or entity (e.g., hospitals, laboratories, or home health agencies). Keep in mind that there may be other policies or guidance that can affect who may report a specific service.

Supplies

Some payers may allow physicians to separately report drugs and other supplies when reporting the place of service as office or other nonfacility setting. Drugs and supplies are to be reported by the facility only when performed in a facility setting.

Professional and Technical Component

Radiology and some pathology codes often have a technical and a professional component. When physicians do not own their own equipment and send their patients to outside testing facilities, they should append modifier 26 to the procedural code to indicate they performed only the professional component.

12020-12021 `1`

12020 Treatment of superficial wound dehiscence; simple closure
12021   with packing

`2`

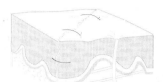

Example of a simple closure
involving only one skin layer

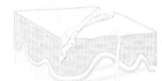

Example of a wound left open
with packing due to infection

Explanation `3`

There has been a breakdown of the healing skin either before or after suture removal. The skin margins have opened. The physician cleanses the wound with irrigation and antimicrobial solutions. The skin margins may be trimmed to initiate bleeding surfaces. Report 12020 if the wound is sutured in a single layer. Report 12021 if the wound is left open and packed with gauze strips due to the presence of infection. This allows infection to drain from the wound and the skin closure will be delayed until the infection is resolved.

Coding Tips `4`

For extensive or complicated secondary wound closure, see 13160. Medicare and some other payers may require G0168 be reported for wound closure by tissue adhesives only. Surgical trays, A4550, are not separately reimbursed by Medicare; however, other third-party payers may cover them. Check with the specific payer to determine coverage.

ICD-10-CM Diagnostic Codes

		`5`
O90.0	Disruption of cesarean delivery wound Ⓜ ♀	
O90.1	Disruption of perineal obstetric wound Ⓜ ♀	
T81.31XA	Disruption of external operation (surgical) wound, not elsewhere classified, initial encounter	
T81.32XA	Disruption of internal operation (surgical) wound, not elsewhere classified, initial encounter	
T81.33XA	Disruption of traumatic injury wound repair, initial encounter	

Associated HCPCS Codes

`6`

G0168   Wound closure utilizing tissue adhesive(s) only

AMA: 12020 2019,Nov,3; 2018,Jan,8; 2017,Jan,8; 2016,Jan,13; 2015,Jan,16; 2014,Jan,11 **12021** 2019,Nov,3; 2018,Jan,8; 2017,Jan,8; 2016,Jan,13; 2015,Jan,16; 2014,Jan,11 `7`

Relative Value Units/Medicare Edits `8`

Non-Facility RVU	Work	PE	MP	Total
12020	2.67	5.31	0.43	8.41
12021	1.89	2.69	0.32	4.9
Facility RVU	**Work**	**PE**	**MP**	**Total**
12020	2.67	2.33	0.43	5.43
12021	1.89	1.8	0.32	4.01

	FUD	Status	MUE	Modifiers				IOM Reference
12020	10	A	2(3)	51	N/A	N/A	N/A	None
12021	10	A	3(3)	51	N/A	N/A	N/A	

* with documentation

Terms To Know `9`

dehiscence. Complication of healing in which the surgical wound ruptures or bursts open, superficially or through multiple layers.

infection. Presence of microorganisms in body tissues that may result in cellular damage.

irrigation. To wash out or cleanse a body cavity, wound, or tissue with water or other fluid.

packing. Material placed into a cavity or wound, such as gels, gauze, pads, and sponges.

perineal. Pertaining to the pelvic floor area between the thighs; the diamond-shaped area bordered by the pubic symphysis in front, the ischial tuberosities on the sides, and the coccyx in back.

subcutaneous. Below the skin.

superficial. On the skin surface or near the surface of any involved structure or field of interest.

wound repair. Surgical closure of a wound is divided into three categories: simple, intermediate, and complex. *simple repair:* Surgical closure of a superficial wound, requiring single layer suturing of the skin epidermis, dermis, or subcutaneous tissue. *intermediate repair:* Surgical closure of a wound requiring closure of one or more of the deeper subcutaneous tissue and non-muscle fascia layers in addition to suturing the skin; contaminated wounds with single layer closure that need extensive cleaning or foreign body removal. *complex repair:* Repair of wounds requiring more than layered closure (debridement, scar revision, stents, retention sutures).

1. CPT Codes and Descriptions

This edition of *Coding Companion* is updated with CPT codes for year 2021.

The following icons are used in *Coding Companion*:

● This CPT code is new for 2021.

▲ This CPT code description is revised for 2021.

✚ This CPT code is an add-on code.

Add-on codes are not subject to bilateral or multiple procedure rules, reimbursement reduction, or appending modifier 50 or 51. Add-on codes describe additional intraservice work associated with the primary procedure performed by the same physician on the same date of service and are not reported as stand-alone procedures. Add-on codes for procedures performed on bilateral structures are reported by listing the add-on code twice.

★ This CPT code is identified by CPT as appropriate for telemedicine services.

The Centers for Medicare and Medicaid Services (CMS) have identified additional services that may be performed via telehealth. Due to the COVID-19 public health emergency (PHE), some services have been designated as temporarily appropriate for telehealth. These CMS approved services are identified in the coding tips where appropriate. Most payers require telehealth/telemedicine to be reported with place of service 02 Telehealth and modifier 95 appended. If specialized equipment is used at the originating site, HCPCS Level II code Q3014 may be reported. Individual payers should be contacted for additional or different guidelines regarding telehealth/telemedicine services. Documentation should include the type of technology used for the treatment in addition to the patient evaluation, treatment, and consents.

[ ] CPT codes enclosed in brackets are resequenced and may not appear in numerical order.

2. Illustrations

The illustrations that accompany the *Coding Companion* series provide coders a better understanding of the medical procedures referenced by the codes and data. The graphics offer coders a visual link between the technical language of the operative report and the cryptic descriptions accompanying the codes. Although most pages will have an illustration, there will be some pages that do not.

3. Explanation

Every CPT code or series of similar codes is presented with its official CPT code description. However, sometimes these descriptions do not provide the coder with sufficient information to make a proper code selection. In *Coding Companion*, an easy-to-understand step-by-step clinical description of the procedure is provided. Technical language that might be used by the physician is included and defined. *Coding Companion* describes the most common method of performing each procedure.

4. Coding Tips

Coding tips provide information on how the code should be used, provides related CPT codes, and offers help concerning common billing errors, modifier usage, and anesthesia. This information comes from consultants and subject matter experts at Optum360 and from the coding guidelines provided in the CPT book and by the Centers for Medicare and Medicaid Services (CMS).

5. ICD-10-CM Diagnostic Codes

ICD-10-CM diagnostic codes listed are common diagnoses or reasons the procedure may be necessary. This list in most cases is inclusive to the specialty. Please note that in some instances the ICD-10-CM codes for only one side of the body (right) have been listed with the CPT code. The associated ICD-10-CM codes for the other side and/or bilateral may also be appropriate. Codes that refer to the right or left are identified with the ☑ icon to alert the user to

check for laterality. In some cases, not every possible code is listed and the ICD-10-CM book should be referenced for other valid codes.

6. Associated HCPCS Codes

Medicare and some other payers require the use of HCPCS Level II codes and not CPT codes when reporting certain services. The HCPCS codes and their description are displayed in this field. If there is not a HCPCS code for this service, this field will not be displayed.

HCPCS codes are current as of time of print. Updated HCPCS codes will be posted at https://www.optum360coding.com/ProductUpdates/. The 2021 edition password is **SPECIALTY21**.

7. AMA References

The AMA references for *CPT Assistant* are listed by CPT code, with the most recent reference listed first. Generally only the last six years of references are listed.

8. Relative Value Units/Medicare Edits

Medicare edits are provided for most codes. These Medicare edits were current as of November 2020.

The 2021 Medicare edits were not available at the time this book went to press. Updated 2021 values will be posted at https://www.optum360coding.com/ProductUpdates/. The 2021 edition password is **SPECIALTY21**.

Relative Value Units

In a resource based relative value scale (RBRVS), services are ranked based on the relative costs of the resources required to provide those services as opposed to the average fee for the service, or average prevailing Medicare charge. The Medicare RBRVS defines three distinct components affecting the value of each service or procedure:

- Physician work component, reflecting the physician's time and skill
- Practice expense (PE) component, reflecting the physician's rent, staff, supplies, equipment, and other overhead
- Malpractice (MP) component, reflecting the relative risk or liability associated with the service
- Total RVUs are a sum of the work, PE, and MP RVUs

There are two groups of RVUs listed for each CPT code. The first RVU group is for facilities (Facility RVU), which includes services provided in hospitals, ambulatory surgical centers, or skilled nursing facilities. The second RVU group is for nonfacilities (Non-Facility RVU), which represents services provided in physician offices, patient's homes, or other nonhospital settings. The appendix includes RVU components for facility and non-facility. Because no values have been established by CMS for the Category III codes, no relative value unit/grids are identified. Refer to the RBRVS tool or guide for the RVUs when the technical (modifier TC) or professional (modifier26) component of a procedure is provided.

Medicare Follow-Up Days (FUD)

Information on the Medicare global period is provided here. The global period is the time following a surgery during which routine care by the physician is considered postoperative and included in the surgical fee. Office visits or other routine care related to the original surgery cannot be separately reported if they occur during the global period.

Status

The Medicare status indicates if the service is separately payable by Medicare. The Medicare RBRVS includes:

A Active code—separate payment may be made

B Bundled code—payment is bundled into other service

C Carrier priced—individual carrier will price the code

I Not valid—Medicare uses another code for this service

N Non-covered—service is not covered by Medicare

R Restricted—special coverage instructions apply

T Paid as only service—These codes are paid only if there are no other services payable under the PFS billed on the same date by the same practitioner. If any other services payable under the PFS are billed on the same date by the same practitioner, these services are bundled into the service(s) for which payment is made.

X Statutory exclusion—no RVUs or payment

Medically Unlikely Edits

This column provides the maximum number of units allowed by Medicare. However, it is also important to note that not every code has a Medically Unlikely Edit (MUE) available. Medicare has assigned some MUE values that are not publicly available. If there is no information in the MUE column for a particular code, this doesn't mean that there is no MUE. It may simply mean that CMS has not released information on that MUE. Watch the remittance advice for possible details on MUE denials related to those codes. If there is not a published MUE, a dash will display in the field.

An additional component of the MUE edit is the MUE Adjudication Indicator (MAI). This edit is the result of an audit by the Office of the Inspector General (OIG) that identified inappropriate billing practices that bypassed the MUE edits. These included inappropriate reporting of bilateral services and split billing.

There are three MUE Adjudication Indicators.

- 1 Line Edit
- 2 Date of Service Edit: Policy
- 3 Date of Service Edit: Clinical

The MUE will be listed following the MAI value. For example code 11446 has a MUE value of 2 and a MAI value of 3. This will display in the MUE field as "2(3)."

Modifiers

Medicare identifies some modifiers that are required or appropriate to report with the CPT code. When the modifiers are not appropriate, it will be indicated with N/A. Four modifiers are included.

51 Multiple Procedure
Medicare and other payers reduce the reimbursement of second and subsequent procedures performed at the same session to 50 percent of the allowable. For endoscopic procedures, the reimbursement is reduced by the value of the endoscopic base code.

50 Bilateral Procedures
This modifier is used to identify when the same procedure is performed bilaterally. Medicare requires one line with modifier 50 and the reimbursement is 50 percent of the allowable. Other payers may require two lines and will reduce the second procedure.

62* Two Surgeons
Medicare identifies procedures that may be performed by co-surgeons. The reimbursement is split between both providers. Both surgeons must report the same code when using this modifier.

80* Assistant Surgeon
An assistant surgeon is allowed if modifier 80 is listed. Reimbursement is usually 20 percent of the allowable. For Medicare it is 16 percent to account for the patient's co-pay amount.

* with documentation

Modifiers 62 and 80 may require supporting documentation to justify the co- or assistant surgeon.

Medicare Official Regulatory Information

Medicare official regulatory information provides official regulatory guidelines. Also known as the CMS Online Manual System, the Internet-only Manuals (IOM) contain official CMS information pertaining to program issuances, instructions, policies, and procedures based on statutes, regulations, guidelines, models, and directives. Optum360 has provided the reference for the surgery codes. The full text of guidelines can be found online at http://www.cms.gov/Regulations-and-Guidance/Guidance/Manuals/.

9. Terms to Know

Some codes are accompanied by general information pertinent to the procedure, labeled "Terms to Know." This information is not critical to code selection, but is a useful supplement to coders hoping to expand their knowledge of the specialty.

99202-99205

▲★**99202** Office or other outpatient visit for the evaluation and management of a new patient, which requires a medically appropriate history and/or examination and straightforward medical decision making. When using time for code selection, 15-29 minutes of total time is spent on the date of the encounter.

▲★**99203** Office or other outpatient visit for the evaluation and management of a new patient, which requires a medically appropriate history and/or examination and low level of medical decision making. When using time for code selection, 30-44 minutes of total time is spent on the date of the encounter.

▲★**99204** Office or other outpatient visit for the evaluation and management of a new patient, which requires a medically appropriate history and/or examination and moderate level of medical decision making. When using time for code selection, 45-59 minutes of total time is spent on the date of the encounter.

▲★**99205** Office or other outpatient visit for the evaluation and management of a new patient, which requires a medically appropriate history and/or examination and high level of medical decision making. When using time for code selection, 60-74 minutes of total time is spent on the date of the encounter.

Explanation

Providers report these codes for new patients being seen in the doctor's office, a multispecialty group clinic, or other outpatient environment. All require a medically appropriate history and/or examination. Code selection is based on the level of medical decision making (MDM) or total time personally spent by the physician and/or other qualified health care professional(s) on the date of the encounter. Factors to be considered in MDM include the number/complexity of problems addressed during the encounter, amount and complexity of data requiring review and analysis, and the risk of complications and/or morbidity or mortality associated with patient management. The most basic service is represented by 99202, which entails straightforward MDM. If time is used for code selection, 15 to 29 minutes of total time is spent on the day of encounter. Report 99203 for a visit requiring a low level of MDM or 30 to 44 minutes of total time; 99204 for a visit requiring a moderate level of MDM or 45 to 59 minutes of total time; and 99205 for a visit requiring a high level of MDM or 60 to 74 minutes of total time.

Coding Tips

These codes are used to report office or other outpatient services for a new patient. A medically appropriate history and physical examination, as determined by the treating provider, should be documented. The level of history and physical examination are no longer used when determining the level of service. Codes should be selected based upon the CPT revised 2021 Medical Decision Making table. Alternately, time alone may be used to select the appropriate level of service. Total time for reporting these services includes face-to-face and non-face-to-face time personally spent by the physician or other qualified health care professional on the date of the encounter. For office or other outpatient services for an established patient, see 99211-99215. For observation care services, see 99217-99226. For patients admitted and discharged from observation or inpatient status on the same date, see 99234-99236. Telemedicine services may be reported by the performing provider by adding modifier 95 to these procedure codes. Services at the origination site are reported with HCPCS Level II code Q3014.

ICD-10-CM Diagnostic Codes

The application of this code is too broad to adequately present ICD-10-CM diagnostic code links here. Refer to your ICD-10-CM book.

AMA: 99202 2020,Sep,3; 2020,Sep,14; 2020,May,3; 2020,Jun,3; 2020,Jan,3; 2020,Feb,3; 2019,Oct,10; 2019,Jan,3; 2019,Feb,3; 2018,Sep,14; 2018,Mar,7; 2018,Jan,8; 2018,Apr,9; 2018,Apr,10; 2017,Jun,6; 2017,Jan,8; 2017,Aug,3; 2016,Sep,6; 2016,Mar,10; 2016,Jan,7; 2016,Jan,13; 2016,Dec,11; 2015,Oct,3; 2015,Jan,16; 2015,Jan,12; 2015,Dec,3; 2014,Oct,8; 2014,Oct,3; 2014,Nov,14; 2014,Jan,11; 2014,Aug,3 **99203** 2020,Sep,3; 2020,Sep,14; 2020,May,3; 2020,Jun,3; 2020,Jan,3; 2020,Feb,3; 2019,Oct,10; 2019,Jan,3; 2019,Feb,3; 2018,Sep,14; 2018,Mar,7; 2018,Jan,8; 2018,Apr,10; 2018,Apr,9; 2017,Jun,6; 2017,Jan,8; 2017,Aug,3; 2016,Sep,6; 2016,Mar,10; 2016,Jan,7; 2016,Jan,13; 2016,Dec,11; 2015,Oct,3; 2015,Jan,12; 2015,Jan,16; 2015,Dec,3; 2014,Oct,3; 2014,Oct,8; 2014,Nov,14; 2014,Jan,11; 2014,Aug,3 **99204** 2020,Sep,14; 2020,Sep,3; 2020,May,3; 2020,Jun,3; 2020,Jan,3; 2020,Feb,3; 2019,Oct,10; 2019,Jan,3; 2019,Feb,3; 2018,Sep,14; 2018,Mar,7; 2018,Jan,8; 2018,Apr,9; 2018,Apr,10; 2017,Jun,6; 2017,Jan,8; 2017,Aug,3; 2016,Sep,6; 2016,Mar,10; 2016,Jan,13; 2016,Jan,7; 2016,Dec,11; 2015,Oct,3; 2015,Jan,12; 2015,Jan,16; 2015,Dec,3; 2014,Oct,3; 2014,Oct,8; 2014,Nov,14; 2014,Jan,11; 2014,Aug,3 **99205** 2020,Sep,3; 2020,Sep,14; 2020,May,3; 2020,Jun,3; 2020,Jan,3; 2020,Feb,3; 2019,Oct,10; 2019,Jan,3; 2019,Feb,3; 2018,Sep,14; 2018,Mar,7; 2018,Jan,8; 2018,Apr,10; 2018,Apr,9; 2017,Jun,6; 2017,Jan,8; 2017,Aug,3; 2016,Sep,6; 2016,Mar,10; 2016,Jan,7; 2016,Jan,13; 2016,Dec,11; 2015,Oct,3; 2015,Jan,12; 2015,Jan,16; 2015,Dec,3; 2014,Oct,8; 2014,Oct,3; 2014,Nov,14; 2014,Jan,11; 2014,Aug,3

Relative Value Units/Medicare Edits

Non-Facility RVU	Work	PE	MP	Total
99202	0.93	1.12	0.09	2.14
99203	1.42	1.48	0.13	3.03
99204	2.43	1.98	0.22	4.63
99205	3.17	2.4	0.28	5.85
Facility RVU	**Work**	**PE**	**MP**	**Total**
99202	0.93	0.41	0.09	1.43
99203	1.42	0.59	0.13	2.14
99204	2.43	1.01	0.22	3.66
99205	3.17	1.33	0.28	4.78

	FUD	Status	MUE	Modifiers				IOM Reference
99202	N/A	A	1(2)	N/A	N/A	N/A	80*	None
99203	N/A	A	1(2)	N/A	N/A	N/A	80*	
99204	N/A	A	1(2)	N/A	N/A	N/A	80*	
99205	N/A	A	1(2)	N/A	N/A	N/A	80*	

* with documentation

Terms To Know

new patient. Patient who is receiving face-to-face care from a provider/qualified health care professional or another physician/qualified health care professional of the exact same specialty and subspecialty who belongs to the same group practice for the first time in three years. For OPPS hospitals, a patient who has not been registered as an inpatient or outpatient, including off-campus provider based clinic or emergency department, within the past three years.

99211-99215

▲ **99211** Office or other outpatient visit for the evaluation and management of an established patient, that may not require the presence of a physician or other qualified health care professional. Usually, the presenting problem(s) are minimal.

▲★**99212** Office or other outpatient visit for the evaluation and management of an established patient, which requires a medically appropriate history and/or examination and straightforward medical decision making. When using time for code selection, 10-19 minutes of total time is spent on the date of the encounter.

▲★**99213** Office or other outpatient visit for the evaluation and management of an established patient, which requires a medically appropriate history and/or examination and low level of medical decision making. When using time for code selection, 20-29 minutes of total time is spent on the date of the encounter.

▲★**99214** Office or other outpatient visit for the evaluation and management of an established patient, which requires a medically appropriate history and/or examination and moderate level of medical decision making. When using time for code selection, 30-39 minutes of total time is spent on the date of the encounter.

▲★**99215** Office or other outpatient visit for the evaluation and management of an established patient, which requires a medically appropriate history and/or examination and high level of medical decision making. When using time for code selection, 40-54 minutes of total time is spent on the date of the encounter.

Explanation

Providers report these codes for established patients being seen in the doctor's office, a multispecialty group clinic, or other outpatient environment. All require a medically appropriate history and/or examination excluding the most basic service represented by 99211 that describes an encounter in which the presenting problems are typically minimal and may not require the presence of a physician or other qualified health care professional. For the remainder of codes within this range, code selection is based on the level of medical decision making (MDM) or total time personally spent by the physician and/or other qualified health care professional(s) on the date of the encounter. Factors to be considered in MDM include the number/complexity of problems addressed during the encounter, amount and complexity of data requiring review and analysis, and the risk of complications and/or morbidity or mortality associated with patient management. Report 99212 for a visit that entails straightforward MDM. If time is used for code selection, 10 to 19 minutes of total time is spent on the day of encounter. Report 99213 for a visit requiring a low level of MDM or 20 to 29 minutes of total time; 99214 for a moderate level of MDM or 30 to 39 minutes of total time; and 99215 for a high level of MDM or 40 to 54 minutes of total time.

Coding Tips

These codes are used to report office or other outpatient services for an established patient. A medically appropriate history and physical examination, as determined by the treating provider, should be documented. The level of history and physical examination are no longer used when determining the level of service. Codes should be selected based upon the CPT revised 2021 Medical Decision Making table. Alternately, time alone may be used to select the appropriate level of service. Total time for reporting these services includes face-to-face and non-face-to-face time personally spent by the physician or other qualified health care professional on the date of the encounter. Code

99211 does not require the presence of a physician or other qualified health care professional. For office or other outpatient services for a new patient, see 99202-99205. For observation care services, see 99217-99226. For patients admitted and discharged from observation or inpatient status on the same date, see 99234-99236. Medicare has identified 99211 as a telehealth/telemedicine service. Commercial payers should be contacted regarding their coverage guidelines. Telemedicine services may be reported by the performing provider by adding modifier 95 to these procedure codes. Services at the origination site are reported with HCPCS Level II code Q3014.

ICD-10-CM Diagnostic Codes

The application of this code is too broad to adequately present ICD-10-CM diagnostic code links here. Refer to your ICD-10-CM book.

AMA: **99211** 2020,Sep,14; 2020,Sep,3; 2020,May,3; 2020,Jun,3; 2020,Jan,3; 2020,Feb,3; 2019,Oct,10; 2019,Jan,3; 2019,Feb,3; 2018,Sep,14; 2018,Mar,7; 2018,Jan,8; 2018,Apr,10; 2018,Apr,9; 2017,Mar,10; 2017,Jun,6; 2017,Jan,8; 2017,Aug,3; 2016,Sep,6; 2016,Mar,10; 2016,Jan,13; 2016,Jan,7; 2016,Dec,11; 2015,Oct,3; 2015,Jan,12; 2015,Jan,16; 2015,Dec,3; 2014,Oct,8; 2014,Oct,3; 2014,Nov,14; 2014,Mar,13; 2014,Jan,11; 2014,Aug,3 **99212** 2020,Sep,14; 2020,Sep,3; 2020,May,3; 2020,Jun,3; 2020,Jan,3; 2020,Feb,3; 2019,Oct,10; 2019,Jan,3; 2019,Feb,3; 2018,Sep,14; 2018,Mar,7; 2018,Jan,8; 2018,Apr,9; 2018,Apr,10; 2017,Oct,5; 2017,Jun,6; 2017,Jan,8; 2017,Aug,3; 2016,Sep,6; 2016,Mar,10; 2016,Jan,13; 2016,Jan,7; 2016,Dec,11; 2015,Oct,3; 2015,Jan,16; 2015,Jan,12; 2015,Dec,3; 2014,Oct,8; 2014,Oct,3; 2014,Nov,14; 2014,Jan,11; 2014,Aug,3 **99213** 2020,Sep,3; 2020,Sep,14; 2020,May,3; 2020,Jun,3; 2020,Jan,3; 2020,Feb,3; 2019,Oct,10; 2019,Jan,3; 2019,Feb,3; 2018,Sep,14; 2018,Mar,7; 2018,Jan,8; 2018,Apr,10; 2018,Apr,9; 2017,Jun,6; 2017,Jan,8; 2017,Aug,3; 2016,Sep,6; 2016,Mar,10; 2016,Jan,7; 2016,Jan,13; 2016,Dec,11; 2015,Oct,3; 2015,Jan,12; 2015,Jan,16; 2015,Dec,3; 2014,Oct,3; 2014,Oct,8; 2014,Nov,14; 2014,Jan,11; 2014,Aug,3 **99214** 2020,Sep,14; 2020,Sep,3; 2020,May,3; 2020,Jun,3; 2020,Jan,3; 2020,Feb,3; 2019,Oct,10; 2019,Jan,3; 2019,Feb,3; 2018,Sep,14; 2018,Mar,7; 2018,Jan,8; 2018,Apr,9; 2018,Apr,10; 2017,Jun,6; 2017,Jan,8; 2017,Aug,3; 2016,Sep,6; 2016,Mar,10; 2016,Jan,13; 2016,Jan,7; 2016,Dec,11; 2015,Oct,3; 2015,Jan,16; 2015,Jan,12; 2015,Dec,3; 2014,Oct,8; 2014,Oct,3; 2014,Nov,14; 2014,Jan,11; 2014,Aug,3 **99215** 2020,Sep,3; 2020,Sep,14; 2020,May,3; 2020,Jun,3; 2020,Jan,3; 2020,Feb,3; 2019,Oct,10; 2019,Jan,3; 2019,Feb,3; 2018,Sep,14; 2018,Mar,7; 2018,Jan,8; 2018,Apr,9; 2018,Apr,10; 2017,Jun,6; 2017,Jan,8; 2017,Aug,3; 2016,Sep,6; 2016,Mar,10; 2016,Jan,13; 2016,Jan,7; 2016,Dec,11; 2015,Oct,3; 2015,Jan,12; 2015,Jan,16; 2015,Dec,3; 2014,Oct,3; 2014,Oct,8; 2014,Nov,14; 2014,Jan,11; 2014,Aug,3

Relative Value Units/Medicare Edits

Non-Facility RVU	Work	PE	MP	Total
99211	0.18	0.46	0.01	0.65
99212	0.48	0.75	0.05	1.28
99213	0.97	1.06	0.08	2.11
99214	1.5	1.45	0.11	3.06
99215	2.11	1.85	0.15	4.11
Facility RVU	Work	PE	MP	Total
99211	0.18	0.07	0.01	0.26
99212	0.48	0.2	0.05	0.73
99213	0.97	0.4	0.08	1.45
99214	1.5	0.62	0.11	2.23
99215	2.11	0.89	0.15	3.15

	FUD	Status	MUE	Modifiers				IOM Reference
99211	N/A	A	1(3)	N/A	N/A	N/A	80*	None
99212	N/A	A	2(3)	N/A	N/A	N/A	80*	
99213	N/A	A	2(3)	N/A	N/A	N/A	80*	
99214	N/A	A	2(3)	N/A	N/A	N/A	80*	
99215	N/A	A	1(3)	N/A	N/A	N/A	80*	

* with documentation

Terms To Know

established patient. Patient who has received professional services in a face-to-face setting within the last three years from the same physician/qualified health care professional or another physician/qualified health care professional of the exact same specialty and subspecialty who belongs to the same group practice. If the patient is seen by a physician/qualified health care professional who is covering for another physician/qualified health care professional, the patient will be considered the same as if seen by the physician/qualified health care professional who is unavailable.

key components. Three components of history, examination, and medical decision making are considered the keys to selecting the correct level of E/M codes. In most cases, all three components must be addressed in the documentation. However, in established, subsequent, and follow-up categories, only two of the three must be met or exceeded for a given code.

qualified health care professional. Educated, licensed or certified, and regulated professional operating under a specified scope of practice to provide patient services that are separate and distinct from other clinical staff.

99217

99217	Observation care discharge day management (This code is to be utilized to report all services provided to a patient on discharge from outpatient hospital "observation status" if the discharge is on other than the initial date of "observation status." To report services to a patient designated as "observation status" or "inpatient status" and discharged on the same date, use the codes for Observation or Inpatient Care Services [including Admission and Discharge Services, 99234-99236 as appropriate.])

Explanation

This code describes the final processes associated with discharging a patient from outpatient hospital observation status and includes a patient exam, a discussion about the hospital stay, instructions for ongoing care, as well as preparing the medical discharge records. Report this code only when the patient has been discharged from observation services on a date other than the initial date of observation care. There are no key components or time estimates associated with this service.

Coding Tips

This code is used to report hospital outpatient observation discharge services. This code includes patient examination, discharge and follow-up care instructions, and preparation of all medical records. Time is not a factor when selecting this E/M service. For patients admitted and discharged from observation or inpatient status on the same date, see 99234-99236; for hospital inpatient discharge services, see 99238-99239. Medicare has provisionally identified this code as a telehealth/telemedicine service. Current Medicare coverage guidelines should be reviewed. Commercial payers should be contacted regarding their coverage guidelines. Telemedicine services may be reported by the performing provider by adding modifier 95 to this procedure code. Services at the origination site are reported with HCPCS Level II code Q3014.

ICD-10-CM Diagnostic Codes

The application of this code is too broad to adequately present ICD-10-CM diagnostic code links here. Refer to your ICD-10-CM book.

AMA: **99217** 2019,Jul,10; 2018,Jan,8; 2017,Jun,6; 2017,Jan,8; 2017,Aug,3; 2016,Jan,13; 2016,Jan,7; 2016,Dec,11; 2015,Jan,16; 2015,Dec,3; 2014,Oct,8; 2014,Nov,14; 2014,Jan,11

Relative Value Units/Medicare Edits

Non-Facility RVU	Work	PE	MP	Total
99217	1.28	0.68	0.09	2.05
Facility RVU	Work	PE	MP	Total
99217	1.28	0.68	0.09	2.05

	FUD	Status	MUE	Modifiers				IOM Reference
99217	N/A	A	1(2)	N/A	N/A	N/A	80*	100-04,11,40.1.3; 100-04,12,30.6.4; 100-04,12,30.6.8; 100-04,12,100; 100-04,32,130.1

* with documentation

Terms To Know

observation patient. Patient who needs to be monitored and assessed for inpatient admission or referral to another site for care.

99218-99220

99218 Initial observation care, per day, for the evaluation and management of a patient which requires these 3 key components: A detailed or comprehensive history; A detailed or comprehensive examination; and Medical decision making that is straightforward or of low complexity. Counseling and/or coordination of care with other physicians, other qualified health care professionals, or agencies are provided consistent with the nature of the problem(s) and the patient's and/or family's needs. Usually, the problem(s) requiring admission to outpatient hospital "observation status" are of low severity. Typically, 30 minutes are spent at the bedside and on the patient's hospital floor or unit.

99219 Initial observation care, per day, for the evaluation and management of a patient, which requires these 3 key components: A comprehensive history; A comprehensive examination; and Medical decision making of moderate complexity. Counseling and/or coordination of care with other physicians, other qualified health care professionals, or agencies are provided consistent with the nature of the problem(s) and the patient's and/or family's needs. Usually, the problem(s) requiring admission to outpatient hospital "observation status" are of moderate severity. Typically, 50 minutes are spent at the bedside and on the patient's hospital floor or unit.

99220 Initial observation care, per day, for the evaluation and management of a patient, which requires these 3 key components: A comprehensive history; A comprehensive examination; and Medical decision making of high complexity. Counseling and/or coordination of care with other physicians, other qualified health care professionals, or agencies are provided consistent with the nature of the problem(s) and the patient's and/or family's needs. Usually, the problem(s) requiring admission to outpatient hospital "observation status" are of high severity. Typically, 70 minutes are spent at the bedside and on the patient's hospital floor or unit.

Explanation

Initial hospital observation service codes describe the first visit of the patient's admission for hospital outpatient observation care by the supervising qualified clinician. Hospital outpatient observation status includes the supervision of the care plan for observation as well as periodic reassessments. The patient is not required to be physically located in a designated observation area within a hospital; however, if such an area is utilized, these codes should be reported. When a patient is admitted to observation status during the course of another encounter from a different site of service, such as the physician's office, a nursing home, or the emergency department, all of the E/M services rendered by the supervising clinician as part of the observation status are considered part of the initial observation care services when they are performed on the same day; the level of initial observation code reported by the clinician should incorporate the other services related to the hospital outpatient observation admission that were provided in any other sites of services as well as those provided in the actual observation setting. Codes are reported per day and do not differentiate between new or established patients. Under the initial observation care category, there are three levels represented by 99218, 99219, and 99220. These levels require all three key components to be documented. The lowest level of care within this category, 99218, requires a detailed or comprehensive history and exam as well as straightforward or low complexity medical decision making (MDM) with approximately 30 minutes time being spent at the patient's bedside and on the patient's floor or unit. For the mid-level and highest level observation care codes, a comprehensive history and examination are required. Medical decision making is the differentiating factor for these two levels. For moderate complexity, report 99219. For observation care requiring MDM of high complexity, report 99220. The clinician

typically spends 50 (99219) to 70 (99220) minutes at the patient's bedside or on the unit accordingly.

Coding Tips

These codes are used to report initial hospital outpatient observation services. All three key components (history, exam, and medical decision making) must be met or exceeded for the level of service selected. Time may be used to select the level of service when counseling and coordination of care are documented as at least half of the time spent face-to-face with the patient. All evaluation and management services provided by the clinician leading up to the initiation of the observation status are considered to be part of the patient's initial observation care when performed on the same date of service. The designation of "observation status" refers to the initiation of observation care and not to a specific area of the facility. CPT guidelines indicate these services are reported only by the admitting/supervising provider; all other providers should report 99224-99226 or 99241-99245. Medicare and some payers may allow providers of different specialties to report initial hospital services and require the admitting/supervising provider to append modifier AI. For observation discharge on a different date of service than the admission, see 99217. For patients admitted and discharged from observation or inpatient status on the same date, see 99234-99236. Medicare has provisionally identified these codes as telehealth/telemedicine services. Current Medicare coverage guidelines should be reviewed. Commercial payers should be contacted regarding their coverage guidelines. Telemedicine services may be reported by the performing provider by adding modifier 95 to these procedure codes. Services at the origination site are reported with HCPCS Level II code Q3014.

ICD-10-CM Diagnostic Codes

The application of this code is too broad to adequately present ICD-10-CM diagnostic code links here. Refer to your ICD-10-CM book.

AMA: 99218 2020,Sep,3; 2019,Jul,10; 2018,Jan,8; 2018,Dec,8; 2018,Dec,8; 2017,Jun,6; 2017,Jan,8; 2017,Aug,3; 2016,Jan,13; 2016,Jan,7; 2016,Dec,11; 2015,Mar,3; 2015,Jul,3; 2015,Jan,16; 2015,Dec,3; 2014,Oct,8; 2014,Nov,14; 2014,Jan,11 **99219** 2020,Sep,3; 2019,Jul,10; 2018,Jan,8; 2018,Dec,8; 2018,Dec,8; 2017,Jun,6; 2017,Jan,8; 2017,Aug,3; 2016,Jan.13; 2016,Jan,7; 2016,Dec,11; 2015,Jul,3; 2015,Jan,16; 2015,Dec,3; 2014,Oct,8; 2014,Nov,14; 2014,Jan,11 **99220** 2020,Sep,3; 2019,Jul,10; 2018,Jan,8; 2018,Dec,8; 2018,Dec,8; 2017,Jun,6; 2017,Jan,8; 2017,Aug,3; 2016,Jan,13; 2016,Jan,7; 2016,Dec,11; 2015,Jul,3; 2015,Jan,16; 2015,Dec,3; 2014,Oct,8; 2014,Nov,14; 2014,Jan,11

Relative Value Units/Medicare Edits

Non-Facility RVU	Work	PE	MP	Total
99218	1.92	0.74	0.16	2.82
99219	2.6	1.05	0.18	3.83
99220	3.56	1.4	0.26	5.22
Facility RVU	Work	PE	MP	Total
99218	1.92	0.74	0.16	2.82
99219	2.6	1.05	0.18	3.83
99220	3.56	1.4	0.26	5.22

	FUD	Status	MUE	Modifiers				IOM Reference
99218	N/A	A	1(2)	N/A	N/A	N/A	80*	100-04,12,100
99219	N/A	A	1(2)	N/A	N/A	N/A	80*	
99220	N/A	A	1(2)	N/A	N/A	N/A	80*	

* with documentation

N Newborn: 0   **P** Pediatric: 0-17   **M** Maternity: 9-64   **A** Adult: 15-124   ♂ **Male Only**   ♀ **Female Only**   CPT © 2020 American Medical Association. All Rights Reserved.

99221-99223

99221 Initial hospital care, per day, for the evaluation and management of a patient, which requires these 3 key components: A detailed or comprehensive history; A detailed or comprehensive examination; and Medical decision making that is straightforward or of low complexity. Counseling and/or coordination of care with other physicians, other qualified health care professionals, or agencies are provided consistent with the nature of the problem(s) and the patient's and/or family's needs. Usually, the problem(s) requiring admission are of low severity. Typically, 30 minutes are spent at the bedside and on the patient's hospital floor or unit.

99222 Initial hospital care, per day, for the evaluation and management of a patient, which requires these 3 key components: A comprehensive history; A comprehensive examination; and Medical decision making of moderate complexity. Counseling and/or coordination of care with other physicians, other qualified health care professionals, or agencies are provided consistent with the nature of the problem(s) and the patient's and/or family's needs. Usually, the problem(s) requiring admission are of moderate severity. Typically, 50 minutes are spent at the bedside and on the patient's hospital floor or unit.

99223 Initial hospital care, per day, for the evaluation and management of a patient, which requires these 3 key components: A comprehensive history; A comprehensive examination; and Medical decision making of high complexity. Counseling and/or coordination of care with other physicians, other qualified health care professionals, or agencies are provided consistent with the nature of the problem(s) and the patient's and/or family's needs. Usually, the problem(s) requiring admission are of high severity. Typically, 70 minutes are spent at the bedside and on the patient's hospital floor or unit.

Explanation

Initial hospital inpatient service codes describe the first encounter with the patient by the admitting physician or qualified clinician. For initial encounters by a physician other than the admitting physician, see the initial inpatient consultation codes or subsequent inpatient care codes. When the patient is admitted to the hospital under inpatient status during the course of another encounter from a different site of service, such as the physician's office, a nursing home, or the emergency department, all of the E/M services rendered by the supervising clinician as part of the inpatient admission status are considered part of the initial inpatient care services when they are performed on the same day. The level of initial inpatient care reported by the clinician should incorporate the other services related to the hospital admission that were provided in any other sites of services as well as those provided in the actual inpatient setting. Codes are reported per day and do not differentiate between new or established patients. Under the initial inpatient care category, there are three levels represented by 99221, 99222, and 99223. All of these levels require all three key components, history, exam, and medical decision-making (MDM), to be documented. The lowest level of care within this category, 99221, requires a detailed or comprehensive history and exam as well as straightforward or low complexity medical decision-making with approximately 30 minutes time being spent at the patient's bedside and on the patient's floor or unit. For the mid-level and highest level initial inpatient care codes, a comprehensive history and examination are required. MDM is the differentiating factor for these two levels; for moderate complexity, report 99222 and for initial inpatient care requiring MDM of high complexity, report 99223. The clinician typically spends 50 (99222) to 70 (99223) minutes at the patient's bedside or on the unit accordingly. Note that these codes include services provided to patients in a "partial hospital" setting.

Coding Tips

These codes are used to report initial hospital inpatient services. All three key components (history, exam, and medical decision making) must be met or exceeded for the level of service selected. Time may be used to select the level of service when counseling and coordination of care are documented as at least half of the floor/unit time spent with the patient. Evaluation and management services provided by the clinician leading up to the initiation of observation status or inpatient admission are considered to be part of the patient's initial hospital care when performed on the same date of service. Codes may be selected based upon the 1995 or the 1997 Evaluation and Management Guidelines. CPT guidelines indicate these services are reported only by the admitting/supervising provider; all other providers should report 99231-99233 or 99251-99255. Medicare and some payers may allow providers of different specialties to report initial hospital services and require the admitting/supervising provider to append modifier AI. For subsequent inpatient care, see 99231-99233. For discharge from an inpatient stay on a different date of service than the admission, see 99238-99239. For patients admitted and discharged from observation or inpatient status on the same date, see 99234-99236. Medicare has provisionally identified these codes as telehealth/telemedicine services. Current Medicare coverage guidelines should be reviewed. Commercial payers should be contacted regarding their coverage guidelines. Telemedicine services may be reported by the performing provider by adding modifier 95 to these procedure codes. Services at the origination site are reported with HCPCS Level II code Q3014.

ICD-10-CM Diagnostic Codes

The application of this code is too broad to adequately present ICD-10-CM diagnostic code links here. Refer to your ICD-10-CM book.

AMA: 99221 2020,Sep,3; 2018,Jan,8; 2018,Dec,8; 2018,Dec,8; 2017,Jun,6; 2017,Jan,8; 2017,Aug,3; 2016,Mar,10; 2016,Jan,13; 2016,Jan,7; 2016,Dec,11; 2015,Jul,3; 2015,Jan,16; 2015,Dec,3; 2015,Dec,18; 2014,Oct,8; 2014,Nov,14; 2014,Jan,11 **99222** 2020,Sep,3; 2018,Jan,8; 2018,Dec,8; 2018,Dec,8; 2017,Jun,6; 2017,Jan,8; 2017,Aug,3; 2016,Mar,10; 2016,Jan,13; 2016,Jan,7; 2016,Dec,11; 2015,Mar,3; 2015,Jul,3; 2015,Jan,16; 2015,Dec,3; 2015,Dec,18; 2014,Oct,8; 2014,Nov,14; 2014,Jan,11 **99223** 2020,Sep,3; 2018,Jan,8; 2018,Dec,8; 2018,Dec,8; 2017,Jun,6; 2017,Jan,8; 2017,Aug,3; 2016,Mar,10; 2016,Jan,13; 2016,Jan,7; 2016,Dec,11; 2015,Jul,3; 2015,Jan,16; 2015,Dec,3; 2015,Dec,18; 2014,Oct,8; 2014,Nov,14; 2014,Jan,11

Relative Value Units/Medicare Edits

Non-Facility RVU	Work	PE	MP	Total
99221	1.92	0.77	0.19	2.88
99222	2.61	1.06	0.22	3.89
99223	3.86	1.57	0.28	5.71
Facility RVU	Work	PE	MP	Total
99221	1.92	0.77	0.19	2.88
99222	2.61	1.06	0.22	3.89
99223	3.86	1.57	0.28	5.71

	FUD	Status	MUE	Modifiers				IOM Reference
99221	N/A	A	1(3)	N/A	N/A	N/A	80*	100-04,12,30.6.4;
99222	N/A	A	1(3)	N/A	N/A	N/A	80*	100-04,12,30.6.9;
99223	N/A	A	1(3)	N/A	N/A	N/A	80*	100-04,12,30.6.9.1;
								100-04,12,30.6.15.1;
								100-04,12,100

* with documentation

99231-99233

★99231 Subsequent hospital care, per day, for the evaluation and management of a patient, which requires at least 2 of these 3 key components: A problem focused interval history; A problem focused examination; Medical decision making that is straightforward or of low complexity. Counseling and/or coordination of care with other physicians, other qualified health care professionals, or agencies are provided consistent with the nature of the problem(s) and the patient's and/or family's needs. Usually, the patient is stable, recovering or improving. Typically, 15 minutes are spent at the bedside and on the patient's hospital floor or unit.

★99232 Subsequent hospital care, per day, for the evaluation and management of a patient, which requires at least 2 of these 3 key components: An expanded problem focused interval history; An expanded problem focused examination; Medical decision making of moderate complexity. Counseling and/or coordination of care with other physicians, other qualified health care professionals, or agencies are provided consistent with the nature of the problem(s) and the patient's and/or family's needs. Usually, the patient is responding inadequately to therapy or has developed a minor complication. Typically, 25 minutes are spent at the bedside and on the patient's hospital floor or unit.

★99233 Subsequent hospital care, per day, for the evaluation and management of a patient, which requires at least 2 of these 3 key components: A detailed interval history; A detailed examination; Medical decision making of high complexity. Counseling and/or coordination of care with other physicians, other qualified health care professionals, or agencies are provided consistent with the nature of the problem(s) and the patient's and/or family's needs. Usually, the patient is unstable or has developed a significant complication or a significant new problem. Typically, 35 minutes are spent at the bedside and on the patient's hospital floor or unit.

Explanation

Subsequent hospital inpatient service codes describe visits that occur after the first encounter of the patient's inpatient hospital admission by the supervising physician or qualified clinician. Codes are reported per day and do not differentiate between new or established patients. Under the subsequent inpatient care category, there are three levels represented by 99231, 99232, and 99233. All of these levels require at least two out of the three key components—history, exam, and medical decision making—to be documented. The lowest level of care within this category, 99231, describes a problem-focused interval history as well as a problem-focused examination with straightforward or low complexity medical decision making and involves approximately 15 minutes of time by the provider at the patient's bedside or on the unit. For the mid-level subsequent inpatient care code, 99232, an expanded problem-focused history and examination are required with moderate medical decision making. Time associated with this level usually involves 25 minutes at the bedside or on the patient's floor. The third and highest level of subsequent inpatient care, 99233, requires a detailed history and exam as well as medical decision making of high complexity. For this level of care, the provider typically spends around 35 minutes with the patient or on the unit. All three levels of subsequent inpatient care involve the clinician reviewing the patient's medical record, results from diagnostic studies, as well as any changes to the patient's status such as physical condition, response to treatments, or changes in health history since the last assessment.

Coding Tips

These codes are used to report subsequent hospital inpatient services. Two of the three key components (history, exam, and medical decision making) must be met or exceeded for the level of service selected. Time may be used to select the level of service when counseling and coordination of care are documented as at least half of the floor/unit time spent with the patient. Codes may be selected based upon the 1995 or the 1997 Evaluation and Management Guidelines. Subsequent inpatient care services include review of the medical record, including all diagnostic studies, as well as changes noted in the patient's condition and response to treatment since the last evaluation. For initial inpatient care, see 99221-99223. For discharge from an inpatient stay on a different date of service than the admission, see 99238-99239. For patients admitted and discharged from observation or inpatient status on the same date, see 99234-99236. Telemedicine services may be reported by the performing provider by adding modifier 95 to these procedure codes. Services at the origination site are reported with HCPCS Level II code Q3014.

ICD-10-CM Diagnostic Codes

The application of this code is too broad to adequately present ICD-10-CM diagnostic code links here. Refer to your ICD-10-CM book.

AMA: **99231** 2020,Sep,3; 2018,Jan,8; 2018,Dec,8; 2018,Dec,8; 2017,Jun,6; 2017,Jan,8; 2017,Aug,3; 2016,Jan,7; 2016,Jan,13; 2016,Dec,11; 2015,Jul,3; 2015,Jan,16; 2015,Dec,3; 2014,Oct,8; 2014,Nov,14; 2014,May,4; 2014,Jan,11 **99232** 2020,Sep,3; 2018,Jan,8; 2018,Dec,8; 2018,Dec,8; 2017,Jun,6; 2017,Jan,8; 2017,Aug,3; 2016,Oct,8; 2016,Jan,13; 2016,Jan,7; 2016,Dec,11; 2015,Jul,3; 2015,Jan,16; 2015,Dec,3; 2014,Oct,8; 2014,Nov,14; 2014,Jan,11 **99233** 2020,Sep,3; 2018,Jan,8; 2018,Dec,8; 2018,Dec,8; 2017,Jun,6; 2017,Jan,8; 2017,Aug,3; 2016,Oct,8; 2016,Jan,13; 2016,Jan,7; 2016,Dec,11; 2015,Jul,3; 2015,Jan,16; 2015,Dec,3; 2014,Oct,8; 2014,Nov,14; 2014,May,4; 2014,Jan,11

Relative Value Units/Medicare Edits

Non-Facility RVU	Work	PE	MP	Total
99231	0.76	0.29	0.06	1.11
99232	1.39	0.56	0.09	2.04
99233	2.0	0.81	0.13	2.94
Facility RVU	Work	PE	MP	Total
99231	0.76	0.29	0.06	1.11
99232	1.39	0.56	0.09	2.04
99233	2.0	0.81	0.13	2.94

	FUD	Status	MUE	Modifiers				IOM Reference
99231	N/A	A	1(3)	N/A	N/A	N/A	80*	100-04,12,30.6.9.2; 100-04,12,100
99232	N/A	A	1(3)	N/A	N/A	N/A	80*	
99233	N/A	A	1(3)	N/A	N/A	N/A	80*	

* with documentation

Terms To Know

key components. Three components of history, examination, and medical decision making are considered the keys to selecting the correct level of E/M codes. In most cases, all three components must be addressed in the documentation. However, in established, subsequent, and follow-up categories, only two of the three must be met or exceeded for a given code.

subsequent care. All evaluation and instructions for care rendered subsequent to the inpatient admission by the admitting provider and all other providers.

99234-99236

99234 Observation or inpatient hospital care, for the evaluation and management of a patient including admission and discharge on the same date, which requires these 3 key components: A detailed or comprehensive history; A detailed or comprehensive examination; and Medical decision making that is straightforward or of low complexity. Counseling and/or coordination of care with other physicians, other qualified health care professionals, or agencies are provided consistent with the nature of the problem(s) and the patient's and/or family's needs. Usually the presenting problem(s) requiring admission are of low severity. Typically, 40 minutes are spent at the bedside and on the patient's hospital floor or unit.

99235 Observation or inpatient hospital care, for the evaluation and management of a patient including admission and discharge on the same date, which requires these 3 key components: A comprehensive history; A comprehensive examination; and Medical decision making of moderate complexity. Counseling and/or coordination of care with other physicians, other qualified health care professionals, or agencies are provided consistent with the nature of the problem(s) and the patient's and/or family's needs. Usually the presenting problem(s) requiring admission are of moderate severity. Typically, 50 minutes are spent at the bedside and on the patient's hospital floor or unit.

99236 Observation or inpatient hospital care, for the evaluation and management of a patient including admission and discharge on the same date, which requires these 3 key components: A comprehensive history; A comprehensive examination; and Medical decision making of high complexity. Counseling and/or coordination of care with other physicians, other qualified health care professionals, or agencies are provided consistent with the nature of the problem(s) and the patient's and/or family's needs. Usually the presenting problem(s) requiring admission are of high severity. Typically, 55 minutes are spent at the bedside and on the patient's hospital floor or unit.

Explanation

Hospital observation or inpatient care service in cases where the patient is admitted and discharged on the same date of service by the supervising or qualified clinician is reported with 99234-99236. Observation status includes the supervision of the care plan for observation, as well as the periodic reassessments. The patient is not required to be physically located in a designated observation area within a hospital; however, if such an area is utilized, these codes should be reported. When a patient is admitted to the hospital from observation status on the same date of service, the clinician should only report the appropriate level of initial hospital care code. The level of care reported should reflect all of the other services from the observation status services the clinician rendered to the patient on the same date of service, as well as those provided in the actual inpatient setting. Codes do not differentiate between new or established patients. Under this care category, there are three levels represented by 99234, 99235, and 99236. All of these levels require all three key components (history, exam, and medical decision-making [MDM]) to be documented. The lowest level of care within this category, 99234, requires a detailed or comprehensive history and exam, as well as straightforward medical decision-making or that of low complexity with approximately 40 minutes time being spent at the patient's bedside and on the patient's floor or unit. For the mid-level and highest level observation or inpatient care codes, a comprehensive history and examination are required. Medical decision-making is the differentiating factor for these two levels; for moderate complexity, report 99235 and for observation or inpatient care requiring MDM of high complexity, report 99236. The clinician typically spends 50 (99235) to 55 (99236) minutes at the patient's bedside or on the unit

accordingly. Note that these codes should be reported only when the patient has been admitted and discharged on the same date of service.

Coding Tips

These codes are used to report observation or initial hospital services for the patient admitted and discharged on the same date of service. All three key components (history, exam, and medical decision making) must be met or exceeded for the level of service selected. Evaluation and management services provided by the clinician leading up to the initiation of observation status or inpatient admission are considered to be part of the patient's initial hospital care when performed on the same date of service. The designation of "observation status" refers to the initiation of observation care and not to a specific area of the facility. For patients admitted to observation status, initial care, see 99218-99220; subsequent observation care, see 99224-99226; for observation discharge on a different date of service than the admission, see 99217. For initial inpatient care, see 99221-99223; subsequent inpatient care, see 99231-99233. For discharge from an inpatient stay on a different date of service than the admission, see 99238-99239. Medicare has provisionally identified these codes as telehealth/telemedicine services. Current Medicare coverage guidelines should be reviewed. Commercial payers should be contacted regarding their coverage guidelines. Telemedicine services may be reported by the performing provider by adding modifier 95 to these procedure codes. Services at the origination site are reported with HCPCS Level II code Q3014.

ICD-10-CM Diagnostic Codes

The application of this code is too broad to adequately present ICD-10-CM diagnostic code links here. Refer to your ICD-10-CM book.

AMA: 99234 2020,Sep,3; 2018,Jan,8; 2018,Dec,8; 2018,Dec,8; 2018,Apr,10; 2017,Jun,6; 2017,Jan,8; 2017,Aug,3; 2016,Jan,13; 2016,Dec,11; 2015,Jul,3; 2015,Jan,16; 2014,Oct,8; 2014,Jan,11 **99235** 2020,Sep,3; 2018,Jan,8; 2018,Dec,8; 2018,Dec,8; 2018,Apr,10; 2017,Jun,6; 2017,Jan,8; 2017,Aug,3; 2016,Jan,13; 2016,Dec,11; 2015,Jul,3; 2015,Jan,16; 2014,Oct,8; 2014,Jan,11 **99236** 2020,Sep,3; 2018,Jan,8; 2018,Dec,8; 2018,Dec,8; 2018,Apr,10; 2017,Jun,6; 2017,Jan,8; 2017,Aug,3; 2016,Jan,13; 2016,Dec,11; 2015,Jul,3; 2015,Jan,16; 2014,Oct,8; 2014,Jan,11

Relative Value Units/Medicare Edits

Non-Facility RVU	Work	PE	MP	Total
99234	2.56	1.0	0.21	3.77
99235	3.24	1.3	0.23	4.77
99236	4.2	1.64	0.3	6.14
Facility RVU	Work	PE	MP	Total
99234	2.56	1.0	0.21	3.77
99235	3.24	1.3	0.23	4.77
99236	4.2	1.64	0.3	6.14

	FUD	Status	MUE	Modifiers				IOM Reference
99234	N/A	A	1(3)	N/A	N/A	N/A	80*	100-04,12,30.6.4;
99235	N/A	A	1(3)	N/A	N/A	N/A	80*	100-04,12,30.6.9;
99236	N/A	A	1(3)	N/A	N/A	N/A	80*	100-04,12,30.6.9.1; 100-04,12,30.6.9.2; 100-04,12,100

* with documentation

99238-99239

99238   Hospital discharge day management; 30 minutes or less
99239   more than 30 minutes

Explanation

Hospital discharge services are time-based codes that, when reported, describe the amount of time spent by the qualified clinician during all final steps involved in the discharge of a patient from the hospital on a date that differs from the date of admission, including the last patient exam, discussing the hospital stay, instructions for ongoing care as it relates to all pertinent caregivers, as well as preparing the medical discharge records, prescriptions, and/or referrals as applicable. Time reported should be for the total duration of time spent by the provider even when the time spent on that date is not continuous. For a hospital discharge duration of 30 minutes or less, report 99238; for a duration of greater than 30 minutes, report 99239. There are no key components associated with these services.

Coding Tips

These codes are used to report all discharge day services for the hospital inpatient, including patient examination, discharge and follow-up care instructions, and preparation of all medical records. These are time-based codes and time spent with the patient must be documented in the medical record. For observation discharge on a different date of service than the admission, see 99217. For patients admitted and discharged from observation or inpatient status on the same date, see 99234-99236. Medicare has provisionally identified these codes as telehealth/telemedicine services. Current Medicare coverage guidelines should be reviewed. Commercial payers should be contacted regarding their coverage guidelines. Telemedicine services may be reported by the performing provider by adding modifier 95 to these procedure codes. Services at the origination site are reported with HCPCS Level II code Q3014.

ICD-10-CM Diagnostic Codes

The application of this code is too broad to adequately present ICD-10-CM diagnostic code links here. Refer to your ICD-10-CM book.

AMA: 99238 2018,Jan,8; 2018,Dec,8; 2018,Dec,8; 2017,Jun,6; 2017,Jan,8; 2017,Aug,3; 2016,Jan,13; 2016,Dec,11; 2015,Jan,16; 2014,Oct,8; 2014,Jan,11 **99239** 2018,Jan,8; 2018,Dec,8; 2018,Dec,8; 2017,Jun,6; 2017,Jan,8; 2017,Aug,3; 2016,Jan,13; 2016,Dec,11; 2015,Jan,16; 2014,Oct,8; 2014,Jan,11

Relative Value Units/Medicare Edits

Non-Facility RVU	Work	PE	MP	Total
99238	1.28	0.69	0.09	2.06
99239	1.9	1.0	0.12	3.02
Facility RVU	**Work**	**PE**	**MP**	**Total**
99238	1.28	0.69	0.09	2.06
99239	1.9	1.0	0.12	3.02

	FUD	Status	MUE	Modifiers				IOM Reference
99238	N/A	A	1(3)	N/A	N/A	N/A	80*	100-04,12,30.6.4;
99239	N/A	A	1(3)	N/A	N/A	N/A	80*	100-04,12,30.6.9;
								100-04,12,30.6.9.1;
								100-04,12,30.6.9.2;
								100-04,12,100

* with documentation

99241-99245

★99241   Office consultation for a new or established patient, which requires these 3 key components: A problem focused history; A problem focused examination; and Straightforward medical decision making. Counseling and/or coordination of care with other physicians, other qualified health care professionals, or agencies are provided consistent with the nature of the problem(s) and the patient's and/or family's needs. Usually, the presenting problem(s) are self limited or minor. Typically, 15 minutes are spent face-to-face with the patient and/or family.

★99242   Office consultation for a new or established patient, which requires these 3 key components: An expanded problem focused history; An expanded problem focused examination; and Straightforward medical decision making. Counseling and/or coordination of care with other physicians, other qualified health care professionals, or agencies are provided consistent with the nature of the problem(s) and the patient's and/or family's needs. Usually, the presenting problem(s) are of low severity. Typically, 30 minutes are spent face-to-face with the patient and/or family.

★99243   Office consultation for a new or established patient, which requires these 3 key components: A detailed history; A detailed examination; and Medical decision making of low complexity. Counseling and/or coordination of care with other physicians, other qualified health care professionals, or agencies are provided consistent with the nature of the problem(s) and the patient's and/or family's needs. Usually, the presenting problem(s) are of moderate severity. Typically, 40 minutes are spent face-to-face with the patient and/or family.

★99244   Office consultation for a new or established patient, which requires these 3 key components: A comprehensive history; A comprehensive examination; and Medical decision making of moderate complexity. Counseling and/or coordination of care with other physicians, other qualified health care professionals, or agencies are provided consistent with the nature of the problem(s) and the patient's and/or family's needs. Usually, the presenting problem(s) are of moderate to high severity. Typically, 60 minutes are spent face-to-face with the patient and/or family.

★99245   Office consultation for a new or established patient, which requires these 3 key components: A comprehensive history; A comprehensive examination; and Medical decision making of high complexity. Counseling and/or coordination of care with other physicians, other qualified health care professionals, or agencies are provided consistent with the nature of the problem(s) and the patient's and/or family's needs. Usually, the presenting problem(s) are of moderate to high severity. Typically, 80 minutes are spent face-to-face with the patient and/or family.

Explanation

Office and other outpatient consultation service codes describe encounters where another qualified clinician's advice or opinion regarding diagnosis and treatment or determination to accept transfer of care of a patient is rendered at the request of the primary treating provider. Consultations may also be requested by another appropriate source; for example, a third-party payer may request a second opinion. The request for a consultation must be documented in the medical record, as well as a written report of the consultation findings. During the course of a consultation, the physician consultant can initiate diagnostic or therapeutic services at the same encounter or at a follow-up visit. Other separately reportable procedures or services performed in conjunction with the consultation may be reported separately. Codes do not differentiate between new or established patients. Services are reported based on meeting all three key components (history, exam, and medical decision-making [MDM]) within each level of service. The most basic service, 99241, describes a problem-focused history and exam with straightforward medical decision-making encompassing approximately 15 minutes of face-to-face time with the patient and/or family discussing a minor or self-limiting complaint. The mid-level services describe problems involving an expanded problem focused history and exam or a detailed history and exam as represented by 99242 and 99243, respectively. Medical decision-making for 99242 is the same as for a level one visit (straightforward) and is designated as low complexity for the level three service (99243). At these levels of service, the encounter can involve face-to-face time of 30 (99242) to 40 (99243) minutes involving minimal to low severity concerns. The last two levels of service in this category represent moderate to high-severity problems and both services involve comprehensive history and examination components. The differentiating factor between the two levels is the medical decision-making; code 99244 involves moderate complexity MDM and approximately 60 minutes of face-to-face time with the patient and/or family, while the highest level of service in this category, 99245, involves MDM of high complexity and approximately 80 minutes of face-to-face time.

Coding Tips

These codes are used to report consultations in the office or outpatient setting. All three key components (history, exam, and medical decision making) must be met or exceeded for the level of service selected. Time may be used to select the level of service when counseling and coordination of care are documented as at least half of the time spent face-to-face with the patient. Codes may be selected based upon the 1995 or the 1997 Evaluation and Management Guidelines. Consultation codes are not covered by Medicare and some payers. Report new or established outpatient E/M codes for consultation services. Consultation services should not be reported when the care and management of a problem or condition is assumed prior to the initial examination of the patient. In these situations, the appropriate initial or subsequent evaluation and management service should be reported. For office or other outpatient services for a new patient, see 99202-99205; for an established patient, see 99211-99215. For inpatient consultation services, see 99251-99255. Telemedicine services may be reported by the performing provider by adding modifier 95 to these procedure codes. Services at the origination site are reported with HCPCS Level II code Q3014.

ICD-10-CM Diagnostic Codes

The application of this code is too broad to adequately present ICD-10-CM diagnostic code links here. Refer to your ICD-10-CM book.

AMA: 99241 2020,Sep,3; 2018,Mar,7; 2018,Jan,8; 2018,Apr,9; 2018,Apr,10; 2017,Jun,6; 2017,Jan,8; 2017,Aug,3; 2016,Sep,6; 2016,Jan,13; 2016,Jan,7; 2016,Dec,11; 2015,Jan,16; 2015,Jan,12; 2014,Sep,13; 2014,Oct,8; 2014,Nov,14; 2014,Jan,11; 2014,Aug,3 **99242** 2020,Sep,3; 2018,Mar,7; 2018,Jan,8; 2018,Apr,9; 2018,Apr,10; 2017,Jun,6; 2017,Jan,8; 2017,Aug,3; 2016,Sep,6; 2016,Jan,13; 2016,Jan,7; 2016,Dec,11; 2015,Jan,16; 2015,Jan,12; 2014,Sep,13; 2014,Oct,8; 2014,Nov,14; 2014,Jan,11; 2014,Aug,3 **99243** 2020,Sep,3; 2018,Mar,7; 2018,Jan,8; 2018,Apr,9; 2018,Apr,10; 2017,Jun,6; 2017,Jan,8; 2017,Aug,3; 2016,Sep,6; 2016,Jan,13; 2016,Jan,7; 2016,Dec,11; 2015,Jan,12; 2015,Jan,16; 2014,Sep,13; 2014,Oct,8; 2014,Nov,14; 2014,Jan,11; 2014,Aug,3 **99244** 2020,Sep,3; 2018,Mar,7; 2018,Jan,8; 2018,Apr,9; 2018,Apr,10; 2017,Jun,6; 2017,Jan,8; 2017,Aug,3; 2016,Sep,6; 2016,Jan,13; 2016,Jan,7; 2016,Dec,11; 2015,Jan,12; 2015,Jan,16; 2014,Sep,13; 2014,Oct,8; 2014,Nov,14; 2014,Jan,11; 2014,Aug,3 **99245** 2020,Sep,3; 2018,Mar,7; 2018,Jan,8; 2018,Apr,9; 2018,Apr,10; 2017,Jun,6; 2017,Jan,8; 2017,Aug,3; 2016,Sep,6; 2016,Jan,13; 2016,Jan,7; 2016,Dec,11; 2015,Jan,16; 2015,Jan,12; 2014,Sep,13; 2014,Oct,8; 2014,Nov,14; 2014,Jan,11; 2014,Aug,3

Relative Value Units/Medicare Edits

Non-Facility RVU	Work	PE	MP	Total
99241	0.64	0.66	0.05	1.35
99242	1.34	1.1	0.11	2.55
99243	1.88	1.46	0.15	3.49
99244	3.02	1.96	0.25	5.23
99245	3.77	2.3	0.3	6.37
Facility RVU	**Work**	**PE**	**MP**	**Total**
99241	0.64	0.24	0.05	0.93
99242	1.34	0.51	0.11	1.96
99243	1.88	0.71	0.15	2.74
99244	3.02	1.14	0.25	4.41
99245	3.77	1.38	0.3	5.45

	FUD	Status	MUE	Modifiers				IOM Reference
99241	N/A	I	0(3)	N/A	N/A	N/A	N/A	100-04,4,160;
99242	N/A	I	0(3)	N/A	N/A	N/A	N/A	100-04,12,30.6.4;
99243	N/A	I	0(3)	N/A	N/A	N/A	N/A	100-04,12,30.6.10;
99244	N/A	I	0(3)	N/A	N/A	N/A	N/A	100-04,12,30.6.15.1;
99245	N/A	I	0(3)	N/A	N/A	N/A	N/A	100-04,12,100

* with documentation

Terms To Know

consultation. Advice or opinion regarding diagnosis and treatment or determination to accept transfer of care of a patient rendered by a medical professional at the request of the primary care provider.

established patient. Patient who has received professional services in a face-to-face setting within the last three years from the same physician/qualified health care professional or another physician/qualified health care professional of the exact same specialty and subspecialty who belongs to the same group practice. If the patient is seen by a physician/qualified health care professional who is covering for another physician/qualified health care professional, the patient will be considered the same as if seen by the physician/qualified health care professional who is unavailable.

key components. Three components of history, examination, and medical decision making are considered the keys to selecting the correct level of E/M codes. In most cases, all three components must be addressed in the documentation. However, in established, subsequent, and follow-up categories, only two of the three must be met or exceeded for a given code.

new patient. Patient who is receiving face-to-face care from a provider/qualified health care professional or another physician/qualified health care professional of the exact same specialty and subspecialty who belongs to the same group practice for the first time in three years. For OPPS hospitals, a patient who has not been registered as an inpatient or outpatient, including off-campus provider based clinic or emergency department, within the past three years.

99251-99255

★**99251** Inpatient consultation for a new or established patient, which requires these 3 key components: A problem focused history; A problem focused examination; and Straightforward medical decision making. Counseling and/or coordination of care with other physicians, other qualified health care professionals, or agencies are provided consistent with the nature of the problem(s) and the patient's and/or family's needs. Usually, the presenting problem(s) are self limited or minor. Typically, 20 minutes are spent at the bedside and on the patient's hospital floor or unit.

★**99252** Inpatient consultation for a new or established patient, which requires these 3 key components: An expanded problem focused history; An expanded problem focused examination; and Straightforward medical decision making. Counseling and/or coordination of care with other physicians, other qualified health care professionals, or agencies are provided consistent with the nature of the problem(s) and the patient's and/or family's needs. Usually, the presenting problem(s) are of low severity. Typically, 40 minutes are spent at the bedside and on the patient's hospital floor or unit.

★**99253** Inpatient consultation for a new or established patient, which requires these 3 key components: A detailed history; A detailed examination; and Medical decision making of low complexity. Counseling and/or coordination of care with other physicians, other qualified health care professionals, or agencies are provided consistent with the nature of the problem(s) and the patient's and/or family's needs. Usually, the presenting problem(s) are of moderate severity. Typically, 55 minutes are spent at the bedside and on the patient's hospital floor or unit.

★**99254** Inpatient consultation for a new or established patient, which requires these 3 key components: A comprehensive history; A comprehensive examination; and Medical decision making of moderate complexity. Counseling and/or coordination of care with other physicians, other qualified health care professionals, or agencies are provided consistent with the nature of the problem(s) and the patient's and/or family's needs. Usually, the presenting problem(s) are of moderate to high severity. Typically, 80 minutes are spent at the bedside and on the patient's hospital floor or unit.

★**99255** Inpatient consultation for a new or established patient, which requires these 3 key components: A comprehensive history; A comprehensive examination; and Medical decision making of high complexity. Counseling and/or coordination of care with other physicians, other qualified health care professionals, or agencies are provided consistent with the nature of the problem(s) and the patient's and/or family's needs. Usually, the presenting problem(s) are of moderate to high severity. Typically, 110 minutes are spent at the bedside and on the patient's hospital floor or unit.

Explanation

Inpatient consultation service codes describe encounters with patients admitted to the hospital, residing in nursing facilities, or to patients in a partial hospital setting where another qualified clinician's advice or opinion regarding diagnosis and treatment or determination to accept transfer of care of a patient is rendered at the request of the primary treating provider. The request for a consultation must be documented in the patient's medical record, as well as a written report of the findings of the consultation to the primary treating physician. During the course of a consultation, the physician consultant can initiate diagnostic or therapeutic services at the same encounter or at a follow-up visit. Other procedures or services performed in conjunction with the consultation may be reported separately. Codes do not differentiate between new or established patients and only one inpatient consultation services code should be reported per admission. Services are reported based on meeting all three key components (history, exam, and medical decision-making [MDM]) within each level of service. The most basic service, as represented by 99251, describes a problem focused history and exam with straightforward medical decision-making for a minor or self-limiting complaint encompassing approximately 20 minutes of time at the patient's bedside or on the unit. The mid-level services describe problems involving an expanded problem focused history and exam or a detailed history and exam as represented by 99252 and 99253, respectively. Medical decision-making for 99252 is the same (straightforward) as for a level one visit (99251) and is designated as low complexity for the level three service (99253). At these levels of service, the encounter can involve time at the patient's bedside or on the unit of 40 (99252) to 55 (99253) minutes involving minimal to low severity concerns. The last two levels of service in this category represent moderate to high-severity problems and both services involve comprehensive history and examination components. The differentiating factor between the two levels is the medical decision-making. Code 99254 involves moderate complexity MDM and approximately 80 minutes of time at the patient's bedside or on the unit, while the highest level of service in this category, 99255, involves MDM of high complexity and approximately 110 minutes at the patient's bedside or on the unit.

Coding Tips

These codes are used to report consultations in the inpatient setting. All three key components (history, exam, and medical decision making) must be met or exceeded for the level of service selected. Time may be used to select the level of service when counseling and coordination of care are documented as at least half of the time spent face-to-face with the patient. Consultation codes are not covered by Medicare and some payers. Report new or established inpatient E/M codes for consultation services. Consultation services should not be reported when the care and management of a problem or condition is assumed prior to the initial examination of the patient. In these situations, the appropriate initial or subsequent evaluation and management service should be reported. Do not report an inpatient and outpatient consultation when both are related to the same inpatient admission. For initial hospital care services, see 99221-99223; for subsequent hospital care services, see 99231-99233. For office or other outpatient consultation services, see 99241-99245. Telemedicine services may be reported by the performing provider by adding modifier 95 to these procedure codes. Services at the origination site are reported with HCPCS Level II code Q3014.

ICD-10-CM Diagnostic Codes

The application of this code is too broad to adequately present ICD-10-CM diagnostic code links here. Refer to your ICD-10-CM book.

AMA: 99251 2020,Sep,3; 2018,Jan,8; 2017,Jun,6; 2017,Jan,8; 2017,Aug,3; 2016,Jan,7; 2016,Jan,13; 2016,Dec,11; 2015,Jan,16; 2014,Oct,8; 2014,Nov,14; 2014,Jan,11 **99252** 2020,Sep,3; 2018,Jan,8; 2017,Jun,6; 2017,Jan,8; 2017,Aug,3; 2016,Jan,7; 2016,Jan,13; 2016,Dec,11; 2015,Jan,16; 2014,Oct,8; 2014,Nov,14; 2014,Jan,11 **99253** 2020,Sep,3; 2018,Jan,8; 2017,Jun,6; 2017,Jan,8; 2017,Aug,3; 2016,Jan,13; 2016,Jan,7; 2016,Dec,11; 2015,Jan,16; 2014,Oct,8; 2014,Nov,14; 2014,Jan,11 **99254** 2020,Sep,3; 2018,Jan,8; 2017,Jun,6; 2017,Jan,8; 2017,Aug,3; 2016,Jan,13; 2016,Jan,7; 2016,Dec,11; 2015,Jan,16; 2014,Oct,8; 2014,Nov,14; 2014,Jan,11 **99255** 2020,Sep,3; 2018,Jan,8; 2017,Jun,6; 2017,Jan,8; 2017,Aug,3; 2016,Jan,13; 2016,Jan,7; 2016,Dec,11; 2015,Jan,16; 2014,Oct,8; 2014,Nov,14; 2014,Jan,11

Relative Value Units/Medicare Edits

Non-Facility RVU	Work	PE	MP	Total
99251	1.0	0.32	0.09	1.41
99252	1.5	0.52	0.11	2.13
99253	2.27	0.84	0.18	3.29
99254	3.29	1.23	0.27	4.79
99255	4.0	1.44	0.32	5.76
Facility RVU	Work	PE	MP	Total
99251	1.0	0.32	0.09	1.41
99252	1.5	0.52	0.11	2.13
99253	2.27	0.84	0.18	3.29
99254	3.29	1.23	0.27	4.79
99255	4.0	1.44	0.32	5.76

	FUD	Status	MUE	Modifiers				IOM Reference
99251	N/A	I	0(3)	N/A	N/A	N/A	N/A	100-04,12,30.6.4;
99252	N/A	I	0(3)	N/A	N/A	N/A	N/A	100-04,12,30.6.10;
99253	N/A	I	0(3)	N/A	N/A	N/A	N/A	100-04,12,100
99254	N/A	I	0(3)	N/A	N/A	N/A	N/A	
99255	N/A	I	0(3)	N/A	N/A	N/A	N/A	

* with documentation

Terms To Know

consultation. Advice or opinion regarding diagnosis and treatment or determination to accept transfer of care of a patient rendered by a medical professional at the request of the primary care provider.

key components. Three components of history, examination, and medical decision making are considered the keys to selecting the correct level of E/M codes. In most cases, all three components must be addressed in the documentation. However, in established, subsequent, and follow-up categories, only two of the three must be met or exceeded for a given code.

other qualified health care professional. Individual who is qualified by education, training, licensure/regulation, and facility privileging to perform a professional service within his or her scope of practice and independently (or as incident-to) report the professional service without requiring physician supervision. Payers may state exemptions in writing or state and local regulations may not follow this definition for performance of some services. Always refer to any relevant plan policies and federal and/or state laws to determine who may perform and report services.

99281-99285

99281 Emergency department visit for the evaluation and management of a patient, which requires these 3 key components: A problem focused history; A problem focused examination; and Straightforward medical decision making. Counseling and/or coordination of care with other physicians, other qualified health care professionals, or agencies are provided consistent with the nature of the problem(s) and the patient's and/or family's needs. Usually, the presenting problem(s) are self limited or minor.

99282 Emergency department visit for the evaluation and management of a patient, which requires these 3 key components: An expanded problem focused history; An expanded problem focused examination; and Medical decision making of low complexity. Counseling and/or coordination of care with other physicians, other qualified health care professionals, or agencies are provided consistent with the nature of the problem(s) and the patient's and/or family's needs. Usually, the presenting problem(s) are of low to moderate severity.

99283 Emergency department visit for the evaluation and management of a patient, which requires these 3 key components: An expanded problem focused history; An expanded problem focused examination; and Medical decision making of moderate complexity. Counseling and/or coordination of care with other physicians, other qualified health care professionals, or agencies are provided consistent with the nature of the problem(s) and the patient's and/or family's needs. Usually, the presenting problem(s) are of moderate severity.

99284 Emergency department visit for the evaluation and management of a patient, which requires these 3 key components: A detailed history; A detailed examination; and Medical decision making of moderate complexity. Counseling and/or coordination of care with other physicians, other qualified health care professionals, or agencies are provided consistent with the nature of the problem(s) and the patient's and/or family's needs. Usually, the presenting problem(s) are of high severity, and require urgent evaluation by the physician, or other qualified health care professionals but do not pose an immediate significant threat to life or physiologic function.

99285 Emergency department visit for the evaluation and management of a patient, which requires these 3 key components within the constraints imposed by the urgency of the patient's clinical condition and/or mental status: A comprehensive history; A comprehensive examination; and Medical decision making of high complexity. Counseling and/or coordination of care with other physicians, other qualified health care professionals, or agencies are provided consistent with the nature of the problem(s) and the patient's and/or family's needs. Usually, the presenting problem(s) are of high severity and pose an immediate significant threat to life or physiologic function.

Explanation

Emergency department services codes describe E/M services provided to patients in the emergency department (ED). ED codes are typically reported per day and do not differentiate between new or established patients. Under the emergency department services category, there are five levels represented by 99281-99285. All levels require the three key components (history, exam, and medical decision-making [MDM]) to be documented. The lowest level of care, 99281, requires a problem-focused history and exam with straightforward medical decision-making involving a minor or self-limiting complaint. Mid-level services describe an expanded problem-focused history and exam with MDM of low or moderate complexity as represented by 99282 and 99283, respectively. At these levels of service, the encounter typically addresses low to moderate severity health concerns. The last two levels of service in this category represent high-severity problems. Code 99284 describes a high-severity health concern that does not pose an immediate threat to life or physiologic function; a detailed history and exam in conjunction with moderate complexity MDM are required for reporting this level of service. The highest level of service, 99285, requires a comprehensive history and examination with high complexity MDM for high-severity health issues that pose an immediate threat to the life or physiologic function of the patient. Time is not listed as a component in the code descriptors for emergency department services as these types of services are provided based on the varying intensity of the patient's condition and may involve emergency providers caring for several patients over an extended period of time involving multiple encounters, making it difficult for the clinician to accurately detail the amount of time spent face-to-face with the patient.

Coding Tips

These codes are used to report emergency department services for the new or established patient. All three key components (history, exam, and medical decision making) must be met or exceeded for the level of service selected. Time is not a factor when selecting this E/M service. An emergency department is typically described as an organized hospital-based facility available 24 hours a day, providing unscheduled episodic services to patients in need of urgent medical attention. For critical care services provided in the emergency department, see 99291-99292. For observation care services provided to a patient located in the emergency department, see 99217-99220. For patients admitted and discharged from observation or inpatient status on the same date, see 99234-99236. Report place of service code 23 for services provided in the hospital emergency room. Medicare has provisionally identified these codes as telehealth/telemedicine services. Current Medicare coverage guidelines should be reviewed. Commercial payers should be contacted regarding their coverage guidelines. Telemedicine services may be reported by the performing provider by adding modifier 95 to these procedure codes. Services at the origination site are reported with HCPCS Level II code Q3014.

ICD-10-CM Diagnostic Codes

The application of this code is too broad to adequately present ICD-10-CM diagnostic code links here. Refer to your ICD-10-CM book.

AMA: 99281 2020,Jul,13; 2019,Jul,10; 2018,Jan,8; 2017,Jun,6; 2017,Jan,8; 2017,Aug,3; 2016,Jan,13; 2016,Jan,7; 2015,Jan,12; 2015,Jan,16; 2014,Oct,8; 2014,Nov,14; 2014,Jan,11 **99282** 2020,Jul,13; 2019,Jul,10; 2018,Jan,8; 2017,Jun,6; 2017,Jan,8; 2017,Aug,3; 2016,Jan,13; 2016,Jan,7; 2015,Jan,16; 2015,Jan,12; 2014,Oct,8; 2014,Nov,14; 2014,Jan,11 **99283** 2020,Jul,13; 2019,Jul,10; 2018,Jan,8; 2017,Jun,6; 2017,Jan,8; 2017,Aug,3; 2016,Jan,13; 2016,Jan,7; 2015,Jan,16; 2015,Jan,12; 2014,Oct,8; 2014,Nov,14; 2014,Jan,11 **99284** 2020,Jul,13; 2019,Jul,10; 2018,Jan,8; 2017,Jun,6; 2017,Jan,8; 2017,Aug,3; 2016,Jan,13; 2016,Jan,7; 2015,Jan,12; 2015,Jan,16; 2014,Oct,8; 2014,Nov,14; 2014,Jan,11 **99285** 2020,Jul,13; 2020,Jan,12; 2019,Jul,10; 2018,Jan,8; 2017,Jun,6; 2017,Jan,8; 2017,Aug,3; 2016,Jan,13; 2016,Jan,7; 2015,Jan,16; 2015,Jan,12; 2014,Oct,8; 2014,Nov,14; 2014,Jan,11

Relative Value Units/Medicare Edits

Non-Facility RVU	Work	PE	MP	Total
99281	0.48	0.11	0.05	0.64
99282	0.93	0.21	0.09	1.23
99283	1.42	0.29	0.13	1.84
99284	2.6	0.51	0.27	3.38
99285	3.8	0.71	0.4	4.91
Facility RVU	**Work**	**PE**	**MP**	**Total**
99281	0.48	0.11	0.05	0.64
99282	0.93	0.21	0.09	1.23
99283	1.42	0.29	0.13	1.84
99284	2.6	0.51	0.27	3.38
99285	3.8	0.71	0.4	4.91

	FUD	Status	MUE	Modifiers				IOM Reference
99281	N/A	A	1(3)	N/A	N/A	N/A	80*	100-04,4,160; 100-04,12,30.6.4; 100-04,12,30.6.11; 100-04,12,100
99282	N/A	A	1(3)	N/A	N/A	N/A	80*	
99283	N/A	A	1(3)	N/A	N/A	N/A	80*	
99284	N/A	A	1(3)	N/A	N/A	N/A	80*	
99285	N/A	A	1(3)	N/A	N/A	N/A	80*	

* with documentation

Terms To Know

emergency. Serious medical condition or symptom (including severe pain) resulting from injury, sickness, or mental illness that arises suddenly and requires immediate care and treatment, generally received within 24 hours of onset, to avoid jeopardy to the life, limb, or health of a covered person.

emergency department. Organized hospital-based facility for the provision of unscheduled episodic services to patients who present for immediate medical attention. The facility must be available 24 hours a day.

established patient. Patient who has received professional services in a face-to-face setting within the last three years from the same physician/qualified health care professional or another physician/qualified health care professional of the exact same specialty and subspecialty who belongs to the same group practice. If the patient is seen by a physician/qualified health care professional who is covering for another physician/qualified health care professional, the patient will be considered the same as if seen by the physician/qualified health care professional who is unavailable.

new patient. Patient who is receiving face-to-face care from a provider/qualified health care professional or another physician/qualified health care professional of the exact same specialty and subspecialty who belongs to the same group practice for the first time in three years. For OPPS hospitals, a patient who has not been registered as an inpatient or outpatient, including off-campus provider based clinic or emergency department, within the past three years.

99291-99292

	99291	Critical care, evaluation and management of the critically ill or critically injured patient; first 30-74 minutes
+	99292	each additional 30 minutes (List separately in addition to code for primary service)

Explanation

Critical care services are reported by a physician or other qualified health care provider for critically ill or injured patients. Critical illnesses or injuries are defined as those with impairment to one or more vital organ systems with an increased risk of rapid or imminent health deterioration. Critical care services require direct patient/provider involvement with highly complex decision making in order to evaluate, control, and support vital systems functions to treat one or more vital organ system failures and/or to avoid further decline of the patient's condition. Vital organ system failure includes, but is not limited to, failure of the central nervous, circulatory, or respiratory systems; kidneys; liver; shock; and other metabolic processes. Generally, critical care services necessitate the interpretation of many physiologic parameters and/or other applications of advanced technology as available in a critical care unit, pediatric intensive care unit, respiratory care unit, in an emergency facility, patient room or other hospital department; however, in emergent situations, critical care may be provided where these elements are not available. Critical care may be provided so long as the patient's condition continues to warrant the level of care according to the criteria described. Care provided to patients residing in a critical care unit but not fitting the criteria for critical care is reported using other E/M codes, as appropriate. These codes are time based codes, meaning the total time spent must be documented and includes direct patient care bedside or time spent on the patient's floor or unit (reviewing laboratory results or imaging studies and discussing the patient's care with medical staff, time spent with family members, caregivers, or other surrogate decision makers to gather information on the patient's medical history, reviewing the patient's condition or prognosis, and discussing various treatment options or limitations of treatment), as long as the clinician is immediately available and not providing services to any other patient during the same time period. Time spent outside of the patient's unit or floor, including telephone calls, caregiver discussions, or time spent in actions that do not directly contribute to the patient's care rendered in the critical unit are not reported as critical care. Report these codes for attendance of the patient during transport for patients 24 months of age or older to or from a facility. Code 99291 represents the first 30 to 74 minutes of critical care and is reported once per day. Additional time beyond the first 74 minutes is reported in 30 minute increments with 99292.

Coding Tips

These codes are used to report critical care services. These are time-based services and the total time spent providing critical care must be documented in the medical record. All time spent providing critical care on the same date of service is added together and does not need to be contiguous. Time is reported for practitioner time spent in care of the critically ill or injured patient at the patient's bedside and on the floor/unit. Time spent off the patient unit, even if related to patient care, is not counted. Do not report critical care for patients who may be in the critical care unit but are not currently critically ill. The following services are considered inclusive to the critical care codes when reported by the clinician: interpretation of cardiac output measurements, chest x-rays, pulse oximetry, blood gases, collection and interpretation of physiologic data, computer data such as ECGs, gastric intubation, vascular access, and ventilation management. Code 99291 is reported once per day. Code 99292 is reported in addition to code 99291. Medicare and some other payers may allow 99292 to be reported alone when critical care is reported by another physician of the same group and specialty the same date as another provider reporting 99291. For care of the critically ill neonate, see 99468-99469;

for patients 29 days through 24 months, see 99471-99472; and for patients 2 through 5 years, see 99475-99476. Medicare has provisionally identified these codes as telehealth/telemedicine services. Current Medicare coverage guidelines should be reviewed. Commercial payers should be contacted regarding their coverage guidelines. Telemedicine services may be reported by the performing provider by adding modifier 95 to these procedure codes. Services at the origination site are reported with HCPCS Level II code Q3014.

ICD-10-CM Diagnostic Codes

The application of this code is too broad to adequately present ICD-10-CM diagnostic code links here. Refer to your ICD-10-CM book.

AMA: 99291 2020,Jan,12; 2020,Feb,7; 2019,Jul,10; 2019,Dec,14; 2019,Aug,8; 2018,Jun,9; 2018,Jan,8; 2018,Dec,8; 2018,Dec,8; 2017,Jun,6; 2017,Jan,8; 2017,Aug,3; 2016,Oct,8; 2016,May,3; 2016,Jan,13; 2016,Aug,9; 2015,Jul,3; 2015,Jan,16; 2015,Feb,10; 2014,Oct,8; 2014,Oct,14; 2014,May,4; 2014,Jan,11; 2014,Aug,5 **99292** 2020,Feb,7; 2019,Jul,10; 2019,Dec,14; 2019,Aug,8; 2018,Jun,9; 2018,Jan,8; 2018,Dec,8; 2018,Dec,8; 2017,Jun,6; 2017,Jan,8; 2017,Aug,3; 2016,May,3; 2016,Jan,13; 2016,Aug,9; 2015,Jul,3; 2015,Jan,16; 2015,Feb,10; 2014,Oct,14; 2014,Oct,8; 2014,May,4; 2014,Jan,11; 2014,Aug,5

Relative Value Units/Medicare Edits

Non-Facility RVU	Work	PE	MP	Total
99291	4.5	2.99	0.4	7.89
99292	2.25	1.03	0.21	3.49
Facility RVU	Work	PE	MP	Total
99291	4.5	1.38	0.4	6.28
99292	2.25	0.7	0.21	3.16

	FUD	Status	MUE	Modifiers				IOM Reference
99291	N/A	A	1(2)	N/A	N/A	N/A	80*	100-04,4,160;
99292	N/A	A	8(3)	N/A	N/A	N/A	80*	100-04,12,30.6.9; 100-04,12,100

* with documentation

Terms To Know

critical care. Treatment of critically ill patients in a variety of medical emergencies that requires the constant attendance of the physician (e.g., cardiac arrest, shock, bleeding, respiratory failure, postoperative complications, critically ill neonate).

established patient. Patient who has received professional services in a face-to-face setting within the last three years from the same physician/qualified health care professional or another physician/qualified health care professional of the exact same specialty and subspecialty who belongs to the same group practice. If the patient is seen by a physician/qualified health care professional who is covering for another physician/qualified health care professional, the patient will be considered the same as if seen by the physician/qualified health care professional who is unavailable.

new patient. Patient who is receiving face-to-face care from a provider/qualified health care professional or another physician/qualified health care professional of the exact same specialty and subspecialty who belongs to the same group practice for the first time in three years. For OPPS hospitals, a patient who has not been registered as an inpatient or outpatient, including off-campus provider based clinic or emergency department, within the past three years.

99354-99359

+▲★	**99354**	Prolonged service(s) in the outpatient setting requiring direct patient contact beyond the time of the usual service; first hour (List separately in addition to code for outpatient Evaluation and Management or psychotherapy service, except with office or other outpatient services [99202, 99203, 99204, 99205, 99212, 99213, 99214, 99215])
+▲★	**99355**	each additional 30 minutes (List separately in addition to code for prolonged service)
+▲	**99356**	Prolonged service in the inpatient or observation setting, requiring unit/floor time beyond the usual service; first hour (List separately in addition to code for inpatient or observation Evaluation and Management service)
+	**99357**	each additional 30 minutes (List separately in addition to code for prolonged service)
	99358	Prolonged evaluation and management service before and/or after direct patient care; first hour
+	**99359**	each additional 30 minutes (List separately in addition to code for prolonged service)

Explanation

Prolonged services involve face-to-face patient contact or psychotherapy services beyond the typical service time and should only be reported once per day. Direct patient contact also includes additional non-face-to-face time, such as time spent on the patient's floor or unit in the hospital or nursing facility setting. For prolonged services rendered in the outpatient setting for the first hour, report 99354; for each additional 30 minutes, report 99355. For prolonged services rendered in the inpatient or observation setting for the first hour, report 99356; for each additional 30 minutes, report 99357. Codes should be reported using the total duration of face-to-face time spent by the clinician on the date of service even when the time spent is not continuous. Report prolonged service without direct patient contact with 99358-99359.

Coding Tips

These codes are used to report prolonged services, with direct patient contact (99354-99357) or without direct patient contact (99358-99359) beyond the usual service. These are time-based codes and time spent with the patient must be documented in the medical record. Codes 99354-99357 are only reported in addition to other time-based E/M services. Time spent on other separately reported services excluding the E/M service should not be counted toward the prolonged service time. Code selection is based on whether the service is provided in the outpatient setting or an inpatient or observation setting. For prolonged services provided by a physician or other qualified health care professional with or without direct patient contact in the office or other outpatient setting (i.e., 99205 or 99215), see 99417. For prolonged services provided by a physician or other qualified health care professional involving total time spent at the patient's bedside and on the floor/unit in the hospital or nursing facility, see 99356-99357. For prolonged services provided by a physician or other qualified health care professional without face-to-face contact or unit/floor time, see 99358-99359. Codes 99358-99359 may be reported on a different date of service than the primary service and do not require the primary service to have an established time. Prolonged service of less than 30 minutes should not be reported separately. Report 99354, 99356, and 99358 only once per day for the initial hour of prolonged service care; for each additional 30-minute block of time beyond the initial hour, see 99355, 99357, and 99359. For prolonged services provided by clinical staff, see 99415-99416. Do not report 99354-99355 with 99202-99205, 99212-99215, or 99415-99417. Report 99354 in addition to 90837, 90847, 99241-99245, 99324-99337, 99341-99350, and 99483. Report 99355 in addition to 99354. Report 99356 in addition to 90837, 90847, 99218-99220, 99221-99223,

99224-99226, 99231-99233, 99234-99236, 99251-99255, and 99304-99310. Report 99357 in addition to 99356. Do not report 99358-99359 on the same date of service as 99202-99205, 99212-99215, or 99417. Do not report 99358 or 99359 for time spent performing the following E/M or monitoring services: 93792-93793, 99339, 99340, 99374-99380, 99366-99368, 99421-99423, 99446-99449, 99451-99452, or 99491. Report 99359 in addition to 99358. Medicare has identified 99356 and 99357 as telehealth/telemedicine services. Commercial payers should be contacted regarding their coverage guidelines. Telemedicine services may be reported by the performing provider by adding modifier 95 to 99354-99357. Services at the origination site are reported with HCPCS Level II code Q3014.

ICD-10-CM Diagnostic Codes

This/these CPT code(s) are add-on code(s). See the primary procedure code that this code is performed with for your ICD-10-CM code selections.

AMA: **99354** 2020,Sep,3; 2020,Feb,3; 2019,Oct,10; 2019,Jun,7; 2018,Jan,8; 2017,Jan,8; 2016,Jan,13; 2016,Dec,11; 2015,Oct,9; 2015,Oct,3; 2015,Jan,16; 2014,Oct,8; 2014,Jun,14; 2014,Jan,11; 2014,Apr,6 **99355** 2020,Sep,3; 2020,Feb,3; 2019,Oct,10; 2019,Jun,7; 2018,Jan,8; 2017,Jan,8; 2016,Jan,13; 2016,Dec,11; 2015,Oct,3; 2015,Oct,9; 2015,Jan,16; 2014,Oct,8; 2014,Jun,14; 2014,Jan,11; 2014,Apr,6 **99356** 2020,Sep,3; 2019,Jun,7; 2018,Jan,8; 2017,Jan,8; 2016,Jan,13; 2016,Dec,11; 2015,Oct,3; 2015,Oct,9; 2015,Jan,16; 2014,Oct,8; 2014,Jun,14; 2014,Jan,11; 2014,Apr,6 **99357** 2020,Sep,3; 2019,Jun,7; 2018,Jan,8; 2017,Jan,8; 2016,Jan,13; 2016,Dec,11; 2015,Oct,3; 2015,Oct,9; 2015,Jan,16; 2014,Oct,8; 2014,Jun,14; 2014,Jan,11; 2014,Apr,6 **99358** 2020,Sep,3; 2020,Feb,3; 2019,Jun,7; 2019,Jan,13; 2018,Oct,9; 2018,Jan,8; 2017,Jan,8; 2016,Jan,13; 2015,Jan,16; 2014,Oct,3; 2014,Oct,8; 2014,Jan,11 **99359** 2020,Sep,3; 2020,Feb,3; 2019,Jun,7; 2019,Jan,13; 2018,Oct,9; 2018,Jan,8; 2017,Jan,8; 2016,Jan,13; 2015,Jan,16; 2014,Oct,3; 2014,Oct,8; 2014,Jan,11

Relative Value Units/Medicare Edits

Non-Facility RVU	Work	PE	MP	Total
99354	2.33	1.18	0.15	3.66
99355	1.77	0.9	0.11	2.78
99356	1.71	0.79	0.11	2.61
99357	1.71	0.81	0.11	2.63
99358	2.1	0.92	0.13	3.15
99359	1.0	0.46	0.08	1.54
Facility RVU	**Work**	**PE**	**MP**	**Total**
99354	2.33	0.96	0.15	3.44
99355	1.77	0.71	0.11	2.59
99356	1.71	0.79	0.11	2.61
99357	1.71	0.81	0.11	2.63
99358	2.1	0.92	0.13	3.15
99359	1.0	0.46	0.08	1.54

	FUD	Status	MUE	Modifiers				IOM Reference
99354	N/A	A	1(2)	N/A	N/A	N/A	80*	100-04,11,40.1.3;
99355	N/A	A	4(3)	N/A	N/A	N/A	80*	100-04,12,30.6.4;
99356	N/A	A	1(2)	N/A	N/A	N/A	80*	100-04,12,30.6.13;
99357	N/A	A	4(3)	N/A	N/A	N/A	80*	100-04,12,30.6.14;
99358	N/A	A	1(2)	N/A	N/A	N/A	80*	100-04,12,30.6.15.1;
99359	N/A	A	2(3)	N/A	N/A	N/A	80*	100-04,12,30.6.15.2; 100-04,12,100

* with documentation

N Newborn: 0   **P** Pediatric: 0-17   **M** Maternity: 9-64   **A** Adult: 15-124   ♂ Male Only   ♀ Female Only

[99415, 99416]

+▲ **99415** Prolonged clinical staff service (the service beyond the highest time in the range of total time of the service) during an evaluation and management service in the office or outpatient setting, direct patient contact with physician supervision; first hour (List separately in addition to code for outpatient Evaluation and Management service)

+▲ **99416** Prolonged clinical staff service (the service beyond the highest time in the range of total time of the service) during an evaluation and management service in the office or outpatient setting, direct patient contact with physician supervision; each additional 30 minutes (List separately in addition to code for prolonged service)

Explanation

Prolonged clinical staff services are reported with resequenced codes that were added to describe special situations in which the physician's staff provided assistance to a patient beyond the usual time associated with circumstances requiring observation of the patient, such as in cases where the patient was administered a new medication or inhaled drug requiring monitoring to ensure patient safety in the office or outpatient setting. Such cases do not necessitate the clinician being face-to-face with the patient throughout the entire time period; observation and monitoring of the patient can be performed by a member of the clinician's staff under the provider's supervision. Report these codes in conjunction with the designated E/M service code along with any other service provided at the same encounter. Codes in this category should report the total amount of face-to-face time spent with the patient by the clinical staff on the same date of service even if the time is not continuous; time spent rendering other separately reportable services other than the E/M service do not count toward the prolonged services time. The highest total time in the time ranges of the code descriptions is used in defining when prolonged services time should begin. Report the first hour of prolonged services on a given date with 99415; for each additional 30 minutes of prolonged services, report 99416.

Coding Tips

These codes are used to report prolonged face-to-face services beyond the highest total time indicated in the code description provided by the clinical staff in the office or outpatient setting. These are time-based codes and time spent with the patient must be documented in the medical record. Time spent on other separately reported services excluding the E/M service should not be counted toward the prolonged service time. These codes are reported in addition to the other E/M service provided on the same date of service. A provider must be available to provide direct supervision of the clinical staff. Report 99415 only once per day for the initial hour of prolonged service care; for each additional 30-minute block of time beyond the initial hour, see 99416. Prolonged service of less than 30 minutes should not be reported separately. For prolonged services with or without direct patient contact provided by the physician or other qualified health care provider in the office or other outpatient setting, see 99417. Do not report 99415-99416 with 99354, 99355, or 99417. Report 99415 in addition to 99202-99205 and 99212-99215. Report 99416 in addition to 99415.

ICD-10-CM Diagnostic Codes

This/these CPT code(s) are add-on code(s). See the primary procedure code that this code is performed with for your ICD-10-CM code selections.

AMA: 99415 2020,Sep,3; 2020,Feb,3; 2019,Oct,10; 2018,Jan,8; 2017,Jan,8; 2016,Mar,8; 2016,Jan,13; 2016,Feb,13; 2015,Oct,3 **99416** 2020,Sep,3; 2020,Feb,3; 2019,Oct,10; 2018,Jan,8; 2017,Jan,8; 2016,Mar,8; 2016,Jan,13; 2016,Feb,13; 2015,Oct,3

Relative Value Units/Medicare Edits

Non-Facility RVU	Work	PE	MP	Total
99415	0.0	0.27	0.01	0.28
99416	0.0	0.12	0.0	0.12
Facility RVU	**Work**	**PE**	**MP**	**Total**
99415	0.0	0.27	0.01	0.28
99416	0.0	0.12	0.0	0.12

	FUD	Status	MUE	Modifiers				IOM Reference
99415	N/A	A	1(2)	N/A	N/A	N/A	80*	None
99416	N/A	A	3(3)	N/A	N/A	N/A	80*	

* with documentation

Terms To Know

clinical staff. Someone who works for, or under, the direction of a physician or qualified health care professional and does not bill services separately. The person may be licensed or regulated to help the physician perform specific duties.

other qualified health care professional. Individual who is qualified by education, training, licensure/regulation, and facility privileging to perform a professional service within his or her scope of practice and independently (or as incident-to) report the professional service without requiring physician supervision. Payers may state exemptions in writing or state and local regulations may not follow this definition for performance of some services. Always refer to any relevant plan policies and federal and/or state laws to determine who may perform and report services.

prolonged physician services. Extended pre- or post-service care provided to a patient whose condition requires services beyond the usual.

[99417]

+●★99417 Prolonged office or other outpatient evaluation and management service(s) beyond the minimum required time of the primary procedure which has been selected using total time, requiring total time with or without direct patient contact beyond the usual service, on the date of the primary service, each 15 minutes of total time (List separately in addition to codes 99205, 99215 for office or other outpatient Evaluation and Management services)

Explanation

Code 99417 reports prolonged total time (time with and without direct patient contact combined) that is provided by the physician or other qualified health care professional on the date of an office visit or other outpatient service. This code is assigned only when the code for the primary E/M service has been selected based solely on total time, and only after exceeding by 15 minutes the minimum time that is required to report the highest-level service. For example, when reporting an established patient encounter (99215), code 99417 would not be reported until at least 15 minutes of time beyond 40 minutes has been accumulated (i.e., 55 minutes) on the day of the encounter.

Coding Tips

This code reports prolonged service time by the physician or other qualified health care professional provided on the same date as 99205 or 99215. The prolonged time may be with or without direct patient contact. This service is reported only when time was the criteria used to select code 99205 or 99215 and the time exceeds the minimum time required to report these levels of service by at least 15 minutes. Code 99417 may be reported once for each additional 15 minutes spent providing prolonged services. Time performing other reportable services is not counted as prolonged service. Prolonged services provided on a date other than the date of the face-to-face encounter may be reported with 99358-99359. Prolonged services provided by clinical staff are reported with 99415-99416. Do not report 99417 with 99354-99355, 99358-99359, or 99415-99416. Telemedicine services may be reported by the performing provider by adding modifier 95 to this procedure code. Services at the origination site are reported with HCPCS Level II code Q3014.

ICD-10-CM Diagnostic Codes

This/these CPT code(s) are add-on code(s). See the primary procedure code that this code is performed with for your ICD-10-CM code selections.

Relative Value Units/Medicare Edits

Non-Facility RVU	Work	PE	MP	Total
99417				
Facility RVU	**Work**	**PE**	**MP**	**Total**
99417				

	FUD	Status	MUE	Modifiers				IOM Reference
99417	N/A		-	N/A	N/A	N/A	N/A	None

* with documentation

99360

99360 Standby service, requiring prolonged attendance, each 30 minutes (eg, operative standby, standby for frozen section, for cesarean/high risk delivery, for monitoring EEG)

Explanation

Standby services are those requested of a qualified clinician that involves prolonged attendance without face-to-face contact with the patient (e.g., operative or cesarean/high-risk delivery standby, EEG monitoring, or standby to obtain a frozen section specimen). The clinician on standby is not permitted to provide care or services to other patients during the standby period. This code should not be used to report time spent proctoring another individual nor should it be used if the standby period ends with the standby clinician performing a procedure that is subject to the surgical package. This code encompasses the total duration of time spent on standby on a given date; standby services of less than 30 minutes total duration are not reported separately. A second and subsequent period of standby, after the initial 30 minutes, may be reported contingent that each unit of standby service equates to a full 30 minutes.

Coding Tips

This code is used to report standby services requested by another clinician for prolonged attendance without face-to-face patient contact. This is a time-based code representing the total duration of time spent providing standby services and must be documented in the medical record. Standby services of less than 30 minutes should not be reported separately. Report each additional 30 minutes of time beyond the initial time only when a full 30-minute period is provided. Report this code with 99460 or 99465, if applicable. Do not report 99360 in addition to 99464.

ICD-10-CM Diagnostic Codes

The application of this code is too broad to adequately present ICD-10-CM diagnostic code links here. Refer to your ICD-10-CM book.

AMA: 99360 2018,Jan,8; 2017,Jan,8; 2016,Jan,13; 2015,Jan,16; 2014,Oct,8; 2014,Jan,11; 2014,Apr,5

Relative Value Units/Medicare Edits

Non-Facility RVU	Work	PE	MP	Total
99360	1.2	0.46	0.09	1.75
Facility RVU	**Work**	**PE**	**MP**	**Total**
99360	1.2	0.46	0.09	1.75

	FUD	Status	MUE	Modifiers				IOM Reference
99360	N/A	X	1(3)	N/A	N/A	N/A	N/A	100-04,12,30.6.4; 100-04,12,30.6.15.3

* with documentation

Terms To Know

other qualified health care professional. Individual who is qualified by education, training, licensure/regulation, and facility privileging to perform a professional service within his or her scope of practice and independently (or as incident-to) report the professional service without requiring physician supervision. Payers may state exemptions in writing or state and local regulations may not follow this definition for performance of some services. Always refer to any relevant plan policies and federal and/or state laws to determine who may perform and report services.

99384-99387

99384 Initial comprehensive preventive medicine evaluation and management of an individual including an age and gender appropriate history, examination, counseling/anticipatory guidance/risk factor reduction interventions, and the ordering of laboratory/diagnostic procedures, new patient; adolescent (age 12 through 17 years)

99385 18-39 years

99386 40-64 years

99387 65 years and older

Explanation

Initial preventive medicine services are typically well-patient examinations for new patients with code selection dependent upon the patient's age. These services include applicable patient history and examination, guidance/recommendation regarding personal risk factors, and any laboratory and/or diagnostic procedures ordered. Clinicians are not required to report minor or self-limiting problems or complaints noted during the course of the preventive examination when those problems do not require any additional work or necessitate performing the key components of a problem oriented E/M service. Report 99384 for adolescents 12 to 17 years of age; 99385 for adult patients 18 to 39 years of age; 99386 for patients 40 to 64 years of age; and 99387 for patients 65 years of age and older.

Coding Tips

These codes are used to report preventive medicine services for a new patient. Time is not a factor when selecting this E/M service. Code selection is determined based on whether the patient is new or established and the age of the patient. When documentation supports that a significant, separately identifiable problem-oriented evaluation and management (E/M) service is rendered, the appropriate code for the E/M service may be reported separately. Append modifier 25 to the service code selected to indicate that a separately identifiable E/M service was provided on the same date of service as the preventive medicine service. Immunizations and ancillary services, including laboratory, radiology, or screening tests, performed at the time of the preventive service may be reported separately. Preventive medicine services are not covered by Medicare. For preventive services provided to an established patient, see 99394-99397.

ICD-10-CM Diagnostic Codes

Z00.00	Encounter for general adult medical examination without abnormal findings ⬛
Z00.01	Encounter for general adult medical examination with abnormal findings ⬛
Z01.411	Encounter for gynecological examination (general) (routine) with abnormal findings ♀
Z01.419	Encounter for gynecological examination (general) (routine) without abnormal findings ♀

AMA: 99384 2018,Jan,8; 2017,Jan,8; 2016,Mar,8; 2016,Jan,13; 2015,Jan,12; 2015,Jan,16; 2014,Oct,8; 2014,Jan,11 **99385** 2018,Jan,8; 2017,Jan,8; 2016,Mar,8; 2016,Jan,13; 2015,Jan,16; 2015,Jan,12; 2014,Oct,8; 2014,Jan,11 **99386** 2018,Jan,8; 2017,Jan,8; 2016,Mar,8; 2016,Jan,13; 2015,Jan,12; 2015,Jan,16; 2014,Oct,8; 2014,Jan,11 **99387** 2018,Jan,8; 2017,Jan,8; 2016,Mar,8; 2016,Jan,13; 2015,Jan,16; 2014,Oct,8; 2014,Jan,11

Relative Value Units/Medicare Edits

Non-Facility RVU	Work	PE	MP	Total
99384	2.0	1.71	0.16	3.87
99385	1.92	1.68	0.15	3.75
99386	2.33	1.83	0.18	4.34
99387	2.5	2.01	0.21	4.72
Facility RVU	**Work**	**PE**	**MP**	**Total**
99384	2.0	0.77	0.16	2.93
99385	1.92	0.74	0.15	2.81
99386	2.33	0.9	0.18	3.41
99387	2.5	0.96	0.21	3.67

	FUD	Status	MUE	Modifiers				IOM Reference
99384	N/A	N	0(3)	N/A	N/A	N/A	N/A	None
99385	N/A	N	0(3)	N/A	N/A	N/A	N/A	
99386	N/A	N	0(3)	N/A	N/A	N/A	N/A	
99387	N/A	N	0(3)	N/A	N/A	N/A	N/A	

* with documentation

Terms To Know

key components. Three components of history, examination, and medical decision making are considered the keys to selecting the correct level of E/M codes. In most cases, all three components must be addressed in the documentation. However, in established, subsequent, and follow-up categories, only two of the three must be met or exceeded for a given code.

new patient. Patient who is receiving face-to-face care from a provider/qualified health care professional or another physician/qualified health care professional of the exact same specialty and subspecialty who belongs to the same group practice for the first time in three years. For OPPS hospitals, a patient who has not been registered as an inpatient or outpatient, including off-campus provider based clinic or emergency department, within the past three years.

preventive medicine service. Evaluation and management service provided as a periodic health screening and/or prophylactic service that does not typically include management of new or existing diagnoses or problems.

99394-99397

99394 Periodic comprehensive preventive medicine reevaluation and management of an individual including an age and gender appropriate history, examination, counseling/anticipatory guidance/risk factor reduction interventions, and the ordering of laboratory/diagnostic procedures, established patient; adolescent (age 12 through 17 years)

99395 18-39 years

99396 40-64 years

99397 65 years and older

Explanation

Periodic comprehensive preventive medicine services are typically well-patient examinations for established patients presenting for reevaluations and/or management of overall health condition with code selection dependent upon the patient's age. These services include applicable patient history and examination, guidance/recommendation regarding personal risk factors, and any laboratory and/or diagnostic procedures ordered. Clinicians are not required to report minor or self-limiting problems or complaints noted during the course of the preventive examination when those problems do not require any additional work or necessitate performing the key components of a problem oriented E/M service. Report 99394 for adolescents 12 to 17 years of age; 99395 for adult patients 18 to 39 years of age; 99396 for patients 40 to 64 years of age; and 99397 for patients 65 years of age and older.

Coding Tips

These codes are used to report preventive medicine services for an established patient. Time is not a factor when selecting this E/M service. Code selection is determined based on whether the patient is new or established and the age of the patient. When documentation supports that a significant, separately identifiable problem-oriented evaluation and management (E/M) service is rendered, the appropriate code for the E/M service may be reported separately. Append modifier 25 to the service code selected to indicate that a separately identifiable E/M service was provided on the same date of service as the preventive medicine service. Immunizations and ancillary services, including laboratory, radiology, or screening tests, performed at the time of the preventive service may be reported separately. Preventive medicine services are not covered by Medicare. For preventive services provided to a new patient, see 99384-99387.

ICD-10-CM Diagnostic Codes

Z00.00	Encounter for general adult medical examination without abnormal findings 🅰
Z00.01	Encounter for general adult medical examination with abnormal findings 🅰
Z01.411	Encounter for gynecological examination (general) (routine) with abnormal findings ♀
Z01.419	Encounter for gynecological examination (general) (routine) without abnormal findings ♀

AMA: **99394** 2018,Jan,8; 2017,Jan,8; 2016,Mar,8; 2016,Jan,13; 2015,Jan,12; 2015,Jan,16; 2014,Oct,8; 2014,Jan,11 **99395** 2018,Jan,8; 2017,Jan,8; 2016,Mar,8; 2016,Jan,13; 2015,Jan,16; 2015,Jan,12; 2014,Oct,8; 2014,Jan,11 **99396** 2018,Jan,8; 2017,Sep,11; 2017,Jan,8; 2016,Mar,8; 2016,Jan,13; 2015,Jan,12; 2015,Jan,16; 2014,Oct,8; 2014,Jan,11 **99397** 2018,Jan,8; 2017,Jan,8; 2016,Mar,8; 2016,Jan,13; 2015,Jan,16; 2014,Oct,8; 2014,Jan,11

Relative Value Units/Medicare Edits

Non-Facility RVU	Work	PE	MP	Total
99394	1.7	1.47	0.13	3.3
99395	1.75	1.5	0.13	3.38
99396	1.9	1.55	0.15	3.6
99397	2.0	1.71	0.16	3.87
Facility RVU	**Work**	**PE**	**MP**	**Total**
99394	1.7	0.65	0.13	2.48
99395	1.75	0.67	0.13	2.55
99396	1.9	0.73	0.15	2.78
99397	2.0	0.77	0.16	2.93

	FUD	Status	MUE	Modifiers				IOM Reference
99394	N/A	N	0(3)	N/A	N/A	N/A	N/A	None
99395	N/A	N	0(3)	N/A	N/A	N/A	N/A	
99396	N/A	N	0(3)	N/A	N/A	N/A	N/A	
99397	N/A	N	0(3)	N/A	N/A	N/A	N/A	

* with documentation

Terms To Know

established patient. Patient who has received professional services in a face-to-face setting within the last three years from the same physician/qualified health care professional or another physician/qualified health care professional of the exact same specialty and subspecialty who belongs to the same group practice. If the patient is seen by a physician/qualified health care professional who is covering for another physician/qualified health care professional, the patient will be considered the same as if seen by the physician/qualified health care professional who is unavailable.

preventive medicine service. Evaluation and management service provided as a periodic health screening and/or prophylactic service that does not typically include management of new or existing diagnoses or problems.

99441-99443

99441 Telephone evaluation and management service by a physician or other qualified health care professional who may report evaluation and management services provided to an established patient, parent, or guardian not originating from a related E/M service provided within the previous 7 days nor leading to an E/M service or procedure within the next 24 hours or soonest available appointment; 5-10 minutes of medical discussion

99442 11-20 minutes of medical discussion

99443 21-30 minutes of medical discussion

Explanation

Telephone services are non-face-to-face encounters originating from the established patient for evaluation or management of a problem provided by a qualified clinician. The problem may not be related to an E/M encounter that occurred within the previous seven days nor can the problem lead to an E/M encounter or other service within the following 24 hours or next available in-office appointment opening. Report 99441 for services lasting five to 10 minutes; 99442 for services lasting 11 to 20 minutes; and 99443 for calls lasting 21 to 30 minutes.

Coding Tips

These codes are used to report non-face-to-face patient services initiated by an established patient via the telephone. These are time-based codes and time spent with the patient must be documented in the medical record. These codes should not be reported if the provider decides to see the patient within 24 hours or by the next available urgent visit appointment, or if the provider performed a related E/M service within the previous seven days or the call is initiated within a postoperative period. Medicare and other payers may not reimburse separately for these services. Check with the specific payer to determine coverage. Do not report 99441-99443 when the same provider has reported 99421-99423 for the same problem in the previous seven days. For nonphysician telephone medical services, see 98966-98968. Do not report these services when performed concurrently with other billable services, such as 99339-99340, 99374-99380, 99487-99489, or 99495-99496. Do not report these services for INR monitoring when reporting 93792 or 93793. Medicare has provisionally identified these codes as telehealth/telemedicine services. Current Medicare coverage guidelines should be reviewed. Commercial payers should be contacted regarding their coverage guidelines. Telemedicine services may be reported by the performing provider by adding modifier 95 to these procedure codes. Services at the origination site are reported with HCPCS Level II code Q3014.

ICD-10-CM Diagnostic Codes

The application of this code is too broad to adequately present ICD-10-CM diagnostic code links here. Refer to your ICD-10-CM book.

AMA: 99441 2020,Jul,1; 2019,Mar,8; 2018,Mar,7; 2018,Jan,8; 2017,Jan,8; 2016,Jan,13; 2015,Jan,16; 2014,Oct,8; 2014,Oct,3; 2014,Jan,11 **99442** 2020,Jul,1; 2019,Mar,8; 2018,Mar,7; 2018,Jan,8; 2017,Jan,8; 2016,Jan,13; 2015,Jan,16; 2014,Oct,3; 2014,Oct,8; 2014,Jan,11 **99443** 2020,Jul,1; 2019,Mar,8; 2018,Mar,7; 2018,Jan,8; 2017,Jan,8; 2016,Jan,13; 2015,Jan,16; 2014,Oct,3; 2014,Oct,8; 2014,Jan,11

Relative Value Units/Medicare Edits

Non-Facility RVU	Work	PE	MP	Total
99441	0.48	0.75	0.05	1.28
99442	0.97	1.06	0.08	2.11
99443	1.5	1.45	0.11	3.06
Facility RVU	**Work**	**PE**	**MP**	**Total**
99441	0.48	0.2	0.05	0.73
99442	0.97	0.4	0.08	1.45
99443	1.5	0.62	0.11	2.23

	FUD	Status	MUE	Modifiers				IOM Reference
99441	N/A	A	1(2)	N/A	N/A	N/A	80*	None
99442	N/A	A	1(2)	N/A	N/A	N/A	80*	
99443	N/A	A	1(2)	N/A	N/A	N/A	80*	

* with documentation

Terms To Know

documentation. Physician's written or transcribed notations about a patient encounter, including a detailed operative report or written notes about a routine encounter. Source documentation must be the treating provider's own account of the encounter and may be transcribed from dictation, dictated by the physician into voice recognition software, or be hand- or typewritten. A signature or authentication accompanies each entry.

noncovered services. Health care services that are not reimbursable according to provisions of a given insurance policy.

qualified health care professional. Educated, licensed or certified, and regulated professional operating under a specified scope of practice to provide patient services that are separate and distinct from other clinical staff.

[99421, 99422, 99423]

99421 Online digital evaluation and management service, for an established patient, for up to 7 days, cumulative time during the 7 days; 5-10 minutes

99422 Online digital evaluation and management service, for an established patient, for up to 7 days, cumulative time during the 7 days; 11-20 minutes

99423 Online digital evaluation and management service, for an established patient, for up to 7 days, cumulative time during the 7 days; 21 or more minutes

Explanation

Online medical evaluation services are non-face-to-face encounters originating from the established patient to the physician or other qualified health care professional for evaluation or management of a problem utilizing internet resources. The service includes all communication, prescription, and laboratory orders with permanent storage in the patient's medical record. The service may include more than one provider responding to the same patient and is only reportable once during seven days for the same encounter. Do not report these codes if the online patient request is related to an E/M service that occurred within the previous seven days or within the global period following a procedure. Report 99421 if the cumulative time during the seven-day period is five to 10 minutes; 99422 for 11 to 20 minutes; and 99423 for 21 or more minutes.

Coding Tips

These codes are used to report non-face-to-face patient services initiated by an established patient via an on-line inquiry. Providers must provide a timely response to the inquiry and the encounter must be stored permanently to report this service. These services are reported once in a seven-day period and are reported for the cumulative time devoted to the service over the seven days. Cumulative time of less than five minutes should not be reported. A new/unrelated problem initiated within seven days of a previous E/M visit that addresses a different problem may be reported separately. Medicare and other payers may not reimburse separately for these services. Check with the specific payer to determine coverage. For nonphysician on-line medical services, see 98970, 98971, and 98972. Do not report these services when performed concurrently with other billable services, such as 99202-99205, 99212-99215, 99241-99245, or when using the following codes for the same communication: 99091, 99339-99340, 99374-99380, or 99487-99489. Do not report these services for INR monitoring when reporting 93792 or 93793.

ICD-10-CM Diagnostic Codes

The application of this code is too broad to adequately present ICD-10-CM diagnostic code links here. Refer to your ICD-10-CM book.

AMA: **99421** 2020,Jan,3 **99422** 2020,Jan,3 **99423** 2020,Jan,3

Relative Value Units/Medicare Edits

Non-Facility RVU	Work	PE	MP	Total
99421	0.25	0.16	0.02	0.43
99422	0.5	0.31	0.05	0.86
99423	0.8	0.51	0.08	1.39
Facility RVU	**Work**	**PE**	**MP**	**Total**
99421	0.25	0.1	0.02	0.37
99422	0.5	0.21	0.05	0.76
99423	0.8	0.33	0.08	1.21

	FUD	Status	MUE	Modifiers				IOM Reference
99421	N/A	A	1(2)	N/A	N/A	N/A	80*	None
99422	N/A	A	1(2)	N/A	N/A	N/A	80*	
99423	N/A	A	1(2)	N/A	N/A	N/A	80*	

* with documentation

Terms To Know

established patient. Patient who has received professional services in a face-to-face setting within the last three years from the same physician/qualified health care professional or another physician/qualified health care professional of the exact same specialty and subspecialty who belongs to the same group practice. If the patient is seen by a physician/qualified health care professional who is covering for another physician/qualified health care professional, the patient will be considered the same as if seen by the physician/qualified health care professional who is unavailable.

evaluation. Dynamic process in which the dentist makes clinical judgments based on data gathered during the examination.

99446-99449 [99451, 99452]

99446 Interprofessional telephone/Internet/electronic health record assessment and management service provided by a consultative physician, including a verbal and written report to the patient's treating/requesting physician or other qualified health care professional; 5-10 minutes of medical consultative discussion and review

99447 11-20 minutes of medical consultative discussion and review

99448 21-30 minutes of medical consultative discussion and review

99449 31 minutes or more of medical consultative discussion and review

99451 Interprofessional telephone/Internet/electronic health record assessment and management service provided by a consultative physician, including a written report to the patient's treating/requesting physician or other qualified health care professional, 5 minutes or more of medical consultative time

99452 Interprofessional telephone/Internet/electronic health record referral service(s) provided by a treating/requesting physician or other qualified health care professional, 30 minutes

Explanation

Interprofessional telephone/internet/electronic health record consultation services are utilized when the attending qualified clinician requests the input of another provider with specific knowledge of the condition. This specialist may assist in diagnosis or treatment of the patient without seeing the patient and often occurs when the situation is urgent and/or complex in nature. The patient may be a new or established patient with a new problem or exacerbation of a current problem in the eyes of the consulting physician; however, the consultant may not have seen the patient within the previous 14 days. This code may not be reported for transfer of care or to schedule a face-to-face with the consultant within the next 14 days or next available appointment opening. This discussion includes appropriate review of medical records, laboratory and radiology results, medication review/tolerance, and pathology results. The consult should account for more than 50 percent of the time in discussion; if more than one discussion is necessary, the time is cumulative with the code reported one time. The patient's medical record should contain a request for consult with an explanation as to the medical necessity of the request and the consulting physician should provide a verbal and written report to the requesting/treating clinician. These codes are not reportable if the discussion requires less than five minutes of time. Report 99446 for encounters of five- to 10 minutes duration; 99447 for 11 to 20 minutes; 99448 for 21 to 30 minutes; and 99449 for encounters of more than 30 minutes duration. Report 99451 for encounters of five or more minutes that include a written report only from the consulting physician. The attending qualified clinician can report 99452 when 16 to 30 minutes of the clinician's time is spent preparing for or communicating with the consultant; 99452 can only be reported once during a 14-day period.

Coding Tips

These codes are used to report an assessment and management service requested by the patient's treating clinician for guidance from a specialist in treating the patient. These are time-based codes and time spent in medical consultation must be documented in the medical record. These codes do not differentiate between a new or established patient. Do not report these codes for the sole purpose of arranging a transfer of care or other face-to-face services. Report 99446-99449 for time spent in telephone/internet/electronic health record assessment and review with verbal and written report of findings. Report 99451 for written report of findings without a verbal report. Report

99452 for the time a provider spends, on a service day, preparing for or communicating with the consultant. Prolonged service codes 99354-99357 may be reported by the treating/requesting provider in addition to these services when the patient is present (on-site) and the telephone/internet/electronic health record discussion with the consultant exceeds 30 minutes. Prolonged service codes 99358-99359 may be reported by the treating/requesting provider in addition to these services when the patient is not present and the telephone/internet discussion with the consultant exceeds 30 minutes. For telephone services conducted by the physician directly with the patient, see 99441-99443. For on-line digital medical evaluation and management services provided by the physician directly with the patient, see 99421-99423. For nonphysician telephone or online medical services, see 98966-98968.

ICD-10-CM Diagnostic Codes

The application of this code is too broad to adequately present ICD-10-CM diagnostic code links here. Refer to your ICD-10-CM book.

AMA: **99446** 2019,Jun,7; 2019,Jan,3; 2018,Jan,8; 2017,Jan,8; 2016,Jan,13; 2015,Jan,16; 2014,Oct,8; 2014,Jun,14 **99447** 2019,Jun,7; 2019,Jan,3; 2018,Jan,8; 2017,Jan,8; 2016,Jan,13; 2015,Jan,16; 2014,Oct,8; 2014,Jun,14 **99448** 2019,Jun,7; 2019,Jan,3; 2018,Jan,8; 2017,Jan,8; 2016,Jan,13; 2015,Jan,16; 2014,Oct,8; 2014,Jun,14 **99449** 2019,Jun,7; 2019,Jan,3; 2018,Jan,8; 2017,Jan,8; 2016,Jan,13; 2015,Jan,16; 2014,Oct,8; 2014,Jun,14 **99451** 2019,Jun,7; 2019,Jan,3 **99452** 2020,Jun,3; 2019,Jun,7; 2019,Jan,3

Relative Value Units/Medicare Edits

Non-Facility RVU	Work	PE	MP	Total
99446	0.35	0.13	0.03	0.51
99447	0.7	0.27	0.06	1.03
99448	1.05	0.4	0.09	1.54
99449	1.4	0.54	0.11	2.05
99451	0.7	0.29	0.05	1.04
99452	0.7	0.29	0.05	1.04
Facility RVU	**Work**	**PE**	**MP**	**Total**
99446	0.35	0.13	0.03	0.51
99447	0.7	0.27	0.06	1.03
99448	1.05	0.4	0.09	1.54
99449	1.4	0.54	0.11	2.05
99451	0.7	0.29	0.05	1.04
99452	0.7	0.29	0.05	1.04

	FUD	Status	MUE	Modifiers				IOM Reference
99446	N/A	A	1(2)	N/A	N/A	N/A	80*	None
99447	N/A	A	1(2)	N/A	N/A	N/A	80*	
99448	N/A	A	1(2)	N/A	N/A	N/A	80*	
99449	N/A	A	1(2)	N/A	N/A	N/A	80*	
99451	N/A	A	1(2)	N/A	N/A	N/A	80*	
99452	N/A	A	1(2)	N/A	N/A	N/A	80*	

* with documentation

Terms To Know

assessment. Process of collecting and studying information and data, such as test values, signs, and symptoms.

consultation. Advice or opinion regarding diagnosis and treatment or determination to accept transfer of care of a patient rendered by a medical professional at the request of the primary care provider.

99464-99465

99464 Attendance at delivery (when requested by the delivering physician or other qualified health care professional) and initial stabilization of newborn

99465 Delivery/birthing room resuscitation, provision of positive pressure ventilation and/or chest compressions in the presence of acute inadequate ventilation and/or cardiac output

Explanation

Delivery/birthing room attendance and resuscitation services are reported when special newborn circumstances require additional attendance and/or care. Report 99464 when attendance during delivery is requested by the delivering health care professional with newborn stabilization. Report 99465 for delivery/birthing room resuscitation, including any positive pressure ventilation and/or chest compression when required due to unsatisfactory ventilation or cardiac output.

Coding Tips

These codes are used to report stabilization or resuscitation services provided to a newborn in the delivery or birthing center. Additional services performed as a necessary part of the resuscitation service, including intubation and vascular lines, may be reported in addition to 99465. These additional services should only be reported when necessary for resuscitation not as a convenience prior to admission to a neonatal intensive care unit. These codes may be reported in addition to 99460, 99468, and 99477. Do not report 99465 with 99464.

ICD-10-CM Diagnostic Codes

The application of this code is too broad to adequately present ICD-10-CM diagnostic code links here. Refer to your ICD-10-CM book.

AMA: 99464 2018,Jan,8; 2017,Jan,8; 2016,Jan,13; 2015,Jan,16; 2014,Oct,8; 2014,Jan,11 **99465** 2018,Jan,8; 2017,Jan,8; 2016,Jan,13; 2015,Jan,16; 2014,Oct,8; 2014,Jan,11

Relative Value Units/Medicare Edits

Non-Facility RVU	Work	PE	MP	Total
99464	1.5	0.52	0.09	2.11
99465	2.93	1.01	0.19	4.13
Facility RVU	Work	PE	MP	Total
99464	1.5	0.52	0.09	2.11
99465	2.93	1.01	0.19	4.13

	FUD	Status	MUE	Modifiers				IOM Reference
99464	N/A	A	1(2)	N/A	N/A	N/A	80*	None
99465	N/A	A	1(2)	N/A	N/A	N/A	80*	

* with documentation

Terms To Know

delivery. Expulsion or extraction of a newborn and the afterbirth.

resuscitation. Restoration to life or consciousness of one apparently dead, it includes such measures as artificial respiration and cardiac massage or electrical shock.

10060-10061

10060 Incision and drainage of abscess (eg, carbuncle, suppurative hidradenitis, cutaneous or subcutaneous abscess, cyst, furuncle, or paronychia); simple or single

10061 complicated or multiple

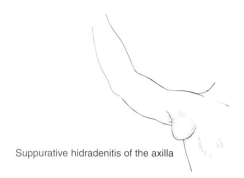

Suppurative hidradenitis of the axilla

Explanation

The physician makes a small incision through the skin overlying an abscess for incision and drainage (e.g., carbuncle, cyst, furuncle, paronychia, hidradenitis). The abscess or cyst is opened with a surgical instrument, allowing the contents to drain. The lesion may be curetted and irrigated. The physician leaves the surgical wound open to allow for continued drainage or the physician may place a Penrose latex drain or gauze strip packing to allow continued drainage. Report 10060 for incision and drainage of a simple or single abscess. Report 10061 for complex or multiple cysts. Complex or multiple cysts may require surgical closure at a later date.

Coding Tips

These codes are not for reporting incision and drainage of a pilonidal cyst, perineal abscess, or postoperative wound infection. For incision and drainage of a pilonidal cyst, see 10080–10081. For incision and drainage of a wound abscess or infection postoperatively, see 10180. For incision and drainage of an abscess on the perineum or vulva, see 56405. For incision and drainage of a vaginal abscess, see 57010. Surgical trays, A4550, are not separately reimbursed by Medicare; however, other third-party payers may cover them. Check with the specific payer to determine coverage.

ICD-10-CM Diagnostic Codes

L02.211	Cutaneous abscess of abdominal wall
L02.212	Cutaneous abscess of back [any part, except buttock]
L02.213	Cutaneous abscess of chest wall
L02.214	Cutaneous abscess of groin
L02.215	Cutaneous abscess of perineum
L02.216	Cutaneous abscess of umbilicus
L02.221	Furuncle of abdominal wall
L02.222	Furuncle of back [any part, except buttock]
L02.223	Furuncle of chest wall
L02.224	Furuncle of groin
L02.225	Furuncle of perineum
L02.226	Furuncle of umbilicus
L02.231	Carbuncle of abdominal wall
L02.232	Carbuncle of back [any part, except buttock]
L02.233	Carbuncle of chest wall
L02.234	Carbuncle of groin
L02.235	Carbuncle of perineum
L02.236	Carbuncle of umbilicus
L02.31	Cutaneous abscess of buttock
L02.32	Furuncle of buttock
L02.33	Carbuncle of buttock
L02.411	Cutaneous abscess of right axilla ☑
L02.412	Cutaneous abscess of left axilla ☑
L02.421	Furuncle of right axilla ☑
L02.422	Furuncle of left axilla ☑
L02.431	Carbuncle of right axilla ☑
L02.432	Carbuncle of left axilla ☑
L02.818	Cutaneous abscess of other sites
L02.828	Furuncle of other sites
L02.838	Carbuncle of other sites
L03.111	Cellulitis of right axilla ☑
L03.112	Cellulitis of left axilla ☑
L03.121	Acute lymphangitis of right axilla ☑
L03.122	Acute lymphangitis of left axilla ☑
L03.311	Cellulitis of abdominal wall
L03.312	Cellulitis of back [any part except buttock]
L03.313	Cellulitis of chest wall
L03.314	Cellulitis of groin
L03.315	Cellulitis of perineum
L03.316	Cellulitis of umbilicus
L03.317	Cellulitis of buttock
L03.321	Acute lymphangitis of abdominal wall
L03.323	Acute lymphangitis of chest wall
L03.325	Acute lymphangitis of perineum
L03.327	Acute lymphangitis of buttock
L03.818	Cellulitis of other sites
L08.0	Pyoderma
L08.81	Pyoderma vegetans
L08.82	Omphalitis not of newborn
L08.89	Other specified local infections of the skin and subcutaneous tissue
L72.3	Sebaceous cyst
L73.2	Hidradenitis suppurativa
L74.8	Other eccrine sweat disorders
L98.0	Pyogenic granuloma
N61.1	Abscess of the breast and nipple
N76.4	Abscess of vulva ♀
O91.011	Infection of nipple associated with pregnancy, first trimester ▥ ♀
O91.012	Infection of nipple associated with pregnancy, second trimester ▥ ♀
O91.013	Infection of nipple associated with pregnancy, third trimester ▥ ♀
O91.02	Infection of nipple associated with the puerperium ▥ ♀
O91.03	Infection of nipple associated with lactation ▥ ♀
O91.111	Abscess of breast associated with pregnancy, first trimester ▥ ♀
O91.112	Abscess of breast associated with pregnancy, second trimester ▥ ♀
O91.113	Abscess of breast associated with pregnancy, third trimester ▥ ♀
O91.12	Abscess of breast associated with the puerperium ▥ ♀
O91.13	Abscess of breast associated with lactation ▥ ♀

O99.711	Diseases of the skin and subcutaneous tissue complicating pregnancy, first trimester Ⓜ ♀
O99.712	Diseases of the skin and subcutaneous tissue complicating pregnancy, second trimester Ⓜ ♀
O99.713	Diseases of the skin and subcutaneous tissue complicating pregnancy, third trimester Ⓜ ♀
O99.73	Diseases of the skin and subcutaneous tissue complicating the puerperium Ⓜ ♀

AMA: 10060 2018,Jan,8; 2017,Jan,8; 2016,Jan,13; 2015,Jan,16; 2014,Jan,11
10061 2018,Jan,8; 2017,Jan,8; 2016,Jan,13; 2015,Jan,16; 2014,Jan,11

Relative Value Units/Medicare Edits

Non-Facility RVU	Work	PE	MP	Total
10060	1.22	2.09	0.13	3.44
10061	2.45	3.2	0.32	5.97
Facility RVU	**Work**	**PE**	**MP**	**Total**
10060	1.22	1.52	0.13	2.87
10061	2.45	2.44	0.32	5.21

	FUD	Status	MUE	Modifiers				IOM Reference
10060	10	A	1(2)	51	N/A	N/A	N/A	None
10061	10	A	1(2)	51	N/A	N/A	N/A	

* with documentation

Terms To Know

abscess. Circumscribed collection of pus resulting from bacteria, frequently associated with swelling and other signs of inflammation.

carbuncle. Infection of the skin that arises from a collection of interconnected infected boils or furuncles, usually from hair follicles infected by staphylococcus. This condition can produce pus and form drainage cavities.

furuncle. Inflamed, painful abscess, cyst, or nodule on the skin caused by bacteria, often Staphylococcus, entering along the hair follicle.

hidradenitis. Infection or inflammation of a sweat gland, usually treated by incision and drainage.

incision and drainage. Cutting open body tissue for the removal of tissue fluids or infected discharge from a wound or cavity.

10080-10081

| 10080 | Incision and drainage of pilonidal cyst; simple |
| 10081 | complicated |

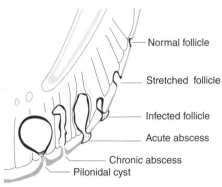

A pilonidal cyst is incised and drained.

Explanation

The physician incises and drains a pilonidal cyst. A pilonidal cyst is an abnormal pocket in the skin and subcutaneous tissue that may contain hair follicles, skin debris, fluid, and exudate. The cyst is usually located in the sacrococcygeal region near the tailbone and cleft of the buttocks. An incision overlying the pocket is made to allow drainage of the contents. The wound may be left open and packed until the cyst heals. Report 10081 if the procedure is more complicated and requires marsupialization, approximation of the wounds edges, and/or primary closure.

Coding Tips

For excision of a pilonidal cyst, see 11770–11772. For incision and drainage of an abscess, other than a pilonidal cyst, simple or single, see 10060; complicated or multiple, see 10061. Surgical trays, A4550, are not separately reimbursed by Medicare; however, other third-party payers may cover them. Check with the specific payer to determine coverage.

ICD-10-CM Diagnostic Codes

L05.01	Pilonidal cyst with abscess
L05.02	Pilonidal sinus with abscess
L05.91	Pilonidal cyst without abscess
L05.92	Pilonidal sinus without abscess

AMA: 10080 2018,Jan,8; 2017,Jan,8; 2016,Jan,13; 2015,Jan,16; 2014,Jan,11
10081 2018,Jan,8; 2017,Jan,8; 2016,Jan,13; 2015,Jan,16; 2014,Jan,11

Relative Value Units/Medicare Edits

Non-Facility RVU	Work	PE	MP	Total
10080	1.22	4.58	0.19	5.99
10081	2.5	5.78	0.39	8.67
Facility RVU	**Work**	**PE**	**MP**	**Total**
10080	1.22	1.54	0.19	2.95
10081	2.5	2.04	0.39	4.93

	FUD	Status	MUE	Modifiers				IOM Reference
10080	10	A	1(3)	51	N/A	N/A	N/A	None
10081	10	A	1(3)	51	N/A	N/A	N/A	

* with documentation

10120-10121

10120 Incision and removal of foreign body, subcutaneous tissues; simple
10121   complicated

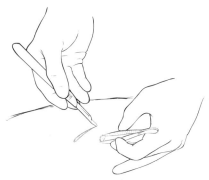

A foreign body is removed through an incision
into subcutaneous tissues

Explanation

The physician removes a foreign body embedded in subcutaneous tissue. The physician makes a simple incision in the skin overlying the foreign body. The foreign body is retrieved using hemostats or forceps. The skin may be sutured or allowed to heal secondarily. Report 10121 if the procedure is more complicated, requiring dissection of underlying tissues.

Coding Tips

These codes may be used when foreign body removal is confined to the skin and/or subcutaneous tissues. For foreign body removal from the vagina, see 57415. Surgical trays, A4550, are not separately reimbursed by Medicare; however, other third-party payers may cover them. Check with the specific payer to determine coverage.

ICD-10-CM Diagnostic Codes

L92.3	Foreign body granuloma of the skin and subcutaneous tissue
M79.5	Residual foreign body in soft tissue
S20.151A	Superficial foreign body of breast, right breast, initial encounter ☑
S20.152A	Superficial foreign body of breast, left breast, initial encounter ☑
S30.850A	Superficial foreign body of lower back and pelvis, initial encounter
S30.851A	Superficial foreign body of abdominal wall, initial encounter
S30.854A	Superficial foreign body of vagina and vulva, initial encounter ♀
S31.020A	Laceration with foreign body of lower back and pelvis without penetration into retroperitoneum, initial encounter
S31.040A	Puncture wound with foreign body of lower back and pelvis without penetration into retroperitoneum, initial encounter
S31.120A	Laceration of abdominal wall with foreign body, right upper quadrant without penetration into peritoneal cavity, initial encounter ☑
S31.121A	Laceration of abdominal wall with foreign body, left upper quadrant without penetration into peritoneal cavity, initial encounter ☑
S31.122A	Laceration of abdominal wall with foreign body, epigastric region without penetration into peritoneal cavity, initial encounter
S31.123A	Laceration of abdominal wall with foreign body, right lower quadrant without penetration into peritoneal cavity, initial encounter ☑
S31.124A	Laceration of abdominal wall with foreign body, left lower quadrant without penetration into peritoneal cavity, initial encounter ☑
S31.125A	Laceration of abdominal wall with foreign body, periumbilic region without penetration into peritoneal cavity, initial encounter
S31.140A	Puncture wound of abdominal wall with foreign body, right upper quadrant without penetration into peritoneal cavity, initial encounter ☑
S31.141A	Puncture wound of abdominal wall with foreign body, left upper quadrant without penetration into peritoneal cavity, initial encounter ☑
S31.142A	Puncture wound of abdominal wall with foreign body, epigastric region without penetration into peritoneal cavity, initial encounter
S31.143A	Puncture wound of abdominal wall with foreign body, right lower quadrant without penetration into peritoneal cavity, initial encounter ☑
S31.144A	Puncture wound of abdominal wall with foreign body, left lower quadrant without penetration into peritoneal cavity, initial encounter ☑
S31.145A	Puncture wound of abdominal wall with foreign body, periumbilic region without penetration into peritoneal cavity, initial encounter
S31.812A	Laceration with foreign body of right buttock, initial encounter ☑
S31.814A	Puncture wound with foreign body of right buttock, initial encounter ☑
S31.822A	Laceration with foreign body of left buttock, initial encounter ☑
S31.824A	Puncture wound with foreign body of left buttock, initial encounter ☑
T81.510A	Adhesions due to foreign body accidentally left in body following surgical operation, initial encounter
T81.511A	Adhesions due to foreign body accidentally left in body following infusion or transfusion, initial encounter
T81.513A	Adhesions due to foreign body accidentally left in body following injection or immunization, initial encounter
T81.516A	Adhesions due to foreign body accidentally left in body following aspiration, puncture or other catheterization, initial encounter
T81.517A	Adhesions due to foreign body accidentally left in body following removal of catheter or packing, initial encounter
T81.518A	Adhesions due to foreign body accidentally left in body following other procedure, initial encounter
T81.520A	Obstruction due to foreign body accidentally left in body following surgical operation, initial encounter
T81.521A	Obstruction due to foreign body accidentally left in body following infusion or transfusion, initial encounter
T81.523A	Obstruction due to foreign body accidentally left in body following injection or immunization, initial encounter
T81.526A	Obstruction due to foreign body accidentally left in body following aspiration, puncture or other catheterization, initial encounter
T81.527A	Obstruction due to foreign body accidentally left in body following removal of catheter or packing, initial encounter
T81.528A	Obstruction due to foreign body accidentally left in body following other procedure, initial encounter
T81.530A	Perforation due to foreign body accidentally left in body following surgical operation, initial encounter

Skin

T81.531A	Perforation due to foreign body accidentally left in body following infusion or transfusion, initial encounter
T81.533A	Perforation due to foreign body accidentally left in body following injection or immunization, initial encounter
T81.536A	Perforation due to foreign body accidentally left in body following aspiration, puncture or other catheterization, initial encounter
T81.537A	Perforation due to foreign body accidentally left in body following removal of catheter or packing, initial encounter
T81.538A	Perforation due to foreign body accidentally left in body following other procedure, initial encounter
T81.590A	Other complications of foreign body accidentally left in body following surgical operation, initial encounter
T81.591A	Other complications of foreign body accidentally left in body following infusion or transfusion, initial encounter
T81.593A	Other complications of foreign body accidentally left in body following injection or immunization, initial encounter
T81.596A	Other complications of foreign body accidentally left in body following aspiration, puncture or other catheterization, initial encounter
T81.597A	Other complications of foreign body accidentally left in body following removal of catheter or packing, initial encounter
T81.598A	Other complications of foreign body accidentally left in body following other procedure, initial encounter

AMA: 10120 2018,Jan,8; 2017,Jan,8; 2016,Jan,13; 2015,Jan,16; 2014,Jan,11
10121 2018,Jan,8; 2017,Jan,8; 2016,Jan,13; 2015,Jan,16; 2014,Jan,11

Relative Value Units/Medicare Edits

Non-Facility RVU	Work	PE	MP	Total
10120	1.22	2.96	0.13	4.31
10121	2.74	4.61	0.41	7.76
Facility RVU	Work	PE	MP	Total
10120	1.22	1.59	0.13	2.94
10121	2.74	2.18	0.41	5.33

	FUD	Status	MUE	Modifiers				IOM Reference
10120	10	A	3(3)	51	N/A	N/A	N/A	None
10121	10	A	2(3)	51	N/A	N/A	N/A	

* with documentation

Terms To Know

foreign body. Any object or substance found in an organ and tissue that does not belong under normal circumstances.

subcutaneous. Below the skin.

10140

10140 Incision and drainage of hematoma, seroma or fluid collection

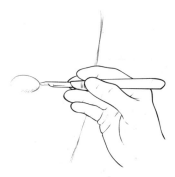

A hematoma, seroma, or fluid collection is incised and drained

Explanation

The physician makes an incision in the skin to decompress and drain a hematoma, seroma, or other collection of fluid. A hemostat bluntly penetrates the fluid pockets, allowing the fluid to evacuate. A latex drain or gauze packing may be placed into the incision site. This will allow the escape of any fluids that may continue to enter the pocket. A pressure dressing may be placed over the region. Any drain or packing is removed within 48 hours. The incision can be closed primarily or may be left to granulate without closure.

Coding Tips

For puncture aspiration of a hematoma, see 10160. Removal of a drain is not reported separately. For imaging guidance, see 76942, 77002, 77012, and 77021. If tissue is transported to an outside laboratory, report 99000 for handling and/or conveyance. Local anesthesia is not reported separately. Surgical trays, A4550, are not separately reimbursed by Medicare; however, other third-party payers may cover them. Check with the specific payer to determine coverage.

ICD-10-CM Diagnostic Codes

L76.02	Intraoperative hemorrhage and hematoma of skin and subcutaneous tissue complicating other procedure
L76.22	Postprocedural hemorrhage of skin and subcutaneous tissue following other procedure
N64.89	Other specified disorders of breast
N90.89	Other specified noninflammatory disorders of vulva and perineum ♀
N94.89	Other specified conditions associated with female genital organs and menstrual cycle ♀
N99.820	Postprocedural hemorrhage of a genitourinary system organ or structure following a genitourinary system procedure
N99.821	Postprocedural hemorrhage of a genitourinary system organ or structure following other procedure
O71.7	Obstetric hematoma of pelvis Ⓜ ♀
O90.2	Hematoma of obstetric wound Ⓜ ♀
S20.01XA	Contusion of right breast, initial encounter ☑
S20.02XA	Contusion of left breast, initial encounter ☑
S30.0XXA	Contusion of lower back and pelvis, initial encounter
S30.1XXA	Contusion of abdominal wall, initial encounter
S30.23XA	Contusion of vagina and vulva, initial encounter ♀
S30.3XXA	Contusion of anus, initial encounter

S39.091A	Other injury of muscle, fascia and tendon of abdomen, initial encounter
S39.093A	Other injury of muscle, fascia and tendon of pelvis, initial encounter
S39.81XA	Other specified injuries of abdomen, initial encounter
S39.83XA	Other specified injuries of pelvis, initial encounter
S39.848A	Other specified injuries of external genitals, initial encounter
S70.11XA	Contusion of right thigh, initial encounter ☑
S70.12XA	Contusion of left thigh, initial encounter ☑
T79.2XXA	Traumatic secondary and recurrent hemorrhage and seroma, initial encounter

AMA: 10140 2018,Jan,8; 2017,Jan,8; 2016,Jan,13; 2015,Jan,16; 2014,Nov,5; 2014,Jan,11

Relative Value Units/Medicare Edits

Non-Facility RVU	Work	PE	MP	Total
10140	1.58	3.05	0.22	4.85
Facility RVU	**Work**	**PE**	**MP**	**Total**
10140	1.58	1.61	0.22	3.41

	FUD	Status	MUE	Modifiers				IOM Reference
10140	10	A	2(3)	51	N/A	N/A	N/A	100-04,13,80.1; 100-04,13,80.2

* with documentation

Terms To Know

contusion. Superficial injury (bruising) produced by impact without a break in the skin.

drain. Device that creates a channel to allow fluid from a cavity, wound, or infected area to exit the body.

granulation. Formation of small, bead-like masses of cytoplasm or granules on the surface of healing wounds of an organ, membrane, or tissue.

hematoma. Tumor-like collection of blood in some part of the body caused by a break in a blood vessel wall, usually as a result of trauma.

hemostat. Tool for clamping vessels and arresting hemorrhaging.

incision and drainage. Cutting open body tissue for the removal of tissue fluids or infected discharge from a wound or cavity.

packing. Material placed into a cavity or wound, such as gels, gauze, pads, and sponges.

seroma. Swelling caused by the collection of serum, or clear fluid, in the tissues.

10160

10160	Puncture aspiration of abscess, hematoma, bulla, or cyst

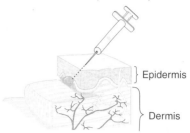

A subcutaneous fluid pocket is aspirated

Epidermis

Dermis

Schematic of layers of the skin

Explanation

The physician performs a puncture aspiration of an abscess, hematoma, bulla, or cyst. The palpable collection of fluid is located subcutaneously. The physician cleanses the overlying skin and introduces a large bore needle on a syringe into the fluid space. The fluid is aspirated into the syringe, decompressing the fluid space. A pressure dressing may be placed over the site.

Coding Tips

For incision and drainage of a cutaneous or subcutaneous abscess, carbuncle, suppurative hidradenitis, cyst, furuncle, or paronychia, see 10060–10061. For incision and drainage of a hematoma, seroma, or fluid collection, see 10140. For incision and drainage of an obstetrical or postpartum vaginal hematoma, see 57022; nonobstetrical, see 57023. For imaging guidance, see 76942, 77002, 77012, and 77021. Surgical trays, A4550, are not separately reimbursed by Medicare; however, other third-party payers may cover them. Check with the specific payer to determine coverage.

ICD-10-CM Diagnostic Codes

L02.211	Cutaneous abscess of abdominal wall
L02.213	Cutaneous abscess of chest wall
L02.214	Cutaneous abscess of groin
L02.215	Cutaneous abscess of perineum
L02.216	Cutaneous abscess of umbilicus
L02.31	Cutaneous abscess of buttock
L02.411	Cutaneous abscess of right axilla ☑
L02.412	Cutaneous abscess of left axilla ☑
L03.111	Cellulitis of right axilla ☑
L03.112	Cellulitis of left axilla ☑
L03.121	Acute lymphangitis of right axilla ☑
L03.122	Acute lymphangitis of left axilla ☑
L03.311	Cellulitis of abdominal wall
L03.313	Cellulitis of chest wall
L03.314	Cellulitis of groin
L03.315	Cellulitis of perineum
L03.316	Cellulitis of umbilicus
L03.317	Cellulitis of buttock
L03.321	Acute lymphangitis of abdominal wall
L03.323	Acute lymphangitis of chest wall
L03.324	Acute lymphangitis of groin
L03.325	Acute lymphangitis of perineum

L03.326	Acute lymphangitis of umbilicus
L03.327	Acute lymphangitis of buttock
L72.0	Epidermal cyst
L72.11	Pilar cyst
L72.12	Trichodermal cyst
L72.3	Sebaceous cyst
L72.8	Other follicular cysts of the skin and subcutaneous tissue
L76.22	Postprocedural hemorrhage of skin and subcutaneous tissue following other procedure
N99.820	Postprocedural hemorrhage of a genitourinary system organ or structure following a genitourinary system procedure
N99.821	Postprocedural hemorrhage of a genitourinary system organ or structure following other procedure
O86.01	Infection of obstetric surgical wound, superficial incisional site 🅜 ♀
O90.2	Hematoma of obstetric wound 🅜 ♀
S20.01XA	Contusion of right breast, initial encounter ☑
S20.02XA	Contusion of left breast, initial encounter ☑
S30.0XXA	Contusion of lower back and pelvis, initial encounter
S30.1XXA	Contusion of abdominal wall, initial encounter
S30.23XA	Contusion of vagina and vulva, initial encounter ♀
S30.3XXA	Contusion of anus, initial encounter
S39.091A	Other injury of muscle, fascia and tendon of abdomen, initial encounter
S39.092A	Other injury of muscle, fascia and tendon of lower back, initial encounter
S39.093A	Other injury of muscle, fascia and tendon of pelvis, initial encounter
S39.81XA	Other specified injuries of abdomen, initial encounter
S39.83XA	Other specified injuries of pelvis, initial encounter
S39.848A	Other specified injuries of external genitals, initial encounter
S70.11XA	Contusion of right thigh, initial encounter ☑
S70.12XA	Contusion of left thigh, initial encounter ☑

AMA: 10160 2018,Jan,8; 2017,Jan,8; 2017,Aug,9; 2016,Jan,13; 2015,Jan,16; 2014,Jan,11

Relative Value Units/Medicare Edits

Non-Facility RVU	Work	PE	MP	Total
10160	1.25	2.31	0.15	3.71
Facility RVU	**Work**	**PE**	**MP**	**Total**
10160	1.25	1.31	0.15	2.71

	FUD	Status	MUE	Modifiers			IOM Reference
10160	10	A	3(3)	51	N/A	N/A N/A	100-04,13,80.1; 100-04,13,80.2

* with documentation

Terms To Know

abscess. Circumscribed collection of pus resulting from bacteria, frequently associated with swelling and other signs of inflammation.

bulla. Large, elevated, membranous sac or blister on the skin containing serous or seropurulent fluid. Bullae are usually treated by incision and drainage or puncture aspiration.

10180

10180   Incision and drainage, complex, postoperative wound infection

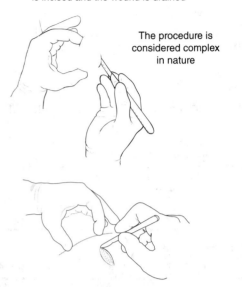

An operation site that has become infected is incised and the wound is drained

The procedure is considered complex in nature

Explanation

This procedure treats an infected postoperative wound. A more complex than usual incision and drainage procedure is necessary to remove the fluid and allow the surgical wound to heal. The physician first removes the surgical sutures or staples and/or makes additional incisions into the skin. The wound is drained of infected fluid. Any necrotic tissue is removed from the surgical site and the wound is irrigated. The wound may be sutured closed or packed open with gauze to allow additional drainage. If closed, the surgical site may have suction or latex drains placed into the wound. If packed open, the wound may be sutured again during a later procedure.

Coding Tips

For secondary closure of a surgical wound or dehiscence, simple or with packing, see 12020–12021, respectively; extensive or complicated, see 13160. Surgical trays, A4550, are not separately reimbursed by Medicare; however, other third-party payers may cover them. Check with the specific payer to determine coverage.

ICD-10-CM Diagnostic Codes

A48.52	Wound botulism
K68.11	Postprocedural retroperitoneal abscess
O86.01	Infection of obstetric surgical wound, superficial incisional site 🅜 ♀
O86.02	Infection of obstetric surgical wound, deep incisional site 🅜 ♀
T81.41XA	Infection following a procedure, superficial incisional surgical site, initial encounter
T81.42XA	Infection following a procedure, deep incisional surgical site, initial encounter

AMA: 10180 2018,Jan,8; 2017,Jan,8; 2016,Jan,13; 2015,Jan,16; 2014,Nov,5; 2014,Jan,11

Relative Value Units/Medicare Edits

Non-Facility RVU	Work	PE	MP	Total
10180	2.3	4.51	0.49	7.3
Facility RVU	Work	PE	MP	Total
10180	2.3	2.32	0.49	5.11

	FUD	Status	MUE	Modifiers				IOM Reference
10180	10	A	2(3)	51	N/A	N/A	N/A	None

* with documentation

Terms To Know

classification of surgical wounds. Surgical wounds fall into four categories that determine treatment methods and outcomes: *1)* Clean wound: No inflammation or contamination; treatment performed with no break in sterile technique; no alimentary, respiratory, or genitourinary tracts involved in the surgery; infection rate = up to 5 percent. *2)* Clean-contaminated wound: No inflammation; treatment performed with minor break in surgical technique; no unusual contamination resulting when alimentary, respiratory, genitourinary, or oropharyngeal cavity is entered; infection rate = up to 11 percent. *3)* Contaminated wound: Less than four hours old with acute, nonpurulent inflammation; treatment performed with major break in surgical technique; gross contamination resulting from the gastrointestinal tract; infection rate = up to 20 percent. *4)* Dirty and infected wound: More than four hours old with existing infection, inflammation, abscess, and nonsterile conditions due to perforated viscus, fecal contamination, necrotic tissue, or foreign body; infection rate = up to 40 percent.

drain. Device that creates a channel to allow fluid from a cavity, wound, or infected area to exit the body.

incision and drainage. Cutting open body tissue for the removal of tissue fluids or infected discharge from a wound or cavity.

infection. Presence of microorganisms in body tissues that may result in cellular damage.

necrosis. Death of cells or tissue within a living organ or structure.

packing. Material placed into a cavity or wound, such as gels, gauze, pads, and sponges.

seroma. Swelling caused by the collection of serum, or clear fluid, in the tissues.

wound. Injury to living tissue often involving a cut or break in the skin.

11004-11006

11004 Debridement of skin, subcutaneous tissue, muscle and fascia for necrotizing soft tissue infection; external genitalia and perineum

11005 abdominal wall, with or without fascial closure

11006 external genitalia, perineum and abdominal wall, with or without fascial closure

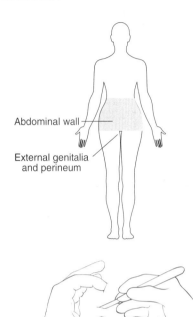

Tissues are debrided of dead and necrotic matter

Explanation

Debridement is carried out for a severe type of tissue infection that causes gangrenous changes, systemic disease, and tissue death. These types of infections are caused by virulent strains of bacteria, such as "flesh-eating" streptococcus, and affect the skin, subcutaneous fat, fascia, and muscle tissue. Surgery is performed immediately upon diagnosis to open and drain the infected area and excise the dead or necrotic tissue. Report 11004 for surgical debridement of necrotic soft tissue of the external genitalia and perineum; 11005 for the abdominal wall, with or without repair of the abdominal fascia; and 11006 for both areas, with or without repair of the abdominal fascia.

Coding Tips

This type of debridement is done on high-risk patients who have a life-threatening infection. Necrosis is often caused by infection from a combination of dangerously virulent microorganisms. Fistulas, herniations, and organ destruction may occur, requiring an extensive level of repair involved with the debridement. Tissue flaps or skin grafting are reported separately when used for repair or closure. For removal of prosthetic material or mesh from the abdominal wall, see 11008. Report skin grafts or flaps separately when performed for closure at the same session as 11004–11006. When reporting debridement of a single wound, the deepest level of tissue removed determines correct code assignment. The debridement of multiple wounds at the same tissue level may be added together to determine the appropriate code. Different tissue depths should not be added together for code selection. According to the AMA, the debridement of skin (epidermis/dermis) is reported with the codes describing active wound care management (97597 or 97598). Surgical trays, A4550, are not separately reimbursed by Medicare; however, other third-party payers may cover them. Check with the specific payer to determine coverage.

ICD-10-CM Diagnostic Codes

A48.0	Gas gangrene
A48.8	Other specified bacterial diseases
I96	Gangrene, not elsewhere classified
M72.6	Necrotizing fasciitis
N49.3	Fournier gangrene ♂
N76.89	Other specified inflammation of vagina and vulva ♀

AMA: 11004 2019,Nov,14; 2018,Jan,8; 2018,Feb,10; 2017,Jan,8; 2016,Jan,13; 2015,Jan,16; 2014,Jan,11 **11005** 2019,Nov,14; 2018,Jan,8; 2018,Feb,10; 2017,Jan,8; 2016,Jan,13; 2015,Jan,16; 2014,Jan,11 **11006** 2019,Nov,14; 2018,Jan,8; 2017,Jan,8; 2016,Jan,13; 2015,Jan,16; 2014,Jan,11

Relative Value Units/Medicare Edits

Non-Facility RVU	Work	PE	MP	Total
11004	10.8	3.9	1.98	16.68
11005	14.24	5.24	3.24	22.72
11006	13.1	4.77	2.62	20.49
Facility RVU	**Work**	**PE**	**MP**	**Total**
11004	10.8	3.9	1.98	16.68
11005	14.24	5.24	3.24	22.72
11006	13.1	4.77	2.62	20.49

	FUD	Status	MUE	Modifiers				IOM Reference
11004	0	A	1(2)	51	N/A	N/A	N/A	None
11005	0	A	1(2)	N/A	N/A	N/A	80*	
11006	0	A	1(2)	51	N/A	N/A	N/A	

* with documentation

Terms To Know

debridement. Removal of dead or contaminated tissue and foreign matter from a wound.

drain. Device that creates a channel to allow fluid from a cavity, wound, or infected area to exit the body.

excise. Remove or cut out.

fascia. Fibrous sheet or band of tissue that envelops organs, muscles, and groupings of muscles.

gangrene. Death of tissue, usually resulting from a loss of vascular supply, followed by a bacterial attack or onset of disease.

infection. Presence of microorganisms in body tissues that may result in cellular damage.

necrotic. Pathological condition of death occurring in a group of cells or tissues within a living part or organism.

soft tissue. Nonepithelial tissues outside of the skeleton.

subcutaneous tissue. Sheet or wide band of adipose (fat) and areolar connective tissue in two layers attached to the dermis.

11008

+ **11008** Removal of prosthetic material or mesh, abdominal wall for infection (eg, for chronic or recurrent mesh infection or necrotizing soft tissue infection) (List separately in addition to code for primary procedure)

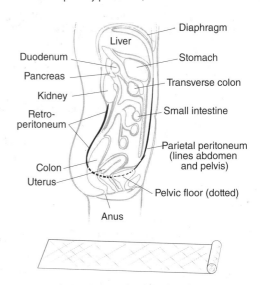

Synthetic mesh is often placed as a surgical wound of the abdominal wall is being closed. The mesh provides support and structure for the healing process.

Explanation

The physician removes prosthetic material or mesh previously placed in the abdominal wall. This may be done due to the presence of a chronic infection, a necrotizing soft tissue infection, or a recurrent mesh infection. Surgery is performed immediately after diagnosis and usually under general anesthesia. The skin is incised and the tissue dissected exposing the prosthetic material. Debridement of the tissue adjacent to or incorporated in the mesh may be performed with instruments or irrigation. Unincorporated or infected areas of the mesh are excised and removed with any remaining areas of infection or necrotic tissue. Incorporated mesh that is not infected may be left in the wound. The area is irrigated and the wound is sutured.

Coding Tips

Report 11008 in conjunction with 10180 and 11004-11006 since the necrotizing soft tissue infection must also be debrided at the same time as the previously placed prosthetic material is removed. Do not report 11008 with 11000-11001 or 11010-11044. Skin grafts or flaps performed at the same operative session as 11004-11008 may be reported separately.

ICD-10-CM Diagnostic Codes

This/these CPT code(s) are add-on code(s). See the primary procedure code that this code is performed with for your ICD-10-CM code selections.

AMA: 11008 2019,Jan,14; 2018,Jan,8; 2017,Jan,8; 2016,Jan,13; 2015,Jan,16; 2014,Jan,11

Skin

Relative Value Units/Medicare Edits

Non-Facility RVU	Work	PE	MP	Total
11008	5.0	1.83	1.16	7.99
Facility RVU	Work	PE	MP	Total
11008	5.0	1.83	1.16	7.99

	FUD	Status	MUE	Modifiers				IOM Reference
11008	N/A	A	1(2)	N/A	N/A	N/A	80*	None

* with documentation

Terms To Know

chronic. Persistent, continuing, or recurring.

debride. To remove all foreign objects and devitalized or infected tissue from a burn or wound to prevent infection and promote healing.

deep fascia. Sheet of dense, fibrous tissue holding muscle groups together below the hypodermis layer or subcutaneous fat layer that lines the extremities and trunk.

dissect. Cut apart or separate tissue for surgical purposes or for visual or microscopic study.

excise. Remove or cut out.

incise. To cut open or into.

infection. Presence of microorganisms in body tissues that may result in cellular damage.

irrigate. Washing out, lavage.

mesh. Synthetic fabric used as a prosthetic patch in hernia repair.

necrotic. Pathological condition of death occurring in a group of cells or tissues within a living part or organism.

prosthetic. Device that replaces all or part of an internal body organ or body part, or that replaces part of the function of a permanently inoperable or malfunctioning internal body organ or body part.

removal. Process of moving out of or away from, or the fact of being removed.

soft tissue. Nonepithelial tissues outside of the skeleton.

11420-11426

11420	Excision, benign lesion including margins, except skin tag (unless listed elsewhere), scalp, neck, hands, feet, genitalia; excised diameter 0.5 cm or less
11421	excised diameter 0.6 to 1.0 cm
11422	excised diameter 1.1 to 2.0 cm
11423	excised diameter 2.1 to 3.0 cm
11424	excised diameter 3.1 to 4.0 cm
11426	excised diameter over 4.0 cm

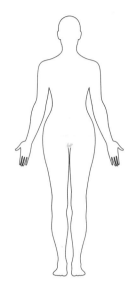

Excision benign lesion of genitalia

Explanation

The physician removes a benign skin lesion located on the genitalia. After administering a local anesthetic, the physician makes a full thickness incision through the dermis with a scalpel, usually in an elliptical shape around and under the lesion. The lesion and a margin of normal tissue are removed. The wound is repaired using a single layer of sutures, chemical or electrocauterization. Complex or layered closure is reported separately, if required. Each lesion removed is reported separately. Report 11420 for an excised diameter 0.5 cm or less; 11421 for 0.6 cm to 1 cm; 11422 for 1.1 cm to 2 cm; 11423 for 2.1 cm to 3 cm; 11424 for 3.1 cm to 4 cm; and 11426 if the excised diameter is greater than 4 cm.

Coding Tips

For excision of a malignant lesion, see 11620–11626. For destruction of benign lesions other than skin tags or cutaneous vascular proliferative lesions, see 17110-17111; premalignant lesions, see 17000, 17003, and 17004; cutaneous vascular proliferative lesions, see 17106, 17107, and 17108; malignant lesions, any method, see 17270–17276. If significant additional time and effort is documented, append modifier 22 and submit a cover letter and operative report. Surgical trays, A4550, are not separately reimbursed by Medicare; however, other third-party payers may cover them. Check with the specific payer to determine coverage.

ICD-10-CM Diagnostic Codes

D17.39	Benign lipomatous neoplasm of skin and subcutaneous tissue of other sites
D17.72	Benign lipomatous neoplasm of other genitourinary organ
D18.01	Hemangioma of skin and subcutaneous tissue
D23.5	Other benign neoplasm of skin of trunk

Skin

D28.0	Benign neoplasm of vulva ♀	
D28.7	Benign neoplasm of other specified female genital organs ♀	
D39.8	Neoplasm of uncertain behavior of other specified female genital organs ♀	
D48.5	Neoplasm of uncertain behavior of skin	
I78.1	Nevus, non-neoplastic	
L72.0	Epidermal cyst	
L72.11	Pilar cyst	
L72.12	Trichodermal cyst	
L72.2	Steatocystoma multiplex	
L72.3	Sebaceous cyst	
L72.8	Other follicular cysts of the skin and subcutaneous tissue	
L82.0	Inflamed seborrheic keratosis	
L82.1	Other seborrheic keratosis	
L91.0	Hypertrophic scar	
L91.8	Other hypertrophic disorders of the skin	
L92.2	Granuloma faciale [eosinophilic granuloma of skin]	
L92.3	Foreign body granuloma of the skin and subcutaneous tissue	
L92.8	Other granulomatous disorders of the skin and subcutaneous tissue	
N90.89	Other specified noninflammatory disorders of vulva and perineum ♀	
Q82.5	Congenital non-neoplastic nevus	

AMA: 11420 2019,Nov,3; 2018,Sep,7; 2018,Jan,8; 2018,Feb,10; 2017,Jan,8; 2016,Jan,13; 2016,Apr,3; 2015,Jan,16; 2014,Mar,12; 2014,Mar,4; 2014,Jan,11
11421 2019,Nov,3; 2018,Sep,7; 2018,Jan,8; 2018,Feb,10; 2017,Jan,8; 2016,Jan,13; 2016,Apr,3; 2015,Jan,16; 2014,Mar,12; 2014,Mar,4; 2014,Jan,11
11422 2019,Nov,3; 2018,Sep,7; 2018,Jan,8; 2018,Feb,10; 2017,Jan,8; 2016,Jan,13; 2016,Apr,3; 2015,Jan,16; 2014,Mar,4; 2014,Mar,12; 2014,Jan,11
11423 2019,Nov,3; 2018,Sep,7; 2018,Jan,8; 2018,Feb,10; 2017,Jan,8; 2016,Jan,13; 2016,Apr,3; 2015,Jan,16; 2014,Mar,12; 2014,Mar,4; 2014,Jan,11
11424 2019,Nov,3; 2018,Sep,7; 2018,Jan,8; 2018,Feb,10; 2017,Jan,8; 2016,Jan,13; 2016,Apr,3; 2015,Jan,16; 2014,Mar,12; 2014,Mar,4; 2014,Jan,11
11426 2019,Nov,3; 2018,Sep,7; 2018,Jan,8; 2018,Feb,10; 2017,Jan,8; 2016,Jan,13; 2016,Apr,3; 2015,Jan,16; 2014,Mar,12; 2014,Mar,4; 2014,Jan,11

Relative Value Units/Medicare Edits

Non-Facility RVU	Work	PE	MP	Total
11420	1.03	2.46	0.11	3.6
11421	1.47	2.89	0.18	4.54
11422	1.68	3.2	0.23	5.11
11423	2.06	3.47	0.28	5.81
11424	2.48	3.86	0.37	6.71
11426	4.09	4.86	0.68	9.63
Facility RVU	**Work**	**PE**	**MP**	**Total**
11420	1.03	1.2	0.11	2.34
11421	1.47	1.48	0.18	3.13
11422	1.68	1.97	0.23	3.88
11423	2.06	2.11	0.28	4.45
11424	2.48	2.26	0.37	5.11
11426	4.09	3.12	0.68	7.89

	FUD	Status	MUE	Modifiers				IOM Reference
11420	10	A	3(3)	51	N/A	N/A	N/A	None
11421	10	A	3(3)	51	N/A	N/A	N/A	
11422	10	A	3(3)	51	N/A	N/A	N/A	
11423	10	A	2(3)	51	N/A	N/A	N/A	
11424	10	A	2(3)	51	N/A	N/A	N/A	
11426	10	A	2(3)	51	N/A	N/A	N/A	

* with documentation

Terms To Know

benign. Mild or nonmalignant in nature.

dermis. Skin layer found under the epidermis that contains a papillary upper layer and the deep reticular layer of collagen, vascular bed, and nerves.

diameter. Straight line connecting two opposite points on the surface of a lesion, spheric, or cylindric body.

electrocautery. Division or cutting of tissue using high-frequency electrical current to produce heat, which destroys cells.

excision. Surgical removal of an organ or tissue.

full thickness. Consisting of skin and subcutaneous tissue.

incision. Act of cutting into tissue or an organ.

lesion. Area of damaged tissue that has lost continuity or function, due to disease or trauma.

margin. Boundary, edge, or border, as of a surface or structure.

11620-11626

11620 Excision, malignant lesion including margins, scalp, neck, hands, feet, genitalia; excised diameter 0.5 cm or less
11621 excised diameter 0.6 to 1.0 cm
11622 excised diameter 1.1 to 2.0 cm
11623 excised diameter 2.1 to 3.0 cm
11624 excised diameter 3.1 to 4.0 cm
11626 excised diameter over 4.0 cm

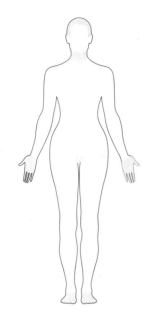

Malignant lesions, including margins, scalp, neck, hands, feet or genitalia are excised

Explanation

The physician removes a malignant lesion located on the genitalia. After administering a local anesthetic, the physician makes a full-thickness incision through the dermis, usually in an elliptical shape around and under the lesion. The lesion and a margin of normal tissue are removed. The wound is repaired using a single layer of sutures, chemical or electrocauterization. Complex, layered, or reconstructive (excluding adjacent tissue transfer) wound repair is reported separately, if required. Each lesion removed is reported separately. Report 11620 for an excised diameter 0.5 cm or less; 11621 for 0.6 cm to 1 cm; 11622 for 1.1 cm to 2 cm; 11623 for 2.1 cm to 3 cm; 11624 for 3.1 cm to 4 cm; and 11626 if the excised diameter is greater than 4 cm.

Coding Tips

For excision of a benign lesion, see 11420–11426. For lesion excision requiring intermediate repair, see 12041–12047; complex repair, see 13131–13133. For any flaps/adjacent tissue transfers, see 14040–14041. For destruction of premalignant lesions, see 17000, 17003, and 17004; cutaneous vascular proliferative lesions, see 17106, 17107, and 17108; malignant lesions, any method, see 17270–17276. If significant additional time and effort is documented, append modifier 22 and submit a cover letter and operative report. Surgical trays, A4550, are not separately reimbursed by Medicare; however, other third-party payers may cover them. Check with the specific payer to determine coverage.

ICD-10-CM Diagnostic Codes

C43.8	Malignant melanoma of overlapping sites of skin
C4A.8	Merkel cell carcinoma of overlapping sites
C51.0	Malignant neoplasm of labium majus ♀
C51.1	Malignant neoplasm of labium minus ♀
C51.2	Malignant neoplasm of clitoris ♀
C51.8	Malignant neoplasm of overlapping sites of vulva ♀
C57.8	Malignant neoplasm of overlapping sites of female genital organs ♀
C79.2	Secondary malignant neoplasm of skin
C79.82	Secondary malignant neoplasm of genital organs
C7B.1	Secondary Merkel cell carcinoma
D03.8	Melanoma in situ of other sites
D07.1	Carcinoma in situ of vulva ♀
D39.8	Neoplasm of uncertain behavior of other specified female genital organs ♀

AMA: **11620** 2019,Nov,3; 2018,Sep,7; 2018,Jan,8; 2017,Jan,8; 2016,Jan,13; 2015,Jan,16; 2014,Mar,4; 2014,Mar,12; 2014,Jan,11 **11621** 2019,Nov,3; 2018,Sep,7; 2018,Jan,8; 2017,Jan,8; 2016,Jan,13; 2015,Jan,16; 2014,Mar,4; 2014,Mar,12; 2014,Jan,11 **11622** 2019,Nov,3; 2018,Sep,7; 2018,Jan,8; 2017,Jan,8; 2016,Jan,13; 2015,Jan,16; 2014,Mar,4; 2014,Mar,12; 2014,Jan,11 **11623** 2019,Nov,3; 2018,Sep,7; 2018,Jan,8; 2017,Jan,8; 2016,Jan,13; 2015,Jan,16; 2014,Mar,12; 2014,Mar,4; 2014,Jan,11 **11624** 2019,Nov,3; 2018,Sep,7; 2018,Jan,8; 2017,Jan,8; 2016,Jan,13; 2015,Jan,16; 2014,Mar,12; 2014,Mar,4; 2014,Jan,11 **11626** 2019,Nov,3; 2018,Sep,7; 2018,Jan,8; 2017,Jan,8; 2016,Jan,13; 2015,Jan,16; 2014,Mar,12; 2014,Mar,4; 2014,Jan,11

Relative Value Units/Medicare Edits

Non-Facility RVU	Work	PE	MP	Total
11620	1.64	3.78	0.22	5.64
11621	2.08	4.21	0.26	6.55
11622	2.41	4.57	0.27	7.25
11623	3.11	5.02	0.39	8.52
11624	3.62	5.54	0.49	9.65
11626	4.61	6.31	0.74	11.66

Facility RVU	Work	PE	MP	Total
11620	1.64	1.64	0.22	3.5
11621	2.08	1.93	0.26	4.27
11622	2.41	2.17	0.27	4.85
11623	3.11	2.53	0.39	6.03
11624	3.62	2.74	0.49	6.85
11626	4.61	3.09	0.74	8.44

	FUD	Status	MUE	Modifiers				IOM Reference
11620	10	A	2(3)	51	N/A	N/A	N/A	None
11621	10	A	2(3)	51	N/A	N/A	N/A	
11622	10	A	2(3)	51	N/A	N/A	N/A	
11623	10	A	2(3)	51	N/A	N/A	N/A	
11624	10	A	2(3)	51	N/A	N/A	N/A	
11626	10	A	2(3)	51	N/A	N/A	N/A	

* with documentation

Terms To Know

malignant neoplasm. Any cancerous tumor or lesion exhibiting uncontrolled tissue growth that can progressively invade other parts of the body with its disease-generating cells.

11770-11772

11770 Excision of pilonidal cyst or sinus; simple
11771   extensive
11772   complicated

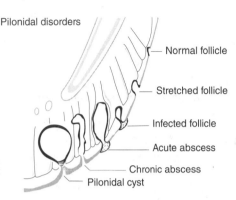

Pilonidal disorders
— Normal follicle
— Stretched follicle
— Infected follicle
— Acute abscess
— Chronic abscess
— Pilonidal cyst

A pilonidal cyst is excised.

Explanation

A pilonidal cyst or sinus is entrapped epithelial tissue located in the sacrococcygeal region above the buttocks. These lesions are usually associated with ingrown hair. A sinus cavity is present and may have a fluid-producing cystic lining. With a small or simple sinus in 11770, the physician uses a scalpel to completely excise the involved tissue. The wound is sutured in a single layer. In 11771, an extensive sinus is present superficial to the fascia overlying the sacrum but with subcutaneous extensions. The physician uses a scalpel to completely excise the cystic tissue. The wound may be sutured in several layers. In 11772, the sinus involves many subcutaneous extensions superficial to the fascia overlying the sacrum. The physician uses a scalpel to completely excise the cystic tissue. Local soft tissue flaps (i.e., Z-plasty, Y-V plasty, myofasciocutaneous flap) may be required for closure of a large defect or the wound may be left open to heal by granulation.

Coding Tips

Closure of the defect is included in this code and should not be reported separately. For incision and drainage of a pilonidal cyst, see 10080–10081. When medically necessary, report moderate (conscious) sedation provided by the performing physician with 99151–99153. When moderate (conscious) sedation is provided by another physician, report 99155–99157. Surgical trays, A4550, are not separately reimbursed by Medicare; however, other third-party payers may cover them. Check with the specific payer to determine coverage.

ICD-10-CM Diagnostic Codes

L05.01	Pilonidal cyst with abscess
L05.02	Pilonidal sinus with abscess
L05.91	Pilonidal cyst without abscess
L05.92	Pilonidal sinus without abscess

AMA: **11772** 2018,Jan,8; 2017,Jan,8; 2016,Jan,13; 2015,Sep,12

Relative Value Units/Medicare Edits

Non-Facility RVU	Work	PE	MP	Total
11770	2.66	5.7	0.56	8.92
11771	6.09	9.84	1.36	17.29
11772	7.35	11.99	1.61	20.95
Facility RVU	**Work**	**PE**	**MP**	**Total**
11770	2.66	2.12	0.56	5.34
11771	6.09	5.29	1.36	12.74
11772	7.35	7.72	1.61	16.68

	FUD	Status	MUE	Modifiers				IOM Reference
11770	10	A	1(3)	51	N/A	N/A	N/A	None
11771	90	A	1(3)	51	N/A	N/A	N/A	
11772	90	A	1(3)	51	N/A	N/A	N/A	

* with documentation

Terms To Know

abscess. Circumscribed collection of pus resulting from bacteria, frequently associated with swelling and other signs of inflammation.

absorbable sutures. Strands used for suture or repair of tissue prepared from collagen or a synthetic polymer and capable of being absorbed by tissue over time.

epithelial tissue. Cells arranged in sheets that cover internal and external body surfaces that can absorb, protect, and/or secrete and includes the protective covering for external surfaces (skin), absorptive linings for internal surfaces such as the intestine, and secreting structures such as salivary or sweat glands.

excision. Surgical removal of an organ or tissue.

granulation. Formation of small, bead-like masses of cytoplasm or granules on the surface of healing wounds of an organ, membrane, or tissue.

nonabsorbable sutures. Strands of natural or synthetic material that resist absorption into living tissue and are removed once healing is under way. Nonabsorbable sutures are commonly used to close skin wounds and repair tendons or collagenous tissue.

pilonidal cyst. Sac or sinus cavity of trapped epithelial tissues in the sacrococcygeal region, usually associated with ingrown hair.

pilonidal sinus. Fistula, tract, or channel that extends from an infected area of ingrown hair to another site within the skin or out to the skin surface.

11976

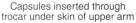

11976   Removal, implantable contraceptive capsules

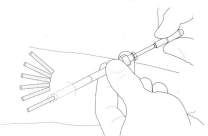

Capsules inserted through
trocar under skin of upper arm

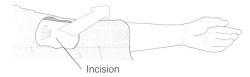

Capsules are surgically removed

Incision

Explanation

The physician makes a small incision in the skin on the inside of the upper arm of a female patient and removes contraceptive capsules previously implanted subdermally. The incision is closed.

Coding Tips

Because this procedure is usually not done out of medical necessity, the patient may be responsible for charges. Verify with the insurance carrier for coverage. Local anesthesia is included in this service. For removal of contraceptive capsules with subsequent reinsertion, report 11976 in conjunction with 11981. The cost of the contraceptive is not included and should be reported separately using the appropriate HCPCS Level II code. Surgical trays, A4550, are not separately reimbursed by Medicare; however, other third-party payers may cover them. Check with the specific payer to determine coverage. Supplies used when providing this service may be reported with 99070 or the appropriate HCPCS Level II code. Check with the specific payer to determine coverage.

ICD-10-CM Diagnostic Codes

Z30.46   Encounter for surveillance of implantable subdermal contraceptive ♀

AMA: **11976** 1992,Win,1

Relative Value Units/Medicare Edits

Non-Facility RVU	Work	PE	MP	Total
11976	1.78	2.09	0.28	4.15
Facility RVU	**Work**	**PE**	**MP**	**Total**
11976	1.78	0.67	0.28	2.73

	FUD	Status	MUE	Modifiers				IOM Reference
11976	0	R	1(2)	51	N/A	N/A	80*	None

* with documentation

11980

11980   Subcutaneous hormone pellet implantation (implantation of estradiol and/or testosterone pellets beneath the skin)

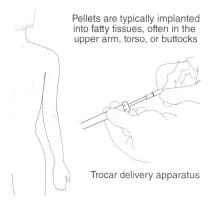

Pellets are typically implanted
into fatty tissues, often in the
upper arm, torso, or buttocks

Trocar delivery apparatus

Explanation

Biodegradable time-release medication pellets are implanted subcutaneously for the slow delivery of hormones. The physician makes a small incision in the skin with a scalpel. A trocar and cannula are inserted into the incised area. Hormone pellets are inserted through the cannula and the cannula is withdrawn. Pressure is applied to the incised area until any bleeding is stopped, and the incision is closed with Steri-strips. The time-release medication is typically used for women who require hormone replacement therapy during menopause. One method is to implant pellets of testosterone and/or estradiol (taken in conjunction with progesterone) into the fatty tissue of the buttocks. New pellets may be inserted whenever symptoms recur, usually in six to nine months.

Coding Tips

When 11980 is performed with another separately identifiable procedure, the highest dollar value code is listed as the primary procedure and subsequent procedures are appended with modifier 51. Report supplies and materials separately using 99070 or the appropriate HCPCS Level II code for the cost of the capsule. Local anesthesia is included in this service. Surgical trays, A4550, are not separately reimbursed by Medicare; however, other third-party payers may cover them. Check with the specific payer to determine coverage. For insertion of implantable contraceptive capsules, see 11981.

ICD-10-CM Diagnostic Codes

E28.310	Symptomatic premature menopause 🅐 ♀
E28.319	Asymptomatic premature menopause 🅐 ♀
E28.39	Other primary ovarian failure ♀
E28.8	Other ovarian dysfunction ♀
E30.0	Delayed puberty
E89.40	Asymptomatic postprocedural ovarian failure ♀
E89.41	Symptomatic postprocedural ovarian failure ♀
N92.4	Excessive bleeding in the premenopausal period ♀
N95.0	Postmenopausal bleeding ♀
N95.1	Menopausal and female climacteric states ♀
N95.2	Postmenopausal atrophic vaginitis ♀
N95.8	Other specified menopausal and perimenopausal disorders ♀
R53.81	Other malaise
R53.83	Other fatigue
R68.82	Decreased libido 🅐

Relative Value Units/Medicare Edits

Non-Facility RVU	Work	PE	MP	Total
11980	1.1	1.46	0.13	2.69
Facility RVU	**Work**	**PE**	**MP**	**Total**
11980	1.1	0.38	0.13	1.61

	FUD	Status	MUE	Modifiers			IOM Reference
11980	0	A	1(2)	51	N/A	N/A	N/A	None

* with documentation

Terms To Know

cannula. Tube inserted into a blood vessel, duct, or body cavity to facilitate passage.

estradiol. Principal and most potent mammalian estrogen produced by the ovaries, which prepares the uterus for implantation after fertilization and is responsible for female reproductive organ maturation.

hormone. Chemical substance produced by the body that has a regulatory effect on the function of its specific target organ(s).

implant. Material or device inserted or placed within the body for therapeutic, reconstructive, or diagnostic purposes.

subcutaneous. Below the skin.

trocar. Cannula or a sharp pointed instrument used to puncture and aspirate fluid from cavities.

11981-11983

11981	Insertion, non-biodegradable drug delivery implant
11982	Removal, non-biodegradable drug delivery implant
11983	Removal with reinsertion, non-biodegradable drug delivery implant

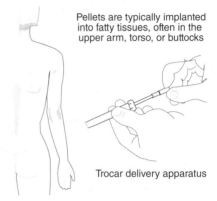

Pellets are typically implanted into fatty tissues, often in the upper arm, torso, or buttocks

Trocar delivery apparatus

Explanation

A nonbiodegradable drug delivery implant is inserted to deliver a therapeutic dose of the drug continuously at a predetermined rate of release. One such system works via a semipermeable membrane at one end of the subcutaneous cylinder that permits the entrance of fluid; the drug is delivered from a port at the other end of the cylinder at a controlled rate appropriate to the specific therapeutic agent. The physician injects local anesthesia and makes a small incision in the skin with a scalpel to insert the miniature drug-containing cylinder, which is held in place with sutures tied by a knot or secured by a single running stitch. The wound is closed with sutures. Various types of medications for different indications may be administered via a nonbiodegradable drug delivery implant system. In 11982, the physician removes a previously implanted miniature drug-containing titanium cylinder through a small incision. In 11983, the physician removes a previously implanted, miniature drug-containing titanium cylinder through a small incision and inserts a replacement cylinder. The cylinders are held in place with sutures tied by a knot or secured by a single running stitch. The wounds are sutured closed.

Coding Tips

The cost of the drug is not included in these codes and should be reported separately using the appropriate HCPCS Level II code. Surgical trays, A4550, are not separately reimbursed by Medicare; however, other third-party payers may cover them. Check with the specific payer to determine coverage. Supplies used when providing this service may be reported with 99070 or the appropriate HCPCS Level II code. Check with the specific payer to determine coverage. Contraceptive capsules are not usually provided out of medical necessity; the patient may be responsible for charges. Verify with the insurance carrier for coverage. Anesthesia is included in these services. For removal of implantable contraceptive capsules, see 11976. For removal and subsequent insertion of implantable contraceptive capsules, report 11976 (for the removal) in conjunction with 11981 (for the insertion of contraceptive capsules). Medicare and some payers may require codes G0516-G0518 be reported for four or more implants.

ICD-10-CM Diagnostic Codes

Z30.017	Encounter for initial prescription of implantable subdermal contraceptive
Z30.46	Encounter for surveillance of implantable subdermal contraceptive ♀

Implant (side tab)

Relative Value Units/Medicare Edits

Non-Facility RVU	Work	PE	MP	Total
11981	1.14	1.6	0.22	2.96
11982	1.34	1.77	0.25	3.36
11983	1.91	1.93	0.31	4.15
Facility RVU	**Work**	**PE**	**MP**	**Total**
11981	1.14	0.5	0.22	1.86
11982	1.34	0.6	0.25	2.19
11983	1.91	0.79	0.31	3.01

	FUD	Status	MUE	Modifiers				IOM Reference
11981	0	A	1(3)	51	N/A	N/A	80*	None
11982	0	A	1(3)	51	N/A	N/A	80*	
11983	0	A	1(3)	51	N/A	N/A	80*	

* with documentation

Terms To Know

drug delivery implant. Device that allows for site-specific drug administration where medication is most needed and may permit lower dosage of drugs reducing potential side effects; sustained, controlled release of the drug; and patient compliance due to the implanted device being less bothersome than oral medications or injections.

implant. Material or device inserted or placed within the body for therapeutic, reconstructive, or diagnostic purposes.

insertion. Placement or implantation into a body part.

levonorgestrel. Drug inhibiting ovulation and preventing sperm from penetrating cervical mucus. It is delivered subcutaneously in polysiloxone capsules. The capsules can be effective for up to five years, and provide a cumulative pregnancy rate of less than 2 percent. The capsules are not biodegradable, and therefore must be removed. Removal is more difficult than insertion of levonorgestrel capsules because fibrosis develops around the capsules. Normal hormonal activity and a return to fertility begins immediately upon removal.

non-biodegradable. Substances, products, and materials that are incapable of decaying through the action of living organisms.

Implant

12001-12007

12001 Simple repair of superficial wounds of scalp, neck, axillae, external genitalia, trunk and/or extremities (including hands and feet); 2.5 cm or less
12002 2.6 cm to 7.5 cm
12004 7.6 cm to 12.5 cm
12005 12.6 cm to 20.0 cm
12006 20.1 cm to 30.0 cm
12007 over 30.0 cm

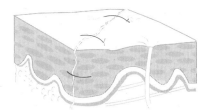

Example of a simple closure
involving only one skin layer, the epidermis

Explanation

The physician performs wound closure of superficial lacerations of the external genitalia, trunk, or extremities using sutures, staples, tissue adhesives, or a combination of these materials. A local anesthetic is injected around the wound and it is cleansed, explored, and often irrigated with a saline solution. The physician performs a simple, one-layer repair of the epidermis, dermis, or subcutaneous tissues. For multiple wounds of the same complexity and in the same anatomical area, the length of all wounds sutured is summed and reported as one total length. Report 12001 for a total length of 2.5 cm or less; 12002 for 2.6 cm to 7.5 cm; 12004 for 7.6 cm to 12.5 cm; 12005 for 12.6 cm to 20 cm; 12006 for 20.1 cm to 30 cm; and 12007 if the total length is greater than 30 cm.

Coding Tips

Wounds treated with tissue glue or staples qualify as a simple repair even if they are not closed with sutures. Suture removal is included in this procedure. Single-layer closure of a wound requiring extensive cleaning or removal of contaminated foreign matter or damaged tissue is classified as an intermediate repair. Surgical trays, A4550, may be separately reimbursed by third-party payers. Check with the specific payer to determine coverage. When medically necessary, report moderate (conscious) sedation provided by the performing physician with 99151–99153. When moderate (conscious) sedation is provided by another physician, report 99155–99157.

ICD-10-CM Diagnostic Codes

S21.011A	Laceration without foreign body of right breast, initial encounter ☑
S21.012A	Laceration without foreign body of left breast, initial encounter ☑
S21.031A	Puncture wound without foreign body of right breast, initial encounter ☑
S21.032A	Puncture wound without foreign body of left breast, initial encounter ☑
S21.051A	Open bite of right breast, initial encounter ☑
S21.052A	Open bite of left breast, initial encounter ☑
S30.810A	Abrasion of lower back and pelvis, initial encounter
S30.811A	Abrasion of abdominal wall, initial encounter
S30.814A	Abrasion of vagina and vulva, initial encounter ♀
S30.817A	Abrasion of anus, initial encounter
S31.010A	Laceration without foreign body of lower back and pelvis without penetration into retroperitoneum, initial encounter
S31.030A	Puncture wound without foreign body of lower back and pelvis without penetration into retroperitoneum, initial encounter
S31.050A	Open bite of lower back and pelvis without penetration into retroperitoneum, initial encounter
S31.110A	Laceration without foreign body of abdominal wall, right upper quadrant without penetration into peritoneal cavity, initial encounter ☑
S31.111A	Laceration without foreign body of abdominal wall, left upper quadrant without penetration into peritoneal cavity, initial encounter ☑
S31.112A	Laceration without foreign body of abdominal wall, epigastric region without penetration into peritoneal cavity, initial encounter
S31.113A	Laceration without foreign body of abdominal wall, right lower quadrant without penetration into peritoneal cavity, initial encounter ☑
S31.114A	Laceration without foreign body of abdominal wall, left lower quadrant without penetration into peritoneal cavity, initial encounter ☑
S31.115A	Laceration without foreign body of abdominal wall, periumbilic region without penetration into peritoneal cavity, initial encounter
S31.130A	Puncture wound of abdominal wall without foreign body, right upper quadrant without penetration into peritoneal cavity, initial encounter ☑
S31.131A	Puncture wound of abdominal wall without foreign body, left upper quadrant without penetration into peritoneal cavity, initial encounter ☑
S31.132A	Puncture wound of abdominal wall without foreign body, epigastric region without penetration into peritoneal cavity, initial encounter
S31.133A	Puncture wound of abdominal wall without foreign body, right lower quadrant without penetration into peritoneal cavity, initial encounter ☑
S31.134A	Puncture wound of abdominal wall without foreign body, left lower quadrant without penetration into peritoneal cavity, initial encounter ☑
S31.135A	Puncture wound of abdominal wall without foreign body, periumbilic region without penetration into peritoneal cavity, initial encounter
S31.150A	Open bite of abdominal wall, right upper quadrant without penetration into peritoneal cavity, initial encounter ☑
S31.151A	Open bite of abdominal wall, left upper quadrant without penetration into peritoneal cavity, initial encounter ☑
S31.152A	Open bite of abdominal wall, epigastric region without penetration into peritoneal cavity, initial encounter
S31.153A	Open bite of abdominal wall, right lower quadrant without penetration into peritoneal cavity, initial encounter ☑
S31.154A	Open bite of abdominal wall, left lower quadrant without penetration into peritoneal cavity, initial encounter ☑
S31.155A	Open bite of abdominal wall, periumbilic region without penetration into peritoneal cavity, initial encounter
S31.41XA	Laceration without foreign body of vagina and vulva, initial encounter ♀

Repair

S31.43XA	Puncture wound without foreign body of vagina and vulva, initial encounter ♀	
S31.45XA	Open bite of vagina and vulva, initial encounter ♀	
S31.831A	Laceration without foreign body of anus, initial encounter	
S31.833A	Puncture wound without foreign body of anus, initial encounter	
S31.835A	Open bite of anus, initial encounter	
S71.011A	Laceration without foreign body, right hip, initial encounter ☑	
S71.012A	Laceration without foreign body, left hip, initial encounter ☑	
S71.031A	Puncture wound without foreign body, right hip, initial encounter ☑	
S71.032A	Puncture wound without foreign body, left hip, initial encounter ☑	
S71.051A	Open bite, right hip, initial encounter ☑	
S71.052A	Open bite, left hip, initial encounter ☑	
S71.111A	Laceration without foreign body, right thigh, initial encounter ☑	
S71.112A	Laceration without foreign body, left thigh, initial encounter ☑	
S71.131A	Puncture wound without foreign body, right thigh, initial encounter ☑	
S71.132A	Puncture wound without foreign body, left thigh, initial encounter ☑	
S71.151A	Open bite, right thigh, initial encounter ☑	
S71.152A	Open bite, left thigh, initial encounter ☑	

Associated HCPCS Codes

G0168   Wound closure utilizing tissue adhesive(s) only

AMA: 12001 2018,Sep,7; 2018,Jan,8; 2017,Jan,8; 2017,Dec,14; 2016,Jan,13; 2015,Jan,16; 2014,Jan,11 **12002** 2018,Sep,7; 2018,Jan,8; 2017,Jan,8; 2016,Jan,13; 2015,Jan,16; 2014,Oct,14; 2014,Jan,11 **12004** 2018,Sep,7; 2018,Jan,8; 2017,Jan,8; 2016,Jan,13; 2015,Jan,16; 2014,Jan,11 **12005** 2018,Sep,7; 2018,Jan,8; 2017,Jan,8; 2016,Jan,13; 2015,Jan,16; 2014,Jan,11 **12006** 2018,Sep,7; 2018,Jan,8; 2017,Jan,8; 2016,Jan,13; 2015,Jan,16; 2014,Jan,11 **12007** 2018,Sep,7; 2018,Jan,8; 2017,Jan,8; 2016,Jan,13; 2015,Jan,16; 2014,Jan,11

Relative Value Units/Medicare Edits

Non-Facility RVU	Work	PE	MP	Total
12001	0.84	1.59	0.15	2.58
12002	1.14	1.8	0.22	3.16
12004	1.44	1.98	0.27	3.69
12005	1.97	2.53	0.38	4.88
12006	2.39	2.91	0.46	5.76
12007	2.9	3.14	0.54	6.58
Facility RVU	Work	PE	MP	Total
12001	0.84	0.31	0.15	1.3
12002	1.14	0.37	0.22	1.73
12004	1.44	0.44	0.27	2.15
12005	1.97	0.45	0.38	2.8
12006	2.39	0.58	0.46	3.43
12007	2.9	0.79	0.54	4.23

	FUD	Status	MUE	Modifiers				IOM Reference
12001	0	A	1(2)	51	N/A	N/A	N/A	None
12002	0	A	1(2)	51	N/A	N/A	N/A	
12004	0	A	1(2)	51	N/A	N/A	N/A	
12005	0	A	1(2)	51	N/A	N/A	N/A	
12006	0	A	1(2)	51	N/A	N/A	N/A	
12007	0	A	1(2)	51	N/A	62*	N/A	

* with documentation

Terms To Know

simple repair. Surgical closure of a superficial wound requiring single layer suturing of the skin (epidermis, dermis, or subcutaneous tissue).

superficial. On the skin surface or near the surface of any involved structure or field of interest.

12020-12021

12020 Treatment of superficial wound dehiscence; simple closure
12021 with packing

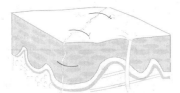

Example of a simple closure
involving only one skin layer

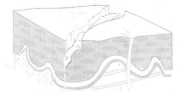

Example of a wound left open
with packing due to infection

Explanation

There has been a breakdown of the healing skin either before or after suture removal. The skin margins have opened. The physician cleanses the wound with irrigation and antimicrobial solutions. The skin margins may be trimmed to initiate bleeding surfaces. Report 12020 if the wound is sutured in a single layer. Report 12021 if the wound is left open and packed with gauze strips due to the presence of infection. This allows infection to drain from the wound and the skin closure will be delayed until the infection is resolved.

Coding Tips

For extensive or complicated secondary wound closure, see 13160. Medicare and some other payers may require G0168 be reported for wound closure by tissue adhesives only. Surgical trays, A4550, are not separately reimbursed by Medicare; however, other third-party payers may cover them. Check with the specific payer to determine coverage.

ICD-10-CM Diagnostic Codes

O90.0	Disruption of cesarean delivery wound Ⓜ ♀
O90.1	Disruption of perineal obstetric wound Ⓜ ♀
T81.31XA	Disruption of external operation (surgical) wound, not elsewhere classified, initial encounter
T81.32XA	Disruption of internal operation (surgical) wound, not elsewhere classified, initial encounter
T81.33XA	Disruption of traumatic injury wound repair, initial encounter

Associated HCPCS Codes

| G0168 | Wound closure utilizing tissue adhesive(s) only |

AMA: 12020 2019,Nov,3; 2018,Jan,8; 2017,Jan,8; 2016,Jan,13; 2015,Jan,16; 2014,Jan,11 **12021** 2019,Nov,3; 2018,Jan,8; 2017,Jan,8; 2016,Jan,13; 2015,Jan,16; 2014,Jan,11

Relative Value Units/Medicare Edits

Non-Facility RVU	Work	PE	MP	Total
12020	2.67	5.31	0.43	8.41
12021	1.89	2.69	0.32	4.9
Facility RVU	**Work**	**PE**	**MP**	**Total**
12020	2.67	2.33	0.43	5.43
12021	1.89	1.8	0.32	4.01

	FUD	Status	MUE	Modifiers			IOM Reference
12020	10	A	2(3)	51	N/A	N/A	N/A	None
12021	10	A	3(3)	51	N/A	N/A	N/A	

* with documentation

Terms To Know

dehiscence. Complication of healing in which the surgical wound ruptures or bursts open, superficially or through multiple layers.

infection. Presence of microorganisms in body tissues that may result in cellular damage.

irrigation. To wash out or cleanse a body cavity, wound, or tissue with water or other fluid.

packing. Material placed into a cavity or wound, such as gels, gauze, pads, and sponges.

perineal. Pertaining to the pelvic floor area between the thighs; the diamond-shaped area bordered by the pubic symphysis in front, the ischial tuberosities on the sides, and the coccyx in back.

subcutaneous. Below the skin.

superficial. On the skin surface or near the surface of any involved structure or field of interest.

wound repair. Surgical closure of a wound is divided into three categories: simple, intermediate, and complex. ***simple repair:*** Surgical closure of a superficial wound, requiring single layer suturing of the skin epidermis, dermis, or subcutaneous tissue. ***intermediate repair:*** Surgical closure of a wound requiring closure of one or more of the deeper subcutaneous tissue and non-muscle fascia layers in addition to suturing the skin; contaminated wounds with single layer closure that need extensive cleaning or foreign body removal. ***complex repair:*** Repair of wounds requiring more than layered closure (debridement, scar revision, stents, retention sutures).

Repair

12031-12037

12031 Repair, intermediate, wounds of scalp, axillae, trunk and/or extremities (excluding hands and feet); 2.5 cm or less
12032 2.6 cm to 7.5 cm
12034 7.6 cm to 12.5 cm
12035 12.6 cm to 20.0 cm
12036 20.1 cm to 30.0 cm
12037 over 30.0 cm

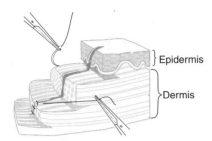

Schematic of layered closure

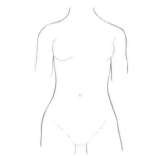

A layered closure is done on the trunk

Explanation

The physician performs a repair of a wound of the trunk using sutures, staples, tissue adhesives, or a combination of these materials to perform a layered closure. Due to deeper or more complex lacerations, deep subcutaneous or layered repair techniques are required. A local anesthetic is injected around the laceration, and the wound is cleansed, explored, and often irrigated with a saline solution. Extensive cleaning or removal of foreign matter from a heavily contaminated wound that is closed with a single layer may also be reported as an intermediate repair. For multiple wounds of the same complexity and in the same anatomical area, the length of all wounds repaired is summed and reported as one total length. Report 12031 for a total length of 2.5 cm or less; 12032 for 2.6 cm to 7.5 cm; 12034 for 7.6 cm to 12.5 cm; 12035 for 12.6 cm to 20 cm; 12036 for 20.1 cm to 30 cm; and 12037 if the total length is greater than 30 cm.

Coding Tips

Intermediate repair includes the repair of wounds that require layered closure of one or more of the deeper layers of subcutaneous tissue and superficial fascia, in addition to skin closure. Single-layer closure of a wound requiring extensive cleaning or removal of contaminated foreign matter or damaged tissue is classified as an intermediate repair. For simple repairs, see 12001–12007; complex repairs, see 13100–13160. Surgical trays, A4550, are not separately reimbursed by Medicare; however, other third-party payers may cover them. Check with the specific payer to determine coverage.

ICD-10-CM Diagnostic Codes

C43.52	Malignant melanoma of skin of breast
C43.59	Malignant melanoma of other part of trunk
C43.8	Malignant melanoma of overlapping sites of skin
C44.511	Basal cell carcinoma of skin of breast
C44.519	Basal cell carcinoma of skin of other part of trunk
C44.521	Squamous cell carcinoma of skin of breast
C44.529	Squamous cell carcinoma of skin of other part of trunk
C44.591	Other specified malignant neoplasm of skin of breast
C44.599	Other specified malignant neoplasm of skin of other part of trunk
C44.81	Basal cell carcinoma of overlapping sites of skin
C44.82	Squamous cell carcinoma of overlapping sites of skin
C44.89	Other specified malignant neoplasm of overlapping sites of skin
C4A.52	Merkel cell carcinoma of skin of breast
C4A.59	Merkel cell carcinoma of other part of trunk
C4A.8	Merkel cell carcinoma of overlapping sites
C7B.1	Secondary Merkel cell carcinoma
D17.1	Benign lipomatous neoplasm of skin and subcutaneous tissue of trunk
D17.39	Benign lipomatous neoplasm of skin and subcutaneous tissue of other sites
D23.4	Other benign neoplasm of skin of scalp and neck
D23.5	Other benign neoplasm of skin of trunk
D48.5	Neoplasm of uncertain behavior of skin
S21.011A	Laceration without foreign body of right breast, initial encounter ☑
S21.012A	Laceration without foreign body of left breast, initial encounter ☑
S21.031A	Puncture wound without foreign body of right breast, initial encounter ☑
S21.032A	Puncture wound without foreign body of left breast, initial encounter ☑
S21.051A	Open bite of right breast, initial encounter ☑
S21.052A	Open bite of left breast, initial encounter ☑
S28.211A	Complete traumatic amputation of right breast, initial encounter ☑
S28.212A	Complete traumatic amputation of left breast, initial encounter ☑
S28.221A	Partial traumatic amputation of right breast, initial encounter ☑
S28.222A	Partial traumatic amputation of left breast, initial encounter ☑
S31.010A	Laceration without foreign body of lower back and pelvis without penetration into retroperitoneum, initial encounter
S31.030A	Puncture wound without foreign body of lower back and pelvis without penetration into retroperitoneum, initial encounter
S31.050A	Open bite of lower back and pelvis without penetration into retroperitoneum, initial encounter
S31.110A	Laceration without foreign body of abdominal wall, right upper quadrant without penetration into peritoneal cavity, initial encounter ☑
S31.111A	Laceration without foreign body of abdominal wall, left upper quadrant without penetration into peritoneal cavity, initial encounter ☑
S31.112A	Laceration without foreign body of abdominal wall, epigastric region without penetration into peritoneal cavity, initial encounter
S31.113A	Laceration without foreign body of abdominal wall, right lower quadrant without penetration into peritoneal cavity, initial encounter ☑

Repair

S31.114A	Laceration without foreign body of abdominal wall, left lower quadrant without penetration into peritoneal cavity, initial encounter ☑
S31.115A	Laceration without foreign body of abdominal wall, periumbilic region without penetration into peritoneal cavity, initial encounter
S31.130A	Puncture wound of abdominal wall without foreign body, right upper quadrant without penetration into peritoneal cavity, initial encounter ☑
S31.131A	Puncture wound of abdominal wall without foreign body, left upper quadrant without penetration into peritoneal cavity, initial encounter ☑
S31.132A	Puncture wound of abdominal wall without foreign body, epigastric region without penetration into peritoneal cavity, initial encounter
S31.133A	Puncture wound of abdominal wall without foreign body, right lower quadrant without penetration into peritoneal cavity, initial encounter ☑
S31.134A	Puncture wound of abdominal wall without foreign body, left lower quadrant without penetration into peritoneal cavity, initial encounter ☑
S31.135A	Puncture wound of abdominal wall without foreign body, periumbilic region without penetration into peritoneal cavity, initial encounter
S31.150A	Open bite of abdominal wall, right upper quadrant without penetration into peritoneal cavity, initial encounter ☑
S31.151A	Open bite of abdominal wall, left upper quadrant without penetration into peritoneal cavity, initial encounter ☑
S31.152A	Open bite of abdominal wall, epigastric region without penetration into peritoneal cavity, initial encounter
S31.153A	Open bite of abdominal wall, right lower quadrant without penetration into peritoneal cavity, initial encounter ☑
S31.154A	Open bite of abdominal wall, left lower quadrant without penetration into peritoneal cavity, initial encounter ☑
S31.155A	Open bite of abdominal wall, periumbilic region without penetration into peritoneal cavity, initial encounter
S31.811A	Laceration without foreign body of right buttock, initial encounter ☑
S31.813A	Puncture wound without foreign body of right buttock, initial encounter ☑
S31.815A	Open bite of right buttock, initial encounter ☑
S31.821A	Laceration without foreign body of left buttock, initial encounter ☑
S31.823A	Puncture wound without foreign body of left buttock, initial encounter ☑
S31.825A	Open bite of left buttock, initial encounter ☑
S71.111A	Laceration without foreign body, right thigh, initial encounter ☑
S71.112A	Laceration without foreign body, left thigh, initial encounter ☑
S71.131A	Puncture wound without foreign body, right thigh, initial encounter ☑
S71.132A	Puncture wound without foreign body, left thigh, initial encounter ☑
S71.151A	Open bite, right thigh, initial encounter ☑
S71.152A	Open bite, left thigh, initial encounter ☑

AMA: **12031** 2019,Nov,3; 2018,Sep,7; 2018,Jan,8; 2017,Jan,8; 2016,Jan,13; 2015,Jan,16; 2014,Jan,11 **12032** 2019,Nov,3; 2018,Sep,7; 2018,Jan,8; 2017,Jan,8;

2016,Jan,13; 2015,Jan,16; 2014,Jan,11 **12034** 2019,Nov,3; 2018,Sep,7; 2018,Jan,8; 2017,Jan,8; 2016,Jan,13; 2015,Jan,16; 2014,Jan,11 **12035** 2019,Nov,3; 2018,Sep,7; 2018,Jan,8; 2017,Jan,8; 2016,Jan,13; 2015,Jan,16; 2014,Jan,11 **12036** 2019,Nov,3; 2018,Sep,7; 2018,Jan,8; 2017,Jan,8; 2016,Jan,13; 2015,Jan,16; 2014,Jan,11 **12037** 2019,Nov,3; 2018,Sep,7; 2018,Jan,8; 2017,Jan,8; 2016,Jan,13; 2015,Jan,16; 2014,Jan,11

Relative Value Units/Medicare Edits

Non-Facility RVU	Work	PE	MP	Total
12031	2.0	4.91	0.26	7.17
12032	2.52	5.8	0.27	8.59
12034	2.97	5.86	0.41	9.24
12035	3.5	6.91	0.62	11.03
12036	4.23	7.27	0.84	12.34
12037	5.0	7.99	1.02	14.01
Facility RVU	Work	PE	MP	Total
12031	2.0	2.1	0.26	4.36
12032	2.52	2.67	0.27	5.46
12034	2.97	2.53	0.41	5.91
12035	3.5	2.82	0.62	6.94
12036	4.23	3.08	0.84	8.15
12037	5.0	3.51	1.02	9.53

	FUD	Status	MUE	Modifiers				IOM Reference
12031	10	A	1(2)	51	N/A	N/A	N/A	None
12032	10	A	1(2)	51	N/A	N/A	N/A	
12034	10	A	1(2)	51	N/A	N/A	N/A	
12035	10	A	1(2)	51	N/A	N/A	N/A	
12036	10	A	1(2)	51	N/A	N/A	N/A	
12037	10	A	1(2)	51	N/A	62*	80*	

* with documentation

Terms To Know

laceration. Tearing injury; a torn, ragged-edged wound.

subcutaneous. Below the skin.

wound repair. Surgical closure of a wound is divided into three categories: simple, intermediate, and complex. *simple repair:* Surgical closure of a superficial wound, requiring single layer suturing of the skin epidermis, dermis, or subcutaneous tissue. *intermediate repair:* Surgical closure of a wound requiring closure of one or more of the deeper subcutaneous tissue and non-muscle fascia layers in addition to suturing the skin; contaminated wounds with single layer closure that need extensive cleaning or foreign body removal. *complex repair:* Repair of wounds requiring more than layered closure (debridement, scar revision, stents, retention sutures).

12041-12047

12041 Repair, intermediate, wounds of neck, hands, feet and/or external genitalia; 2.5 cm or less
12042 2.6 cm to 7.5 cm
12044 7.6 cm to 12.5 cm
12045 12.6 cm to 20.0 cm
12046 20.1 cm to 30.0 cm
12047 over 30.0 cm

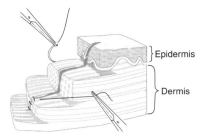

Schematic of layered closure

Explanation

The physician performs a repair of a wound located on the external genitalia. A local anesthetic is injected around the laceration, and the wound is cleansed, explored, and often irrigated with a saline solution. Due to deeper or more complex lacerations, deep subcutaneous or layered suturing techniques are required. The physician closes tissue layers under the skin with dissolvable sutures before suturing the skin. Extensive cleaning or removal of foreign matter from a heavily contaminated wound that is closed with a single layer may also be reported as an intermediate repair. With multiple wounds of the same complexity and in the same anatomical area, the length of all wounds sutured is summed and reported as one total length. Report 12041 for a total length of 2.5 cm or less; 12042 for 2.6 cm to 7.5 cm; 12044 for 7.6 cm to 12.5 cm; 12045 for 12.6 cm to 20 cm; 12046 for 20.1 cm to 30 cm; and 12047 if the total length is greater than 30 cm.

Coding Tips

Intermediate repair includes the repair of wounds that require layered closure of one or more of the deeper layers of subcutaneous tissue and superficial fascia, in addition to skin closure. Single-layer closure of a wound requiring extensive cleaning or removal of contaminated foreign matter or damaged tissue is classified as an intermediate repair. For simple repairs, see 12001–12007; complex repairs, see 13100–13160. Surgical trays, A4550, are not separately reimbursed by Medicare; however, other third-party payers may cover them. Check with the specific payer to determine coverage.

ICD-10-CM Diagnostic Codes

C44.81	Basal cell carcinoma of overlapping sites of skin
C44.82	Squamous cell carcinoma of overlapping sites of skin
C4A.8	Merkel cell carcinoma of overlapping sites
C51.0	Malignant neoplasm of labium majus ♀
C51.1	Malignant neoplasm of labium minus ♀
C79.2	Secondary malignant neoplasm of skin
C79.82	Secondary malignant neoplasm of genital organs
C7B.1	Secondary Merkel cell carcinoma
D03.8	Melanoma in situ of other sites
D04.8	Carcinoma in situ of skin of other sites
D07.1	Carcinoma in situ of vulva ♀
D07.2	Carcinoma in situ of vagina ♀
D07.39	Carcinoma in situ of other female genital organs ♀
D17.39	Benign lipomatous neoplasm of skin and subcutaneous tissue of other sites
D18.01	Hemangioma of skin and subcutaneous tissue
D28.0	Benign neoplasm of vulva ♀
D48.5	Neoplasm of uncertain behavior of skin
S31.41XA	Laceration without foreign body of vagina and vulva, initial encounter ♀
S31.42XA	Laceration with foreign body of vagina and vulva, initial encounter ♀
S31.43XA	Puncture wound without foreign body of vagina and vulva, initial encounter ♀
S31.44XA	Puncture wound with foreign body of vagina and vulva, initial encounter ♀
S31.45XA	Open bite of vagina and vulva, initial encounter ♀

AMA: 12041 2019,Nov,3; 2018,Sep,7; 2018,Jan,8; 2017,Jan,8; 2016,Jan,13; 2015,Jan,16; 2014,Jan,11 **12042** 2019,Nov,3; 2018,Sep,7; 2018,Jan,8; 2017,Jan,8; 2016,Jan,13; 2015,Jan,16; 2014,Jan,11 **12044** 2019,Nov,3; 2018,Sep,7; 2018,Jan,8; 2017,Jan,8; 2016,Jan,13; 2015,Jan,16; 2014,Jan,11 **12045** 2019,Nov,3; 2018,Sep,7; 2018,Jan,8; 2017,Jan,8; 2016,Jan,13; 2015,Jan,16; 2014,Jan,11 **12046** 2019,Nov,3; 2018,Sep,7; 2018,Jan,8; 2017,Jan,8; 2016,Jan,13; 2015,Jan,16; 2014,Jan,11 **12047** 2019,Nov,3; 2018,Sep,7; 2018,Jan,8; 2017,Jan,8; 2016,Jan,13; 2015,Jan,16; 2014,Jan,11

Relative Value Units/Medicare Edits

Non-Facility RVU	Work	PE	MP	Total
12041	2.1	4.82	0.27	7.19
12042	2.79	5.44	0.31	8.54
12044	3.19	6.95	0.46	10.6
12045	3.75	7.24	0.64	11.63
12046	4.3	8.71	1.04	14.05
12047	4.95	9.27	1.21	15.43
Facility RVU	**Work**	**PE**	**MP**	**Total**
12041	2.1	1.85	0.27	4.22
12042	2.79	2.54	0.31	5.64
12044	3.19	2.51	0.46	6.16
12045	3.75	3.37	0.64	7.76
12046	4.3	3.74	1.04	9.08
12047	4.95	3.97	1.21	10.13

	FUD	Status	MUE		Modifiers			IOM Reference
12041	10	A	1(2)	51	N/A	N/A	N/A	None
12042	10	A	1(2)	51	N/A	N/A	N/A	
12044	10	A	1(2)	51	N/A	N/A	N/A	
12045	10	A	1(2)	51	N/A	N/A	N/A	
12046	10	A	1(2)	51	N/A	N/A	80*	
12047	10	A	1(2)	51	N/A	62*	80	

* with documentation

Repair

13100-13102

13100 Repair, complex, trunk; 1.1 cm to 2.5 cm
13101 2.6 cm to 7.5 cm
+ 13102 each additional 5 cm or less (List separately in addition to code for primary procedure)

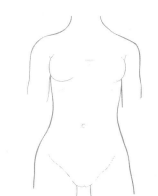

A complex repair in the general region of the trunk is performed

Explanation

The physician repairs complex wounds of the trunk. The physician performs complex, layered suturing of torn, crushed, or deeply lacerated tissue. The physician debrides the wound by removing foreign material or damaged tissue. Irrigation of the wound is performed and antimicrobial solutions are used to decontaminate and cleanse the wound. The physician may trim skin margins with a scalpel or scissors to allow for proper closure. The wound is closed in layers. The physician may perform scar revision, which creates a complex defect requiring repair. Stents or retention sutures may also be used in complex repair of a wound. Reconstructive procedures, such as utilization of local flaps, may be required and are reported separately. Report 13100 for wounds 1.1 cm to 2.5 cm; 13101 for 2.6 cm to 7.5 cm; and 13102 for each additional 5 cm or less.

Coding Tips

Report 13102 in addition to 13101. When reporting the repair of wounds, the sum of the lengths of repair are added together and are listed as a total for each anatomical site. For wounds 1 cm or less, see simple or intermediate repair codes. Complex wounds require additional special treatment, such as the use of stent dressings, retention sutures, or extensive revision, which may involve removing sizable portions of skin or extensive undermining of the skin to loosen the tissues to close a defect. In addition, at least one of the following is required: 1) exposure of bone, cartilage, tendon, or a named neurovascular structure, 2) extensive undermining that is at least one entire edge of the defect but a distance greater than or equal to the maximum width of the defect, measured perpendicular to the closure line, 3) involvement of free margins of helical rim, nostril rim, or vermilion border in which retention sutures are placed. When more than one repair and/or another separately identifiable procedure is performed, the highest dollar value code is listed as the primary procedure and subsequent procedures are appended with modifier 51. Surgical trays, A4550, are not separately reimbursed by Medicare; however, other third-party payers may cover them. Check with the specific payer to determine coverage.

ICD-10-CM Diagnostic Codes

C43.52	Malignant melanoma of skin of breast
C43.59	Malignant melanoma of other part of trunk
C44.511	Basal cell carcinoma of skin of breast
C44.519	Basal cell carcinoma of skin of other part of trunk
C44.521	Squamous cell carcinoma of skin of breast
C44.529	Squamous cell carcinoma of skin of other part of trunk
C44.591	Other specified malignant neoplasm of skin of breast
C44.599	Other specified malignant neoplasm of skin of other part of trunk
C4A.52	Merkel cell carcinoma of skin of breast
C4A.59	Merkel cell carcinoma of other part of trunk
D03.52	Melanoma in situ of breast (skin) (soft tissue)
D03.59	Melanoma in situ of other part of trunk
D04.5	Carcinoma in situ of skin of trunk
D17.1	Benign lipomatous neoplasm of skin and subcutaneous tissue of trunk
D22.5	Melanocytic nevi of trunk
D23.5	Other benign neoplasm of skin of trunk
D24.1	Benign neoplasm of right breast ☑
D24.2	Benign neoplasm of left breast ☑
R22.2	Localized swelling, mass and lump, trunk
S21.011A	Laceration without foreign body of right breast, initial encounter ☑
S21.012A	Laceration without foreign body of left breast, initial encounter ☑
S21.021A	Laceration with foreign body of right breast, initial encounter ☑
S21.022A	Laceration with foreign body of left breast, initial encounter ☑
S21.031A	Puncture wound without foreign body of right breast, initial encounter ☑
S21.032A	Puncture wound without foreign body of left breast, initial encounter ☑
S21.041A	Puncture wound with foreign body of right breast, initial encounter ☑
S21.042A	Puncture wound with foreign body of left breast, initial encounter ☑
S21.051A	Open bite of right breast, initial encounter ☑
S21.052A	Open bite of left breast, initial encounter ☑
S28.211A	Complete traumatic amputation of right breast, initial encounter ☑
S28.212A	Complete traumatic amputation of left breast, initial encounter ☑
S28.221A	Partial traumatic amputation of right breast, initial encounter ☑
S28.222A	Partial traumatic amputation of left breast, initial encounter ☑
S31.010A	Laceration without foreign body of lower back and pelvis without penetration into retroperitoneum, initial encounter
S31.020A	Laceration with foreign body of lower back and pelvis without penetration into retroperitoneum, initial encounter
S31.030A	Puncture wound without foreign body of lower back and pelvis without penetration into retroperitoneum, initial encounter
S31.040A	Puncture wound with foreign body of lower back and pelvis without penetration into retroperitoneum, initial encounter
S31.050A	Open bite of lower back and pelvis without penetration into retroperitoneum, initial encounter
S31.112A	Laceration without foreign body of abdominal wall, epigastric region without penetration into peritoneal cavity, initial encounter
S31.113A	Laceration without foreign body of abdominal wall, right lower quadrant without penetration into peritoneal cavity, initial encounter ☑

Repair

S31.114A   Laceration without foreign body of abdominal wall, left lower quadrant without penetration into peritoneal cavity, initial encounter ☑

S31.115A   Laceration without foreign body of abdominal wall, periumbilic region without penetration into peritoneal cavity, initial encounter

S31.122A   Laceration of abdominal wall with foreign body, epigastric region without penetration into peritoneal cavity, initial encounter

S31.123A   Laceration of abdominal wall with foreign body, right lower quadrant without penetration into peritoneal cavity, initial encounter ☑

S31.124A   Laceration of abdominal wall with foreign body, left lower quadrant without penetration into peritoneal cavity, initial encounter ☑

S31.125A   Laceration of abdominal wall with foreign body, periumbilic region without penetration into peritoneal cavity, initial encounter

S31.132A   Puncture wound of abdominal wall without foreign body, epigastric region without penetration into peritoneal cavity, initial encounter

S31.133A   Puncture wound of abdominal wall without foreign body, right lower quadrant without penetration into peritoneal cavity, initial encounter ☑

S31.134A   Puncture wound of abdominal wall without foreign body, left lower quadrant without penetration into peritoneal cavity, initial encounter ☑

S31.135A   Puncture wound of abdominal wall without foreign body, periumbilic region without penetration into peritoneal cavity, initial encounter

S31.142A   Puncture wound of abdominal wall with foreign body, epigastric region without penetration into peritoneal cavity, initial encounter

S31.143A   Puncture wound of abdominal wall with foreign body, right lower quadrant without penetration into peritoneal cavity, initial encounter ☑

S31.144A   Puncture wound of abdominal wall with foreign body, left lower quadrant without penetration into peritoneal cavity, initial encounter ☑

S31.145A   Puncture wound of abdominal wall with foreign body, periumbilic region without penetration into peritoneal cavity, initial encounter

S31.152A   Open bite of abdominal wall, epigastric region without penetration into peritoneal cavity, initial encounter

S31.153A   Open bite of abdominal wall, right lower quadrant without penetration into peritoneal cavity, initial encounter ☑

S31.154A   Open bite of abdominal wall, left lower quadrant without penetration into peritoneal cavity, initial encounter ☑

S31.155A   Open bite of abdominal wall, periumbilic region without penetration into peritoneal cavity, initial encounter

S31.811A   Laceration without foreign body of right buttock, initial encounter ☑

S31.812A   Laceration with foreign body of right buttock, initial encounter ☑

S31.813A   Puncture wound without foreign body of right buttock, initial encounter ☑

S31.814A   Puncture wound with foreign body of right buttock, initial encounter ☑

S31.815A   Open bite of right buttock, initial encounter ☑

S31.821A   Laceration without foreign body of left buttock, initial encounter ☑

S31.822A   Laceration with foreign body of left buttock, initial encounter ☑

S31.823A   Puncture wound without foreign body of left buttock, initial encounter ☑

S31.824A   Puncture wound with foreign body of left buttock, initial encounter ☑

S31.825A   Open bite of left buttock, initial encounter ☑

S31.831A   Laceration without foreign body of anus, initial encounter

S31.832A   Laceration with foreign body of anus, initial encounter

S31.833A   Puncture wound without foreign body of anus, initial encounter

S31.834A   Puncture wound with foreign body of anus, initial encounter

S31.835A   Open bite of anus, initial encounter

AMA: 13100 2019,Nov,3; 2019,Nov,14; 2018,Sep,7; 2018,Jan,8; 2017,Jan,8; 2017,Apr,9; 2016,Jan,13; 2015,Jan,16; 2014,Jan,11 **13101** 2019,Nov,3; 2019,Dec,14; 2018,Sep,7; 2018,Jan,8; 2017,Jan,8; 2017,Apr,9; 2016,Jan,13; 2015,Jan,16; 2014,Jan,11 **13102** 2019,Nov,14; 2019,Nov,3; 2018,Sep,7; 2018,Jan,8; 2017,Jan,8; 2017,Apr,9; 2016,Jan,13; 2015,Jan,16; 2014,Jan,11

Relative Value Units/Medicare Edits

Non-Facility RVU	Work	PE	MP	Total
13100	3.0	6.37	0.35	9.72
13101	3.5	7.52	0.39	11.41
13102	1.24	2.01	0.18	3.43
Facility RVU	**Work**	**PE**	**MP**	**Total**
13100	3.0	2.46	0.35	5.81
13101	3.5	3.25	0.39	7.14
13102	1.24	0.68	0.18	2.1

	FUD	Status	MUE	Modifiers				IOM Reference
13100	10	A	1(2)	51	N/A	N/A	N/A	None
13101	10	A	1(2)	51	N/A	N/A	N/A	
13102	N/A	A	9(3)	N/A	N/A	N/A	N/A	

* with documentation

Terms To Know

complex repair. Surgical closure of a wound requiring more than layered closure of the deeper subcutaneous tissue and fascia.

defect. Imperfection, flaw, or absence.

irrigation. To wash out or cleanse a body cavity, wound, or tissue with water or other fluid.

laceration. Tearing injury; a torn, ragged-edged wound.

margin. Boundary, edge, or border, as of a surface or structure.

wound. Injury to living tissue often involving a cut or break in the skin.

Repair

13131-13133

13131 Repair, complex, forehead, cheeks, chin, mouth, neck, axillae, genitalia, hands and/or feet; 1.1 cm to 2.5 cm
13132 2.6 cm to 7.5 cm
+ **13133** each additional 5 cm or less (List separately in addition to code for primary procedure)

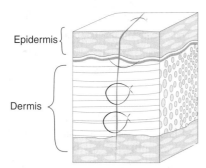

Epidermis
Dermis

Schematic of complex layered suturing
of torn or deeply lacerated tissue

Explanation

The physician repairs wounds located on the genitalia. The physician performs complex, layered suturing of torn, crushed, or deeply lacerated tissue. The physician debrides the wound by removing foreign material or damaged tissue. Irrigation of the wound is performed and antimicrobial solutions are used to decontaminate and cleanse the wound. The physician may trim skin margins with a scalpel or scissors to allow for proper closure. The wound is closed in layers. The physician may perform scar revision, which creates a complex defect requiring repair. Stents or retention sutures may also be used in complex repair of a wound. Reconstructive procedures, such as utilization of local flaps, may be required and are reported separately. Report 13131 for wounds 1.1 cm to 2.5 cm; 13132 for 2.6 cm to 7.5 cm; and 13133 for each additional 5 cm or less.

Coding Tips

Report 13133 in addition to 13132. When reporting the repair of wounds, the sum of the lengths of repair are added together and are listed as a total for each anatomical site. For wounds 1 cm or less, see simple or intermediate repair codes. Complex wounds require additional special treatment, such as the use of stent dressings, retention sutures, or extensive revision, which may involve removing sizable portions of skin or extensive undermining of the skin to loosen the tissues to close a defect. In addition, at least one of the following is required: 1) exposure of bone, cartilage, tendon, or a named neurovascular structure, 2) extensive undermining that is at least one entire edge of the defect but a distance greater than or equal to the maximum width of the defect, measured perpendicular to the closure line, 3) involvement of free margins of helical rim, nostril rim, or vermilion border in which retention sutures are placed. When more than one repair and/or another separately identifiable procedure is performed, the highest dollar value code is listed as the primary procedure and subsequent procedures are appended with modifier 51. Surgical trays, A4550, are not separately reimbursed by Medicare; however, other third-party payers may cover them. Check with the specific payer to determine coverage.

ICD-10-CM Diagnostic Codes

C43.59	Malignant melanoma of other part of trunk
C79.82	Secondary malignant neoplasm of genital organs
D07.1	Carcinoma in situ of vulva ♀
D07.2	Carcinoma in situ of vagina ♀
D07.39	Carcinoma in situ of other female genital organs ♀
D28.0	Benign neoplasm of vulva ♀
D39.8	Neoplasm of uncertain behavior of other specified female genital organs ♀
N90.811	Female genital mutilation Type I status ♀
N90.812	Female genital mutilation Type II status ♀
N90.813	Female genital mutilation Type III status ♀
N90.818	Other female genital mutilation status ♀
S31.41XA	Laceration without foreign body of vagina and vulva, initial encounter ♀
S31.42XA	Laceration with foreign body of vagina and vulva, initial encounter ♀
S31.43XA	Puncture wound without foreign body of vagina and vulva, initial encounter ♀
S31.44XA	Puncture wound with foreign body of vagina and vulva, initial encounter ♀
S31.45XA	Open bite of vagina and vulva, initial encounter ♀
S38.211A	Complete traumatic amputation of female external genital organs, initial encounter ♀
S38.212A	Partial traumatic amputation of female external genital organs, initial encounter ♀

AMA: 13131 2019,Nov,3; 2018,Sep,7; 2018,Jan,8; 2017,Jan,8; 2017,Apr,9; 2016,Jan,13; 2015,Jan,16; 2014,Jan,11 **13132** 2019,Nov,3; 2018,Sep,7; 2018,Jan,8; 2017,Jan,8; 2017,Apr,9; 2016,Jan,13; 2015,Jan,16; 2014,Oct,14; 2014,Jan,11 **13133** 2019,Nov,3; 2018,Sep,7; 2018,Jan,8; 2017,Jan,8; 2017,Apr,9; 2016,Jan,13; 2015,Jan,16; 2014,Jan,11

Relative Value Units/Medicare Edits

Non-Facility RVU	Work	PE	MP	Total
13131	3.73	6.95	0.43	11.11
13132	4.78	8.3	0.51	13.59
13133	2.19	2.52	0.27	4.98
Facility RVU	**Work**	**PE**	**MP**	**Total**
13131	3.73	2.88	0.43	7.04
13132	4.78	3.52	0.51	8.81
13133	2.19	1.23	0.27	3.69

	FUD	Status	MUE	Modifiers				IOM Reference
13131	10	A	1(2)	51	N/A	N/A	N/A	None
13132	10	A	1(2)	51	N/A	N/A	N/A	
13133	N/A	A	7(3)	N/A	N/A	N/A	N/A	

* with documentation

Terms To Know

complex repair. Surgical closure of a wound requiring more than layered closure of the deeper subcutaneous tissue and fascia.

debride. To remove all foreign objects and devitalized or infected tissue from a burn or wound to prevent infection and promote healing.

irrigation. To wash out or cleanse a body cavity, wound, or tissue with water or other fluid.

margin. Boundary, edge, or border, as of a surface or structure.

Repair

13160

13160 Secondary closure of surgical wound or dehiscence, extensive or complicated

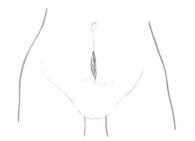

An extensive or complicated surgical wound is closed secondarily or an extensive or complicated dehiscence is treated and closed

Explanation

The physician secondarily repairs a surgical skin closure after an infectious breakdown of the healing skin. After resolution of the infection, the wound is now ready for closure. The physician uses a scalpel to excise granulation and scar tissue. Skin margins are trimmed to bleeding edges. The wound is sutured in several layers.

Coding Tips

For simple closure of secondary wound dehiscence, see 12020; with packing, see 12021. If incision and drainage of a hematoma, seroma, or fluid collection is performed, see 10140. Do not report 13160 with 11960. Surgical trays, A4550, are not separately reimbursed by Medicare; however, other third-party payers may cover them. Check with the specific payer to determine coverage.

ICD-10-CM Diagnostic Codes

O90.0	Disruption of cesarean delivery wound Ⓜ ♀
O90.1	Disruption of perineal obstetric wound Ⓜ ♀
T81.31XA	Disruption of external operation (surgical) wound, not elsewhere classified, initial encounter
T81.32XA	Disruption of internal operation (surgical) wound, not elsewhere classified, initial encounter
Z48.1	Encounter for planned postprocedural wound closure

AMA: 13160 2019,Nov,3; 2018,Jan,8; 2017,Jan,8; 2016,Jan,13; 2015,Jan,16; 2014,Jan,11

Relative Value Units/Medicare Edits

Non-Facility RVU	Work	PE	MP	Total
13160	12.04	8.89	2.06	22.99
Facility RVU	**Work**	**PE**	**MP**	**Total**
13160	12.04	8.89	2.06	22.99

	FUD	Status	MUE	Modifiers				IOM Reference
13160	90	A	2(3)	51	N/A	N/A	N/A	None

* with documentation

Terms To Know

dehiscence. Complication of healing in which the surgical wound ruptures or bursts open, superficially or through multiple layers.

14040-14041

14040 Adjacent tissue transfer or rearrangement, forehead, cheeks, chin, mouth, neck, axillae, genitalia, hands and/or feet; defect 10 sq cm or less

14041 defect 10.1 sq cm to 30.0 sq cm

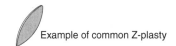
Example of common Z-plasty

Defect is removed with oval-shaped incision

 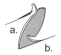

Two additional incisions intersect the removal area

Skin of each incision is reflected back

 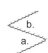

The flaps are then transposed

And the repair is closed

Explanation

The physician transfers or rearranges adjacent tissue to repair traumatic or surgical wounds on the genitalia. This includes, but is not limited to, such rearrangement procedures as Z-plasty, W-plasty, ZY-plasty, or tissue transfers such as rotational flaps or advancement flaps. Report 14040 for defects that are 10 sq cm or less and 14041 for defects that are 10.1 sq cm to 30 sq cm.

Coding Tips

When adjacent tissue transfer or rearrangement is performed in conjunction with excision of a lesion, the lesion excision is not reported separately. When these codes are used to report repair of traumatic wounds, the procedure must have been previously planned and developed by the physician to constitute the repair. These codes do not apply when direct closure or rearrangement of the traumatized tissue itself incidentally results in these configurations. Any skin grafting required to close the secondary defect is reported separately. For intralesional injection to limit scarring, see 11900. Surgical trays, A4550, are not separately reimbursed by Medicare; however, other third-party payers may cover them. Check with the specific payer to determine coverage.

ICD-10-CM Diagnostic Codes

C51.0	Malignant neoplasm of labium majus ♀
C51.1	Malignant neoplasm of labium minus ♀
C51.2	Malignant neoplasm of clitoris ♀
C51.8	Malignant neoplasm of overlapping sites of vulva ♀
C52	Malignant neoplasm of vagina ♀
C57.7	Malignant neoplasm of other specified female genital organs ♀
C57.8	Malignant neoplasm of overlapping sites of female genital organs ♀
S31.41XA	Laceration without foreign body of vagina and vulva, initial encounter ♀
S31.42XA	Laceration with foreign body of vagina and vulva, initial encounter ♀
S31.43XA	Puncture wound without foreign body of vagina and vulva, initial encounter ♀

Repair

S31.44XA	Puncture wound with foreign body of vagina and vulva, initial encounter ♀
S31.45XA	Open bite of vagina and vulva, initial encounter ♀
S38.211A	Complete traumatic amputation of female external genital organs, initial encounter ♀
S38.212A	Partial traumatic amputation of female external genital organs, initial encounter ♀
T21.37XA	Burn of third degree of female genital region, initial encounter ♀
T21.77XA	Corrosion of third degree of female genital region, initial encounter ♀

AMA: **14040** 2018,Jan,8; 2017,Nov,6; 2017,Jan,8; 2016,Jan,13; 2015,Jan,16; 2014,Jan,11 **14041** 2018,Jan,8; 2017,Nov,6; 2017,Jan,8; 2016,Jan,13; 2015,Jan,16; 2014,Jan,11

Relative Value Units/Medicare Edits

Non-Facility RVU	Work	PE	MP	Total
14040	8.6	11.95	1.01	21.56
14041	10.83	14.32	1.22	26.37
Facility RVU	**Work**	**PE**	**MP**	**Total**
14040	8.6	8.22	1.01	17.83
14041	10.83	9.81	1.22	21.86

	FUD	Status	MUE	Modifiers				IOM Reference
14040	90	A	2(3)	51	N/A	N/A	N/A	None
14041	90	A	3(3)	51	N/A	N/A	N/A	

* with documentation

Terms To Know

adjacent tissue transfer. Rotation or advancement of skin from an adjacent area to repair or fill in a defect while maintaining attachment to original blood supply.

defect. Imperfection, flaw, or absence.

tissue. Group of similar cells with a similar function that form definite structures and organs. Tissue types include epithelial tissue, muscle tissue, connective tissue, and nervous tissue.

wound. Injury to living tissue often involving a cut or break in the skin.

z-plasty. Plastic surgery technique used primarily to release tension or elongate contracted scar tissue in which a Z-shaped incision is made with the middle line of the Z crossing the area of greatest tension. The triangular flaps are then rotated so that they cross the incision line in the opposite direction, creating a reversed Z.

17270-17276

17270 Destruction, malignant lesion (eg, laser surgery, electrosurgery, cryosurgery, chemosurgery, surgical curettement), scalp, neck, hands, feet, genitalia; lesion diameter 0.5 cm or less
17271 lesion diameter 0.6 to 1.0 cm
17272 lesion diameter 1.1 to 2.0 cm
17273 lesion diameter 2.1 to 3.0 cm
17274 lesion diameter 3.1 to 4.0 cm
17276 lesion diameter over 4.0 cm

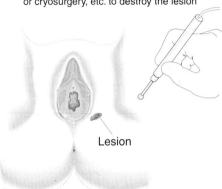

The physician may use laser, fulguration, or cryosurgery, etc. to destroy the lesion

Lesion

Report according to the area of destruction

Explanation

The physician destroys a malignant lesion of the genitalia. Destruction may be accomplished by using a laser or electrocautery to burn the lesion, cryotherapy to freeze the lesion, chemicals to destroy the lesion, or surgical curettement to remove the lesion. Report 17270 for a lesion diameter 0.5 cm or less; 17271 for 0.6 cm to 1 cm; 17272 for 1.1 cm to 2 cm; 17273 for 2.1 cm to 3 cm; 17274 for 3.1 cm to 4 cm; and 17276 if the lesion diameter is greater than 4 cm.

Coding Tips

These codes are appropriate for reporting this procedure when performed with any technique or combination of techniques (e.g., laser, hot cautery). Local anesthesia is included in these services. For destruction of benign lesions other than skin tags or cutaneous vascular lesions, see 17110–17111. For excision of a malignant lesion, see 11620–11626.

ICD-10-CM Diagnostic Codes

C4A.8	Merkel cell carcinoma of overlapping sites
C51.0	Malignant neoplasm of labium majus ♀
C51.1	Malignant neoplasm of labium minus ♀
C51.2	Malignant neoplasm of clitoris ♀
C51.8	Malignant neoplasm of overlapping sites of vulva ♀
C52	Malignant neoplasm of vagina ♀
C57.7	Malignant neoplasm of other specified female genital organs ♀
C57.8	Malignant neoplasm of overlapping sites of female genital organs ♀
C7B.1	Secondary Merkel cell carcinoma

AMA: **17270** 2018,Jan,8; 2017,Jan,8; 2017,Dec,14; 2016,Jan,13; 2015,Jan,16; 2014,Jan,11 **17271** 2018,Jan,8; 2017,Jan,8; 2017,Dec,14; 2016,Jan,13; 2015,Jan,16; 2014,Jan,11 **17272** 2018,Jan,8; 2017,Jan,8; 2017,Dec,14; 2016,Jan,13; 2015,Jan,16; 2014,Jan,11 **17273** 2018,Jan,8; 2017,Jan,8; 2017,Dec,14; 2016,Jan,13; 2015,Jan,16; 2014,Jan,11 **17274** 2018,Jan,8; 2017,Jan,8; 2017,Dec,14; 2016,Jan,13; 2015,Jan,16; 2014,Jan,11 **17276** 2018,Jan,8; 2017,Jan,8; 2017,Dec,14; 2016,Jan,13; 2015,Jan,16; 2014,Jan,11

Relative Value Units/Medicare Edits

Non-Facility RVU	Work	PE	MP	Total
17270	1.37	2.72	0.13	4.22
17271	1.54	2.98	0.13	4.65
17272	1.82	3.32	0.18	5.32
17273	2.1	3.61	0.21	5.92
17274	2.64	4.07	0.26	6.97
17276	3.25	4.51	0.31	8.07
Facility RVU	**Work**	**PE**	**MP**	**Total**
17270	1.37	1.24	0.13	2.74
17271	1.54	1.35	0.13	3.02
17272	1.82	1.52	0.18	3.52
17273	2.1	1.68	0.21	3.99
17274	2.64	1.98	0.26	4.88
17276	3.25	2.3	0.31	5.86

	FUD	Status	MUE	Modifiers				IOM Reference
17270	10	A	6(3)	51	N/A	N/A	N/A	None
17271	10	A	4(3)	51	N/A	N/A	N/A	
17272	10	A	5(3)	51	N/A	N/A	N/A	
17273	10	A	4(3)	51	N/A	N/A	N/A	
17274	10	A	2(3)	51	N/A	N/A	N/A	
17276	10	A	2(3)	51	N/A	N/A	N/A	

* with documentation

Terms To Know

chemosurgery. Application of chemical agents to destroy tissue, originally referring to the in situ chemical fixation of premalignant or malignant lesions to facilitate surgical excision.

cryosurgery. Application of intense cold, usually produced using liquid nitrogen, to locally freeze diseased or unwanted tissue and induce tissue necrosis without causing harm to adjacent tissue.

destruction. Ablation or eradication of a structure or tissue.

electrocautery. Division or cutting of tissue using high-frequency electrical current to produce heat, which destroys cells.

electrosurgery. Use of electric currents to generate heat in performing surgery.

fulguration. Destruction of living tissue by using sparks from a high-frequency electric current.

lesion. Area of damaged tissue that has lost continuity or function, due to disease or trauma.

malignant. Any condition tending to progress toward death, specifically an invasive tumor with a loss of cellular differentiation that has the ability to spread or metastasize to other body areas.

neoplasm. New abnormal growth, tumor.

Destruction

35840

35840 Exploration for postoperative hemorrhage, thrombosis or infection; abdomen

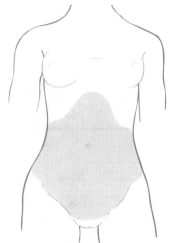

A surgical exploration is performed in the abdominal cavity for the purpose of finding and identifying postoperative hemorrhage, thrombosis (clotting), or infection

Explanation

The physician reopens the original incision site and inspects the operative area for active bleeding, hematoma, thrombus, and exudate. The physician removes or debrides any observed hematoma, thrombus, and infected tissues. The physician looks for and corrects any active bleeding sites using electrocautery or ligation of bleeding vessels. The physician may leave an infected wound open, but generally closes the incision, leaving drains in place.

Coding Tips

This code is used to report exploration for postoperative hemorrhage, thrombosis, or infection of veins and arteries of the abdomen only.

ICD-10-CM Diagnostic Codes

G89.18	Other acute postprocedural pain
G89.28	Other chronic postprocedural pain
I77.2	Rupture of artery
K68.11	Postprocedural retroperitoneal abscess
K91.31	Postprocedural partial intestinal obstruction
K91.32	Postprocedural complete intestinal obstruction
K91.840	Postprocedural hemorrhage of a digestive system organ or structure following a digestive system procedure
K91.841	Postprocedural hemorrhage of a digestive system organ or structure following other procedure
N99.0	Postprocedural (acute) (chronic) kidney failure
N99.820	Postprocedural hemorrhage of a genitourinary system organ or structure following a genitourinary system procedure
N99.821	Postprocedural hemorrhage of a genitourinary system organ or structure following other procedure
N99.89	Other postprocedural complications and disorders of genitourinary system
T81.31XA	Disruption of external operation (surgical) wound, not elsewhere classified, initial encounter
T81.32XA	Disruption of internal operation (surgical) wound, not elsewhere classified, initial encounter
T81.43XA	Infection following a procedure, organ and space surgical site, initial encounter
T81.711A	Complication of renal artery following a procedure, not elsewhere classified, initial encounter
T81.718A	Complication of other artery following a procedure, not elsewhere classified, initial encounter
T81.72XA	Complication of vein following a procedure, not elsewhere classified, initial encounter
T88.8XXA	Other specified complications of surgical and medical care, not elsewhere classified, initial encounter

AMA: 35840 1997,Nov,1; 1997,May,4

Relative Value Units/Medicare Edits

Non-Facility RVU	Work	PE	MP	Total
35840	20.75	9.38	4.73	34.86
Facility RVU	**Work**	**PE**	**MP**	**Total**
35840	20.75	9.38	4.73	34.86

	FUD	Status	MUE	Modifiers				IOM Reference
35840	90	A	2(3)	51	N/A	62*	80	None

* with documentation

Terms To Know

debride. To remove all foreign objects and devitalized or infected tissue from a burn or wound to prevent infection and promote healing.

electrocautery. Division or cutting of tissue using high-frequency electrical current to produce heat, which destroys cells.

embolism. Obstruction of a blood vessel resulting from a clot or foreign substance.

exploration. Examination for diagnostic purposes.

exudate. Fluid or other material, such as debris from cells, that has escaped blood vessel circulation and is deposited in or on tissues and usually occurs due to inflammation.

hematoma. Tumor-like collection of blood in some part of the body caused by a break in a blood vessel wall, usually as a result of trauma.

hemorrhage. Internal or external bleeding with loss of significant amounts of blood.

infection. Presence of microorganisms in body tissues that may result in cellular damage.

ligation. Tying off a blood vessel or duct with a suture or a soft, thin wire.

seroma. Swelling caused by the collection of serum, or clear fluid, in the tissues.

thrombosis. Condition arising from the presence or formation of blood clots within a blood vessel that may cause vascular obstruction and insufficient oxygenation.

Arteries and Veins

36415-36416

36415 Collection of venous blood by venipuncture
36416 Collection of capillary blood specimen (eg, finger, heel, ear stick)

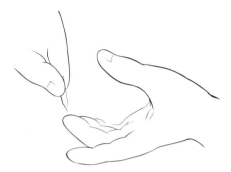

Capillary blood is collected. The specimen is typically collected by finger stick

Explanation

A needle is inserted into the skin over a vein to puncture the blood vessel and withdraw blood for venous collection in 36415. In 36416, a prick is made into the finger, heel, or ear and capillary blood that pools at the puncture site is collected in a pipette. In either case, the blood is used for diagnostic study and no catheter is placed.

Coding Tips

These procedures do not include laboratory analysis. If a specimen is transported to an outside laboratory, report 99000. Modifier 63 should not be reported with 36415. Medicare and some payers may require HCPCS Level II code G0471 to report this service when provided in a federally qualified health center (FQHC).

ICD-10-CM Diagnostic Codes

The application of this code is too broad to adequately present ICD-10-CM diagnostic code links here. Refer to your ICD-10-CM book.

Associated HCPCS Codes

G0471   Collection of venous blood by venipuncture or urine sample by catheterization from an individual in a skilled nursing facility (SNF) or by a laboratory on behalf of a home health agency (HHA)

AMA: 36415 2019,Aug,8; 2018,Jan,8; 2017,Jan,8; 2016,Jan,13; 2015,Jan,16; 2014,May,4; 2014,Jan,11

Relative Value Units/Medicare Edits

Non-Facility RVU	Work	PE	MP	Total
36415	0.0	0.0	0.0	0.0
36416	0.0	0.0	0.0	0.0
Facility RVU	Work	PE	MP	Total
36415	0.0	0.0	0.0	0.0
36416	0.0	0.0	0.0	0.0

	FUD	Status	MUE	Modifiers				IOM Reference
36415	N/A	X	2(3)	N/A	N/A	N/A	N/A	None
36416	N/A	B	0(3)	N/A	N/A	N/A	N/A	

* with documentation

36460

36460 Transfusion, intrauterine, fetal

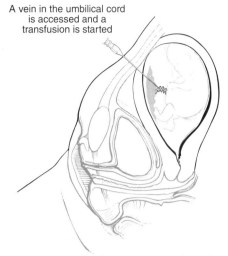

A vein in the umbilical cord is accessed and a transfusion is started

An intrauterine transfusion is performed on a fetus

Explanation

The physician performs a blood transfusion to a fetus. The physician uses separately reportable ultrasound guidance to locate the umbilical vein. A needle is directed through the abdominal wall into the amniotic cavity. The umbilical vein is pierced and fetal blood is exchanged with transfused blood. The needle is withdrawn and the fetus is observed under separately reportable ultrasound.

Coding Tips

Radiological supervision and interpretation is reported with 76941. Modifier 63 should not be reported with 36460.

ICD-10-CM Diagnostic Codes

O35.3XX1	Maternal care for (suspected) damage to fetus from viral disease in mother, fetus 1 🅜 ♀
O35.3XX2	Maternal care for (suspected) damage to fetus from viral disease in mother, fetus 2 🅜 ♀
O35.3XX3	Maternal care for (suspected) damage to fetus from viral disease in mother, fetus 3 🅜 ♀
O36.0111	Maternal care for anti-D [Rh] antibodies, first trimester, fetus 1 🅜 ♀
O36.0112	Maternal care for anti-D [Rh] antibodies, first trimester, fetus 2 🅜 ♀
O36.0113	Maternal care for anti-D [Rh] antibodies, first trimester, fetus 3 🅜 ♀
O36.0121	Maternal care for anti-D [Rh] antibodies, second trimester, fetus 1 🅜 ♀
O36.0122	Maternal care for anti-D [Rh] antibodies, second trimester, fetus 2 🅜 ♀
O36.0123	Maternal care for anti-D [Rh] antibodies, second trimester, fetus 3 🅜 ♀
O36.0131	Maternal care for anti-D [Rh] antibodies, third trimester, fetus 1 🅜 ♀
O36.0132	Maternal care for anti-D [Rh] antibodies, third trimester, fetus 2 🅜 ♀

Arteries and Veins

O36.0133	Maternal care for anti-D [Rh] antibodies, third trimester, fetus 3 ▣ ♀
O36.0911	Maternal care for other rhesus isoimmunization, first trimester, fetus 1 ▣ ♀
O36.0912	Maternal care for other rhesus isoimmunization, first trimester, fetus 2 ▣ ♀
O36.0913	Maternal care for other rhesus isoimmunization, first trimester, fetus 3 ▣ ♀
O36.0921	Maternal care for other rhesus isoimmunization, second trimester, fetus 1 ▣ ♀
O36.0922	Maternal care for other rhesus isoimmunization, second trimester, fetus 2 ▣ ♀
O36.0923	Maternal care for other rhesus isoimmunization, second trimester, fetus 3 ▣ ♀
O36.0931	Maternal care for other rhesus isoimmunization, third trimester, fetus 1 ▣ ♀
O36.0932	Maternal care for other rhesus isoimmunization, third trimester, fetus 2 ▣ ♀
O36.0933	Maternal care for other rhesus isoimmunization, third trimester, fetus 3 ▣ ♀
O36.1111	Maternal care for Anti-A sensitization, first trimester, fetus 1 ▣ ♀
O36.1112	Maternal care for Anti-A sensitization, first trimester, fetus 2 ▣ ♀
O36.1113	Maternal care for Anti-A sensitization, first trimester, fetus 3 ▣ ♀
O36.1121	Maternal care for Anti-A sensitization, second trimester, fetus 1 ▣ ♀
O36.1122	Maternal care for Anti-A sensitization, second trimester, fetus 2 ▣ ♀
O36.1123	Maternal care for Anti-A sensitization, second trimester, fetus 3 ▣ ♀
O36.1131	Maternal care for Anti-A sensitization, third trimester, fetus 1 ▣ ♀
O36.1132	Maternal care for Anti-A sensitization, third trimester, fetus 2 ▣ ♀
O36.1133	Maternal care for Anti-A sensitization, third trimester, fetus 3 ▣ ♀
O36.1911	Maternal care for other isoimmunization, first trimester, fetus 1 ▣ ♀
O36.1912	Maternal care for other isoimmunization, first trimester, fetus 2 ▣ ♀
O36.1913	Maternal care for other isoimmunization, first trimester, fetus 3 ▣ ♀
O36.1921	Maternal care for other isoimmunization, second trimester, fetus 1 ▣ ♀
O36.1922	Maternal care for other isoimmunization, second trimester, fetus 2 ▣ ♀
O36.1923	Maternal care for other isoimmunization, second trimester, fetus 3 ▣ ♀
O36.1931	Maternal care for other isoimmunization, third trimester, fetus 1 ▣ ♀
O36.1932	Maternal care for other isoimmunization, third trimester, fetus 2 ▣ ♀
O36.1933	Maternal care for other isoimmunization, third trimester, fetus 3 ▣ ♀
O36.21X1	Maternal care for hydrops fetalis, first trimester, fetus 1 ▣ ♀
O36.21X2	Maternal care for hydrops fetalis, first trimester, fetus 2 ▣ ♀
O36.21X3	Maternal care for hydrops fetalis, first trimester, fetus 3 ▣ ♀
O36.22X1	Maternal care for hydrops fetalis, second trimester, fetus 1 ▣ ♀
O36.22X2	Maternal care for hydrops fetalis, second trimester, fetus 2 ▣ ♀
O36.22X3	Maternal care for hydrops fetalis, second trimester, fetus 3 ▣ ♀
O36.23X1	Maternal care for hydrops fetalis, third trimester, fetus 1 ▣ ♀
O36.23X2	Maternal care for hydrops fetalis, third trimester, fetus 2 ▣ ♀
O36.23X3	Maternal care for hydrops fetalis, third trimester, fetus 3 ▣ ♀
O36.8211	Fetal anemia and thrombocytopenia, first trimester, fetus 1 ▣ ♀
O36.8212	Fetal anemia and thrombocytopenia, first trimester, fetus 2 ▣ ♀
O36.8213	Fetal anemia and thrombocytopenia, first trimester, fetus 3 ▣ ♀
O36.8221	Fetal anemia and thrombocytopenia, second trimester, fetus 1 ▣ ♀
O36.8222	Fetal anemia and thrombocytopenia, second trimester, fetus 2 ▣ ♀
O36.8223	Fetal anemia and thrombocytopenia, second trimester, fetus 3 ▣ ♀
O36.8231	Fetal anemia and thrombocytopenia, third trimester, fetus 1 ▣ ♀
O36.8232	Fetal anemia and thrombocytopenia, third trimester, fetus 2 ▣ ♀
O36.8233	Fetal anemia and thrombocytopenia, third trimester, fetus 3 ▣ ♀
O36.8911	Maternal care for other specified fetal problems, first trimester, fetus 1 ▣ ♀
O36.8912	Maternal care for other specified fetal problems, first trimester, fetus 2 ▣ ♀
O36.8913	Maternal care for other specified fetal problems, first trimester, fetus 3 ▣ ♀
O36.8921	Maternal care for other specified fetal problems, second trimester, fetus 1 ▣ ♀
O36.8922	Maternal care for other specified fetal problems, second trimester, fetus 2 ▣ ♀
O36.8923	Maternal care for other specified fetal problems, second trimester, fetus 3 ▣ ♀
O36.8931	Maternal care for other specified fetal problems, third trimester, fetus 1 ▣ ♀
O36.8932	Maternal care for other specified fetal problems, third trimester, fetus 2 ▣ ♀
O36.8933	Maternal care for other specified fetal problems, third trimester, fetus 3 ▣ ♀

AMA: **36460** 2003,Apr,7

Relative Value Units/Medicare Edits

Non-Facility RVU	Work	PE	MP	Total
36460	6.58	2.48	1.04	10.1
Facility RVU	**Work**	**PE**	**MP**	**Total**
36460	6.58	2.48	1.04	10.1

	FUD	Status	MUE	Modifiers				IOM Reference
36460	N/A	A	2(3)	51	N/A	N/A	80	100-01,3,20.5.2; 100-04,3,40.2.2

* with documentation

Terms To Know

blood transfusion. Introduction of blood or blood products from another source into a vein or an artery.

fetus. Unborn offspring past the embryonic stage that has developed major structures. It is the period defined from nine weeks after fertilization until birth.

ultrasound. Imaging using ultra-high sound frequency bounced off body structures.

38562

38562 Limited lymphadenectomy for staging (separate procedure); pelvic and para-aortic

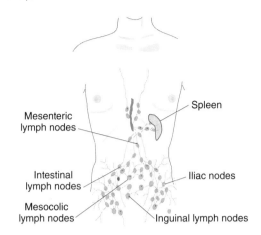

Mesenteric lymph nodes

Spleen

Intestinal lymph nodes

Iliac nodes

Mesocolic lymph nodes

Inguinal lymph nodes

Explanation

The physician makes a midline abdominal incision just below the navel. The surrounding tissue, nerves, and blood vessels are dissected away, and the pelvic and/or para-aortic lymph nodes are visualized. The nodes are removed. The wound is closed with sutures or staples.

Coding Tips

This separate procedure by definition is usually a component of a more complex service and is not identified separately. When performed alone or with other unrelated procedures or services it may be reported. If performed alone, list the code; if performed with other procedures/services, list the code and append modifier 59 or an X{EPSU} modifier. For extensive retroperitoneal transabdominal lymphadenectomy, see 38780.

ICD-10-CM Diagnostic Codes

C19	Malignant neoplasm of rectosigmoid junction
C20	Malignant neoplasm of rectum
C45.1	Mesothelioma of peritoneum
C48.0	Malignant neoplasm of retroperitoneum
C48.1	Malignant neoplasm of specified parts of peritoneum
C48.8	Malignant neoplasm of overlapping sites of retroperitoneum and peritoneum
C53.0	Malignant neoplasm of endocervix ♀
C53.1	Malignant neoplasm of exocervix ♀
C53.8	Malignant neoplasm of overlapping sites of cervix uteri ♀
C54.0	Malignant neoplasm of isthmus uteri ♀
C54.1	Malignant neoplasm of endometrium ♀
C54.2	Malignant neoplasm of myometrium ♀
C54.3	Malignant neoplasm of fundus uteri ♀
C54.8	Malignant neoplasm of overlapping sites of corpus uteri ♀
C56.1	Malignant neoplasm of right ovary ♀ ☑
C56.2	Malignant neoplasm of left ovary ♀ ☑
C57.01	Malignant neoplasm of right fallopian tube ♀ ☑
C57.02	Malignant neoplasm of left fallopian tube ♀ ☑
C57.11	Malignant neoplasm of right broad ligament ♀ ☑
C57.12	Malignant neoplasm of left broad ligament ♀ ☑
C57.21	Malignant neoplasm of right round ligament ♀ ☑
C57.22	Malignant neoplasm of left round ligament ♀ ☑
C57.3	Malignant neoplasm of parametrium ♀
C58	Malignant neoplasm of placenta Ⓜ ♀
C66.1	Malignant neoplasm of right ureter ☑
C66.2	Malignant neoplasm of left ureter ☑
C67.0	Malignant neoplasm of trigone of bladder
C67.1	Malignant neoplasm of dome of bladder
C67.2	Malignant neoplasm of lateral wall of bladder
C67.3	Malignant neoplasm of anterior wall of bladder
C67.4	Malignant neoplasm of posterior wall of bladder
C67.5	Malignant neoplasm of bladder neck
C67.6	Malignant neoplasm of ureteric orifice
C67.8	Malignant neoplasm of overlapping sites of bladder
C68.0	Malignant neoplasm of urethra
C68.1	Malignant neoplasm of paraurethral glands
C68.8	Malignant neoplasm of overlapping sites of urinary organs
C76.3	Malignant neoplasm of pelvis
C7B.04	Secondary carcinoid tumors of peritoneum
C81.46	Lymphocyte-rich Hodgkin lymphoma, intrapelvic lymph nodes
C81.76	Other Hodgkin lymphoma, intrapelvic lymph nodes
C82.06	Follicular lymphoma grade I, intrapelvic lymph nodes
C82.16	Follicular lymphoma grade II, intrapelvic lymph nodes
C82.36	Follicular lymphoma grade IIIa, intrapelvic lymph nodes
C82.46	Follicular lymphoma grade IIIb, intrapelvic lymph nodes
C82.56	Diffuse follicle center lymphoma, intrapelvic lymph nodes
C82.66	Cutaneous follicle center lymphoma, intrapelvic lymph nodes
C82.86	Other types of follicular lymphoma, intrapelvic lymph nodes
C83.06	Small cell B-cell lymphoma, intrapelvic lymph nodes
C83.16	Mantle cell lymphoma, intrapelvic lymph nodes
C83.36	Diffuse large B-cell lymphoma, intrapelvic lymph nodes
C83.56	Lymphoblastic (diffuse) lymphoma, intrapelvic lymph nodes
C83.76	Burkitt lymphoma, intrapelvic lymph nodes
C83.86	Other non-follicular lymphoma, intrapelvic lymph nodes
C84.06	Mycosis fungoides, intrapelvic lymph nodes
C84.16	Sezary disease, intrapelvic lymph nodes
C84.46	Peripheral T-cell lymphoma, not classified, intrapelvic lymph nodes
C84.66	Anaplastic large cell lymphoma, ALK-positive, intrapelvic lymph nodes
C84.76	Anaplastic large cell lymphoma, ALK-negative, intrapelvic lymph nodes
C84.Z6	Other mature T/NK-cell lymphomas, intrapelvic lymph nodes
C85.26	Mediastinal (thymic) large B-cell lymphoma, intrapelvic lymph nodes
C85.86	Other specified types of non-Hodgkin lymphoma, intrapelvic lymph nodes
C85.89	Other specified types of non-Hodgkin lymphoma, extranodal and solid organ sites
D01.1	Carcinoma in situ of rectosigmoid junction
D01.2	Carcinoma in situ of rectum
D12.7	Benign neoplasm of rectosigmoid junction
D12.8	Benign neoplasm of rectum
D12.9	Benign neoplasm of anus and anal canal
D37.5	Neoplasm of uncertain behavior of rectum

Lymph Nodes

D3A.026	Benign carcinoid tumor of the rectum
D48.3	Neoplasm of uncertain behavior of retroperitoneum
D48.4	Neoplasm of uncertain behavior of peritoneum

AMA: 38562 2019,Feb,8; 2018,Jan,8; 2017,Jan,8; 2016,Jan,13; 2015,Jan,16; 2014,Jan,11

Relative Value Units/Medicare Edits

Non-Facility RVU	Work	PE	MP	Total
38562	11.06	7.39	1.96	20.41
Facility RVU	**Work**	**PE**	**MP**	**Total**
38562	11.06	7.39	1.96	20.41

	FUD	Status	MUE	Modifiers				IOM Reference
38562	90	A	1(2)	51	N/A	62*	80	None

* with documentation

Terms To Know

dissect. Cut apart or separate tissue for surgical purposes or for visual or microscopic study.

lymph nodes. Bean-shaped structures along the lymphatic vessels that intercept and destroy foreign materials in the tissue and bloodstream.

lymphadenectomy. Dissection of lymph nodes free from the vessels and removal for examination by frozen section in a separate procedure to detect early-stage metastases.

para-. Indicates near, similar, beside, or past.

staging. Determination of the course of a disease, as in the case of a malignancy, to determine whether the malignancy is confined to the primary tumor, has spread to one or more lymph nodes, or has metastasized.

38747

+ **38747** Abdominal lymphadenectomy, regional, including celiac, gastric, portal, peripancreatic, with or without para-aortic and vena caval nodes (List separately in addition to code for primary procedure)

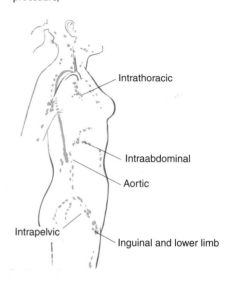

Intrathoracic
Intraabdominal
Aortic
Intrapelvic
Inguinal and lower limb

Explanation

The physician makes a midline abdominal incision. The abdominal contents are exposed, allowing the physician to locate the lymph nodes. Each lymph node grouping, with or without para-aortic and vena caval nodes, is dissected away from the surrounding tissue, nerves, and blood vessels, and removed. The incision is closed with sutures or staples.

Coding Tips

Report 38747 in addition to the code for the primary procedure. For extensive retroperitoneal transabdominal lymphadenectomy, see 38780.

ICD-10-CM Diagnostic Codes

This/these CPT code(s) are add-on code(s). See the primary procedure code that this code is performed with for your ICD-10-CM code selections.

AMA: 38747 2020,Apr,10; 2019,Feb,8; 2014,Jan,11

Relative Value Units/Medicare Edits

Non-Facility RVU	Work	PE	MP	Total
38747	4.88	1.78	1.12	7.78
Facility RVU	**Work**	**PE**	**MP**	**Total**
38747	4.88	1.78	1.12	7.78

	FUD	Status	MUE	Modifiers				IOM Reference
38747	N/A	A	1(2)	N/A	N/A	62*	80	None

* with documentation

Terms To Know

lymph nodes. Bean-shaped structures along the lymphatic vessels that intercept and destroy foreign materials in the tissue and bloodstream.

lymphadenectomy. Dissection of lymph nodes free from the vessels and removal for examination by frozen section in a separate procedure to detect early-stage metastases.

38760-38765

38760 Inguinofemoral lymphadenectomy, superficial, including Cloquet's node (separate procedure)

38765 Inguinofemoral lymphadenectomy, superficial, in continuity with pelvic lymphadenectomy, including external iliac, hypogastric, and obturator nodes (separate procedure)

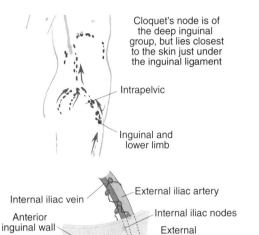

Cloquet's node is of the deep inguinal group, but lies closest to the skin just under the inguinal ligament

Intrapelvic

Inguinal and lower limb

Internal iliac vein

External iliac artery

Anterior inguinal wall

Internal iliac nodes

External iliac nodes

Femoral ligament

Deep inguinal nodes

Superficial inguinal nodes

Explanation

The physician makes an incision across the groin area. The surrounding tissue, nerves, and blood vessels are dissected away, and the inguinal and femoral lymph nodes are visualized. The nodes are removed by group. The wound is closed with sutures or staples. Report 38765 if performing pelvic lymphadenectomy concurrently.

Coding Tips

These separate procedures by definition are usually a component of a more complex service and are not identified separately. When performed alone or with other unrelated procedures/services they may be reported. Append modifier 59 or an X{EPSU} modifier. These are unilateral procedures. If performed bilaterally, some payers require that the service be reported twice with modifier 50 appended to the second code while others require identification of the service only once with modifier 50 appended. Check with individual payers. Modifier 50 identifies a procedure performed identically on the opposite side of the body (mirror image).

ICD-10-CM Diagnostic Codes

C19	Malignant neoplasm of rectosigmoid junction
C20	Malignant neoplasm of rectum
C46.3	Kaposi's sarcoma of lymph nodes
C4A.51	Merkel cell carcinoma of anal skin
C4A.59	Merkel cell carcinoma of other part of trunk
C4A.8	Merkel cell carcinoma of overlapping sites
C51.0	Malignant neoplasm of labium majus ♀
C51.1	Malignant neoplasm of labium minus ♀
C51.2	Malignant neoplasm of clitoris ♀
C51.8	Malignant neoplasm of overlapping sites of vulva ♀

C52	Malignant neoplasm of vagina ♀
C53.0	Malignant neoplasm of endocervix ♀
C53.1	Malignant neoplasm of exocervix ♀
C53.8	Malignant neoplasm of overlapping sites of cervix uteri ♀
C54.0	Malignant neoplasm of isthmus uteri ♀
C54.1	Malignant neoplasm of endometrium ♀
C54.2	Malignant neoplasm of myometrium ♀
C54.3	Malignant neoplasm of fundus uteri ♀
C54.8	Malignant neoplasm of overlapping sites of corpus uteri ♀
C56.1	Malignant neoplasm of right ovary ♀ ☑
C56.2	Malignant neoplasm of left ovary ♀ ☑
C57.01	Malignant neoplasm of right fallopian tube ♀ ☑
C57.02	Malignant neoplasm of left fallopian tube ♀ ☑
C57.11	Malignant neoplasm of right broad ligament ♀ ☑
C57.12	Malignant neoplasm of left broad ligament ♀ ☑
C57.21	Malignant neoplasm of right round ligament ♀ ☑
C57.22	Malignant neoplasm of left round ligament ♀ ☑
C57.3	Malignant neoplasm of parametrium ♀
C57.7	Malignant neoplasm of other specified female genital organs ♀
C57.8	Malignant neoplasm of overlapping sites of female genital organs ♀
C66.1	Malignant neoplasm of right ureter ☑
C66.2	Malignant neoplasm of left ureter ☑
C67.0	Malignant neoplasm of trigone of bladder
C67.1	Malignant neoplasm of dome of bladder
C67.2	Malignant neoplasm of lateral wall of bladder
C67.3	Malignant neoplasm of anterior wall of bladder
C67.4	Malignant neoplasm of posterior wall of bladder
C67.5	Malignant neoplasm of bladder neck
C67.6	Malignant neoplasm of ureteric orifice
C67.7	Malignant neoplasm of urachus
C67.8	Malignant neoplasm of overlapping sites of bladder
C68.0	Malignant neoplasm of urethra
C68.1	Malignant neoplasm of paraurethral glands
C77.4	Secondary and unspecified malignant neoplasm of inguinal and lower limb lymph nodes
C78.5	Secondary malignant neoplasm of large intestine and rectum
C7B.01	Secondary carcinoid tumors of distant lymph nodes
C7B.09	Secondary carcinoid tumors of other sites
C82.55	Diffuse follicle center lymphoma, lymph nodes of inguinal region and lower limb
C84.Z5	Other mature T/NK-cell lymphomas, lymph nodes of inguinal region and lower limb
C85.25	Mediastinal (thymic) large B-cell lymphoma, lymph nodes of inguinal region and lower limb
C85.85	Other specified types of non-Hodgkin lymphoma, lymph nodes of inguinal region and lower limb
D01.1	Carcinoma in situ of rectosigmoid junction
D01.2	Carcinoma in situ of rectum
D12.7	Benign neoplasm of rectosigmoid junction
D12.8	Benign neoplasm of rectum
D12.9	Benign neoplasm of anus and anal canal
D36.0	Benign neoplasm of lymph nodes
D37.5	Neoplasm of uncertain behavior of rectum

Lymph Nodes

D3A.026	Benign carcinoid tumor of the rectum
D49.89	Neoplasm of unspecified behavior of other specified sites
I88.8	Other nonspecific lymphadenitis
R59.0	Localized enlarged lymph nodes
R59.1	Generalized enlarged lymph nodes

AMA: **38760** 2019,Feb,8; 2018,Jan,8; 2017,Jan,8; 2016,Jan,13; 2015,Jan,16; 2014,Jan,11 **38765** 2019,Feb,8; 2018,Jan,8; 2017,Jan,8; 2016,Jan,13; 2015,Jan,16; 2014,Jan,11

Relative Value Units/Medicare Edits

Non-Facility RVU	Work	PE	MP	Total
38760	13.62	7.85	2.82	24.29
38765	21.91	11.38	4.43	37.72
Facility RVU	**Work**	**PE**	**MP**	**Total**
38760	13.62	7.85	2.82	24.29
38765	21.91	11.38	4.43	37.72

	FUD	Status	MUE	Modifiers				IOM Reference
38760	90	A	1(2)	51	50	62*	80	None
38765	90	A	1(2)	51	50	62*	80	

* with documentation

Terms To Know

Cloquet's node. Highest deep inguinofemoral lymph node.

dissect. Cut apart or separate tissue for surgical purposes or for visual or microscopic study.

incision. Act of cutting into tissue or an organ.

lymph nodes. Bean-shaped structures along the lymphatic vessels that intercept and destroy foreign materials in the tissue and bloodstream.

lymphadenectomy. Dissection of lymph nodes free from the vessels and removal for examination by frozen section in a separate procedure to detect early-stage metastases.

superficial. On the skin surface or near the surface of any involved structure or field of interest.

wound. Injury to living tissue often involving a cut or break in the skin.

38770

38770 Pelvic lymphadenectomy, including external iliac, hypogastric, and obturator nodes (separate procedure)

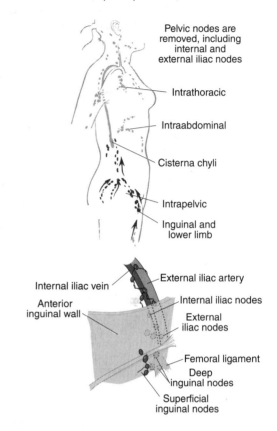

Pelvic nodes are removed, including internal and external iliac nodes

Intrathoracic

Intraabdominal

Cisterna chyli

Intrapelvic

Inguinal and lower limb

Internal iliac vein

External iliac artery

Anterior inguinal wall

Internal iliac nodes

External iliac nodes

Femoral ligament

Deep inguinal nodes

Superficial inguinal nodes

Explanation

The physician makes a low abdominal vertical incision. The surrounding tissue, nerves, and blood vessels are dissected away, and the pelvic lymph nodes are visualized. The nodes are removed by group. The wound is closed with sutures or staples.

Coding Tips

This separate procedure by definition is usually a component of a more complex service and is not identified separately. When performed alone or with other unrelated procedures/services it may be reported. If performed alone, list the code; if performed with other procedures/services, list the code and append modifier 59 or an X{EPSU} modifier. This is a unilateral procedure. If performed bilaterally, some payers require that the service be reported twice with modifier 50 appended to the second code while others require identification of the service only once with modifier 50 appended. Check with individual payers. Modifier 50 identifies a procedure performed identically on the opposite side of the body (mirror image). For limited pelvic and para-aortic lymphadenectomy staging procedure, see 38562.

ICD-10-CM Diagnostic Codes

C51.0	Malignant neoplasm of labium majus ♀
C51.1	Malignant neoplasm of labium minus ♀
C51.2	Malignant neoplasm of clitoris ♀
C51.8	Malignant neoplasm of overlapping sites of vulva ♀
C52	Malignant neoplasm of vagina ♀
C53.0	Malignant neoplasm of endocervix ♀

C53.1	Malignant neoplasm of exocervix ♀
C53.8	Malignant neoplasm of overlapping sites of cervix uteri ♀
C54.0	Malignant neoplasm of isthmus uteri ♀
C54.1	Malignant neoplasm of endometrium ♀
C54.2	Malignant neoplasm of myometrium ♀
C54.3	Malignant neoplasm of fundus uteri ♀
C54.8	Malignant neoplasm of overlapping sites of corpus uteri ♀
C56.1	Malignant neoplasm of right ovary ♀ ☑
C56.2	Malignant neoplasm of left ovary ♀ ☑
C57.01	Malignant neoplasm of right fallopian tube ♀ ☑
C57.02	Malignant neoplasm of left fallopian tube ♀ ☑
C57.11	Malignant neoplasm of right broad ligament ♀ ☑
C57.12	Malignant neoplasm of left broad ligament ♀ ☑
C57.21	Malignant neoplasm of right round ligament ♀ ☑
C57.22	Malignant neoplasm of left round ligament ♀ ☑
C57.3	Malignant neoplasm of parametrium ♀
C57.7	Malignant neoplasm of other specified female genital organs ♀
C57.8	Malignant neoplasm of overlapping sites of female genital organs ♀
C66.1	Malignant neoplasm of right ureter ☑
C66.2	Malignant neoplasm of left ureter ☑
C67.0	Malignant neoplasm of trigone of bladder
C67.1	Malignant neoplasm of dome of bladder
C67.2	Malignant neoplasm of lateral wall of bladder
C67.3	Malignant neoplasm of anterior wall of bladder
C67.4	Malignant neoplasm of posterior wall of bladder
C67.5	Malignant neoplasm of bladder neck
C67.6	Malignant neoplasm of ureteric orifice
C67.7	Malignant neoplasm of urachus
C67.8	Malignant neoplasm of overlapping sites of bladder
C68.0	Malignant neoplasm of urethra
C68.1	Malignant neoplasm of paraurethral glands
C77.5	Secondary and unspecified malignant neoplasm of intrapelvic lymph nodes
C79.89	Secondary malignant neoplasm of other specified sites
C7A.098	Malignant carcinoid tumors of other sites
C7B.01	Secondary carcinoid tumors of distant lymph nodes
C7B.09	Secondary carcinoid tumors of other sites
D48.7	Neoplasm of uncertain behavior of other specified sites

AMA: **38770** 2019,Feb,8; 2014,Jan,11

Relative Value Units/Medicare Edits

Non-Facility RVU	Work	PE	MP	Total
38770	14.06	7.21	1.95	23.22
Facility RVU	**Work**	**PE**	**MP**	**Total**
38770	14.06	7.21	1.95	23.22

	FUD	Status	MUE	Modifiers				IOM Reference
38770	90	A	1(2)	51	50	62*	80	None

* with documentation

38780

38780 Retroperitoneal transabdominal lymphadenectomy, extensive, including pelvic, aortic, and renal nodes (separate procedure)

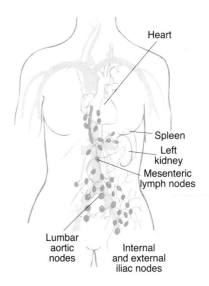

Extensive removal of lymph nodes of the retroperitoneal area is performed by a transabdominal approach

Explanation

The physician makes a large midline abdominal incision. The surrounding tissue, nerves, and blood vessels are dissected away, and the lymph nodes are visualized. The nodes are removed by group. Some surrounding tissues may also be removed. The wound is closed with sutures or staples.

Coding Tips

This separate procedure by definition is usually a component of a more complex service and is not identified separately. When performed alone or with other unrelated procedures or services it may be reported. If performed alone, list the code; if performed with other procedures/services, list the code and append modifier 59 or an X{EPSU} modifier. For pelvic lymphadenectomy, see 38770. For a limited pelvic and para-aortic lymphadenectomy staging procedure, see 38562. For excision and repair of lymphedematous skin and subcutaneous tissue, see 15004–15005 or 15570–15650.

ICD-10-CM Diagnostic Codes

C20	Malignant neoplasm of rectum
C45.1	Mesothelioma of peritoneum
C48.0	Malignant neoplasm of retroperitoneum
C48.1	Malignant neoplasm of specified parts of peritoneum
C48.8	Malignant neoplasm of overlapping sites of retroperitoneum and peritoneum
C4A.51	Merkel cell carcinoma of anal skin
C4A.52	Merkel cell carcinoma of skin of breast
C4A.59	Merkel cell carcinoma of other part of trunk
C4A.8	Merkel cell carcinoma of overlapping sites

Lymph Nodes

C53.0	Malignant neoplasm of endocervix ♀
C53.1	Malignant neoplasm of exocervix ♀
C53.8	Malignant neoplasm of overlapping sites of cervix uteri ♀
C54.0	Malignant neoplasm of isthmus uteri ♀
C54.1	Malignant neoplasm of endometrium ♀
C54.2	Malignant neoplasm of myometrium ♀
C54.3	Malignant neoplasm of fundus uteri ♀
C54.8	Malignant neoplasm of overlapping sites of corpus uteri ♀
C56.1	Malignant neoplasm of right ovary ♀ ☑
C56.2	Malignant neoplasm of left ovary ♀ ☑
C57.01	Malignant neoplasm of right fallopian tube ♀ ☑
C57.02	Malignant neoplasm of left fallopian tube ♀ ☑
C57.11	Malignant neoplasm of right broad ligament ♀ ☑
C57.12	Malignant neoplasm of left broad ligament ♀ ☑
C57.21	Malignant neoplasm of right round ligament ♀ ☑
C57.22	Malignant neoplasm of left round ligament ♀ ☑
C57.3	Malignant neoplasm of parametrium ♀
C65.1	Malignant neoplasm of right renal pelvis ☑
C65.2	Malignant neoplasm of left renal pelvis ☑
C66.1	Malignant neoplasm of right ureter ☑
C66.2	Malignant neoplasm of left ureter ☑
C67.0	Malignant neoplasm of trigone of bladder
C67.1	Malignant neoplasm of dome of bladder
C67.2	Malignant neoplasm of lateral wall of bladder
C67.3	Malignant neoplasm of anterior wall of bladder
C67.4	Malignant neoplasm of posterior wall of bladder
C67.5	Malignant neoplasm of bladder neck
C67.6	Malignant neoplasm of ureteric orifice
C67.8	Malignant neoplasm of overlapping sites of bladder
C68.0	Malignant neoplasm of urethra
C68.1	Malignant neoplasm of paraurethral glands
C68.8	Malignant neoplasm of overlapping sites of urinary organs
C77.2	Secondary and unspecified malignant neoplasm of intra-abdominal lymph nodes
C78.5	Secondary malignant neoplasm of large intestine and rectum
C78.6	Secondary malignant neoplasm of retroperitoneum and peritoneum
C7B.01	Secondary carcinoid tumors of distant lymph nodes
C7B.04	Secondary carcinoid tumors of peritoneum
C7B.09	Secondary carcinoid tumors of other sites
C7B.1	Secondary Merkel cell carcinoma
C7B.8	Other secondary neuroendocrine tumors
D48.3	Neoplasm of uncertain behavior of retroperitoneum
D48.4	Neoplasm of uncertain behavior of peritoneum

AMA: 38780 2019,Feb,8; 2014,Jan,11

Relative Value Units/Medicare Edits

Non-Facility RVU	Work	PE	MP	Total
38780	17.7	9.33	2.89	29.92
Facility RVU	**Work**	**PE**	**MP**	**Total**
38780	17.7	9.33	2.89	29.92

	FUD	Status	MUE	Modifiers				IOM Reference
38780	90	A	1(2)	51	N/A	62*	80	None

* with documentation

Terms To Know

approach. Method or anatomical location used to gain access to a body organ or specific area for procedures.

blood vessel. Tubular channel consisting of arteries, veins, and capillaries that transports blood throughout the body.

dissect. Cut apart or separate tissue for surgical purposes or for visual or microscopic study.

lymph nodes. Bean-shaped structures along the lymphatic vessels that intercept and destroy foreign materials in the tissue and bloodstream.

malignant neoplasm. Any cancerous tumor or lesion exhibiting uncontrolled tissue growth that can progressively invade other parts of the body with its disease-generating cells.

Merkel cell carcinoma. Rare form of skin cancer that typically presents on the face, head, or neck as a flesh-colored or bluish-red lesion. This neoplasm is fast growing and can metastasize quickly to other areas of the body. Risk factors include older patients with weakened immune systems and/or long-term exposure to the sun.

retroperitoneal. Located behind the peritoneum, the membrane that lines the abdominopelvic walls and forms a covering for the internal organs.

secondary. Second in order of occurrence or importance, or appearing during the course of another disease or condition.

transabdominal. Across or through the belly or abdomen.

wound. Injury to living tissue often involving a cut or break in the skin.

44180

44180 Laparoscopy, surgical, enterolysis (freeing of intestinal adhesion) (separate procedure)

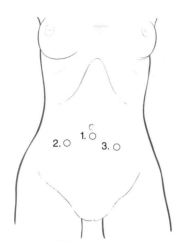

1. Laparoscope is inserted near the umbilicus
2. and 3. Ports for trocars and surgical instruments

Explanation

The physician performs laparoscopic enterolysis to free intestinal adhesions. With the patient under anesthesia, the physician places a trocar at the umbilicus into the abdominal or retroperitoneal space and insufflates the abdominal cavity. The physician places a laparoscope through the umbilical incision and additional trocars are placed into the abdomen. Intestinal adhesions are identified and instruments are passed through to dissect and remove the adhesions. The trocars are removed and the incisions are closed with sutures.

Coding Tips

This separate procedure by definition is usually a component of a more complex service and is not identified separately. When performed alone or with other unrelated procedures/services it may be reported. If performed alone, list the code; if performed with other procedures/services, list the code and append modifier 59 or an X{EPSU} modifier. Surgical laparoscopy always includes diagnostic laparoscopy. For diagnostic laparoscopy only, see 49320. To report laparoscopic salpingolysis, ovariolysis, see 58660.

ICD-10-CM Diagnostic Codes

C21.8	Malignant neoplasm of overlapping sites of rectum, anus and anal canal
D12.8	Benign neoplasm of rectum
D12.9	Benign neoplasm of anus and anal canal
K56.51	Intestinal adhesions [bands], with partial obstruction
K56.52	Intestinal adhesions [bands] with complete obstruction
K91.31	Postprocedural partial intestinal obstruction
K91.32	Postprocedural complete intestinal obstruction
N80.5	Endometriosis of intestine ♀
R10.0	Acute abdomen
R10.31	Right lower quadrant pain
R10.32	Left lower quadrant pain
R10.33	Periumbilical pain
R10.84	Generalized abdominal pain
R19.01	Right upper quadrant abdominal swelling, mass and lump
R19.02	Left upper quadrant abdominal swelling, mass and lump
R19.03	Right lower quadrant abdominal swelling, mass and lump
R19.04	Left lower quadrant abdominal swelling, mass and lump
R19.05	Periumbilic swelling, mass or lump
R19.06	Epigastric swelling, mass or lump
R19.07	Generalized intra-abdominal and pelvic swelling, mass and lump
R19.09	Other intra-abdominal and pelvic swelling, mass and lump

AMA: 44180 2018,Jan,8; 2018,Feb,11; 2017,Jan,8; 2016,Jan,13; 2015,Jan,16; 2014,Jan,11

Relative Value Units/Medicare Edits

Non-Facility RVU	Work	PE	MP	Total
44180	15.27	8.0	3.52	26.79
Facility RVU	**Work**	**PE**	**MP**	**Total**
44180	15.27	8.0	3.52	26.79

	FUD	Status	MUE	Modifiers				IOM Reference
44180	90	A	1(2)	51	N/A	62*	80	None

* with documentation

Terms To Know

adhesion. Abnormal fibrous connection between two structures, soft tissue or bony structures, that may occur as the result of surgery, infection, or trauma.

dissect. Cut apart or separate tissue for surgical purposes or for visual or microscopic study.

endometriosis. Aberrant uterine mucosal tissue appearing in areas of the pelvic cavity outside of its normal location, lining the uterus, and inflaming surrounding tissues often resulting in infertility or spontaneous abortion.

enterolysis. Division of intestinal adhesions.

insufflation. Blowing air or gas into a body cavity.

laparoscopy. Direct visualization of the peritoneal cavity, outer fallopian tubes, uterus, and ovaries utilizing a laparoscope, a thin, flexible fiberoptic tube.

retroperitoneal. Located behind the peritoneum, the membrane that lines the abdominopelvic walls and forms a covering for the internal organs.

trocar. Cannula or a sharp pointed instrument used to puncture and aspirate fluid from cavities.

Intestines

45560

45560   Repair of rectocele (separate procedure)

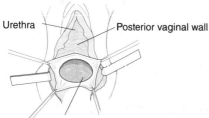

The posterior wall of the vagina is opened directly over the rectocele. The walls of both structures are repaired. A rectocele is a herniated protrusion of part of the rectum into the vagina

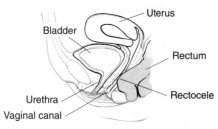

Rectum descends and protrudes through posterior wall of vagina

Explanation

The physician repairs a rectocele, a herniation of the rectum against the vaginal wall. The physician makes an incision in the mucosa of the posterior vaginal wall over the rectocele. The rectocele is dissected free of surrounding structures and the levator muscles are identified. The rectum is plicated to surrounding fascia with multiple sutures and the levator muscles are reapproximated. The vaginal mucosa is excised and the incision is closed.

Coding Tips

This separate procedure by definition is usually a component of a more complex service and is not identified separately. When performed alone or with other unrelated procedures or services it may be reported. If performed alone, list the code; if performed with other procedures/services, list the code and append modifier 59 or an X{EPSU} modifier. For posterior colporrhaphy with repair of a rectocele, with or without perineorrhaphy, see 57250. For combined anteroposterior colporrhaphy, see 57260; with enterocele repair, see 57265.

ICD-10-CM Diagnostic Codes

N81.2   Incomplete uterovaginal prolapse ♀
N81.3   Complete uterovaginal prolapse ♀
N81.6   Rectocele ♀
N99.3   Prolapse of vaginal vault after hysterectomy ♀

AMA: **45560** 2014,Jan,11

Relative Value Units/Medicare Edits

Non-Facility RVU	Work	PE	MP	Total
45560	11.5	6.82	1.7	20.02
Facility RVU	**Work**	**PE**	**MP**	**Total**
45560	11.5	6.82	1.7	20.02

	FUD	Status	MUE	Modifiers				IOM Reference
45560	90	A	1(2)	51	N/A	62*	80	None

* with documentation

Terms To Know

closure. Repairing an incision or wound by suture or other means.

dissection. Separating by cutting tissue or body structures apart.

excision. Surgical removal of an organ or tissue.

fascia. Fibrous sheet or band of tissue that envelops organs, muscles, and groupings of muscles.

idiopathic. Having no known cause.

incision. Act of cutting into tissue or an organ.

mucous membranes. Thin sheets of tissue that secrete mucous and absorb water, salt, and other solutes. Mucous membranes cover or line cavities or canals of the body that open to the outside, such as linings of the mouth, respiratory and genitourinary passages, and the digestive tube.

plication. Surgical technique involving folding, tucking, or pleating to reduce the size of a hollow structure or organ.

posterior. Located in the back part or caudal end of the body.

prolapse. Falling, sliding, or sinking of an organ from its normal location in the body.

rectocele. Rectal tissue herniation into the vaginal wall.

separate procedures. Services commonly carried out as a fundamental part of a total service and, as such, do not usually warrant separate identification. These services are identified in CPT with the parenthetical phrase (separate procedure) at the end of the description and are payable only when performed alone.

urethra. Small tube lined with mucous membrane that leads from the bladder to the exterior of the body.

uterovaginal prolapse. Uterus displaced downward and exposed in the external genitalia.

46900-46916

46900 Destruction of lesion(s), anus (eg, condyloma, papilloma, molluscum contagiosum, herpetic vesicle), simple; chemical
46910 electrodesiccation
46916 cryosurgery

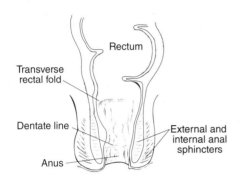

Explanation

The physician performs destruction of anal lesions with chemicals in 46900. The physician exposes the perianal skin and identifies the lesions. The lesions are painted with destructive chemicals. In 46910, the physician performs destruction of anal lesions with electrodesiccation. The physician exposes the perianal skin and identifies the lesions. The lesions are destroyed with cautery. In 46916, the physician performs destruction of anal lesions with cryosurgery. The physician exposes the perianal skin and identifies the lesions. The lesions are frozen and destroyed, usually with liquid nitrogen.

Coding Tips

Select the code based on the method of destruction (chemical, electrodesiccation, cryosurgery, laser, surgical excision) and the extent of the procedure (simple, extensive). For simple destruction of anal lesions by laser, see 46917; surgical excision, see 46922; extensive, by any method, see 46924. Destruction of internal hemorrhoids by thermal energy is reported with 46930.

ICD-10-CM Diagnostic Codes

A54.6	Gonococcal infection of anus and rectum
A56.3	Chlamydial infection of anus and rectum
A60.1	Herpesviral infection of perianal skin and rectum
A63.0	Anogenital (venereal) warts
A63.8	Other specified predominantly sexually transmitted diseases
A66.1	Multiple papillomata and wet crab yaws
B00.89	Other herpesviral infection
B07.8	Other viral warts
B08.1	Molluscum contagiosum
B08.8	Other specified viral infections characterized by skin and mucous membrane lesions
C21.1	Malignant neoplasm of anal canal
C21.2	Malignant neoplasm of cloacogenic zone
C21.8	Malignant neoplasm of overlapping sites of rectum, anus and anal canal
C44.520	Squamous cell carcinoma of anal skin
C44.590	Other specified malignant neoplasm of anal skin
C78.5	Secondary malignant neoplasm of large intestine and rectum
D01.3	Carcinoma in situ of anus and anal canal
D12.9	Benign neoplasm of anus and anal canal

K62.5	Hemorrhage of anus and rectum
K62.6	Ulcer of anus and rectum
K62.82	Dysplasia of anus
K62.89	Other specified diseases of anus and rectum
K92.1	Melena
S30.827A	Blister (nonthermal) of anus, initial encounter

AMA: 46900 2014,Jan,11 **46910** 2019,Dec,12; 2014,Jan,11 **46916** 2014,Jan,11

Relative Value Units/Medicare Edits

Non-Facility RVU	Work	PE	MP	Total
46900	1.91	4.59	0.27	6.77
46910	1.91	5.18	0.3	7.39
46916	1.91	4.91	0.18	7.0
Facility RVU	**Work**	**PE**	**MP**	**Total**
46900	1.91	1.74	0.27	3.92
46910	1.91	1.63	0.3	3.84
46916	1.91	1.97	0.18	4.06

	FUD	Status	MUE		Modifiers			IOM Reference
46900	10	A	1(2)	51	N/A	N/A	N/A	None
46910	10	A	1(2)	51	N/A	N/A	N/A	
46916	10	A	1(2)	51	N/A	N/A	N/A	

* with documentation

Terms To Know

cautery. Destruction or burning of tissue by means of a hot instrument, an electric current, or a caustic chemical, such as silver nitrate.

condyloma. Infectious tumor-like growth caused by the human papilloma virus, with a branching connective tissue core and epithelial covering that occurs on the skin and mucous membranes of the perianal region and external genitalia.

destruction. Ablation or eradication of a structure or tissue.

herpes. Inflammatory diseases of the skin caused by the herpes virus.

lesion. Area of damaged tissue that has lost continuity or function, due to disease or trauma.

molluscum contagiosum. Common, benign, viral skin infection, usually self-limiting, that appears as a gray or flesh-colored umbilicated lesion by itself or in groups, and later becomes white with an expulsable core containing the replication bodies. It is often transmitted sexually in adults, by autoinoculation, or close contact in children.

papilloma. Benign skin neoplasm with small branchings from the epithelial surface.

peri-. About, around, or in the vicinity.

46917-46922

46917 Destruction of lesion(s), anus (eg, condyloma, papilloma, molluscum contagiosum, herpetic vesicle), simple; laser surgery

46922 surgical excision

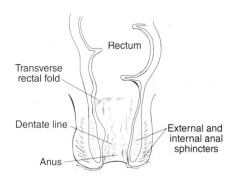

Explanation

The physician performs destruction of anal lesions with laser therapy in 46917. The physician exposes the perianal skin and identifies the lesions. The lesions are destroyed by laser ablation or laser excision. In 46922, the physician performs destruction of anal lesions by excision. The physician exposes the perianal skin and identifies the lesions. The lesions are surgically excised. The incisions are closed.

Coding Tips

Select the code based on the method of destruction (chemical, electrodesiccation, cryosurgery, laser, or surgical excision). For simple destruction, chemical, see 46900; electrodesiccation, see 46910; cryosurgery, see 46916; extensive, by any method, see 46924. Destruction of internal hemorrhoids by thermal energy is reported with 46930.

ICD-10-CM Diagnostic Codes

A54.6	Gonococcal infection of anus and rectum
A56.3	Chlamydial infection of anus and rectum
A60.1	Herpesviral infection of perianal skin and rectum
A63.0	Anogenital (venereal) warts
A63.8	Other specified predominantly sexually transmitted diseases
A66.1	Multiple papillomata and wet crab yaws
B00.89	Other herpesviral infection
B07.8	Other viral warts
B08.1	Molluscum contagiosum
B08.8	Other specified viral infections characterized by skin and mucous membrane lesions
C21.1	Malignant neoplasm of anal canal
C21.2	Malignant neoplasm of cloacogenic zone
C21.8	Malignant neoplasm of overlapping sites of rectum, anus and anal canal
C44.520	Squamous cell carcinoma of anal skin
C44.590	Other specified malignant neoplasm of anal skin
C78.5	Secondary malignant neoplasm of large intestine and rectum
D01.3	Carcinoma in situ of anus and anal canal
D12.9	Benign neoplasm of anus and anal canal
K62.5	Hemorrhage of anus and rectum
K62.82	Dysplasia of anus
K62.89	Other specified diseases of anus and rectum

AMA: **46917** 2014,Jan,11 **46922** 2014,Jan,11

Relative Value Units/Medicare Edits

Non-Facility RVU	Work	PE	MP	Total
46917	1.91	9.77	0.3	11.98
46922	1.91	6.13	0.35	8.39
Facility RVU	**Work**	**PE**	**MP**	**Total**
46917	1.91	1.47	0.3	3.68
46922	1.91	1.67	0.35	3.93

	FUD	Status	MUE	Modifiers				IOM Reference
46917	10	A	1(2)	51	N/A	N/A	N/A	100-03,140.5
46922	10	A	1(2)	51	N/A	N/A	N/A	

* with documentation

Terms To Know

ablation. Removal or destruction of tissue by cutting, electrical energy, chemical substances, or excessive heat application.

condyloma. Infectious tumor-like growth caused by the human papilloma virus, with a branching connective tissue core and epithelial covering that occurs on the skin and mucous membranes of the perianal region and external genitalia.

destruction. Ablation or eradication of a structure or tissue.

excision. Surgical removal of an organ or tissue.

herpes. Inflammatory diseases of the skin caused by the herpes virus.

laser surgery. Use of concentrated, sharply defined light beams to cut, cauterize, coagulate, seal, or vaporize tissue.

lesion. Area of damaged tissue that has lost continuity or function, due to disease or trauma. Lesions may be located on internal structures such as the brain, nerves, or kidneys, or visible on the skin.

molluscum contagiosum. Common, benign, viral skin infection, usually self-limiting, that appears as a gray or flesh-colored umbilicated lesion by itself or in groups, and later becomes white with an expulsable core containing the replication bodies. It is often transmitted sexually in adults, by autoinoculation, or close contact in children.

papilloma. Benign skin neoplasm with small branchings from the epithelial surface.

N Newborn: 0 **P** Pediatric: 0-17 **M** Maternity: 9-64 **A** Adult: 15-124 ♂ Male Only ♀ Female Only

49000

49000 Exploratory laparotomy, exploratory celiotomy with or without biopsy(s) (separate procedure)

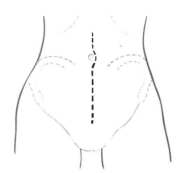

Typical incision for laparotomy

An access incision is made into the abdominal cavity for exploratory purposes.

Explanation

To explore the intra-abdominal organs and structures, the physician makes a large incision extending from just above the pubic hairline to the rib cage. The abdominal cavity is opened for a systematic examination of all organs. The physician may take tissue samples of any or all intra-abdominal organs for diagnosis. The incision is closed with sutures.

Coding Tips

This separate procedure by definition is usually a component of a more complex service and is not identified separately. When performed alone or with other unrelated procedures or services it may be reported. If performed alone, list the code; if performed with other procedures/services, list the code and append modifier 59 or an X{EPSU} modifier. When 49000 is performed with another separately identifiable procedure, the highest dollar value code is listed as the primary procedure and subsequent procedures are appended with modifier 51. For diagnostic laparoscopy, see 49320. For exploration of a wound resulting from penetrating trauma without laparotomy, see 20102.

ICD-10-CM Diagnostic Codes

The application of this code is too broad to adequately present ICD-10-CM diagnostic code links here. Refer to your ICD-10-CM book.

AMA: 49000 2020,Jan,6; 2019,Dec,5; 2018,Jan,8; 2017,Jan,8; 2017,Dec,3; 2016,Jan,13; 2015,Jan,16; 2014,Jan,11

Relative Value Units/Medicare Edits

Non-Facility RVU	Work	PE	MP	Total
49000	12.54	7.01	2.83	22.38
Facility RVU	Work	PE	MP	Total
49000	12.54	7.01	2.83	22.38

	FUD	Status	MUE	Modifiers				IOM Reference
49000	90	A	1(2)	51	N/A	62*	80	None

* with documentation

Terms To Know

biopsy. Tissue or fluid removed for diagnostic purposes through analysis of the cells in the biopsy material.

exploration. Examination for diagnostic purposes.

49002

49002 Reopening of recent laparotomy

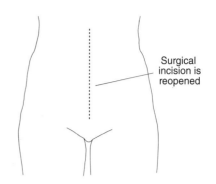

Surgical incision is reopened

Explanation

The physician reopens the incision of a recent laparotomy before the incision has fully healed to control bleeding, remove packing, or drain a postoperative infection.

Coding Tips

Diagnosis codes should support the reason for reopening the laparotomy. For exploratory laparotomy, exploratory celiotomy, with or without biopsies, see 49000. For re-exploration of a pelvic wound to remove preperitoneal pelvic packing, see 49014.

ICD-10-CM Diagnostic Codes

N73.6	Female pelvic peritoneal adhesions (postinfective) ♀
O86.01	Infection of obstetric surgical wound, superficial incisional site 🄼 ♀
O86.02	Infection of obstetric surgical wound, deep incisional site 🄼 ♀
O86.03	Infection of obstetric surgical wound, organ and space site 🄼 ♀
O86.04	Sepsis following an obstetrical procedure 🄼 ♀
O86.09	Infection of obstetric surgical wound, other surgical site 🄼 ♀
O90.2	Hematoma of obstetric wound 🄼 ♀
R10.0	Acute abdomen
R10.11	Right upper quadrant pain
R10.12	Left upper quadrant pain
R10.2	Pelvic and perineal pain
R10.31	Right lower quadrant pain
R10.32	Left lower quadrant pain
R10.33	Periumbilical pain
R10.84	Generalized abdominal pain
R19.01	Right upper quadrant abdominal swelling, mass and lump
R19.02	Left upper quadrant abdominal swelling, mass and lump
R19.03	Right lower quadrant abdominal swelling, mass and lump
R19.04	Left lower quadrant abdominal swelling, mass and lump
R19.05	Periumbilic swelling, mass or lump
R19.07	Generalized intra-abdominal and pelvic swelling, mass and lump
R19.09	Other intra-abdominal and pelvic swelling, mass and lump
T81.510A	Adhesions due to foreign body accidentally left in body following surgical operation, initial encounter
T81.514A	Adhesions due to foreign body accidentally left in body following endoscopic examination, initial encounter
T81.516A	Adhesions due to foreign body accidentally left in body following aspiration, puncture or other catheterization, initial encounter

T81.517A	Adhesions due to foreign body accidentally left in body following removal of catheter or packing, initial encounter
T81.518A	Adhesions due to foreign body accidentally left in body following other procedure, initial encounter
T81.520A	Obstruction due to foreign body accidentally left in body following surgical operation, initial encounter
T81.527A	Obstruction due to foreign body accidentally left in body following removal of catheter or packing, initial encounter
T81.528A	Obstruction due to foreign body accidentally left in body following other procedure, initial encounter
T81.530A	Perforation due to foreign body accidentally left in body following surgical operation, initial encounter
T81.534A	Perforation due to foreign body accidentally left in body following endoscopic examination, initial encounter
T81.536A	Perforation due to foreign body accidentally left in body following aspiration, puncture or other catheterization, initial encounter
T81.537A	Perforation due to foreign body accidentally left in body following removal of catheter or packing, initial encounter
T81.538A	Perforation due to foreign body accidentally left in body following other procedure, initial encounter
T81.590A	Other complications of foreign body accidentally left in body following surgical operation, initial encounter
T81.593A	Other complications of foreign body accidentally left in body following injection or immunization, initial encounter
T81.596A	Other complications of foreign body accidentally left in body following aspiration, puncture or other catheterization, initial encounter
T81.597A	Other complications of foreign body accidentally left in body following removal of catheter or packing, initial encounter
T81.598A	Other complications of foreign body accidentally left in body following other procedure, initial encounter

AMA: **49002** 2020,Jan,6; 2018,Jan,8; 2017,Jan,8; 2016,Jan,13; 2015,Jan,16; 2014,Jan,11

Relative Value Units/Medicare Edits

Non-Facility RVU	Work	PE	MP	Total
49002	17.63	8.81	4.0	30.44
Facility RVU	**Work**	**PE**	**MP**	**Total**
49002	17.63	8.81	4.0	30.44

	FUD	Status	MUE	Modifiers				IOM Reference
49002	90	A	1(3)	51	N/A	62*	80	None

* with documentation

49020

49020	Drainage of peritoneal abscess or localized peritonitis, exclusive of appendiceal abscess, open

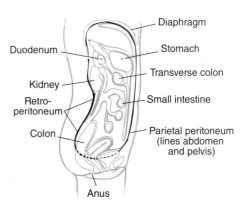

Explanation

The physician makes an open abdominal or flank incision (laparotomy) to gain access to the peritoneal cavity. The peritoneum is explored and the abscess or isolated area of peritoneal inflammation is identified. The abscess is incised and drained and inflamed peritoneal tissue may be excised. The abscess and surrounding peritoneal cavity may be irrigated. A drain may be placed whereby a separate abdominal incision is made and the drain is drawn through it and sutured in place. The physician may completely reapproximate the abdominal incision or leave a portion of the incision open to allow for further drainage. Specimens taken during the procedure are typically sent to microbiology for identification and to determine antibiotic suitability. If a drain is placed, it is removed at a later date.

Coding Tips

For image guided, percutaneous drainage, via catheter, of peritoneal abscess or localized peritonitis, see 49406; transrectal or transvaginal image-guided peritoneal or retroperitoneal fluid collection drainage, via catheter, see 49407.

ICD-10-CM Diagnostic Codes

K65.1	Peritoneal abscess
K65.2	Spontaneous bacterial peritonitis
K65.3	Choleperitonitis
K65.4	Sclerosing mesenteritis
K65.8	Other peritonitis
K66.1	Hemoperitoneum
K66.8	Other specified disorders of peritoneum
K68.11	Postprocedural retroperitoneal abscess
K68.12	Psoas muscle abscess
K68.19	Other retroperitoneal abscess
K68.9	Other disorders of retroperitoneum

AMA: **49020** 2014,Jan,11

Coding Companion for Ob/Gyn

Relative Value Units/Medicare Edits

Non-Facility RVU	Work	PE	MP	Total
49020	26.67	13.74	5.95	46.36
Facility RVU	Work	PE	MP	Total
49020	26.67	13.74	5.95	46.36

	FUD	Status	MUE	Modifiers				IOM Reference
49020	90	A	2(3)	51	N/A	N/A	80	None

* with documentation

Terms To Know

abscess. Circumscribed collection of pus resulting from bacteria, frequently associated with swelling and other signs of inflammation.

approach. Method or anatomical location used to gain access to a body organ or specific area for procedures.

drainage. Releasing, taking, or letting out fluids and/or gases from a body part.

exploration. Examination for diagnostic purposes.

flank. Part of the body found between the posterior ribs and the uppermost crest of the ilium, or the lateral side of the hip, thigh, and buttock.

inflammation. Cytologic and chemical reactions that occur in affected blood vessels and adjacent tissues in response to injury or abnormal stimulation from a physical, chemical, or biologic agent.

irrigation. To wash out or cleanse a body cavity, wound, or tissue with water or other fluid.

laparotomy. Incision through the flank or abdomen for therapeutic or diagnostic purposes.

peritoneal cavity. Space between the lining of the abdominal wall, or parietal peritoneum, and the surface layer of the abdominal organs, or visceral peritoneum. It contains a thin, watery fluid that keeps the peritoneal surfaces moist.

peritoneum. Strong, continuous membrane that forms the lining of the abdominal and pelvic cavity. The parietal peritoneum, or outer layer, is attached to the abdominopelvic walls and the visceral peritoneum, or inner layer, surrounds the organs inside the abdominal cavity.

peritonitis. Inflammation and infection within the peritoneal cavity, the space between the membrane lining the abdominopelvic walls and covering the internal organs.

specimen. Tissue cells or sample of fluid taken for analysis, pathologic examination, and diagnosis.

49082-49083

49082 Abdominal paracentesis (diagnostic or therapeutic); without imaging guidance
49083 with imaging guidance

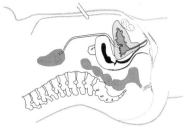

The peritoneum is accessed by a nick incision and a catheter is introduced into the cavity

Explanation

The physician inserts a needle or catheter into the abdominal cavity and withdraws and drains fluid for diagnostic or therapeutic purposes. The needle or catheter is removed at the completion of the procedure. Report 49082 if imaging guidance is not used and 49083 if imaging guidance is used.

Coding Tips

Code 49083 includes imaging guidance. Do not report 76942, 77002, 77012, or 77021 with 49083. For peritoneal lavage, see 49084. For image guided, percutaneous drainage, via catheter, of peritoneal abscess or localized peritonitis, see 49406.

ICD-10-CM Diagnostic Codes

C78.6	Secondary malignant neoplasm of retroperitoneum and peritoneum
E87.2	Acidosis
E87.79	Other fluid overload
E87.8	Other disorders of electrolyte and fluid balance, not elsewhere classified
I89.8	Other specified noninfective disorders of lymphatic vessels and lymph nodes
K56.51	Intestinal adhesions [bands], with partial obstruction
K56.52	Intestinal adhesions [bands] with complete obstruction
K56.690	Other partial intestinal obstruction
K56.691	Other complete intestinal obstruction
K65.0	Generalized (acute) peritonitis
K65.1	Peritoneal abscess
K65.2	Spontaneous bacterial peritonitis
K65.8	Other peritonitis
K66.1	Hemoperitoneum
K66.8	Other specified disorders of peritoneum
K91.31	Postprocedural partial intestinal obstruction
K91.32	Postprocedural complete intestinal obstruction
S36.81XA	Injury of peritoneum, initial encounter
S36.892A	Contusion of other intra-abdominal organs, initial encounter
S36.893A	Laceration of other intra-abdominal organs, initial encounter
S36.898A	Other injury of other intra-abdominal organs, initial encounter

AMA: **49082** 2018,Jan,8; 2017,Jan,8; 2016,Jan,13; 2015,Jan,16; 2014,Jan,11
49083 2018,Jan,8; 2017,Jan,8; 2016,Jan,13; 2015,Jan,16; 2014,Mar,13; 2014,Jan,11

Relative Value Units/Medicare Edits

Non-Facility RVU	Work	PE	MP	Total
49082	1.24	4.4	0.18	5.82
49083	2.0	6.38	0.18	8.56
Facility RVU	**Work**	**PE**	**MP**	**Total**
49082	1.24	0.72	0.18	2.14
49083	2.0	0.93	0.18	3.11

	FUD	Status	MUE	Modifiers				IOM Reference
49082	0	A	1(3)	51	N/A	N/A	N/A	None
49083	0	A	2(3)	51	N/A	N/A	N/A	

* with documentation

Terms To Know

catheter. Flexible tube inserted into an area of the body for introducing or withdrawing fluid.

diagnostic. Examination or procedure to which the patient is subjected, or which is performed on materials derived from a hospital outpatient, to obtain information to aid in the assessment of a medical condition or the identification of a disease. Among these examinations and tests are diagnostic laboratory services such as hematology and chemistry, diagnostic x-rays, isotope studies, EKGs, pulmonary function studies, thyroid function tests, psychological tests, and other tests given to determine the nature and severity of an ailment or injury.

drainage. Releasing, taking, or letting out fluids and/or gases from a body part.

imaging. Radiologic means of producing pictures for clinical study of the internal structures and functions of the body, such as x-ray, ultrasound, magnetic resonance, or positron emission tomography.

paracentesis. Surgical puncture of a body cavity with a specialized needle or hollow tubing to aspirate fluid for diagnostic or therapeutic reasons.

peritoneum. Strong, continuous membrane that forms the lining of the abdominal and pelvic cavity. The parietal peritoneum, or outer layer, is attached to the abdominopelvic walls and the visceral peritoneum, or inner layer, surrounds the organs inside the abdominal cavity.

therapeutic. Act meant to alleviate a medical or mental condition.

49084

49084   Peritoneal lavage, including imaging guidance, when performed

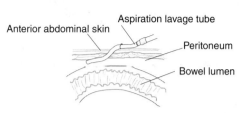

The peritoneum is accessed by a nick incision and a catheter is introduced into the cavity

Explanation

Peritoneal lavage is usually performed to determine the presence and/or extent of internal bleeding within the peritoneum. The physician makes a small incision to insert a catheter into the abdominal cavity. Fluids are infused into the cavity and subsequently aspirated for diagnostic testing. The catheter is removed at the completion of the procedure and the incision is closed.

Coding Tips

Do not report 49084 with 76942, 77002, 77012, or 77021. To report percutaneous, image-guided drainage of a retroperitoneal abscess, via catheter, see 49406.

ICD-10-CM Diagnostic Codes

C78.6	Secondary malignant neoplasm of retroperitoneum and peritoneum
E87.2	Acidosis
E87.79	Other fluid overload
E87.8	Other disorders of electrolyte and fluid balance, not elsewhere classified
I89.8	Other specified noninfective disorders of lymphatic vessels and lymph nodes
K56.51	Intestinal adhesions [bands], with partial obstruction
K56.52	Intestinal adhesions [bands] with complete obstruction
K56.690	Other partial intestinal obstruction
K56.691	Other complete intestinal obstruction
K65.0	Generalized (acute) peritonitis
K65.1	Peritoneal abscess
K65.2	Spontaneous bacterial peritonitis
K65.8	Other peritonitis
K66.1	Hemoperitoneum
K66.8	Other specified disorders of peritoneum
K91.31	Postprocedural partial intestinal obstruction
K91.32	Postprocedural complete intestinal obstruction
S36.81XA	Injury of peritoneum, initial encounter
S36.892A	Contusion of other intra-abdominal organs, initial encounter
S36.893A	Laceration of other intra-abdominal organs, initial encounter
S36.898A	Other injury of other intra-abdominal organs, initial encounter

AMA: **49084** 2018,Jan,8; 2017,Jan,8; 2016,Jan,13; 2015,Jan,16; 2014,Jan,11

Relative Value Units/Medicare Edits

Non-Facility RVU	Work	PE	MP	Total
49084	2.0	0.73	0.43	3.16
Facility RVU	**Work**	**PE**	**MP**	**Total**
49084	2.0	0.73	0.43	3.16

	FUD	Status	MUE	Modifiers				IOM Reference
49084	0	A	1(3)	51	N/A	N/A	N/A	None

* with documentation

Terms To Know

aspirate. To withdraw fluid or air from a body cavity by suction.

catheter. Flexible tube inserted into an area of the body for introducing or withdrawing fluid.

diagnostic. Examination or procedure to which the patient is subjected, or which is performed on materials derived from a hospital outpatient, to obtain information to aid in the assessment of a medical condition or the identification of a disease. Among these examinations and tests are diagnostic laboratory services such as hematology and chemistry, diagnostic x-rays, isotope studies, EKGs, pulmonary function studies, thyroid function tests, psychological tests, and other tests given to determine the nature and severity of an ailment or injury.

imaging. Radiologic means of producing pictures for clinical study of the internal structures and functions of the body, such as x-ray, ultrasound, magnetic resonance, or positron emission tomography.

lavage. Washing.

peritoneal. Space between the lining of the abdominal wall, or parietal peritoneum, and the surface layer of the abdominal organs, or visceral peritoneum. It contains a thin, watery fluid that keeps the peritoneal surfaces moist.

peritoneum. Strong, continuous membrane that forms the lining of the abdominal and pelvic cavity. The parietal peritoneum, or outer layer, is attached to the abdominopelvic walls and the visceral peritoneum, or inner layer, surrounds the organs inside the abdominal cavity.

49180

49180 Biopsy, abdominal or retroperitoneal mass, percutaneous needle

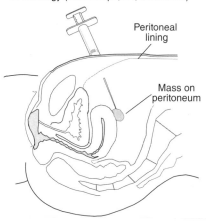

Biopsy needle guided to mass with aid of radiology (fluoroscope, CT, ultrasound)

Peritoneal lining

Mass on peritoneum

Explanation

Using radiological supervision, the physician locates the mass within or immediately outside the peritoneal lining of the abdominal cavity. A biopsy needle is passed into the mass, a tissue sample is removed, and the needle is withdrawn. This may be repeated several times. No incision is necessary.

Coding Tips

If multiple areas are biopsied, report 49180 for each site taken and append modifier 51 to additional codes. Report radiology services separately. For radiological supervision and interpretation, see 77002, 77012, 77021, and 76942; code choice is dependent on the type of radiological guidance used. Report final needle aspiration (FNA) with 10004–10012 or 10021. For evaluation of fine needle aspirate, see 88172–88173. Local anesthesia is included in this service. However, general anesthesia may be administered depending on the age or condition of the patient.

ICD-10-CM Diagnostic Codes

C48.0	Malignant neoplasm of retroperitoneum
C76.2	Malignant neoplasm of abdomen
C77.2	Secondary and unspecified malignant neoplasm of intra-abdominal lymph nodes
C78.6	Secondary malignant neoplasm of retroperitoneum and peritoneum
D20.0	Benign neoplasm of soft tissue of retroperitoneum
D48.3	Neoplasm of uncertain behavior of retroperitoneum
D48.4	Neoplasm of uncertain behavior of peritoneum
D48.7	Neoplasm of uncertain behavior of other specified sites
D49.0	Neoplasm of unspecified behavior of digestive system
D49.89	Neoplasm of unspecified behavior of other specified sites
R10.817	Generalized abdominal tenderness
R10.827	Generalized rebound abdominal tenderness
R10.84	Generalized abdominal pain
R19.01	Right upper quadrant abdominal swelling, mass and lump
R19.02	Left upper quadrant abdominal swelling, mass and lump
R19.03	Right lower quadrant abdominal swelling, mass and lump
R19.04	Left lower quadrant abdominal swelling, mass and lump

R19.05	Periumbilic swelling, mass or lump
R19.06	Epigastric swelling, mass or lump
R19.07	Generalized intra-abdominal and pelvic swelling, mass and lump
R19.09	Other intra-abdominal and pelvic swelling, mass and lump
R19.8	Other specified symptoms and signs involving the digestive system and abdomen
R59.0	Localized enlarged lymph nodes
R59.1	Generalized enlarged lymph nodes

AMA: **49180** 2019,Feb,8; 2019,Apr,4; 2018,Jan,8; 2017,Jan,8; 2016,Jan,13; 2015,Jan,16; 2014,Jan,11

Relative Value Units/Medicare Edits

Non-Facility RVU	Work	PE	MP	Total
49180	1.73	3.0	0.13	4.86
Facility RVU	**Work**	**PE**	**MP**	**Total**
49180	1.73	0.57	0.13	2.43

	FUD	Status	MUE	Modifiers				IOM Reference
49180	0	A	2(3)	51	N/A	N/A	N/A	None

* with documentation

Terms To Know

biopsy. Tissue or fluid removed for diagnostic purposes through analysis of the cells in the biopsy material.

percutaneous approach. Method used to gain access to a body organ or specific area by puncture or minor incision through the skin or mucous membrane and/or any other body layers necessary to reach the procedure site.

peritoneum. Strong, continuous membrane that forms the lining of the abdominal and pelvic cavity. The parietal peritoneum, or outer layer, is attached to the abdominopelvic walls and the visceral peritoneum, or inner layer, surrounds the organs inside the abdominal cavity.

retroperitoneal. Located behind the peritoneum, the membrane that lines the abdominopelvic walls and forms a covering for the internal organs.

specimen. Tissue cells or sample of fluid taken for analysis, pathologic examination, and diagnosis.

supervision and interpretation. Radiology services that usually contain an invasive component and are reported by the radiologist for supervision of the procedure and the personnel involved with performing the examination, reading the film, and preparing the written report.

tissue. Group of similar cells with a similar function that form definite structures and organs. Tissue types include epithelial tissue, muscle tissue, connective tissue, and nervous tissue.

49203-49205

49203	Excision or destruction, open, intra-abdominal tumors, cysts or endometriomas, 1 or more peritoneal, mesenteric, or retroperitoneal primary or secondary tumors; largest tumor 5 cm diameter or less
49204	largest tumor 5.1-10.0 cm diameter
49205	largest tumor greater than 10.0 cm diameter

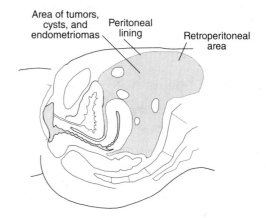

Area of tumors, cysts, and endometriomas / Peritoneal lining / Retroperitoneal area

Explanation

The physician removes or destroys intraabdominal tumors, cysts, or endometriomas (displaced endometrial tissue) or primary or secondary mesenteric, peritoneal, or retroperitoneal tumors. The physician makes a large incision extending from just above the pubic hairline to the rib cage. The growths are removed using a laser, electric cautery, or a scalpel. The incision is closed with sutures. Report 49203 when the diameter of the largest tumor is 5 cm or smaller, 49204 when the diameter is 5.1 to 10 cm, and 49205 when the diameter is larger than 10 cm.

Coding Tips

For laparoscopic fulguration (destruction) or excision of lesions of the ovary, pelvic viscera, or peritoneal surface, any method, see 58662. For resection of recurrent ovarian, tubal, primary peritoneal, or uterine malignancy, see 58957–58958. Do not report these codes with 38770, 38780, 49000, 49010, 49215, 50010, 50205, 50225, 50236, 50250, 50290, or 58920-58960.

ICD-10-CM Diagnostic Codes

C48.0	Malignant neoplasm of retroperitoneum
C48.1	Malignant neoplasm of specified parts of peritoneum
C48.8	Malignant neoplasm of overlapping sites of retroperitoneum and peritoneum
C49.4	Malignant neoplasm of connective and soft tissue of abdomen
C49.5	Malignant neoplasm of connective and soft tissue of pelvis
C54.0	Malignant neoplasm of isthmus uteri ♀
C54.1	Malignant neoplasm of endometrium ♀
C54.2	Malignant neoplasm of myometrium ♀
C54.3	Malignant neoplasm of fundus uteri ♀
C54.8	Malignant neoplasm of overlapping sites of corpus uteri ♀
C56.1	Malignant neoplasm of right ovary ♀ ☑
C56.2	Malignant neoplasm of left ovary ♀ ☑
C57.01	Malignant neoplasm of right fallopian tube ♀ ☑
C57.02	Malignant neoplasm of left fallopian tube ♀ ☑
C57.11	Malignant neoplasm of right broad ligament ♀ ☑
C57.12	Malignant neoplasm of left broad ligament ♀ ☑

C57.21	Malignant neoplasm of right round ligament ♀ ☑
C57.22	Malignant neoplasm of left round ligament ♀ ☑
C57.3	Malignant neoplasm of parametrium ♀
C57.7	Malignant neoplasm of other specified female genital organs ♀
C57.8	Malignant neoplasm of overlapping sites of female genital organs ♀
C76.2	Malignant neoplasm of abdomen
C78.6	Secondary malignant neoplasm of retroperitoneum and peritoneum
C7B.04	Secondary carcinoid tumors of peritoneum
D19.1	Benign neoplasm of mesothelial tissue of peritoneum
D20.0	Benign neoplasm of soft tissue of retroperitoneum
D20.1	Benign neoplasm of soft tissue of peritoneum
D25.0	Submucous leiomyoma of uterus ♀
D25.1	Intramural leiomyoma of uterus ♀
D25.2	Subserosal leiomyoma of uterus ♀
D30.8	Benign neoplasm of other specified urinary organs
D37.5	Neoplasm of uncertain behavior of rectum
D48.3	Neoplasm of uncertain behavior of retroperitoneum
D48.4	Neoplasm of uncertain behavior of peritoneum
K66.8	Other specified disorders of peritoneum
K68.9	Other disorders of retroperitoneum
N73.6	Female pelvic peritoneal adhesions (postinfective) ♀
N80.0	Endometriosis of uterus ♀
N80.1	Endometriosis of ovary ♀
N80.2	Endometriosis of fallopian tube ♀
N80.3	Endometriosis of pelvic peritoneum ♀
N80.8	Other endometriosis ♀
N83.01	Follicular cyst of right ovary ♀ ☑
N83.02	Follicular cyst of left ovary ♀ ☑
N83.291	Other ovarian cyst, right side ♀ ☑
N83.292	Other ovarian cyst, left side ♀ ☑

AMA: 49203 2018,Jan,8; 2017,Jan,8; 2016,Jan,13; 2015,Jan,16; 2014,Jan,11
49204 2018,Jan,8; 2017,Jan,8; 2016,Jan,13; 2015,Jan,16; 2014,Jan,11 **49205**
2018,Jan,8; 2017,Jan,8; 2016,Jan,13; 2015,Jan,16; 2014,Jan,11

Relative Value Units/Medicare Edits

Non-Facility RVU	Work	PE	MP	Total
49203	20.13	10.38	4.17	34.68
49204	26.13	12.75	5.33	44.21
49205	30.13	14.39	6.12	50.64
Facility RVU	Work	PE	MP	Total
49203	20.13	10.38	4.17	34.68
49204	26.13	12.75	5.33	44.21
49205	30.13	14.39	6.12	50.64

	FUD	Status	MUE	Modifiers				IOM Reference
49203	90	A	1(2)	51	N/A	62*	80	None
49204	90	A	1(2)	51	N/A	62*	80	
49205	90	A	1(2)	51	N/A	62*	80	

* with documentation

49320

49320	Laparoscopy, abdomen, peritoneum, and omentum, diagnostic, with or without collection of specimen(s) by brushing or washing (separate procedure)

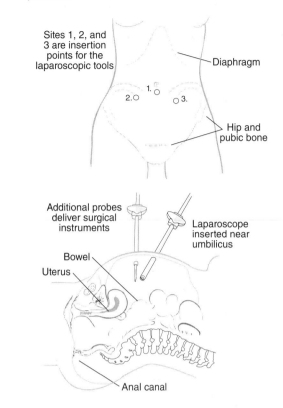

Sites 1, 2, and 3 are insertion points for the laparoscopic tools

Diaphragm

Hip and pubic bone

Additional probes deliver surgical instruments

Laparoscope inserted near umbilicus

Bowel

Uterus

Anal canal

Explanation

The physician makes a 1.0-centimeter incision in the umbilicus through which the abdomen is inflated and a fiberoptic laparoscope is inserted. Other incisions are also made through which trocars can be passed into the abdominal cavity to deliver instruments, a video camera, and when needed an additional light source. The physician manipulates the tools so that the pelvic organs, peritoneum, abdomen, and omentum can be viewed through the laparoscope and/or video monitor. Biopsy from any or all of the areas observed are obtained by brushing the surface and collecting the cells or by washing (bathing) the area with a saline solution, and suctioning out the cell rich solution. When the procedure is complete, the laparoscope, instruments, and light source are removed and the incisions are closed with sutures. If biopsy of pelvic organs is performed, the physician may also insert an instrument through the vagina to grasp the cervix and pass another instrument through the cervix, into the uterus to manipulate the uterus.

Coding Tips

Surgical laparoscopy always includes diagnostic laparoscopy. This separate procedure by definition is usually a component of a more complex service and is not identified separately. When performed alone or with other unrelated procedures or services it may be report. If performed alone, list the code; if performed with other procedures/services, list the code and append modifier 59 or an X{EPSU} modifier. For exploratory laparotomy (open approach), exploratory celiotomy, with or without biopsies, see 49000. For surgical laparoscopy, report a code from the appropriate anatomical section in CPT. For fulguration or excision of lesions of the ovary, pelvic viscera, or peritoneal surface via laparoscopy, see 58662.

ICD-10-CM Diagnostic Codes

C26.9	Malignant neoplasm of ill-defined sites within the digestive system
C48.1	Malignant neoplasm of specified parts of peritoneum
C48.2	Malignant neoplasm of peritoneum, unspecified
C48.8	Malignant neoplasm of overlapping sites of retroperitoneum and peritoneum
C57.3	Malignant neoplasm of parametrium ♀
C67.0	Malignant neoplasm of trigone of bladder
C67.1	Malignant neoplasm of dome of bladder
C67.2	Malignant neoplasm of lateral wall of bladder
C67.3	Malignant neoplasm of anterior wall of bladder
C67.4	Malignant neoplasm of posterior wall of bladder
C67.5	Malignant neoplasm of bladder neck
C76.2	Malignant neoplasm of abdomen
C78.6	Secondary malignant neoplasm of retroperitoneum and peritoneum
C79.11	Secondary malignant neoplasm of bladder
C79.19	Secondary malignant neoplasm of other urinary organs
C79.89	Secondary malignant neoplasm of other specified sites
D09.8	Carcinoma in situ of other specified sites
D20.1	Benign neoplasm of soft tissue of peritoneum
D36.7	Benign neoplasm of other specified sites
D48.4	Neoplasm of uncertain behavior of peritoneum
D48.7	Neoplasm of uncertain behavior of other specified sites
D49.0	Neoplasm of unspecified behavior of digestive system
D49.89	Neoplasm of unspecified behavior of other specified sites

AMA: 49320 2018,Jan,8; 2017,Jan,8; 2017,Apr,7; 2016,Jan,13; 2015,Jan,16; 2015,Dec,16; 2014,Jan,11

Relative Value Units/Medicare Edits

Non-Facility RVU	Work	PE	MP	Total
49320	5.14	3.26	1.14	9.54
Facility RVU	Work	PE	MP	Total
49320	5.14	3.26	1.14	9.54

	FUD	Status	MUE	Modifiers				IOM Reference
49320	10	A	1(3)	51	N/A	N/A	80	None

* with documentation

Terms To Know

biopsy. Tissue or fluid removed for diagnostic purposes through analysis of the cells in the biopsy material.

omentum. Fold of peritoneal tissue suspended between the stomach and neighboring visceral organs of the abdominal cavity.

peritoneum. Strong, continuous membrane that forms the lining of the abdominal and pelvic cavity. The parietal peritoneum, or outer layer, is attached to the abdominopelvic walls and the visceral peritoneum, or inner layer, surrounds the organs inside the abdominal cavity.

49321

49321 Laparoscopy, surgical; with biopsy (single or multiple)

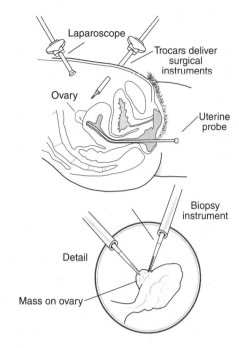

Explanation

The physician makes a 1.0 centimeter incision in the umbilicus through which the abdomen is inflated and a fiberoptic laparoscope is inserted. Other incisions are also made through which trocars can be passed into the abdominal cavity to deliver instruments, a video camera, and, when needed, an additional light source. The physician manipulates the tools so that the pelvic organs, peritoneum, abdomen, and omentum can be viewed through the laparoscope and/or video monitor. Biopsy from any or all of the areas observed are obtained by grasping a sample with a biopsy forceps that is capable of "biting off" small pieces of tissue. When the procedure is complete, the laparoscope, instruments, and light source are removed and the incisions are closed with sutures. If a biopsy of female pelvic organs is performed, the physician may also insert an instrument through the vagina to grasp the cervix and pass another instrument through the cervix and into the uterus to manipulate the uterus.

Coding Tips

Surgical laparoscopy always includes diagnostic laparoscopy. To report a diagnostic laparoscopy (peritoneoscopy), see 49320. For laparoscopic aspiration of a cavity or cyst (single or multiple), see 49322. For exploratory laparotomy (open approach), exploratory celiotomy, with or without biopsies, see 49000.

ICD-10-CM Diagnostic Codes

C48.0	Malignant neoplasm of retroperitoneum
C48.1	Malignant neoplasm of specified parts of peritoneum
C48.8	Malignant neoplasm of overlapping sites of retroperitoneum and peritoneum
C66.1	Malignant neoplasm of right ureter ☑
C66.2	Malignant neoplasm of left ureter ☑
C67.8	Malignant neoplasm of overlapping sites of bladder
C79.11	Secondary malignant neoplasm of bladder
C79.19	Secondary malignant neoplasm of other urinary organs
D09.19	Carcinoma in situ of other urinary organs

AMA: **49321** 2018,Jan,8; 2018,Aug,10; 2017,Jan,8; 2016,Jan,13; 2015,Jan,16; 2014,Jan,11

Relative Value Units/Medicare Edits

Non-Facility RVU	Work	PE	MP	Total
49321	5.44	3.4	1.18	10.02
Facility RVU	**Work**	**PE**	**MP**	**Total**
49321	5.44	3.4	1.18	10.02

	FUD	Status	MUE	Modifiers				IOM Reference
49321	10	A	1(2)	51	N/A	62	80	None

* with documentation

Terms To Know

biopsy. Tissue or fluid removed for diagnostic purposes through analysis of the cells in the biopsy material.

forceps. Tool used for grasping or compressing tissue.

laparoscopy. Direct visualization of the peritoneal cavity, outer fallopian tubes, uterus, and ovaries utilizing a laparoscope, a thin, flexible fiberoptic tube.

omentum. Fold of peritoneal tissue suspended between the stomach and neighboring visceral organs of the abdominal cavity.

peritoneum. Strong, continuous membrane that forms the lining of the abdominal and pelvic cavity. The parietal peritoneum, or outer layer, is attached to the abdominopelvic walls and the visceral peritoneum, or inner layer, surrounds the organs inside the abdominal cavity.

trocar. Cannula or a sharp pointed instrument used to puncture and aspirate fluid from cavities.

49322

49322   Laparoscopy, surgical; with aspiration of cavity or cyst (eg, ovarian cyst) (single or multiple)

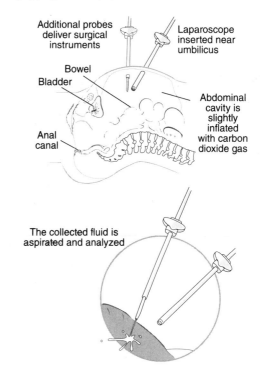

The collected fluid is aspirated and analyzed

Explanation

The physician makes a 1.0-centimeter incision in the umbilicus through which the abdomen is inflated and a fiberoptic laparoscope is inserted. A second incision is made directly below the umbilicus, just above the pubic hairline, through which a trocar can be passed into the abdominal cavity to deliver instruments. The physician manipulates the tools to view the pelvic organs through the laparoscope. An additional incision may be needed for a second light source. Once the biopsy site is viewed through the laparoscope, a 5.0-centimeter incision is made just above the site. Through this incision, the physician uses an aspirating probe to aspirate a cavity or cyst or to collect fluid for culture. The instruments are removed and the incisions are sutured.

Coding Tips

Surgical laparoscopy always includes diagnostic laparoscopy. For diagnostic laparoscopy only, see 49320. For laparoscopic fulguration or excision of lesions of the ovary, pelvic viscera, or peritoneal surface by any method, see 58662.

ICD-10-CM Diagnostic Codes

N70.01	Acute salpingitis ♀
N70.02	Acute oophoritis ♀
N70.03	Acute salpingitis and oophoritis ♀
N70.11	Chronic salpingitis ♀
N70.12	Chronic oophoritis ♀
N70.13	Chronic salpingitis and oophoritis ♀
N73.0	Acute parametritis and pelvic cellulitis ♀
N73.1	Chronic parametritis and pelvic cellulitis ♀
N73.4	Female chronic pelvic peritonitis ♀
N73.8	Other specified female pelvic inflammatory diseases ♀
N83.01	Follicular cyst of right ovary ♀ ☑

Abdomen

N83.02	Follicular cyst of left ovary ♀ ☑
N83.11	Corpus luteum cyst of right ovary ♀ ☑
N83.12	Corpus luteum cyst of left ovary ♀ ☑
N83.291	Other ovarian cyst, right side ♀ ☑
N83.292	Other ovarian cyst, left side ♀ ☑
N83.6	Hematosalpinx ♀

AMA: 49322 2018,Jan,8; 2017,Jan,8; 2016,Jan,13; 2015,Jan,16; 2014,Jan,11

Relative Value Units/Medicare Edits

Non-Facility RVU	Work	PE	MP	Total
49322	6.01	3.55	1.29	10.85
Facility RVU	**Work**	**PE**	**MP**	**Total**
49322	6.01	3.55	1.29	10.85

	FUD	Status	MUE	Modifiers				IOM Reference
49322	10	A	1(2)	51	N/A	62	80	None

* with documentation

Terms To Know

aspiration. Drawing fluid out by suction.

cyst. Elevated encapsulated mass containing fluid, semisolid, or solid material with a membranous lining.

insufflation. Blowing air or gas into a body cavity.

laparoscopy. Direct visualization of the peritoneal cavity, outer fallopian tubes, uterus, and ovaries utilizing a laparoscope, a thin, flexible fiberoptic tube.

trocar. Cannula or a sharp pointed instrument used to puncture and aspirate fluid from cavities.

49324-49325

49324 Laparoscopy, surgical; with insertion of tunneled intraperitoneal catheter

49325   with revision of previously placed intraperitoneal cannula or catheter, with removal of intraluminal obstructive material if performed

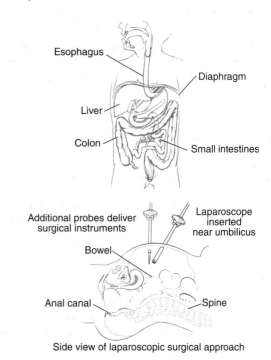

Side view of laparoscopic surgical approach

Explanation

A permanent intraperitoneal catheter is inserted laparoscopically using a tunneling technique. The physician makes a 1 cm incision in the umbilicus through which the abdomen is inflated and a fiberoptic laparoscope is inserted. Other incisions are also made through which trocars can be passed into the abdominal cavity to deliver additional instruments. The physician manipulates the tools so that the pelvic organs, peritoneum, abdomen, and omentum can be viewed through the laparoscope and/or video monitor. Using various tunneling techniques, the physician inserts the intraperitoneal catheter, positioning the tip inside the peritoneal cavity. A separately reportable subcutaneous extension of the catheter with a remote chest exit site may also be performed. If the physician is revising an intraperitoneal catheter, the catheter is inspected and freed of occlusion or blockage. When either procedure is complete, the laparoscope and other instruments are removed and the incisions are closed with sutures. Report 49324 for the tunneled insertion of an intraperitoneal cannula or catheter and 49325 for its revision.

Coding Tips

Surgical laparoscopy always includes diagnostic laparoscopy. To report a diagnostic laparoscopy (peritoneoscopy), see 49320. Subcutaneous extension of an intraperitoneal catheter with remote chest exit site is reported separately, see 49435. For open insertion of permanent tunneled intraperitoneal cannula or catheter, see 49421.

ICD-10-CM Diagnostic Codes

C48.0	Malignant neoplasm of retroperitoneum
C48.1	Malignant neoplasm of specified parts of peritoneum
C48.8	Malignant neoplasm of overlapping sites of retroperitoneum and peritoneum

C51.8	Malignant neoplasm of overlapping sites of vulva ♀
C54.0	Malignant neoplasm of isthmus uteri ♀
C54.1	Malignant neoplasm of endometrium ♀
C54.2	Malignant neoplasm of myometrium ♀
C54.3	Malignant neoplasm of fundus uteri ♀
C54.8	Malignant neoplasm of overlapping sites of corpus uteri ♀
C56.1	Malignant neoplasm of right ovary ♀ ☑
C56.2	Malignant neoplasm of left ovary ♀ ☑
C57.01	Malignant neoplasm of right fallopian tube ♀ ☑
C57.02	Malignant neoplasm of left fallopian tube ♀ ☑
C57.21	Malignant neoplasm of right round ligament ♀ ☑
C57.22	Malignant neoplasm of left round ligament ♀ ☑
C57.7	Malignant neoplasm of other specified female genital organs ♀
C57.8	Malignant neoplasm of overlapping sites of female genital organs ♀
C78.6	Secondary malignant neoplasm of retroperitoneum and peritoneum
C78.7	Secondary malignant neoplasm of liver and intrahepatic bile duct
C79.61	Secondary malignant neoplasm of right ovary ♀ ☑
C79.62	Secondary malignant neoplasm of left ovary ♀ ☑
R10.31	Right lower quadrant pain
R10.32	Left lower quadrant pain
R10.33	Periumbilical pain
R10.84	Generalized abdominal pain

AMA: **49324** 2014,Jan,11 **49325** 2014,Jan,11

Relative Value Units/Medicare Edits

Non-Facility RVU	Work	PE	MP	Total
49324	6.32	3.52	1.5	11.34
49325	6.82	3.65	1.63	12.1
Facility RVU	Work	PE	MP	Total
49324	6.32	3.52	1.5	11.34
49325	6.82	3.65	1.63	12.1

	FUD	Status	MUE	Modifiers				IOM Reference
49324	10	A	1(2)	51	N/A	62	80	None
49325	10	A	1(2)	51	N/A	62	80	

* with documentation

Terms To Know

cannula. Tube inserted into a blood vessel, duct, or body cavity to facilitate passage.

catheter. Flexible tube inserted into an area of the body for introducing or withdrawing fluid.

intraperitoneal. Within the cavity or space created by the double-layered sac that lines the abdominopelvic walls and forms a covering for the internal organs.

49326-49327

+ **49326** Laparoscopy, surgical; with omentopexy (omental tacking procedure) (List separately in addition to code for primary procedure)

+ **49327** with placement of interstitial device(s) for radiation therapy guidance (eg, fiducial markers, dosimeter), intra-abdominal, intrapelvic, and/or retroperitoneum, including imaging guidance, if performed, single or multiple (List separately in addition to code for primary procedure)

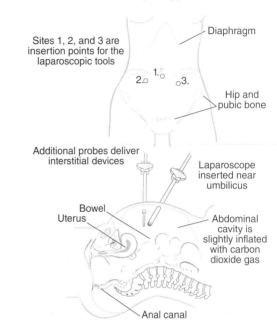

Sites 1, 2, and 3 are insertion points for the laparoscopic tools

Diaphragm

Hip and pubic bone

Additional probes deliver interstitial devices

Laparoscope inserted near umbilicus

Bowel
Uterus

Abdominal cavity is slightly inflated with carbon dioxide gas

Anal canal

Explanation

Omentum is a strong and highly vascularized serous membrane in the abdomen. The physician makes a 1 cm incision in the umbilicus through which the abdomen is inflated and a fiberoptic laparoscope is inserted. Other incisions are also made through which trocars can be passed into the abdominal cavity to deliver instruments, a video camera, and, when needed, an additional light source. The physician manipulates the tools so the pelvic organs, peritoneum, abdomen, and omentum can be viewed through the laparoscope and/or video monitor. In 49326, the physician isolates the omentum at the stomach and intestine and may cut, suture, or plicate omental tissue to achieve the desired effect. When the procedure is complete, the laparoscope, instruments, and light source are removed and the incisions are closed with sutures. In 49327, the physician, using image guidance if necessary, places one or more interstitial devices such as gold seeds (fiducial markers) for radiation therapy guidance or a dosimeter to gauge the amount of radiation received into the targeted soft tissue tumor. Allowing for precision in targeting radiation and/or for measuring the radiation doses received, a fiducial marker is visible by ultrasound and fluoroscopy and permits accurate triangulation of the tissue to be treated. A capsule dosimeter relays radiation dose information so that the clinical team can monitor for any deviation between the radiation plan and the actual radiation received. When the procedure is complete, the laparoscope, instruments, and light source are removed and the incisions are closed with sutures.

Coding Tips

Report 49326 in addition to 49324 and 49325. Report 49327 in addition to laparoscopic abdominal, pelvic, or retroperitoneal procedures performed at the same session. Surgical laparoscopy always includes diagnostic laparoscopy.

For a diagnostic laparoscopy (peritoneoscopy), see 49320. For placement of interstitial devices percutaneously, see 49411; for placement by open method, see 49412.

ICD-10-CM Diagnostic Codes

This/these CPT code(s) are add-on code(s). See the primary procedure code that this code is performed with for your ICD-10-CM code selections.

AMA: 49326 2014,Jan,11 **49327** 2014,Jan,11

Relative Value Units/Medicare Edits

Non-Facility RVU	Work	PE	MP	Total
49326	3.5	1.18	0.84	5.52
49327	2.38	0.86	0.57	3.81
Facility RVU	**Work**	**PE**	**MP**	**Total**
49326	3.5	1.18	0.84	5.52
49327	2.38	0.86	0.57	3.81

	FUD	Status	MUE	Modifiers				IOM Reference
49326	N/A	A	1(2)	N/A	N/A	62*	80	None
49327	N/A	A	1(2)	N/A	N/A	62*	80	

* with documentation

Terms To Know

interstitial. Within the small spaces or gaps occurring in tissue or organs.

laparoscopy. Direct visualization of the peritoneal cavity, including outer fallopian tubes, uterus, ovaries, and other structures, utilizing a laparoscope, which is a thin, flexible fiberoptic tube. Laparoscopy can be performed for diagnostic purposes alone or included as part of other surgical procedures accomplished by this approach.

omentum. Fold of peritoneal tissue suspended between the stomach and neighboring visceral organs of the abdominal cavity.

trocar. Cannula or a sharp pointed instrument used to puncture and aspirate fluid from cavities.

49402

49402   Removal of peritoneal foreign body from peritoneal cavity

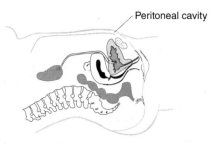

Peritoneal cavity

Explanation

The physician removes a foreign body from the abdominal cavity. The physician makes an abdominal incision and explores the abdominal cavity. The foreign body is identified and removed. The incision is closed.

Coding Tips

For lysis of intestinal adhesions, see 44005. For peritoneal drainage or lavage, open or percutaneous approach, see 49406, 49020, 49040, or 49082–49084, as appropriate. For percutaneous insertion of a tunneled intraperitoneal catheter without subcutaneous port, see 49418.

ICD-10-CM Diagnostic Codes

S31.620A	Laceration with foreign body of abdominal wall, right upper quadrant with penetration into peritoneal cavity, initial encounter ☑
S31.621A	Laceration with foreign body of abdominal wall, left upper quadrant with penetration into peritoneal cavity, initial encounter ☑
S31.623A	Laceration with foreign body of abdominal wall, right lower quadrant with penetration into peritoneal cavity, initial encounter ☑
S31.624A	Laceration with foreign body of abdominal wall, left lower quadrant with penetration into peritoneal cavity, initial encounter ☑
S31.625A	Laceration with foreign body of abdominal wall, periumbilic region with penetration into peritoneal cavity, initial encounter
S31.640A	Puncture wound with foreign body of abdominal wall, right upper quadrant with penetration into peritoneal cavity, initial encounter ☑
S31.641A	Puncture wound with foreign body of abdominal wall, left upper quadrant with penetration into peritoneal cavity, initial encounter ☑
S31.643A	Puncture wound with foreign body of abdominal wall, right lower quadrant with penetration into peritoneal cavity, initial encounter ☑
S31.644A	Puncture wound with foreign body of abdominal wall, left lower quadrant with penetration into peritoneal cavity, initial encounter ☑
S31.645A	Puncture wound with foreign body of abdominal wall, periumbilic region with penetration into peritoneal cavity, initial encounter
T81.510A	Adhesions due to foreign body accidentally left in body following surgical operation, initial encounter
T81.516A	Adhesions due to foreign body accidentally left in body following aspiration, puncture or other catheterization, initial encounter

T81.517A	Adhesions due to foreign body accidentally left in body following removal of catheter or packing, initial encounter
T81.518A	Adhesions due to foreign body accidentally left in body following other procedure, initial encounter
T81.520A	Obstruction due to foreign body accidentally left in body following surgical operation, initial encounter
T81.526A	Obstruction due to foreign body accidentally left in body following aspiration, puncture or other catheterization, initial encounter
T81.527A	Obstruction due to foreign body accidentally left in body following removal of catheter or packing, initial encounter
T81.528A	Obstruction due to foreign body accidentally left in body following other procedure, initial encounter
T81.530A	Perforation due to foreign body accidentally left in body following surgical operation, initial encounter
T81.536A	Perforation due to foreign body accidentally left in body following aspiration, puncture or other catheterization, initial encounter
T81.537A	Perforation due to foreign body accidentally left in body following removal of catheter or packing, initial encounter
T81.538A	Perforation due to foreign body accidentally left in body following other procedure, initial encounter
T81.590A	Other complications of foreign body accidentally left in body following surgical operation, initial encounter
T81.596A	Other complications of foreign body accidentally left in body following aspiration, puncture or other catheterization, initial encounter
T81.597A	Other complications of foreign body accidentally left in body following removal of catheter or packing, initial encounter
T81.598A	Other complications of foreign body accidentally left in body following other procedure, initial encounter

AMA: 49402 2014,Jan,11

Relative Value Units/Medicare Edits

Non-Facility RVU	Work	PE	MP	Total
49402	14.09	7.62	3.22	24.93
Facility RVU	Work	PE	MP	Total
49402	14.09	7.62	3.22	24.93

	FUD	Status	MUE	Modifiers				IOM Reference
49402	90	A	1(3)	51	N/A	62*	N/A	None

* with documentation

Terms To Know

foreign body. Any object or substance found in an organ and tissue that does not belong under normal circumstances.

peritoneal cavity. Space between the lining of the abdominal wall, or parietal peritoneum, and the surface layer of the abdominal organs, or visceral peritoneum. It contains a thin, watery fluid that keeps the peritoneal surfaces moist.

removal. Process of moving out of or away from, or the fact of being removed.

49406

49406 Image-guided fluid collection drainage by catheter (eg, abscess, hematoma, seroma, lymphocele, cyst); peritoneal or retroperitoneal, percutaneous

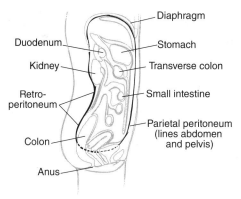

Percutaneous drainage of peritoneal or retroperitoneal abscess, hematoma, seroma, or lymphocele using image guidance

Explanation

A fluid collection in the peritoneum or retroperitoneum, such as a hematoma, a seroma, an abscess, a lymphocele, or a cyst, is drained using a catheter. The area over the affected site is cleansed and local anesthesia is administered. Imaging is performed to assist in the insertion of a needle or guidewire into the fluid collection. Small tissue samples may be collected from the site for pathological examination. A catheter is inserted to drain and collect the fluid for analysis and is then removed. More imaging may be performed to ensure hemostasis. A bandage is applied. In some cases, the catheter may be attached to a bag to allow for further drainage over the course of days.

Coding Tips

This code should be reported for each individual collection drained using a separate catheter. For transrectal or transvaginal image-guided peritoneal or retroperitoneal fluid collection drainage, via catheter, see 49407. Open transrectal drainage of a pelvic abscess is reported with 45000. For open peritoneal or retroperitoneal drainage of an appendiceal abscess, see 44900; peritoneal abscess or localized peritonitis, see 49020; subdiaphragmatic or subphrenic abscess, see 49040; retroperitoneal abscess, see 49060; extraperitoneal lymphocele, see 49062; peritoneal lavage, see 49084; perirenal or renal abscess, see 50020; ovarian cyst, see 58805; and for an ovarian abscess, see 58822. Percutaneous paracentesis is reported with 49082 and/or 49083. Do not report 49406 with 75989, 76942, 77002–77003, 77012, or 77021.

ICD-10-CM Diagnostic Codes

K65.1	Peritoneal abscess
K68.11	Postprocedural retroperitoneal abscess
K68.19	Other retroperitoneal abscess

AMA: 49406 2020,Feb,13; 2018,Jan,8; 2017,Jan,8; 2016,Jan,13; 2015,Jan,16; 2014,May,9; 2014,Jan,11

Relative Value Units/Medicare Edits

Non-Facility RVU	Work	PE	MP	Total
49406	4.0	20.79	0.34	25.13
Facility RVU	Work	PE	MP	Total
49406	4.0	1.36	0.34	5.7

	FUD	Status	MUE	Modifiers				IOM Reference
49406	0	A	2(3)	51	N/A	N/A	N/A	None

* with documentation

Terms To Know

abscess. Circumscribed collection of pus resulting from bacteria, frequently associated with swelling and other signs of inflammation.

catheter. Flexible tube inserted into an area of the body for introducing or withdrawing fluid.

cyst. Elevated encapsulated mass containing fluid, semisolid, or solid material with a membranous lining.

drainage. Releasing, taking, or letting out fluids and/or gases from a body part.

hematoma. Tumor-like collection of blood in some part of the body caused by a break in a blood vessel wall, usually as a result of trauma.

imaging. Radiologic means of producing pictures for clinical study of the internal structures and functions of the body, such as x-ray, ultrasound, magnetic resonance, or positron emission tomography.

lymph. Clear, sometimes yellow fluid that flows through the tissues in the body, through the lymphatic system, and into the blood stream.

lymphocele. Cyst that contains lymph.

percutaneous. Through the skin.

peritoneal. Space between the lining of the abdominal wall, or parietal peritoneum, and the surface layer of the abdominal organs, or visceral peritoneum. It contains a thin, watery fluid that keeps the peritoneal surfaces moist.

retroperitoneal. Located behind the peritoneum, the membrane that lines the abdominopelvic walls and forms a covering for the internal organs.

seroma. Swelling caused by the collection of serum, or clear fluid, in the tissues.

49407

49407 Image-guided fluid collection drainage by catheter (eg, abscess, hematoma, seroma, lymphocele, cyst); peritoneal or retroperitoneal, transvaginal or transrectal

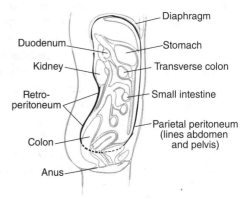

Transrectal or transvaginal approach is used to drain abscess, hematoma, seroma, or lymphocele using image guidance

Explanation

A fluid collection in the peritoneum or retroperitoneum, such as a hematoma, a seroma, an abscess, a lymphocele, or a cyst, is drained via a vaginal or rectal approach. An intracavitary probe is used to create access through the rectal or vaginal wall. Imaging is performed to assist in the insertion of a needle or guidewire into the fluid collection. Small tissue samples may be collected from the site for pathological examination. A catheter is inserted to drain and collect the fluid for analysis and is then removed. In some cases, the catheter may be attached to a bag to allow for further drainage over the course of days.

Coding Tips

This code should be reported for each individual collection drained using a separate catheter. For open transrectal or transvaginal drainage of an abscess or a cyst, pelvic, see 45000; ovarian cyst, see 58800; ovarian abscess, see 58820. For peritoneal drainage or lavage, open, see 49020, 49040, or 49082. For image guided percutaneous drainage of an abscess or cyst of the soft tissue via catheter, see 10030. Do not report 49407 with 75989, 76942, 77002–77003, 77012, or 77021.

ICD-10-CM Diagnostic Codes

K65.1	Peritoneal abscess
K68.11	Postprocedural retroperitoneal abscess
K68.19	Other retroperitoneal abscess

AMA: **49407** 2018,Jan,8; 2017,Jan,8; 2016,Jan,13; 2015,Jan,16; 2014,May,9; 2014,Jan,11

Relative Value Units/Medicare Edits

Non-Facility RVU	Work	PE	MP	Total
49407	4.25	15.99	0.41	20.65
Facility RVU	Work	PE	MP	Total
49407	4.25	1.39	0.41	6.05

	FUD	Status	MUE	Modifiers				IOM Reference
49407	0	A	1(3)	51	N/A	N/A	N/A	None

* with documentation

Coding Companion for Ob/Gyn

50722

50722 Ureterolysis for ovarian vein syndrome

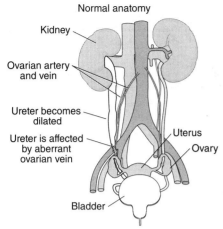

Normal anatomy

Kidney

Ovarian artery
and vein

Ureter becomes
dilated

Ureter is affected
by aberrant
ovarian vein

Uterus

Ovary

Bladder

Physician surgically frees ureter from obstruction

Explanation

The physician surgically frees the ureter from ureteral obstruction caused by aberrant ovarian veins (ovarian vein syndrome). To access the ureter, the physician makes an incision in the skin above the pubic hairline, and cuts the muscles, fat, and fibrous membranes (fascia) overlying the ureter. The physician incises surrounding adhesions to free the ureter from the obstructing ovarian veins. The physician places a drain tube, bringing it out through a separate stab incision in the skin, and performs a layered closure.

Coding Tips

For excision of urethral diverticulum, see 53230. For excision of urethral polyps, see 53260.

ICD-10-CM Diagnostic Codes

N13.8   Other obstructive and reflux uropathy

AMA: 50722 2014,Jan,11

Relative Value Units/Medicare Edits

Non-Facility RVU	Work	PE	MP	Total
50722	17.95	9.04	2.83	29.82
Facility RVU	**Work**	**PE**	**MP**	**Total**
50722	17.95	9.04	2.83	29.82

	FUD	Status	MUE	Modifiers				IOM Reference
50722	90	A	1(2)	51	N/A	62*	80	None

* with documentation

Terms To Know

aberrant. Deviation or departure from the normal or usual course, condition, or pattern.

ovarian vein syndrome. Retroperitoneal structures involving and often obstructing the ureters following certain types of chemical treatment; there is no identified cause.

● New   ▲ Revised   + Add On   ★ Telemedicine   AMA: CPT Assist   [Resequenced]   ☑ Laterality   © 2020 Optum360, LLC

51020-51030

51020 Cystotomy or cystostomy; with fulguration and/or insertion of radioactive material
51030 with cryosurgical destruction of intravesical lesion

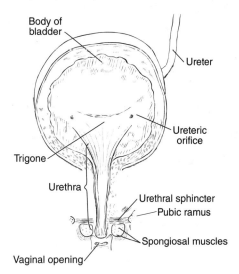

Frontal section of the female bladder, urethra, and select bone and musculature

Explanation

The physician makes an incision (cystotomy) or creates an opening (cystostomy) into the bladder to destroy abnormal tissue. To access the bladder, the physician makes an incision in the skin of the lower abdomen and cuts the corresponding muscles, fat, fibrous membranes (fascia), and bladder wall. Report 51020 if the physician uses electric current (fulguration) or inserts radioactive material to destroy a lesion on the bladder (usually with the aid of a radiation oncologist). Report 51030 if the physician uses cryosurgery to destroy the lesion. The bladder wall and lower abdomen is sutured closed. If a cystostomy is made, the cystostomy tube is sutured in place and the bladder and abdominal wall is closed.

Coding Tips

For a cystotomy with insertion of a ureteral catheter or stent, see 51045.

ICD-10-CM Diagnostic Codes

C67.0	Malignant neoplasm of trigone of bladder
C67.1	Malignant neoplasm of dome of bladder
C67.2	Malignant neoplasm of lateral wall of bladder
C67.3	Malignant neoplasm of anterior wall of bladder
C67.4	Malignant neoplasm of posterior wall of bladder
C67.5	Malignant neoplasm of bladder neck
C67.6	Malignant neoplasm of ureteric orifice
C67.7	Malignant neoplasm of urachus
C67.8	Malignant neoplasm of overlapping sites of bladder
C79.11	Secondary malignant neoplasm of bladder
D09.0	Carcinoma in situ of bladder
D30.3	Benign neoplasm of bladder
D41.4	Neoplasm of uncertain behavior of bladder
D49.4	Neoplasm of unspecified behavior of bladder
N21.0	Calculus in bladder
N30.10	Interstitial cystitis (chronic) without hematuria
N30.11	Interstitial cystitis (chronic) with hematuria
N32.89	Other specified disorders of bladder

AMA: 51020 2014,Jan,11 **51030** 2014,Jan,11

Relative Value Units/Medicare Edits

Non-Facility RVU	Work	PE	MP	Total
51020	7.69	4.94	0.88	13.51
51030	7.81	4.91	0.89	13.61
Facility RVU	**Work**	**PE**	**MP**	**Total**
51020	7.69	4.94	0.88	13.51
51030	7.81	4.91	0.89	13.61

	FUD	Status	MUE		Modifiers			IOM Reference
51020	90	A	1(2)	51	N/A	62*	80	None
51030	90	A	1(2)	51	N/A	N/A	80*	

* with documentation

Terms To Know

benign. Mild or nonmalignant in nature.

carcinoma in situ. Malignancy that arises from the cells of the vessel, gland, or organ of origin that remains confined to that site or has not invaded neighboring tissue.

cryosurgery. Application of intense cold, usually produced using liquid nitrogen, to locally freeze diseased or unwanted tissue and induce tissue necrosis without causing harm to adjacent tissue.

cystostomy. Formation of an opening through the abdominal wall into the bladder.

cystotomy. Surgical incision into the gallbladder or urinary bladder.

destruction. Ablation or eradication of a structure or tissue.

electrocautery. Division or cutting of tissue using high-frequency electrical current to produce heat, which destroys cells.

fulguration. Destruction of living tissue by using sparks from a high-frequency electric current.

malignant. Any condition tending to progress toward death, specifically an invasive tumor with a loss of cellular differentiation that has the ability to spread or metastasize to other body areas.

Bladder

51045

51045 Cystotomy, with insertion of ureteral catheter or stent (separate procedure)

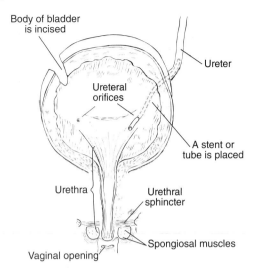

Body of bladder is incised

Ureter

Ureteral orifices

A stent or tube is placed

Urethra

Urethral sphincter

Spongiosal muscles

Vaginal opening

Explanation

The physician makes an incision in the bladder to insert a catheter or slender tube (stent) into the ureter. To access the bladder and ureters, the physician makes a midline incision in the skin of the abdomen and cuts the corresponding muscles, fat, and fibrous membranes (fascia). The physician incises the bladder (cystotomy) and inserts a stent or catheter in the ureter. Insertion of a ureteral catheter requires that the physician bring the tube end out through the urethra or bladder incision. The physician inserts a drain tube and performs a layered closure.

Coding Tips

This separate procedure by definition is usually a component of a more complex service and is not identified separately. When performed alone or with other unrelated procedures or services it may be reported. If performed alone, list the code; if performed with other procedures/services, list the code and append modifier 59 or an X{EPSU} modifier. For a bladder incision for drainage, fulguration, insertion of radioactive material, and/or cryosurgical destruction of lesions, see 51020–51030.

ICD-10-CM Diagnostic Codes

C66.1	Malignant neoplasm of right ureter ☑
C66.2	Malignant neoplasm of left ureter ☑
D30.21	Benign neoplasm of right ureter ☑
D30.22	Benign neoplasm of left ureter ☑
D41.21	Neoplasm of uncertain behavior of right ureter ☑
D41.22	Neoplasm of uncertain behavior of left ureter ☑
N11.1	Chronic obstructive pyelonephritis
N13.4	Hydroureter
N13.5	Crossing vessel and stricture of ureter without hydronephrosis
N13.8	Other obstructive and reflux uropathy
N20.1	Calculus of ureter
N28.89	Other specified disorders of kidney and ureter
Q62.0	Congenital hydronephrosis
Q62.11	Congenital occlusion of ureteropelvic junction
Q62.12	Congenital occlusion of ureterovesical orifice
Q62.2	Congenital megaureter
Q62.31	Congenital ureterocele, orthotopic
Q62.32	Cecoureterocele
Q62.39	Other obstructive defects of renal pelvis and ureter
S37.12XA	Contusion of ureter, initial encounter
S37.13XA	Laceration of ureter, initial encounter
S37.19XA	Other injury of ureter, initial encounter

AMA: 51045 2014,Jan,11

Relative Value Units/Medicare Edits

Non-Facility RVU	Work	PE	MP	Total
51045	7.81	5.33	1.29	14.43
Facility RVU	**Work**	**PE**	**MP**	**Total**
51045	7.81	5.33	1.29	14.43

	FUD	Status	MUE	Modifiers				IOM Reference
51045	90	A	2(3)	51	N/A	N/A	80	None

* with documentation

Terms To Know

calculus. Abnormal, stone-like concretion of calcium, cholesterol, mineral salts, or other substances that forms in any part of the body.

catheter. Flexible tube inserted into an area of the body for introducing or withdrawing fluid.

cystotomy. Surgical incision into the gallbladder or urinary bladder.

drain. Device that creates a channel to allow fluid from a cavity, wound, or infected area to exit the body.

fascia. Fibrous sheet or band of tissue that envelops organs, muscles, and groupings of muscles.

fistula. Abnormal tube-like passage between two body cavities or organs or from an organ to the outside surface.

hematuria. Blood in urine, which may present as gross visible blood or as the presence of red blood cells visible only under a microscope.

hydroureter. Abnormal enlargement or distension of the ureter with water or urine caused by an obstruction.

stent. Tube to provide support in a body cavity or lumen.

stricture. Narrowing of an anatomical structure.

ureter. Tube leading from the kidney to the urinary bladder made up of three layers of tissue: the mucous lining of the inner layer; the smooth, muscular middle layer that propels the urine from the kidney to the bladder by peristalsis; and the outer layer made of fibrous connective tissue. Each ureter leaves the kidney from the hilum, a concave notch on the middle surface, and enters the bladder through a narrow valve-like orifice that prevents the backflow of urine to the kidney.

Bladder

51100-51102

51100 Aspiration of bladder; by needle
51101   by trocar or intracatheter
51102   with insertion of suprapubic catheter

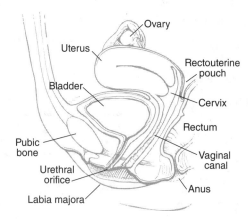

Explanation

In 51100, the physician inserts a needle through the skin into the bladder to withdraw urine. In 51101, the physician inserts a trocar or intracatheter through the skin into the bladder. In 51102, a suprapubic catheter is placed into the bladder. This procedure may also be performed after the abdomen has been surgically incised.

Coding Tips

Local anesthesia is included in these services. However, these procedures may be performed under general anesthesia, depending on the age and/or condition of the patient. If a specimen is transported to an outside laboratory, report 99000 for handling or conveyance. Imaging guidance is reported with 76942, 77002, or 77012.

ICD-10-CM Diagnostic Codes

A56.01	Chlamydial cystitis and urethritis
C67.0	Malignant neoplasm of trigone of bladder
C67.2	Malignant neoplasm of lateral wall of bladder
C67.3	Malignant neoplasm of anterior wall of bladder
C67.4	Malignant neoplasm of posterior wall of bladder
C67.5	Malignant neoplasm of bladder neck
C67.6	Malignant neoplasm of ureteric orifice
G83.4	Cauda equina syndrome
N11.8	Other chronic tubulo-interstitial nephritis
N13.71	Vesicoureteral-reflux without reflux nephropathy
N28.86	Ureteritis cystica
N30.00	Acute cystitis without hematuria
N30.01	Acute cystitis with hematuria
N30.10	Interstitial cystitis (chronic) without hematuria
N30.11	Interstitial cystitis (chronic) with hematuria
N30.30	Trigonitis without hematuria
N30.31	Trigonitis with hematuria
N30.80	Other cystitis without hematuria
N30.81	Other cystitis with hematuria
N32.0	Bladder-neck obstruction
N32.1	Vesicointestinal fistula
N32.3	Diverticulum of bladder

N32.81	Overactive bladder
N32.89	Other specified disorders of bladder
N36.0	Urethral fistula
N39.3	Stress incontinence (female) (male)
N99.81	Other intraoperative complications of genitourinary system
N99.89	Other postprocedural complications and disorders of genitourinary system
Q64.2	Congenital posterior urethral valves
Q64.31	Congenital bladder neck obstruction
Q64.32	Congenital stricture of urethra
Q64.33	Congenital stricture of urinary meatus
Q64.39	Other atresia and stenosis of urethra and bladder neck
R82.71	Bacteriuria
R82.79	Other abnormal findings on microbiological examination of urine
S37.22XA	Contusion of bladder, initial encounter
S37.23XA	Laceration of bladder, initial encounter
S37.29XA	Other injury of bladder, initial encounter
S37.32XA	Contusion of urethra, initial encounter
S37.33XA	Laceration of urethra, initial encounter
S37.39XA	Other injury of urethra, initial encounter

AMA: 51100 2018,Jan,8; 2017,Jan,8; 2016,Jan,13; 2015,Jan,16; 2014,Jan,11 **51101** 2018,Jan,8; 2017,Jan,8; 2016,Jan,13; 2015,Jan,16; 2014,Jan,11 **51102** 2018,Jan,8; 2017,Jan,8; 2016,Jan,13; 2015,Jan,16; 2014,Jan,11

Relative Value Units/Medicare Edits

Non-Facility RVU	Work	PE	MP	Total
51100	0.78	1.08	0.09	1.95
51101	1.02	2.92	0.12	4.06
51102	2.7	3.78	0.3	6.78

Facility RVU	Work	PE	MP	Total
51100	0.78	0.25	0.09	1.12
51101	1.02	0.35	0.12	1.49
51102	2.7	1.2	0.3	4.2

	FUD	Status	MUE		Modifiers			IOM Reference
51100	0	A	1(3)	51	N/A	N/A	N/A	None
51101	0	A	1(3)	51	N/A	N/A	N/A	
51102	0	A	1(3)	51	N/A	N/A	N/A	

* with documentation

Terms To Know

aspiration. Drawing fluid out by suction.

catheter. Flexible tube inserted into an area of the body for introducing or withdrawing fluid.

intra. Within.

trocar. Cannula or a sharp pointed instrument used to puncture and aspirate fluid from cavities.

Bladder

51597

51597 Pelvic exenteration, complete, for vesical, prostatic or urethral malignancy, with removal of bladder and ureteral transplantations, with or without hysterectomy and/or abdominoperineal resection of rectum and colon and colostomy, or any combination thereof

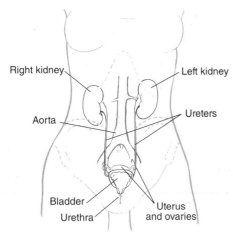

A complete pelvic exenteration is performed

Explanation

The physician removes the bladder, lower ureters, lymph nodes, urethra, colon, and rectum due to a vesical or urethral malignancy. To access the bladder and ureters, the physician makes a midline incision in the skin of the abdomen and cuts the corresponding muscles, fat, and fibrous membranes (fascia). The physician dissects and ligates the hypogastric and vesical vessels, and severs the bladder, urethra, lower ureters, and lymph nodes from surrounding structures. The physician removes the bladder and diverts urine flow by transplanting the ureters to the skin or colon. The vagina and uterus and/or rectum and part of the colon may be removed and an artificial abdominal opening in the skin surface created for waste (colostomy). After completing the urinary diversion procedure, the physician inserts drain tubes and performs a layered closure.

Coding Tips

Pelvic exenteration for a gynecological malignancy is reported with 58240.

ICD-10-CM Diagnostic Codes

C67.0	Malignant neoplasm of trigone of bladder
C67.1	Malignant neoplasm of dome of bladder
C67.2	Malignant neoplasm of lateral wall of bladder
C67.3	Malignant neoplasm of anterior wall of bladder
C67.4	Malignant neoplasm of posterior wall of bladder
C67.5	Malignant neoplasm of bladder neck
C67.6	Malignant neoplasm of ureteric orifice
C67.8	Malignant neoplasm of overlapping sites of bladder
C68.0	Malignant neoplasm of urethra
C79.11	Secondary malignant neoplasm of bladder
C79.19	Secondary malignant neoplasm of other urinary organs

AMA: **51597** 2014,Jan,11

Relative Value Units/Medicare Edits

Non-Facility RVU	Work	PE	MP	Total
51597	42.86	18.26	5.16	66.28
Facility RVU	**Work**	**PE**	**MP**	**Total**
51597	42.86	18.26	5.16	66.28

	FUD	Status	MUE	Modifiers				IOM Reference
51597	90	A	1(2)	51	N/A	62*	80	None

* with documentation

Terms To Know

dissect. Cut apart or separate tissue for surgical purposes or for visual or microscopic study.

exenteration. Surgical removal of the entire contents of a body cavity, such as the pelvis or orbit.

ligate. To tie off a blood vessel or duct with a suture or a soft, thin wire (ligature wire).

malignant neoplasm. Any cancerous tumor or lesion exhibiting uncontrolled tissue growth that can progressively invade other parts of the body with its disease-generating cells.

resection. Surgical removal of a part or all of an organ or body part.

secondary. Second in order of occurrence or importance, or appearing during the course of another disease or condition.

Bladder

51701-51703

51701 Insertion of non-indwelling bladder catheter (eg, straight catheterization for residual urine)
51702 Insertion of temporary indwelling bladder catheter; simple (eg, Foley)
51703 complicated (eg, altered anatomy, fractured catheter/balloon)

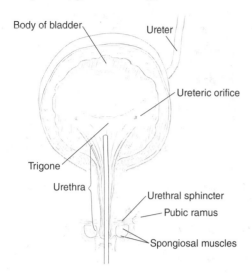

Explanation

The patient is catheterized with a non-indwelling bladder catheter (e.g., for residual urine) in 51701; simple catheterization with a temporary indwelling bladder catheter (Foley) is performed in 51702. The area is properly cleaned and sterilized. A water-soluble lubricant may be injected into the urethra before catheterization begins. The distal part of the catheter is coated with lubricant. The catheter is gently inserted until urine is noted. With an indwelling catheter, insertion continues into the bladder until the retention balloon can be inflated. The catheter is gently pulled until the retention balloon is snuggled against the neck of the bladder. The catheter is secured to the abdomen or thigh and the drainage bag is secured below bladder level. Report 51703 if a circumstance (i.e., change in anatomy or fractured catheter/balloon) occurs to complicate the catheterization process.

Coding Tips

Codes 51701 and 51702 should not be reported in addition to any other procedure that includes catheter insertion as a component. Report 51701 and 51702 only when performed independently. Do not report 51702 with CPT Category III code 0071T or 0072T. Supplies used when providing these procedures may be reported with the appropriate HCPCS Level II code. Check with the specific payer to determine coverage.

ICD-10-CM Diagnostic Codes

C67.5	Malignant neoplasm of bladder neck
C68.0	Malignant neoplasm of urethra
N32.89	Other specified disorders of bladder
N35.021	Urethral stricture due to childbirth ♀
N35.028	Other post-traumatic urethral stricture, female ♀
N35.82	Other urethral stricture, female ♀
N39.3	Stress incontinence (female) (male)
N39.45	Continuous leakage
N39.490	Overflow incontinence
N99.12	Postprocedural urethral stricture, female ♀
R30.0	Dysuria
R30.1	Vesical tenesmus
R31.0	Gross hematuria
R31.1	Benign essential microscopic hematuria
R31.21	Asymptomatic microscopic hematuria
R31.29	Other microscopic hematuria
R33.8	Other retention of urine
R35.0	Frequency of micturition
R35.8	Other polyuria
R39.14	Feeling of incomplete bladder emptying
R39.81	Functional urinary incontinence

AMA: 51701 2018,Jan,8; 2017,Jan,8; 2016,Jan,13; 2015,Jan,16; 2014,Jan,11 **51702** 2018,Jan,8; 2017,Jan,8; 2016,Jan,13; 2015,Jan,16; 2014,May,3; 2014,Jan,11 **51703** 2018,Jan,8; 2017,Jan,8; 2016,Jan,13; 2015,Jan,16; 2014,Jan,11

Relative Value Units/Medicare Edits

Non-Facility RVU	Work	PE	MP	Total
51701	0.5	0.7	0.08	1.28
51702	0.5	1.18	0.06	1.74
51703	1.47	2.33	0.18	3.98
Facility RVU	Work	PE	MP	Total
51701	0.5	0.18	0.08	0.76
51702	0.5	0.18	0.06	0.74
51703	1.47	0.58	0.18	2.23

	FUD	Status	MUE	Modifiers				IOM Reference
51701	0	A	2(3)	51	N/A	N/A	N/A	None
51702	0	A	2(3)	51	N/A	N/A	N/A	
51703	0	A	2(3)	51	N/A	N/A	N/A	

* with documentation

Terms To Know

catheterization. Use or insertion of a tubular device into a duct, blood vessel, hollow organ, or body cavity for injecting or withdrawing fluids for diagnostic or therapeutic purposes.

distal. Located farther away from a specified reference point or the trunk.

dysuria. Pain upon urination.

Foley catheter. Temporary indwelling urethral catheter held in place in the bladder by an inflated balloon containing fluid or air.

hematuria. Blood in urine, which may present as gross visible blood or as the presence of red blood cells visible only under a microscope.

polyuria. Excessive urination.

stress incontinence. Involuntary escape of urine at times of minor stress against the bladder, such as coughing, sneezing, or laughing.

Bladder

51725-51729

51725 Simple cystometrogram (CMG) (eg, spinal manometer)
51726 Complex cystometrogram (ie, calibrated electronic equipment);
51727   with urethral pressure profile studies (ie, urethral closure pressure profile), any technique
51728   with voiding pressure studies (ie, bladder voiding pressure), any technique
51729   with voiding pressure studies (ie, bladder voiding pressure) and urethral pressure profile studies (ie, urethral closure pressure profile), any technique

Body of bladder

Ureter

Orifice

Pressure catheter

Frontal section of the bladder

Explanation

A cystometrogram (a graphic record of urinary bladder pressure at different volumes) is used to distinguish bladder outlet obstruction from other voiding dysfunctions. For a simple cystometrogram (51725), the physician inserts a pressure catheter into the bladder and connects it to a manometer line filled with fluid to measure pressure and flow in the lower urinary tract. For a complex cystometrogram (51726), the physician typically uses a transurethral catheter to fill the bladder with water or gas while simultaneously obtaining rectal pressure. As the bladder is being filled, intravesical pressure is measured by a microtip transducer or fluid-filled catheter attached to the transducer. Code 51727 reports a complex cystometrogram performed in conjunction with a study for measuring urethral pressure. In one technique, the bladder is filled with fluid and the catheter withdrawn into the urethra while bladder sensations and volume are recorded. Urethral pressure changes are recorded as the patient follows specific instructions (Valsalva maneuver, cough). For voiding pressure studies performed in conjunction with a complex cystometrogram (51728), a transducer is placed into the bladder and the bladder is filled with fluid. The patient is instructed to attempt to void upon the feeling of bladder fullness, and recordings are taken of bladder sensation and volume at specific times. Report 51729 if complex cystometrogram is combined with both voiding pressure studies and urethral pressure profile studies.

Coding Tips

These codes imply that the service is performed by, or under the direct supervision of, a physician or other qualified health care professional. All instruments, equipment, fluids, gases, probes, catheters, technician fees, medications, gloves, trays, tubing, and other sterile supplies are presumed to be provided by the physician. To claim only the professional component of a code, append modifier 26 or for the technical component, append modifier TC. To claim the complete procedure (i.e., both the professional and technical components), submit without a modifier. When multiple procedures are performed during the same operative session, modifier 51 should be reported on all subsequent procedures beyond the primary service.

ICD-10-CM Diagnostic Codes

N30.10	Interstitial cystitis (chronic) without hematuria
N30.11	Interstitial cystitis (chronic) with hematuria
N31.8	Other neuromuscular dysfunction of bladder
N32.0	Bladder-neck obstruction
N32.81	Overactive bladder
N36.41	Hypermobility of urethra
N36.42	Intrinsic sphincter deficiency (ISD)
N36.43	Combined hypermobility of urethra and intrinsic sphincter deficiency
N36.44	Muscular disorders of urethra
N39.3	Stress incontinence (female) (male)
N39.41	Urge incontinence
N39.42	Incontinence without sensory awareness
N39.43	Post-void dribbling
N39.44	Nocturnal enuresis
N39.45	Continuous leakage
N39.46	Mixed incontinence
N39.490	Overflow incontinence
N39.491	Coital incontinence
N39.492	Postural (urinary) incontinence
N39.498	Other specified urinary incontinence
Q64.74	Double urethra
Q64.79	Other congenital malformations of bladder and urethra
R30.0	Dysuria
R33.0	Drug induced retention of urine
R33.8	Other retention of urine
R35.0	Frequency of micturition
R35.1	Nocturia
R35.8	Other polyuria
R39.11	Hesitancy of micturition
R39.12	Poor urinary stream
R39.13	Splitting of urinary stream
R39.14	Feeling of incomplete bladder emptying
R39.15	Urgency of urination
R39.16	Straining to void
R39.191	Need to immediately re-void
R39.192	Position dependent micturition
R39.198	Other difficulties with micturition
R39.81	Functional urinary incontinence
R39.89	Other symptoms and signs involving the genitourinary system

AMA: 51725 2018,Jan,8; 2017,Jan,8; 2016,Jan,13; 2015,Jan,16; 2014,Jan,11 **51726** 2018,Jan,8; 2017,Jan,8; 2016,Jan,13; 2015,Jan,16; 2014,Jan,11 **51727** 2018,Jan,8; 2017,Jan,8; 2016,Jan,13; 2015,Jan,16; 2014,Jan,11 **51728** 2018,Jan,8; 2017,Jan,8; 2016,Jan,13; 2015,Jan,16; 2014,Jan,11 **51729** 2018,Jan,8; 2017,Jan,8; 2016,Jan,13; 2015,Jan,16; 2014,Jan,11

Bladder

Relative Value Units/Medicare Edits

Non-Facility RVU	Work	PE	MP	Total
51725	1.51	4.38	0.15	6.04
51726	1.71	6.37	0.15	8.23
51727	2.11	7.54	0.23	9.88
51728	2.11	7.69	0.2	10.0
51729	2.51	7.89	0.27	10.67
Facility RVU	**Work**	**PE**	**MP**	**Total**
51725	1.51	4.38	0.15	6.04
51726	1.71	6.37	0.15	8.23
51727	2.11	7.54	0.23	9.88
51728	2.11	7.69	0.2	10.0
51729	2.51	7.89	0.27	10.67

	FUD	Status	MUE	Modifiers				IOM Reference
51725	0	A	1(3)	51	N/A	N/A	80*	None
51726	0	A	1(3)	51	N/A	N/A	N/A	
51727	0	A	1(3)	51	N/A	N/A	80*	
51728	0	A	1(3)	51	N/A	N/A	80*	
51729	0	A	1(3)	51	N/A	N/A	80*	

* with documentation

Terms To Know

catheter. Flexible tube inserted into an area of the body for introducing or withdrawing fluid.

CMG. Cystometrogram. Graphic recording of urinary bladder pressure at various volumes, which is useful in differentiating bladder outlet obstruction from other voiding dysfunctions. A simple CMG utilizes a pressure catheter inserted into the bladder connected to a manometer line filled with fluid to measure pressure through the changes in the height of the water column. A complex CMG utilizes calibrated electronic equipment with a microtipped pressure catheter.

cystometrogram. Recorded measurement of bladder pressure from multiple volume amounts.

LUTS. Lower urinary tract symptoms.

micturition. Urination.

transducer. Apparatus that transfers or translates one type of energy into another, such as converting pressure to an electrical signal.

urethral pressure profile. Measures urethral pressure by pulling a transducer through the urethra and noting the pressure change.

voiding pressure study. Voiding pressure produced by the bladder and the resultant flow of urine is determined.

51736-51741

51736   Simple uroflowmetry (UFR) (eg, stop-watch flow rate, mechanical uroflowmeter)

51741   Complex uroflowmetry (eg, calibrated electronic equipment)

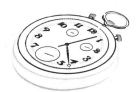

Simple uroflowmetry is performed. Typically, a stopwatch is used to measure the amount of time a patient needs to urinate into a calibrated vessel. The physician assesses the ratio

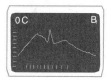

Complex uroflowmetry is performed. Typically, electronic equipment is used to record the volume of urine and elapsed time. The physician assesses the ratio

Explanation

For simple uroflowmetry (51736), the physician assesses the rate of emptying the bladder by stopwatch, recording the volume of urine per time. For complex uroflowmetry, (51741), the physician assesses the rate of emptying of the bladder by electronic equipment, recording the volume of urine per time.

Coding Tips

These codes imply that the service is performed by, or under the direct supervision of, a physician, and that all instruments, equipment, fluids, gases, probes, catheters, technician's fee, medications, gloves, trays, tubing, and other sterile supplies be provided by the physician. Procedures 51736 and 51741 have both a technical and professional component. To claim only the professional component, append modifier 26. To claim only the technical component, append modifier TC. To claim the complete procedure (i.e., both the professional and technical components), submit without a modifier.

ICD-10-CM Diagnostic Codes

A56.01	Chlamydial cystitis and urethritis
N30.10	Interstitial cystitis (chronic) without hematuria
N30.11	Interstitial cystitis (chronic) with hematuria
N30.20	Other chronic cystitis without hematuria
N30.21	Other chronic cystitis with hematuria
N30.30	Trigonitis without hematuria
N30.31	Trigonitis with hematuria
N30.40	Irradiation cystitis without hematuria
N30.41	Irradiation cystitis with hematuria
N30.80	Other cystitis without hematuria
N30.81	Other cystitis with hematuria
N31.8	Other neuromuscular dysfunction of bladder
N32.0	Bladder-neck obstruction
N32.81	Overactive bladder
N32.89	Other specified disorders of bladder
N35.021	Urethral stricture due to childbirth ♀

Bladder

N35.028	Other post-traumatic urethral stricture, female ♀
N35.12	Postinfective urethral stricture, not elsewhere classified, female ♀
N35.82	Other urethral stricture, female ♀
N36.41	Hypermobility of urethra
N36.42	Intrinsic sphincter deficiency (ISD)
N36.43	Combined hypermobility of urethra and intrinsic sphincter deficiency
N36.44	Muscular disorders of urethra
N36.8	Other specified disorders of urethra
N39.3	Stress incontinence (female) (male)
N39.41	Urge incontinence
N39.42	Incontinence without sensory awareness
N39.43	Post-void dribbling
N39.46	Mixed incontinence
N39.490	Overflow incontinence
N39.491	Coital incontinence
N39.492	Postural (urinary) incontinence
N39.498	Other specified urinary incontinence
N39.8	Other specified disorders of urinary system
N81.84	Pelvic muscle wasting ♀
N99.12	Postprocedural urethral stricture, female ♀
Q62.2	Congenital megaureter
Q64.2	Congenital posterior urethral valves
Q64.31	Congenital bladder neck obstruction
Q64.32	Congenital stricture of urethra
Q64.33	Congenital stricture of urinary meatus
Q64.39	Other atresia and stenosis of urethra and bladder neck
R30.0	Dysuria
R33.0	Drug induced retention of urine
R33.8	Other retention of urine
R35.0	Frequency of micturition
R39.11	Hesitancy of micturition
R39.12	Poor urinary stream
R39.13	Splitting of urinary stream
R39.14	Feeling of incomplete bladder emptying
R39.15	Urgency of urination
R39.16	Straining to void

AMA: 51736 2018,Jan,8; 2017,Jan,8; 2016,Jan,13; 2015,Jan,16; 2014,Jan,11
51741 2018,Jan,8; 2017,Jan,8; 2016,Jan,13; 2015,Jan,16; 2014,Sep,13; 2014,Jan,11

Relative Value Units/Medicare Edits

Non-Facility RVU	Work	PE	MP	Total
51736	0.17	0.2	0.02	0.39
51741	0.17	0.21	0.03	0.41
Facility RVU	Work	PE	MP	Total
51736	0.17	0.2	0.02	0.39
51741	0.17	0.21	0.03	0.41

	FUD	Status	MUE	Modifiers				IOM Reference
51736	N/A	A	1(3)	51	N/A	N/A	80*	None
51741	N/A	A	1(3)	51	N/A	N/A	N/A	

* with documentation

51840-51841

51840 Anterior vesicourethropexy, or urethropexy (eg, Marshall-Marchetti-Krantz, Burch); simple
51841 complicated (eg, secondary repair)

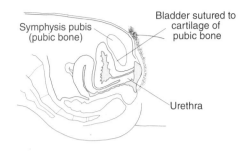

Symphysis pubis (pubic bone)
Bladder sutured to cartilage of pubic bone
Urethra

Explanation

The physician performs a vesicourethropexy or urethropexy in the Marshall-Marchetti-Krantz or Burch style. The physician makes a small horizontal incision in the abdomen above the symphysis pubis, which is the midline junction of the pubic bones at the front. The bladder is suspended by placing several sutures through the tissue surrounding the urethra and into the vaginal wall. The sutures are pulled tight so that the tissues are tacked to the symphysis pubis and the urethra is moved forward. The incision is closed by suturing. 51841 is used when the procedure is performed for the second time or if some other factor increases the time or level of complexity.

Coding Tips

When 51840 or 51841 is performed with another separately identifiable procedure, the highest dollar value code is listed as the primary procedure and subsequent procedures are appended with modifier 51. When reporting 51841, the operative and diagnostic documentation should support the complicated procedure. For a urethropexy with a hysterectomy, see 58152 or 58267. Use 57289, 58152, or 58267 if suspension of the urethra is performed with a hysterectomy. For plastic repair and reconstruction of the female urethra only, see 53430.

ICD-10-CM Diagnostic Codes

N39.3	Stress incontinence (female) (male)

AMA: 51840 2018,Jan,8; 2017,Jan,8; 2016,Jan,13; 2015,Jan,16; 2014,Jan,11
51841 2018,Jan,8; 2017,Jan,8; 2016,Jan,13; 2015,Jan,16; 2014,Jan,11

Relative Value Units/Medicare Edits

Non-Facility RVU	Work	PE	MP	Total
51840	11.36	6.87	1.47	19.7
51841	13.68	7.56	1.57	22.81
Facility RVU	Work	PE	MP	Total
51840	11.36	6.87	1.47	19.7
51841	13.68	7.56	1.57	22.81

	FUD	Status	MUE	Modifiers				IOM Reference
51840	90	A	1(2)	51	N/A	62*	80	None
51841	90	A	1(2)	51	N/A	62*	80	

* with documentation

Bladder

51845

51845 Abdomino-vaginal vesical neck suspension, with or without endoscopic control (eg, Stamey, Raz, modified Pereyra)

1. A common approach involves placing sutures from the pubic bone on both sides of the bladder neck through the vagina

2. The bladder neck and continence are restored, vagina is suspended

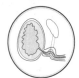

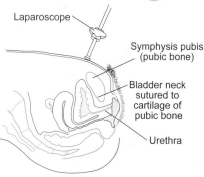

Laparoscope

Symphysis pubis (pubic bone)

Bladder neck sutured to cartilage of pubic bone

Urethra

Explanation

The physician surgically suspends the bladder neck by suturing surrounding tissue to the fibrous membranes (fascia) of the abdomen in a female patient. After inserting a catheter through the urethra to visualize the bladder neck, the physician makes an incision in the vagina, extending it upward toward the base of the bladder. On both sides of the vesical neck, the physician passes a needle through a small incision in the skin above the pubic bone down through the vaginal incision. The physician threads the needle in the vagina and pulls the needle back through the suprapubic incision. Dacron tubing may be threaded onto the sutures to provide extra periurethral support. The physician repeats this process, using an endoscope to ensure proper placement of the suspending sutures. After placing sutures on both sides of the bladder neck, the physician uses moderate upward traction to tighten the bladder neck. The physician inserts a drain tube, bringing it out through a stab incision in the skin, and performs a layered closure.

Coding Tips

Report 51840–51841 if the urethra is suspended from the pubic bone by sutures through the vaginal wall and pubic bone. Use 57289 if a Pereyra type operation is done. For laparoscopic repair of stress incontinence only, see 51990 and 51992.

ICD-10-CM Diagnostic Codes

N39.3   Stress incontinence (female) (male)

AMA: 51845 2018,Jan,8; 2017,Jan,8; 2016,Jan,13; 2015,Jan,16; 2014,Jan,11

Relative Value Units/Medicare Edits

Non-Facility RVU	Work	PE	MP	Total
51845	10.15	5.49	1.16	16.8
Facility RVU	Work	PE	MP	Total
51845	10.15	5.49	1.16	16.8

	FUD	Status	MUE	Modifiers				IOM Reference
51845	90	A	1(2)	51	N/A	62*	80	None

* with documentation

Terms To Know

Raz procedure. Abdominovaginal vesicle neck suspension procedure to control female urinary stress incontinence. The bladder neck is suspended by suturing surrounding tissue through an incision in the vagina near the base of the bladder to the fibrous membranes (fascia) of the abdomen.

Stamey procedure. Abdomino-vaginal vesicle neck suspension procedure to control female urinary stress incontinence. The bladder neck is suspended by suturing surrounding tissue through an incision in the vagina near the base of the bladder to the fibrous membranes (fascia) of the abdomen.

stress incontinence. Involuntary escape of urine at times of minor stress against the bladder, such as coughing, sneezing, or laughing.

suspension. Fixation of an organ for support; temporary state of cessation of an activity, process, or experience.

Bladder

51900

51900 Closure of vesicovaginal fistula, abdominal approach

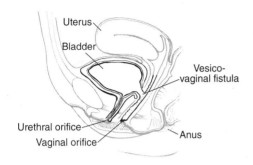

Explanation

The physician closes a vesicovaginal fistula, which is an abnormal passage between the bladder and the vagina. This procedure is done through the abdomen. The fistula and surrounding scar tissue of the vaginal wall are usually excised. The physician makes an incision in the skin, muscle, and fascia of the abdomen. The bladder wall is opened and the bladder explored. The fistula is excised along with the surrounding tissue. The resulting defect is closed with sutures in multiple layers. In some cases, a pedicle graft of tissue may be sutured between the bladder and the vagina. A urethral or suprapubic catheter is left in the bladder to prevent distension of the bladder and tension to the sutured areas.

Coding Tips

For a vaginal approach, see 57320 and 57330. For closure of a vesicouterine fistula, see 51920 or 51925.

ICD-10-CM Diagnostic Codes

N82.0   Vesicovaginal fistula ♀

AMA: 51900 2014,Jan,11

Relative Value Units/Medicare Edits

Non-Facility RVU	Work	PE	MP	Total
51900	14.63	7.49	1.68	23.8
Facility RVU	**Work**	**PE**	**MP**	**Total**
51900	14.63	7.49	1.68	23.8

	FUD	Status	MUE	Modifiers				IOM Reference
51900	90	A	1(3)	51	N/A	62*	80	None

*with documentation

Terms To Know

approach. Method or anatomical location used to gain access to a body organ or specific area for procedures. The approach is not coded separately although it may be a specified component of the procedure, such as laparoscopic versus incisional, or spinal procedures in which the amount of dissection required to expose the spine significantly alters with the site of approach.

vesicovaginal fistula. Abnormal communication between the bladder and the vagina that is the most common genital fistula, often with urinary leakage causing skin irritation of the vulva and thighs, or total incontinence.

51920-51925

51920 Closure of vesicouterine fistula;
51925   with hysterectomy

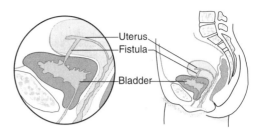

Fistula between uterus and bladder

Explanation

The physician excises an abnormal opening between the uterus and the bladder, then sutures the clean tissues together closing the resulting defect and creating a smooth surface. In 51920, the procedure is done through the bladder with a small abdominal incision or during a laparotomy. In 51925, the physician completes the fistula closure and also removes the uterus through a small horizontal incision just above the pubic hairline. To remove the uterus, the supporting pedicles containing the tubes, ligaments, and arteries are clamped and cut free. The uterus and cervix are removed along with a narrow rim or cuff of vaginal lining. The vaginal defect may be left open for drainage. The abdominal incision is closed by suturing.

Coding Tips

When both a vesicouterine fistula closure and a hysterectomy are performed, only 51925 should be reported. When 51920 or 51925 is performed with another separately identifiable procedure, the highest dollar value code is listed as the primary procedure and subsequent procedures are appended with modifier 51. For closure of a vesicovaginal fistula, abdominal approach, see 51900; by vaginal approach, see 57320 and 57330.

ICD-10-CM Diagnostic Codes

N82.1   Other female urinary-genital tract fistulae ♀

AMA: 51920 2014,Jan,11 **51925** 2014,Jan,11

Relative Value Units/Medicare Edits

Non-Facility RVU	Work	PE	MP	Total
51920	13.41	7.09	1.53	22.03
51925	17.53	10.45	2.75	30.73
Facility RVU	**Work**	**PE**	**MP**	**Total**
51920	13.41	7.09	1.53	22.03
51925	17.53	10.45	2.75	30.73

	FUD	Status	MUE	Modifiers				IOM Reference
51920	90	A	1(3)	51	N/A	62*	80	None
51925	90	A	1(2)	51	N/A	62*	80	

*with documentation

51990-51992

51990 Laparoscopy, surgical; urethral suspension for stress incontinence
51992 sling operation for stress incontinence (eg, fascia or synthetic)

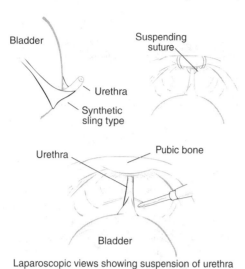

Laparoscopic views showing suspension of urethra

Explanation

The physician makes a 1 cm incision just below the umbilicus through which a fiberoptic laparoscope is inserted. A second incision is made on the left or right side of the abdomen and a second instrument is passed into the abdomen. The physician manipulates the tools so that the pelvic organs can be observed through the laparoscope. The bladder is suspended by placing several sutures through the tissue surrounding the urethra and into support structures. The sutures are pulled tight so that the urethra is elevated and moved forward. In 51992, a sling is placed under the junction of the urethra and bladder. A catheter is inserted into the bladder and an incision is made in the anterior wall of the vagina. Tissue is folded and tacked around the urethra. A sling is formed out of synthetic material or from fascia harvested from the sheath of the rectus abdominis muscle. The loop end of the sling is sutured around the junction of the urethra. An incision is made into the lower abdomen and the ends of the sling are grasped with a clamp and pulled into the incision and sutured to the rectus abdominis sheath. The instruments are removed and incisions are closed with sutures.

Coding Tips

Surgical laparoscopy always includes diagnostic laparoscopy. For removal or revision of sling for stress incontinence, see 57287; open approach for sling procedure, see 57288.

ICD-10-CM Diagnostic Codes

N39.3   Stress incontinence (female) (male)
N39.46   Mixed incontinence

AMA: 51990 2019,Feb,10; 2018,Jan,8; 2017,Jan,8; 2016,Jan,13; 2015,Jan,16; 2014,Jan,11 **51992** 2019,Feb,10; 2018,Jan,8; 2017,Jan,8; 2016,Jan,13; 2015,Jan,16; 2014,Jan,11

Relative Value Units/Medicare Edits

Non-Facility RVU	Work	PE	MP	Total
51990	13.36	6.62	1.61	21.59
51992	14.87	7.31	2.12	24.3
Facility RVU	Work	PE	MP	Total
51990	13.36	6.62	1.61	21.59
51992	14.87	7.31	2.12	24.3

	FUD	Status	MUE	Modifiers				IOM Reference
51990	90	A	1(2)	51	N/A	62*	80	100-03,230.10
51992	90	A	1(2)	51	N/A	62*	80	

* with documentation

Terms To Know

mixed incontinence. Type of incontinence that reflects a combination of symptoms from two different types of incontinence: stress and urge incontinence. Stress urinary incontinence results from an increase of pressure on the bladder from actions such as coughing, laughing, or sneezing and urge incontinence is characterized by a sudden and strong need to urinate.

sling operation. Procedure to correct urinary incontinence. A sling of fascia or synthetic material is placed under the junction of the urethra and bladder in females, or across the muscles surrounding the urethra in males.

stress incontinence. Involuntary escape of urine at times of minor stress against the bladder, such as coughing, sneezing, or laughing.

suspension. Fixation of an organ for support; temporary state of cessation of an activity, process, or experience.

52000

52000 Cystourethroscopy (separate procedure)

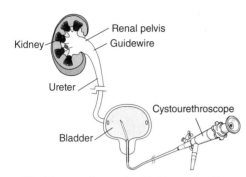

Physician examines ureter, bladder, and urethra

Explanation

The physician examines the urethra, bladder, and ureteric openings into the bladder with a cystourethroscope passed through the urethra and bladder. No other procedure is performed at this time. After examination, the physician removes the cystourethroscope.

Coding Tips

This separate procedure by definition is usually a component of a more complex service and is not identified separately. When performed alone or with other unrelated procedures/services it may be reported. If performed alone, list the code; if performed with other procedures/services, list the code and append modifier 59 or an X{EPSU} modifier. When 52000 is performed with another separately identifiable procedure, the highest dollar value code is listed as the primary procedure and subsequent procedures are appended with modifier 51. If a microscope is attached to the cystourethroscope, it is not reported separately. Do not report 52000 with 52001, 52320, 52325, 52327, 52330, 52332, 52334, 52341, 52342, 52343, 52356, 57240, 57260, or 57265 when the services are performed together on the same side. Local anesthesia is included in this service. However, this procedure may be performed under general anesthesia, depending on the age and/or condition of the patient.

ICD-10-CM Diagnostic Codes

C67.0	Malignant neoplasm of trigone of bladder
C67.1	Malignant neoplasm of dome of bladder
C67.2	Malignant neoplasm of lateral wall of bladder
C67.3	Malignant neoplasm of anterior wall of bladder
C67.4	Malignant neoplasm of posterior wall of bladder
C67.5	Malignant neoplasm of bladder neck
C67.6	Malignant neoplasm of ureteric orifice
C67.8	Malignant neoplasm of overlapping sites of bladder
C68.0	Malignant neoplasm of urethra
C79.11	Secondary malignant neoplasm of bladder
C79.19	Secondary malignant neoplasm of other urinary organs
D09.0	Carcinoma in situ of bladder
D09.19	Carcinoma in situ of other urinary organs
D30.3	Benign neoplasm of bladder
D30.4	Benign neoplasm of urethra
D41.3	Neoplasm of uncertain behavior of urethra
D41.4	Neoplasm of uncertain behavior of bladder
D49.4	Neoplasm of unspecified behavior of bladder

D49.59	Neoplasm of unspecified behavior of other genitourinary organ
N11.8	Other chronic tubulo-interstitial nephritis
N30.10	Interstitial cystitis (chronic) without hematuria
N30.11	Interstitial cystitis (chronic) with hematuria
N30.20	Other chronic cystitis without hematuria
N30.21	Other chronic cystitis with hematuria
N30.30	Trigonitis without hematuria
N30.31	Trigonitis with hematuria
N30.40	Irradiation cystitis without hematuria
N30.41	Irradiation cystitis with hematuria
N30.80	Other cystitis without hematuria
N30.81	Other cystitis with hematuria
N31.8	Other neuromuscular dysfunction of bladder
N32.0	Bladder-neck obstruction
N32.1	Vesicointestinal fistula
N32.3	Diverticulum of bladder
N32.81	Overactive bladder
N32.89	Other specified disorders of bladder
N34.0	Urethral abscess
N34.1	Nonspecific urethritis
N34.2	Other urethritis
N35.021	Urethral stricture due to childbirth ♀
N35.028	Other post-traumatic urethral stricture, female ♀
N35.12	Postinfective urethral stricture, not elsewhere classified, female ♀
N35.82	Other urethral stricture, female ♀
N36.0	Urethral fistula
N36.1	Urethral diverticulum
N36.2	Urethral caruncle
N36.41	Hypermobility of urethra
N36.42	Intrinsic sphincter deficiency (ISD)
N36.43	Combined hypermobility of urethra and intrinsic sphincter deficiency
N36.44	Muscular disorders of urethra
N36.5	Urethral false passage
N36.8	Other specified disorders of urethra
N39.3	Stress incontinence (female) (male)
N39.41	Urge incontinence
N39.42	Incontinence without sensory awareness
N39.43	Post-void dribbling
N39.44	Nocturnal enuresis
N39.45	Continuous leakage
N39.46	Mixed incontinence
N39.490	Overflow incontinence
N39.491	Coital incontinence
N39.492	Postural (urinary) incontinence
N39.498	Other specified urinary incontinence
N39.8	Other specified disorders of urinary system
N82.0	Vesicovaginal fistula ♀
N82.1	Other female urinary-genital tract fistulae ♀
N99.12	Postprocedural urethral stricture, female ♀
Q64.11	Supravesical fissure of urinary bladder
Q64.12	Cloacal exstrophy of urinary bladder
Q64.19	Other exstrophy of urinary bladder

Bladder

Q64.2	Congenital posterior urethral valves
Q64.31	Congenital bladder neck obstruction
Q64.32	Congenital stricture of urethra
Q64.33	Congenital stricture of urinary meatus
Q64.39	Other atresia and stenosis of urethra and bladder neck
Q64.5	Congenital absence of bladder and urethra
Q64.6	Congenital diverticulum of bladder
Q64.71	Congenital prolapse of urethra
Q64.72	Congenital prolapse of urinary meatus
Q64.73	Congenital urethrorectal fistula
Q64.74	Double urethra
Q64.75	Double urinary meatus
Q64.79	Other congenital malformations of bladder and urethra
R30.0	Dysuria
R30.1	Vesical tenesmus
R31.0	Gross hematuria
R31.1	Benign essential microscopic hematuria
R31.21	Asymptomatic microscopic hematuria
R31.29	Other microscopic hematuria
R33.8	Other retention of urine
R34	Anuria and oliguria
R82.71	Bacteriuria
R82.79	Other abnormal findings on microbiological examination of urine
S37.29XA	Other injury of bladder, initial encounter
S37.39XA	Other injury of urethra, initial encounter
T19.0XXA	Foreign body in urethra, initial encounter
T19.1XXA	Foreign body in bladder, initial encounter
Z03.823	Encounter for observation for suspected inserted (injected) foreign body ruled out

AMA: 52000 2019,Feb,10; 2018,Nov,10; 2018,Jan,8; 2017,Oct,9; 2017,Jan,8; 2016,Jan,13; 2015,Jan,16; 2014,May,3; 2014,Jan,11

Relative Value Units/Medicare Edits

Non-Facility RVU	Work	PE	MP	Total
52000	1.53	4.28	0.18	5.99
Facility RVU	**Work**	**PE**	**MP**	**Total**
52000	1.53	0.62	0.18	2.33

	FUD	Status	MUE	Modifiers			IOM Reference
52000	0	A	1(3)	51	N/A	N/A	N/A	None

* with documentation

53060

53060   Drainage of Skene's gland abscess or cyst

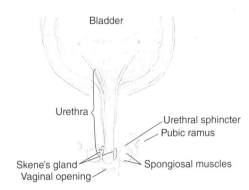

Frontal section of the female bladder and urethra
showing Skene's (or paraurethral) gland

Explanation

The physician drains an abscess or a cyst of the Skene's gland, the paraurethral glands in the female. The physician makes an incision through the skin, subcutaneous tissue, and overlying layers of muscle, fat, and tissue (fascia) over the site of the abscess. By blunt or sharp dissection, the incision is carried into the abscess or cyst. Several drains are inserted and the incision is closed in layers.

Coding Tips

For removal or destruction by electric current (fulguration) of Skene's glands, see 53270. Local anesthesia is included in this service. However, this procedure may be performed under general anesthesia, depending on the age and/or condition of the patient. For drainage of a subcutaneous abscess, see 10060–10061. Dilation or manipulation of the urethra is not separately identified. Surgical trays, A4550, are not separately reimbursed by Medicare; however, other third-party payers may cover them. Check with the specific payer to determine coverage.

ICD-10-CM Diagnostic Codes

N34.0   Urethral abscess
N36.8   Other specified disorders of urethra

AMA: 53060 2014,Jan,11

Relative Value Units/Medicare Edits

Non-Facility RVU	Work	PE	MP	Total
53060	2.68	2.27	0.43	5.38
Facility RVU	**Work**	**PE**	**MP**	**Total**
53060	2.68	1.69	0.43	4.8

	FUD	Status	MUE	Modifiers			IOM Reference
53060	10	A	1(3)	51	N/A	N/A	N/A	None

* with documentation

Terms To Know

abscess. Circumscribed collection of pus resulting from bacteria, frequently associated with swelling and other signs of inflammation.

Skene's gland. Paraurethral ducts that drain a group of the female urethral glands into the vestibule.

53230

53230   Excision of urethral diverticulum (separate procedure); female

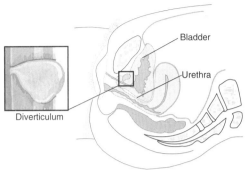

A diverticulum of the urethra is excised. Typically the
urethra is reconstructed around a temporary catheter

Explanation

The physician removes a urethral diverticulum. A longitudinal incision is made in the anterior vaginal wall and the urethral diverticulum is separated from the vaginal wall by a combination of blunt and sharp dissection. The urethra may be opened back to the orifice of the diverticulum in order to facilitate identification. A balloon catheter may be inserted and inflated. Once the diverticulum has been excised, the urethra is closed over a catheter and the vaginal wall is repaired with a layered closure.

Coding Tips

This separate procedure by definition is usually a component of a more complex service and is not identified separately. When performed alone or with other unrelated procedures or services it may be reported. If performed alone, list the code; if performed with other procedures/services, list the code and append modifier 59 or an X{EPSU} modifier. Dilation or manipulation of the urethra is not reported separately. For marsupialization of the urethral diverticulum, see 53240. For excision or fulguration of urethral polyps, see 53260. Surgical trays, A4550, are not separately reimbursed by Medicare; however, other third-party payers may cover them. Check with the specific payer to determine coverage.

ICD-10-CM Diagnostic Codes

N36.1   Urethral diverticulum

AMA: 53230 2014,Jan,11

Relative Value Units/Medicare Edits

Non-Facility RVU	Work	PE	MP	Total
53230	10.44	5.86	1.28	17.58
Facility RVU	**Work**	**PE**	**MP**	**Total**
53230	10.44	5.86	1.28	17.58

	FUD	Status	MUE	Modifiers			IOM Reference
53230	90	A	1(3)	51	N/A	62*	80	None

* with documentation

Terms To Know

diverticulum. Pouch or sac in the walls of an organ or canal.

excision. Surgical removal of an organ or tissue.

Urethra

53240

53240 Marsupialization of urethral diverticulum, male or female

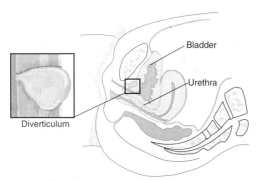

Physician converts the diverticulum
into a depression (marsupialization)

Explanation

The physician repairs a urethral diverticulum by creating a pouch
(marsupialization). In a female patient, a longitudinal incision is made in the
anterior vaginal wall of the female and the borders of the urethral diverticulum
are raised and sutured to create a pouch. The interior of the sac separates and
gradually closes by granulation. The urethra is closed over a catheter and the
vaginal wall is repaired with a layered closure.

Coding Tips

Dilation or manipulation of the urethra and vagina is not reported separately.
For excision of urethral diverticulum, see 53230. For excision or fulguration of
urethral polyps, or urethral caruncle, see 53260 or 53265.

ICD-10-CM Diagnostic Codes

N36.1   Urethral diverticulum

AMA: 53240 2014,Jan,11

Relative Value Units/Medicare Edits

Non-Facility RVU	Work	PE	MP	Total
53240	7.08	4.35	0.79	12.22
Facility RVU	**Work**	**PE**	**MP**	**Total**
53240	7.08	4.35	0.79	12.22

	FUD	Status	MUE	Modifiers				IOM Reference
53240	90	A	1(3)	51	N/A	N/A	N/A	None

* with documentation

Terms To Know

diverticulum. Pouch or sac in the walls of an organ or canal.

marsupialization. Creation of a pouch in surgical treatment of a cyst in which
one wall is resected and the remaining cut edges are sutured to adjacent tissue
creating an open pouch of the previously enclosed cyst.

urethra. Small tube lined with mucous membrane that leads from the bladder
to the exterior of the body.

urethral diverticulum. Abnormal outpouching in the urethral wall that
causes urinary urgency and frequency, persistent urinary tract infections, a
weak stream with post-void dribbling, discomfort, or incontinence.

92

53260-53275

53260 Excision or fulguration; urethral polyp(s), distal urethra
53265   urethral caruncle
53270   Skene's glands
53275   urethral prolapse

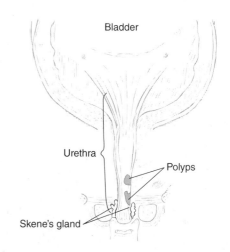

Explanation

The physician removes urethral polyps, caruncles, Skene's glands or treats
urethral prolapse. The physician separates the urethra from the vaginal wall.
The urethra is incised. A circular excision is made around the lesion and the
targeted tissue is resected. The urethra and vaginal mucosa are reattached in
layers. Report 53260 if removing distal urethral polyps; 53265 if removing a
urethral caruncle; 53270 if removing the Skene's glands; or 53275 if treating
urethral prolapse.

Coding Tips

Report 52285 if fulguration of urethral polyps is part of the treatment for
female urethral syndrome. For drainage of an abscess or a cyst of the Skene's
gland, see 53060. For fulguration via an endoscopic approach, see 52214 and
52224.

ICD-10-CM Diagnostic Codes

C68.1   Malignant neoplasm of paraurethral glands
C79.19   Secondary malignant neoplasm of other urinary organs
D09.19   Carcinoma in situ of other urinary organs
D30.8   Benign neoplasm of other specified urinary organs
D41.8   Neoplasm of uncertain behavior of other specified urinary organs
D49.59   Neoplasm of unspecified behavior of other genitourinary organ
N34.0   Urethral abscess
N36.2   Urethral caruncle
N36.8   Other specified disorders of urethra
Q64.71   Congenital prolapse of urethra

AMA: 53260 2014,Jan,11 **53265** 2014,Jan,11 **53270** 2014,Jan,11 **53275**
2014,Jan,11

Relative Value Units/Medicare Edits

Non-Facility RVU	Work	PE	MP	Total
53260	3.03	2.45	0.39	5.87
53265	3.17	2.87	0.41	6.45
53270	3.14	2.49	0.35	5.98
53275	4.57	2.47	0.54	7.58
Facility RVU	**Work**	**PE**	**MP**	**Total**
53260	3.03	1.8	0.39	5.22
53265	3.17	1.84	0.41	5.42
53270	3.14	1.81	0.35	5.3
53275	4.57	2.47	0.54	7.58

	FUD	Status	MUE	Modifiers				IOM Reference
53260	10	A	1(2)	51	N/A	N/A	N/A	None
53265	10	A	1(3)	51	N/A	N/A	N/A	
53270	10	A	1(2)	51	N/A	N/A	N/A	
53275	10	A	1(2)	51	N/A	N/A	N/A	

* with documentation

Terms To Know

abscess. Circumscribed collection of pus resulting from bacteria, frequently associated with swelling and other signs of inflammation.

anomaly. Irregularity in the structure or position of an organ or tissue.

congenital. Present at birth, occurring through heredity or an influence during gestation up to the moment of birth.

distal. Located farther away from a specified reference point or the trunk.

excision. Surgical removal of an organ or tissue.

fulguration. Destruction of living tissue by using sparks from a high-frequency electric current.

polyp. Small growth on a stalk-like attachment projecting from a mucous membrane.

prolapse. Falling, sliding, or sinking of an organ from its normal location in the body.

resect. Cutting out or removing a portion or all of a bone, organ, or other structure.

Skene's gland. Paraurethral ducts that drain a group of the female urethral glands into the vestibule.

urethra. Small tube lined with mucous membrane that leads from the bladder to the exterior of the body.

urethral caruncle. Small, polyp-like growth of a deep red color found in women on the mucous membrane of the urethral opening.

53430

53430   Urethroplasty, reconstruction of female urethra

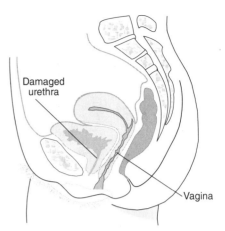

A flap of vaginal tissue is used to construct a new urethra

Explanation

The physician uses perineal or vaginal tissue to reconstruct the female urethra. With the patient in the lithotomy position and a catheter in the urethra, the physician cuts an inverted U-shaped flap above the urethral meatus and extending on the anterior vaginal wall. This flap is undermined with sharp dissection and spreading of the scissors around the upper portion of the urethral meatus, leaving a strip attached. The flap is sutured into a tube shape, reconstructing the distal urethra. The vaginal wall on each side is brought together in several layers to cover the new urethra. Small submucosal vessels are cauterized and a drain may be placed for one to two days.

Coding Tips

For suture of a urethral wound or injury, see 53502.

ICD-10-CM Diagnostic Codes

N35.021	Urethral stricture due to childbirth ♀
N35.028	Other post-traumatic urethral stricture, female ♀
N35.12	Postinfective urethral stricture, not elsewhere classified, female ♀
N35.82	Other urethral stricture, female ♀
N99.12	Postprocedural urethral stricture, female ♀

AMA: 53430 2014,Jan,11

Relative Value Units/Medicare Edits

Non-Facility RVU	Work	PE	MP	Total
53430	17.43	8.41	2.23	28.07
Facility RVU	**Work**	**PE**	**MP**	**Total**
53430	17.43	8.41	2.23	28.07

	FUD	Status	MUE	Modifiers				IOM Reference
53430	90	A	1(2)	51	N/A	62*	80	None

* with documentation

Terms To Know

reconstruction. Recreating, restoring, or rebuilding a body part or organ.

Urethra

53500

53500 Urethrolysis, transvaginal, secondary, open, including cystourethroscopy (eg, postsurgical obstruction, scarring)

Scar tissue or an obstruction of the urethra is removed

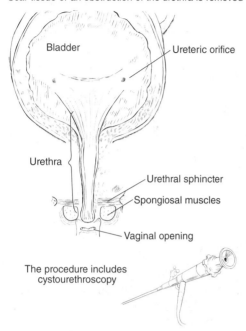

The procedure includes cystourethroscopy

Explanation

Transvaginal, secondary, open urethrolysis is performed in cases when voiding is obstructed due to excessive periurethral scarring caused by previous surgical repair of stress incontinence, procedures such as bladder neck suspension. Urethrolysis involves cutting obstructive adhesions or bands of fibrous tissue that have grown to fix the urethra to the pubic bone. An incision is made through the vagina. The adhering fibrous bands and periurethral scar tissue are visualized and dissected. Lysis and removal continues until the urethra is mobilized away from the surrounding fibrous tissue. Some correction to vaginal abnormalities may be accomplished before closure of the incision. Postsurgical cystourethroscopy is included in this procedure to examine the urethra following urethrolysis.

Coding Tips

Postsurgical diagnostic cystourethroscopy is included in this procedure to examine the urethra following urethrolysis. Urethrolysis performed by retropubic approach is reported with 53899. Do not report 53500 with 52000.

ICD-10-CM Diagnostic Codes

N35.021	Urethral stricture due to childbirth ♀
N35.028	Other post-traumatic urethral stricture, female ♀
N35.12	Postinfective urethral stricture, not elsewhere classified, female ♀
N35.82	Other urethral stricture, female ♀
N36.8	Other specified disorders of urethra
N99.12	Postprocedural urethral stricture, female ♀

AMA: 53500 2018,Jan,8; 2017,Jan,8; 2016,Jan,13; 2015,Jan,16; 2014,Jan,11

Relative Value Units/Medicare Edits

Non-Facility RVU	Work	PE	MP	Total
53500	13.0	6.96	1.69	21.65
Facility RVU	**Work**	**PE**	**MP**	**Total**
53500	13.0	6.96	1.69	21.65

	FUD	Status	MUE	Modifiers				IOM Reference
53500	90	A	1(2)	51	N/A	62*	80	None

* with documentation

Terms To Know

adhesion. Abnormal fibrous connection between two structures, soft tissue or bony structures, that may occur as the result of surgery, infection, or trauma.

connective tissue. Body tissue made from fibroblasts, collagen, and elastic fibrils that connects, supports, and holds together other tissues and cells and includes cartilage, collagenous, fibrous, elastic, and osseous tissue.

dissect. Cut apart or separate tissue for surgical purposes or for visual or microscopic study.

fibrous tissue. Connective tissues.

lysis. Destruction, breakdown, dissolution, or decomposition of cells or substances by a specific catalyzing agent.

obstruction. Blockage that prevents normal function of the valve or structure.

scar tissue. Fibrous connective tissue that forms around a wounded area or injury, composed mainly of fibroblasts or collagenous fibers.

secondary. Second in order of occurrence or importance, or appearing during the course of another disease or condition.

stricture. Narrowing of an anatomical structure.

urethra. Small tube lined with mucous membrane that leads from the bladder to the exterior of the body.

urethrolysis. Procedure performed to cut obstructive adhesions, fibrous bands, or periurethral scar tissue that affix the urethra to the pubic bone, obstructing voiding. This is often caused by previous surgical repair of stress incontinence, such as bladder neck suspension.

53502

53502 Urethrorrhaphy, suture of urethral wound or injury, female

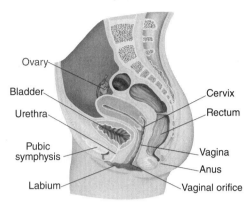

Side view of female anatomy

Explanation

The physician repairs a urethral wound or injury, including the skin and even more traumatic wounds requiring more than a layered closure. Examples include debridement of cuts (lacerations) or tears (avulsion). Suturing of the urethra is done in layers to prevent later complications and fistula formations. The tissue can be constructed around a catheter.

Coding Tips

For plastic repair and reconstruction of the female urethra, see 53430.

ICD-10-CM Diagnostic Codes

N99.71	Accidental puncture and laceration of a genitourinary system organ or structure during a genitourinary system procedure
N99.72	Accidental puncture and laceration of a genitourinary system organ or structure during other procedure
O71.5	Other obstetric injury to pelvic organs ᴹ ♀
S37.32XA	Contusion of urethra, initial encounter
S37.33XA	Laceration of urethra, initial encounter
S37.39XA	Other injury of urethra, initial encounter

AMA: **53502** 2014,Jan,11

Relative Value Units/Medicare Edits

Non-Facility RVU	Work	PE	MP	Total
53502	8.26	4.82	0.93	14.01
Facility RVU	**Work**	**PE**	**MP**	**Total**
53502	8.26	4.82	0.93	14.01

	FUD	Status	MUE	Modifiers				IOM Reference
53502	90	A	1(3)	51	N/A	N/A	N/A	None

* with documentation

Terms To Know

laceration. Tearing injury; a torn, ragged-edged wound.

urethra. Small tube lined with mucous membrane that leads from the bladder to the exterior of the body.

wound. Injury to living tissue often involving a cut or break in the skin.

53660-53665

53660 Dilation of female urethra including suppository and/or instillation; initial
53661   subsequent
53665 Dilation of female urethra, general or conduction (spinal) anesthesia

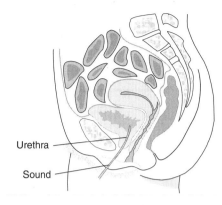

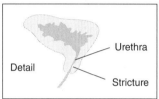

Physician passes a sound through a stricture in the urethra

Explanation

The physician uses dilators of increasing size to widen the female urethra. A suppository or instillation of a saline solution may be used. Report 53660 for initial dilation, and 53661 for subsequent dilation. Use 53665 if general or spinal anesthesia is administered for dilation of female urethral stricture.

Coding Tips

These procedures include insertion of a suppository and/or instillation of a saline solution and are usually performed with local anesthesia. For urethral catheterization, see 51701–51703.

ICD-10-CM Diagnostic Codes

N35.021	Urethral stricture due to childbirth ♀
N35.028	Other post-traumatic urethral stricture, female ♀
N35.12	Postinfective urethral stricture, not elsewhere classified, female ♀
N35.82	Other urethral stricture, female ♀
N99.12	Postprocedural urethral stricture, female ♀
Q64.31	Congenital bladder neck obstruction
Q64.32	Congenital stricture of urethra
Q64.39	Other atresia and stenosis of urethra and bladder neck

AMA: **53660** 2014,Jan,11 **53661** 2014,Jan,11 **53665** 2014,Jan,11

Urethra

Relative Value Units/Medicare Edits

Non-Facility RVU	Work	PE	MP	Total
53660	0.71	1.22	0.09	2.02
53661	0.72	1.18	0.09	1.99
53665	0.76	0.26	0.09	1.11
Facility RVU	Work	PE	MP	Total
53660	0.71	0.4	0.09	1.2
53661	0.72	0.36	0.09	1.17
53665	0.76	0.26	0.09	1.11

	FUD	Status	MUE	Modifiers				IOM Reference
53660	0	A	1(2)	51	N/A	N/A	N/A	None
53661	0	A	1(3)	51	N/A	N/A	N/A	
53665	0	A	1(3)	51	N/A	N/A	N/A	

* with documentation

Terms To Know

atresia. Congenital closure or absence of a tubular organ or an opening to the body surface.

cystitis. Inflammation of the urinary bladder. Symptoms include dysuria, frequency of urination, urgency, and hematuria.

dilation. Artificial increase in the diameter of an opening or lumen made by medication or by instrumentation.

initial. First stage in a series of events.

instillation. Administering a liquid slowly over time, drop by drop.

stenosis. Narrowing or constriction of a passage.

suppository. Medication in the form of a solid mass at room temperature that dissolves at body temperature, for insertion into a body orifice such as the rectal, vaginal, or urethral opening.

trigonitis. Inflammation of the triangular area of mucous membrane at the base of the bladder, called the trigonum vesicae.

53860

53860   Transurethral radiofrequency micro-remodeling of the female bladder neck and proximal urethra for stress urinary incontinence

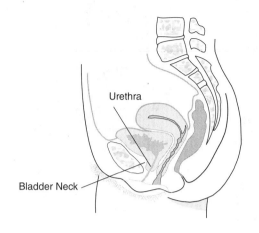

Urethra

Bladder Neck

Explanation

The physician uses radiofrequency energy to treat female stress urinary incontinence, the involuntary loss of urine from the urethra due to increased intra-abdominal pressure. Using a small transurethral probe, the physician applies low temperature radiofrequency energy to targeted submucosal areas of the bladder neck and urethra. This results in minute structural alterations to the collagen that, upon healing, makes the tissues firmer and increases the resistance to involuntary leakage.

Coding Tips

When this procedure is performed with another separately identifiable procedure, the highest dollar value code is listed as the primary procedure and the subsequent procedures are appended with modifier 51.

ICD-10-CM Diagnostic Codes

N39.3   Stress incontinence (female) (male)
N39.46   Mixed incontinence

AMA: 53860 2014,Jan,11

Relative Value Units/Medicare Edits

Non-Facility RVU	Work	PE	MP	Total
53860	3.97	55.34	0.46	59.77
Facility RVU	Work	PE	MP	Total
53860	3.97	2.02	0.46	6.45

	FUD	Status	MUE	Modifiers				IOM Reference
53860	90	A	1(2)	51	N/A	N/A	80*	None

* with documentation

Terms To Know

mixed incontinence. Type of incontinence that reflects a combination of symptoms from two different types of incontinence: stress and urge incontinence. Stress urinary incontinence results from an increase of pressure on the bladder from actions such as coughing, laughing, or sneezing and urge incontinence is characterized by a sudden and strong need to urinate.

Urethra

55920

55920 Placement of needles or catheters into pelvic organs and/or genitalia (except prostate) for subsequent interstitial radioelement application

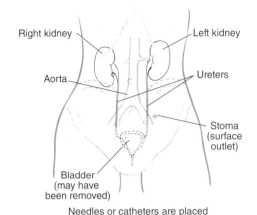

Needles or catheters are placed in the genitalia or pelvic organs

Explanation

The physician places needles or catheters into the pelvic organs and/or genitalia for subsequent interstitial radioelement application. The radioactive isotopes that are introduced subsequently, such as iodine-125 or palladium-103, are contained within tiny seeds that are left in place to deliver radiation over a period of months. They do not cause any harm after becoming inert. This method provides radiation to the prescribed body area while minimizing exposure to normal tissue.

Coding Tips

For insertion of a uterine tandem and/or vaginal ovoids for clinical brachytherapy, see 57155. For insertion of Heyman capsules for clinical brachytherapy, see 58346.

ICD-10-CM Diagnostic Codes

C20	Malignant neoplasm of rectum
C21.1	Malignant neoplasm of anal canal
C21.2	Malignant neoplasm of cloacogenic zone
C21.8	Malignant neoplasm of overlapping sites of rectum, anus and anal canal
C49.8	Malignant neoplasm of overlapping sites of connective and soft tissue
C49.A5	Gastrointestinal stromal tumor of rectum
C51.0	Malignant neoplasm of labium majus ♀
C51.1	Malignant neoplasm of labium minus ♀
C51.2	Malignant neoplasm of clitoris ♀
C51.8	Malignant neoplasm of overlapping sites of vulva ♀
C52	Malignant neoplasm of vagina ♀
C53.0	Malignant neoplasm of endocervix ♀
C53.1	Malignant neoplasm of exocervix ♀
C53.8	Malignant neoplasm of overlapping sites of cervix uteri ♀
C54.0	Malignant neoplasm of isthmus uteri ♀
C54.1	Malignant neoplasm of endometrium ♀
C54.2	Malignant neoplasm of myometrium ♀
C54.3	Malignant neoplasm of fundus uteri ♀
C54.8	Malignant neoplasm of overlapping sites of corpus uteri ♀
C56.1	Malignant neoplasm of right ovary ♀ ☑
C56.2	Malignant neoplasm of left ovary ♀ ☑
C57.01	Malignant neoplasm of right fallopian tube ♀ ☑
C57.02	Malignant neoplasm of left fallopian tube ♀ ☑
C57.11	Malignant neoplasm of right broad ligament ♀ ☑
C57.12	Malignant neoplasm of left broad ligament ♀ ☑
C57.21	Malignant neoplasm of right round ligament ♀ ☑
C57.22	Malignant neoplasm of left round ligament ♀ ☑
C57.3	Malignant neoplasm of parametrium ♀
C57.7	Malignant neoplasm of other specified female genital organs ♀
C57.8	Malignant neoplasm of overlapping sites of female genital organs ♀
C58	Malignant neoplasm of placenta ⓜ ♀
C76.3	Malignant neoplasm of pelvis
C79.82	Secondary malignant neoplasm of genital organs
C7A.026	Malignant carcinoid tumor of the rectum
D01.2	Carcinoma in situ of rectum
D01.3	Carcinoma in situ of anus and anal canal

AMA: **55920** 2018,Jan,8; 2017,Jan,8; 2016,Jan,13; 2015,Jan,16; 2014,Jan,11

Relative Value Units/Medicare Edits

Non-Facility RVU	Work	PE	MP	Total
55920	8.31	4.14	0.64	13.09
Facility RVU	**Work**	**PE**	**MP**	**Total**
55920	8.31	4.14	0.64	13.09

	FUD	Status	MUE	Modifiers				IOM Reference
55920	0	A	1(2)	51	N/A	N/A	80*	None

* with documentation

Terms To Know

catheter. Flexible tube inserted into an area of the body for introducing or withdrawing fluid.

interstitial radiation. Radioactive source placed into the tissue being treated.

isotope. Chemical element possessing the same atomic number (protons in the nucleus) as another, but with a different atomic weight (number of neutrons).

radioelement. Any element that emits particle or electromagnetic radiations from nuclear disintegration, occurring naturally in any element with an atomic number above 83.

Reproductive

56405

56405   Incision and drainage of vulva or perineal abscess

An abscess of the vulva or perineum is drained

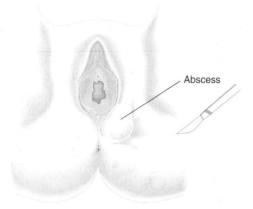

The wound may be packed with gauze

Explanation

The vulva includes the labia majora, labia minora, mons pubis, bulb of the vestibule, vestibule of the vagina, greater and lesser vestibular glands, and vaginal orifice. The perineum is the area between the vulva and the anus. The physician makes an incision into the abscess at its softest point and drains the purulent contents. The cavity of the abscess is flushed and often packed with medicated gauze to facilitate drainage.

Coding Tips

For incision and drainage of a sebaceous, cutaneous, or subcutaneous cyst, furuncle, or abscess, see 10040, 10060, and 10061. For drainage of a Skene's gland abscess or cyst, see 53060.

ICD-10-CM Diagnostic Codes

L02.215   Cutaneous abscess of perineum
N76.4   Abscess of vulva ♀

AMA: 56405 2019,Jul,6; 2014,Jan,11

Relative Value Units/Medicare Edits

Non-Facility RVU	Work	PE	MP	Total
56405	1.49	1.94	0.26	3.69
Facility RVU	Work	PE	MP	Total
56405	1.49	1.68	0.26	3.43

	FUD	Status	MUE	Modifiers				IOM Reference
56405	10	A	2(3)	51	N/A	62	N/A	None

* with documentation

Terms To Know

abscess. Circumscribed collection of pus resulting from bacteria, frequently associated with swelling and other signs of inflammation.

perineal. Pertaining to the pelvic floor area between the thighs; the diamond-shaped area bordered by the pubic symphysis in front, the ischial tuberosities on the sides, and the coccyx in back.

purulent. Cyst, wound, or any other sore or condition full of or discharging pus.

56420

56420   Incision and drainage of Bartholin's gland abscess

The physician incises and drains
the Bartholin's gland abscess

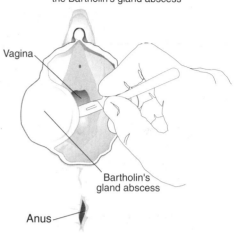

Vagina

Bartholin's
gland abscess

Anus

Explanation

The physician incises and drains a Bartholin's gland abscess. Bartholin's gland is at the end of the bulb of the vestibule of the vagina and is connected by a duct to the mucosa at the opening of the vagina. The physician makes an incision just inside the opening of the vagina through the mucosal surface into the cavity of the abscess to flush and drain it. A small wick or catheter may be left in the cavity to facilitate drainage.

Coding Tips

This is a unilateral procedure. If performed bilaterally, some payers require that the service be reported twice with modifier 50 appended to the second code while others require identification of the service only once with modifier 50 appended. Check with individual payers. Modifier 50 identifies a procedure performed identically on the opposite side of the body (mirror image). For marsupialization of Bartholin's gland, see 56440. For incision and drainage of a vulvar or perineal abscess, see 56405. For incision and drainage of a sebaceous, cutaneous, or subcutaneous cyst, furuncle, or abscess, see 10040 and 10060–10061. If a specimen is transported to an outside laboratory, report 99000 for conveyance.

ICD-10-CM Diagnostic Codes

N75.1   Abscess of Bartholin's gland ♀

AMA: 56420 2019,Jul,6; 2014,Jan,11

Relative Value Units/Medicare Edits

Non-Facility RVU	Work	PE	MP	Total
56420	1.44	2.78	0.25	4.47
Facility RVU	Work	PE	MP	Total
56420	1.44	1.28	0.25	2.97

	FUD	Status	MUE	Modifiers				IOM Reference
56420	10	A	1(3)	51	N/A	N/A	N/A	None

* with documentation

Vulva

56440

56440   Marsupialization of Bartholin's gland cyst

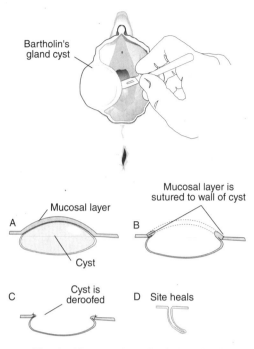

The physician unroofs the Bartholin's gland cyst and sutures the edges of the gland site

A   Mucosal layer / Cyst

B   Mucosal layer is sutured to wall of cyst

C   Cyst is deroofed

D   Site heals

Explanation

The physician treats a Bartholin's gland cyst with marsupialization. Bartholin's gland is at the end of the bulb of the vestibule of the vagina and is connected by a duct to the mucosa at the opening of the vagina. The physician makes an elliptical excision over the center of the Bartholin's gland cyst and drains it. The lining of the cyst is everted and approximated to the vaginal mucosa with sutures creating a pouch. Marsupialization prevents recurrent cysts and infections.

Coding Tips

This is a unilateral procedure. If performed bilaterally, some payers require that the service be reported twice with modifier 50 appended to the second code while others require identification of the service only once with modifier 50 appended. Check with individual payers. Modifier 50 identifies a procedure performed identically on the opposite side of the body (mirror image). For incision and drainage of a Bartholin's gland abscess, see 56420. For incision and drainage of a sebaceous, cutaneous, or subcutaneous cyst, furuncle, or abscess, see 10040, 10060, and 10061. For drainage of a Skene's gland abscess or cyst, see 53060.

ICD-10-CM Diagnostic Codes

N75.0   Cyst of Bartholin's gland ♀

AMA: **56440** 2019,Jul,6; 2014,Jan,11

Relative Value Units/Medicare Edits

Non-Facility RVU	Work	PE	MP	Total
56440	2.89	1.89	0.47	5.25
Facility RVU	**Work**	**PE**	**MP**	**Total**
56440	2.89	1.89	0.47	5.25

	FUD	Status	MUE	Modifiers			IOM Reference
56440	10	A	1(3)	51	N/A	N/A	N/A	None

* with documentation

Terms To Know

Bartholin's gland. Mucous-producing gland found in the vestibular bulbs on either side of the vaginal orifice and connected to the mucosal membrane at the opening by a duct.

cyst. Elevated encapsulated mass containing fluid, semisolid, or solid material with a membranous lining.

incision. Act of cutting into tissue or an organ.

infection. Presence of microorganisms in body tissues that may result in cellular damage.

marsupialization. Creation of a pouch in surgical treatment of a cyst in which one wall is resected and the remaining cut edges are sutured to adjacent tissue creating an open pouch of the previously enclosed cyst.

Vulva

56441

56441   Lysis of labial adhesions

Adhesions between the labial folds are lysed

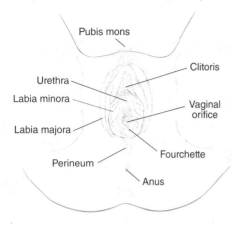

Explanation

The labia majora and minora are the greater and lesser folds of skin on the pudendum on either side of the vagina. The physician separates the labia majora from the labia minora, which are fused by fibrous bands of scar tissue. Using a blunt instrument, probe, scissors, and/or clamp, the labia are separated by breaking or cutting the fibrous tissue. The procedure is accomplished using general or local anesthesia.

Coding Tips

This is a bilateral procedure and as such is reported once even if the procedure is performed on both sides. This is a pediatric surgical procedure commonly performed on young girls who have had adhesions form between the labia minora. For destruction of lesions of the vulva, see 56501–56515.

ICD-10-CM Diagnostic Codes

N90.89	Other specified noninflammatory disorders of vulva and perineum ♀
Q52.5	Fusion of labia ♀

AMA: 56441 2019,Jul,6; 2014,Jan,11

Relative Value Units/Medicare Edits

Non-Facility RVU	Work	PE	MP	Total
56441	2.02	2.42	0.28	4.72
Facility RVU	**Work**	**PE**	**MP**	**Total**
56441	2.02	1.94	0.28	4.24

	FUD	Status	MUE	Modifiers				IOM Reference
56441	10	A	1(2)	51	N/A	N/A	80*	None

* with documentation

Terms To Know

adhesion. Abnormal fibrous connection between two structures, soft tissue or bony structures, that may occur as the result of surgery, infection, or trauma.

scar tissue. Fibrous connective tissue that forms around a wounded area or injury, composed mainly of fibroblasts or collagenous fibers.

56442

56442   Hymenotomy, simple incision

The physician incises the hymen

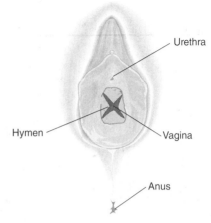

No tissue is removed

Explanation

The physician performs a hymenotomy. A hymen is a membrane that partially or wholly occludes the vaginal opening. Following local injection of an anesthetic, the physician incises the hymenal membrane with a stellate (star-shaped) incision. This procedure is sometimes preceded by aspiration of the intact membrane with a needle and syringe.

Coding Tips

Local anesthesia is included in this service. However, this procedure may be performed under general anesthesia, depending on the age and/or condition of the patient. For partial hymenectomy or revision of the hymenal ring, see 56700. Surgical trays, A4550, are not separately reimbursed by Medicare; however, other third-party payers may cover them. Check with the specific payer to determine coverage.

ICD-10-CM Diagnostic Codes

N89.6	Tight hymenal ring ♀
Q52.3	Imperforate hymen ♀

AMA: 56442 2019,Jul,6; 2014,Jan,11

Relative Value Units/Medicare Edits

Non-Facility RVU	Work	PE	MP	Total
56442	0.68	0.57	0.11	1.36
Facility RVU	**Work**	**PE**	**MP**	**Total**
56442	0.68	0.57	0.11	1.36

	FUD	Status	MUE	Modifiers				IOM Reference
56442	0	A	1(2)	51	N/A	N/A	80*	None

* with documentation

Terms To Know

hymen. Thin, often half-moon shaped membrane that surrounds and partially closes the opening to the vagina. The shape permits the flow of menstrual blood out of the vagina, though hymens can be different shapes.

Vulva

56501-56515

56501 Destruction of lesion(s), vulva; simple (eg, laser surgery, electrosurgery, cryosurgery, chemosurgery)

56515 extensive (eg, laser surgery, electrosurgery, cryosurgery, chemosurgery)

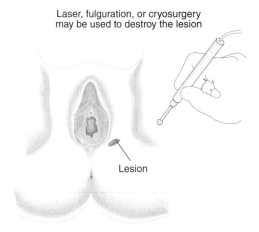

Laser, fulguration, or cryosurgery may be used to destroy the lesion

Lesion

Explanation

The vulva includes the labia majora, labia minora, mons pubis, bulb of the vestibule, vestibule of the vagina, greater and lesser vestibular glands, and vaginal orifice. After examination of the lower genital tract and perianal area, the physician destroys one or more lesions of the vulva by any method including laser surgery, electrosurgery, chemosurgery, or cryosurgery. Use 56501 to report single, simple lesion destruction, or 56515 to report multiple or complicated destruction of extensive vulvar lesions.

Coding Tips

For removal or destruction by electric current (fulguration) of Skene's glands, see 53270. For destruction of vaginal lesions, see 57061–57065. For lysis of labial adhesions, see 56441.

ICD-10-CM Diagnostic Codes

A60.04	Herpesviral vulvovaginitis ♀
A63.0	Anogenital (venereal) warts
C79.82	Secondary malignant neoplasm of genital organs
D07.1	Carcinoma in situ of vulva ♀
D28.0	Benign neoplasm of vulva ♀
D39.8	Neoplasm of uncertain behavior of other specified female genital organs ♀
D49.59	Neoplasm of unspecified behavior of other genitourinary organ
I86.3	Vulval varices ♀
N76.6	Ulceration of vulva ♀
N76.81	Mucositis (ulcerative) of vagina and vulva ♀
N90.0	Mild vulvar dysplasia ♀
N90.1	Moderate vulvar dysplasia ♀
N90.4	Leukoplakia of vulva ♀
N90.7	Vulvar cyst ♀
N90.89	Other specified noninflammatory disorders of vulva and perineum ♀
Q52.79	Other congenital malformations of vulva ♀

AMA: **56501** 2019,Jul,6; 2019,Aug,10; 2014,Jan,11 **56515** 2019,Jul,6; 2019,Aug,10; 2014,Jan,11

Relative Value Units/Medicare Edits

Non-Facility RVU	Work	PE	MP	Total
56501	1.58	2.87	0.24	4.69
56515	3.08	3.69	0.48	7.25
Facility RVU	**Work**	**PE**	**MP**	**Total**
56501	1.58	1.78	0.24	3.6
56515	3.08	2.41	0.48	5.97

	FUD	Status	MUE	Modifiers				IOM Reference
56501	10	A	1(2)	51	N/A	N/A	N/A	100-03,140.5
56515	10	A	1(2)	51	N/A	N/A	N/A	

* with documentation

Terms To Know

carcinoma in situ. Malignancy that arises from the cells of the vessel, gland, or organ of origin that remains confined to that site or has not invaded neighboring tissue. ·

chemosurgery. Application of chemical agents to destroy tissue, originally referring to the in situ chemical fixation of premalignant or malignant lesions to facilitate surgical excision.

condyloma. Infectious tumor-like growth caused by the human papilloma virus, with a branching connective tissue core and epithelial covering that occurs on the skin and mucous membranes of the perianal region and external genitalia.

cryosurgery. Application of intense cold, usually produced using liquid nitrogen, to locally freeze diseased or unwanted tissue and induce tissue necrosis without causing harm to adjacent tissue.

destruction. Ablation or eradication of a structure or tissue.

electrocautery. Division or cutting of tissue using high-frequency electrical current to produce heat, which destroys cells.

electrosurgery. Use of electric currents to generate heat in performing surgery.

laser surgery. Use of concentrated, sharply defined light beams to cut, cauterize, coagulate, seal, or vaporize tissue.

lesion. Area of damaged tissue that has lost continuity or function, due to disease or trauma.

varices. Enlarged, dilated, or twisted turning veins.

vulva. Area on the female external genitalia that includes the labia majora and minora, mons pubis, clitoris, bulb of the vestibule, vaginal vestibule and orifice, and the greater and lesser vestibular glands.

Vulva

56605-56606

56605 Biopsy of vulva or perineum (separate procedure); 1 lesion
+ 56606 each separate additional lesion (List separately in addition to code for primary procedure)

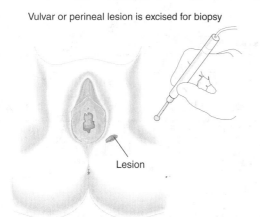

Vulvar or perineal lesion is excised for biopsy

Lesion

Explanation

The vulva includes the labia majora, labia minora, mons pubis, bulb of the vestibule, vestibule of the vagina, greater and lesser vestibular glands, and vaginal orifice. The perineum is the area between the vulva and the anus. The physician removes a sample of tissue from the vulva or perineum. After injecting a local anesthetic around the suspect tissue, the physician obtains a sample using a skin punch or sharp scalpel. A clip or suture can be used to control bleeding if pressure is not successful. Use 56605 for the biopsy of one lesion and 56606 for each additional lesion.

Coding Tips

Note that 56605, a separate procedure by definition, is usually a component of a more complex service and is not identified separately. When performed alone or with other unrelated procedures/services it may be reported. If performed alone, list the code; if performed with other procedures/services, list the code and append 59 or an X{EPSU} modifier. Report 56606 in addition to 56605. These codes report the excision of a portion of a lesion for biopsy. If the entire lesion is excised, see 11420–11426 and 11620–11626. If a specimen is transported to an outside laboratory, report 99000 for conveyance.

ICD-10-CM Diagnostic Codes

A60.04	Herpesviral vulvovaginitis ♀
A63.0	Anogenital (venereal) warts
C51.0	Malignant neoplasm of labium majus ♀
C51.1	Malignant neoplasm of labium minus ♀
C51.2	Malignant neoplasm of clitoris ♀
C51.8	Malignant neoplasm of overlapping sites of vulva ♀
C76.3	Malignant neoplasm of pelvis
C79.82	Secondary malignant neoplasm of genital organs
C79.89	Secondary malignant neoplasm of other specified sites
D07.1	Carcinoma in situ of vulva ♀
D09.8	Carcinoma in situ of other specified sites
D28.0	Benign neoplasm of vulva ♀
D36.7	Benign neoplasm of other specified sites
D39.8	Neoplasm of uncertain behavior of other specified female genital organs ♀
D48.7	Neoplasm of uncertain behavior of other specified sites
D49.59	Neoplasm of unspecified behavior of other genitourinary organ
D49.89	Neoplasm of unspecified behavior of other specified sites
I86.3	Vulval varices ♀
N76.2	Acute vulvitis ♀
N76.3	Subacute and chronic vulvitis ♀
N76.6	Ulceration of vulva ♀
N76.81	Mucositis (ulcerative) of vagina and vulva ♀
N76.89	Other specified inflammation of vagina and vulva ♀
N90.0	Mild vulvar dysplasia ♀
N90.4	Leukoplakia of vulva ♀
N90.7	Vulvar cyst ♀
N90.89	Other specified noninflammatory disorders of vulva and perineum ♀
Q52.79	Other congenital malformations of vulva ♀

AMA: 56605 2019,Jul,6; 2019,Jan,9; 2018,Jan,8; 2017,Jan,8; 2016,Jan,13; 2015,Jan,16; 2014,Jan,11 **56606** 2019,Jul,6; 2019,Jan,9; 2014,Jan,11

Relative Value Units/Medicare Edits

Non-Facility RVU	Work	PE	MP	Total
56605	1.1	1.32	0.18	2.6
56606	0.55	0.47	0.09	1.11
Facility RVU	**Work**	**PE**	**MP**	**Total**
56605	1.1	0.47	0.18	1.75
56606	0.55	0.22	0.09	0.86

	FUD	Status	MUE	Modifiers				IOM Reference
56605	0	A	1(2)	51	N/A	62	N/A	None
56606	N/A	A	6(3)	N/A	N/A	62	N/A	

* with documentation

Terms To Know

biopsy. Tissue or fluid removed for diagnostic purposes through analysis of the cells in the biopsy material.

carcinoma in situ. Malignancy that arises from the cells of the vessel, gland, or organ of origin that remains confined to that site or has not invaded neighboring tissue.

dystrophy of vulva. Abnormal cell growth of the fleshy external female genitalia.

lesion. Area of damaged tissue that has lost continuity or function, due to disease or trauma.

neoplasm. New abnormal growth, tumor.

specimen. Tissue cells or sample of fluid taken for analysis, pathologic examination, and diagnosis.

tissue. Group of similar cells with a similar function that form definite structures and organs. Tissue types include epithelial tissue, muscle tissue, connective tissue, and nervous tissue.

vulva. Area on the female external genitalia that includes the labia majora and minora, mons pubis, clitoris, bulb of the vestibule, vaginal vestibule and orifice, and the greater and lesser vestibular glands.

Vulva

56620-56625

56620 Vulvectomy simple; partial
56625   complete

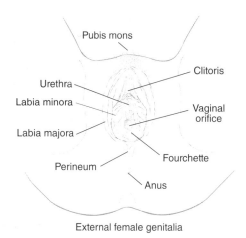

External female genitalia

Labels: Pubis mons, Clitoris, Urethra, Labia minora, Vaginal orifice, Labia majora, Fourchette, Perineum, Anus

Explanation

The physician removes part or all of the vulva to treat premalignant or malignant lesions. A simple complete vulvectomy includes removal of all of the labia majora, labia minora, and clitoris, while a simple, partial vulvectomy may include removal of part or all of the labia majora and labia minora on one side and the clitoris. The physician examines the lower genital tract and the perianal skin through a colposcope. In 56620, a wide semi-elliptical incision that contains the diseased area is made. In 56625, two wide elliptical incisions encompassing the vulvar area are made. One elliptical incision extends from well above the clitoris around both labia majora to a point just in front of the anus. The second elliptical incision starts at a point between the clitoris and the opening of the urethra and is carried around both sides of the opening of the vagina. The underlying subcutaneous fatty tissue is removed along with the large portion of excised skin. Vessels are clamped and tied off with sutures or are electrocoagulated to control bleeding. The considerable defect is usually closed in layers using separately reportable plastic techniques. Vaginal gauze packing may be placed in the vagina.

Coding Tips

Simple complete vulvectomy encompasses all of the labia majora and labia minora on both sides. Report skin grafts separately, see 15004-15005, 15120-15121, and 15240-15241, when performed. If significant additional time and effort is documented, append modifier 22 and submit a cover letter and operative report.

ICD-10-CM Diagnostic Codes

C51.0	Malignant neoplasm of labium majus ♀
C51.1	Malignant neoplasm of labium minus ♀
C51.2	Malignant neoplasm of clitoris ♀
C51.8	Malignant neoplasm of overlapping sites of vulva ♀
C79.82	Secondary malignant neoplasm of genital organs
D07.1	Carcinoma in situ of vulva ♀
D28.0	Benign neoplasm of vulva ♀
D39.8	Neoplasm of uncertain behavior of other specified female genital organs ♀
D49.59	Neoplasm of unspecified behavior of other genitourinary organ
N90.0	Mild vulvar dysplasia ♀
N90.1	Moderate vulvar dysplasia ♀
N90.4	Leukoplakia of vulva ♀

AMA: **56620** 2019,Jul,6; 2019,Jan,14; 2018,Jan,8; 2017,Jan,8; 2016,Jan,13; 2015,Jan,16; 2014,Jan,11 **56625** 2019,Jul,6; 2014,Jan,11

Relative Value Units/Medicare Edits

Non-Facility RVU	Work	PE	MP	Total
56620	7.53	7.21	1.18	15.92
56625	9.68	7.41	1.52	18.61
Facility RVU	**Work**	**PE**	**MP**	**Total**
56620	7.53	7.21	1.18	15.92
56625	9.68	7.41	1.52	18.61

	FUD	Status	MUE	Modifiers				IOM Reference
56620	90	A	1(2)	51	N/A	62*	80	None
56625	90	A	1(2)	51	N/A	62*	80	

* with documentation

Terms To Know

benign. Mild or nonmalignant in nature.

carcinoma in situ. Malignancy that arises from the cells of the vessel, gland, or organ of origin that remains confined to that site or has not invaded neighboring tissue.

defect. Imperfection, flaw, or absence.

dysplasia. Abnormality or alteration in the size, shape, and organization of cells from their normal pattern of development.

leukoplakia. Thickened white patches or lesions appearing on a mucous membrane, such as oral mucosa or tongue.

malignant. Any condition tending to progress toward death, specifically an invasive tumor with a loss of cellular differentiation that has the ability to spread or metastasize to other body areas.

neoplasm. New abnormal growth, tumor.

secondary. Second in order of occurrence or importance, or appearing during the course of another disease or condition.

vulva. Area on the female external genitalia that includes the labia majora and minora, mons pubis, clitoris, bulb of the vestibule, vaginal vestibule and orifice, and the greater and lesser vestibular glands.

Vulva

56630

56630   Vulvectomy, radical, partial;

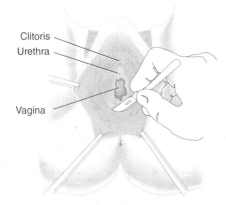

Clitoris
Urethra
Vagina

Vulva is partially removed

Explanation

The physician removes part of the vulva to treat malignancy. A partial radical vulvectomy includes partial or complete removal of a large, deep segment of skin from the following structures: abdomen and groin, labia majora, labia minora, clitoris, mons veneris, and terminal portions of the urethra, vagina, and other vulvar organs. The clitoris may or may not be included in the partial vulvectomy. Through incisions in the lower abdomen, thighs, and vulvar area, the physician removes skin, subcutaneous fatty tissue, and deeper tissue. Also included in the en bloc removal of tissue are portions of the saphenous veins and ligaments and the target lesion. The resulting large and disfiguring defect is usually closed using separately reported plastic surgical techniques, which may include pedicle flaps or free skin grafts. Subcutaneous rubber drains may be left in the surgical site, and vaginal gauze packing may be placed in the vagina.

Coding Tips

This procedure does not include removal of the inguinal and femoral lymph nodes. For a partial radical vulvectomy, including inguinofemoral lymph node biopsy without complete inguinofemoral lymphadenectomy, report 56630 with 38531; for a partial radical vulvectomy with inguinofemoral lymphadenectomy, unilateral, see 56631; bilateral, see 56632. For a simple vulvectomy, partial, see 56620; complete, see 56625. Report skin grafts, when used, with 15004-15005, 15120-15121, and 15240-15241. If significant additional time and effort is documented, append modifier 22 and submit a cover letter and operative report.

ICD-10-CM Diagnostic Codes

C51.0	Malignant neoplasm of labium majus ♀
C51.1	Malignant neoplasm of labium minus ♀
C51.2	Malignant neoplasm of clitoris ♀
C51.8	Malignant neoplasm of overlapping sites of vulva ♀
C79.82	Secondary malignant neoplasm of genital organs
D03.8	Melanoma in situ of other sites
D07.1	Carcinoma in situ of vulva ♀
D39.8	Neoplasm of uncertain behavior of other specified female genital organs ♀
D49.59	Neoplasm of unspecified behavior of other genitourinary organ
N90.1	Moderate vulvar dysplasia ♀
Q52.79	Other congenital malformations of vulva ♀

AMA: **56630** 2019,Jul,6; 2019,Feb,8; 2014,Jan,11

Relative Value Units/Medicare Edits

Non-Facility RVU	Work	PE	MP	Total
56630	14.8	9.93	2.35	27.08
Facility RVU	**Work**	**PE**	**MP**	**Total**
56630	14.8	9.93	2.35	27.08

	FUD	Status	MUE	Modifiers				IOM Reference
56630	90	A	1(2)	51	N/A	62*	80	None

* with documentation

Terms To Know

carcinoma in situ. Malignancy that arises from the cells of the vessel, gland, or organ of origin that remains confined to that site or has not invaded neighboring tissue.

defect. Imperfection, flaw, or absence.

drain. Device that creates a channel to allow fluid from a cavity, wound, or infected area to exit the body.

dysplasia. Abnormality or alteration in the size, shape, and organization of cells from their normal pattern of development.

en bloc. In total.

malignant. Any condition tending to progress toward death, specifically an invasive tumor with a loss of cellular differentiation that has the ability to spread or metastasize to other body areas.

melanoma. Highly metastatic malignant neoplasm composed of melanocytes that occur most often on the skin from a preexisting mole or nevus but may also occur in the mouth, esophagus, anal canal, or vagina.

neoplasm. New abnormal growth, tumor.

packing. Material placed into a cavity or wound, such as gels, gauze, pads, and sponges.

pedicle flap. Full-thickness skin and subcutaneous tissue for grafting that remains partially attached to the donor site by a pedicle or stem in which the blood vessels supplying the flap remain intact.

radical. Extensive surgery.

secondary. Second in order of occurrence or importance, or appearing during the course of another disease or condition.

vulvectomy. Surgical removal of all or part of the vulva, often performed to treat malignant or premalignant lesions. Lymph nodes may be removed at the same surgical session.

Vulva

56631-56632

56631   Vulvectomy, radical, partial; with unilateral inguinofemoral lymphadenectomy
56632   with bilateral inguinofemoral lymphadenectomy

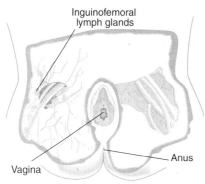

Inguinofemoral
lymph glands

Vagina
Anus

Vulva is partially removed

Explanation

The physician removes part of the vulva to treat malignancy. A partial radical vulvectomy includes the partial or complete removal of a large, deep segment of skin and tissue from the abdomen and groin, labia majora and minora, clitoris, mons veneris, and terminal portions of the urethra, vagina, and other vulvar organs. Through incisions in the lower abdomen, thighs, and vulvar area, the physician removes skin, subcutaneous fatty tissue, and deeper tissue. The physician also removes superficial and deep inguinal lymph nodes and adjacent femoral lymph nodes on one side in 56631 and on both sides in 56632. Also included in the en bloc removal of tissue are portions of the saphenous veins and ligaments and the target lesion. The resulting large and disfiguring defect is usually closed in layers using plastic surgical techniques, which may include pedicle flaps or free skin grafts. Subcutaneous rubber drains may be left in the surgical site, and vaginal gauze packing may be placed in the vagina.

Coding Tips

For a simple vulvectomy, see 56620 or 56625. For a partial radical vulvectomy, see 56630; partial radical vulvectomy, including inguinofemoral lymph node biopsy, without complete inguinofemoral lymphadenectomy, report 56630 with 38531. For a complete radical vulvectomy, see 56633; with inguinofemoral lymphadenectomy, unilateral see 56634; bilateral inguinofemoral lymphadenectomy, see 56637. Report skin grafts with 15004-15005, 15120-15121, and 15240-15241, when performed.

ICD-10-CM Diagnostic Codes

C51.0	Malignant neoplasm of labium majus ♀
C51.1	Malignant neoplasm of labium minus ♀
C51.2	Malignant neoplasm of clitoris ♀
C51.8	Malignant neoplasm of overlapping sites of vulva ♀
C77.4	Secondary and unspecified malignant neoplasm of inguinal and lower limb lymph nodes
C79.82	Secondary malignant neoplasm of genital organs
D03.8	Melanoma in situ of other sites
D07.1	Carcinoma in situ of vulva ♀
D39.8	Neoplasm of uncertain behavior of other specified female genital organs ♀
D49.59	Neoplasm of unspecified behavior of other genitourinary organ

AMA: **56631** 2019,Jul,6; 2019,Feb,8; 2014,Jan,11 **56632** 2019,Jul,6; 2019,Feb,8; 2014,Jan,11

Relative Value Units/Medicare Edits

Non-Facility RVU	Work	PE	MP	Total
56631	18.99	11.84	3.0	33.83
56632	21.86	14.97	3.45	40.28
Facility RVU	**Work**	**PE**	**MP**	**Total**
56631	18.99	11.84	3.0	33.83
56632	21.86	14.97	3.45	40.28

	FUD	Status	MUE	Modifiers				IOM Reference
56631	90	A	1(2)	51	N/A	62	80	None
56632	90	A	1(2)	51	N/A	62	80	

* with documentation

Terms To Know

bilateral. Consisting of or affecting two sides.

defect. Imperfection, flaw, or absence.

inguinal. Within the groin region.

lymph nodes. Bean-shaped structures along the lymphatic vessels that intercept and destroy foreign materials in the tissue and bloodstream.

lymphadenectomy. Dissection of lymph nodes free from the vessels and removal for examination by frozen section in a separate procedure to detect early-stage metastases.

malignant. Any condition tending to progress toward death, specifically an invasive tumor with a loss of cellular differentiation that has the ability to spread or metastasize to other body areas.

pedicle flap. Full-thickness skin and subcutaneous tissue for grafting that remains partially attached to the donor site by a pedicle or stem in which the blood vessels supplying the flap remain intact.

radical. Extensive surgery.

unilateral. Located on or affecting one side.

vulvectomy. Surgical removal of all or part of the vulva, often performed to treat malignant or premalignant lesions. Lymph nodes may be removed at the same surgical session.

Vulva

56633

56633 Vulvectomy, radical, complete;

The distal portions of the urethra and vagina are excised with the labia

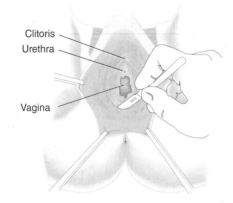

- Clitoris
- Urethra
- Vagina

Explanation

The physician removes the vulva to treat malignancy. A complete radical vulvectomy includes the removal of a large, deep segment of skin and tissue from the following structures: abdomen and groin, labia majora, labia minora, clitoris, mons veneris, and terminal portions of the urethra, vagina, and other vulvar organs. Deep tissue from more than 80 percent of the vulva is excised. Through incisions in the lower abdomen, thighs, and vulvar area, the physician removes skin, subcutaneous fatty tissue, and deeper tissues. Also included in the en bloc removal of tissue are portions of the saphenous veins and ligaments and the target lesion. The resulting large and disfiguring defect is usually closed in layers using separately reported plastic surgical techniques, which may include pedicle flaps or free skin grafts. Subcutaneous rubber drains may be used, and vaginal gauze packing may be placed in the vagina.

Coding Tips

This procedure does not include removal of the inguinal and femoral lymph nodes. For a complete radical vulvectomy, including inguinofemoral lymph node biopsy without complete inguinofemoral lymphadenectomy, report 56633 with 38531; for a simple vulvectomy, see 56620 or 56625. For a partial radical vulvectomy, see 56630; partial radical vulvectomy, including inguinofemoral lymph node biopsy, without complete inguinofemoral lymphadenectomy, report 56630 with 38531. For a partial radical vulvectomy with inguinofemoral lymphadenectomy, unilateral, see 56631; bilateral, see 56632. For a complete radical vulvectomy with inguinofemoral lymphadenectomy, unilateral see 56634; bilateral inguinofemoral lymphadenectomy, see 56637. Report a radial complete vulvectomy with inguinofemoral, iliac, and pelvic lymphadenectomy with 56640. Report skin grafts with 15004-15005, 15120-15121, and 15240-15241, when performed.

ICD-10-CM Diagnostic Codes

C51.0	Malignant neoplasm of labium majus ♀
C51.1	Malignant neoplasm of labium minus ♀
C51.2	Malignant neoplasm of clitoris ♀
C51.8	Malignant neoplasm of overlapping sites of vulva ♀
C79.82	Secondary malignant neoplasm of genital organs
D03.8	Melanoma in situ of other sites
D07.1	Carcinoma in situ of vulva ♀
D39.8	Neoplasm of uncertain behavior of other specified female genital organs ♀

D49.59	Neoplasm of unspecified behavior of other genitourinary organ

AMA: **56633** 2019,Jul,6; 2019,Feb,8; 2014,Jan,11

Relative Value Units/Medicare Edits

Non-Facility RVU	Work	PE	MP	Total
56633	19.62	12.24	3.1	34.96
Facility RVU	**Work**	**PE**	**MP**	**Total**
56633	19.62	12.24	3.1	34.96

	FUD	Status	MUE	Modifiers				IOM Reference
56633	90	A	1(2)	51	N/A	62	80	None

* with documentation

Terms To Know

en bloc. In total.

malignant. Any condition tending to progress toward death, specifically an invasive tumor with a loss of cellular differentiation that has the ability to spread or metastasize to other body areas.

packing. Material placed into a cavity or wound, such as gels, gauze, pads, and sponges.

pedicle flap. Full-thickness skin and subcutaneous tissue for grafting that remains partially attached to the donor site by a pedicle or stem in which the blood vessels supplying the flap remain intact.

radical. Extensive surgery.

staging of carcinoma of the vulva.

Carcinoma of the vulva is classified by stage:

Stage 0: Carcinoma in situ.

Stage 1: Tumor 2.0 cm or smaller confined to vulva; nodes not palpable.

Stage 2: Tumor larger than 2.0 cm confined to vulva; nodes not palpable.

Stage 3: Tumor of any size infiltrating urethra, vagina, anus, or perineum; two nodes palpable but not fixed.

Stage 4: Tumor of any size infiltrating anal or bladder mucosa; fixed to bone or metastases; fixed nodes.

Note: This staging does not apply to melanoma or secondary malignancies.

vulvectomy. Surgical removal of all or part of the vulva, often performed to treat malignant or premalignant lesions. Lymph nodes may be removed at the same surgical session.

Vulva

56634-56637

56634 Vulvectomy, radical, complete; with unilateral inguinofemoral lymphadenectomy

56637 with bilateral inguinofemoral lymphadenectomy

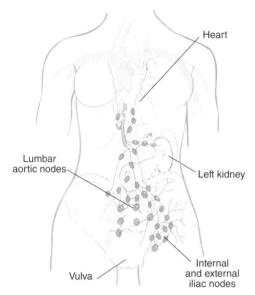

The vulva is removed in a radical procedure

Explanation

The physician removes the vulva to treat malignancy. A complete radical vulvectomy includes the removal of a large, deep segment of skin and tissue from the lower abdomen and groin, labia majora and minora, clitoris, mons veneris, and terminal portions of the urethra, vagina, and other vulvar organs. Deep tissue from more than 80 percent of the vulva is removed. Through incisions in the lower abdomen, thighs, and vulvar area, the physician removes skin, subcutaneous fatty tissue, and deeper tissues. The physician also removes the inguinal and femoral lymph nodes on one side in 56634 and on both sides in 56637. Also included in the en bloc removal of tissue are portions of the saphenous veins and ligaments and the target lesion. The resulting large and disfiguring defect is usually closed in layers using plastic surgical techniques, which may include pedicle flaps or free skin grafts. Subcutaneous rubber drains may be used, and vaginal gauze packing may be placed in the vagina.

Coding Tips

For a complete radical vulvectomy, including inguinofemoral lymph node biopsy without complete inguinofemoral lymphadenectomy, report 56633 with 38531; For a simple vulvectomy, see 56620 or 56625. For a partial radical vulvectomy, see 56630; partial radical vulvectomy, including inguinofemoral lymph node biopsy, without complete inguinofemoral lymphadenectomy, report 56630 with 38531. For a partial radical vulvectomy with inguinofemoral lymphadenectomy, unilateral, see 56631; bilateral, see 56632. Report a radical complete vulvectomy with inguinofemoral, iliac, and pelvic lymphadenectomy with 56640. Report skin grafts with 15004-15005, 15120-15121, and 15240-15241, when performed.

ICD-10-CM Diagnostic Codes

C51.0	Malignant neoplasm of labium majus ♀
C51.1	Malignant neoplasm of labium minus ♀
C51.2	Malignant neoplasm of clitoris ♀
C51.8	Malignant neoplasm of overlapping sites of vulva ♀
C77.4	Secondary and unspecified malignant neoplasm of inguinal and lower limb lymph nodes
C79.82	Secondary malignant neoplasm of genital organs
D03.8	Melanoma in situ of other sites
D07.1	Carcinoma in situ of vulva ♀
D39.8	Neoplasm of uncertain behavior of other specified female genital organs ♀
D49.59	Neoplasm of unspecified behavior of other genitourinary organ

AMA: 56634 2019,Jul,6; 2019,Feb,8; 2014,Jan,11 **56637** 2019,Jul,6; 2019,Feb,8; 2014,Jan,11

Relative Value Units/Medicare Edits

Non-Facility RVU	Work	PE	MP	Total
56634	20.66	12.96	3.26	36.88
56637	24.75	14.2	3.89	42.84
Facility RVU	**Work**	**PE**	**MP**	**Total**
56634	20.66	12.96	3.26	36.88
56637	24.75	14.2	3.89	42.84

	FUD	Status	MUE	Modifiers				IOM Reference
56634	90	A	1(2)	51	N/A	62	80	None
56637	90	A	1(2)	51	N/A	62	80	

* with documentation

Terms To Know

femoral lymph node. Lymphatic, right lower extremity, left lower extremity.

inguinal. Within the groin region.

lymph nodes. Bean-shaped structures along the lymphatic vessels that intercept and destroy foreign materials in the tissue and bloodstream.

lymphadenectomy. Dissection of lymph nodes free from the vessels and removal for examination by frozen section in a separate procedure to detect early-stage metastases.

malignant. Any condition tending to progress toward death, specifically an invasive tumor with a loss of cellular differentiation that has the ability to spread or metastasize to other body areas.

radical. Extensive surgery.

vulvectomy. Surgical removal of all or part of the vulva, often performed to treat malignant or premalignant lesions. Lymph nodes may be removed at the same surgical session.

Vulva

56640

56640 Vulvectomy, radical, complete, with inguinofemoral, iliac, and pelvic lymphadenectomy

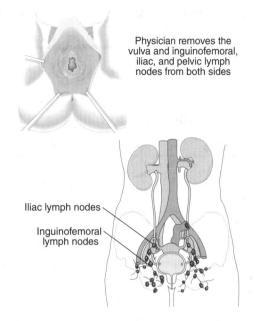

Physician removes the vulva and inguinofemoral, iliac, and pelvic lymph nodes from both sides

Iliac lymph nodes

Inguinofemoral lymph nodes

Explanation

The physician removes the entire vulva to treat malignancy. A complete radical vulvectomy includes the removal of a large, deep segment of skin and tissue from the following structures: lower abdomen and groin, labia majora, labia minora, clitoris, mons veneris, and terminal portions of the urethra, vagina, and other vulvar organs. Through incisions in the lower abdomen, thighs, and vulvar area, the physician removes skin, subcutaneous fatty tissue, and deeper tissue. The physician also removes the inguinal and femoral lymph nodes on both sides as well as the iliac and pelvic lymph nodes in the pelvic cavity, which is entered through an abdominal incision. Also included in the en bloc removal of tissue are portions of the saphenous veins and ligaments and the target lesion. The resulting large and disfiguring defect is usually closed in layers using separately reported plastic surgical techniques, which may include pedicle flaps or free skin grafts. Subcutaneous rubber drains may be used, and vaginal gauze packing may be placed in the vagina.

Coding Tips

For a simple vulvectomy, see 56620 or 56625. For a partial radical vulvectomy, see 56630; partial radical vulvectomy, including inguinofemoral lymph node biopsy, without complete inguinofemoral lymphadenectomy, report 56630 with 38531. For a partial radical vulvectomy with inguinofemoral lymphadenectomy, unilateral, see 56631; bilateral, see 56632. For a complete radical vulvectomy, see 56633; including inguinofemoral lymph node biopsy without complete inguinofemoral lymphadenectomy, report 56633 with 38531. For a complete radical vulvectomy with inguinofemoral lymphadenectomy, unilateral see 56634; bilateral, see 56637. Report skin grafts with 15004-15005, 15120-15121, and 15240-15241, when performed. This is a unilateral procedure. If performed bilaterally, some payers require that the service be reported twice with modifier 50 appended to the second code while others require identification of the service only once with modifier 50 appended. Check with individual payers. Modifier 50 identifies a procedure performed identically on the opposite side of the body (mirror image).

ICD-10-CM Diagnostic Codes

C51.0	Malignant neoplasm of labium majus ♀
C51.1	Malignant neoplasm of labium minus ♀
C51.2	Malignant neoplasm of clitoris ♀
C51.8	Malignant neoplasm of overlapping sites of vulva ♀
C77.4	Secondary and unspecified malignant neoplasm of inguinal and lower limb lymph nodes
C77.5	Secondary and unspecified malignant neoplasm of intrapelvic lymph nodes
C79.82	Secondary malignant neoplasm of genital organs
D03.8	Melanoma in situ of other sites
D07.1	Carcinoma in situ of vulva ♀
D39.8	Neoplasm of uncertain behavior of other specified female genital organs ♀
D49.59	Neoplasm of unspecified behavior of other genitourinary organ

AMA: 56640 2019,Jul,6; 2019,Feb,8; 2014,Jan,11

Relative Value Units/Medicare Edits

Non-Facility RVU	Work	PE	MP	Total
56640	24.78	14.69	3.9	43.37
Facility RVU	**Work**	**PE**	**MP**	**Total**
56640	24.78	14.69	3.9	43.37

	FUD	Status	MUE	Modifiers				IOM Reference
56640	90	A	1(2)	51	50	62*	80	None

* with documentation

Terms To Know

defect. Imperfection, flaw, or absence.

femoral lymph node. Lymphatic, right lower extremity, left lower extremity.

inguinal. Within the groin region.

lymph nodes. Bean-shaped structures along the lymphatic vessels that intercept and destroy foreign materials in the tissue and bloodstream.

malignant. Any condition tending to progress toward death, specifically an invasive tumor with a loss of cellular differentiation that has the ability to spread or metastasize to other body areas.

radical. Extensive surgery.

staging of carcinoma of the vulva.

Carcinoma of the vulva is classified by stage:

Stage 0: Carcinoma in situ.

Stage 1: Tumor 2.0 cm or smaller confined to vulva; nodes not palpable.

Stage 2: Tumor larger than 2.0 cm confined to vulva; nodes not palpable.

Stage 3: Tumor of any size infiltrating urethra, vagina, anus, or perineum; two nodes palpable but not fixed.

Stage 4: Tumor of any size infiltrating anal or bladder mucosa; fixed to bone or metastases; fixed nodes.

Note: This staging does not apply to melanoma or secondary malignancies.

vulvectomy. Surgical removal of all or part of the vulva, often performed to treat malignant or premalignant lesions. Lymph nodes may be removed at the same surgical session.

N Newborn: 0 **P** Pediatric: 0-17 **M** Maternity: 9-64 **A** Adult: 15-124 ♂ Male Only ♀ Female Only

Coding Companion for Ob/Gyn

Vulva

56700

56700   Partial hymenectomy or revision of hymenal ring

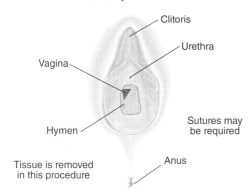

The physician uses a scalpel or scissors
to remove the hymenal membrane

Clitoris

Urethra

Vagina

Hymen

Sutures may
be required

Tissue is removed
in this procedure

Anus

Explanation

A hymen is a membrane that partially or wholly occludes the vaginal opening. Following local injection of an anesthetic, the physician excises a portion of the hymenal membrane. Using a scalpel or scissors, the physician removes the membrane at its junction with the opening of the vagina. The cut margins of the vaginal mucosa are sutured with fine, absorbable material.

Coding Tips

Local anesthesia is included in this service. However, this procedure may be performed under general anesthesia, depending on the age and/or condition of the patient. If a specimen is transported to an outside laboratory, report 99000 for conveyance. For hymenotomy via simple excision, see 56442. Surgical trays, A4550, are not separately reimbursed by Medicare; however, other third-party payers may cover them. Check with the specific payer to determine coverage.

ICD-10-CM Diagnostic Codes

N89.6   Tight hymenal ring ♀
Q52.3   Imperforate hymen ♀

AMA: 56700 2019,Jul,6; 2014,Jan,11

Relative Value Units/Medicare Edits

Non-Facility RVU	Work	PE	MP	Total
56700	2.84	2.38	0.46	5.68
Facility RVU	**Work**	**PE**	**MP**	**Total**
56700	2.84	2.38	0.46	5.68

	FUD	Status	MUE	Modifiers				IOM Reference
56700	10	A	1(2)	51	N/A	62*	80	None

* with documentation

Terms To Know

membrane. Thin, flexible tissue layer that covers or functions to separate or connect anatomic areas, structures, or organs. May also be described as having the characteristic of allowing certain substances to permeate or pass through but not others (semipermeable).

56740

56740   Excision of Bartholin's gland or cyst

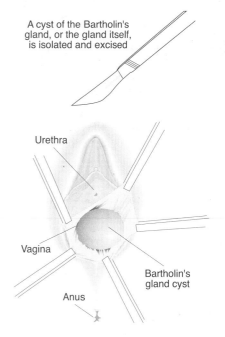

A cyst of the Bartholin's
gland, or the gland itself,
is isolated and excised

Urethra

Vagina

Bartholin's
gland cyst

Anus

The operative site is closed
with layered sutures

Explanation

The physician removes a cystic Bartholin's gland, which lies at the tail end of the bulb of the vestibular opening just inside of the vagina. The physician makes an incision through the vaginal mucosa. The cyst is isolated through the vaginal incision by dissecting the deeper fatty tissues and excised. The remaining cavity and skin are closed in layers using absorbable material.

Coding Tips

For excision of Skene's gland, see 53270. For marsupialization of Bartholin's gland, see 56440. For incision and drainage of Bartholin's gland abscess, see 56420. For excision of urethral caruncle, see 53265. For excision or marsupialization of urethral diverticulum, see 53230 and 53240, respectively. Surgical trays, A4550, are not separately reimbursed by Medicare; however, other third-party payers may cover them. Check with the specific payer to determine coverage.

ICD-10-CM Diagnostic Codes

N75.0   Cyst of Bartholin's gland ♀
N75.1   Abscess of Bartholin's gland ♀
N75.8   Other diseases of Bartholin's gland ♀

AMA: 56740 2019,Jul,6; 2014,Jan,11

Vulva

Relative Value Units/Medicare Edits

Non-Facility RVU	Work	PE	MP	Total
56740	4.88	3.25	0.79	8.92
Facility RVU	**Work**	**PE**	**MP**	**Total**
56740	4.88	3.25	0.79	8.92

	FUD	Status	MUE	Modifiers				IOM Reference
56740	10	A	1(3)	51	50	N/A	N/A	None

* with documentation

Terms To Know

absorbable sutures. Strands used for suture or repair of tissue prepared from collagen or a synthetic polymer and capable of being absorbed by tissue over time.

Bartholin's gland. Mucous-producing gland found in the vestibular bulbs on either side of the vaginal orifice and connected to the mucosal membrane at the opening by a duct.

cyst. Elevated encapsulated mass containing fluid, semisolid, or solid material with a membranous lining.

dissect. Cut apart or separate tissue for surgical purposes or for visual or microscopic study.

excision. Surgical removal of an organ or tissue.

nonabsorbable sutures. Strands of natural or synthetic material that resist absorption into living tissue and are removed once healing is under way. Nonabsorbable sutures are commonly used to close skin wounds and repair tendons or collagenous tissue.

56800

56800   Plastic repair of introitus

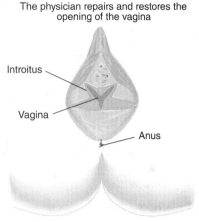

The physician repairs and restores the opening of the vagina

Introitus

Vagina

Anus

The introitus is the entrance to the vagina

Explanation

The physician repairs and restores the anatomy of the opening of the vagina by excising scar tissue and strengthening the supporting tissues using tissue flaps and suturing techniques. This procedure varies greatly from patient to patient, depending on the defect to be corrected.

Coding Tips

This code is associated with congenital anomalies of the female genital system. Report genital wound repair with 12001-12007, 12041-12047, and 13131-13133. For suture of a non-obstetrical injury of the vagina or perineum, see 57200–57210.

ICD-10-CM Diagnostic Codes

N89.5	Stricture and atresia of vagina ♀
N90.811	Female genital mutilation Type I status ♀
N90.812	Female genital mutilation Type II status ♀
N90.813	Female genital mutilation Type III status ♀
N90.818	Other female genital mutilation status ♀
N90.89	Other specified noninflammatory disorders of vulva and perineum ♀
N99.2	Postprocedural adhesions of vagina ♀
O94	Sequelae of complication of pregnancy, childbirth, and the puerperium Ⓜ ♀
Q52.11	Transverse vaginal septum ♀
Q52.120	Longitudinal vaginal septum, nonobstructing ♀
Q52.121	Longitudinal vaginal septum, obstructing, right side ♀ ☑
Q52.122	Longitudinal vaginal septum, obstructing, left side ♀ ☑
Q52.123	Longitudinal vaginal septum, microperforate, right side ♀ ☑
Q52.124	Longitudinal vaginal septum, microperforate, left side ♀ ☑
Q52.2	Congenital rectovaginal fistula ♀
Q52.4	Other congenital malformations of vagina ♀
Q52.5	Fusion of labia ♀
Q52.79	Other congenital malformations of vulva ♀
Q52.8	Other specified congenital malformations of female genitalia ♀
S31.41XA	Laceration without foreign body of vagina and vulva, initial encounter ♀

Vulva

Coding Companion for Ob/Gyn

S31.42XA	Laceration with foreign body of vagina and vulva, initial encounter ♀
S31.43XA	Puncture wound without foreign body of vagina and vulva, initial encounter ♀
S31.44XA	Puncture wound with foreign body of vagina and vulva, initial encounter ♀
S31.45XA	Open bite of vagina and vulva, initial encounter ♀
S38.211A	Complete traumatic amputation of female external genital organs, initial encounter ♀
S38.212A	Partial traumatic amputation of female external genital organs, initial encounter ♀
S39.023A	Laceration of muscle, fascia and tendon of pelvis, initial encounter

AMA: 56800 2019,Jul,6; 2014,Jan,11

Relative Value Units/Medicare Edits

Non-Facility RVU	Work	PE	MP	Total
56800	3.93	2.64	0.6	7.17
Facility RVU	**Work**	**PE**	**MP**	**Total**
56800	3.93	2.64	0.6	7.17

	FUD	Status	MUE	Modifiers				IOM Reference
56800	10	A	1(2)	51	N/A	62*	80	None

* with documentation

Terms To Know

anomaly. Irregularity in the structure or position of an organ or tissue.

atresia. Congenital closure or absence of a tubular organ or an opening to the body surface.

congenital. Present at birth, occurring through heredity or an influence during gestation up to the moment of birth.

defect. Imperfection, flaw, or absence.

excise. Remove or cut out.

genitalia. External organs related to reproduction.

introitus. Entrance into the vagina.

scar tissue. Fibrous connective tissue that forms around a wounded area or injury, composed mainly of fibroblasts or collagenous fibers.

stricture. Narrowing of an anatomical structure.

56805

56805 Clitoroplasty for intersex state

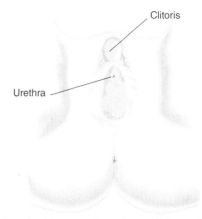

The physician corrects an abnormally large clitoris

Explanation

The physician reduces the size of an enlarged clitoris, which has been masculinized by the production of male hormones from an abnormal adrenal gland. A portion of the body of the clitoris is resected with care to ensure preservation of vital nerves and blood vessels to the glans of the clitoris. The incisions are closed using plastic surgical techniques.

Coding Tips

For creation of a labia minora from excised clitoral tissue, report 58999 and include the operative report and a cover letter. Report a nonobstetrical repair of the perineum with 56810. Report genital wound repair with 12001-12007, 12041-12047, and 13131-13133. For suture of a nonobstetrical injury of the vagina or perineum, see 57200–57210.

ICD-10-CM Diagnostic Codes

N90.89	Other specified noninflammatory disorders of vulva and perineum ♀
Q52.6	Congenital malformation of clitoris ♀
Q56.4	Indeterminate sex, unspecified

AMA: 56805 2019,Jul,6; 2014,Jan,11

Relative Value Units/Medicare Edits

Non-Facility RVU	Work	PE	MP	Total
56805	19.88	10.64	3.11	33.63
Facility RVU	**Work**	**PE**	**MP**	**Total**
56805	19.88	10.64	3.11	33.63

	FUD	Status	MUE	Modifiers				IOM Reference
56805	90	A	1(2)	51	N/A	62*	80	None

* with documentation

Terms To Know

adrenal gland. Specialized group of secretory cells located above the kidneys that produce hormones that regulate the metabolism, maintain fluid balance, and control blood pressure. The adrenal glands also produce slight amounts of androgens, estrogens, and progesterone.

56810

56810 Perineoplasty, repair of perineum, nonobstetrical (separate procedure)

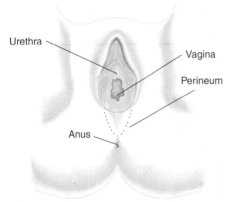

Urethra

Vagina

Perineum

Anus

Repair of the perineum

Explanation

With upward traction on the vagina, the physician makes an incision from the lower vaginal opening to a point just in front of the anus. The underlying weakened tissues are dissected and repaired and tightened by suturing. This restores strength to the pelvic floor, closes tissue defects, and improves function of the perineal muscles.

Coding Tips

This procedure is also known as perineorrhaphy. This separate procedure by definition is usually a component of a more complex service and is not identified separately. When performed alone or with other unrelated procedures/services it may be reported. If performed alone, list the code; if performed with other procedures/services, list the code and append modifier 59 or an X{EPSU} modifier. For suture of a nonobstetrical injury of the vagina and/or perineum, see 57200–57210. For repair of genital wounds, see 12001-12007, 12041-12047, and 13131-13133. For plastic repair of introitus, see 56800.

ICD-10-CM Diagnostic Codes

C76.3	Malignant neoplasm of pelvis
C79.89	Secondary malignant neoplasm of other specified sites
D09.8	Carcinoma in situ of other specified sites
D36.7	Benign neoplasm of other specified sites
D48.7	Neoplasm of uncertain behavior of other specified sites
D49.89	Neoplasm of unspecified behavior of other specified sites
N94.11	Superficial (introital) dyspareunia ♀
N94.12	Deep dyspareunia ♀
N94.19	Other specified dyspareunia ♀
N94.2	Vaginismus ♀
N94.810	Vulvar vestibulitis ♀
S31.41XA	Laceration without foreign body of vagina and vulva, initial encounter ♀
S31.42XA	Laceration with foreign body of vagina and vulva, initial encounter ♀
S31.43XA	Puncture wound without foreign body of vagina and vulva, initial encounter ♀
S31.44XA	Puncture wound with foreign body of vagina and vulva, initial encounter ♀
S31.45XA	Open bite of vagina and vulva, initial encounter ♀
S39.848A	Other specified injuries of external genitals, initial encounter

AMA: 56810 2019,Jul,6; 2014,Jan,11

Relative Value Units/Medicare Edits

Non-Facility RVU	Work	PE	MP	Total
56810	4.29	2.79	0.64	7.72
Facility RVU	**Work**	**PE**	**MP**	**Total**
56810	4.29	2.79	0.64	7.72

	FUD	Status	MUE	Modifiers				IOM Reference
56810	10	A	1(2)	51	N/A	62	80	None

* with documentation

Terms To Know

defect. Imperfection, flaw, or absence.

dissect. Cut apart or separate tissue for surgical purposes or for visual or microscopic study.

dyspareunia. Pain experienced during or after intercourse, commonly occurring in the clitoris, vagina, or labia.

foreign body. Any object or substance found in an organ and tissue that does not belong under normal circumstances.

incision. Act of cutting into tissue or an organ.

laceration. Tearing injury; a torn, ragged-edged wound.

perineal. Pertaining to the pelvic floor area between the thighs; the diamond-shaped area bordered by the pubic symphysis in front, the ischial tuberosities on the sides, and the coccyx in back.

prolapse. Falling, sliding, or sinking of an organ from its normal location in the body.

vaginismus. Spontaneous contractions of the muscles surrounding the vagina, causing it to constrict or close.

Coding Companion for Ob/Gyn

Vulva

56820-56821

56820 Colposcopy of the vulva;
56821 with biopsy(s)

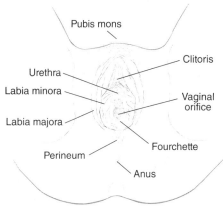

The region of the vulva is viewed by colposcopy

Explanation

The physician performs a colposcopy of the vulva, the external genitalia region of the female that includes the labia, clitoris, mons pubis, vaginal vestibule, bulb and glands, and the vaginal orifice. The patient is placed in the lithotomy position and the vulva is inspected through the colposcope, a binocular microscope used for direct visualization of the vagina and cervix. The bright light of the colposcope is directed so as to inspect the vulva and perianal area for any lesions or ulceration. In 56821, a biopsy is taken of any vulvar tissue in question under direct vision. The number and size of the biopsy will depend on the lesions. Pressure is applied and hemostasis of the biopsy site is achieved.

Coding Tips

For colposcopy performed on the vagina, see 57420–57421. For colposcopy performed on the cervix, see 57452–57461.

ICD-10-CM Diagnostic Codes

A56.02	Chlamydial vulvovaginitis ♀
A60.04	Herpesviral vulvovaginitis ♀
A63.0	Anogenital (venereal) warts
C51.0	Malignant neoplasm of labium majus ♀
C51.1	Malignant neoplasm of labium minus ♀
C51.2	Malignant neoplasm of clitoris ♀
C79.82	Secondary malignant neoplasm of genital organs
D07.1	Carcinoma in situ of vulva ♀
D28.0	Benign neoplasm of vulva ♀
D39.8	Neoplasm of uncertain behavior of other specified female genital organs ♀
D49.59	Neoplasm of unspecified behavior of other genitourinary organ ♀
I86.3	Vulval varices ♀
L29.2	Pruritus vulvae ♀
N76.0	Acute vaginitis ♀
N76.1	Subacute and chronic vaginitis ♀
N76.2	Acute vulvitis ♀
N76.3	Subacute and chronic vulvitis ♀
N76.4	Abscess of vulva ♀
N76.5	Ulceration of vagina ♀
N76.6	Ulceration of vulva ♀
N76.81	Mucositis (ulcerative) of vagina and vulva ♀
N76.89	Other specified inflammation of vagina and vulva ♀
N84.3	Polyp of vulva ♀
N90.0	Mild vulvar dysplasia ♀
N90.1	Moderate vulvar dysplasia ♀
N90.4	Leukoplakia of vulva ♀
N90.5	Atrophy of vulva ♀
N90.61	Childhood asymmetric labium majus enlargement ♀
N90.69	Other specified hypertrophy of vulva ♀
N90.7	Vulvar cyst ♀
N90.89	Other specified noninflammatory disorders of vulva and perineum ♀
O34.71	Maternal care for abnormality of vulva and perineum, first trimester Ⓜ ♀
O34.72	Maternal care for abnormality of vulva and perineum, second trimester Ⓜ ♀
O34.73	Maternal care for abnormality of vulva and perineum, third trimester Ⓜ ♀
Q52.3	Imperforate hymen ♀
Q52.5	Fusion of labia ♀
Q52.6	Congenital malformation of clitoris ♀
Q52.79	Other congenital malformations of vulva ♀
Q52.8	Other specified congenital malformations of female genitalia ♀

AMA: 56820 2019,Jul,6; 2018,Jan,8; 2017,Jan,8; 2016,Jan,13; 2015,Jan,16; 2014,Jan,11 **56821** 2019,Jul,6; 2018,Jan,8; 2017,Jan,8; 2016,Jan,13; 2015,Jan,16; 2014,Jan,11

Relative Value Units/Medicare Edits

Non-Facility RVU	Work	PE	MP	Total
56820	1.5	1.69	0.24	3.43
56821	2.05	2.2	0.32	4.57
Facility RVU	**Work**	**PE**	**MP**	**Total**
56820	1.5	0.73	0.24	2.47
56821	2.05	0.93	0.32	3.3

	FUD	Status	MUE	Modifiers				IOM Reference
56820	0	A	1(2)	51	N/A	N/A	N/A	None
56821	0	A	1(2)	51	N/A	N/A	N/A	

* with documentation

Terms To Know

biopsy. Tissue or fluid removed for diagnostic purposes through analysis of the cells in the biopsy material.

colposcopy. Procedure in which the physician views the cervix and vagina through a colposcope, which is a binocular microscope used for direct visualization of the vagina, ectocervix, and endocervix.

hemostasis. Interruption of blood flow or the cessation or arrest of bleeding.

Vulva

57000

57000   Colpotomy; with exploration

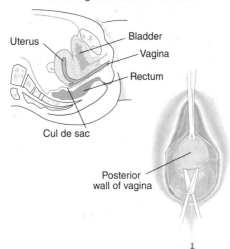

The physician cuts the posterior wall of the vagina to view the cul de sac

Uterus

Bladder

Vagina

Rectum

Cul de sac

Posterior wall of vagina

Explanation

Colpotomy is an incision in the wall of the vagina, usually to access a recess between the rectum and uterus formed by a fold in the peritoneum (cul-de-sac). Through a speculum inserted in the vagina, the physician grasps the posterior lip of the cervix with a toothed instrument called a tenaculum. The cervix is lifted, exposing the posterior vaginal pouch. An incision is made through the back wall of the vagina into the posterior pelvic cavity. Through this opening, the pelvic cavity can be explored using instruments. After exploration, the physician closes the incision with absorbable sutures.

Coding Tips

For colpotomy with drainage of a pelvic abscess, see 57010. Surgical trays, A4550, are not separately reimbursed by Medicare; however, other third-party payers may cover them. Check with the specific payer to determine coverage.

ICD-10-CM Diagnostic Codes

C45.1	Mesothelioma of peritoneum
C48.1	Malignant neoplasm of specified parts of peritoneum
C48.8	Malignant neoplasm of overlapping sites of retroperitoneum and peritoneum
C52	Malignant neoplasm of vagina ♀
C78.6	Secondary malignant neoplasm of retroperitoneum and peritoneum
C79.82	Secondary malignant neoplasm of genital organs
C7B.04	Secondary carcinoid tumors of peritoneum
D19.1	Benign neoplasm of mesothelial tissue of peritoneum
D20.0	Benign neoplasm of soft tissue of retroperitoneum
D20.1	Benign neoplasm of soft tissue of peritoneum
D28.1	Benign neoplasm of vagina ♀
D39.8	Neoplasm of uncertain behavior of other specified female genital organs ♀
D48.3	Neoplasm of uncertain behavior of retroperitoneum
D48.4	Neoplasm of uncertain behavior of peritoneum
D49.59	Neoplasm of unspecified behavior of other genitourinary organ
N76.0	Acute vaginitis ♀
N76.1	Subacute and chronic vaginitis ♀
N76.2	Acute vulvitis ♀
N76.3	Subacute and chronic vulvitis ♀
N89.8	Other specified noninflammatory disorders of vagina ♀
N94.4	Primary dysmenorrhea ♀
N94.5	Secondary dysmenorrhea ♀

AMA: 57000 2019,Jul,6; 2018,Jan,8; 2017,Jan,8; 2016,Jan,13; 2015,Jan,16; 2014,Jan,11

Relative Value Units/Medicare Edits

Non-Facility RVU	Work	PE	MP	Total
57000	3.02	2.19	0.48	5.69
Facility RVU	**Work**	**PE**	**MP**	**Total**
57000	3.02	2.19	0.48	5.69

	FUD	Status	MUE	Modifiers				IOM Reference
57000	10	A	1(3)	51	N/A	N/A	80*	None

* with documentation

Terms To Know

absorbable sutures. Strands used for suture or repair of tissue prepared from collagen or a synthetic polymer and capable of being absorbed by tissue over time.

benign. Mild or nonmalignant in nature.

culdotomy/colpotomy. Incision through the vaginal wall into the cul-de-sac of Douglas (retro uterine pouch).

dysmenorrhea. Painful menstruation that may be primary, or essential, due to prostaglandin production and the onset of menstruation; secondary due to uterine, tubal, or ovarian abnormality or disease; spasmodic arising uterine contractions; or obstructive due to some mechanical blockage or interference with the menstrual flow.

incision. Act of cutting into tissue or an organ.

malignant neoplasm. Any cancerous tumor or lesion exhibiting uncontrolled tissue growth that can progressively invade other parts of the body with its disease-generating cells.

peritoneum. Strong, continuous membrane that forms the lining of the abdominal and pelvic cavity. The parietal peritoneum, or outer layer, is attached to the abdominopelvic walls and the visceral peritoneum, or inner layer, surrounds the organs inside the abdominal cavity.

secondary. Second in order of occurrence or importance, or appearing during the course of another disease or condition.

speculum. Tool used to enlarge the opening of any canal or cavity.

Vagina

57010

57010   Colpotomy; with drainage of pelvic abscess

Pelvic abscess is drained

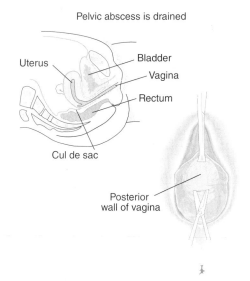

Uterus — Bladder — Vagina — Rectum

Cul de sac

Posterior wall of vagina

Explanation

Colpotomy is an incision in the wall of the vagina, usually to access a recess between the rectum and uterus formed by a fold in the peritoneum (cul de sac). Through a speculum inserted in the vagina, the physician grasps the posterior lip of the cervix with a toothed instrument called a tenaculum. The cervix is lifted, exposing the posterior vaginal pouch. An incision is made through the back wall of the vagina into the posterior pelvic cavity. Through this opening, the pelvic cavity can be explored. The abscess in the cavity is located, entered, and drained through the vaginal incision. Rubber drains are often inserted and left in place for several days. The physician closes the incision with absorbable sutures.

Coding Tips

For a colpotomy with exploration, see 57000.

ICD-10-CM Diagnostic Codes

K65.1	Peritoneal abscess
N73.0	Acute parametritis and pelvic cellulitis ♀
N73.1	Chronic parametritis and pelvic cellulitis ♀
N73.2	Unspecified parametritis and pelvic cellulitis ♀
N73.9	Female pelvic inflammatory disease, unspecified ♀

AMA: 57010 2019,Jul,6; 2014,Jan,11

Relative Value Units/Medicare Edits

Non-Facility RVU	Work	PE	MP	Total
57010	6.84	5.04	1.07	12.95
Facility RVU	**Work**	**PE**	**MP**	**Total**
57010	6.84	5.04	1.07	12.95

	FUD	Status	MUE	Modifiers				IOM Reference
57010	90	A	1(3)	51	N/A	N/A	80*	None

* with documentation

57020

57020   Colpocentesis (separate procedure)

Matter from the pelvis is aspirated through a needle inserted through the vaginal wall

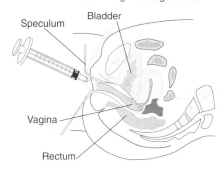

Speculum — Bladder

Vagina

Rectum

Explanation

Colpocentesis is the aspiration of fluid in the peritoneum through the wall of the vagina. Through a speculum inserted in the vagina, the physician grasps the posterior lip of the cervix with a toothed instrument called a tenaculum. The cervix is lifted, exposing the posterior vaginal pouch and deep back wall of the vagina. A long needle attached to a syringe is inserted through the exposed vaginal wall and the posterior pelvic cavity is entered. Fluid is aspirated through the needle into the syringe.

Coding Tips

This separate procedure by definition is usually a component of a more complex service and is not identified separately. When performed alone or with other unrelated procedures or services it may be reported. If performed alone, list the code; if performed with other procedures/services, list the code and append modifier 59 or an X{EPSU} modifier. If the aspirated fluid is transported to an outside laboratory, report 99000 for conveyance of the specimen.

ICD-10-CM Diagnostic Codes

A56.11	Chlamydial female pelvic inflammatory disease ♀
C52	Malignant neoplasm of vagina ♀
C79.82	Secondary malignant neoplasm of genital organs
D07.1	Carcinoma in situ of vulva ♀
D07.2	Carcinoma in situ of vagina ♀
D07.39	Carcinoma in situ of other female genital organs ♀
D28.1	Benign neoplasm of vagina ♀
D39.8	Neoplasm of uncertain behavior of other specified female genital organs ♀
D49.59	Neoplasm of unspecified behavior of other genitourinary organ
N73.0	Acute parametritis and pelvic cellulitis ♀
N73.1	Chronic parametritis and pelvic cellulitis ♀
N73.3	Female acute pelvic peritonitis ♀
N73.4	Female chronic pelvic peritonitis ♀
N73.8	Other specified female pelvic inflammatory diseases ♀
Q51.0	Agenesis and aplasia of uterus ♀
Q51.5	Agenesis and aplasia of cervix ♀
Q51.6	Embryonic cyst of cervix ♀
Q51.7	Congenital fistulae between uterus and digestive and urinary tracts ♀
Q51.821	Hypoplasia of cervix ♀

AMA: 57020 2019,Jul,6; 2014,Jan,11

Relative Value Units/Medicare Edits

Non-Facility RVU	Work	PE	MP	Total
57020	1.5	1.42	0.25	3.17
Facility RVU	**Work**	**PE**	**MP**	**Total**
57020	1.5	0.6	0.25	2.35

	FUD	Status	MUE	Modifiers				IOM Reference
57020	0	A	1(3)	51	N/A	N/A	80*	None

* with documentation

Terms To Know

aspiration. Drawing fluid out by suction.

benign. Mild or nonmalignant in nature.

carcinoma in situ. Malignancy that arises from the cells of the vessel, gland, or organ of origin that remains confined to that site or has not invaded neighboring tissue.

malignant neoplasm. Any cancerous tumor or lesion exhibiting uncontrolled tissue growth that can progressively invade other parts of the body with its disease-generating cells.

peritoneum. Strong, continuous membrane that forms the lining of the abdominal and pelvic cavity. The parietal peritoneum, or outer layer, is attached to the abdominopelvic walls and the visceral peritoneum, or inner layer, surrounds the organs inside the abdominal cavity.

57022-57023

57022   Incision and drainage of vaginal hematoma; obstetrical/postpartum
57023   non-obstetrical (eg, post-trauma, spontaneous bleeding)

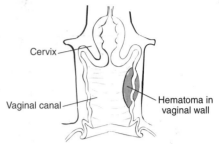

Cervix

Vaginal canal

Hematoma in vaginal wall

The hematoma may be post obstetrical or nonobstetrical

Explanation

The physician incises and drains a vaginal hematoma in an obstetrical or postpartum patient. The patient is placed in a dorso-lithotomy position. The physician inserts a speculum into the vagina. The hematoma is visualized, and incised. Blood and clot are drained from the hematoma. Electrocautery or suture is used to control bleeding. When needed, a Hemovac drain is placed. The vagina is irrigated, and the area of hematoma is sponged with dressings. When hemostasis is achieved, the speculum is removed. Report 57022 when the procedure is performed on an obstetrical patient and 57023 when the procedure is performed on a non-obstetrical patient. Hemovac drains may be placed if the hematoma bed is still oozing.

Coding Tips

When 57022 or 57023 is performed with another separately identifiable procedure, the highest dollar value code is listed as the primary procedure and subsequent procedures are appended with modifier 51. Surgical trays, A4550, are not separately reimbursed by Medicare; however, other third-party payers may cover them. Check with the specific payer to determine coverage.

ICD-10-CM Diagnostic Codes

N89.8   Other specified noninflammatory disorders of vagina ♀
O71.7   Obstetric hematoma of pelvis 🅼 ♀

AMA: 57022 2019,Jul,6; 2014,Jan,11 57023 2019,Jul,6; 2014,Jan,11

Relative Value Units/Medicare Edits

Non-Facility RVU	Work	PE	MP	Total
57022	2.73	1.93	0.44	5.1
57023	5.18	3.17	0.81	9.16
Facility RVU	**Work**	**PE**	**MP**	**Total**
57022	2.73	1.93	0.44	5.1
57023	5.18	3.17	0.81	9.16

	FUD	Status	MUE	Modifiers				IOM Reference
57022	10	A	1(3)	51	N/A	N/A	80*	None
57023	10	A	1(3)	51	N/A	N/A	80*	

* with documentation

Terms To Know

hematoma. Tumor-like collection of blood in some part of the body caused by a break in a blood vessel wall, usually as a result of trauma.

57061-57065

57061 Destruction of vaginal lesion(s); simple (eg, laser surgery, electrosurgery, cryosurgery, chemosurgery)

57065 extensive (eg, laser surgery, electrosurgery, cryosurgery, chemosurgery)

Vaginal lesions are destroyed
with electrocautery, laser or cryoprobe

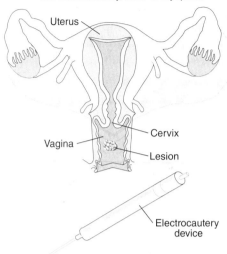

Uterus

Cervix

Vagina

Lesion

Electrocautery
device

Explanation

Using a colposcope, a binocular microscope used for direct visualization of the vagina and cervix, the physician identifies lesion(s) in and/or around the vagina. The physician destroys the abnormal tissue by chemosurgery, electrosurgery, laser surgery, or cryotherapy. Use 57061 if the lesions are few in number, small, or simple. Use 57065 if the lesions are numerous, large, or difficult.

Coding Tips

For excision of a vaginal cyst or tumor, see 57135. For biopsy of a vaginal mucosa, see 57100–57105. Destruction of vulvar lesions is reported with 56501–56515.

ICD-10-CM Diagnostic Codes

A63.0	Anogenital (venereal) warts
C52	Malignant neoplasm of vagina ♀
C79.82	Secondary malignant neoplasm of genital organs
D07.2	Carcinoma in situ of vagina ♀
D28.1	Benign neoplasm of vagina ♀
D39.8	Neoplasm of uncertain behavior of other specified female genital organs ♀
D49.59	Neoplasm of unspecified behavior of other genitourinary organ
N76.5	Ulceration of vagina ♀
N76.81	Mucositis (ulcerative) of vagina and vulva ♀
N76.89	Other specified inflammation of vagina and vulva ♀
N84.2	Polyp of vagina ♀
N89.0	Mild vaginal dysplasia ♀
N89.1	Moderate vaginal dysplasia ♀
N89.4	Leukoplakia of vagina ♀
N89.8	Other specified noninflammatory disorders of vagina ♀
N90.89	Other specified noninflammatory disorders of vulva and perineum ♀

AMA: 57061 2019,Jul,6; 2018,Jan,8; 2017,Jan,8; 2016,Jan,13; 2015,Jan,16; 2014,Jan,11 **57065** 2019,Jul,6; 2018,Jan,8; 2017,Jan,8; 2016,Jan,13; 2015,Jan,16; 2014,Jan,11

Relative Value Units/Medicare Edits

Non-Facility RVU	Work	PE	MP	Total
57061	1.3	2.54	0.21	4.05
57065	2.66	3.29	0.42	6.37
Facility RVU	**Work**	**PE**	**MP**	**Total**
57061	1.3	1.58	0.21	3.09
57065	2.66	2.12	0.42	5.2

	FUD	Status	MUE	Modifiers				IOM Reference
57061	10	A	1(2)	51	N/A	N/A	N/A	100-03,140.5
57065	10	A	1(2)	51	N/A	N/A	N/A	

* with documentation

Terms To Know

chemosurgery. Application of chemical agents to destroy tissue, originally referring to the in situ chemical fixation of premalignant or malignant lesions to facilitate surgical excision.

condyloma. Infectious tumor-like growth caused by the human papilloma virus, with a branching connective tissue core and epithelial covering that occurs on the skin and mucous membranes of the perianal region and external genitalia.

cryosurgery. Application of intense cold, usually produced using liquid nitrogen, to locally freeze diseased or unwanted tissue and induce tissue necrosis without causing harm to adjacent tissue.

destruction. Ablation or eradication of a structure or tissue.

electrocautery. Division or cutting of tissue using high-frequency electrical current to produce heat, which destroys cells.

laser surgery. Use of concentrated, sharply defined light beams to cut, cauterize, coagulate, seal, or vaporize tissue.

lesion. Area of damaged tissue that has lost continuity or function, due to disease or trauma.

polyp. Small growth on a stalk-like attachment projecting from a mucous membrane.

Vagina

57100-57105

57100 Biopsy of vaginal mucosa; simple (separate procedure)
57105 extensive, requiring suture (including cysts)

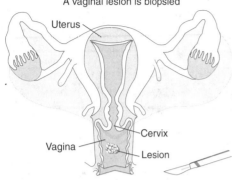

A vaginal lesion is biopsied

Uterus

Cervix

Vagina

Lesion

Explanation

The physician takes a sample of vaginal mucosa for examination. After injecting a local anesthetic into the suspect area, the physician obtains a sample with a skin punch or sharp scalpel. In 57100, the biopsy is simple and no sutures are required. In 57105, sutures are required as the excision site is extensive and bleeding may need to be controlled.

Coding Tips

Note that 57100, a separate procedure by definition, is usually a component of a more complex service and is not identified separately. When performed alone or with other unrelated procedures/services it may be reported. If performed alone, list the code; if performed with other procedures/services, list the code and append modifier 59 or an X{EPSU} modifier. If the excised tissue is transported to an outside laboratory, report 99000 for conveyance of the specimen. Any local or topical anesthetic is not reported separately.

ICD-10-CM Diagnostic Codes

A54.1	Gonococcal infection of lower genitourinary tract with periurethral and accessory gland abscess
A60.04	Herpesviral vulvovaginitis ♀
A63.0	Anogenital (venereal) warts
C52	Malignant neoplasm of vagina ♀
C79.82	Secondary malignant neoplasm of genital organs
D07.2	Carcinoma in situ of vagina ♀
D28.1	Benign neoplasm of vagina ♀
D39.8	Neoplasm of uncertain behavior of other specified female genital organs ♀
D49.59	Neoplasm of unspecified behavior of other genitourinary organ
N76.0	Acute vaginitis ♀
N76.1	Subacute and chronic vaginitis ♀
N76.5	Ulceration of vagina ♀
N76.81	Mucositis (ulcerative) of vagina and vulva ♀
N76.89	Other specified inflammation of vagina and vulva ♀
N84.2	Polyp of vagina ♀
N89.0	Mild vaginal dysplasia ♀
N89.1	Moderate vaginal dysplasia ♀
N89.4	Leukoplakia of vagina ♀
N89.8	Other specified noninflammatory disorders of vagina ♀
N95.2	Postmenopausal atrophic vaginitis ♀

Q52.2	Congenital rectovaginal fistula ♀
Q52.4	Other congenital malformations of vagina ♀
Z08	Encounter for follow-up examination after completed treatment for malignant neoplasm
Z09	Encounter for follow-up examination after completed treatment for conditions other than malignant neoplasm

AMA: **57100** 2019,Jul,6; 2014,Jan,11 **57105** 2019,Jul,6; 2014,Jan,11

Relative Value Units/Medicare Edits

Non-Facility RVU	Work	PE	MP	Total
57100	1.2	1.38	0.18	2.76
57105	1.74	2.55	0.27	4.56
Facility RVU	**Work**	**PE**	**MP**	**Total**
57100	1.2	0.52	0.18	1.9
57105	1.74	1.92	0.27	3.93

	FUD	Status	MUE	Modifiers				IOM Reference
57100	0	A	2(3)	51	N/A	N/A	N/A	None
57105	10	A	2(3)	51	N/A	N/A	N/A	

* with documentation

Terms To Know

biopsy. Tissue or fluid removed for diagnostic purposes through analysis of the cells in the biopsy material.

carcinoma in situ. Malignancy that arises from the cells of the vessel, gland, or organ of origin that remains confined to that site or has not invaded neighboring tissue.

cyst. Elevated encapsulated mass containing fluid, semisolid, or solid material with a membranous lining.

dysplasia. Abnormality or alteration in the size, shape, and organization of cells from their normal pattern of development.

leukoplakia. Thickened white patches or lesions appearing on a mucous membrane, such as oral mucosa or tongue.

malignant. Any condition tending to progress toward death, specifically an invasive tumor with a loss of cellular differentiation that has the ability to spread or metastasize to other body areas.

neoplasm. New abnormal growth, tumor.

polyp. Small growth on a stalk-like attachment projecting from a mucous membrane.

Coding Companion for Ob/Gyn

Vagina

57106-57109

57106 Vaginectomy, partial removal of vaginal wall;
57107 with removal of paravaginal tissue (radical vaginectomy)
57109 with removal of paravaginal tissue (radical vaginectomy) with bilateral total pelvic lymphadenectomy and para-aortic lymph node sampling (biopsy)

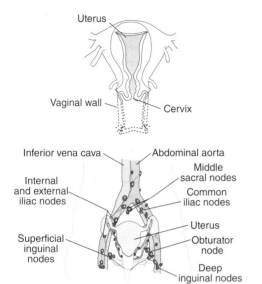

Explanation

The physician excises part of the vagina. This is sometimes preceded by injection of medication to constrict blood vessels to control bleeding. The vagina is everted and sizeable sections are removed by sharp and blunt dissection. In 57107, the physician removes surrounding diseased and/or damaged tissue. In 57109, the physician removes surrounding diseased and/or damaged tissue, in addition to removing the pelvic lymph nodes, and performing biopsy of the lymph nodes of the aorta to check for the extent of disease. Remaining vaginal and/or support tissue is inverted and sutured in place to obliterate some or all of the space formerly occupied by the vagina. The perineum is closed over the former vaginal opening.

Coding Tips

Lymph node removal is included in 57109 and should not be reported separately. For vaginectomy with complete removal of the vaginal wall, see 57110; with removal of paravaginal tissue (radical vaginectomy), see 57111.

ICD-10-CM Diagnostic Codes

C52	Malignant neoplasm of vagina ♀
C77.2	Secondary and unspecified malignant neoplasm of intra-abdominal lymph nodes
C77.5	Secondary and unspecified malignant neoplasm of intrapelvic lymph nodes
C79.82	Secondary malignant neoplasm of genital organs
D07.2	Carcinoma in situ of vagina ♀
D28.1	Benign neoplasm of vagina ♀
D39.8	Neoplasm of uncertain behavior of other specified female genital organs ♀
D49.59	Neoplasm of unspecified behavior of other genitourinary organ
N89.0	Mild vaginal dysplasia ♀
N89.1	Moderate vaginal dysplasia ♀
N89.4	Leukoplakia of vagina ♀

AMA: **57106** 2019,Jul,6; 2018,Jan,8; 2017,Jan,8; 2016,Jan,13; 2015,Jan,16; 2014,Jan,11 **57107** 2019,Jul,6; 2018,Jan,8; 2017,Jan,8; 2016,Jan,13; 2015,Jan,16; 2014,Jan,11 **57109** 2019,Jul,6; 2018,Jan,8; 2017,Jan,8; 2016,Jan,13; 2015,Jan,16; 2014,Jan,11

Relative Value Units/Medicare Edits

Non-Facility RVU	Work	PE	MP	Total
57106	7.5	6.24	1.15	14.89
57107	24.56	13.33	3.64	41.53
57109	28.4	16.48	4.46	49.34
Facility RVU	**Work**	**PE**	**MP**	**Total**
57106	7.5	6.24	1.15	14.89
57107	24.56	13.33	3.64	41.53
57109	28.4	16.48	4.46	49.34

	FUD	Status	MUE	Modifiers				IOM Reference
57106	90	A	1(2)	51	N/A	62*	80	None
57107	90	A	1(2)	51	N/A	62*	80	
57109	90	A	1(2)	51	N/A	62*	80	

* with documentation

Terms To Know

biopsy. Tissue or fluid removed for diagnostic purposes through analysis of the cells in the biopsy material.

blunt dissection. Surgical technique used to expose an underlying area by separating along natural cleavage lines of tissue, without cutting.

excise. Remove or cut out.

lymph nodes. Bean-shaped structures along the lymphatic vessels that intercept and destroy foreign materials in the tissue and bloodstream.

lymphadenectomy. Dissection of lymph nodes free from the vessels and removal for examination by frozen section in a separate procedure to detect early-stage metastases.

malignant neoplasm. Any cancerous tumor or lesion exhibiting uncontrolled tissue growth that can progressively invade other parts of the body with its disease-generating cells.

radical. Extensive surgery.

Vagina

57110-57111

57110 Vaginectomy, complete removal of vaginal wall;
57111 with removal of paravaginal tissue (radical vaginectomy)

The physician excises the entire vagina

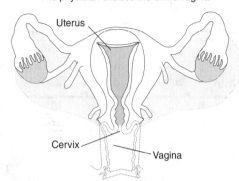

The perineum is closed over the operative wound

Explanation

The physician performs a complete removal of the vaginal wall in 57110. This is sometimes proceeded by injection of medication to constrict blood vessels to control bleeding. The vagina is everted. An incision circumscribes the hymen, and the vagina is marked into four quadrants. Each quadrant of vaginal wall is removed by sharp and blunt dissection. In 57111, the physician also removes surrounding diseased and/or damaged tissue. The remaining support tissues are inverted and sutured in place obliterating the space formerly occupied by the vagina. The perineum is closed over the former vaginal opening.

Coding Tips

For vaginectomy with partial removal of the vaginal wall, see 57106; with removal of paravaginal tissue (radical vaginectomy), see 57107; with removal of paravaginal tissue (radical vaginectomy) with bilateral total pelvic lymphadenectomy and para-aortic lymph node sampling, see 57109.

ICD-10-CM Diagnostic Codes

C52	Malignant neoplasm of vagina ♀
C79.82	Secondary malignant neoplasm of genital organs
D07.2	Carcinoma in situ of vagina ♀
D28.1	Benign neoplasm of vagina ♀
D39.8	Neoplasm of uncertain behavior of other specified female genital organs ♀
D49.59	Neoplasm of unspecified behavior of other genitourinary organ
N89.0	Mild vaginal dysplasia ♀
N89.1	Moderate vaginal dysplasia ♀
N89.4	Leukoplakia of vagina ♀

AMA: **57110** 2019,Jul,6; 2018,Jan,8; 2017,Jan,8; 2016,Jan,13; 2015,Jan,16; 2014,Jan,11 **57111** 2019,Jul,6; 2018,Jan,8; 2017,Jan,8; 2016,Jan,13; 2015,Jan,16; 2014,Jan,11

Relative Value Units/Medicare Edits

Non-Facility RVU	Work	PE	MP	Total
57110	15.48	8.29	2.37	26.14
57111	28.4	16.48	4.46	49.34
Facility RVU	**Work**	**PE**	**MP**	**Total**
57110	15.48	8.29	2.37	26.14
57111	28.4	16.48	4.46	49.34

	FUD	Status	MUE	Modifiers				IOM Reference
57110	90	A	1(2)	51	N/A	62*	80	None
57111	90	A	1(2)	51	N/A	62*	80	

* with documentation

Terms To Know

biopsy. Tissue or fluid removed for diagnostic purposes through analysis of the cells in the biopsy material.

blunt dissection. Surgical technique used to expose an underlying area by separating along natural cleavage lines of tissue, without cutting.

dysplasia. Abnormality or alteration in the size, shape, and organization of cells from their normal pattern of development.

malignant neoplasm. Any cancerous tumor or lesion exhibiting uncontrolled tissue growth that can progressively invade other parts of the body with its disease-generating cells.

radical. Extensive surgery.

secondary. Second in order of occurrence or importance, or appearing during the course of another disease or condition.

vaginectomy. Surgical excision of all or a portion of the vagina.

Vagina

57120

57120   Colpocleisis (Le Fort type)

The vagina is surgically closed

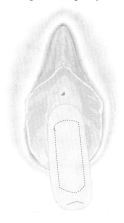

Explanation

The physician grasps the deepest portion of the vaginal vault and everts the vagina. Two large flaps of vaginal wall are removed from opposite sides of the prolapsed vagina. The vaginal walls are sutured to one another and this structure is inverted back inside the body. The former vaginal opening is closed with sutures obliterating the vagina and preventing uterine prolapse.

Coding Tips

This procedure is rarely used: code with caution. For vaginectomy other than Le Fort, see 57106–57109 and 57110–57111.

ICD-10-CM Diagnostic Codes

N81.2   Incomplete uterovaginal prolapse ♀
N81.3   Complete uterovaginal prolapse ♀
N99.3   Prolapse of vaginal vault after hysterectomy ♀

AMA: **57120** 2019,Jul,6; 2014,Jan,11

Relative Value Units/Medicare Edits

Non-Facility RVU	Work	PE	MP	Total
57120	8.28	5.58	1.25	15.11
Facility RVU	**Work**	**PE**	**MP**	**Total**
57120	8.28	5.58	1.25	15.11

	FUD	Status	MUE	Modifiers				IOM Reference
57120	90	A	1(2)	51	N/A	62*	80	None

* with documentation

Terms To Know

colpocleisis. Surgical procedure in which the vaginal canal is closed in order to prevent uterine prolapse.

obliterate. Get rid or do away with completely.

uterovaginal prolapse. Uterus displaced downward and exposed in the external genitalia.

57130

57130   Excision of vaginal septum

The physician excises a septum that bisects the vagina

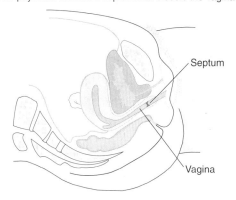

Septum

Vagina

Explanation

The physician excises a vaginal septum, an anomaly that separates the vagina into two portions. The septum can be longitudinal, creating two vaginal canals, or transverse, blocking the vagina and preventing menstrual flow. For a small, thin septum, the procedure is often done by injecting a local anesthetic in the tissues around the septum and making an incision through the narrowest portion of the septum. The divided tissue is tied off with suture material and the tissue is excised. For a thicker and more extensive septum, the procedure may be done under general anesthesia. The tissue is excised, and the resulting vaginal lining defects are closed. The vagina is packed with medicated gauze or a support device.

Coding Tips

Local anesthesia is included in this service. However, this procedure may be performed under general anesthesia, depending on the age and/or condition of the patient. Report any free grafts or flaps separately. For excision of a vaginal cyst or tumor, see 57135.

ICD-10-CM Diagnostic Codes

Q52.11   Transverse vaginal septum ♀
Q52.120   Longitudinal vaginal septum, nonobstructing ♀
Q52.121   Longitudinal vaginal septum, obstructing, right side ♀ ☑
Q52.122   Longitudinal vaginal septum, obstructing, left side ♀ ☑
Q52.123   Longitudinal vaginal septum, microperforate, right side ♀ ☑
Q52.124   Longitudinal vaginal septum, microperforate, left side ♀ ☑

AMA: **57130** 2019,Jul,6; 2014,Jan,11

Relative Value Units/Medicare Edits

Non-Facility RVU	Work	PE	MP	Total
57130	2.46	3.08	0.39	5.93
Facility RVU	**Work**	**PE**	**MP**	**Total**
57130	2.46	1.98	0.39	4.83

	FUD	Status	MUE	Modifiers				IOM Reference
57130	10	A	1(2)	51	N/A	62*	80	None

* with documentation

Vagina

57135

57135   Excision of vaginal cyst or tumor

The physician removes a vaginal cyst or tumor

Uterus

Vagina

Cervix

Cyst or tumor

Explanation

Through a speculum inserted in the vagina, the physician uses a forceps or hemostat clamp to grasp and elongate the vaginal tissue containing the cyst or tumor, causing the mucosa to tent. With a scalpel or scissors, the physician excises an ellipse of tissue containing the lesion. The defect is closed with absorbable sutures.

Coding Tips

If the excised tissue is transported to an outside laboratory, report 99000 for conveyance of the specimen. For excision of a vaginal septum, see 57130. For destruction of a vaginal lesion(s), see 57061–57065. For excision with partial or complete removal of the vagina, see 57106–57111.

ICD-10-CM Diagnostic Codes

C52	Malignant neoplasm of vagina ♀
C79.82	Secondary malignant neoplasm of genital organs
D07.2	Carcinoma in situ of vagina ♀
D28.1	Benign neoplasm of vagina ♀
D39.8	Neoplasm of uncertain behavior of other specified female genital organs ♀
D49.59	Neoplasm of unspecified behavior of other genitourinary organ
N84.2	Polyp of vagina ♀
N89.8	Other specified noninflammatory disorders of vagina ♀
Q52.4	Other congenital malformations of vagina ♀

AMA: **57135** 2019,Jul,6; 2014,Jan,11

Relative Value Units/Medicare Edits

Non-Facility RVU	Work	PE	MP	Total
57135	2.7	3.26	0.42	6.38
Facility RVU	**Work**	**PE**	**MP**	**Total**
57135	2.7	2.12	0.42	5.24

	FUD	Status	MUE	Modifiers				IOM Reference
57135	10	A	2(3)	51	N/A	N/A	N/A	None

* with documentation

57150

57150   Irrigation of vagina and/or application of medicament for treatment of bacterial, parasitic, or fungoid disease

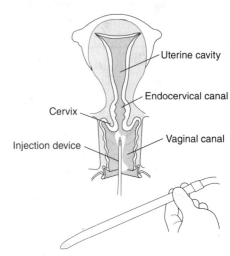

Uterine cavity

Endocervical canal

Cervix

Vaginal canal

Injection device

Explanation

The physician passes a catheter or similar tube high into the vaginal canal and flushes the canal with medicated solution from a large syringe. The physician also paints infected areas with medication using a cotton-tipped applicator or similar device.

Coding Tips

For clinical brachytherapy to treat cancerous conditions via insertion of vaginal ovoids and/or a uterine tandem, see 57155. For introduction of packing or hemostatic agent to stop nonobstetrical vaginal hemorrhaging, see 57180. Surgical trays, A4550, are not separately reimbursed by Medicare; however, other third-party payers may cover them. Check with the specific payer to determine coverage.

ICD-10-CM Diagnostic Codes

A56.02	Chlamydial vulvovaginitis ♀
A59.01	Trichomonal vulvovaginitis ♀
A60.04	Herpesviral vulvovaginitis ♀
B37.3	Candidiasis of vulva and vagina ♀
B80	Enterobiasis
N72	Inflammatory disease of cervix uteri ♀
N76.0	Acute vaginitis ♀
N76.1	Subacute and chronic vaginitis ♀
N76.2	Acute vulvitis ♀
N76.3	Subacute and chronic vulvitis ♀
N76.81	Mucositis (ulcerative) of vagina and vulva ♀
N76.89	Other specified inflammation of vagina and vulva ♀
N89.8	Other specified noninflammatory disorders of vagina ♀

AMA: **57150** 2019,Jul,6; 2014,Jan,11

N Newborn: 0   **P** Pediatric: 0-17   **M** Maternity: 9-64   **A** Adult: 15-124   ♂ Male Only   ♀ Female Only

Coding Companion for Ob/Gyn

Vagina

Relative Value Units/Medicare Edits

Non-Facility RVU	Work	PE	MP	Total
57150	0.5	0.95	0.09	1.54
Facility RVU	**Work**	**PE**	**MP**	**Total**
57150	0.5	0.19	0.09	0.78

	FUD	Status	MUE	Modifiers				IOM Reference
57150	0	A	1(3)	51	N/A	N/A	N/A	None

* with documentation

Terms To Know

acute. Sudden, severe.

candida. Genus of yeast-like fungi that are commonly found in the mouth, skin, intestinal tract, and vagina. It may cause a white, cheesy discharge.

catheter. Flexible tube inserted into an area of the body for introducing or withdrawing fluid.

enterobiasis. Infection with pinworms, especially nematodes of the genus E. vermicularis, usually located in portions of the intestine.

inflammation. Cytologic and chemical reactions that occur in affected blood vessels and adjacent tissues in response to injury or abnormal stimulation from a physical, chemical, or biologic agent.

irrigation. To wash out or cleanse a body cavity, wound, or tissue with water or other fluid.

leukorrhea. White mucousy vaginal discharge.

medicament. Medical and therapeutic compound, drug, substance, or remedy.

trichomonas vaginalis. Vaginal infection by a single-celled, flagellate protozoan causing discharge, inflammation, and itching.

57155

57155   Insertion of uterine tandem and/or vaginal ovoids for clinical brachytherapy

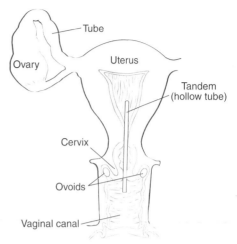

A hollow metal tube, or tandem, is placed through the cervical os

Explanation

The physician places a brachytherapy applicator (also called a tandem and ovoids) prior to the first brachytherapy treatment for cervical cancer. Under appropriate anesthesia, a hollow plastic sleeve that has been custom fitted to the uterine cavity is inserted into the uterus through the cervical opening and sutured into place onto the cervix. This sleeve remains in the uterus for the duration of the brachytherapy treatments, keeping the cervix open to allow for comfortable positioning of the tandem (a hollow metal tube that is inserted into the sleeve). Two ovoids, containing small radiation shields that reduce radiation doses to the bladder and rectum, are then positioned on either side of the cervix. Separately reportable brachytherapy follows, after which the tandem and ovoids are removed.

Coding Tips

The tandem holds radiotherapy doses. Additionally, in some instances, ovoids are placed high in the vaginal cavity and around the cervix. Any insertions may have shields to protect the bladder and/or rectum. For insertion of radioelement sources or ribbons, see 77761–77763 or 77770–77772. To report placement of needles or catheters into pelvic organs and/or genitalia for interstitial radioelement application, see 55920.

ICD-10-CM Diagnostic Codes

C53.0	Malignant neoplasm of endocervix ♀
C53.1	Malignant neoplasm of exocervix ♀
C53.8	Malignant neoplasm of overlapping sites of cervix uteri ♀
C54.0	Malignant neoplasm of isthmus uteri ♀
C54.1	Malignant neoplasm of endometrium ♀
C54.2	Malignant neoplasm of myometrium ♀
C54.3	Malignant neoplasm of fundus uteri ♀
C54.8	Malignant neoplasm of overlapping sites of corpus uteri ♀
C79.82	Secondary malignant neoplasm of genital organs
D06.0	Carcinoma in situ of endocervix ♀
D06.1	Carcinoma in situ of exocervix ♀
D06.7	Carcinoma in situ of other parts of cervix ♀
D07.0	Carcinoma in situ of endometrium ♀

Vagina

D39.0   Neoplasm of uncertain behavior of uterus ♀

D39.8   Neoplasm of uncertain behavior of other specified female genital organs ♀

AMA: **57155** 2019,Jul,6; 2018,Jan,8; 2017,Jan,8; 2016,Jan,13; 2015,Jan,16; 2014,Jan,11

Relative Value Units/Medicare Edits

Non-Facility RVU	Work	PE	MP	Total
57155	5.15	5.33	0.42	10.9
Facility RVU	**Work**	**PE**	**MP**	**Total**
57155	5.15	2.56	0.42	8.13

	FUD	Status	MUE	Modifiers				IOM Reference
57155	0	A	1(3)	51	N/A	62	N/A	None

* with documentation

Terms To Know

brachytherapy. Form of radiation therapy in which radioactive pellets or seeds are implanted directly into the tissue being treated to deliver their dose of radiation in a more directed fashion. Brachytherapy provides radiation to the prescribed body area while minimizing exposure to normal tissue.

carcinoma in situ. Malignancy that arises from the cells of the vessel, gland, or organ of origin that remains confined to that site or has not invaded neighboring tissue.

endometrial carcinoma. Cancer of the inner lining of the uterine wall.

insertion. Placement or implantation into a body part.

internal os. Opening through the cervix into the uterus.

malignant. Any condition tending to progress toward death, specifically an invasive tumor with a loss of cellular differentiation that has the ability to spread or metastasize to other body areas.

neoplasm. New abnormal growth, tumor.

ovoid. Round, hollow metal holder implants placed next to, or on the side of, the cervix for the purpose of administering clinical brachytherapy. The implants may be stabilized in place with the use of packing to ensure no movement during treatment. Radiation is placed into the implants.

secondary. Second in order of occurrence or importance, or appearing during the course of another disease or condition.

tandem. Small, metal tube inserts placed into the vagina and uterus (in women who have not had a hysterectomy) for the purpose of administering clinical brachytherapy. The inserts are stabilized in place with the use of packing to ensure no movement during treatment. The tube endings remain outside the vagina to allow radiation to be inserted into the tube.

57156

57156   Insertion of a vaginal radiation afterloading apparatus for clinical brachytherapy

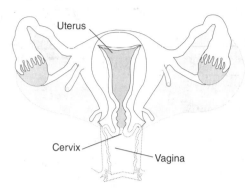

Radiation afterloading apparatus is inserted into the vagina

Explanation

A non-radioactive applicator or cylinder is placed into the uterine cavity and vagina in preparation for clinical brachytherapy. Under appropriate anesthesia, the physician inserts the applicator/cylinder and secures it into position, often using radiological guidance. The applicator is subsequently loaded with the radiation sources, often using a remote system in which the applicators are connected to an "afterloader" machine via a series of guide tubes. Remote afterloading systems provide radiation exposure protection to health care professionals by delivering radiation sources along the guide tubes into the prespecified positions within the applicator without staff presence in the treatment room. Separately reportable vaginal brachytherapy is then administered using low-dose rate (LDR) or high-dose rate (HDR) radiotherapy. Code 57156 reports insertion of the afterloading apparatus only.

Coding Tips

For insertion of a uterine tandem and/or vaginal ovoids, see 57155.

ICD-10-CM Diagnostic Codes

C53.0	Malignant neoplasm of endocervix ♀
C53.1	Malignant neoplasm of exocervix ♀
C53.8	Malignant neoplasm of overlapping sites of cervix uteri ♀
C54.0	Malignant neoplasm of isthmus uteri ♀
C54.1	Malignant neoplasm of endometrium ♀
C54.2	Malignant neoplasm of myometrium ♀
C54.3	Malignant neoplasm of fundus uteri ♀
C54.8	Malignant neoplasm of overlapping sites of corpus uteri ♀
C79.82	Secondary malignant neoplasm of genital organs
D06.0	Carcinoma in situ of endocervix ♀
D06.1	Carcinoma in situ of exocervix ♀
D06.7	Carcinoma in situ of other parts of cervix ♀
D07.0	Carcinoma in situ of endometrium ♀
D39.0	Neoplasm of uncertain behavior of uterus ♀
D39.8	Neoplasm of uncertain behavior of other specified female genital organs ♀

AMA: **57156** 2019,Jul,6; 2014,Jan,11

Vagina

Relative Value Units/Medicare Edits

Non-Facility RVU	Work	PE	MP	Total
57156	2.69	3.25	0.19	6.13
Facility RVU	Work	PE	MP	Total
57156	2.69	1.42	0.19	4.3

	FUD	Status	MUE	Modifiers				IOM Reference
57156	0	A	1(3)	51	N/A	N/A	80*	None

* with documentation

Terms To Know

apparatus. Equipment, devices, gear, or machinery required for a specific procedure or service.

brachytherapy. Form of radiation therapy in which radioactive pellets or seeds are implanted directly into the tissue being treated to deliver their dose of radiation in a more directed fashion. Brachytherapy provides radiation to the prescribed body area while minimizing exposure to normal tissue.

carcinoma in situ. Malignancy that arises from the cells of the vessel, gland, or organ of origin that remains confined to that site or has not invaded neighboring tissue.

endometrial carcinoma. Cancer of the inner lining of the uterine wall.

imaging. Radiologic means of producing pictures for clinical study of the internal structures and functions of the body, such as x-ray, ultrasound, magnetic resonance, or positron emission tomography.

insertion. Placement or implantation into a body part.

malignant. Any condition tending to progress toward death, specifically an invasive tumor with a loss of cellular differentiation that has the ability to spread or metastasize to other body areas.

neoplasm. New abnormal growth, tumor.

secondary. Second in order of occurrence or importance, or appearing during the course of another disease or condition.

57160

57160 Fitting and insertion of pessary or other intravaginal support device

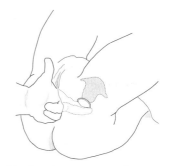

The physician inserts a pessary or other support device

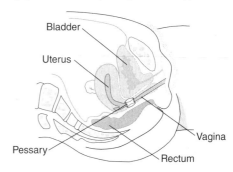

Explanation

The physician fits a pessary to a patient, provides instructions for its use, and inserts it into the vagina. A pessary is a prosthesis that comes in different shapes and styles and is used to support the uterus, cervical stump, or hernias of the pelvic floor. The pessary selection and fitting will depend on the patient's symptoms and anatomy.

Coding Tips

Supplies used when providing this service may be reported with 99070 or with the appropriate HCPCS Level II code. Check with the specific payer to determine coverage.

ICD-10-CM Diagnostic Codes

N39.3	Stress incontinence (female) (male)
N81.0	Urethrocele ♀
N81.11	Cystocele, midline ♀
N81.12	Cystocele, lateral ♀
N81.2	Incomplete uterovaginal prolapse ♀
N81.3	Complete uterovaginal prolapse ♀
N81.5	Vaginal enterocele ♀
N81.6	Rectocele ♀
N81.81	Perineocele ♀
N81.82	Incompetence or weakening of pubocervical tissue ♀
N81.83	Incompetence or weakening of rectovaginal tissue ♀
N81.84	Pelvic muscle wasting ♀
N81.85	Cervical stump prolapse ♀
N81.89	Other female genital prolapse ♀
N99.3	Prolapse of vaginal vault after hysterectomy ♀

AMA: 57160 2019,Jul,6; 2018,Jan,8; 2017,Jan,8; 2016,Jan,13; 2015,Jan,16; 2014,Jan,11

Vagina

Relative Value Units/Medicare Edits

Non-Facility RVU	Work	PE	MP	Total
57160	0.89	0.94	0.13	1.96
Facility RVU	Work	PE	MP	Total
57160	0.89	0.33	0.13	1.35

	FUD	Status	MUE	Modifiers				IOM Reference
57160	0	A	1(2)	51	N/A	N/A	N/A	None

* with documentation

Terms To Know

enterocele. Intestinal herniation into the vaginal wall.

insertion. Placement or implantation into a body part.

pessary. Device placed in the vagina to support and reposition a prolapsing or retropositioned uterus, rectum, or vagina.

prolapse. Falling, sliding, or sinking of an organ from its normal location in the body.

prosthesis. Device that replaces all or part of an internal body organ or replaces all or part of the function of a permanently inoperative or malfunctioning internal body organ.

rectocele. Rectal tissue herniation into the vaginal wall.

stress incontinence. Involuntary escape of urine at times of minor stress against the bladder, such as coughing, sneezing, or laughing.

57170

57170   Diaphragm or cervical cap fitting with instructions

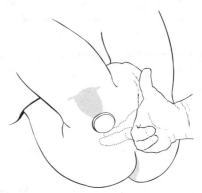

Fitting of cervical cap or diaphragm

Explanation

The physician fits a diaphragm or cervical cap and provides instructions for use. A diaphragm is a device that acts as a mechanical barrier between the vagina and the cervical canal. Cervical caps are larger, cup-like diaphragms pressed up against the cervix to form a snug seal. Either device can be used to prevent pregnancy.

Coding Tips

This procedure may also be performed by a registered nurse, physician assistant, nurse practitioner, or other trained paramedical person under the supervision of a physician. Because this procedure is usually not done out of medical necessity, the patient may be responsible for charges. Verify with the insurance carrier for coverage. Supplies used when providing this service may be reported with the appropriate HCPCS Level II code. Check with the specific payer to determine coverage.

ICD-10-CM Diagnostic Codes

Z30.018	Encounter for initial prescription of other contraceptives ♀
Z30.09	Encounter for other general counseling and advice on contraception
Z30.49	Encounter for surveillance of other contraceptives ♀

AMA: **57170** 2019,Jul,6; 2014,Jan,11

Relative Value Units/Medicare Edits

Non-Facility RVU	Work	PE	MP	Total
57170	0.91	0.98	0.13	2.02
Facility RVU	Work	PE	MP	Total
57170	0.91	0.34	0.13	1.38

	FUD	Status	MUE	Modifiers				IOM Reference
57170	0	A	1(2)	51	N/A	N/A	80*	None

* with documentation

Terms To Know

cervical cap. Contraceptive device similar in form and function to the diaphragm but that can be left in place for 48 hours.

diaphragm. Flexible disk inserted into the vagina and against the cervix as a method of birth control.

57180

57180 Introduction of any hemostatic agent or pack for spontaneous or traumatic nonobstetrical vaginal hemorrhage (separate procedure)

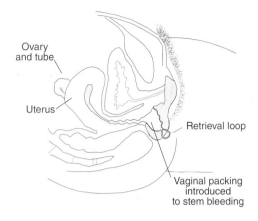

Ovary and tube
Uterus
Retrieval loop
Vaginal packing introduced to stem bleeding

Explanation

The physician pushes gauze packing into the vagina to put pressure on bleeding that is not related to childbirth or pregnancy. The packing may be coated with a chemical to make the blood clot and stop hemorrhaging.

Coding Tips

This separate procedure by definition is usually a component of a more complex service and is not identified separately. When performed alone or with other unrelated procedures/services it may be reported. If performed alone, list the code; if performed with other procedures/services, list the code and append modifier 59 or an X{EPSU} modifier. When 57180 is performed with another separately identifiable procedure, the highest dollar value code is listed as the primary procedure and subsequent procedures are appended with modifier 51. This procedure might be performed by a registered nurse, physician assistant, nurse practitioner, or other trained paramedical person under the supervision of a physician. Removal of packing is not reported separately. Ablation or cauterization required to stop vaginal hemorrhage may be reported separately. Surgical trays, A4550, are not separately reimbursed by Medicare; however, other third-party payers may cover them. Check with the specific payer to determine coverage.

ICD-10-CM Diagnostic Codes

N93.8	Other specified abnormal uterine and vaginal bleeding ♀
N93.9	Abnormal uterine and vaginal bleeding, unspecified ♀
N99.61	Intraoperative hemorrhage and hematoma of a genitourinary system organ or structure complicating a genitourinary system procedure
N99.62	Intraoperative hemorrhage and hematoma of a genitourinary system organ or structure complicating other procedure
N99.820	Postprocedural hemorrhage of a genitourinary system organ or structure following a genitourinary system procedure
N99.821	Postprocedural hemorrhage of a genitourinary system organ or structure following other procedure
S31.41XA	Laceration without foreign body of vagina and vulva, initial encounter ♀
S31.42XA	Laceration with foreign body of vagina and vulva, initial encounter ♀
S31.43XA	Puncture wound without foreign body of vagina and vulva, initial encounter ♀
S31.44XA	Puncture wound with foreign body of vagina and vulva, initial encounter ♀
S31.45XA	Open bite of vagina and vulva, initial encounter ♀
T83.83XA	Hemorrhage due to genitourinary prosthetic devices, implants and grafts, initial encounter

AMA: 57180 2019,Jul,6; 2018,Jan,8; 2017,Jan,8; 2016,Jan,13; 2015,Jan,16; 2014,Jan,11

Relative Value Units/Medicare Edits

Non-Facility RVU	Work	PE	MP	Total
57180	1.63	3.08	0.26	4.97
Facility RVU	**Work**	**PE**	**MP**	**Total**
57180	1.63	1.43	0.26	3.32

	FUD	Status	MUE	Modifiers				IOM Reference
57180	10	A	1(3)	51	N/A	N/A	N/A	None

* with documentation

Terms To Know

complication. Condition arising after the beginning of observation and treatment that modifies the course of the patient's illness or the medical care required, or an undesired result or misadventure in medical care.

hemorrhage. Internal or external bleeding with loss of significant amounts of blood.

hemostasis. Interruption of blood flow or the cessation or arrest of bleeding.

intra. Within.

introduction. Induction of an instrument, such as a catheter, needle, or endotracheal tube.

packing. Material placed into a cavity or wound, such as gels, gauze, pads, and sponges.

Vagina

57200-57210

57200 Colporrhaphy, suture of injury of vagina (nonobstetrical)
57210 Colpoperineorrhaphy, suture of injury of vagina and/or perineum (nonobstetrical)

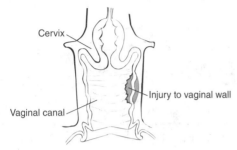

Cervix
Injury to vaginal wall
Vaginal canal

The laceration or injury is non-obstetrical in nature

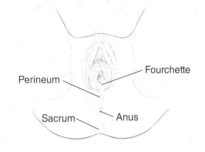

Perineum
Fourchette
Sacrum
Anus

Explanation

The physician inserts a speculum into the vagina and identifies the extent of the vaginal laceration or wound that is not related to childbirth or pregnancy. Usually a local anesthetic is used; however, some instances may require general anesthesia. The wound is closed with absorbable sutures. In 57210, after the speculum is removed, the perineal laceration is closed in layers with sutures.

Coding Tips

These are nonobstetrical procedures and should not be used if the injury is a result of delivery. Local anesthesia is included in this service. However, these procedures may be performed under general anesthesia, depending on the age and/or condition of the patient. For episiotomy or vaginal repair following delivery, see 59300.

ICD-10-CM Diagnostic Codes

N90.811	Female genital mutilation Type I status ♀
N90.812	Female genital mutilation Type II status ♀
N90.813	Female genital mutilation Type III status ♀
N90.818	Other female genital mutilation status ♀
S30.854A	Superficial foreign body of vagina and vulva, initial encounter ♀
S31.41XA	Laceration without foreign body of vagina and vulva, initial encounter ♀
S31.42XA	Laceration with foreign body of vagina and vulva, initial encounter ♀
S31.43XA	Puncture wound without foreign body of vagina and vulva, initial encounter ♀
S31.44XA	Puncture wound with foreign body of vagina and vulva, initial encounter ♀
S31.45XA	Open bite of vagina and vulva, initial encounter ♀
S38.03XA	Crushing injury of vulva, initial encounter ♀
T19.2XXA	Foreign body in vulva and vagina, initial encounter ♀

T74.21XA	Adult sexual abuse, confirmed, initial encounter △
T74.22XA	Child sexual abuse, confirmed, initial encounter ℗
T76.21XA	Adult sexual abuse, suspected, initial encounter △
T76.22XA	Child sexual abuse, suspected, initial encounter ℗

AMA: 57200 2019,Jul,6; 2014,Jan,11 **57210** 2019,Jul,6; 2014,Jan,11

Relative Value Units/Medicare Edits

Non-Facility RVU	Work	PE	MP	Total
57200	4.42	4.07	0.68	9.17
57210	5.71	4.47	0.89	11.07
Facility RVU	**Work**	**PE**	**MP**	**Total**
57200	4.42	4.07	0.68	9.17
57210	5.71	4.47	0.89	11.07

	FUD	Status	MUE	Modifiers				IOM Reference
57200	90	A	1(3)	51	N/A	62*	80	None
57210	90	A	1(3)	51	N/A	62*	80	

* with documentation

Terms To Know

absorbable sutures. Strands used for suture or repair of tissue prepared from collagen or a synthetic polymer and capable of being absorbed by tissue over time.

foreign body. Any object or substance found in an organ and tissue that does not belong under normal circumstances.

laceration. Tearing injury; a torn, ragged-edged wound.

perineal. Pertaining to the pelvic floor area between the thighs; the diamond-shaped area bordered by the pubic symphysis in front, the ischial tuberosities on the sides, and the coccyx in back.

speculum. Tool used to enlarge the opening of any canal or cavity.

wound. Injury to living tissue often involving a cut or break in the skin.

Coding Companion for Ob/Gyn

Vagina

57220

57220 Plastic operation on urethral sphincter, vaginal approach (eg, Kelly urethral plication)

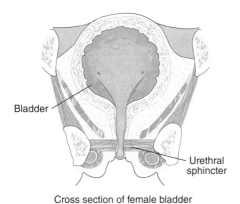

Bladder

Urethral sphincter

Cross section of female bladder

Explanation

The physician accesses the urethral sphincter from the vagina. With a catheter in the urethra, the physician dissects the midline vaginal wall separating it from the bladder and the proximal urethra. Sutures are placed at the junction of the bladder and urethra on each side of the urethra. This supports the area. Excess vaginal tissue is excised and the vaginal wall is closed.

Coding Tips

For a Marshall-Marchetti-Krantz urethral suspension, abdominal approach, see 51840-51841. For laparoscopic repair of stress incontinence only, see 51990-51992.

ICD-10-CM Diagnostic Codes

N39.3   Stress incontinence (female) (male)

AMA: 57220 2019,Jul,6; 2014,Jan,11

Relative Value Units/Medicare Edits

Non-Facility RVU	Work	PE	MP	Total
57220	4.85	4.08	0.74	9.67
Facility RVU	Work	PE	MP	Total
57220	4.85	4.08	0.74	9.67

	FUD	Status	MUE	Modifiers				IOM Reference
57220	90	A	1(2)	51	N/A	62*	80	None

* with documentation

Terms To Know

approach. Method or anatomical location used to gain access to a body organ or specific area for procedures.

plication. Surgical technique involving folding, tucking, or pleating to reduce the size of a hollow structure or organ.

stress incontinence. Involuntary escape of urine at times of minor stress against the bladder, such as coughing, sneezing, or laughing.

57230

57230 Plastic repair of urethrocele

Physician repairs urethrocele via vagina

Urethra

Bladder

Vagina

Urethrocele

Explanation

The physician repairs a urethrocele, which is a sagging or prolapse of the urethra through its opening or a bulging of the posterior wall of the urethra against the vaginal canal. The prolapsed urethral tissue is excised from the meatus in a circular manner. The cut edges of urethral mucosa and vaginal mucosa are sutured.

Coding Tips

For a Marshall-Marchetti-Krantz urethral suspension, abdominal approach, see 51840-51841. For laparoscopic repair of stress incontinence only, see 51990-51992.

ICD-10-CM Diagnostic Codes

N36.8	Other specified disorders of urethra
N81.0	Urethrocele ♀
N81.10	Cystocele, unspecified ♀
N81.11	Cystocele, midline ♀
N81.12	Cystocele, lateral ♀
Q64.71	Congenital prolapse of urethra

AMA: 57230 2019,Jul,6; 2014,Jan,11

Relative Value Units/Medicare Edits

Non-Facility RVU	Work	PE	MP	Total
57230	6.3	4.56	0.99	11.85
Facility RVU	Work	PE	MP	Total
57230	6.3	4.56	0.99	11.85

	FUD	Status	MUE	Modifiers				IOM Reference
57230	90	A	1(2)	51	N/A	62*	80	None

* with documentation

Terms To Know

prolapse. Falling, sliding, or sinking of an organ from its normal location in the body.

urethrocele. Urethral herniation into the vaginal wall.

Vagina

57240

57240   Anterior colporrhaphy, repair of cystocele with or without repair of urethrocele, including cystourethroscopy, when performed

Through an incision in the anterior wall of the vagina, the physician repairs a cystocele

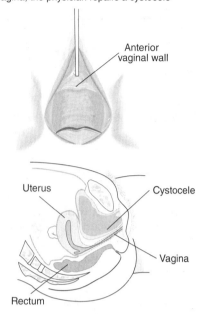

Any urethrocele may also be repaired

Explanation

The physician repairs a cystocele, which is a herniation of the bladder through its support tissues and against the anterior vaginal wall causing it to bulge downward. The physician may also repair a urethrocele, which is a prolapse of the urethra. An incision is made from the apex of the vagina to within 1 cm of the urethral meatus. Plication sutures are placed along the urethral course from the meatus to the bladder neck. A suture is placed through the pubourethral ligament to the posterior symphysis pubis on each side of the urethra. The sutures are tied (ligated) and the posterior urethra is pulled upward to a retropubic position. If a cystocele is repaired, mattress sutures are placed in the mobilized perivesical tissue. The vaginal mucosa is closed. Cystourethroscopy is included when performed with this procedure.

Coding Tips

This procedure includes any repair of a urethrocele the physician may perform together with the cystocele repair. For a Marshall-Marchetti-Krantz urethral suspension, abdominal approach, see 51840-51841. For plastic repair of a urethrocele, see 57230. Do not report 57240 with 52000.

ICD-10-CM Diagnostic Codes

N36.8	Other specified disorders of urethra
N81.0	Urethrocele ♀
N81.10	Cystocele, unspecified ♀
N81.11	Cystocele, midline ♀
N81.12	Cystocele, lateral ♀
Q64.71	Congenital prolapse of urethra

AMA: **57240** 2019,Jul,6; 2018,Jan,8; 2017,Jan,8; 2016,Jan,13; 2015,Jan,16; 2014,Jan,11

Relative Value Units/Medicare Edits

Non-Facility RVU	Work	PE	MP	Total
57240	10.08	5.96	1.45	17.49
Facility RVU	**Work**	**PE**	**MP**	**Total**
57240	10.08	5.96	1.45	17.49

	FUD	Status	MUE	Modifiers				IOM Reference
57240	90	A	1(2)	51	N/A	62*	80	None

* with documentation

Terms To Know

anterior. Situated in the front area or toward the belly surface of the body.

colporrhaphy. Plastic repair or reconstruction of the vagina by suturing the vaginal wall and surrounding fibrous tissue.

cystocele. Herniation of the bladder into the vagina.

meatus. Opening or passage into the body.

plication. Surgical technique involving folding, tucking, or pleating to reduce the size of a hollow structure or organ.

prolapse. Falling, sliding, or sinking of an organ from its normal location in the body.

urethrocele. Urethral herniation into the vaginal wall.

uterovaginal prolapse. Uterus displaced downward and exposed in the external genitalia.

Coding Companion for Ob/Gyn

Vagina

57250

57250 Posterior colporrhaphy, repair of rectocele with or without perineorrhaphy

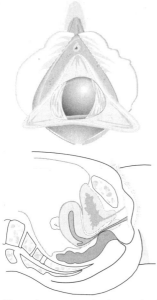

Through an incision in the posterior wall of the vagina, the physician repairs the rectocele

The perineum may also be repaired

Explanation

The physician repairs a rectocele by colporrhaphy. A rectocele is a protrusion of part of the rectum through its supporting tissues against the vagina causing a bulging in the vagina. Colporrhaphy involves a plastic repair of the vagina and the fibrous tissue separating the vagina and rectum. The physician makes a posterior midline incision that includes the perineum and posterior vaginal wall. In order to strengthen the area, the rectovaginal fascia is plicated by folding and tacking, and it is closed with layered sutures. The physician may also perform a perineorrhaphy, which is a plastic repair of the perineum, including midline approximation of the levator and perineal muscles. Excess fascia in the posterior vaginal wall is excised. The incisions are closed with sutures.

Coding Tips

This procedure includes any perineorrhaphy the physician may perform. For repair of a rectocele (separate procedure) without posterior colporrhaphy, see 45560. For combined anteroposterior colporrhaphy, see 57260–57265.

ICD-10-CM Diagnostic Codes

K62.3	Rectal prolapse
N81.2	Incomplete uterovaginal prolapse ♀
N81.3	Complete uterovaginal prolapse ♀
N81.6	Rectocele ♀
N81.81	Perineocele ♀

AMA: **57250** 2019,Jul,6; 2018,Jan,8; 2017,Jan,8; 2016,Jan,13; 2015,Jan,16; 2014,Jan,11

Relative Value Units/Medicare Edits

Non-Facility RVU	Work	PE	MP	Total
57250	10.08	6.0	1.52	17.6
Facility RVU	**Work**	**PE**	**MP**	**Total**
57250	10.08	6.0	1.52	17.6

	FUD	Status	MUE	Modifiers				IOM Reference
57250	90	A	1(2)	51	N/A	62*	80	None

* with documentation

Terms To Know

colporrhaphy. Plastic repair or reconstruction of the vagina by suturing the vaginal wall and surrounding fibrous tissue.

enterocele. Intestinal herniation into the vaginal wall.

female stress incontinence. Involuntary escape of urine at times of minor stress against the female bladder, such as coughing, sneezing, or laughing.

perineocele. Uncommon condition in which herniation occurs in the perineal area between the rectum and vagina, the rectum and bladder, or beside the rectum.

posterior. Located in the back part or caudal end of the body.

rectocele. Rectal tissue herniation into the vaginal wall.

uterovaginal prolapse. Uterus displaced downward and exposed in the external genitalia.

Vagina

57260-57265

57260 Combined anteroposterior colporrhaphy, including cystourethroscopy, when performed;

57265 with enterocele repair

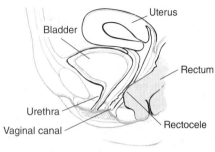

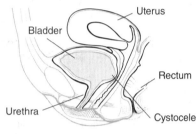

A repair of the vaginal canal is performed

Explanation

The physician repairs a cystocele and rectocele by colporrhaphy. Colporrhaphy involves a plastic repair of the vagina and the fibrous tissue separating the bladder, vagina, and rectum. A cystocele is a herniation of the bladder through its support tissues causing the anterior vaginal wall to bulge downward. A rectocele is a protrusion of part of the rectum through its support tissues causing the posterior vaginal wall to bulge. Using a combined vaginal approach and a posterior midline incision that includes the perineum and posterior vaginal wall, the physician dissects the tissues between the bladder, urethra, vagina, and rectum. The specific tissue weaknesses are repaired and strengthened using tissue transfer techniques and layered and plication suturing. In 57260, the physician may also repair a urethrocele, which is a prolapse of the urethra, and perform a perineorrhaphy, which is plastic repair of the perineum, including midline approximation of the levator and perineal muscles. In 57265, the physician performs all of the same services and also repairs an enterocele, which is a herniation of the bowel contents of the rectouterine pouch that protrudes into the septum of tissue between the bladder and vagina or between the vagina and rectum. Through the vagina, the enterocele sac is incised and ligated and the uterosacral ligaments and endopelvic fascia anterior to the rectum are approximated. In both procedures, incisions are closed with sutures. Cystourethroscopy is included when performed with these procedures.

Coding Tips

For vaginal repair of an enterocele without anteroposterior repair, see 57268. For a Marshall-Marchetti-Krantz urethral suspension, abdominal approach, see 51840-51841. For laparoscopic repair of stress incontinence only, see 51990-51992. Do not report these codes with 52000.

ICD-10-CM Diagnostic Codes

K62.3	Rectal prolapse
N36.8	Other specified disorders of urethra
N81.0	Urethrocele ♀
N81.11	Cystocele, midline ♀
N81.12	Cystocele, lateral ♀
N81.2	Incomplete uterovaginal prolapse ♀
N81.3	Complete uterovaginal prolapse ♀
N81.5	Vaginal enterocele ♀
N81.6	Rectocele ♀
N81.81	Perineocele ♀
Q64.71	Congenital prolapse of urethra

AMA: **57260** 2019,Jul,6; 2018,Jan,8; 2017,Jan,8; 2016,Jan,13; 2015,Jan,16; 2014,Jan,11 **57265** 2019,Jul,6; 2018,Jan,8; 2017,Jan,8; 2016,Jan,13; 2015,Jan,16; 2014,Jan,11

Relative Value Units/Medicare Edits

Non-Facility RVU	Work	PE	MP	Total
57260	13.25	7.18	2.0	22.43
57265	15.0	7.86	2.32	25.18
Facility RVU	**Work**	**PE**	**MP**	**Total**
57260	13.25	7.18	2.0	22.43
57265	15.0	7.86	2.32	25.18

	FUD	Status	MUE	Modifiers				IOM Reference
57260	90	A	1(2)	51	N/A	62*	80	None
57265	90	A	1(2)	51	N/A	62*	80	

* with documentation

Terms To Know

anterior. Situated in the front area or toward the belly surface of the body.

colporrhaphy. Plastic repair or reconstruction of the vagina by suturing the vaginal wall and surrounding fibrous tissue.

cystocele. Herniation of the bladder into the vagina.

enterocele. Intestinal herniation into the vaginal wall.

perineocele. Uncommon condition in which herniation occurs in the perineal area between the rectum and vagina, the rectum and bladder, or beside the rectum.

posterior. Located in the back part or caudal end of the body.

repair. Surgical closure of a wound. The wound may be a result of injury/trauma or it may be a surgically created defect. Repairs are divided into three categories: simple, intermediate, and complex.

Vagina

57267

+ **57267** Insertion of mesh or other prosthesis for repair of pelvic floor defect, each site (anterior, posterior compartment), vaginal approach (List separately in addition to code for primary procedure)

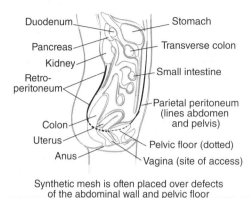

Synthetic mesh is often placed over defects of the abdominal wall and pelvic floor

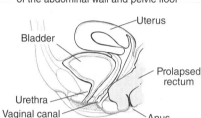

Explanation

The physician inserts mesh or other prosthetic support material to repair a pelvic floor defect using a vaginal approach. Pelvic floor defects resulting in prolapse of the pelvic viscera occur when the pelvic fascia weakens or is damaged. The physician selects the appropriate type of prosthetic support material. Some mesh supports, such as horseshoe shaped mesh, are purchased preformed in the desired configuration. Other types of mesh supports, such as tension free tapes, are cut and fashioned by the physician during surgery into the required shapes and sizes. The mesh is inserted through the vagina and placed at the site requiring support. The exact placement of the mesh is determined by the type of pelvic floor defect being repaired. For example, horseshoe mesh is placed between the pubis and sacrum to close the area between the pelvic viscera and the inferior pelvic hiatus. Report 57267 in addition to the primary procedure for each site requiring insertion of mesh or other prosthesis, such as an anterior repair for cystocele or a posterior repair for a rectocele.

Coding Tips

Report 57267 in addition to the codes for the primary vaginal or rectocele repair: 45560, 57240–57265, or 57285.

ICD-10-CM Diagnostic Codes

This/these CPT code(s) are add-on code(s). See the primary procedure code that this code is performed with for your ICD-10-CM code selections.

AMA: **57267** 2019,Jul,6; 2018,Jan,8; 2017,Jan,8; 2016,Jan,13; 2015,Jan,16; 2014,Jan,11

Relative Value Units/Medicare Edits

Non-Facility RVU	Work	PE	MP	Total
57267	4.88	1.78	0.68	7.34
Facility RVU	**Work**	**PE**	**MP**	**Total**
57267	4.88	1.78	0.68	7.34

	FUD	Status	MUE	Modifiers				IOM Reference
57267	N/A	A	2(3)	N/A	N/A	62*	80	None

* with documentation

Terms To Know

anterior. Situated in the front area or toward the belly surface of the body.

approach. Method or anatomical location used to gain access to a body organ or specific area for procedures. The approach is not coded separately although it may be a specified component of the procedure, such as laparoscopic versus incisional, or spinal procedures in which the amount of dissection required to expose the spine significantly alters with the site of approach.

cystocele. Herniation of the bladder into the vagina.

fascia. Fibrous sheet or band of tissue that envelops organs, muscles, and groupings of muscles.

insertion. Placement or implantation into a body part.

mesh. Synthetic fabric used as a prosthetic patch in hernia repair.

pelvis. Distal anterior portion of the trunk that lies between the hipbones, sacrum, and coccyx bones; the inferior portion of the abdominal cavity.

posterior. Located in the back part or caudal end of the body.

prolapse. Falling, sliding, or sinking of an organ from its normal location in the body.

prosthesis. Man-made substitute for a missing body part.

rectocele. Rectal tissue herniation into the vaginal wall.

viscera. Large interior organs enclosed within a cavity, generally referring to the abdominal organs.

Vagina

57268-57270

57268 Repair of enterocele, vaginal approach (separate procedure)
57270 Repair of enterocele, abdominal approach (separate procedure)

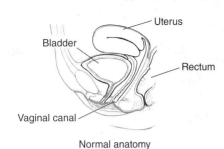

Normal anatomy

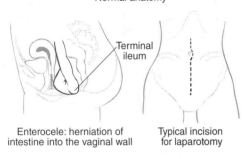

Enterocele: herniation of intestine into the vaginal wall

Typical incision for laparotomy

Explanation

The physician repairs an enterocele, which is a herniation of the bowel contents of the rectouterine pouch that protrudes into the septum of tissue between the bladder and vagina or between the vagina and rectum. Through the vaginal approach in 57268, the physician incises and ligates the enterocele sac and approximates the uterosacral ligaments and endopelvic fascia anterior to the rectum. In 57270, the approach is made through an incision in the lower abdominal wall. A vaginal hysterectomy, anterior (cystocele) and posterior (rectocele) colporrhaphy, and perineorrhaphy may also be performed to augment the support.

Coding Tips

These separate procedures by definition are usually a component of a more complex service and are not identified separately. When performed alone or with other unrelated procedures/services they may be reported. If performed alone, list the code; if performed with other procedures/services, list the code and append modifier 59 or an X{EPSU} modifier. If anteroposterior colporrhaphy is performed with enterocele repair, report 57265. For laparoscopic repair of stress incontinence only, see 51990-51992.

ICD-10-CM Diagnostic Codes

N81.5   Vaginal enterocele ♀

AMA: 57268 2019,Jul,6; 2018,Jan,8; 2017,Jan,8; 2016,Jan,13; 2015,Jan,16; 2014,Jan,11 **57270** 2019,Jul,6; 2018,Jan,8; 2017,Jan,8; 2016,Jan,13; 2015,Jan,16; 2014,Jan,11

Relative Value Units/Medicare Edits

Non-Facility RVU	Work	PE	MP	Total
57268	7.57	5.64	1.15	14.36
57270	13.67	7.67	2.1	23.44
Facility RVU	**Work**	**PE**	**MP**	**Total**
57268	7.57	5.64	1.15	14.36
57270	13.67	7.67	2.1	23.44

	FUD	Status	MUE	Modifiers				IOM Reference
57268	90	A	1(2)	51	N/A	62*	80	None
57270	90	A	1(2)	51	N/A	62*	80	

* with documentation

Terms To Know

anterior. Situated in the front area or toward the belly surface of the body.

approach. Method or anatomical location used to gain access to a body organ or specific area for procedures. The approach is not coded separately although it may be a specified component of the procedure, such as laparoscopic versus incisional, or spinal procedures in which the amount of dissection required to expose the spine significantly alters with the site of approach.

enterocele. Intestinal herniation into the vaginal wall.

fascia. Fibrous sheet or band of tissue that envelops organs, muscles, and groupings of muscles.

female stress incontinence. Involuntary escape of urine at times of minor stress against the female bladder, such as coughing, sneezing, or laughing.

incise. To cut open or into.

ligate. To tie off a blood vessel or duct with a suture or a soft, thin wire (ligature wire).

posterior. Located in the back part or caudal end of the body.

septum. Anatomical partition or dividing wall.

Vagina

57280

57280 Colpopexy, abdominal approach

The physician sutures vaginal supports in the pelvic cavity

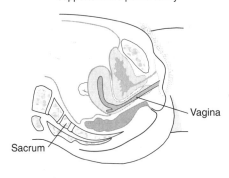

Vagina

Sacrum

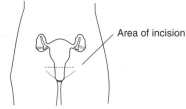

Area of incision

Explanation

Through a lower abdominal incision, the physician attaches the vault of the vagina to the prominent point of the sacrum. This is accomplished by suturing surgical fabric or a strip of abdominal wall fascia to the tissue in front of the internal sacral wall inside the pelvic cavity forming a bridge. The apex of the vagina is firmly sutured to this bridge. This stabilizes the vaginal vault and prevents prolapse of the vagina. The abdominal incision is closed with sutures.

Coding Tips

Transvaginal colporrhaphy often accompanies this procedure and should not be reported separately. For laparoscopic repair of stress incontinence only, see 51990-51992. For colpopexy by extraperitoneal approach, see 57282. For colpopexy by intraperitoneal approach, see 57283.

ICD-10-CM Diagnostic Codes

N81.0	Urethrocele ♀
N81.11	Cystocele, midline ♀
N81.12	Cystocele, lateral ♀
N81.2	Incomplete uterovaginal prolapse ♀
N81.3	Complete uterovaginal prolapse ♀
N81.6	Rectocele ♀
N81.81	Perineocele ♀
N81.82	Incompetence or weakening of pubocervical tissue ♀
N81.83	Incompetence or weakening of rectovaginal tissue ♀
N81.85	Cervical stump prolapse ♀
N81.89	Other female genital prolapse ♀
N99.3	Prolapse of vaginal vault after hysterectomy ♀

AMA: 57280 2019,Jul,6; 2018,Jan,8; 2017,Jan,8; 2016,Jan,13; 2015,Jan,16; 2014,Jan,11

Relative Value Units/Medicare Edits

Non-Facility RVU	Work	PE	MP	Total
57280	16.72	8.71	2.44	27.87
Facility RVU	**Work**	**PE**	**MP**	**Total**
57280	16.72	8.71	2.44	27.87

	FUD	Status	MUE	Modifiers				IOM Reference
57280	90	A	1(2)	51	N/A	62*	80	None

* with documentation

Terms To Know

approach. Method or anatomical location used to gain access to a body organ or specific area for procedures.

colpopexy. Suturing a prolapsed vagina to its surrounding structures for vaginal fixation.

colporrhaphy. Plastic repair or reconstruction of the vagina by suturing the vaginal wall and surrounding fibrous tissue.

fascia. Fibrous sheet or band of tissue that envelops organs, muscles, and groupings of muscles.

female stress incontinence. Involuntary escape of urine at times of minor stress against the female bladder, such as coughing, sneezing, or laughing.

prolapse. Falling, sliding, or sinking of an organ from its normal location in the body.

sacrum. Lower portion of the spine composed of five fused vertebrae designated as S1-S5.

uterovaginal prolapse. Uterus displaced downward and exposed in the external genitalia.

Vagina

57282

57282 Colpopexy, vaginal; extra-peritoneal approach (sacrospinous, iliococcygeus)

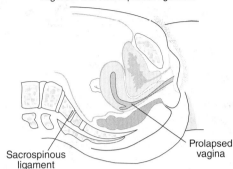

The physician uses sutures to fix the vagina to the sacrospinous ligament

Sacrospinous ligament

Prolapsed vagina

Explanation

Colpopexy is performed by transvaginal, extraperitoneal approach to restore the apex or vault of the vagina to its anatomic position in cases of prolapse. Extraperitoneal transvaginal approach is used to perform a sacrospinous ligament fixation or iliococcygeus fascial suspension. Sacrospinous ligament fixation is performed using an anterior transvaginal approach through the paravaginal space or a posterior transvaginal approach by perforation of the rectal pillar. A pair of sutures are placed approximately 1 to 2 cm apart in the sacrospinous ligaments. After placing the sutures in the sacrospinous ligaments, the apex of the vagina is identified and the sutures in the sacrospinous ligaments are incorporated into the apex of the vagina allowing for maximal suspension of the vaginal vault. Iliococcygeus fascial suspension is performed by extraperitoneal transvaginal approach. The rectum is first retracted medially. The iliococcygeus muscle is located lateral to the rectum and anterior to the ischial spine. A single suture is placed in both sides of the apex of the vaginal vault to provide bilateral fixation of the vault to the iliococcygeus fascia.

Coding Tips

Transvaginal colporrhaphy performed at the same surgical session may be reported separately. For colpopexy by abdominal approach, see 57280. For colpopexy by intra-peritoneal approach, see 57283.

ICD-10-CM Diagnostic Codes

N81.0	Urethrocele ♀
N81.11	Cystocele, midline ♀
N81.12	Cystocele, lateral ♀
N81.2	Incomplete uterovaginal prolapse ♀
N81.3	Complete uterovaginal prolapse ♀
N81.6	Rectocele ♀
N81.81	Perineocele ♀
N81.82	Incompetence or weakening of pubocervical tissue ♀
N81.83	Incompetence or weakening of rectovaginal tissue ♀
N81.85	Cervical stump prolapse ♀
N81.89	Other female genital prolapse ♀
N99.3	Prolapse of vaginal vault after hysterectomy ♀

AMA: 57282 2019,Jul,6; 2018,Jan,8; 2017,Jan,8; 2016,Jan,13; 2015,Jan,16; 2014,Jan,11

Relative Value Units/Medicare Edits

Non-Facility RVU	Work	PE	MP	Total
57282	7.97	6.03	1.18	15.18
Facility RVU	**Work**	**PE**	**MP**	**Total**
57282	7.97	6.03	1.18	15.18

	FUD	Status	MUE	Modifiers				IOM Reference
57282	90	A	1(2)	51	N/A	62*	80	None

* with documentation

Terms To Know

apex. Highest point of a root end of a tooth, or the end of any organ.

approach. Method or anatomical location used to gain access to a body organ or specific area for procedures.

cystocele. Herniation of the bladder into the vagina.

perineocele. Uncommon condition in which herniation occurs in the perineal area between the rectum and vagina, the rectum and bladder, or beside the rectum.

prolapse. Falling, sliding, or sinking of an organ from its normal location in the body.

rectocele. Rectal tissue herniation into the vaginal wall.

57283

57283   Colpopexy, vaginal; intra-peritoneal approach (uterosacral, levator myorrhaphy)

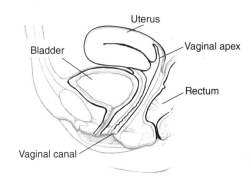

Normal anatomy

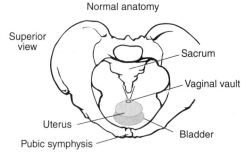

The vaginal column may be attached to ligaments of the sacral spine or other areas to support it anatomically

Explanation

Colpopexy is performed by transvaginal, intraperitoneal approach to restore the apex or vault of the vagina to its anatomic position in cases of prolapse. Intraperitoneal technique is used to perform a uterosacral ligament suspension or a levator myorrhaphy, which are performed using a posterior transvaginal approach. Uterosacral ligament suspension is performed by first locating the uterosacral ligament remnant with the use of Allis clamps posterior and medial to the ischial spine. Prior to placement of sutures in the ligaments, the ureters are located by palpation. Two to three nonabsorbable sutures are placed in each ligament and tied together. The ligaments are placated and brought together in the midline. Sutures are placed in the apical portion of the anterior and posterior vaginal walls to secure and anchor the vaginal walls to the plicated uterosacral ligaments. Levator myorrhaphy uses the levator musculature to repair the vaginal vault prolapse. The levator musculature is brought together and a high levator shelf created. The shelf is created by tagging and tying together the levator muscles at a site slightly above the junction of the levator and rectum. The vaginal vault is anchored to the shelf.

Coding Tips

Do not report 57283 with 57556, 58263, 58270, 58280, 58292, or 58294. For colpopexy via abdominal approach, see 57280; vaginal via extraperitoneal approach, see 57282.

ICD-10-CM Diagnostic Codes

N81.0	Urethrocele ♀
N81.11	Cystocele, midline ♀
N81.12	Cystocele, lateral ♀
N81.2	Incomplete uterovaginal prolapse ♀
N81.3	Complete uterovaginal prolapse ♀
N81.6	Rectocele ♀
N81.81	Perineocele ♀
N81.82	Incompetence or weakening of pubocervical tissue ♀
N81.83	Incompetence or weakening of rectovaginal tissue ♀
N81.85	Cervical stump prolapse ♀
N81.89	Other female genital prolapse ♀
N99.3	Prolapse of vaginal vault after hysterectomy ♀

AMA: 57283 2019,Jul,6; 2018,Jan,8; 2017,Jan,8; 2016,Jan,13; 2015,Jan,16; 2014,Jan,11

Relative Value Units/Medicare Edits

Non-Facility RVU	Work	PE	MP	Total
57283	11.66	6.81	1.78	20.25
Facility RVU	**Work**	**PE**	**MP**	**Total**
57283	11.66	6.81	1.78	20.25

	FUD	Status	MUE	Modifiers				IOM Reference
57283	90	A	1(2)	51	N/A	62*	80	None

* with documentation

Terms To Know

anterior. Situated in the front area or toward the belly surface of the body.

apex. Highest point of a root end of a tooth, or the end of any organ.

apical. At the top, tip or end of a structure; the opposite of basal.

approach. Method or anatomical location used to gain access to a body organ or specific area for procedures.

colpopexy. Suturing a prolapsed vagina to its surrounding structures for vaginal fixation.

intra. Within.

perineocele. Uncommon condition in which herniation occurs in the perineal area between the rectum and vagina, the rectum and bladder, or beside the rectum.

posterior. Located in the back part or caudal end of the body.

prolapse. Falling, sliding, or sinking of an organ from its normal location in the body.

Vagina

57284-57285

57284 Paravaginal defect repair (including repair of cystocele, if performed); open abdominal approach

57285 vaginal approach

The physician repairs paravaginal defects

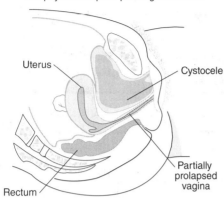

Explanation

The physician repairs a paravaginal defect, in which there is loss of the lateral vaginal attachment to the pelvic sidewall, by dissecting the tissues between the vagina and the bladder and urethra. The specific tissue weaknesses are found, repaired, and strengthened using tissue transfer techniques and plication suturing. The paravaginal repair may be performed alone or in conjunction with cystocele repair, in which a herniation of the bladder through its support tissues into the anterior vaginal wall causes it to bulge downward. These procedures help restore the normal anatomic relationships of the urethra, bladder, and vagina. Report 57284 if access is achieved via laparotomy (open abdominal approach) and 57285 if a vaginal approach is utilized.

Coding Tips

If only one of the components of these procedures is performed, see other codes in this section of CPT. For example, if repair of a cystocele with anterior colporrhaphy is performed by itself, report 57240. For a Marshall-Marchetti-Krantz urethral suspension, abdominal approach, see 51840-51841. For laparoscopic repair of stress incontinence, see 51990-51992. For sling operation for stress incontinence, see 57288. Do not report 57284-57285 with 51990, 57240, 57260, 57265, or 58267. Code 57284 should also not be reported with 51840-51841 or 58152.

ICD-10-CM Diagnostic Codes

N81.0	Urethrocele ♀
N81.11	Cystocele, midline ♀
N81.12	Cystocele, lateral ♀
N81.2	Incomplete uterovaginal prolapse ♀
N81.3	Complete uterovaginal prolapse ♀
N81.6	Rectocele ♀
N81.81	Perineocele ♀
N81.83	Incompetence or weakening of rectovaginal tissue ♀
N81.85	Cervical stump prolapse ♀
N81.89	Other female genital prolapse ♀
N99.3	Prolapse of vaginal vault after hysterectomy ♀

AMA: 57284 2019,Jul,6; 2018,Jan,8; 2017,Jan,8; 2016,Jan,13; 2015,Jan,16; 2014,Jan,11 **57285** 2019,Jul,6; 2018,Jan,8; 2017,Jan,8; 2016,Jan,13; 2015,Jan,16; 2014,Jan,11

Relative Value Units/Medicare Edits

Non-Facility RVU	Work	PE	MP	Total
57284	14.33	7.56	1.99	23.88
57285	11.6	6.59	1.69	19.88
Facility RVU	**Work**	**PE**	**MP**	**Total**
57284	14.33	7.56	1.99	23.88
57285	11.6	6.59	1.69	19.88

	FUD	Status	MUE	Modifiers				IOM Reference
57284	90	A	1(2)	51	N/A	62	80	100-03,230.10
57285	90	A	1(2)	51	N/A	62	80	

* with documentation

Terms To Know

approach. Method or anatomical location used to gain access to a body organ or specific area for procedures.

cystocele. Herniation of the bladder into the vagina.

defect. Imperfection, flaw, or absence.

dissect. Cut apart or separate tissue for surgical purposes or for visual or microscopic study.

para-. Indicates near, similar, beside, or past.

perineocele. Uncommon condition in which herniation occurs in the perineal area between the rectum and vagina, the rectum and bladder, or beside the rectum.

prolapse. Falling, sliding, or sinking of an organ from its normal location in the body.

rectocele. Rectal tissue herniation into the vaginal wall.

repair. Surgical closure of a wound. The wound may be a result of injury/trauma or it may be a surgically created defect. Repairs are divided into three categories: simple, intermediate, and complex.

urethrocele. Urethral herniation into the vaginal wall.

57287

57287   Removal or revision of sling for stress incontinence (eg, fascia or synthetic)

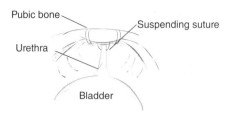

Overhead schematic showing suspension sutures (fascial suspension may also be found)

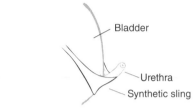

A synthetic or fascial sling for stress incontinence is revisited and either revised or removed

Explanation

The physician removes or revises a fascial or synthetic sling previously placed to correct urinary stress incontinence. To remove a sling, the physician makes a small abdominal skin incision to the level of the rectus fascia and releases the arm of the sling from the rectus abdominis. The physician releases the sling's attachment to the junction of the urethra via canals or tunnels formed by an instrument or a finger placed through a vertical or flap incision in the vaginal wall. In revision of a sling the physician may remove and partially or completely replace the sling using fascia or a synthetic graft through an abdominal and vaginal approach. The sling may be revised by increasing the tension on the sling using suture at one or both of the attachment sites at the junction of the urethra and/or to the rectus abdominis muscle. At the end of the procedure the area is irrigated, and hemostasis is achieved. The abdominal and/or vaginal incisions are closed with layered sutures.

Coding Tips

When 57287 is performed with another separately identifiable procedure, the highest dollar value code is listed as the primary procedure and subsequent procedures are appended with modifier 51. For initial sling operation, see 57288. For laparoscopic sling operation for stress incontinence, see 51992.

ICD-10-CM Diagnostic Codes

N39.3   Stress incontinence (female) (male)
T83.118A   Breakdown (mechanical) of other urinary devices and implants, initial encounter
T83.128A   Displacement of other urinary devices and implants, initial encounter
T83.198A   Other mechanical complication of other urinary devices and implants, initial encounter
T83.21XA   Breakdown (mechanical) of graft of urinary organ, initial encounter
T83.22XA   Displacement of graft of urinary organ, initial encounter
T83.23XA   Leakage of graft of urinary organ, initial encounter
T83.24XA   Erosion of graft of urinary organ, initial encounter
T83.25XA   Exposure of graft of urinary organ, initial encounter
T83.29XA   Other mechanical complication of graft of urinary organ, initial encounter
T83.711A   Erosion of implanted vaginal mesh to surrounding organ or tissue, initial encounter ♀
T83.721A   Exposure of implanted vaginal mesh into vagina, initial encounter ♀
T83.81XA   Embolism due to genitourinary prosthetic devices, implants and grafts, initial encounter
T83.82XA   Fibrosis due to genitourinary prosthetic devices, implants and grafts, initial encounter
T83.83XA   Hemorrhage due to genitourinary prosthetic devices, implants and grafts, initial encounter
T83.84XA   Pain due to genitourinary prosthetic devices, implants and grafts, initial encounter
T83.85XA   Stenosis due to genitourinary prosthetic devices, implants and grafts, initial encounter
T83.86XA   Thrombosis due to genitourinary prosthetic devices, implants and grafts, initial encounter
T83.89XA   Other specified complication of genitourinary prosthetic devices, implants and grafts, initial encounter
Z46.6   Encounter for fitting and adjustment of urinary device

AMA: 57287 2019,Jul,6; 2018,Jan,8; 2017,Jan,8; 2016,Jan,13; 2015,Jan,16; 2014,Jan,11

Relative Value Units/Medicare Edits

Non-Facility RVU	Work	PE	MP	Total
57287	11.15	8.02	1.51	20.68
Facility RVU	Work	PE	MP	Total
57287	11.15	8.02	1.51	20.68

	FUD	Status	MUE	Modifiers				IOM Reference
57287	90	A	1(2)	51	N/A	62*	80	100-03,230.10

* with documentation

Terms To Know

complication. Condition arising after the beginning of observation and treatment that modifies the course of the patient's illness or the medical care required, or an undesired result or misadventure in medical care.

fascia. Fibrous sheet or band of tissue that envelops organs, muscles, and groupings of muscles.

female stress incontinence. Involuntary escape of urine at times of minor stress against the female bladder, such as coughing, sneezing, or laughing.

hemostasis. Interruption of blood flow or the cessation or arrest of bleeding.

infection. Presence of microorganisms in body tissues that may result in cellular damage.

removal. Process of moving out of or away from, or the fact of being removed.

sling operation. Procedure to correct urinary incontinence. A sling of fascia or synthetic material is placed under the junction of the urethra and bladder in females, or across the muscles surrounding the urethra in males.

Vagina

57288

57288   Sling operation for stress incontinence (eg, fascia or synthetic)

The physician places a support sling
to eliminate stress incontinence

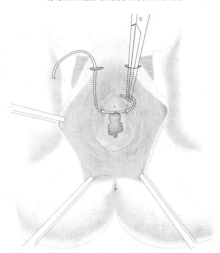

The sling can be synthetic or fascial

Explanation

Through vaginal and abdominal incisions, the physician places a sling under the junction of the urethra and bladder. The physician places a catheter in the bladder, makes an incision in the anterior wall of the vagina, and folds and tacks the tissues around the urethra. A sling is formed out of synthetic material or from fascia harvested from the sheath of the rectus abdominis muscle. The loop end of the sling is sutured around the junction of the urethra. An incision is made in the lower abdomen and the ends of the sling are grasped with a clamp and pulled into the incision and sutured to the rectus abdominis sheath. The abdominal and vaginal incisions are closed in layers by suturing.

Coding Tips

For removal or revision of a sling, see 57287. For a Marshall-Marchetti-Krantz urethral suspension, abdominal approach, see 51840-51841. For laparoscopic sling operation for stress incontinence, see 51992. Supplies used when providing this procedure may be reported with the appropriate HCPCS Level II code. Check with the specific payer to determine coverage.

ICD-10-CM Diagnostic Codes

N39.3   Stress incontinence (female) (male)

AMA: **57288** 2019,Jul,6; 2019,Feb,10; 2018,Jan,8; 2017,Jan,8; 2016,Jan,13; 2015,Jan,16; 2014,Jan,11

Relative Value Units/Medicare Edits

Non-Facility RVU	Work	PE	MP	Total
57288	12.13	7.37	1.69	21.19
Facility RVU	Work	PE	MP	Total
57288	12.13	7.37	1.69	21.19

	FUD	Status	MUE	Modifiers				IOM Reference
57288	90	A	1(2)	51	N/A	62*	80	None

* with documentation

57289

57289   Pereyra procedure, including anterior colporrhaphy

Pereyra ligature carrier

The physician guides the
ligature with a finger
inserted in the vagina

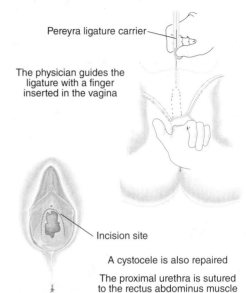

Incision site

A cystocele is also repaired

The proximal urethra is sutured
to the rectus abdominus muscle

Explanation

The physician makes an inverted U-shaped incision in the area between the vagina and the urethra. By blunt and sharp dissection, the physician creates an opening in the space on each side of the urethra as it passes into the bladder. Using a continuous suture for each side, the physician stitches the fascial tissues along the urethra to the urethrovesical junction. The physician makes an incision in the abdomen above the pubis and, doing each side in turn, drives a Pereyra ligature carrier through the tissues just lateral to the midline and takes it down to the sutured tissue. The sutures are threaded into the instrument and brought back through the abdominal incision. The urethrovesical junction is elevated by pulling on the sutures and fixing them around the rectus abdominis muscle. In addition, the physician performs an anterior colporrhaphy using a vaginal approach, which corrects a cystocele and repairs the tissues between the vagina, bladder, and urethra.

Coding Tips

For a Marshall-Marchetti-Krantz urethral suspension, abdominal approach, see 51840-51841. For laparoscopic repair of stress incontinence, see 51990-51992. For anterior colporrhaphy with repair of cystocele, see 57240.

ICD-10-CM Diagnostic Codes

N39.3   Stress incontinence (female) (male)
N81.10   Cystocele, unspecified ♀
N81.11   Cystocele, midline ♀
N81.12   Cystocele, lateral ♀

AMA: **57289** 2019,Jul,6; 2018,Jan,8; 2017,Jan,8; 2016,Jan,13; 2015,Jan,16; 2014,Jan,11

Vagina

Relative Value Units/Medicare Edits

Non-Facility RVU	Work	PE	MP	Total
57289	12.8	7.85	2.0	22.65
Facility RVU	Work	PE	MP	Total
57289	12.8	7.85	2.0	22.65

	FUD	Status	MUE	Modifiers				IOM Reference
57289	90	A	1(2)	51	N/A	62*	80	None

* with documentation

Terms To Know

anterior. Situated in the front area or toward the belly surface of the body.

colporrhaphy. Plastic repair or reconstruction of the vagina by suturing the vaginal wall and surrounding fibrous tissue.

cystocele. Herniation of the bladder into the vagina.

dissect. Cut apart or separate tissue for surgical purposes or for visual or microscopic study.

female stress incontinence. Involuntary escape of urine at times of minor stress against the female bladder, such as coughing, sneezing, or laughing.

prolapse. Falling, sliding, or sinking of an organ from its normal location in the body.

urethrocele. Urethral herniation into the vaginal wall.

uterovaginal prolapse. Uterus displaced downward and exposed in the external genitalia.

57291-57292

57291 Construction of artificial vagina; without graft
57292   with graft

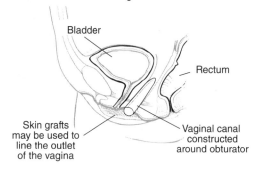

An artificial vagina is constructed

Bladder

Rectum

Skin grafts may be used to line the outlet of the vagina

Vaginal canal constructed around obturator

Explanation

For construction of an artificial vagina without graft, the physician develops a vagina by a program of perineal pressure using progressively longer and wider firm obturators. Pressure is applied to the soft area between the urethra and rectum with an obturator. Over several months of consistent, daily use by the patient, a sexually functional vagina can be created. In 57292, the physician creates or enlarges the vagina using one or more skin grafts. Through a midline episiotomy incision, the physician creates a space between the urethra and rectum. Using split thickness or full thickness skin grafts, the space is lined and the vagina created. An obturator or mold is inserted into the vagina and a catheter is passed into the bladder and left for several days. The full thickness skin donor sites are closed using plastic surgical techniques. The split thickness sites are dressed with medicated gauze.

Coding Tips

For repair of an injury of the vagina and perineum, see 57210. For vaginoplasty, see 57335.

ICD-10-CM Diagnostic Codes

Q52.0   Congenital absence of vagina ♀

AMA: **57291** 2019,Jul,6; 2014,Jan,11 **57292** 2019,Jul,6; 2014,Jan,11

Relative Value Units/Medicare Edits

Non-Facility RVU	Work	PE	MP	Total
57291	8.64	5.7	1.34	15.68
57292	14.01	7.72	2.2	23.93
Facility RVU	Work	PE	MP	Total
57291	8.64	5.7	1.34	15.68
57292	14.01	7.72	2.2	23.93

	FUD	Status	MUE	Modifiers				IOM Reference
57291	90	A	1(2)	51	N/A	N/A	80	None
57292	90	A	1(2)	51	N/A	62*	80	

* with documentation

Terms To Know

obturate. To occlude or close off an opening.

Vagina

57295

57295 Revision (including removal) of prosthetic vaginal graft; vaginal approach

An artificial vagina is revised using a vaginal approach

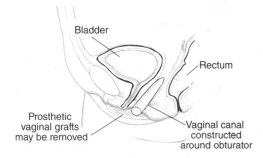

Bladder

Rectum

Prosthetic vaginal grafts may be removed

Vaginal canal constructed around obturator

Explanation

The physician revises or removes a previously placed prosthetic vaginal graft via a vaginal approach. The patient is placed in the lithotomy position and a speculum is inserted. The physician visualizes the vagina. The apex of the vagina is accessed with deep retractors. Dissection is carried out to reach the affected graft material. Depending upon the type of complication (i.e., stricture or infection), the vaginal graft may be completely or partially excised to remove eroding mesh or revisions may be made in the graft and surrounding tissue. The vaginal epithelial layers and pelvic fascia are rearranged or reapproximated and closed. Vaginal packing is put in place.

Coding Tips

Revision of prosthetic vaginal graft is done for complications, such as infection, that require surgical intervention. Complete removal of the graft is included. For initial construction of an artificial vagina using a graft, see 57292.

ICD-10-CM Diagnostic Codes

T83.418A	Breakdown (mechanical) of other prosthetic devices, implants and grafts of genital tract, initial encounter
T83.428A	Displacement of other prosthetic devices, implants and grafts of genital tract, initial encounter
T83.498A	Other mechanical complication of other prosthetic devices, implants and grafts of genital tract, initial encounter
T83.69XA	Infection and inflammatory reaction due to other prosthetic device, implant and graft in genital tract, initial encounter
T83.711A	Erosion of implanted vaginal mesh to surrounding organ or tissue, initial encounter ♀
T83.721A	Exposure of implanted vaginal mesh into vagina, initial encounter ♀
T83.81XA	Embolism due to genitourinary prosthetic devices, implants and grafts, initial encounter
T83.82XA	Fibrosis due to genitourinary prosthetic devices, implants and grafts, initial encounter
T83.83XA	Hemorrhage due to genitourinary prosthetic devices, implants and grafts, initial encounter
T83.84XA	Pain due to genitourinary prosthetic devices, implants and grafts, initial encounter
T83.85XA	Stenosis due to genitourinary prosthetic devices, implants and grafts, initial encounter
T83.86XA	Thrombosis due to genitourinary prosthetic devices, implants and grafts, initial encounter

T83.89XA	Other specified complication of genitourinary prosthetic devices, implants and grafts, initial encounter

AMA: **57295** 2019,Jul,6; 2014,Jan,11

Relative Value Units/Medicare Edits

Non-Facility RVU	Work	PE	MP	Total
57295	7.82	5.28	1.13	14.23
Facility RVU	**Work**	**PE**	**MP**	**Total**
57295	7.82	5.28	1.13	14.23

	FUD	Status	MUE	Modifiers				IOM Reference
57295	90	A	1(2)	51	N/A	62*	80	None

* with documentation

Terms To Know

apex. Highest point of a root end of a tooth, or the end of any organ.

approach. Method or anatomical location used to gain access to a body organ or specific area for procedures.

dissection. (dis. apart; -section, act of cutting) Separating by cutting tissue or body structures apart.

excise. Remove or cut out.

graft. Tissue implant from another part of the body or another person.

lithotomy position. Common position patients may be placed in for some surgical procedures and examinations involving the pelvis and/or lower abdomen. The patient is placed supine (on their back), hips and knees flexed, thighs apart, with feet supported in raised stirrups.

mesh. Synthetic fabric used as a prosthetic patch in hernia repair.

packing. Material placed into a cavity or wound, such as gels, gauze, pads, and sponges.

revision. Reordering or rearrangement of tissue to suit a particular need or function.

Vagina

57296

57296 Revision (including removal) of prosthetic vaginal graft; open abdominal approach

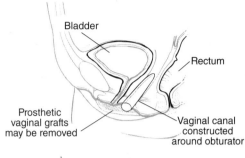

Bladder

Rectum

Prosthetic vaginal grafts may be removed

Vaginal canal constructed around obturator

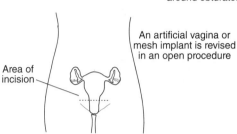

An artificial vagina or mesh implant is revised in an open procedure

Area of incision

Explanation

The physician revises or removes a previously placed prosthetic vaginal graft using an open abdominal approach in conjunction with a vaginal approach. A laparotomy incision is made and the physician dissects into the pelvis. The vagina is elevated with tools or with the physician's hand. The graft is located, the peritoneum is opened over it, and the graft is dissected free and removed. Depending upon the type of complication (i.e., stricture or infection), the vaginal graft may be completely or partially excised to remove eroding mesh or revisions may be made in the graft and surrounding tissue. Endopelvic fascia is reapproximated and the vaginal epithelial layers and pelvic fascia are rearranged or reapproximated and closed. The abdominal incision is repaired in layers. Vaginal packing is put in place.

Coding Tips

Revision of prosthetic vaginal graft is done for complications, such as infection, that require surgical intervention. 57296 is performed by open abdominal approach. Complete removal of the graft is included. For laparoscopic approach, see 57426. For vaginal approach, see 57295.

ICD-10-CM Diagnostic Codes

T83.418A	Breakdown (mechanical) of other prosthetic devices, implants and grafts of genital tract, initial encounter
T83.428A	Displacement of other prosthetic devices, implants and grafts of genital tract, initial encounter
T83.498A	Other mechanical complication of other prosthetic devices, implants and grafts of genital tract, initial encounter
T83.69XA	Infection and inflammatory reaction due to other prosthetic device, implant and graft in genital tract, initial encounter
T83.711A	Erosion of implanted vaginal mesh to surrounding organ or tissue, initial encounter ♀
T83.721A	Exposure of implanted vaginal mesh into vagina, initial encounter ♀
T83.81XA	Embolism due to genitourinary prosthetic devices, implants and grafts, initial encounter

T83.82XA	Fibrosis due to genitourinary prosthetic devices, implants and grafts, initial encounter
T83.83XA	Hemorrhage due to genitourinary prosthetic devices, implants and grafts, initial encounter
T83.84XA	Pain due to genitourinary prosthetic devices, implants and grafts, initial encounter
T83.85XA	Stenosis due to genitourinary prosthetic devices, implants and grafts, initial encounter
T83.86XA	Thrombosis due to genitourinary prosthetic devices, implants and grafts, initial encounter
T83.89XA	Other specified complication of genitourinary prosthetic devices, implants and grafts, initial encounter

AMA: 57296 2019,Jul,6; 2014,Jan,11

Relative Value Units/Medicare Edits

Non-Facility RVU	Work	PE	MP	Total
57296	16.56	8.46	2.38	27.4
Facility RVU	**Work**	**PE**	**MP**	**Total**
57296	16.56	8.46	2.38	27.4

	FUD	Status	MUE	Modifiers				IOM Reference
57296	90	A	1(2)	51	N/A	62*	80	None

* with documentation

Terms To Know

approach. Method or anatomical location used to gain access to a body organ or specific area for procedures.

graft. Tissue implant from another part of the body or another person.

hemorrhage. Internal or external bleeding with loss of significant amounts of blood.

infection. Presence of microorganisms in body tissues that may result in cellular damage.

laparotomy. Incision through the flank or abdomen for therapeutic or diagnostic purposes.

prosthetic. Device that replaces all or part of an internal body organ or body part, or that replaces part of the function of a permanently inoperable or malfunctioning internal body organ or body part.

revision. Reordering or rearrangement of tissue to suit a particular need or function.

stenosis. Narrowing or constriction of a passage.

stricture. Narrowing of an anatomical structure.

thrombosis. Condition arising from the presence or formation of blood clots within a blood vessel that may cause vascular obstruction and insufficient oxygenation.

Vagina

57300

57300   Closure of rectovaginal fistula; vaginal or transanal approach

The repair is made transvaginally or transanally

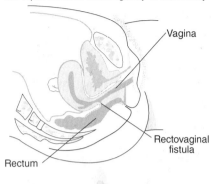

Vagina

Rectovaginal fistula

Rectum

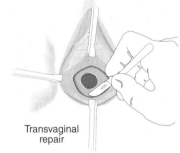

Transvaginal repair

Explanation

The physician closes a rectovaginal fistula, which is an abnormal passage between the rectum and the vagina. The physician also repairs the perineum, fascia, and muscle-supporting structures between the rectum and vagina. The scar tissue and tract between the rectum and vagina are excised and the clean edges sutured together. Often a flap of tissue is transplanted between the vagina and the rectum and the area is closed in layers. The rectal wall opening is closed by inverting the mucosa into the rectal canal. The vaginal wall opening is closed by inverting the mucosal layer into the vaginal wall. Sometimes the vaginal side is left open for drainage.

Coding Tips

For closure of a rectovaginal fistula, abdominal approach, see 57305. For closure of a rectovaginal fistula, abdominal approach with concomitant colostomy, see 57307; via transperineal approach including perineal body reconstruction, with or without levator plication, see 57308. For closure of a urethrovaginal fistula, see 57310 and 57311. For vaginal closure of a vesicovaginal fistula, see 57320 and 57330; abdominal closure, see 51900.

ICD-10-CM Diagnostic Codes

N82.3   Fistula of vagina to large intestine ♀

AMA: **57300** 2019,Jul,6; 2014,Jan,11

Relative Value Units/Medicare Edits

Non-Facility RVU	Work	PE	MP	Total
57300	8.71	6.88	1.46	17.05
Facility RVU	**Work**	**PE**	**MP**	**Total**
57300	8.71	6.88	1.46	17.05

	FUD	Status	MUE	Modifiers				IOM Reference
57300	90	A	1(3)	51	N/A	62*	80	None

* with documentation

Terms To Know

approach. Method or anatomical location used to gain access to a body organ or specific area for procedures. The approach is not coded separately although it may be a specified component of the procedure, such as laparoscopic versus incisional, or spinal procedures in which the amount of dissection required to expose the spine significantly alters with the site of approach.

closure. Repairing an incision or wound by suture or other means.

drainage. Releasing, taking, or letting out fluids and/or gases from a body part.

excise. Remove or cut out.

flap. Mass of flesh and skin partially excised from its location but retaining its blood supply that is moved to another site to repair adjacent or distant defects.

free flap. Tissue that is completely detached from the donor site and transplanted to the recipient site, receiving its blood supply from capillary ingrowth at the recipient site.

rectovaginal fistula. Abnormal communication between the rectum and the vagina that may follow obstetrical laceration repair, vaginal or rectal surgery, radiation therapy, trauma, or infection with fecal incontinence or leakage into the vaginal canal.

scar tissue. Fibrous connective tissue that forms around a wounded area or injury, composed mainly of fibroblasts or collagenous fibers.

Vagina

57305

57305   Closure of rectovaginal fistula; abdominal approach

The fistula is repaired through an abdominal incision

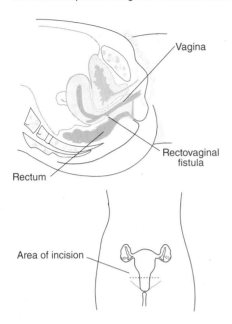

Vagina

Rectovaginal fistula

Rectum

Area of incision

Explanation

Through a lower abdominal incision, the physician closes a rectovaginal fistula, which is an abnormal passage between the rectum and the vagina. The physician also repairs the perineum, fascia, and muscle-supporting structures between the rectum and vagina. The scar tissue and tract between the rectum and vagina are excised and the clean edges sutured together. Often a flap of tissue is transplanted between the vagina and the rectum and the area is closed in layers. The rectal wall opening is closed by inverting the mucosa into the rectal canal. The vaginal wall opening is closed by inverting the mucosal layer into the vaginal wall. Sometimes the vaginal side is left open for drainage. The abdominal incision is closed with sutures.

Coding Tips

For closure of a rectovaginal fistula, vaginal or transanal approach, see 57300. For closure of a rectovaginal fistula, abdominal approach with concomitant colostomy, see 57307; via transperineal approach including perineal body reconstruction, with or without levator plication, see 57308. For closure of a urethrovaginal fistula, see 57310 and 57311. For vaginal closure of a vesicovaginal fistula, see 57320 and 57330; abdominal approach, see 51900.

ICD-10-CM Diagnostic Codes

N82.3   Fistula of vagina to large intestine ♀

AMA: **57305** 2019,Jul,6; 2014,Jan,11

Relative Value Units/Medicare Edits

Non-Facility RVU	Work	PE	MP	Total
57305	15.35	9.75	2.86	27.96
Facility RVU	**Work**	**PE**	**MP**	**Total**
57305	15.35	9.75	2.86	27.96

	FUD	Status	MUE	Modifiers				IOM Reference
57305	90	A	1(3)	51	N/A	62*	80	None

* with documentation

Terms To Know

approach. Method or anatomical location used to gain access to a body organ or specific area for procedures. The approach is not coded separately although it may be a specified component of the procedure, such as laparoscopic versus incisional, or spinal procedures in which the amount of dissection required to expose the spine significantly alters with the site of approach.

closure. Repairing an incision or wound by suture or other means.

concomitant. Occurring at the same time, accompanying.

drainage. Releasing, taking, or letting out fluids and/or gases from a body part.

fascia. Fibrous sheet or band of tissue that envelops organs, muscles, and groupings of muscles.

mucosa. Moist tissue lining the mouth (buccal mucosa), stomach (gastric mucosa), intestines, and respiratory tract.

rectovaginal fistula. Abnormal communication between the rectum and the vagina that may follow obstetrical laceration repair, vaginal or rectal surgery, radiation therapy, trauma, or infection with fecal incontinence or leakage into the vaginal canal.

scar tissue. Fibrous connective tissue that forms around a wounded area or injury, composed mainly of fibroblasts or collagenous fibers.

Vagina

57307

57307 Closure of rectovaginal fistula; abdominal approach, with concomitant colostomy

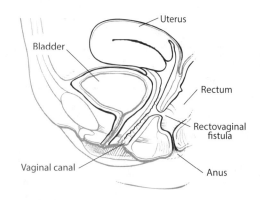

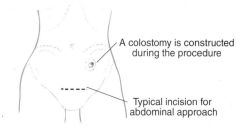

A colostomy is constructed during the procedure

Typical incision for abdominal approach

Explanation

Through a lower abdominal incision, the physician closes a rectovaginal fistula, which is an abnormal passage between the rectum and vagina. The physician also repairs the perineum, fascia, and muscle-supporting structures between the rectum and vagina. The scar tissue and tract between the rectum and vagina are excised and the clean edges sutured together. Often a flap of tissue is transplanted between the vagina and rectum and the area is closed in layers. The rectal wall opening created during the excision is closed by inverting the mucosa into the rectal canal. The vaginal wall opening is closed by inverting the mucosal layer into the vaginal canal. The vaginal side may be left open for drainage. A transverse colostomy is done to divert the flow of feces and to allow healing of the rectal colon repair. The abdominal incision is closed with sutures.

Coding Tips

After the fistula repair has healed, a second operation is done to take down the colostomy and re-establish normal function of the bowel. For closure of a rectovaginal fistula, vaginal or transanal approach, see 57300. For closure of a rectovaginal fistula, abdominal approach, without colostomy, see 57305; via transperineal approach including perineal body reconstruction, with or without levator plication, see 57308. For closure of a urethrovaginal fistula, see 57310 and 57311. For vaginal closure of a vesicovaginal fistula, see 57320 and 57330; abdominal approach, see 51900.

ICD-10-CM Diagnostic Codes

N82.3　　　Fistula of vagina to large intestine ♀

AMA: 57307 2019,Jul,6; 2014,Jan,11

Relative Value Units/Medicare Edits

Non-Facility RVU	Work	PE	MP	Total
57307	17.17	11.05	2.17	30.39
Facility RVU	Work	PE	MP	Total
57307	17.17	11.05	2.17	30.39

	FUD	Status	MUE	Modifiers				IOM Reference
57307	90	A	1(3)	51	N/A	62*	80	None

* with documentation

Terms To Know

approach. Method or anatomical location used to gain access to a body organ or specific area for procedures. The approach is not coded separately although it may be a specified component of the procedure, such as laparoscopic versus incisional, or spinal procedures in which the amount of dissection required to expose the spine significantly alters with the site of approach.

colostomy. Artificial surgical opening anywhere along the length of the colon to the skin surface for the diversion of feces.

concomitant. Occurring at the same time, accompanying.

rectovaginal fistula. Abnormal communication between the rectum and the vagina that may follow obstetrical laceration repair, vaginal or rectal surgery, radiation therapy, trauma, or infection with fecal incontinence or leakage into the vaginal canal.

scar tissue. Fibrous connective tissue that forms around a wounded area or injury, composed mainly of fibroblasts or collagenous fibers.

transverse. Crosswise at right angles to the long axis of a structure or part.

Vagina

57308

57308 Closure of rectovaginal fistula; transperineal approach, with perineal body reconstruction, with or without levator plication

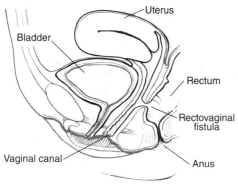

A rectovaginal fistula is surgically closed by transperineal approach

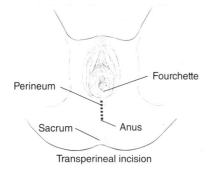

Transperineal incision

Explanation

Through a transperineal approach, the physician closes a rectovaginal fistula, which is an abnormal passage between the rectum and vagina. The physician also repairs the perineum, fascia, and muscle-supporting structures between the rectum and vagina. The scar tissue and tract between the rectum and vagina are excised and the clean edges sutured together. Often a flap of tissue is transplanted in between the vagina and rectum and the area is closed in multiple layers. The rectal wall opening created during the excision is closed by inverting the mucosa into the rectal canal. The vaginal wall opening is closed by inverting the mucosal layer into the vaginal canal. The vaginal side may be left open for drainage. The perineal body is reconstructed with or without a levator plication.

Coding Tips

For closure of a rectovaginal fistula, abdominal approach, with concomitant colostomy, see 57307; without colostomy, see 57305. For closure of a rectovaginal fistula, vaginal or transanal approach, see 57300. For closure of a urethrovaginal fistula, see 57310 and 57311. For vaginal closure of a vesicovaginal fistula, see 57320 and 57330; abdominal approach, see 51900.

ICD-10-CM Diagnostic Codes

N82.3   Fistula of vagina to large intestine ♀

AMA: **57308** 2019,Jul,6; 2014,Jan,11

Relative Value Units/Medicare Edits

Non-Facility RVU	Work	PE	MP	Total
57308	10.59	7.08	1.33	19.0
Facility RVU	**Work**	**PE**	**MP**	**Total**
57308	10.59	7.08	1.33	19.0

	FUD	Status	MUE	Modifiers				IOM Reference
57308	90	A	1(3)	51	N/A	62*	80	None

* with documentation

Terms To Know

approach. Method or anatomical location used to gain access to a body organ or specific area for procedures. The approach is not coded separately although it may be a specified component of the procedure, such as laparoscopic versus incisional, or spinal procedures in which the amount of dissection required to expose the spine significantly alters with the site of approach.

perineal. Pertaining to the pelvic floor area between the thighs; the diamond-shaped area bordered by the pubic symphysis in front, the ischial tuberosities on the sides, and the coccyx in back.

plication. Surgical technique involving folding, tucking, or pleating to reduce the size of a hollow structure or organ.

reconstruction. Recreating, restoring, or rebuilding a body part or organ.

rectovaginal fistula. Abnormal communication between the rectum and the vagina that may follow obstetrical laceration repair, vaginal or rectal surgery, radiation therapy, trauma, or infection with fecal incontinence or leakage into the vaginal canal.

scar tissue. Fibrous connective tissue that forms around a wounded area or injury, composed mainly of fibroblasts or collagenous fibers.

Vagina

57310-57311

57310 Closure of urethrovaginal fistula;
57311 with bulbocavernosus transplant

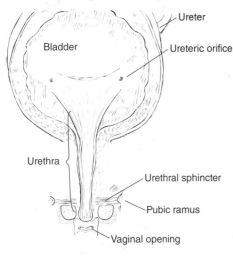
A fistula between the urethra and vagina is surgically closed

Ureter
Bladder
Ureteric orifice
Urethra
Urethral sphincter
Pubic ramus
Vaginal opening

Explanation

The physician closes a urethrovaginal fistula, which is an abnormal passage between the urethra and vagina. With a catheter in the urethra, the fistula tract is excised and the defect in the urethra is sutured closed. A pad of fatty tissue is sutured between the repaired urethral defect and the vaginal defect in 57310. In 57311, a pad of fatty tissue and a strip of the bulbocavernosus muscle are brought through a tunnel created between the vagina and one labium. The fat and muscle flap are sutured between the repaired urethral defect and the vaginal defect. In either case, the involved area in the vagina is excised and the defect is sutured closed. The catheter is left in place for several days to allow healing of the urethra.

Coding Tips

For closure of a rectovaginal fistula, vaginal or transanal approach, see 57300. For closure of a rectovaginal fistula, abdominal approach, see 57305. For closure of a rectovaginal fistula, abdominal approach, with concomitant colostomy, see 57307; via transperineal approach including perineal body reconstruction, with or without levator plication, see 57308. For vaginal closure of a vesicovaginal fistula, see 57320 and 57330; abdominal approach, see 51900.

ICD-10-CM Diagnostic Codes

N82.1   Other female urinary-genital tract fistulae ♀

AMA: 57310 2019,Jul,6; 2014,Jan,11 **57311** 2019,Jul,6; 2014,Jan,11

Relative Value Units/Medicare Edits

Non-Facility RVU	Work	PE	MP	Total
57310	7.65	5.33	0.87	13.85
57311	8.91	5.75	1.02	15.68
Facility RVU	**Work**	**PE**	**MP**	**Total**
57310	7.65	5.33	0.87	13.85
57311	8.91	5.75	1.02	15.68

	FUD	Status	MUE	Modifiers				IOM Reference
57310	90	A	1(3)	51	N/A	62*	80	None
57311	90	A	1(3)	51	N/A	62*	80	

* with documentation

Terms To Know

absorbable sutures. Strands used for suture or repair of tissue prepared from collagen or a synthetic polymer and capable of being absorbed by tissue over time.

closure. Repairing an incision or wound by suture or other means.

complication. Condition arising after the beginning of observation and treatment that modifies the course of the patient's illness or the medical care required, or an undesired result or misadventure in medical care.

defect. Imperfection, flaw, or absence.

excise. Remove or cut out.

transplant. Insertion of an organ or tissue from one person or site into another.

urethrovaginal fistula. Abnormal communication between the urethra and the vagina resulting in urinary leakage from the vagina.

Vagina

57320-57330

57320 Closure of vesicovaginal fistula; vaginal approach
57330 transvesical and vaginal approach

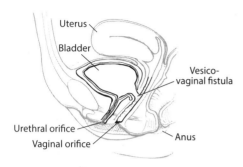

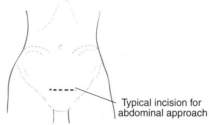

Typical incision for abdominal approach

A fistula between the bladder and the vagina is surgically closed

Explanation

The physician closes a vesicovaginal fistula, which is an abnormal passage between the bladder and the vagina. In 57320, this procedure is performed through the vagina, with catheters through the urethra into both ureters. The fistula and surrounding scar tissue of the vaginal wall are usually excised. Using a vaginal approach, the bladder wall is opened and the bladder explored. The fistula is excised along with the surrounding tissue. The resulting defect is closed with sutures in layers, starting with the bladder wall and ending with the vaginal mucosa. In some cases, a pedicle graft of tissue may be sutured between the bladder and the vagina. In 57330, the procedure is performed through the vagina and lower abdomen, with catheters through the urethra into both ureters. The physician opens the bladder wall through the lower abdominal incision and excises the fistula. The resulting defect is closed with sutures in layers, starting with the bladder wall and ending with the abdominal wall. Through the vagina, the physician excises the fistula and surrounding scar tissue of the vaginal wall. In some cases, a pedicle graft of tissue may be sutured between the bladder and the vagina. A urethral or suprapubic catheter is left in the bladder to prevent distension of the bladder and tension to the sutured areas.

Coding Tips

For closure of a vesicovaginal fistula, abdominal approach, see 51900. For closure of a urethrovaginal fistula, see 57310 and 57311. For closure of a rectovaginal fistula, vaginal or transanal approach, see 57300. For closure of a rectovaginal fistula, abdominal approach, see 57305. For closure of a rectovaginal fistula, abdominal approach with colostomy, see 57307; via transperineal approach including perineal body reconstruction, with or without levator plication, see 57308.

ICD-10-CM Diagnostic Codes

N82.0   Vesicovaginal fistula ♀

AMA: **57320** 2019,Jul,6; 2014,Jan,11 **57330** 2019,Jul,6; 2014,Jan,11

Relative Value Units/Medicare Edits

Non-Facility RVU	Work	PE	MP	Total
57320	8.88	5.81	1.16	15.85
57330	13.21	7.16	1.5	21.87
Facility RVU	**Work**	**PE**	**MP**	**Total**
57320	8.88	5.81	1.16	15.85
57330	13.21	7.16	1.5	21.87

	FUD	Status	MUE	Modifiers				IOM Reference
57320	90	A	1(3)	51	N/A	62*	80	None
57330	90	A	1(3)	51	N/A	62*	80	

* with documentation

Terms To Know

approach. Method or anatomical location used to gain access to a body organ or specific area for procedures. The approach is not coded separately although it may be a specified component of the procedure, such as laparoscopic versus incisional, or spinal procedures in which the amount of dissection required to expose the spine significantly alters with the site of approach.

closure. Repairing an incision or wound by suture or other means.

complication. Condition arising after the beginning of observation and treatment that modifies the course of the patient's illness or the medical care required, or an undesired result or misadventure in medical care.

scar tissue. Fibrous connective tissue that forms around a wounded area or injury, composed mainly of fibroblasts or collagenous fibers.

vesicovaginal fistula. Abnormal communication between the bladder and the vagina that is the most common genital fistula, often with urinary leakage causing skin irritation of the vulva and thighs, or total incontinence.

Vagina

57335

57335   Vaginoplasty for intersex state

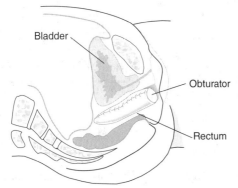

This is for congenital absence of a vagina

The vagina is created between the urethra and rectum. An obturator mold is placed in the newly created vagina

Explanation
The physician uses various plastic surgical techniques to correct a small, underdeveloped vagina due to the overproduction of male hormones. The physician constructs a larger and more functional vagina using carefully placed incisions and skin grafts.

Coding Tips
For construction of an artificial vagina without graft, see 57291; with graft, see 57292. For clitoroplasty, see 56805.

ICD-10-CM Diagnostic Codes
Q52.0   Congenital absence of vagina ♀
Q52.4   Other congenital malformations of vagina ♀

AMA: 57335 2019,Jul,6; 2014,Jan,11

Relative Value Units/Medicare Edits

Non-Facility RVU	Work	PE	MP	Total
57335	20.02	10.81	3.13	33.96
Facility RVU	**Work**	**PE**	**MP**	**Total**
57335	20.02	10.81	3.13	33.96

	FUD	Status	MUE	Modifiers				IOM Reference
57335	90	A	1(2)	51	N/A	62*	80	None

* with documentation

Terms To Know

congenital. Present at birth, occurring through heredity or an influence during gestation up to the moment of birth.

graft. Tissue implant from another part of the body or another person.

obturate. To occlude or close off an opening.

57400

57400   Dilation of vagina under anesthesia (other than local)

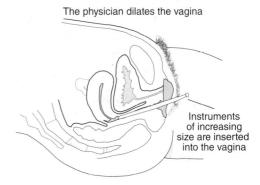

The physician dilates the vagina

Instruments of increasing size are inserted into the vagina

Explanation
The physician enlarges the vagina by using a set of progressively longer and wider vaginal obturator dilators. The physician inserts the vaginal dilators sequentially from smaller to larger with firm and gentle pressure while the patient is under anesthesia (other than local).

Coding Tips
For pelvic exam under anesthesia, see 57410. For removal of an impacted foreign body of the vagina, under anesthesia, see 57415.

ICD-10-CM Diagnostic Codes
N76.5   Ulceration of vagina ♀
N76.81   Mucositis (ulcerative) of vagina and vulva ♀
N76.89   Other specified inflammation of vagina and vulva ♀
N89.5   Stricture and atresia of vagina ♀
N99.2   Postprocedural adhesions of vagina ♀
Q51.0   Agenesis and aplasia of uterus ♀
Q51.5   Agenesis and aplasia of cervix ♀
Q51.7   Congenital fistulae between uterus and digestive and urinary tracts ♀
Q51.821   Hypoplasia of cervix ♀
Q51.828   Other congenital malformations of cervix ♀
Q52.2   Congenital rectovaginal fistula ♀
Q52.4   Other congenital malformations of vagina ♀
Q52.5   Fusion of labia ♀
Q52.6   Congenital malformation of clitoris ♀
Q52.70   Unspecified congenital malformations of vulva ♀
Q52.71   Congenital absence of vulva ♀
Q52.79   Other congenital malformations of vulva ♀
Q52.8   Other specified congenital malformations of female genitalia ♀

AMA: 57400 2019,Jul,6; 2014,Jan,11

Vagina

Relative Value Units/Medicare Edits

Non-Facility RVU	Work	PE	MP	Total
57400	2.27	1.19	0.35	3.81
Facility RVU	Work	PE	MP	Total
57400	2.27	1.19	0.35	3.81

	FUD	Status	MUE	Modifiers				IOM Reference
57400	0	A	1(2)	51	N/A	N/A	80*	None

* with documentation

Terms To Know

anomaly. Irregularity in the structure or position of an organ or tissue.

atresia. Congenital closure or absence of a tubular organ or an opening to the body surface.

colpalgia. Pain in the vagina.

congenital. Present at birth, occurring through heredity or an influence during gestation up to the moment of birth.

dilation. Artificial increase in the diameter of an opening or lumen made by medication or by instrumentation.

stricture. Narrowing of an anatomical structure.

57410

57410   Pelvic examination under anesthesia (other than local)

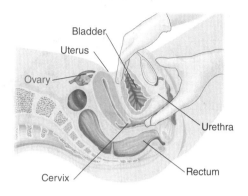

Explanation

Prior to the examination, the patient is placed under anesthesia, other than local, for a bimanual examination of the pelvic organs. The physician places two fingers inside the vagina to palpate the cervix, uterus, and ovaries while using the other hand to gently palpate the top of the uterus with pressure on the abdomen noting the organs' size, shape, and/or any abnormality.

Coding Tips

When 57410 is performed with another separately identifiable procedure, the highest dollar value code is listed as the primary procedure and subsequent procedures are appended with modifier 51. A pelvic exam under anesthesia done with other gynecological surgical procedures is generally an integral portion of the surgical procedure and is not identified separately. For removal of an impacted foreign body of the vagina, under anesthesia, see 57415.

ICD-10-CM Diagnostic Codes

The application of this code is too broad to adequately present ICD-10-CM diagnostic code links here. Refer to your ICD-10-CM book.

AMA: 57410 2019,Jul,6; 2018,Jan,8; 2017,Jan,8; 2016,Jan,13; 2015,Jan,16; 2014,Jan,11

Relative Value Units/Medicare Edits

Non-Facility RVU	Work	PE	MP	Total
57410	1.75	1.05	0.27	3.07
Facility RVU	Work	PE	MP	Total
57410	1.75	1.05	0.27	3.07

	FUD	Status	MUE	Modifiers				IOM Reference
57410	0	A	1(2)	51	N/A	N/A	N/A	None

* with documentation

Terms To Know

examination. Comprehensive visual and tactile screening and specific testing leading to diagnosis or, as appropriate, to a referral to another practitioner.

general anesthesia. State of unconsciousness produced by an anesthetic agent or agents, inducing amnesia by blocking the awareness center in the brain, and rendering the patient unable to control protective reflexes, such as breathing.

palpate. Examination by feeling with the hand.

Vagina

57415

57415 Removal of impacted vaginal foreign body (separate procedure) under anesthesia (other than local)

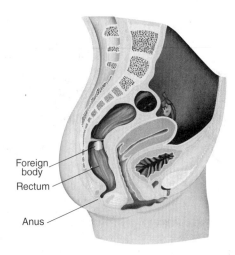

Foreign body
Rectum
Anus

Explanation

Using a vaginal speculum, the physician removes a foreign body lodged in the vagina. During the procedure, the patient is under anesthesia (other than local) because of the patient's inability to tolerate the procedure while fully alert or awake, as in the case of a young child or due to the type or size of the object being removed.

Coding Tips

This separate procedure by definition is usually a component of a more complex service and is not identified separately. When performed alone or with other unrelated procedures or services it may be reported. If performed alone, list the code; if performed with other procedures/services, list the code and append modifier 59 or an X{EPSU} modifier. For removal of an impacted vaginal foreign body without anesthesia, see the appropriate evaluation and management code.

ICD-10-CM Diagnostic Codes

S31.42XA	Laceration with foreign body of vagina and vulva, initial encounter ♀
S31.44XA	Puncture wound with foreign body of vagina and vulva, initial encounter ♀
T19.2XXA	Foreign body in vulva and vagina, initial encounter ♀

AMA: 57415 2019,Jul,6; 2014,Jan,11

Relative Value Units/Medicare Edits

Non-Facility RVU	Work	PE	MP	Total
57415	2.49	2.03	0.37	4.89
Facility RVU	**Work**	**PE**	**MP**	**Total**
57415	2.49	2.03	0.37	4.89

	FUD	Status	MUE	Modifiers				IOM Reference
57415	10	A	1(3)	51	N/A	N/A	80*	None

* with documentation

57420-57421

57420 Colposcopy of the entire vagina, with cervix if present;
57421   with biopsy(s) of vagina/cervix

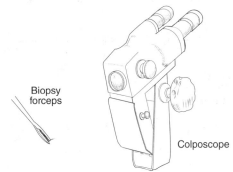

Biopsy forceps
Colposcope

The entire vagina and cervix (if present) are viewed by colposcopy

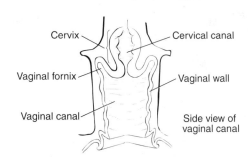

Cervix — Cervical canal
Vaginal fornix — Vaginal wall
Vaginal canal — Side view of vaginal canal

Explanation

The physician performs a colposcopy of the vagina and the cervix, if present. The patient is placed in the lithotomy position and a speculum is inserted into the vagina. The vagina is inspected through the colposcope, a binocular microscope providing direct, magnified visualization of the vagina and cervix. The physician examines the tissue for discharge, inflammation, ulceration, and lesions. The cervix is exposed, cleansed, and inspected for any ulceration or lesions. Acetic acid may be applied to help enhance visualization of the columnar villi and any lesions. In 57421, the area is examined and questionable tissue is removed from the vagina and/or cervix under direct visualization. The number and size of the biopsy(ies) is variable; multiple biopsies may be taken. Pressure is applied with a cotton swab as silver nitrate or other solution is applied with another applicator directly onto the biopsy site(s) for hemostasis. The instruments are removed.

Coding Tips

For colposcopy performed on the vulva, see 56820–56821; cervix and adjoining portion of upper vagina, see 57452. Report computer-aided mapping of cervix uteri at the time of colposcopy with 57465, when performed. Surgical trays, A4550, are not separately reimbursed by Medicare; however, other third-party payers may cover them. Check with the specific payer to determine coverage.

ICD-10-CM Diagnostic Codes

A56.02	Chlamydial vulvovaginitis ♀
A60.04	Herpesviral vulvovaginitis ♀
A63.0	Anogenital (venereal) warts
C51.8	Malignant neoplasm of overlapping sites of vulva ♀
C52	Malignant neoplasm of vagina ♀
C53.0	Malignant neoplasm of endocervix ♀
C53.1	Malignant neoplasm of exocervix ♀

Vagina

C53.8	Malignant neoplasm of overlapping sites of cervix uteri ♀
D06.0	Carcinoma in situ of endocervix ♀
D06.1	Carcinoma in situ of exocervix ♀
D06.7	Carcinoma in situ of other parts of cervix ♀
D07.2	Carcinoma in situ of vagina ♀
D26.0	Other benign neoplasm of cervix uteri ♀
D28.1	Benign neoplasm of vagina ♀
D39.0	Neoplasm of uncertain behavior of uterus ♀
D39.8	Neoplasm of uncertain behavior of other specified female genital organs ♀
D49.59	Neoplasm of unspecified behavior of other genitourinary organ
N72	Inflammatory disease of cervix uteri ♀
N75.0	Cyst of Bartholin's gland ♀
N75.1	Abscess of Bartholin's gland ♀
N75.8	Other diseases of Bartholin's gland ♀
N76.0	Acute vaginitis ♀
N76.1	Subacute and chronic vaginitis ♀
N76.5	Ulceration of vagina ♀
N76.81	Mucositis (ulcerative) of vagina and vulva ♀
N76.89	Other specified inflammation of vagina and vulva ♀
N80.4	Endometriosis of rectovaginal septum and vagina ♀
N84.1	Polyp of cervix uteri ♀
N84.2	Polyp of vagina ♀
N86	Erosion and ectropion of cervix uteri ♀
N87.0	Mild cervical dysplasia ♀
N87.1	Moderate cervical dysplasia ♀
N88.0	Leukoplakia of cervix uteri ♀
N88.1	Old laceration of cervix uteri ♀
N88.2	Stricture and stenosis of cervix uteri ♀
N88.3	Incompetence of cervix uteri ♀
N88.4	Hypertrophic elongation of cervix uteri ♀
N88.8	Other specified noninflammatory disorders of cervix uteri ♀
N89.0	Mild vaginal dysplasia ♀
N89.1	Moderate vaginal dysplasia ♀
N89.4	Leukoplakia of vagina ♀
N89.5	Stricture and atresia of vagina ♀
N89.7	Hematocolpos ♀
N89.8	Other specified noninflammatory disorders of vagina ♀
N92.4	Excessive bleeding in the premenopausal period ♀
N93.0	Postcoital and contact bleeding ♀
N93.1	Pre-pubertal vaginal bleeding ♀
N93.8	Other specified abnormal uterine and vaginal bleeding ♀
N94.2	Vaginismus ♀
N94.89	Other specified conditions associated with female genital organs and menstrual cycle ♀
N95.2	Postmenopausal atrophic vaginitis ♀
N99.2	Postprocedural adhesions of vagina ♀
Q51.6	Embryonic cyst of cervix ♀

AMA: **57420** 2019,Jul,6; 2018,Jan,8; 2017,Jan,8; 2016,Jan,13; 2015,Jan,16; 2014,Jan,11 **57421** 2019,Jul,6; 2018,Jan,8; 2017,Jan,8; 2016,Jan,13; 2015,Jan,16; 2014,Jan,11

Relative Value Units/Medicare Edits

Non-Facility RVU	Work	PE	MP	Total
57420	1.6	1.75	0.26	3.61
57421	2.2	2.31	0.35	4.86
Facility RVU	**Work**	**PE**	**MP**	**Total**
57420	1.6	0.76	0.26	2.62
57421	2.2	1.0	0.35	3.55

	FUD	Status	MUE	Modifiers				IOM Reference
57420	0	A	1(3)	51	N/A	N/A	N/A	None
57421	0	A	1(3)	51	N/A	N/A	N/A	

* with documentation

Terms To Know

biopsy. Tissue or fluid removed for diagnostic purposes through analysis of the cells in the biopsy material.

colposcopy. Procedure in which the physician views the cervix and vagina through a colposcope, which is a binocular microscope used for direct visualization of the vagina, ectocervix, and endocervix.

discharge. Secretion, flow, or evacuation.

hemostasis. Interruption of blood flow or the cessation or arrest of bleeding.

inflammation. Cytologic and chemical reactions that occur in affected blood vessels and adjacent tissues in response to injury or abnormal stimulation from a physical, chemical, or biologic agent.

lithotomy position. Common position patients may be placed in for some surgical procedures and examinations involving the pelvis and/or lower abdomen. The patient is placed supine (on their back), hips and knees flexed, thighs apart, with feet supported in raised stirrups.

ulceration. Destruction of epithelial tissue associated with the loss of surface tissue.

Vagina

57423

57423 Paravaginal defect repair (including repair of cystocele, if performed), laparoscopic approach

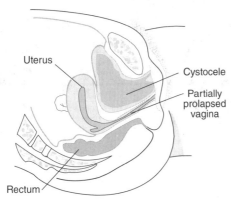

Uterus
Cystocele
Partially prolapsed vagina
Rectum

The physician repairs paravaginal defects

Explanation

The physician performs laparoscopic repair of a paravaginal defect, in which there is loss of the lateral vaginal attachment to the pelvic sidewall. Through small stab incisions in the abdomen, a fiberoptic laparoscope and trocars are inserted into the abdominal/pelvic space and the abdomen is insufflated. The bladder may be filled with sterile water to allow the surgeon to identify the superior border of the bladder's edge and then drained to prevent injury after the space of Retzius has been entered and the pubic ramus visualized. Following identification of the defect, the surgeon inserts the nondominant hand into the vagina in order to elevate the anterior vaginal wall and pubocervical fascia to their normal positions. Nonabsorbable sutures with attached needles are introduced through the laparoscopy port and grasped using a laparoscopic needle driver. A series of four to six sutures are placed and tied sequentially along the defects from the ischial spine toward the urethra. The procedure is repeated on the opposite side if a bilateral defect is present. The paravaginal defect repair may be performed alone or in conjunction with cystocele repair, in which a herniation of the bladder through its support tissues into the anterior vaginal wall causes it to bulge downward. These procedures help restore the normal anatomic relationships of the urethra, bladder, and vagina. At completion of the procedure, laparoscopic tools are removed, excess gas expelled, and fascial defects and skin edges are sutured.

Coding Tips

If only one of the components of this procedure is performed, see other codes in this section of CPT. For example, if repair of cystocele with anterior colporrhaphy is performed by itself, report 57240. For a Marshall-Marchetti-Krantz urethral suspension, abdominal approach, see 51840 and 51841. For laparoscopic repair of stress incontinence, see 51990 and 51992. For sling operation for stress incontinence, see 57288. Do not report 57423 with 49320, 51840-51841, 51990, 57240, 57260, 58152, or 58267.

ICD-10-CM Diagnostic Codes

N81.0	Urethrocele ♀
N81.11	Cystocele, midline ♀
N81.12	Cystocele, lateral ♀
N81.2	Incomplete uterovaginal prolapse ♀
N81.3	Complete uterovaginal prolapse ♀
N81.6	Rectocele ♀
N81.81	Perineocele ♀
N81.83	Incompetence or weakening of rectovaginal tissue ♀
N81.85	Cervical stump prolapse ♀
N81.89	Other female genital prolapse ♀
N99.3	Prolapse of vaginal vault after hysterectomy ♀

AMA: 57423 2019,Jul,6; 2018,Jan,8; 2017,Jan,8; 2016,Jan,13; 2015,Jan,16; 2014,Jan,11

Relative Value Units/Medicare Edits

Non-Facility RVU	Work	PE	MP	Total
57423	16.08	8.33	2.42	26.83
Facility RVU	**Work**	**PE**	**MP**	**Total**
57423	16.08	8.33	2.42	26.83

	FUD	Status	MUE	Modifiers				IOM Reference
57423	90	A	1(2)	51	N/A	62	80	None

* with documentation

Terms To Know

approach. Method or anatomical location used to gain access to a body organ or specific area for procedures.

cystocele, lateral. Detachment of the lateral support connections of the vagina at the arcus tendineus fasciae pelvis (ATFP) that results in bladder drop. The bladder herniates into the vagina laterally.

defect. Imperfection, flaw, or absence.

insufflation. Blowing air or gas into a body cavity.

midline cystocele. Form of hernia of the vagina in which a weakness in the midline supporting tissue between the bladder and vagina allows the bladder to protrude into the vaginal wall (central defect) with anterior disruption or bulging of the vagina.

repair. Surgical closure of a wound. The wound may be a result of injury/trauma or it may be a surgically created defect. Repairs are divided into three categories: simple, intermediate, and complex.

uterovaginal prolapse. Uterus displaced downward and exposed in the external genitalia.

Vagina

57425

57425　Laparoscopy, surgical, colpopexy (suspension of vaginal apex)

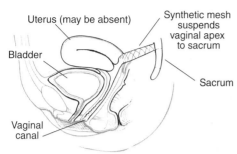

The top of the vagina is surgically suspended, often from tissues surrounding the sacrum

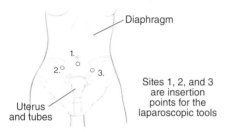

Sites 1, 2, and 3 are insertion points for the laparoscopic tools

Explanation

The physician performs a laparoscopic colpopexy and suspends or reattaches the apex of the vagina to the uterosacral ligaments to correct a uterovaginal prolapse and restore the vaginal apex to its normal anatomic position, often post-hysterectomy. Through small stab incisions in the abdomen, a fiberoptic laparoscope and trocars are inserted into the abdominal/pelvic space. The bowel is mobilized or moved aside to provide a better view and easier access to the uterosacral ligaments. A vaginal probe is placed for manipulation and to help ensure the cul-de-sac is properly closed. The peritoneum is incised over the vaginal apex. After the vaginal vault is elevated into its normal position, and the cul-de-sac is obliterated, if necessary, a suture is placed through the base of the right uterosacral ligament and through the apex of the vagina-securing it posteriorly to the top of the rectovaginal fascia and anteriorly to the pubocervical fascia (to a dermal or mesh graft, if placed) and secured. Four total sutures are used to elevate the vagina, this being done twice through each ligament and the vaginal apex on each side.

Coding Tips

A surgical laparoscopy always includes a diagnostic laparoscopy; the diagnostic laparoscopy should not be reported separately. For open colpopexy by abdominal approach, see 57280. For colposcopic diagnostic visualization of the vagina, see 57420.

ICD-10-CM Diagnostic Codes

N81.2	Incomplete uterovaginal prolapse ♀
N81.3	Complete uterovaginal prolapse ♀
N99.3	Prolapse of vaginal vault after hysterectomy ♀

AMA: **57425** 2019,Jul,6; 2014,Jan,11

Relative Value Units/Medicare Edits

Non-Facility RVU	Work	PE	MP	Total
57425	17.03	8.8	2.48	28.31
Facility RVU	**Work**	**PE**	**MP**	**Total**
57425	17.03	8.8	2.48	28.31

	FUD	Status	MUE	Modifiers			IOM Reference
57425	90	A	1(2)	51	N/A	62*	80	None

* with documentation

Terms To Know

apex. Highest point of a root end of a tooth, or the end of any organ.

colpopexy. Suturing a prolapsed vagina to its surrounding structures for vaginal fixation.

fascia. Fibrous sheet or band of tissue that envelops organs, muscles, and groupings of muscles.

female stress incontinence. Involuntary escape of urine at times of minor stress against the female bladder, such as coughing, sneezing, or laughing.

laparoscopic. Minimally invasive procedure used for intraabdominal inspection; surgery that uses an endoscopic instrument inserted through small access incisions into the peritoneum for video-controlled imaging.

suspension. Fixation of an organ for support; temporary state of cessation of an activity, process, or experience.

trocar. Cannula or a sharp pointed instrument used to puncture and aspirate fluid from cavities.

uterovaginal prolapse. Uterus displaced downward and exposed in the external genitalia.

Vagina

57426

57426 Revision (including removal) of prosthetic vaginal graft, laparoscopic approach

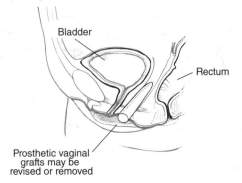

Prosthetic vaginal grafts may be revised or removed

Explanation

The physician revises or removes a previously placed prosthetic vaginal graft via a laparoscopic approach. Through small stab incisions in the umbilicus and/or abdomen, a fiberoptic laparoscope and trocars are inserted into the peritoneal cavity. Depending upon the type of complication (e.g., mesh erosion into the bladder or persistent vaginal/pelvic pain), the vaginal graft may be completely or partially excised to remove eroding mesh or revisions may be made in the graft and surrounding tissue.

Coding Tips

For revision, including removal, of a prosthetic vaginal graft, vaginal approach, see 57295; abdominal approach, see 57296.

ICD-10-CM Diagnostic Codes

T83.418A	Breakdown (mechanical) of other prosthetic devices, implants and grafts of genital tract, initial encounter
T83.428A	Displacement of other prosthetic devices, implants and grafts of genital tract, initial encounter
T83.498A	Other mechanical complication of other prosthetic devices, implants and grafts of genital tract, initial encounter
T83.711A	Erosion of implanted vaginal mesh to surrounding organ or tissue, initial encounter ♀
T83.721A	Exposure of implanted vaginal mesh into vagina, initial encounter ♀
T83.81XA	Embolism due to genitourinary prosthetic devices, implants and grafts, initial encounter
T83.82XA	Fibrosis due to genitourinary prosthetic devices, implants and grafts, initial encounter
T83.83XA	Hemorrhage due to genitourinary prosthetic devices, implants and grafts, initial encounter
T83.84XA	Pain due to genitourinary prosthetic devices, implants and grafts, initial encounter
T83.85XA	Stenosis due to genitourinary prosthetic devices, implants and grafts, initial encounter
T83.86XA	Thrombosis due to genitourinary prosthetic devices, implants and grafts, initial encounter
T83.89XA	Other specified complication of genitourinary prosthetic devices, implants and grafts, initial encounter

AMA: **57426** 2019,Jul,6; 2014,Jan,11

Relative Value Units/Medicare Edits

Non-Facility RVU	Work	PE	MP	Total
57426	14.3	8.47	2.1	24.87
Facility RVU	**Work**	**PE**	**MP**	**Total**
57426	14.3	8.47	2.1	24.87

	FUD	Status	MUE	Modifiers				IOM Reference
57426	90	A	1(2)	51	N/A	62*	80	None

* with documentation

Terms To Know

approach. Method or anatomical location used to gain access to a body organ or specific area for procedures. The approach is not coded separately although it may be a specified component of the procedure, such as laparoscopic versus incisional, or spinal procedures in which the amount of dissection required to expose the spine significantly alters with the site of approach.

graft. Tissue implant from another part of the body or another person.

prosthesis. Device that replaces all or part of an internal body organ or replaces all or part of the function of a permanently inoperative or malfunctioning internal body organ.

revision. Reordering or rearrangement of tissue to suit a particular need or function.

N Newborn: 0   **P** Pediatric: 0-17   **M** Maternity: 9-64   **A** Adult: 15-124   ♂ Male Only   ♀ Female Only

Coding Companion for Ob/Gyn

Vagina

57452

57452 Colposcopy of the cervix including upper/adjacent vagina;

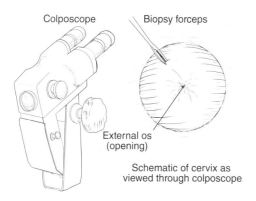

Colposcope

Biopsy forceps

External os (opening)

Schematic of cervix as viewed through colposcope

Explanation

The physician inserts a speculum into the vagina to fully expose and examine the cervix to identify abnormal cells. The upper/adjacent portion of the vagina is examined through a colposcope and a binocular microscope is used for direct visualization of the vagina, ectocervix, and endocervix. This procedure is usually performed when the patient has had an abnormal Pap test. The physician swabs the vaginal walls and cervix with vinegar, iodine, or another type of solution to remove mucus and highlight abnormal cells by turning them white, making them more easily identifiable for possible biopsy. The solution may cause a slight tingling or burning sensation.

Coding Tips

Do not report 57452 in addition to 57454-57461. For colposcopy with biopsy and endocervical curettage, see 57454; biopsy, see 57455; with endocervical curettage, see 57456; with loop electrode biopsy(s) of the cervix, see 57460; with loop electrode conization of the cervix, see 57461. For colposcopic procedures on the vulva, see 56820–56821; on the vagina, see 57420–57421.

ICD-10-CM Diagnostic Codes

A56.02	Chlamydial vulvovaginitis ♀
A60.04	Herpesviral vulvovaginitis ♀
A63.0	Anogenital (venereal) warts
C52	Malignant neoplasm of vagina ♀
C53.0	Malignant neoplasm of endocervix ♀
C53.1	Malignant neoplasm of exocervix ♀
C53.8	Malignant neoplasm of overlapping sites of cervix uteri ♀
C54.0	Malignant neoplasm of isthmus uteri ♀
C54.1	Malignant neoplasm of endometrium ♀
C54.2	Malignant neoplasm of myometrium ♀
C54.3	Malignant neoplasm of fundus uteri ♀
C54.8	Malignant neoplasm of overlapping sites of corpus uteri ♀
D06.0	Carcinoma in situ of endocervix ♀
D06.1	Carcinoma in situ of exocervix ♀
D06.7	Carcinoma in situ of other parts of cervix ♀
D07.1	Carcinoma in situ of vulva ♀
D07.2	Carcinoma in situ of vagina ♀
D26.0	Other benign neoplasm of cervix uteri ♀
D28.1	Benign neoplasm of vagina ♀
D39.0	Neoplasm of uncertain behavior of uterus ♀
D39.8	Neoplasm of uncertain behavior of other specified female genital organs ♀

D49.59	Neoplasm of unspecified behavior of other genitourinary organ
N72	Inflammatory disease of cervix uteri ♀
N75.0	Cyst of Bartholin's gland ♀
N75.1	Abscess of Bartholin's gland ♀
N75.8	Other diseases of Bartholin's gland ♀
N76.0	Acute vaginitis ♀
N76.1	Subacute and chronic vaginitis ♀
N76.5	Ulceration of vagina ♀
N76.81	Mucositis (ulcerative) of vagina and vulva ♀
N76.89	Other specified inflammation of vagina and vulva ♀
N80.4	Endometriosis of rectovaginal septum and vagina ♀
N84.1	Polyp of cervix uteri ♀
N84.2	Polyp of vagina ♀
N86	Erosion and ectropion of cervix uteri ♀
N87.0	Mild cervical dysplasia ♀
N87.1	Moderate cervical dysplasia ♀
N88.0	Leukoplakia of cervix uteri ♀
N88.1	Old laceration of cervix uteri ♀
N88.2	Stricture and stenosis of cervix uteri ♀
N88.3	Incompetence of cervix uteri ♀
N88.4	Hypertrophic elongation of cervix uteri ♀
N88.8	Other specified noninflammatory disorders of cervix uteri ♀
N89.0	Mild vaginal dysplasia ♀
N89.1	Moderate vaginal dysplasia ♀
N89.4	Leukoplakia of vagina ♀
N89.5	Stricture and atresia of vagina ♀
N89.7	Hematocolpos ♀
N89.8	Other specified noninflammatory disorders of vagina ♀
N92.4	Excessive bleeding in the premenopausal period ♀
N93.0	Postcoital and contact bleeding ♀
N93.1	Pre-pubertal vaginal bleeding ♀
N93.8	Other specified abnormal uterine and vaginal bleeding ♀
N94.2	Vaginismus ♀
N94.89	Other specified conditions associated with female genital organs and menstrual cycle ♀
N95.0	Postmenopausal bleeding ♀
N95.2	Postmenopausal atrophic vaginitis ♀
N99.2	Postprocedural adhesions of vagina ♀
Q51.6	Embryonic cyst of cervix ♀
Z12.4	Encounter for screening for malignant neoplasm of cervix ♀

AMA: 57452 2019,Jul,6; 2018,Jan,8; 2017,Jan,8; 2016,Jan,13; 2015,Jan,16; 2014,Jan,11

Relative Value Units/Medicare Edits

Non-Facility RVU	Work	PE	MP	Total
57452	1.5	1.71	0.24	3.45
Facility RVU	**Work**	**PE**	**MP**	**Total**
57452	1.5	0.9	0.24	2.64

	FUD	Status	MUE	Modifiers				IOM Reference
57452	0	A	1(3)	51	N/A	N/A	N/A	None

* with documentation

Cervix Uteri

57454-57456

57454 Colposcopy of the cervix including upper/adjacent vagina; with biopsy(s) of the cervix and endocervical curettage
57455 with biopsy(s) of the cervix
57456 with endocervical curettage

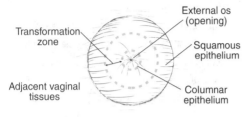

Schematic of cervix as viewed through colposcope

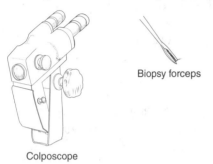

Colposcope

Explanation

The physician inserts a speculum into the vagina to fully expose and examine the cervix to identify abnormal cells. The upper/adjacent portion of the vagina is examined through a colposcope and a binocular microscope is used for direct visualization of the vagina, ectocervix, and endocervix. The physician swabs the vaginal walls and cervix with vinegar, iodine, or another type of solution to remove mucus and highlight abnormal cells by turning them white, making them more easily identifiable for biopsy. In 57455, the physician biopsies the cervix by inserting an instrument into the vagina and removing one or more small tissue samples. In 57456, endocervical curettage is performed by passing a small curette into the endocervical canal, the passage between the external cervical os and the uterine cavity. A specimen is obtained by scraping in the canal with the curette. In 57454, the physician performs biopsy and endocervical curettage procedures. The instrument is removed.

Coding Tips

For colposcopy performed on the vulva, see 56820–56821; on the vagina, see 57420–57421. For colposcopy with loop electrode biopsy(s) of the cervix, see 57460; with loop electrode conization of the cervix, see 57461. Endometrial biopsy performed at the same time as a colposcopy is reported with 58110. Do not report 57454-57456 with 57452.

ICD-10-CM Diagnostic Codes

A56.02	Chlamydial vulvovaginitis ♀
A60.04	Herpesviral vulvovaginitis ♀
A63.0	Anogenital (venereal) warts
C52	Malignant neoplasm of vagina ♀
C53.0	Malignant neoplasm of endocervix ♀
C53.1	Malignant neoplasm of exocervix ♀
C53.8	Malignant neoplasm of overlapping sites of cervix uteri ♀
C54.0	Malignant neoplasm of isthmus uteri ♀
C54.1	Malignant neoplasm of endometrium ♀
C54.2	Malignant neoplasm of myometrium ♀
C54.3	Malignant neoplasm of fundus uteri ♀
C54.8	Malignant neoplasm of overlapping sites of corpus uteri ♀
D06.0	Carcinoma in situ of endocervix ♀
D06.1	Carcinoma in situ of exocervix ♀
D06.7	Carcinoma in situ of other parts of cervix ♀
D07.1	Carcinoma in situ of vulva ♀
D07.2	Carcinoma in situ of vagina ♀
D26.0	Other benign neoplasm of cervix uteri ♀
D28.1	Benign neoplasm of vagina ♀
D39.0	Neoplasm of uncertain behavior of uterus ♀
D39.8	Neoplasm of uncertain behavior of other specified female genital organs ♀
N72	Inflammatory disease of cervix uteri ♀
N75.0	Cyst of Bartholin's gland ♀
N75.1	Abscess of Bartholin's gland ♀
N75.8	Other diseases of Bartholin's gland ♀
N76.0	Acute vaginitis ♀
N76.1	Subacute and chronic vaginitis ♀
N76.5	Ulceration of vagina ♀
N76.81	Mucositis (ulcerative) of vagina and vulva ♀
N76.89	Other specified inflammation of vagina and vulva ♀
N80.4	Endometriosis of rectovaginal septum and vagina ♀
N84.1	Polyp of cervix uteri ♀
N84.2	Polyp of vagina ♀
N86	Erosion and ectropion of cervix uteri ♀
N87.0	Mild cervical dysplasia ♀
N87.1	Moderate cervical dysplasia ♀
N88.0	Leukoplakia of cervix uteri ♀
N88.1	Old laceration of cervix uteri ♀
N88.2	Stricture and stenosis of cervix uteri ♀
N88.3	Incompetence of cervix uteri ♀
N88.4	Hypertrophic elongation of cervix uteri ♀
N88.8	Other specified noninflammatory disorders of cervix uteri ♀
N89.0	Mild vaginal dysplasia ♀
N89.1	Moderate vaginal dysplasia ♀
N89.4	Leukoplakia of vagina ♀
N89.5	Stricture and atresia of vagina ♀
N89.7	Hematocolpos ♀
N89.8	Other specified noninflammatory disorders of vagina ♀
N92.4	Excessive bleeding in the premenopausal period ♀
N93.0	Postcoital and contact bleeding ♀
N93.1	Pre-pubertal vaginal bleeding ♀
N93.8	Other specified abnormal uterine and vaginal bleeding ♀
N94.2	Vaginismus ♀
N94.89	Other specified conditions associated with female genital organs and menstrual cycle ♀
N95.0	Postmenopausal bleeding ♀
N95.2	Postmenopausal atrophic vaginitis ♀
N99.2	Postprocedural adhesions of vagina ♀
Q51.6	Embryonic cyst of cervix ♀
Z12.4	Encounter for screening for malignant neoplasm of cervix ♀

Cervix Uteri

AMA: **57454** 2019,Jul,6; 2018,Jan,8; 2017,Jan,8; 2016,Jan,13; 2015,Jan,16; 2014,Jan,11 **57455** 2019,Jul,6; 2018,Jan,8; 2017,Jan,8; 2016,Jan,13; 2015,Jan,16; 2014,Jan,11 **57456** 2019,Jul,6; 2018,Jan,8; 2017,Jan,8; 2016,Jan,13; 2015,Jan,16; 2014,Jan,11

Relative Value Units/Medicare Edits

Non-Facility RVU	Work	PE	MP	Total
57454	2.33	2.01	0.37	4.71
57455	1.99	2.14	0.31	4.44
57456	1.85	2.04	0.28	4.17
Facility RVU	**Work**	**PE**	**MP**	**Total**
57454	2.33	1.19	0.37	3.89
57455	1.99	0.89	0.31	3.19
57456	1.85	0.82	0.28	2.95

	FUD	Status	MUE	Modifiers				IOM Reference
57454	0	A	1(3)	51	N/A	N/A	N/A	None
57455	0	A	1(3)	51	N/A	N/A	N/A	
57456	0	A	1(3)	51	N/A	N/A	N/A	

* with documentation

Terms To Know

biopsy. Tissue or fluid removed for diagnostic purposes through analysis of the cells in the biopsy material.

curettage. Removal of tissue by scraping.

dysplasia. Abnormality or alteration in the size, shape, and organization of cells from their normal pattern of development.

leukoplakia. Thickened white patches or lesions appearing on a mucous membrane, such as oral mucosa or tongue.

ulceration. Destruction of epithelial tissue associated with the loss of surface tissue.

57460

57460	Colposcopy of the cervix including upper/adjacent vagina; with loop electrode biopsy(s) of the cervix

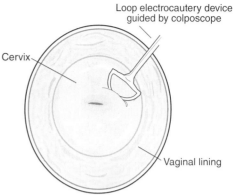

The cervix is examined by colposcopy and a biopsy specimen is collected by loop electrode.

Explanation

The physician inserts a speculum into the vagina to fully expose and examine the cervix to identify abnormal cells. The upper/adjacent portion of the vagina is examined through a colposcope and a binocular microscope is used for direct visualization of the vagina, ectocervix, and endocervix. The physician swabs the vaginal walls and cervix with vinegar or another type of solution (acetic acid) to remove mucus and highlight abnormal cells by turning them white, making them more easily identifiable for possible biopsy. Sometimes a Schiller test, iodine solution used to coat the cervix, is performed. The solution may cause a slight tingling or burning sensation. Local anesthesia may be used to numb the area. A biopsy specimen of cervical tissue is removed by the loop electrode excision procedure (LEEP). LEEP uses a thin wire loop carrying an electrical cutting current that acts as a cutting instrument to remove abnormal cells. Due to the electrical current, a grounding pad is attached to the patient's leg during the procedure. The physician may apply Monsel's solution, a special type of paste that helps to seal blood vessels to prevent bleeding.

Coding Tips

When 57460 is performed with another separately identifiable procedure, the highest dollar value code is listed as the primary procedure and subsequent procedures are appended with modifier 51. For cauterization of the cervix, see 57510–57513. If conization of the cervix is performed, see 57520–57522. For loop electrode conization of the cervix by colposcopy, report 57461. Local anesthesia is included in the service. However, this procedure may be performed under general anesthesia, depending on the age and/or condition of the patient.

ICD-10-CM Diagnostic Codes

A56.02	Chlamydial vulvovaginitis ♀
A60.04	Herpesviral vulvovaginitis ♀
A63.0	Anogenital (venereal) warts
C52	Malignant neoplasm of vagina ♀
C53.0	Malignant neoplasm of endocervix ♀
C53.1	Malignant neoplasm of exocervix ♀
C53.8	Malignant neoplasm of overlapping sites of cervix uteri ♀
C54.0	Malignant neoplasm of isthmus uteri ♀
C54.1	Malignant neoplasm of endometrium ♀

Cervix Uteri

C54.2	Malignant neoplasm of myometrium ♀
C54.3	Malignant neoplasm of fundus uteri ♀
C54.8	Malignant neoplasm of overlapping sites of corpus uteri ♀
D06.0	Carcinoma in situ of endocervix ♀
D06.1	Carcinoma in situ of exocervix ♀
D06.7	Carcinoma in situ of other parts of cervix ♀
D07.1	Carcinoma in situ of vulva ♀
D07.2	Carcinoma in situ of vagina ♀
D26.0	Other benign neoplasm of cervix uteri ♀
D28.1	Benign neoplasm of vagina ♀
D39.0	Neoplasm of uncertain behavior of uterus ♀
D39.8	Neoplasm of uncertain behavior of other specified female genital organs ♀
D49.59	Neoplasm of unspecified behavior of other genitourinary organ
N72	Inflammatory disease of cervix uteri ♀
N75.0	Cyst of Bartholin's gland ♀
N75.1	Abscess of Bartholin's gland ♀
N75.8	Other diseases of Bartholin's gland ♀
N76.0	Acute vaginitis ♀
N76.1	Subacute and chronic vaginitis ♀
N76.5	Ulceration of vagina ♀
N76.81	Mucositis (ulcerative) of vagina and vulva ♀
N76.89	Other specified inflammation of vagina and vulva ♀
N80.4	Endometriosis of rectovaginal septum and vagina ♀
N84.1	Polyp of cervix uteri ♀
N84.2	Polyp of vagina ♀
N86	Erosion and ectropion of cervix uteri ♀
N87.0	Mild cervical dysplasia ♀
N87.1	Moderate cervical dysplasia ♀
N88.0	Leukoplakia of cervix uteri ♀
N88.1	Old laceration of cervix uteri ♀
N88.2	Stricture and stenosis of cervix uteri ♀
N88.3	Incompetence of cervix uteri ♀
N88.4	Hypertrophic elongation of cervix uteri ♀
N88.8	Other specified noninflammatory disorders of cervix uteri ♀
N89.0	Mild vaginal dysplasia ♀
N89.1	Moderate vaginal dysplasia ♀
N89.4	Leukoplakia of vagina ♀
N89.5	Stricture and atresia of vagina ♀
N89.7	Hematocolpos ♀
N89.8	Other specified noninflammatory disorders of vagina ♀
N92.4	Excessive bleeding in the premenopausal period ♀
N93.0	Postcoital and contact bleeding ♀
N93.1	Pre-pubertal vaginal bleeding ♀
N93.8	Other specified abnormal uterine and vaginal bleeding ♀
N94.2	Vaginismus ♀
N94.89	Other specified conditions associated with female genital organs and menstrual cycle ♀
N95.0	Postmenopausal bleeding ♀
N95.2	Postmenopausal atrophic vaginitis ♀
N99.2	Postprocedural adhesions of vagina ♀
Q51.6	Embryonic cyst of cervix ♀
Z12.4	Encounter for screening for malignant neoplasm of cervix ♀

AMA: **57460** 2019,Jul,6; 2018,Jan,8; 2017,Jan,8; 2016,Jan,13; 2015,Jan,16; 2014,Jan,11

Relative Value Units/Medicare Edits

Non-Facility RVU	Work	PE	MP	Total
57460	2.83	5.51	0.44	8.78
Facility RVU	**Work**	**PE**	**MP**	**Total**
57460	2.83	1.39	0.44	4.66

	FUD	Status	MUE	Modifiers				IOM Reference
57460	0	A	1(3)	51	N/A	N/A	N/A	None

* with documentation

Terms To Know

biopsy. Tissue or fluid removed for diagnostic purposes through analysis of the cells in the biopsy material.

LEEP. Loop electrode excision procedure. Biopsy specimen or cone shaped wedge of cervical tissue is removed using a hot cautery wire loop with an electrical current running through it.

malignant neoplasm. Any cancerous tumor or lesion exhibiting uncontrolled tissue growth that can progressively invade other parts of the body with its disease-generating cells.

microsurgery. Surgical procedures performed under magnification using a surgical microscope.

specimen. Tissue cells or sample of fluid taken for analysis, pathologic examination, and diagnosis.

Cervix Uteri

57461

57461 Colposcopy of the cervix including upper/adjacent vagina; with loop electrode conization of the cervix

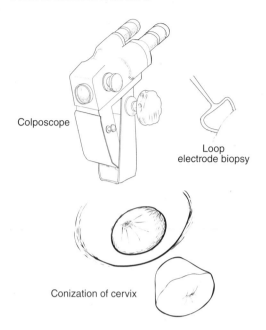

Colposcope

Loop electrode biopsy

Conization of cervix

Explanation

The physician inserts a speculum into the vagina to fully expose and examine the cervix to identify abnormal cells. The upper/adjacent portion of the vagina is examined through a colposcope and a binocular microscope is used for direct visualization of the vagina, ectocervix, and endocervix. The physician swabs the vaginal walls and cervix with vinegar or another type solution (acetic acid) to remove mucus and highlight abnormal cells by turning them white, making them more easily identifiable for possible biopsy. Sometimes a Schiller test, iodine solution used to coat the cervix, is performed. The solution may cause a slight tingling or burning sensation. Local anesthesia may be used to numb the area. LEEP uses a thin wire loop carrying an electrical cutting current that acts as a cutting instrument to remove abnormal cells. Due to the electrical current, a grounding pad is attached to the patient's leg during the procedure. The cutting current is set. Using the loop, the lesion and transformation zone (the boundary of the excision to assure complete removal of the dysplasia) is removed as one specimen. If the lesion is large and another pass is required, two equal specimens are removed and labeled for the axis of orientation. The same procedure is done again with a smaller loop if an endocervical excision is necessary. The physician may apply Monsel's solution, a special type of paste that helps to seal blood vessels to prevent bleeding or bleeding vessels are cauterized. The vagina is inspected for any accidental injury and the instruments are removed.

Coding Tips

For colposcopy performed on the vulva, see 56820–56821; on the vagina, see 57420–57421. For colposcopy of the cervix with a biopsy of the cervix and endocervical curettage, see 57454. For a loop electrode biopsy of the cervix by colposcopy, see 57460. Do not report 57461 with 57456. For endometrial biopsy performed with colposcopy, see 58110.

ICD-10-CM Diagnostic Codes

A56.02	Chlamydial vulvovaginitis ♀
A60.04	Herpesviral vulvovaginitis ♀
A63.0	Anogenital (venereal) warts
C52	Malignant neoplasm of vagina ♀
C53.0	Malignant neoplasm of endocervix ♀
C53.1	Malignant neoplasm of exocervix ♀
C53.8	Malignant neoplasm of overlapping sites of cervix uteri ♀
C54.0	Malignant neoplasm of isthmus uteri ♀
C54.1	Malignant neoplasm of endometrium ♀
C54.2	Malignant neoplasm of myometrium ♀
C54.3	Malignant neoplasm of fundus uteri ♀
C54.8	Malignant neoplasm of overlapping sites of corpus uteri ♀
D06.0	Carcinoma in situ of endocervix ♀
D06.1	Carcinoma in situ of exocervix ♀
D06.7	Carcinoma in situ of other parts of cervix ♀
D07.1	Carcinoma in situ of vulva ♀
D07.2	Carcinoma in situ of vagina ♀
D26.0	Other benign neoplasm of cervix uteri ♀
D28.1	Benign neoplasm of vagina ♀
D39.0	Neoplasm of uncertain behavior of uterus ♀
D39.8	Neoplasm of uncertain behavior of other specified female genital organs ♀
D49.59	Neoplasm of unspecified behavior of other genitourinary organ
N72	Inflammatory disease of cervix uteri ♀
N75.0	Cyst of Bartholin's gland ♀
N75.1	Abscess of Bartholin's gland ♀
N75.8	Other diseases of Bartholin's gland ♀
N76.0	Acute vaginitis ♀
N76.1	Subacute and chronic vaginitis ♀
N76.5	Ulceration of vagina ♀
N76.81	Mucositis (ulcerative) of vagina and vulva ♀
N76.89	Other specified inflammation of vagina and vulva ♀
N80.4	Endometriosis of rectovaginal septum and vagina ♀
N84.1	Polyp of cervix uteri ♀
N84.2	Polyp of vagina ♀
N86	Erosion and ectropion of cervix uteri ♀
N87.0	Mild cervical dysplasia ♀
N87.1	Moderate cervical dysplasia ♀
N88.0	Leukoplakia of cervix uteri ♀
N88.1	Old laceration of cervix uteri ♀
N88.2	Stricture and stenosis of cervix uteri ♀
N88.3	Incompetence of cervix uteri ♀
N88.4	Hypertrophic elongation of cervix uteri ♀
N88.8	Other specified noninflammatory disorders of cervix uteri ♀
N89.0	Mild vaginal dysplasia ♀
N89.1	Moderate vaginal dysplasia ♀
N89.4	Leukoplakia of vagina ♀
N89.5	Stricture and atresia of vagina ♀
N89.7	Hematocolpos ♀
N89.8	Other specified noninflammatory disorders of vagina ♀
N92.4	Excessive bleeding in the premenopausal period ♀
N93.0	Postcoital and contact bleeding ♀
N93.1	Pre-pubertal vaginal bleeding ♀
N93.8	Other specified abnormal uterine and vaginal bleeding ♀
N94.2	Vaginismus ♀

N94.89	Other specified conditions associated with female genital organs and menstrual cycle ♀
N95.0	Postmenopausal bleeding ♀
N95.2	Postmenopausal atrophic vaginitis ♀
N99.2	Postprocedural adhesions of vagina ♀
Q51.6	Embryonic cyst of cervix ♀
Z12.4	Encounter for screening for malignant neoplasm of cervix ♀

AMA: 57461 2019,Jul,6; 2018,Jan,8; 2017,Jan,8; 2016,Jan,13; 2015,Jan,16; 2014,Jan,11

Relative Value Units/Medicare Edits

Non-Facility RVU	Work	PE	MP	Total
57461	3.43	5.88	0.54	9.85
Facility RVU	**Work**	**PE**	**MP**	**Total**
57461	3.43	1.42	0.54	5.39

	FUD	Status	MUE	Modifiers				IOM Reference
57461	0	A	1(3)	51	N/A	N/A	N/A	None

* with documentation

Terms To Know

cauterization. Tissue destruction by means of a hot instrument, an electric current, or a caustic chemical.

LEEP. Loop electrode excision procedure. Biopsy specimen or cone shaped wedge of cervical tissue is removed using a hot cautery wire loop with an electrical current running through it.

lesion. Area of damaged tissue that has lost continuity or function, due to disease or trauma.

microsurgery. Surgical procedures performed under magnification using a surgical microscope.

57465

+● **57465** Computer-aided mapping of cervix uteri during colposcopy, including optical dynamic spectral imaging and algorithmic quantification of the acetowhitening effect (List separately in addition to code for primary procedure)

Explanation

The physician performs computer-aided mapping of the cervix uteri during colposcopy, which is reported separately. Colposcopy includes the application of an acetic acid solution to differentiate between normal and abnormal tissue. This reaction, known as acetowhitening, produces a perceptible variance when compared to the normal pinkish color of the surrounding epithelia found in the cervix. By measuring the reaction of the cervical epithelium using proprietary dynamic spectral imaging (DSI), identification of cervical disease may be aided by highlighting suspicious areas, providing more accurate biopsy site selection, and ensuring a more accurate diagnosis.

Coding Tips

Report 57465 in addition to 57420-57421 and 57452-57461.

ICD-10-CM Diagnostic Codes

This/these CPT code(s) are add-on code(s). See the primary procedure code that this code is performed with for your ICD-10-CM code selections.

Relative Value Units/Medicare Edits

Non-Facility RVU	Work	PE	MP	Total
57465				
Facility RVU	**Work**	**PE**	**MP**	**Total**
57465				

	FUD	Status	MUE	Modifiers				IOM Reference
57465	N/A		-	N/A	N/A	N/A	N/A	None

* with documentation

Terms To Know

biopsy. Tissue or fluid removed for diagnostic purposes through analysis of the cells in the biopsy material.

colposcopy. Procedure in which the physician views the cervix and vagina through a colposcope, which is a binocular microscope used for direct visualization of the vagina, ectocervix, and endocervix.

epithelial tissue. Cells arranged in sheets that cover internal and external body surfaces that can absorb, protect, and/or secrete and includes the protective covering for external surfaces (skin), absorptive linings for internal surfaces such as the intestine, and secreting structures such as salivary or sweat glands.

57500

57500 Biopsy of cervix, single or multiple, or local excision of lesion, with or without fulguration (separate procedure)

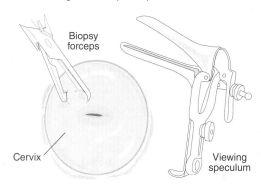

Explanation

The physician inserts a speculum into the vagina to view the cervix. A small cut is made in the cervix and biopsy forceps are used to remove a piece or multiple pieces of tissue, or to completely remove a lesion. Bleeding, usually minimal, may be stopped by electric current (fulguration).

Coding Tips

This separate procedure by definition is usually a component of a more complex service and is not identified separately. When performed alone or with other unrelated procedures/services it may be reported. If performed alone, list the code; if performed with other procedures/services, list the code and append modifier 59 or an X{EPSU} modifier. When 57500 is performed with another separately identifiable procedure, the highest dollar value code is listed as the primary procedure and subsequent procedures are appended with modifier 51. Local anesthesia is included in the service. However, this procedure may be performed under general anesthesia, depending on the age and/or condition of the patient.

ICD-10-CM Diagnostic Codes

A63.0	Anogenital (venereal) warts
C53.0	Malignant neoplasm of endocervix ♀
C53.1	Malignant neoplasm of exocervix ♀
C53.8	Malignant neoplasm of overlapping sites of cervix uteri ♀
D06.0	Carcinoma in situ of endocervix ♀
D06.1	Carcinoma in situ of exocervix ♀
D06.7	Carcinoma in situ of other parts of cervix ♀
D26.0	Other benign neoplasm of cervix uteri ♀
D28.7	Benign neoplasm of other specified female genital organs ♀
D49.59	Neoplasm of unspecified behavior of other genitourinary organ
N72	Inflammatory disease of cervix uteri ♀
N84.1	Polyp of cervix uteri ♀
N86	Erosion and ectropion of cervix uteri ♀
N87.0	Mild cervical dysplasia ♀
N87.1	Moderate cervical dysplasia ♀
N88.0	Leukoplakia of cervix uteri ♀
N88.1	Old laceration of cervix uteri ♀
N88.4	Hypertrophic elongation of cervix uteri ♀
N88.8	Other specified noninflammatory disorders of cervix uteri ♀
Q51.6	Embryonic cyst of cervix ♀
Z12.4	Encounter for screening for malignant neoplasm of cervix ♀

AMA: **57500** 2019,Jul,6; 2014,Jan,11

Relative Value Units/Medicare Edits

Non-Facility RVU	Work	PE	MP	Total
57500	1.2	2.72	0.19	4.11
Facility RVU	**Work**	**PE**	**MP**	**Total**
57500	1.2	0.78	0.19	2.17

	FUD	Status	MUE	Modifiers				IOM Reference
57500	0	A	1(3)	51	N/A	N/A	N/A	None

* with documentation

Terms To Know

biopsy. Tissue or fluid removed for diagnostic purposes through analysis of the cells in the biopsy material.

excision. Surgical removal of an organ or tissue.

forceps. Tool used for grasping or compressing tissue.

fulguration. Destruction of living tissue by using sparks from a high-frequency electric current.

speculum. Tool used to enlarge the opening of any canal or cavity.

Cervix Uteri

57505

57505   Endocervical curettage (not done as part of a dilation and curettage)

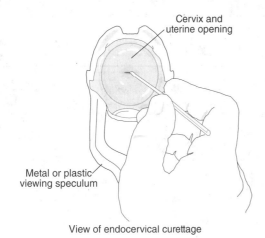

Cervix and
uterine opening

Metal or plastic
viewing speculum

View of endocervical curettage

Explanation

The physician inserts a speculum into the vagina to view the cervix. A small curette is used to scrape tissue from the endocervix, which is the region of the opening of the cervix into the uterine cavity.

Coding Tips

When 57505 is performed with another separately identifiable procedure, the highest dollar value code is listed as the primary procedure and subsequent procedures are appended with modifier 51. This procedure is usually performed with a local anesthesia. A paracervical anesthetic block is considered an inherent part of the surgical package. For colposcopy with biopsy of the cervix and endocervical curettage, see 57454; endocervical curettage only, see 57456.

ICD-10-CM Diagnostic Codes

A63.0	Anogenital (venereal) warts
C53.0	Malignant neoplasm of endocervix ♀
C53.8	Malignant neoplasm of overlapping sites of cervix uteri ♀
D06.0	Carcinoma in situ of endocervix ♀
D26.0	Other benign neoplasm of cervix uteri ♀
D28.7	Benign neoplasm of other specified female genital organs ♀
D39.0	Neoplasm of uncertain behavior of uterus ♀
D49.59	Neoplasm of unspecified behavior of other genitourinary organ
N72	Inflammatory disease of cervix uteri ♀
N84.1	Polyp of cervix uteri ♀
N86	Erosion and ectropion of cervix uteri ♀
N87.0	Mild cervical dysplasia ♀
N87.1	Moderate cervical dysplasia ♀
N88.0	Leukoplakia of cervix uteri ♀
N88.4	Hypertrophic elongation of cervix uteri ♀
N88.8	Other specified noninflammatory disorders of cervix uteri ♀
Q51.6	Embryonic cyst of cervix ♀

AMA: 57505 2019,Jul,6; 2018,Jan,8; 2017,Jan,8; 2016,Jan,13; 2015,Jan,16; 2014,Jan,11

Relative Value Units/Medicare Edits

Non-Facility RVU	Work	PE	MP	Total
57505	1.19	2.32	0.18	3.69
Facility RVU	**Work**	**PE**	**MP**	**Total**
57505	1.19	1.53	0.18	2.9

	FUD	Status	MUE	Modifiers				IOM Reference
57505	10	A	1(3)	51	N/A	N/A	N/A	None

* with documentation

Terms To Know

curettage. Removal of tissue by scraping.

curette. Spoon-shaped instrument used to scrape out abnormal tissue from a cavity or bone.

endocervix. Region of the cervix uteri that opens into the uterus or the mucous membrane lining the cervical canal.

speculum. Tool used to enlarge the opening of any canal or cavity.

57510-57513

57510 Cautery of cervix; electro or thermal
57511 cryocautery, initial or repeat
57513 laser ablation

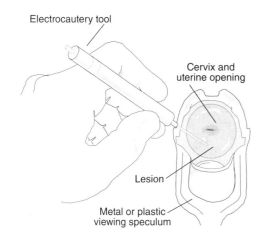

Electrocautery tool

Cervix and uterine opening

Lesion

Metal or plastic viewing speculum

Explanation

The physician inserts a speculum into the vagina to view the cervix. In 57510, electric current or heat is used to destroy the outer layers of the cervix causing them to slough off. In 57511, the outer layers of the cervix are destroyed by freezing using a liquid such as carbon dioxide, freon, nitrous oxide, or nitrogen, or a low temperature instrument. The outer layers of the cervix slough off. This code can be used for a first-time or repeat procedure. In 57513, a laser is directed at the cervix to vaporize the outer cells.

Coding Tips

The code choice for cauterization is determined by the equipment/method of cautery used. When 57510, 57511, or 57513 is performed with another separately identifiable procedure, the highest dollar value code is listed as the primary procedure and subsequent procedures are appended with modifier 51. Local anesthesia is included in the service.

ICD-10-CM Diagnostic Codes

A63.0	Anogenital (venereal) warts
C53.0	Malignant neoplasm of endocervix ♀
C53.1	Malignant neoplasm of exocervix ♀
C53.8	Malignant neoplasm of overlapping sites of cervix uteri ♀
D06.0	Carcinoma in situ of endocervix ♀
D06.1	Carcinoma in situ of exocervix ♀
D06.7	Carcinoma in situ of other parts of cervix ♀
D26.0	Other benign neoplasm of cervix uteri ♀
D28.7	Benign neoplasm of other specified female genital organs ♀
D49.59	Neoplasm of unspecified behavior of other genitourinary organ
N72	Inflammatory disease of cervix uteri ♀
N80.0	Endometriosis of uterus ♀
N84.1	Polyp of cervix uteri ♀
N86	Erosion and ectropion of cervix uteri ♀
N87.0	Mild cervical dysplasia ♀
N87.1	Moderate cervical dysplasia ♀
N88.0	Leukoplakia of cervix uteri ♀
N88.1	Old laceration of cervix uteri ♀
N88.4	Hypertrophic elongation of cervix uteri ♀

N88.8	Other specified noninflammatory disorders of cervix uteri ♀
Q51.6	Embryonic cyst of cervix ♀
Q51.821	Hypoplasia of cervix ♀
Q51.828	Other congenital malformations of cervix ♀

AMA: 57510 2019,Jul,6; 2014,Jan,11 **57511** 2019,Jul,6; 2014,Jan,11 **57513** 2019,Jul,6; 2014,Jan,11

Relative Value Units/Medicare Edits

Non-Facility RVU	Work	PE	MP	Total
57510	1.9	2.13	0.3	4.33
57511	1.95	2.74	0.31	5.0
57513	1.95	2.82	0.31	5.08
Facility RVU	**Work**	**PE**	**MP**	**Total**
57510	1.9	1.09	0.3	3.29
57511	1.95	1.8	0.31	4.06
57513	1.95	1.79	0.31	4.05

	FUD	Status	MUE	Modifiers				IOM Reference
57510	10	A	1(3)	51	N/A	N/A	N/A	None
57511	10	A	1(3)	51	N/A	N/A	N/A	
57513	10	A	1(3)	51	N/A	N/A	N/A	

* with documentation

Terms To Know

ablation. Removal or destruction of tissue by cutting, electrical energy, chemical substances, or excessive heat application.

cautery. Destruction or burning of tissue by means of a hot instrument, an electric current, or a caustic chemical, such as silver nitrate.

cryosurgery. Application of intense cold, usually produced using liquid nitrogen, to locally freeze diseased or unwanted tissue and induce tissue necrosis without causing harm to adjacent tissue.

laser surgery. Use of concentrated, sharply defined light beams to cut, cauterize, coagulate, seal, or vaporize tissue.

speculum. Tool used to enlarge the opening of any canal or cavity.

Cervix Uteri

57520-57522

57520 Conization of cervix, with or without fulguration, with or without dilation and curettage, with or without repair; cold knife or laser
57522   loop electrode excision

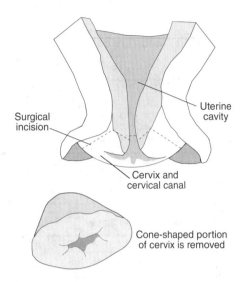

Surgical incision

Uterine cavity

Cervix and cervical canal

Cone-shaped portion of cervix is removed

Explanation

The physician performs a conization of the cervix, with or without fulguration, with or without dilation and curettage, with or without repair by using the cold knife or laser technique in 57520 or by using a loop electrode excision (LEEP) in 57522. The physician inserts a speculum into the vagina to view and fully expose the cervix. For most cases, the appropriate local anesthesia is administered as opposed to forms of premedication. In 57520, using a scalpel or laser instrument, a cone or slice of tissue, including about 1 to 2 cm of the endocervix and exocervical cells, is cut from the end of the cervix with the axis of the cone parallel to the axis of the cervix. In 57522, the electric grounding pad is placed and safety checks are run. The cutting current is set. Using a loop that encompasses the lesion, an excision of the ectocervix is done with every effort made to remove the lesion in one specimen. If the lesion is large and another pass is required, two equal specimens are removed and labeled for the axis of orientation. The same procedure is done again with a smaller loop if an endocervical excision is necessary. Following either procedure, the cervix may be dilated and an endocervical curettage collected, bleeding vessels may be cauterized or sutured to achieve hemostasis, and the speculum is removed.

Coding Tips

If the cervical stump is excised (following supracervical hysterectomy), see 57540 and 57550. When 57520 is performed with another separately identifiable procedure, the highest dollar value code is listed as the primary procedure and subsequent procedures are appended with modifier 51. Local anesthesia is included in the service. However, this procedure may be performed under general anesthesia, depending on the age and/or condition of the patient. For dilation and curettage only, see 58120.

ICD-10-CM Diagnostic Codes

C53.0	Malignant neoplasm of endocervix ♀
C53.1	Malignant neoplasm of exocervix ♀
C53.8	Malignant neoplasm of overlapping sites of cervix uteri ♀
D06.0	Carcinoma in situ of endocervix ♀
D06.1	Carcinoma in situ of exocervix ♀
D06.7	Carcinoma in situ of other parts of cervix ♀

D26.0	Other benign neoplasm of cervix uteri ♀
D28.7	Benign neoplasm of other specified female genital organs ♀
D49.59	Neoplasm of unspecified behavior of other genitourinary organ
N72	Inflammatory disease of cervix uteri ♀
N84.1	Polyp of cervix uteri ♀
N86	Erosion and ectropion of cervix uteri ♀
N87.0	Mild cervical dysplasia ♀
N87.1	Moderate cervical dysplasia ♀
N88.4	Hypertrophic elongation of cervix uteri ♀
N88.8	Other specified noninflammatory disorders of cervix uteri ♀

AMA: 57520 2019,Jul,6; 2018,Jan,8; 2017,Jan,8; 2016,Jan,13; 2015,Jan,16; 2014,Jan,11 **57522** 2019,Jul,6; 2018,Jan,8; 2017,Jan,8; 2016,Jan,13; 2015,Jan,16; 2014,Jan,11

Relative Value Units/Medicare Edits

Non-Facility RVU	Work	PE	MP	Total
57520	4.11	4.85	0.63	9.59
57522	3.67	4.01	0.57	8.25
Facility RVU	**Work**	**PE**	**MP**	**Total**
57520	4.11	3.49	0.63	8.23
57522	3.67	2.97	0.57	7.21

	FUD	Status	MUE	Modifiers				IOM Reference
57520	90	A	1(3)	51	N/A	N/A	N/A	None
57522	90	A	1(3)	51	N/A	N/A	N/A	

* with documentation

Terms To Know

conization. Excision of a cone-shaped piece of tissue.

curettage. Removal of tissue by scraping.

dilation. Artificial increase in the diameter of an opening or lumen made by medication or by instrumentation.

fulguration. Destruction of living tissue by using sparks from a high-frequency electric current.

LEEP. Loop electrode excision procedure. Biopsy specimen or cone shaped wedge of cervical tissue is removed using a hot cautery wire loop with an electrical current running through it.

Cervix Uteri

57530

57530 Trachelectomy (cervicectomy), amputation of cervix (separate procedure)

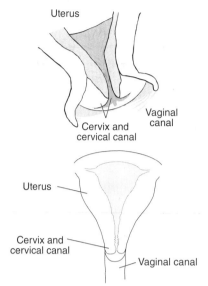

Uterus

Vaginal canal

Cervix and cervical canal

Uterus

Cervix and cervical canal

Vaginal canal

The cervix is surgically removed

Explanation

The physician inserts a speculum into the vagina to view the cervix and perform an amputation of the cervix. A tool is used to pull down the cervix. A scalpel is used to divide the cervix from the uterus just after it enters the vagina. The physician removes the cervix through the vagina and stops the bleeding with cautery and sutures.

Coding Tips

This separate procedure by definition is usually a component of a more complex service and is not identified separately. When performed alone or with other unrelated procedures/services it may be reported. If performed alone, list the code; if performed with other procedures/services, list the code and append modifier 59 or an X{EPSU} modifier. When 57530 is performed with another separately identifiable procedure, the highest dollar value code is listed as the primary procedure and subsequent procedures are appended with modifier 51. Local anesthesia is included in the service. For radical trachelectomy with lymphadenectomy, with or without the removal of a tube and/or ovary, see 57531. For radical abdominal hysterectomy, see 58210.

ICD-10-CM Diagnostic Codes

C53.0	Malignant neoplasm of endocervix ♀
C53.1	Malignant neoplasm of exocervix ♀
C53.8	Malignant neoplasm of overlapping sites of cervix uteri ♀
D06.0	Carcinoma in situ of endocervix ♀
D06.1	Carcinoma in situ of exocervix ♀
D06.7	Carcinoma in situ of other parts of cervix ♀
D26.0	Other benign neoplasm of cervix uteri ♀
D49.59	Neoplasm of unspecified behavior of other genitourinary organ
N87.0	Mild cervical dysplasia ♀
N87.1	Moderate cervical dysplasia ♀

AMA: 57530 2019,Jul,6; 2014,Jan,11

Relative Value Units/Medicare Edits

Non-Facility RVU	Work	PE	MP	Total
57530	5.27	4.33	0.82	10.42
Facility RVU	**Work**	**PE**	**MP**	**Total**
57530	5.27	4.33	0.82	10.42

	FUD	Status	MUE	Modifiers				IOM Reference
57530	90	A	1(3)	51	N/A	62*	80	None

* with documentation

Terms To Know

cautery. Destruction or burning of tissue by means of a hot instrument, an electric current, or a caustic chemical, such as silver nitrate.

endocervical canal. Opening between the uterus and the vagina, through the cervix, lined with mucous membrane.

separate procedures. Services commonly carried out as a fundamental part of a total service and, as such, do not usually warrant separate identification. These services are identified in CPT with the parenthetical phrase (separate procedure) at the end of the description and are payable only when performed alone.

speculum. Tool used to enlarge the opening of any canal or cavity.

57531

57531 Radical trachelectomy, with bilateral total pelvic lymphadenectomy and para-aortic lymph node sampling biopsy, with or without removal of tube(s), with or without removal of ovary(s)

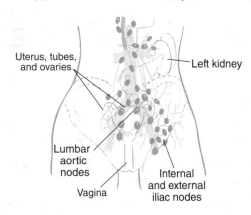

Uterus, tubes, and ovaries
Left kidney
Lumbar aortic nodes
Vagina
Internal and external iliac nodes

Explanation

The physician inserts a speculum into the vagina to view the cervix and perform a radical excision of the cervix, including removal of local lymph nodes. A tool is used to pull down the cervix. A scalpel is used to divide the cervix from the uterus just after it enters the vagina. The physician removes the cervix through the vagina, stops the bleeding with cautery, and also removes the pelvic lymph nodes bilaterally, performs a para-aortic lymph node biopsy, and may remove one or both tubes and/or ovaries.

Coding Tips

This procedure includes bilateral total pelvic lymphadenectomy, para-aortic lymph node sampling biopsy, and removal of a tube(s), with removal of an ovary(s). For trachelectomy (cervicectomy), amputation of the cervix alone, see 57530. For radical vaginal hysterectomy, see 58285. For radical abdominal hysterectomy, see 58210.

ICD-10-CM Diagnostic Codes

C53.0	Malignant neoplasm of endocervix ♀
C53.1	Malignant neoplasm of exocervix ♀
C53.8	Malignant neoplasm of overlapping sites of cervix uteri ♀
C77.2	Secondary and unspecified malignant neoplasm of intra-abdominal lymph nodes
C77.5	Secondary and unspecified malignant neoplasm of intrapelvic lymph nodes
D06.0	Carcinoma in situ of endocervix ♀
D06.1	Carcinoma in situ of exocervix ♀
D06.7	Carcinoma in situ of other parts of cervix ♀
D26.0	Other benign neoplasm of cervix uteri ♀
D49.59	Neoplasm of unspecified behavior of other genitourinary organ
N87.0	Mild cervical dysplasia ♀
N87.1	Moderate cervical dysplasia ♀

AMA: **57531** 2019,Jul,6; 2014,Jan,11

Relative Value Units/Medicare Edits

Non-Facility RVU	Work	PE	MP	Total
57531	29.95	14.72	8.26	52.93
Facility RVU	Work	PE	MP	Total
57531	29.95	14.72	8.26	52.93

	FUD	Status	MUE	Modifiers				IOM Reference
57531	90	A	1(2)	51	N/A	62*	80	None

* with documentation

Terms To Know

bilateral. Consisting of or affecting two sides.

biopsy. Tissue or fluid removed for diagnostic purposes through analysis of the cells in the biopsy material.

excision. Surgical removal of an organ or tissue.

lymphadenectomy. Dissection of lymph nodes free from the vessels and removal for examination by frozen section in a separate procedure to detect early-stage metastases.

radical. Extensive surgery.

speculum. Tool used to enlarge the opening of any canal or cavity.

57540-57545

57540 Excision of cervical stump, abdominal approach;
57545 with pelvic floor repair

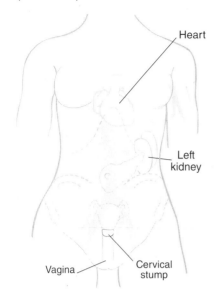

A cervical stump (remnant from a previous hysterectomy) is excised

Explanation

The physician makes an incision horizontally just within the pubic hairline. In 57540, the physician removes the cervical stump, which is the part of the cervix left after the supracervical uterus has been removed. The incision is closed by suturing. In 57545, the physician removes the cervical stump and repairs the muscular floor of the pelvis where the cervix rests using suture plication. This involves folding the tissues on top of each other and suturing. The incision is sutured.

Coding Tips

This service is performed on patients who have had a supracervical abdominal hysterectomy. When either of these procedures are performed with another separately identifiable procedure, the highest dollar value code is listed as the primary procedure and subsequent procedures are appended with modifier 51. For the initial supracervical abdominal hysterectomy, report 58180. For excision of a cervical stump, vaginal approach, report 57550.

ICD-10-CM Diagnostic Codes

C53.8	Malignant neoplasm of overlapping sites of cervix uteri ♀
C79.82	Secondary malignant neoplasm of genital organs
D06.7	Carcinoma in situ of other parts of cervix ♀
D26.0	Other benign neoplasm of cervix uteri ♀
D39.0	Neoplasm of uncertain behavior of uterus ♀
D49.59	Neoplasm of unspecified behavior of other genitourinary organ
N72	Inflammatory disease of cervix uteri ♀
N81.85	Cervical stump prolapse ♀
N86	Erosion and ectropion of cervix uteri ♀
N87.0	Mild cervical dysplasia ♀
N87.1	Moderate cervical dysplasia ♀

AMA: **57540** 2019,Jul,6; 2014,Jan,11 **57545** 2019,Jul,6; 2014,Jan,11

Relative Value Units/Medicare Edits

Non-Facility RVU	Work	PE	MP	Total
57540	13.29	7.47	2.08	22.84
57545	14.1	7.77	2.21	24.08
Facility RVU	**Work**	**PE**	**MP**	**Total**
57540	13.29	7.47	2.08	22.84
57545	14.1	7.77	2.21	24.08

	FUD	Status	MUE	Modifiers				IOM Reference
57540	90	A	1(2)	51	N/A	62*	80	None
57545	90	A	1(3)	51	N/A	62*	80	

* with documentation

Terms To Know

approach. Method or anatomical location used to gain access to a body organ or specific area for procedures.

excision. Surgical removal of an organ or tissue.

incision. Act of cutting into tissue or an organ.

plication. Surgical technique involving folding, tucking, or pleating to reduce the size of a hollow structure or organ.

supra. Above.

57550

57550   Excision of cervical stump, vaginal approach;

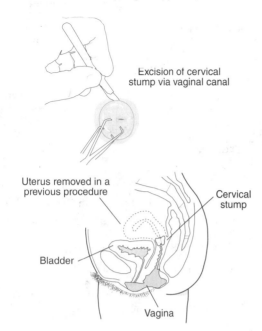

Excision of cervical stump via vaginal canal

Uterus removed in a previous procedure

Cervical stump

Bladder

Vagina

Explanation

Through an incision at the apex of the vagina, the physician removes the cervical stump, which is the part of the cervix left after the supracervical uterus has been removed. The vaginal incision is closed with sutures.

Coding Tips

This service is performed on patients who have had a supracervical abdominal hysterectomy. In some cases, scar tissue is an additional complication. Any manipulation or dilation of the vagina is not reported separately. When 57550 is performed with another separately identifiable procedure, the highest dollar value code is listed as the primary procedure and subsequent procedures are appended with modifier 51. For the initial supracervical abdominal hysterectomy, report 58180. For excision of a cervical stump, vaginal approach, with anterior and/or posterior repair, see 57555; with repair of enterocele, see 57556. For excision of a cervical stump, abdominal approach, see 57540–57545.

ICD-10-CM Diagnostic Codes

C53.8	Malignant neoplasm of overlapping sites of cervix uteri ♀
C79.82	Secondary malignant neoplasm of genital organs
D06.7	Carcinoma in situ of other parts of cervix ♀
D26.0	Other benign neoplasm of cervix uteri ♀
D39.0	Neoplasm of uncertain behavior of uterus ♀
D49.59	Neoplasm of unspecified behavior of other genitourinary organ
N72	Inflammatory disease of cervix uteri ♀
N81.85	Cervical stump prolapse ♀
N86	Erosion and ectropion of cervix uteri ♀
N87.0	Mild cervical dysplasia ♀
N87.1	Moderate cervical dysplasia ♀

AMA: 57550 2019,Jul,6; 2014,Jan,11

Relative Value Units/Medicare Edits

Non-Facility RVU	Work	PE	MP	Total
57550	6.34	4.85	1.0	12.19
Facility RVU	**Work**	**PE**	**MP**	**Total**
57550	6.34	4.85	1.0	12.19

	FUD	Status	MUE	Modifiers				IOM Reference
57550	90	A	1(3)	51	N/A	62*	80	None

* with documentation

Terms To Know

apex. Highest point of a root end of a tooth, or the end of any organ.

approach. Method or anatomical location used to gain access to a body organ or specific area for procedures.

cervical intraepithelial neoplasia. Classification system used to report abnormalities in the epithelial cells of the cervix uteri: *1)* CIN I: Cervical intraepithelial neoplasia I, low-grade abnormality, mild dysplasia. *2)* CIN II: Cervical intraepithelial neoplasia II, high-grade abnormality, moderate dysplasia. *3)* CIN III: Cervical intraepithelial neoplasia III, carcinoma in situ, severe dysplasia.

excision. Surgical removal of an organ or tissue.

57555-57556

57555 Excision of cervical stump, vaginal approach; with anterior and/or posterior repair
57556 with repair of enterocele

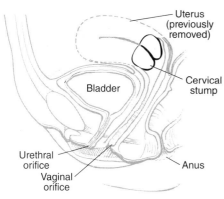

A cervical stump is excised by vaginal approach and anterior and/or posterior repair is performed at the same session

Explanation

Through an incision in the apex of the vagina, the physician removes the cervical stump. In 57555, the physician also repairs the relaxed or herniated tissues in the front or back wall of the vagina. Through the vaginal incision, the physician dissects the tissues between the bladder, urethra, vagina, and rectum. The specific tissue weaknesses are repaired and strengthened using tissue transfer techniques and layered and plication suturing. The incisions are closed with sutures. In 57556, the physician also repairs an enterocele, which is a herniation of the bowel against the rectouterine pouch. Through the vaginal incision, the physician incises and ligates the enterocele sac and approximates the uterosacral ligaments and endopelvic fascia anterior to the rectum. The incisions are closed with sutures.

Coding Tips

This service is performed on patients who have had a supracervical abdominal hysterectomy. When either of these procedures are performed with another separately identifiable procedure, the highest dollar value code is listed as the primary procedure and subsequent procedures are appended with modifier 51. For the initial supracervical abdominal hysterectomy, see 58180. For excision of the cervical stump only, vaginal approach, see 57550. If performing a repair of the vagina without surgical excision of the cervical stump, see 57200–57210 and 57240–57265. Insertion of an intrauterine device is reported with 58300. Insertion of any hemostatic agent or pack for the control of nonobstetrical, spontaneous hemorrhage is reported with 57180.

ICD-10-CM Diagnostic Codes

C53.8	Malignant neoplasm of overlapping sites of cervix uteri ♀
C79.82	Secondary malignant neoplasm of genital organs
D06.7	Carcinoma in situ of other parts of cervix ♀
D26.0	Other benign neoplasm of cervix uteri ♀
D39.0	Neoplasm of uncertain behavior of uterus ♀
D49.59	Neoplasm of unspecified behavior of other genitourinary organ
N72	Inflammatory disease of cervix uteri ♀
N81.5	Vaginal enterocele ♀
N81.82	Incompetence or weakening of pubocervical tissue ♀
N81.83	Incompetence or weakening of rectovaginal tissue ♀
N81.85	Cervical stump prolapse ♀
N86	Erosion and ectropion of cervix uteri ♀
N87.0	Mild cervical dysplasia ♀
N87.1	Moderate cervical dysplasia ♀
N99.3	Prolapse of vaginal vault after hysterectomy ♀

AMA: **57555** 2019,Jul,6; 2014,Jan,11 **57556** 2019,Jul,6; 2014,Jan,11

Relative Value Units/Medicare Edits

Non-Facility RVU	Work	PE	MP	Total
57555	9.94	6.24	1.57	17.75
57556	9.36	5.99	1.46	16.81
Facility RVU	**Work**	**PE**	**MP**	**Total**
57555	9.94	6.24	1.57	17.75
57556	9.36	5.99	1.46	16.81

	FUD	Status	MUE	Modifiers				IOM Reference
57555	90	A	1(2)	51	N/A	62*	80	None
57556	90	A	1(2)	51	N/A	62*	80	

* with documentation

Terms To Know

dissect. Cut apart or separate tissue for surgical purposes or for visual or microscopic study.

dysplasia. Abnormality or alteration in the size, shape, and organization of cells from their normal pattern of development.

enterocele. Intestinal herniation into the vaginal wall.

prolapse. Falling, sliding, or sinking of an organ from its normal location in the body.

Cervix Uteri

57558

57558   Dilation and curettage of cervical stump

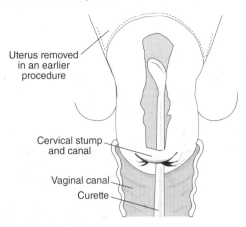

Uterus removed in an earlier procedure

Cervical stump and canal

Vaginal canal

Curette

Explanation

The physician performs a dilation and curettage of the cervical stump. The physician inserts a speculum into the vagina to view the cervix. The physician enlarges the cervix using a dilator and scrapes tissue from the lining of the cervical stump, which is the part of the cervix left after removal of the uterus.

Coding Tips

This code is used for the dilation and curettage of the cervical stump, and should not be confused with 58120. When 57558 is performed with another separately identifiable procedure, the highest dollar value code is listed as the primary procedure and subsequent procedures are appended with modifier 51. However, this code is often misused when larger invasive procedures are performed, in which case it is not reported separately. Local anesthesia is included in this service. However, this procedure may be performed under general anesthesia, depending on the age and/or condition of the patient. Surgical trays, A4550, are not separately reimbursed by Medicare; however, other third-party payers may cover them. Check with the specific payer to determine coverage.

ICD-10-CM Diagnostic Codes

C53.8	Malignant neoplasm of overlapping sites of cervix uteri ♀
C79.82	Secondary malignant neoplasm of genital organs
D06.7	Carcinoma in situ of other parts of cervix ♀
D26.0	Other benign neoplasm of cervix uteri ♀
D39.0	Neoplasm of uncertain behavior of uterus ♀
D49.59	Neoplasm of unspecified behavior of other genitourinary organ
N72	Inflammatory disease of cervix uteri ♀
N84.1	Polyp of cervix uteri ♀
N86	Erosion and ectropion of cervix uteri ♀
N87.0	Mild cervical dysplasia ♀
N87.1	Moderate cervical dysplasia ♀
N88.0	Leukoplakia of cervix uteri ♀
N88.1	Old laceration of cervix uteri ♀
N88.2	Stricture and stenosis of cervix uteri ♀
N88.4	Hypertrophic elongation of cervix uteri ♀
N88.8	Other specified noninflammatory disorders of cervix uteri ♀
Q51.6	Embryonic cyst of cervix ♀

AMA: **57558** 2019,Jul,6; 2014,Jan,11

Relative Value Units/Medicare Edits

Non-Facility RVU	Work	PE	MP	Total
57558	1.72	2.15	0.27	4.14
Facility RVU	**Work**	**PE**	**MP**	**Total**
57558	1.72	1.54	0.27	3.53

	FUD	Status	MUE	Modifiers				IOM Reference
57558	10	A	1(3)	51	N/A	N/A	N/A	None

* with documentation

Terms To Know

cervical ectropion. Eversion or turning outward of the cervical canal with epithelium extending further out of the external os of the cervix.

curettage. Removal of tissue by scraping.

dilation. Artificial increase in the diameter of an opening or lumen made by medication or by instrumentation.

dysplasia. Abnormality or alteration in the size, shape, and organization of cells from their normal pattern of development.

endometriosis. Aberrant uterine mucosal tissue appearing in areas of the pelvic cavity outside of its normal location, lining the uterus, and inflaming surrounding tissues often resulting in infertility or spontaneous abortion.

leukoplakia. Thickened white patches or lesions appearing on a mucous membrane, such as oral mucosa or tongue.

malignant. Any condition tending to progress toward death, specifically an invasive tumor with a loss of cellular differentiation that has the ability to spread or metastasize to other body areas.

mucous polyp. Outgrowth or projection of the mucous membrane tissue lining a body cavity.

polyp. Small growth on a stalk-like attachment projecting from a mucous membrane.

stenosis. Narrowing or constriction of a passage.

stricture. Narrowing of an anatomical structure.

57700

57700   Cerclage of uterine cervix, nonobstetrical

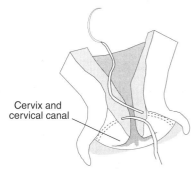

Cervix and
cervical canal

Suture material inserted around cervix

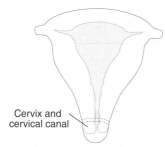

Cervix and
cervical canal

Suture material is tightened

Explanation

The physician inserts a speculum into the vagina to view the cervix of a nonpregnant patient. Suture or wire is threaded around the cervix and pulled in pursestring fashion to make the opening smaller.

Coding Tips

Depending on the patient's anatomy, there may be additional complications. When 57700 is performed with another separately identifiable procedure, the highest dollar value code is listed as the primary procedure and subsequent procedures are appended with modifier 51. If the patient is pregnant, see 59320 or 59325. Surgical trays, A4550, are not separately reimbursed by Medicare; however, other third-party payers may cover them. Check with the specific payer to determine coverage.

ICD-10-CM Diagnostic Codes

N88.3   Incompetence of cervix uteri ♀
S37.60XA   Unspecified injury of uterus, initial encounter ♀
S37.69XA   Other injury of uterus, initial encounter ♀

AMA: 57700 2019,Jul,6; 2014,Jan,11

Relative Value Units/Medicare Edits

Non-Facility RVU	Work	PE	MP	Total
57700	4.35	4.67	0.66	9.68
Facility RVU	Work	PE	MP	Total
57700	4.35	4.67	0.66	9.68

	FUD	Status	MUE	Modifiers				IOM Reference
57700	90	A	1(3)	51	N/A	N/A	80*	None

* with documentation

57720

57720   Trachelorrhaphy, plastic repair of uterine cervix, vaginal approach

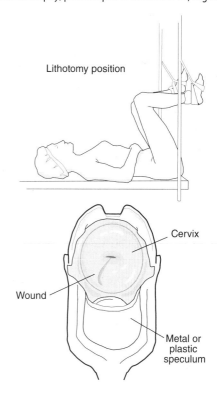

Lithotomy position

Cervix

Wound

Metal or
plastic
speculum

Explanation

The physician inserts a speculum into the vagina to view the cervix. The physician performs a plastic suture repair of a laceration or wound on the cervix. A plastic repair also can encompass excising scar tissue or tightening an incompetent cervix.

Coding Tips

A more complex plastic repair may also encompass an excision of scar tissue or tightening of the cervix. Any manipulation or dilation of the vagina is not reported separately. Electrocautery may be used to stop small bleeding points. When 57720 is performed with another separately identifiable procedure, the highest dollar value code is listed as the primary procedure and subsequent procedures are appended with modifier 51. For repairs of the vagina, see 57200–57270.

ICD-10-CM Diagnostic Codes

N88.1   Old laceration of cervix uteri ♀
N88.3   Incompetence of cervix uteri ♀
O71.3   Obstetric laceration of cervix Ⓜ ♀
S37.62XA   Contusion of uterus, initial encounter ♀
S37.63XA   Laceration of uterus, initial encounter ♀
S37.69XA   Other injury of uterus, initial encounter ♀

AMA: 57720 2019,Jul,6; 2014,Jan,11

Cervix Uteri

Relative Value Units/Medicare Edits

Non-Facility RVU	Work	PE	MP	Total
57720	4.61	4.0	0.72	9.33
Facility RVU	**Work**	**PE**	**MP**	**Total**
57720	4.61	4.0	0.72	9.33

	FUD	Status	MUE	Modifiers				IOM Reference
57720	90	A	1(3)	51	N/A	N/A	80	None

* with documentation

Terms To Know

approach. Method or anatomical location used to gain access to a body organ or specific area for procedures. The approach is not coded separately although it may be a specified component of the procedure, such as laparoscopic versus incisional, or spinal procedures in which the amount of dissection required to expose the spine significantly alters with the site of approach.

endocervical canal. Opening between the uterus and the vagina, through the cervix, lined with mucous membrane.

external os. Uterine opening through the cervix and into the vagina.

incompetent cervix. Narrow end of the uterus opening into the birth canal that abnormally dilates during the second trimester of the pregnancy and can lead to a miscarriage or premature delivery.

internal os. Opening through the cervix into the uterus.

laceration. Tearing injury; a torn, ragged-edged wound.

scar tissue. Fibrous connective tissue that forms around a wounded area or injury, composed mainly of fibroblasts or collagenous fibers.

speculum. Tool used to enlarge the opening of any canal or cavity.

57800

57800   Dilation of cervical canal, instrumental (separate procedure)

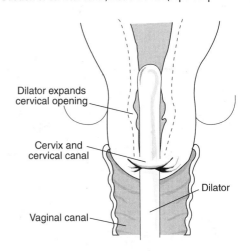

Dilator expands cervical opening

Cervix and cervical canal

Dilator

Vaginal canal

Explanation

The physician inserts a speculum into the vagina to view the cervix. A tool is used to grasp the cervix and pull it down. A dilator or series of dilators is inserted into the endocervix and passed through the cervical canal.

Coding Tips

This separate procedure by definition is usually a component of a more complex service and is not identified separately. When performed alone or with other unrelated procedures/services it may be reported. If performed alone, list the code; if performed with other procedures/services, list the code and append modifier 59 or an X{EPSU} modifier. For dilation and curettage of cervical stump, see 57558. For endometrial and/or endocervical sampling (biopsy), without cervical dilation, any method, see 58100. For dilation and curettage, diagnostic and/or therapeutic (nonobstetrical), see 58120. For treatment of a missed abortion, see 59820–59821. Surgical trays, A4550, are not separately reimbursed by Medicare; however, other third-party payers may cover them. Check with the specific payer to determine coverage.

ICD-10-CM Diagnostic Codes

N88.2   Stricture and stenosis of cervix uteri ♀

AMA: 57800 2019,Jul,6; 2014,Jan,11

Relative Value Units/Medicare Edits

Non-Facility RVU	Work	PE	MP	Total
57800	0.77	1.12	0.12	2.01
Facility RVU	**Work**	**PE**	**MP**	**Total**
57800	0.77	0.5	0.12	1.39

	FUD	Status	MUE	Modifiers				IOM Reference
57800	0	A	1(3)	51	N/A	N/A	N/A	None

* with documentation

Terms To Know

dilation. Artificial increase in the diameter of an opening or lumen made by medication or by instrumentation.

endocervix. Region of the cervix uteri that opens into the uterus or the mucous membrane lining the cervical canal.

58100

58100 Endometrial sampling (biopsy) with or without endocervical sampling (biopsy), without cervical dilation, any method (separate procedure)

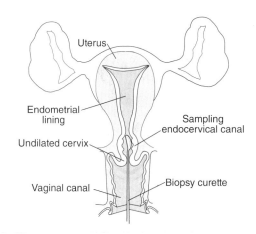

Uterus

Endometrial lining

Undilated cervix

Vaginal canal

Sampling endocervical canal

Biopsy curette

Explanation

The physician inserts a speculum into the vagina to view the cervix. A tool is used to grasp the cervix and pull it down. The physician places a curette in the endocervical canal and passes it into the uterus. The endometrial lining of the uterus is scraped on all sides to obtain tissue for diagnosis. Biopsy(ies) may also be taken from the endocervix. Cervical dilation is not required.

Coding Tips

This separate procedure by definition is usually a component of a more complex service and is not identified separately. When performed alone or with other unrelated procedures/services it may be reported. If performed alone, list the code; if performed with other procedures/services, list the code and append modifier 59 or an X{EPSU} modifier. If a specimen is transported to an outside laboratory, report 99000 for handling or conveyance. For endometrial sampling/biopsy performed with a colposcopy (57420-57421, 57452-57461), see 58110. For endocervical curettage (not done as part of a dilation and curettage), see 57505. For dilation and curettage, diagnostic and/or therapeutic (nonobstetrical), see 58120. For curettage for postpartum hemorrhage, see 59160.

ICD-10-CM Diagnostic Codes

C53.0	Malignant neoplasm of endocervix ♀
C54.1	Malignant neoplasm of endometrium ♀
C79.82	Secondary malignant neoplasm of genital organs
D06.0	Carcinoma in situ of endocervix ♀
D07.0	Carcinoma in situ of endometrium ♀
D25.0	Submucous leiomyoma of uterus ♀
D25.1	Intramural leiomyoma of uterus ♀
D25.2	Subserosal leiomyoma of uterus ♀
D26.0	Other benign neoplasm of cervix uteri ♀
D26.1	Other benign neoplasm of corpus uteri ♀
D39.0	Neoplasm of uncertain behavior of uterus ♀
D49.59	Neoplasm of unspecified behavior of other genitourinary organ
E28.2	Polycystic ovarian syndrome ♀
N71.0	Acute inflammatory disease of uterus ♀
N71.1	Chronic inflammatory disease of uterus ♀
N72	Inflammatory disease of cervix uteri ♀
N80.0	Endometriosis of uterus ♀

N84.0	Polyp of corpus uteri ♀
N84.1	Polyp of cervix uteri ♀
N85.01	Benign endometrial hyperplasia ♀
N85.02	Endometrial intraepithelial neoplasia [EIN] ♀
N85.2	Hypertrophy of uterus ♀
N85.6	Intrauterine synechiae ♀
N85.7	Hematometra ♀
N85.8	Other specified noninflammatory disorders of uterus ♀
N87.0	Mild cervical dysplasia ♀
N87.1	Moderate cervical dysplasia ♀
N88.2	Stricture and stenosis of cervix uteri ♀
N89.7	Hematocolpos ♀
N89.8	Other specified noninflammatory disorders of vagina ♀
N91.0	Primary amenorrhea ♀
N91.1	Secondary amenorrhea ♀
N91.3	Primary oligomenorrhea ♀
N91.4	Secondary oligomenorrhea ♀
N92.0	Excessive and frequent menstruation with regular cycle ♀
N92.1	Excessive and frequent menstruation with irregular cycle ♀
N92.2	Excessive menstruation at puberty ▣ ♀
N92.3	Ovulation bleeding ♀
N92.4	Excessive bleeding in the premenopausal period ♀
N92.5	Other specified irregular menstruation ♀
N93.8	Other specified abnormal uterine and vaginal bleeding ♀
N94.89	Other specified conditions associated with female genital organs and menstrual cycle ♀
N95.0	Postmenopausal bleeding ♀
N95.8	Other specified menopausal and perimenopausal disorders ♀
N97.0	Female infertility associated with anovulation ♀
N97.2	Female infertility of uterine origin ♀

AMA: **58100** 2019,Jul,6; 2014,Jan,11

Relative Value Units/Medicare Edits

Non-Facility RVU	Work	PE	MP	Total
58100	1.21	1.4	0.19	2.8
Facility RVU	**Work**	**PE**	**MP**	**Total**
58100	1.21	0.46	0.19	1.86

	FUD	Status	MUE		Modifiers			IOM Reference
58100	0	A	1(3)	51	N/A	N/A	N/A	100-03,240.4

* with documentation

Terms To Know

biopsy. Tissue or fluid removed for diagnostic purposes through analysis of the cells in the biopsy material.

curette. Spoon-shaped instrument used to scrape out abnormal tissue from a cavity or bone.

endocervix. Region of the cervix uteri that opens into the uterus or the mucous membrane lining the cervical canal.

58110

+ **58110** Endometrial sampling (biopsy) performed in conjunction with colposcopy (List separately in addition to code for primary procedure)

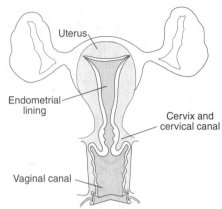

The endometrial lining of the uterus is sampled

Explanation

A tool is used to grasp the cervix and pull it down. The physician places a curette in the endocervical canal and passes it into the uterus. The endometrial lining of the uterus is scraped in several places to obtain tissue for a biopsy sample. The endometrial sampling is performed in conjunction with direct visualization of the vagina and cervix and is reported in addition to the separately reportable primary colposcopy.

Coding Tips

Report 58110 in addition to 57420–57421 and 57452–57461.

ICD-10-CM Diagnostic Codes

This/these CPT code(s) are add-on code(s). See the primary procedure code that this code is performed with for your ICD-10-CM code selections. Diagnostic code(s) would be the same as the actual procedure performed.

AMA: **58110** 2019,Jul,6; 2018,Jan,8; 2017,Jan,8; 2016,Jan,13; 2015,Jan,16; 2014,Jan,11

Relative Value Units/Medicare Edits

Non-Facility RVU	Work	PE	MP	Total
58110	0.77	0.57	0.12	1.46
Facility RVU	Work	PE	MP	Total
58110	0.77	0.3	0.12	1.19

	FUD	Status	MUE	Modifiers				IOM Reference
58110	N/A	A	1(3)	N/A	N/A	N/A	80*	None

* with documentation

Terms To Know

biopsy. Tissue or fluid removed for diagnostic purposes through analysis of the cells in the biopsy material.

colposcopy. Procedure in which the physician views the cervix and vagina through a colposcope, which is a binocular microscope used for direct visualization of the vagina, ectocervix, and endocervix.

58120

58120 Dilation and curettage, diagnostic and/or therapeutic (nonobstetrical)

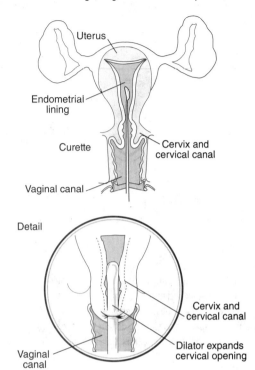

Explanation

The physician inserts a speculum into the vagina to view the cervix. A tool is used to grasp the cervix and pull it down. A dilator is inserted into the endocervix and through the cervical canal to enlarge the opening. The physician places a curette in the endocervical canal and passes it into the uterus. The endometrial lining of the uterus is scraped on all sides for diagnostic or therapeutic purposes.

Coding Tips

This code includes a biopsy, single or multiple, whether being performed with a curette or another method. This procedure should not be separately identified when being used in conjunction with the hysterectomy procedures. When 58120 is performed with another separately identifiable procedure, the highest dollar value code is listed as the primary procedure and subsequent procedures are appended with modifier 51. Local anesthesia is included in this service. However, this procedure may be performed under general anesthesia, depending on the age and/or condition of the patient. For curettage due to postpartum hemorrhage, see 59160.

ICD-10-CM Diagnostic Codes

C53.0	Malignant neoplasm of endocervix ♀
C54.1	Malignant neoplasm of endometrium ♀
C79.82	Secondary malignant neoplasm of genital organs
D06.0	Carcinoma in situ of endocervix ♀
D07.0	Carcinoma in situ of endometrium ♀
D25.0	Submucous leiomyoma of uterus ♀
D25.1	Intramural leiomyoma of uterus ♀
D25.2	Subserosal leiomyoma of uterus ♀
D26.0	Other benign neoplasm of cervix uteri ♀
D26.1	Other benign neoplasm of corpus uteri ♀

N Newborn: 0 **P** Pediatric: 0-17 **M** Maternity: 9-64 **A** Adult: 15-124 ♂ Male Only ♀ Female Only

<table>
D39.0	Neoplasm of uncertain behavior of uterus ♀
D49.59	Neoplasm of unspecified behavior of other genitourinary organ
E28.2	Polycystic ovarian syndrome ♀
N71.0	Acute inflammatory disease of uterus ♀
N71.1	Chronic inflammatory disease of uterus ♀
N72	Inflammatory disease of cervix uteri ♀
N80.0	Endometriosis of uterus ♀
N84.0	Polyp of corpus uteri ♀
N84.1	Polyp of cervix uteri ♀
N85.01	Benign endometrial hyperplasia ♀
N85.02	Endometrial intraepithelial neoplasia [EIN] ♀
N85.2	Hypertrophy of uterus ♀
N85.6	Intrauterine synechiae ♀
N85.7	Hematometra ♀
N85.8	Other specified noninflammatory disorders of uterus ♀
N87.0	Mild cervical dysplasia ♀
N87.1	Moderate cervical dysplasia ♀
N88.2	Stricture and stenosis of cervix uteri ♀
N89.7	Hematocolpos ♀
N89.8	Other specified noninflammatory disorders of vagina ♀
N91.0	Primary amenorrhea ♀
N91.1	Secondary amenorrhea ♀
N91.3	Primary oligomenorrhea ♀
N91.4	Secondary oligomenorrhea ♀
N92.0	Excessive and frequent menstruation with regular cycle ♀
N92.1	Excessive and frequent menstruation with irregular cycle ♀
N92.2	Excessive menstruation at puberty 🅿 ♀
N92.3	Ovulation bleeding ♀
N92.4	Excessive bleeding in the premenopausal period ♀
N92.5	Other specified irregular menstruation ♀
N93.8	Other specified abnormal uterine and vaginal bleeding ♀
N94.89	Other specified conditions associated with female genital organs and menstrual cycle ♀
N95.0	Postmenopausal bleeding ♀
N95.8	Other specified menopausal and perimenopausal disorders ♀
N97.0	Female infertility associated with anovulation ♀
N97.2	Female infertility of uterine origin ♀
</table>

AMA: **58120** 2019,Jul,6; 2018,Jan,8; 2017,Jan,8; 2016,Jan,13; 2015,Jan,16; 2014,Jan,11

Relative Value Units/Medicare Edits

Non-Facility RVU	Work	PE	MP	Total
58120	3.59	3.93	0.56	8.08
Facility RVU	**Work**	**PE**	**MP**	**Total**
58120	3.59	2.41	0.56	6.56

	FUD	Status	MUE	Modifiers				IOM Reference
58120	10	A	1(3)	51	N/A	N/A	N/A	None

* with documentation

58140

58140   Myomectomy, excision of fibroid tumor(s) of uterus, 1 to 4 intramural myoma(s) with total weight of 250 g or less and/or removal of surface myomas; abdominal approach

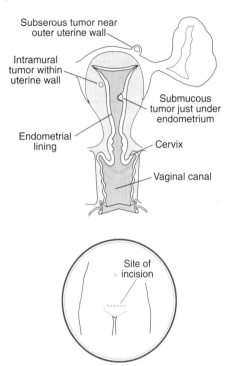

Subserous tumor near outer uterine wall
Intramural tumor within uterine wall
Submucous tumor just under endometrium
Endometrial lining
Cervix
Vaginal canal

Site of incision

Explanation

The physician removes one to four fibroid tumors from the wall of the uterus (intramural myomas) with a total weight of 250 gm or less and/or removes surface myomas by abdominal approach. A transverse incision is made in the abdomen, the anterior sheath of the rectus abdominis muscle is dissected, and muscles are retracted. Vasoconstrictors are injected and a tourniquet is applied to encompass the uterine mass and the adnexa to limit blood flow. A scalpel, electrocautery, and/or laser may be used to remove small surface myomas. The physician incises the uterus through the myometrium to expose the myoma, which is grasped with a clamp and dissected free from the surrounding myometrium with sharp and blunt dissection. The pedicle is isolated, clamped, and ligated and the myoma is dissected down to the pedicular blood supply. Other myomas are identified by palpating the uterine wall through the defect created by the already excised myoma. Adjacent myomas are reached and removed by tunneling further through the initial incision to avoid additional uterine trauma. The uterine wall defects are repaired by approximating the tissues to restore previous anatomy. The serosa is closed so as to minimize adhesion formation. Antiadhesion prophylaxis may be instilled in the abdominal cavity and the wound is closed.

Coding Tips

This code is often misused when the fibroid tumor is excised through laparoscopy or hysteroscopy. For removal of 5 or more intramural myomas with a total weight greater than 250 grams, see 58146. For the laparoscopic removal of intramural myomas, see 58545–58546. If removal of leiomyomata is performed through hysteroscopy, report 58561. If myomectomy is performed through a vaginal approach, see 58145.

ICD-10-CM Diagnostic Codes

D25.0   Submucous leiomyoma of uterus ♀

D25.1	Intramural leiomyoma of uterus ♀
D25.2	Subserosal leiomyoma of uterus ♀
D25.9	Leiomyoma of uterus, unspecified ♀

AMA: 58140 2019,Jul,6; 2018,Jan,8; 2017,Jan,8; 2016,Jan,13; 2015,Jan,16; 2014,Jan,11

Relative Value Units/Medicare Edits

Non-Facility RVU	Work	PE	MP	Total
58140	15.79	8.53	2.6	26.92
Facility RVU	**Work**	**PE**	**MP**	**Total**
58140	15.79	8.53	2.6	26.92

	FUD	Status	MUE	Modifiers				IOM Reference
58140	90	A	1(3)	51	N/A	62*	80	None

* with documentation

Terms To Know

adhesion. Abnormal fibrous connection between two structures, soft tissue or bony structures, that may occur as the result of surgery, infection, or trauma.

approach. Method or anatomical location used to gain access to a body organ or specific area for procedures. The approach is not coded separately although it may be a specified component of the procedure, such as laparoscopic versus incisional, or spinal procedures in which the amount of dissection required to expose the spine significantly alters with the site of approach.

defect. Imperfection, flaw, or absence.

intramural uterine leiomyoma. Benign, smooth muscle tumor within the wall of the uterus.

myometrium. Muscular middle layer of the uterine wall responsible for contractions associated with childbirth.

prophylaxis. Intervention or protective therapy intended to prevent a disease.

submucous uterine leiomyoma. Benign, smooth muscle tumor beneath the inner lining of the uterus.

subserous uterine leiomyoma. Benign, smooth muscle tumor beneath the serous membrane lining of the uterus.

58145

| 58145 | Myomectomy, excision of fibroid tumor(s) of uterus, 1 to 4 intramural myoma(s) with total weight of 250 g or less and/or removal of surface myomas; vaginal approach |

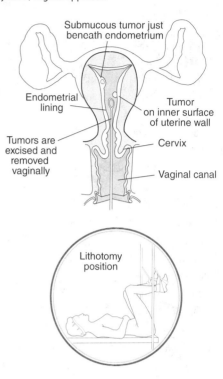

Explanation

The physician removes one to four fibroid tumors from the wall of the uterus (intramural myomas) with a total weight of 250 gm or less and/or removes surface myomas by vaginal approach. This approach is used for pedunculated myomas protruding through the cervix and for prolapsed myomas. The cervix is dilated with laminaria to facilitate exposure and a tonsil snare or other appropriate device is passed through to reach the myoma. Prolapsed myomas are usually attached to the cervical or endometrial cavity by a stalk. The tumor is removed by ligating or twisting the stalk or a tonsil snare is employed to encircle the tumor, cut it from its stalk, and remove it. The instruments are removed.

Coding Tips

Any manipulation or dilation of the vagina is not reported separately. This code is often misused when the fibroid tumor is excised through laparoscopy or hysteroscopy. For laparoscopic removal of intramural myomas, see 58545–58546. If removal of leiomyomata is performed through a hysteroscopy, see 58561. If myomectomy is performed through an abdominal approach, see 58140 and 58146.

ICD-10-CM Diagnostic Codes

D25.0	Submucous leiomyoma of uterus ♀
D25.1	Intramural leiomyoma of uterus ♀
D25.2	Subserosal leiomyoma of uterus ♀
D25.9	Leiomyoma of uterus, unspecified ♀

AMA: 58145 2019,Jul,6; 2014,Jan,11

Relative Value Units/Medicare Edits

Non-Facility RVU	Work	PE	MP	Total
58145	8.91	5.94	1.39	16.24
Facility RVU	Work	PE	MP	Total
58145	8.91	5.94	1.39	16.24

	FUD	Status	MUE	Modifiers				IOM Reference
58145	90	A	1(3)	51	N/A	62*	80	None

* with documentation

Terms To Know

approach. Method or anatomical location used to gain access to a body organ or specific area for procedures. The approach is not coded separately although it may be a specified component of the procedure, such as laparoscopic versus incisional, or spinal procedures in which the amount of dissection required to expose the spine significantly alters with the site of approach.

corpus uteri. Main body of the uterus, which is located above the isthmus and below the openings of the fallopian tubes.

dilation. Artificial increase in the diameter of an opening or lumen made by medication or by instrumentation.

endometrium. Lining of the uterus, which thickens in preparation for fertilization. A fertilized ovum embeds into the thickened endometrium. When no fertilization takes place, the endometrial lining sheds during the process of menstruation.

intramural uterine leiomyoma. Benign, smooth muscle tumor within the wall of the uterus.

ligate. To tie off a blood vessel or duct with a suture or a soft, thin wire (ligature wire).

myometrium. Muscular middle layer of the uterine wall responsible for contractions associated with childbirth.

parametrium. Connective tissue between the uterus and the broad ligament.

snare. Wire used as a loop to excise a polyp or lesion.

submucous uterine leiomyoma. Benign, smooth muscle tumor beneath the inner lining of the uterus.

58146

58146 Myomectomy, excision of fibroid tumor(s) of uterus, 5 or more intramural myomas and/or intramural myomas with total weight greater than 250 g, abdominal approach

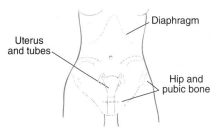

The approach is by abdominal incision

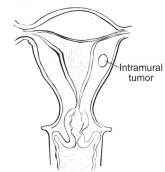

An abdominal myomectomy is performed

Explanation

The physician removes five or more fibroid tumors from the wall of the uterus and/or intramural myomas with a total weight greater than 250 gm by abdominal approach. A transverse incision is made in the abdomen (a midline incision is made for large myomas) and the anterior sheath of the rectus abdominis muscle is dissected and muscles are retracted. Vasoconstrictors are injected and a tourniquet is applied to encompass the uterine mass and the adnexa to limit blood flow. The physician incises the uterus down through the myometrium to expose the myoma, which is grasped with a clamp and dissected free from the surrounding myometrium with sharp and blunt dissection. For deep intramural myomas, the endometrial cavity may be exposed. The pedicle is isolated, clamped, and ligated and the myoma is dissected down to the pedicular blood supply. Other myomas are identified by palpating the uterine wall through the defect created by the already excised myoma. Adjacent myomas are reached and removed by tunneling further through the initial incision to avoid additional uterine trauma. The uterine wall defects are repaired by approximating the tissues to restore previous anatomy. The serosa is closed so as to minimize adhesion formation. Antiadhesion prophylaxis may be instilled in the abdominal cavity and the wound is closed.

Coding Tips

This code is often misused when fibroid tumors are excised through laparoscopy or hysteroscopy. For the laparoscopic removal of intramural myomas, see 58545–58546. If removal of leiomyomata is performed through a hysteroscopy, see 58561. For removal of one to four intramural myomas with a total weight of 250 grams or less, see 58140. If a myomectomy is performed through a vaginal approach, see 58145. Do not report 58146 with 51840–58145 or 58150–58240.

ICD-10-CM Diagnostic Codes

D25.0   Submucous leiomyoma of uterus ♀

D25.1	Intramural leiomyoma of uterus ♀
D25.2	Subserosal leiomyoma of uterus ♀
D25.9	Leiomyoma of uterus, unspecified ♀

AMA: 58146 2019,Jul,6; 2018,Jan,8; 2017,Jan,8; 2016,Jan,13; 2015,Jan,16; 2014,Jan,11

Relative Value Units/Medicare Edits

Non-Facility RVU	Work	PE	MP	Total
58146	20.34	10.05	3.19	33.58
Facility RVU	**Work**	**PE**	**MP**	**Total**
58146	20.34	10.05	3.19	33.58

	FUD	Status	MUE	Modifiers				IOM Reference
58146	90	A	1(3)	51	N/A	62*	80	None

* with documentation

Terms To Know

approach. Method or anatomical location used to gain access to a body organ or specific area for procedures. The approach is not coded separately although it may be a specified component of the procedure, such as laparoscopic versus incisional, or spinal procedures in which the amount of dissection required to expose the spine significantly alters with the site of approach.

defect. Imperfection, flaw, or absence.

dissect. Cut apart or separate tissue for surgical purposes or for visual or microscopic study.

intramural uterine leiomyoma. Benign, smooth muscle tumor within the wall of the uterus.

ligate. To tie off a blood vessel or duct with a suture or a soft, thin wire (ligature wire).

myometrium. Muscular middle layer of the uterine wall responsible for contractions associated with childbirth.

prophylaxis. Intervention or protective therapy intended to prevent a disease.

submucous uterine leiomyoma. Benign, smooth muscle tumor beneath the inner lining of the uterus.

subserous uterine leiomyoma. Benign, smooth muscle tumor beneath the serous membrane lining of the uterus.

transverse. Crosswise at right angles to the long axis of a structure or part.

58150

| 58150 | Total abdominal hysterectomy (corpus and cervix), with or without removal of tube(s), with or without removal of ovary(s); |

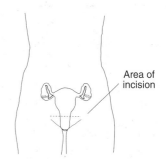

Area of incision

Surgeon may elect to leave any combination of tubes and ovaries

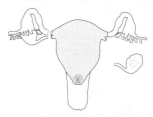

Explanation

Through a horizontal incision just within the pubic hairline, the physician removes the uterus including the cervix and may elect to remove one or both of the ovaries and one or both of the fallopian tubes (salpingo-oophorectomy). The supporting pedicles containing the tubes, ligaments, and arteries are clamped and cut free. The uterus and cervix are removed along with a narrow rim or cuff of vaginal lining. The vaginal defect may be left open for drainage. The abdominal incision is closed by suturing.

Coding Tips

If a colpourethrocystopexy (Marshall-Marchetti-Krantz or Burch type) is performed in conjunction with the total abdominal hysterectomy, report 58152.

ICD-10-CM Diagnostic Codes

C53.0	Malignant neoplasm of endocervix ♀
C53.1	Malignant neoplasm of exocervix ♀
C53.8	Malignant neoplasm of overlapping sites of cervix uteri ♀
C54.0	Malignant neoplasm of isthmus uteri ♀
C54.1	Malignant neoplasm of endometrium ♀
C54.2	Malignant neoplasm of myometrium ♀
C54.3	Malignant neoplasm of fundus uteri ♀
C54.8	Malignant neoplasm of overlapping sites of corpus uteri ♀
C56.1	Malignant neoplasm of right ovary ♀ ☑
C56.2	Malignant neoplasm of left ovary ♀ ☑
C57.01	Malignant neoplasm of right fallopian tube ♀ ☑
C57.02	Malignant neoplasm of left fallopian tube ♀ ☑
C57.11	Malignant neoplasm of right broad ligament ♀ ☑
C57.12	Malignant neoplasm of left broad ligament ♀ ☑
C57.21	Malignant neoplasm of right round ligament ♀ ☑
C57.22	Malignant neoplasm of left round ligament ♀ ☑
C57.3	Malignant neoplasm of parametrium ♀

C57.7	Malignant neoplasm of other specified female genital organs ♀
C57.8	Malignant neoplasm of overlapping sites of female genital organs ♀
C79.61	Secondary malignant neoplasm of right ovary ♀ ☑
C79.62	Secondary malignant neoplasm of left ovary ♀ ☑
C79.82	Secondary malignant neoplasm of genital organs
D06.0	Carcinoma in situ of endocervix ♀
D06.1	Carcinoma in situ of exocervix ♀
D06.7	Carcinoma in situ of other parts of cervix ♀
D07.0	Carcinoma in situ of endometrium ♀
D07.39	Carcinoma in situ of other female genital organs ♀
D25.0	Submucous leiomyoma of uterus ♀
D25.1	Intramural leiomyoma of uterus ♀
D25.2	Subserosal leiomyoma of uterus ♀
D39.0	Neoplasm of uncertain behavior of uterus ♀
D39.11	Neoplasm of uncertain behavior of right ovary ♀ ☑
D39.12	Neoplasm of uncertain behavior of left ovary ♀ ☑
D39.2	Neoplasm of uncertain behavior of placenta Ⓜ ♀
D39.8	Neoplasm of uncertain behavior of other specified female genital organs ♀
D49.59	Neoplasm of unspecified behavior of other genitourinary organ ♀
N70.11	Chronic salpingitis ♀
N70.12	Chronic oophoritis ♀
N70.13	Chronic salpingitis and oophoritis ♀
N71.0	Acute inflammatory disease of uterus ♀
N71.1	Chronic inflammatory disease of uterus ♀
N72	Inflammatory disease of cervix uteri ♀
N73.0	Acute parametritis and pelvic cellulitis ♀
N73.1	Chronic parametritis and pelvic cellulitis ♀
N73.3	Female acute pelvic peritonitis ♀
N73.4	Female chronic pelvic peritonitis ♀
N73.6	Female pelvic peritoneal adhesions (postinfective) ♀
N73.8	Other specified female pelvic inflammatory diseases ♀
N80.0	Endometriosis of uterus ♀
N80.1	Endometriosis of ovary ♀
N80.2	Endometriosis of fallopian tube ♀
N81.2	Incomplete uterovaginal prolapse ♀
N81.3	Complete uterovaginal prolapse ♀
N81.89	Other female genital prolapse ♀
N83.01	Follicular cyst of right ovary ♀ ☑
N83.02	Follicular cyst of left ovary ♀ ☑
N83.11	Corpus luteum cyst of right ovary ♀ ☑
N83.12	Corpus luteum cyst of left ovary ♀ ☑
N83.291	Other ovarian cyst, right side ♀ ☑
N83.292	Other ovarian cyst, left side ♀ ☑
N83.6	Hematosalpinx ♀
N83.8	Other noninflammatory disorders of ovary, fallopian tube and broad ligament ♀
N84.0	Polyp of corpus uteri ♀
N84.8	Polyp of other parts of female genital tract ♀
N85.01	Benign endometrial hyperplasia ♀
N85.02	Endometrial intraepithelial neoplasia [EIN] ♀
N85.2	Hypertrophy of uterus ♀

N85.7	Hematometra ♀
N85.8	Other specified noninflammatory disorders of uterus ♀
N87.0	Mild cervical dysplasia ♀
N87.1	Moderate cervical dysplasia ♀
N92.0	Excessive and frequent menstruation with regular cycle ♀
N92.1	Excessive and frequent menstruation with irregular cycle ♀
N92.5	Other specified irregular menstruation ♀
N93.8	Other specified abnormal uterine and vaginal bleeding ♀
N94.89	Other specified conditions associated with female genital organs and menstrual cycle ♀
N95.0	Postmenopausal bleeding ♀

AMA: **58150** 2019,Jul,6; 2018,Jan,8; 2017,Jan,8; 2016,Jan,13; 2015,Jan,16; 2014,Jan,11

Relative Value Units/Medicare Edits

Non-Facility RVU	Work	PE	MP	Total
58150	17.31	9.2	2.74	29.25
Facility RVU	Work	PE	MP	Total
58150	17.31	9.2	2.74	29.25

	FUD	Status	MUE	Modifiers				IOM Reference
58150	90	A	1(3)	51	N/A	62*	80	100-03,230.3

* with documentation

Terms To Know

adhesion. Abnormal fibrous connection between two structures, soft tissue or bony structures, that may occur as the result of surgery, infection, or trauma.

dysplasia. Abnormality or alteration in the size, shape, and organization of cells from their normal pattern of development.

endometriosis. Aberrant uterine mucosal tissue appearing in areas of the pelvic cavity outside of its normal location, lining the uterus, and inflaming surrounding tissues often resulting in infertility or spontaneous abortion.

hematometra. Accumulation of blood within the uterus.

hyperplasia. Abnormal proliferation in the number of normal cells in regular tissue arrangement.

peritonitis. Inflammation and infection within the peritoneal cavity, the space between the membrane lining the abdominopelvic walls and covering the internal organs.

polyp. Small growth on a stalk-like attachment projecting from a mucous membrane.

58152

58152 Total abdominal hysterectomy (corpus and cervix), with or without removal of tube(s), with or without removal of ovary(s); with colpo-urethrocystopexy (eg, Marshall-Marchetti-Krantz, Burch)

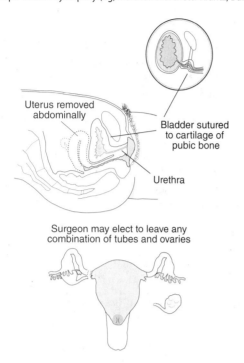

Uterus removed abdominally

Bladder sutured to cartilage of pubic bone

Urethra

Surgeon may elect to leave any combination of tubes and ovaries

Explanation

Through a horizontal incision just within the pubic hairline, the physician removes the uterus including the cervix and may elect to remove one or both of the ovaries and one or both of the fallopian tubes (salpingo-oophorectomy). The supporting pedicles containing the tubes, ligaments, and arteries are clamped and cut free. The uterus and cervix are removed. The bladder neck is suspended by placing sutures through the tissue surrounding the urethra and into the back of the symphysis pubis, which is the midline junction of the pubic bones in the front (Marshall-Marchetti-Krantz). The sutures are pulled tight so that the tissues are tacked to the symphysis pubis and the urethra is moved forward. The abdominal incision is closed by suturing.

Coding Tips

For a urethrocystopexy without hysterectomy, see 51840 and 51841.

ICD-10-CM Diagnostic Codes

C53.0	Malignant neoplasm of endocervix ♀
C53.1	Malignant neoplasm of exocervix ♀
C53.8	Malignant neoplasm of overlapping sites of cervix uteri ♀
C54.0	Malignant neoplasm of isthmus uteri ♀
C54.1	Malignant neoplasm of endometrium ♀
C54.2	Malignant neoplasm of myometrium ♀
C54.3	Malignant neoplasm of fundus uteri ♀
C54.8	Malignant neoplasm of overlapping sites of corpus uteri ♀
C56.1	Malignant neoplasm of right ovary ♀ ☑
C56.2	Malignant neoplasm of left ovary ♀ ☑
C57.01	Malignant neoplasm of right fallopian tube ♀ ☑
C57.02	Malignant neoplasm of left fallopian tube ♀ ☑
C57.11	Malignant neoplasm of right broad ligament ♀ ☑
C57.12	Malignant neoplasm of left broad ligament ♀ ☑
C57.21	Malignant neoplasm of right round ligament ♀ ☑
C57.22	Malignant neoplasm of left round ligament ♀ ☑
C57.3	Malignant neoplasm of parametrium ♀
C57.7	Malignant neoplasm of other specified female genital organs ♀
C57.8	Malignant neoplasm of overlapping sites of female genital organs ♀
C79.61	Secondary malignant neoplasm of right ovary ♀ ☑
C79.62	Secondary malignant neoplasm of left ovary ♀ ☑
C79.82	Secondary malignant neoplasm of genital organs
D06.0	Carcinoma in situ of endocervix ♀
D06.1	Carcinoma in situ of exocervix ♀
D06.7	Carcinoma in situ of other parts of cervix ♀
D07.0	Carcinoma in situ of endometrium ♀
D07.39	Carcinoma in situ of other female genital organs ♀
D25.0	Submucous leiomyoma of uterus ♀
D25.1	Intramural leiomyoma of uterus ♀
D25.2	Subserosal leiomyoma of uterus ♀
D39.0	Neoplasm of uncertain behavior of uterus ♀
D39.11	Neoplasm of uncertain behavior of right ovary ♀ ☑
D39.12	Neoplasm of uncertain behavior of left ovary ♀ ☑
D39.2	Neoplasm of uncertain behavior of placenta Ⓜ ♀
D39.8	Neoplasm of uncertain behavior of other specified female genital organs ♀
D49.59	Neoplasm of unspecified behavior of other genitourinary organ
N39.3	Stress incontinence (female) (male)
N70.01	Acute salpingitis ♀
N70.02	Acute oophoritis ♀
N70.03	Acute salpingitis and oophoritis ♀
N70.11	Chronic salpingitis ♀
N70.12	Chronic oophoritis ♀
N70.13	Chronic salpingitis and oophoritis ♀
N71.0	Acute inflammatory disease of uterus ♀
N71.1	Chronic inflammatory disease of uterus ♀
N72	Inflammatory disease of cervix uteri ♀
N73.0	Acute parametritis and pelvic cellulitis ♀
N73.1	Chronic parametritis and pelvic cellulitis ♀
N73.3	Female acute pelvic peritonitis ♀
N73.4	Female chronic pelvic peritonitis ♀
N73.6	Female pelvic peritoneal adhesions (postinfective) ♀
N73.8	Other specified female pelvic inflammatory diseases ♀
N80.0	Endometriosis of uterus ♀
N80.1	Endometriosis of ovary ♀
N80.2	Endometriosis of fallopian tube ♀
N81.2	Incomplete uterovaginal prolapse ♀
N81.3	Complete uterovaginal prolapse ♀
N81.89	Other female genital prolapse ♀
N83.01	Follicular cyst of right ovary ♀ ☑
N83.02	Follicular cyst of left ovary ♀ ☑
N83.11	Corpus luteum cyst of right ovary ♀ ☑
N83.12	Corpus luteum cyst of left ovary ♀ ☑
N83.291	Other ovarian cyst, right side ♀ ☑
N83.292	Other ovarian cyst, left side ♀ ☑

N83.6	Hematosalpinx ♀
N83.8	Other noninflammatory disorders of ovary, fallopian tube and broad ligament ♀
N84.0	Polyp of corpus uteri ♀
N84.8	Polyp of other parts of female genital tract ♀
N85.01	Benign endometrial hyperplasia ♀
N85.02	Endometrial intraepithelial neoplasia [EIN] ♀
N85.2	Hypertrophy of uterus ♀
N85.7	Hematometra ♀
N85.8	Other specified noninflammatory disorders of uterus ♀
N87.0	Mild cervical dysplasia ♀
N87.1	Moderate cervical dysplasia ♀
N92.0	Excessive and frequent menstruation with regular cycle ♀
N92.1	Excessive and frequent menstruation with irregular cycle ♀
N92.5	Other specified irregular menstruation ♀
N93.8	Other specified abnormal uterine and vaginal bleeding ♀
N94.89	Other specified conditions associated with female genital organs and menstrual cycle ♀
N95.0	Postmenopausal bleeding ♀

AMA: 58152 2019,Jul,6; 2018,Jan,8; 2017,Jan,8; 2016,Jan,13; 2015,Jan,16; 2014,Jan,11

Relative Value Units/Medicare Edits

Non-Facility RVU	Work	PE	MP	Total
58152	21.86	10.97	3.51	36.34
Facility RVU	**Work**	**PE**	**MP**	**Total**
58152	21.86	10.97	3.51	36.34

	FUD	Status	MUE	Modifiers				IOM Reference
58152	90	A	1(2)	51	N/A	62*	80	None

* with documentation

Terms To Know

carcinoma in situ. Malignancy that arises from the cells of the vessel, gland, or organ of origin that remains confined to that site or has not invaded neighboring tissue.

intramural. Within the wall of an organ.

leiomyoma. Benign tumor consisting of smooth muscle in the uterus.

malignant neoplasm. Any cancerous tumor or lesion exhibiting uncontrolled tissue growth that can progressively invade other parts of the body with its disease-generating cells.

secondary. Second in order of occurrence or importance, or appearing during the course of another disease or condition.

58180

58180   Supracervical abdominal hysterectomy (subtotal hysterectomy), with or without removal of tube(s), with or without removal of ovary(s)

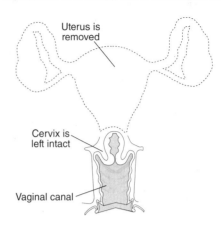

Uterus is removed

Cervix is left intact

Vaginal canal

Surgeon may elect to leave any combination of tubes and ovaries

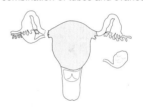

Explanation

Through a horizontal incision just within the pubic hairline, the physician removes the uterus above the cervix and may elect to remove one or both of the ovaries and one or both of the fallopian tubes (salpingo-oophorectomy). The supporting pedicles containing the tubes, ligaments, and arteries are clamped and cut free. The uterus is cut free from the cervix leaving the cervix still attached to the vagina. The abdominal incision is closed by suturing.

Coding Tips

When 58180 is performed with another separately identifiable procedure, the highest dollar value code is listed as the primary procedure and subsequent procedures are appended with modifier 51. For excision of a remaining cervical stump, see 57540–57556.

ICD-10-CM Diagnostic Codes

C54.0	Malignant neoplasm of isthmus uteri ♀
C54.1	Malignant neoplasm of endometrium ♀
C54.2	Malignant neoplasm of myometrium ♀
C54.3	Malignant neoplasm of fundus uteri ♀
C54.8	Malignant neoplasm of overlapping sites of corpus uteri ♀
C56.1	Malignant neoplasm of right ovary ♀ ☑
C56.2	Malignant neoplasm of left ovary ♀ ☑
C57.01	Malignant neoplasm of right fallopian tube ♀ ☑
C57.02	Malignant neoplasm of left fallopian tube ♀ ☑
C57.11	Malignant neoplasm of right broad ligament ♀ ☑
C57.12	Malignant neoplasm of left broad ligament ♀ ☑
C57.21	Malignant neoplasm of right round ligament ♀ ☑
C57.22	Malignant neoplasm of left round ligament ♀ ☑
C57.3	Malignant neoplasm of parametrium ♀
C57.7	Malignant neoplasm of other specified female genital organs ♀

C57.8	Malignant neoplasm of overlapping sites of female genital organs ♀
C79.61	Secondary malignant neoplasm of right ovary ♀ ☑
C79.62	Secondary malignant neoplasm of left ovary ♀ ☑
C79.82	Secondary malignant neoplasm of genital organs
D07.0	Carcinoma in situ of endometrium ♀
D07.39	Carcinoma in situ of other female genital organs ♀
D25.0	Submucous leiomyoma of uterus ♀
D25.1	Intramural leiomyoma of uterus ♀
D25.2	Subserosal leiomyoma of uterus ♀
D39.0	Neoplasm of uncertain behavior of uterus ♀
D39.11	Neoplasm of uncertain behavior of right ovary ♀ ☑
D39.12	Neoplasm of uncertain behavior of left ovary ♀ ☑
D39.2	Neoplasm of uncertain behavior of placenta Ⓜ ♀
D39.8	Neoplasm of uncertain behavior of other specified female genital organs ♀
D49.59	Neoplasm of unspecified behavior of other genitourinary organ
N39.3	Stress incontinence (female) (male)
N70.01	Acute salpingitis ♀
N70.02	Acute oophoritis ♀
N70.03	Acute salpingitis and oophoritis ♀
N70.11	Chronic salpingitis ♀
N70.12	Chronic oophoritis ♀
N70.13	Chronic salpingitis and oophoritis ♀
N71.0	Acute inflammatory disease of uterus ♀
N71.1	Chronic inflammatory disease of uterus ♀
N73.0	Acute parametritis and pelvic cellulitis ♀
N73.1	Chronic parametritis and pelvic cellulitis ♀
N73.3	Female acute pelvic peritonitis ♀
N73.4	Female chronic pelvic peritonitis ♀
N73.6	Female pelvic peritoneal adhesions (postinfective) ♀
N73.8	Other specified female pelvic inflammatory diseases ♀
N80.0	Endometriosis of uterus ♀
N80.1	Endometriosis of ovary ♀
N80.2	Endometriosis of fallopian tube ♀
N81.2	Incomplete uterovaginal prolapse ♀
N81.3	Complete uterovaginal prolapse ♀
N81.89	Other female genital prolapse ♀
N83.01	Follicular cyst of right ovary ♀ ☑
N83.02	Follicular cyst of left ovary ♀ ☑
N83.11	Corpus luteum cyst of right ovary ♀ ☑
N83.12	Corpus luteum cyst of left ovary ♀ ☑
N83.291	Other ovarian cyst, right side ♀ ☑
N83.292	Other ovarian cyst, left side ♀ ☑
N83.6	Hematosalpinx ♀
N83.8	Other noninflammatory disorders of ovary, fallopian tube and broad ligament ♀
N84.0	Polyp of corpus uteri ♀
N84.8	Polyp of other parts of female genital tract ♀
N85.01	Benign endometrial hyperplasia ♀
N85.02	Endometrial intraepithelial neoplasia [EIN] ♀
N85.2	Hypertrophy of uterus ♀
N85.7	Hematometra ♀
N85.8	Other specified noninflammatory disorders of uterus ♀
N87.0	Mild cervical dysplasia ♀
N87.1	Moderate cervical dysplasia ♀
N92.0	Excessive and frequent menstruation with regular cycle ♀
N92.1	Excessive and frequent menstruation with irregular cycle ♀
N92.5	Other specified irregular menstruation ♀
N93.8	Other specified abnormal uterine and vaginal bleeding ♀
N94.89	Other specified conditions associated with female genital organs and menstrual cycle ♀
N95.0	Postmenopausal bleeding ♀

AMA: **58180** 2019,Jul,6; 2014,Jan,11

Relative Value Units/Medicare Edits

Non-Facility RVU	Work	PE	MP	Total
58180	16.6	8.63	2.61	27.84
Facility RVU	**Work**	**PE**	**MP**	**Total**
58180	16.6	8.63	2.61	27.84

	FUD	Status	MUE	Modifiers				IOM Reference
58180	90	A	1(3)	51	N/A	62*	80	None

* with documentation

Terms To Know

submucous uterine leiomyoma. Benign, smooth muscle tumor beneath the inner lining of the uterus.

subserous uterine leiomyoma. Benign, smooth muscle tumor beneath the serous membrane lining of the uterus.

58200

58200 Total abdominal hysterectomy, including partial vaginectomy, with para-aortic and pelvic lymph node sampling, with or without removal of tube(s), with or without removal of ovary(s)

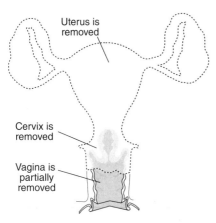

Uterus is removed

Cervix is removed

Vagina is partially removed

Surgeon may elect to leave any combination of tubes and ovaries

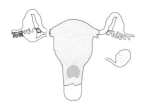

Explanation

Through a horizontal incision just within the pubic hairline, the physician removes the uterus, including the cervix and part of the vagina. The supporting pedicles containing the tubes, ligaments and arteries are clamped and cut free and the uterus, cervix, and part of the vagina are removed. A biopsy is taken of the para-aortic and pelvic lymph nodes. The physician may elect to remove one or both of the ovaries and one or both of the fallopian tubes (salpingo-oophorectomy). The abdominal incision is closed by suturing.

Coding Tips

Removal of the tubes and ovaries is included in this procedure and should not be reported separately. For a hysterectomy with pelvic lymphadenectomy, see 58210. Several hysterectomy codes exist, see 58150–58294 for open procedures and 58541–58554 and 58570–58575 for a laparoscopic vaginal hysterectomy.

ICD-10-CM Diagnostic Codes

C52	Malignant neoplasm of vagina ♀
C53.0	Malignant neoplasm of endocervix ♀
C53.1	Malignant neoplasm of exocervix ♀
C53.8	Malignant neoplasm of overlapping sites of cervix uteri ♀
C54.0	Malignant neoplasm of isthmus uteri ♀
C54.1	Malignant neoplasm of endometrium ♀
C54.2	Malignant neoplasm of myometrium ♀
C54.3	Malignant neoplasm of fundus uteri ♀
C54.8	Malignant neoplasm of overlapping sites of corpus uteri ♀
C56.1	Malignant neoplasm of right ovary ♀ ☑
C56.2	Malignant neoplasm of left ovary ♀ ☑
C57.01	Malignant neoplasm of right fallopian tube ♀ ☑
C57.02	Malignant neoplasm of left fallopian tube ♀ ☑
C57.11	Malignant neoplasm of right broad ligament ♀ ☑
C57.12	Malignant neoplasm of left broad ligament ♀ ☑
C57.21	Malignant neoplasm of right round ligament ♀ ☑
C57.22	Malignant neoplasm of left round ligament ♀ ☑
C57.3	Malignant neoplasm of parametrium ♀
C57.7	Malignant neoplasm of other specified female genital organs ♀
C57.8	Malignant neoplasm of overlapping sites of female genital organs ♀
C77.2	Secondary and unspecified malignant neoplasm of intra-abdominal lymph nodes
C77.5	Secondary and unspecified malignant neoplasm of intrapelvic lymph nodes
C79.61	Secondary malignant neoplasm of right ovary ♀ ☑
C79.62	Secondary malignant neoplasm of left ovary ♀ ☑
C79.82	Secondary malignant neoplasm of genital organs
D06.0	Carcinoma in situ of endocervix ♀
D06.1	Carcinoma in situ of exocervix ♀
D06.7	Carcinoma in situ of other parts of cervix ♀
D07.0	Carcinoma in situ of endometrium ♀
D07.39	Carcinoma in situ of other female genital organs ♀
D25.0	Submucous leiomyoma of uterus ♀
D25.1	Intramural leiomyoma of uterus ♀
D25.2	Subserosal leiomyoma of uterus ♀
D39.0	Neoplasm of uncertain behavior of uterus ♀
D39.11	Neoplasm of uncertain behavior of right ovary ♀ ☑
D39.12	Neoplasm of uncertain behavior of left ovary ♀ ☑
D39.2	Neoplasm of uncertain behavior of placenta Ⓜ ♀
D39.8	Neoplasm of uncertain behavior of other specified female genital organs ♀
D49.59	Neoplasm of unspecified behavior of other genitourinary organ
N70.01	Acute salpingitis ♀
N70.02	Acute oophoritis ♀
N70.03	Acute salpingitis and oophoritis ♀
N70.11	Chronic salpingitis ♀
N70.12	Chronic oophoritis ♀
N70.13	Chronic salpingitis and oophoritis ♀
N71.0	Acute inflammatory disease of uterus ♀
N71.1	Chronic inflammatory disease of uterus ♀
N72	Inflammatory disease of cervix uteri ♀
N73.0	Acute parametritis and pelvic cellulitis ♀
N73.1	Chronic parametritis and pelvic cellulitis ♀
N73.3	Female acute pelvic peritonitis ♀
N73.4	Female chronic pelvic peritonitis ♀
N73.6	Female pelvic peritoneal adhesions (postinfective) ♀
N73.8	Other specified female pelvic inflammatory diseases ♀
N80.0	Endometriosis of uterus ♀
N80.1	Endometriosis of ovary ♀
N80.2	Endometriosis of fallopian tube ♀
N81.2	Incomplete uterovaginal prolapse ♀
N81.3	Complete uterovaginal prolapse ♀
N81.89	Other female genital prolapse ♀
N83.01	Follicular cyst of right ovary ♀ ☑

N83.02	Follicular cyst of left ovary ♀ ☑	
N83.11	Corpus luteum cyst of right ovary ♀ ☑	
N83.12	Corpus luteum cyst of left ovary ♀ ☑	
N83.291	Other ovarian cyst, right side ♀ ☑	
N83.292	Other ovarian cyst, left side ♀ ☑	
N83.6	Hematosalpinx ♀	
N83.8	Other noninflammatory disorders of ovary, fallopian tube and broad ligament ♀	
N84.0	Polyp of corpus uteri ♀	
N84.8	Polyp of other parts of female genital tract ♀	
N85.01	Benign endometrial hyperplasia ♀	
N85.02	Endometrial intraepithelial neoplasia [EIN] ♀	
N85.2	Hypertrophy of uterus ♀	
N85.7	Hematometra ♀	
N85.8	Other specified noninflammatory disorders of uterus ♀	
N87.0	Mild cervical dysplasia ♀	
N87.1	Moderate cervical dysplasia ♀	
N92.0	Excessive and frequent menstruation with regular cycle ♀	
N92.1	Excessive and frequent menstruation with irregular cycle ♀	
N92.5	Other specified irregular menstruation ♀	
N93.8	Other specified abnormal uterine and vaginal bleeding ♀	
N94.89	Other specified conditions associated with female genital organs and menstrual cycle ♀	
N95.0	Postmenopausal bleeding ♀	

AMA: 58200 2019,Jul,6; 2014,Jan,11

Relative Value Units/Medicare Edits

Non-Facility RVU	Work	PE	MP	Total
58200	23.1	12.31	3.62	39.03
Facility RVU	**Work**	**PE**	**MP**	**Total**
58200	23.1	12.31	3.62	39.03

	FUD	Status	MUE	Modifiers				IOM Reference
58200	90	A	1(2)	51	N/A	62*	80	None

* with documentation

Terms To Know

lymph nodes. Bean-shaped structures along the lymphatic vessels that intercept and destroy foreign materials in the tissue and bloodstream.

salpingo-oophorectomy. Surgical removal of both the fallopian tube and ovary.

vaginectomy. Surgical excision of all or a portion of the vagina.

58210

58210 Radical abdominal hysterectomy, with bilateral total pelvic lymphadenectomy and para-aortic lymph node sampling (biopsy), with or without removal of tube(s), with or without removal of ovary(s)

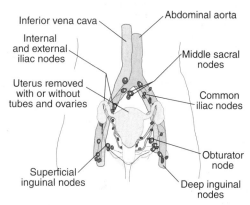

Explanation

Through a horizontal incision just within the pubic hairline, the physician removes the uterus, including the cervix and the pelvic lymph nodes on both sides and takes a biopsy of the para-aortic lymph nodes. The supporting pedicles containing the tubes, ligaments, and arteries are clamped and cut free and the uterus, cervix, all or part of the vagina, and all pelvic lymph nodes are removed. The physician may elect to remove one or both of the ovaries and one or both of the fallopian tubes (salpingo-oophorectomy). The abdominal incision is closed by suturing.

Coding Tips

For total abdominal hysterectomy, with or without removal of a tube(s) and/or ovary(s), see 58150. Report ovarian transposition with 58825, when performed.

ICD-10-CM Diagnostic Codes

C51.8	Malignant neoplasm of overlapping sites of vulva ♀
C52	Malignant neoplasm of vagina ♀
C53.0	Malignant neoplasm of endocervix ♀
C53.1	Malignant neoplasm of exocervix ♀
C53.8	Malignant neoplasm of overlapping sites of cervix uteri ♀
C54.0	Malignant neoplasm of isthmus uteri ♀
C54.1	Malignant neoplasm of endometrium ♀
C54.2	Malignant neoplasm of myometrium ♀
C54.3	Malignant neoplasm of fundus uteri ♀
C54.8	Malignant neoplasm of overlapping sites of corpus uteri ♀
C56.1	Malignant neoplasm of right ovary ♀ ☑
C56.2	Malignant neoplasm of left ovary ♀ ☑
C57.01	Malignant neoplasm of right fallopian tube ♀ ☑
C57.02	Malignant neoplasm of left fallopian tube ♀ ☑
C57.11	Malignant neoplasm of right broad ligament ♀ ☑
C57.12	Malignant neoplasm of left broad ligament ♀ ☑
C57.21	Malignant neoplasm of right round ligament ♀ ☑
C57.22	Malignant neoplasm of left round ligament ♀ ☑
C57.3	Malignant neoplasm of parametrium ♀
C57.7	Malignant neoplasm of other specified female genital organs ♀

C57.8	Malignant neoplasm of overlapping sites of female genital organs ♀	
C77.2	Secondary and unspecified malignant neoplasm of intra-abdominal lymph nodes	
C77.5	Secondary and unspecified malignant neoplasm of intrapelvic lymph nodes	
C79.61	Secondary malignant neoplasm of right ovary ♀ ☑	
C79.62	Secondary malignant neoplasm of left ovary ♀ ☑	
C79.82	Secondary malignant neoplasm of genital organs	
D06.0	Carcinoma in situ of endocervix ♀	
D06.1	Carcinoma in situ of exocervix ♀	
D06.7	Carcinoma in situ of other parts of cervix ♀	
D07.0	Carcinoma in situ of endometrium ♀	
D07.39	Carcinoma in situ of other female genital organs ♀	
D25.0	Submucous leiomyoma of uterus ♀	
D25.1	Intramural leiomyoma of uterus ♀	
D25.2	Subserosal leiomyoma of uterus ♀	
D39.0	Neoplasm of uncertain behavior of uterus ♀	
D39.11	Neoplasm of uncertain behavior of right ovary ♀ ☑	
D39.12	Neoplasm of uncertain behavior of left ovary ♀ ☑	
D39.2	Neoplasm of uncertain behavior of placenta 🔲 ♀	
D39.8	Neoplasm of uncertain behavior of other specified female genital organs ♀	
D49.59	Neoplasm of unspecified behavior of other genitourinary organ	
N70.01	Acute salpingitis ♀	
N70.02	Acute oophoritis ♀	
N70.03	Acute salpingitis and oophoritis ♀	
N70.11	Chronic salpingitis ♀	
N70.12	Chronic oophoritis ♀	
N70.13	Chronic salpingitis and oophoritis ♀	
N71.0	Acute inflammatory disease of uterus ♀	
N71.1	Chronic inflammatory disease of uterus ♀	
N72	Inflammatory disease of cervix uteri ♀	
N73.0	Acute parametritis and pelvic cellulitis ♀	
N73.1	Chronic parametritis and pelvic cellulitis ♀	
N73.3	Female acute pelvic peritonitis ♀	
N73.4	Female chronic pelvic peritonitis ♀	
N73.6	Female pelvic peritoneal adhesions (postinfective) ♀	
N73.8	Other specified female pelvic inflammatory diseases ♀	
N80.0	Endometriosis of uterus ♀	
N80.1	Endometriosis of ovary ♀	
N80.2	Endometriosis of fallopian tube ♀	
N81.2	Incomplete uterovaginal prolapse ♀	
N81.3	Complete uterovaginal prolapse ♀	
N81.89	Other female genital prolapse ♀	
N83.01	Follicular cyst of right ovary ♀ ☑	
N83.02	Follicular cyst of left ovary ♀ ☑	
N83.11	Corpus luteum cyst of right ovary ♀ ☑	
N83.12	Corpus luteum cyst of left ovary ♀ ☑	
N83.291	Other ovarian cyst, right side ♀ ☑	
N83.292	Other ovarian cyst, left side ♀ ☑	
N83.6	Hematosalpinx ♀	

N83.8	Other noninflammatory disorders of ovary, fallopian tube and broad ligament ♀	
N84.0	Polyp of corpus uteri ♀	
N84.8	Polyp of other parts of female genital tract ♀	
N85.01	Benign endometrial hyperplasia ♀	
N85.02	Endometrial intraepithelial neoplasia [EIN] ♀	
N85.2	Hypertrophy of uterus ♀	
N85.7	Hematometra ♀	
N85.8	Other specified noninflammatory disorders of uterus ♀	
N87.0	Mild cervical dysplasia ♀	
N87.1	Moderate cervical dysplasia ♀	
N92.0	Excessive and frequent menstruation with regular cycle ♀	
N92.1	Excessive and frequent menstruation with irregular cycle ♀	
N92.5	Other specified irregular menstruation ♀	
N93.8	Other specified abnormal uterine and vaginal bleeding ♀	
N94.89	Other specified conditions associated with female genital organs and menstrual cycle ♀	
N95.0	Postmenopausal bleeding ♀	

AMA: **58210** 2019,Jul,6; 2018,Jan,8; 2017,Jan,8; 2016,Jan,13; 2015,Jan,16; 2014,Jan,11

Relative Value Units/Medicare Edits

Non-Facility RVU	Work	PE	MP	Total
58210	30.91	16.54	4.92	52.37
Facility RVU	**Work**	**PE**	**MP**	**Total**
58210	30.91	16.54	4.92	52.37

	FUD	Status	MUE	Modifiers				IOM Reference
58210	90	A	1(2)	51	N/A	62*	80	None

* with documentation

Terms To Know

benign. Mild or nonmalignant in nature.

biopsy. Tissue or fluid removed for diagnostic purposes through analysis of the cells in the biopsy material.

dysplasia. Abnormality or alteration in the size, shape, and organization of cells from their normal pattern of development.

hyperplasia. Abnormal proliferation in the number of normal cells in regular tissue arrangement.

lymph nodes. Bean-shaped structures along the lymphatic vessels that intercept and destroy foreign materials in the tissue and bloodstream.

malignant neoplasm. Any cancerous tumor or lesion exhibiting uncontrolled tissue growth that can progressively invade other parts of the body with its disease-generating cells.

58240

58240 Pelvic exenteration for gynecologic malignancy, with total abdominal hysterectomy or cervicectomy, with or without removal of tube(s), with or without removal of ovary(s), with removal of bladder and ureteral transplantations, and/or abdominoperineal resection of rectum and colon and colostomy, or any combination thereof

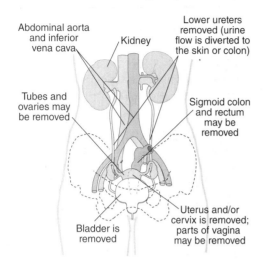

Abdominal aorta and inferior vena cava

Kidney

Lower ureters removed (urine flow is diverted to the skin or colon)

Tubes and ovaries may be removed

Sigmoid colon and rectum may be removed

Bladder is removed

Uterus and/or cervix is removed; parts of vagina may be removed

Explanation

Through a horizontal incision just within the pubic hairline, the physician removes all of the organs and adjacent structures of the pelvis including the cervix, uterus, and all or part of the vagina. The supporting pedicles containing the tubes, ligaments, and arteries are clamped and cut free and the uterus, cervix, and all or part of the vagina are removed. The physician may remove one or both of the ovaries and one or both of the fallopian tubes (salpingo-oophorectomy). The physician removes the bladder and diverts urine flow by transplanting the ureters to the skin or colon. The rectum and part of the colon may be removed and an artificial abdominal opening in the skin surface created for waste (colostomy). The abdominal incision is closed by suturing.

Coding Tips

Report 51597 for a pelvic exenteration for malignancy of the lower urinary tract. Check diagnoses carefully to ensure metastases are reported correctly.

ICD-10-CM Diagnostic Codes

C51.8	Malignant neoplasm of overlapping sites of vulva ♀
C52	Malignant neoplasm of vagina ♀
C53.0	Malignant neoplasm of endocervix ♀
C53.1	Malignant neoplasm of exocervix ♀
C53.8	Malignant neoplasm of overlapping sites of cervix uteri ♀
C54.0	Malignant neoplasm of isthmus uteri ♀
C54.1	Malignant neoplasm of endometrium ♀
C54.2	Malignant neoplasm of myometrium ♀
C54.3	Malignant neoplasm of fundus uteri ♀
C54.8	Malignant neoplasm of overlapping sites of corpus uteri ♀
C56.1	Malignant neoplasm of right ovary ♀ ☑
C56.2	Malignant neoplasm of left ovary ♀ ☑
C57.01	Malignant neoplasm of right fallopian tube ♀ ☑
C57.02	Malignant neoplasm of left fallopian tube ♀ ☑
C57.11	Malignant neoplasm of right broad ligament ♀ ☑
C57.12	Malignant neoplasm of left broad ligament ♀ ☑
C57.21	Malignant neoplasm of right round ligament ♀ ☑
C57.22	Malignant neoplasm of left round ligament ♀ ☑
C57.3	Malignant neoplasm of parametrium ♀
C57.7	Malignant neoplasm of other specified female genital organs ♀
C57.8	Malignant neoplasm of overlapping sites of female genital organs ♀
C79.61	Secondary malignant neoplasm of right ovary ♀ ☑
C79.62	Secondary malignant neoplasm of left ovary ♀ ☑
C79.82	Secondary malignant neoplasm of genital organs

AMA: **58240** 2019,Jul,6; 2014,Jan,11

Relative Value Units/Medicare Edits

Non-Facility RVU	Work	PE	MP	Total
58240	49.33	26.73	7.75	83.81
Facility RVU	**Work**	**PE**	**MP**	**Total**
58240	49.33	26.73	7.75	83.81

	FUD	Status	MUE	Modifiers				IOM Reference
58240	90	A	1(2)	51	N/A	62*	80	None

* with documentation

Terms To Know

exenteration. Surgical removal of the entire contents of a body cavity, such as the pelvis or orbit.

hysterectomy. Surgical removal of the uterus. A complete hysterectomy may also include removal of tubes and ovaries.

malignant. Any condition tending to progress toward death, specifically an invasive tumor with a loss of cellular differentiation that has the ability to spread or metastasize to other body areas.

resection. Surgical removal of a part or all of an organ or body part.

58260

58260 Vaginal hysterectomy, for uterus 250 g or less;

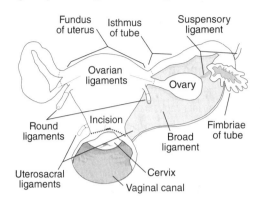

Explanation

The physician performs a vaginal hysterectomy for a uterus 250 gm or less. An incision is made around the cervix through the full thickness of the vaginal membrane. The cut vaginal edge is pulled toward the lower cervix and vaginal dissection is continued with countertraction. The posterior peritoneum is opened to admit a finger examination of the pelvis. The uterosacral ligaments are clamped and possibly shortened, cut from the uterus, and secured to the vagina. The vesicovaginal space is entered. The connective tissue fusing the bladder and vagina is dissected and the bladder is separated from the cervix. The bladder pillars are clamped, cut, and ligated near their cervical attachments, as well as the cardinal ligament tissue on each side of the cervix and the left and right uterine vessels. The physician clamps, cuts, and ligates the upper cardinal and lower broad ligament complex. Traction applied to the cervix moves the uterus down until the fundus is low in the pelvis. Hemostats are applied to the angle of the uterus on each side and the uterus is removed. The peritoneum is closed with purse-string sutures that incorporate the proximal part of the uterosacral ligaments.

Coding Tips

When the tubes and ovaries are also removed, see 58262–58263. For vaginal hysterectomy for a uterus greater than 250 grams, see 58290–58294. For laparoscopy with vaginal hysterectomy for a uterus 250 grams or less, see 58550.

ICD-10-CM Diagnostic Codes

C53.0	Malignant neoplasm of endocervix ♀
C53.1	Malignant neoplasm of exocervix ♀
C53.8	Malignant neoplasm of overlapping sites of cervix uteri ♀
C54.0	Malignant neoplasm of isthmus uteri ♀
C54.1	Malignant neoplasm of endometrium ♀
C54.2	Malignant neoplasm of myometrium ♀
C54.3	Malignant neoplasm of fundus uteri ♀
C54.8	Malignant neoplasm of overlapping sites of corpus uteri ♀
C57.11	Malignant neoplasm of right broad ligament ♀ ☑
C57.12	Malignant neoplasm of left broad ligament ♀ ☑
C57.21	Malignant neoplasm of right round ligament ♀ ☑
C57.22	Malignant neoplasm of left round ligament ♀ ☑
C57.3	Malignant neoplasm of parametrium ♀
C79.82	Secondary malignant neoplasm of genital organs
D06.0	Carcinoma in situ of endocervix ♀
D06.1	Carcinoma in situ of exocervix ♀
D06.7	Carcinoma in situ of other parts of cervix ♀
D07.0	Carcinoma in situ of endometrium ♀
D25.0	Submucous leiomyoma of uterus ♀
D25.1	Intramural leiomyoma of uterus ♀
D25.2	Subserosal leiomyoma of uterus ♀
D39.0	Neoplasm of uncertain behavior of uterus ♀
D39.2	Neoplasm of uncertain behavior of placenta Ⓜ ♀
N71.0	Acute inflammatory disease of uterus ♀
N71.1	Chronic inflammatory disease of uterus ♀
N72	Inflammatory disease of cervix uteri ♀
N73.0	Acute parametritis and pelvic cellulitis ♀
N73.1	Chronic parametritis and pelvic cellulitis ♀
N73.3	Female acute pelvic peritonitis ♀
N73.4	Female chronic pelvic peritonitis ♀
N73.6	Female pelvic peritoneal adhesions (postinfective) ♀
N80.0	Endometriosis of uterus ♀
N81.2	Incomplete uterovaginal prolapse ♀
N81.3	Complete uterovaginal prolapse ♀
N84.0	Polyp of corpus uteri ♀
N84.8	Polyp of other parts of female genital tract ♀
N85.01	Benign endometrial hyperplasia ♀
N85.02	Endometrial intraepithelial neoplasia [EIN] ♀
N85.2	Hypertrophy of uterus ♀
N85.7	Hematometra ♀
N87.0	Mild cervical dysplasia ♀
N87.1	Moderate cervical dysplasia ♀
N92.0	Excessive and frequent menstruation with regular cycle ♀
N92.1	Excessive and frequent menstruation with irregular cycle ♀
N95.0	Postmenopausal bleeding ♀

AMA: 58260 2019,Jul,6; 2018,Jan,8; 2017,Jan,8; 2016,Jan,13; 2015,Jan,16; 2014,Jan,11

Relative Value Units/Medicare Edits

Non-Facility RVU	Work	PE	MP	Total
58260	14.15	7.85	2.2	24.2
Facility RVU	**Work**	**PE**	**MP**	**Total**
58260	14.15	7.85	2.2	24.2

	FUD	Status	MUE	Modifiers				IOM Reference
58260	90	A	1(3)	51	N/A	62*	80	None

* with documentation

Terms To Know

carcinoma in situ. Malignancy that arises from the cells of the vessel, gland, or organ of origin that remains confined to that site or has not invaded neighboring tissue.

endometriosis. Aberrant uterine mucosal tissue appearing in areas of the pelvic cavity outside of its normal location, lining the uterus, and inflaming surrounding tissues often resulting in infertility or spontaneous abortion.

58262-58263

58262 Vaginal hysterectomy, for uterus 250 g or less; with removal of tube(s), and/or ovary(s)

58263 with removal of tube(s), and/or ovary(s), with repair of enterocele

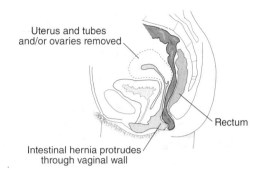

Uterus and tubes and/or ovaries removed

Rectum

Intestinal hernia protrudes through vaginal wall

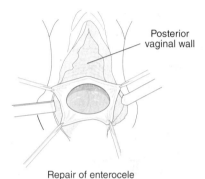

Posterior vaginal wall

Repair of enterocele

Explanation

The physician performs a vaginal hysterectomy for a uterus 250 gm or less and removes the tubes and/or ovaries. An incision is made around the cervix through the full thickness of the vaginal membrane. The cut vaginal edge is pulled toward the lower cervix and vaginal dissection is continued with countertraction. The posterior peritoneum is opened to admit a finger examination of the pelvis. The uterosacral ligaments are clamped and possibly shortened, cut from the uterus, and secured to the vagina. The vesicovaginal space is entered. The connective tissue fusing the bladder and vagina is dissected and the bladder is separated from the cervix. The bladder pillars are clamped, cut, and ligated near their cervical attachments, as well as the cardinal ligament tissue on each side of the cervix and the left and right uterine vessels. The physician clamps, cuts, and ligates the upper cardinal and lower broad ligament complex. Traction applied to the cervix moves the uterus down until the fundus is low in the pelvis. Hemostats are applied to the angle of the uterus on each side and the uterus is removed. After the uterus is exteriorized, care is taken to ensure ligation of the ovarian vessels. The ovary is excised under direct vision. For removal of both tubes and ovaries, the round ligament on one side at a time is clamped and divided. A tunnel is made through the layers of the uterine broad ligament that enclose the tube and the tube and ovary are clamped together. The structure is pulled forward, the two sheets of the broad ligament are each cut, and the broad ligament is opened completely. The whole specimen is separated from its attaching ligament, which is clamped, and the tube and ovary on that side are removed. Report 58263 if an enterocele is repaired in addition to removing the tube and/or ovary. An enterocele is a hernia of the intestine protruding against the vaginal wall. The hernia sac is bluntly and sharply dissected from the surrounding connective tissue, excised and ligated, and the surrounding tissues are strengthened and sutured. The peritoneal and vaginal wall incisions of the hysterectomy procedure are closed.

Coding Tips

These codes include removal of tubes and ovaries and should not be reported separately. Enterocele repair is included in 58263 and should not be reported separately. For a hysterectomy only, see 58260. For other vaginal hysterectomy codes, see 58267–58294. For laparoscopy with vaginal hysterectomy for a uterus 250 grams or less, see 58550; with removal of tubes and/or ovaries, see 58552.

ICD-10-CM Diagnostic Codes

C53.0	Malignant neoplasm of endocervix ♀
C53.1	Malignant neoplasm of exocervix ♀
C53.8	Malignant neoplasm of overlapping sites of cervix uteri ♀
C54.0	Malignant neoplasm of isthmus uteri ♀
C54.1	Malignant neoplasm of endometrium ♀
C54.2	Malignant neoplasm of myometrium ♀
C54.3	Malignant neoplasm of fundus uteri ♀
C54.8	Malignant neoplasm of overlapping sites of corpus uteri ♀
C56.1	Malignant neoplasm of right ovary ♀ ☑
C56.2	Malignant neoplasm of left ovary ♀ ☑
C57.01	Malignant neoplasm of right fallopian tube ♀ ☑
C57.02	Malignant neoplasm of left fallopian tube ♀ ☑
C57.11	Malignant neoplasm of right broad ligament ♀ ☑
C57.12	Malignant neoplasm of left broad ligament ♀ ☑
C57.21	Malignant neoplasm of right round ligament ♀ ☑
C57.22	Malignant neoplasm of left round ligament ♀ ☑
C57.3	Malignant neoplasm of parametrium ♀
C57.7	Malignant neoplasm of other specified female genital organs ♀
C57.8	Malignant neoplasm of overlapping sites of female genital organs ♀
C79.61	Secondary malignant neoplasm of right ovary ♀ ☑
C79.62	Secondary malignant neoplasm of left ovary ♀ ☑
C79.82	Secondary malignant neoplasm of genital organs
D06.0	Carcinoma in situ of endocervix ♀
D06.1	Carcinoma in situ of exocervix ♀
D06.7	Carcinoma in situ of other parts of cervix ♀
D07.0	Carcinoma in situ of endometrium ♀
D07.39	Carcinoma in situ of other female genital organs ♀
D25.0	Submucous leiomyoma of uterus ♀
D25.1	Intramural leiomyoma of uterus ♀
D25.2	Subserosal leiomyoma of uterus ♀
D39.0	Neoplasm of uncertain behavior of uterus ♀
D39.11	Neoplasm of uncertain behavior of right ovary ♀ ☑
D39.12	Neoplasm of uncertain behavior of left ovary ♀ ☑
D39.2	Neoplasm of uncertain behavior of placenta Ⓜ ♀
D39.8	Neoplasm of uncertain behavior of other specified female genital organs ♀
D49.59	Neoplasm of unspecified behavior of other genitourinary organ
N70.01	Acute salpingitis ♀
N70.02	Acute oophoritis ♀
N70.03	Acute salpingitis and oophoritis ♀
N70.11	Chronic salpingitis ♀
N70.12	Chronic oophoritis ♀
N70.13	Chronic salpingitis and oophoritis ♀
N71.0	Acute inflammatory disease of uterus ♀

N71.1	Chronic inflammatory disease of uterus ♀			
N72	Inflammatory disease of cervix uteri ♀			
N73.0	Acute parametritis and pelvic cellulitis ♀			
N73.1	Chronic parametritis and pelvic cellulitis ♀			
N73.3	Female acute pelvic peritonitis ♀			
N73.4	Female chronic pelvic peritonitis ♀			
N73.6	Female pelvic peritoneal adhesions (postinfective) ♀			
N73.8	Other specified female pelvic inflammatory diseases ♀			
N80.0	Endometriosis of uterus ♀			
N80.1	Endometriosis of ovary ♀			
N80.2	Endometriosis of fallopian tube ♀			
N81.2	Incomplete uterovaginal prolapse ♀			
N81.3	Complete uterovaginal prolapse ♀			
N81.5	Vaginal enterocele ♀			
N81.89	Other female genital prolapse ♀			
N83.01	Follicular cyst of right ovary ♀ ☑			
N83.02	Follicular cyst of left ovary ♀ ☑			
N83.11	Corpus luteum cyst of right ovary ♀ ☑			
N83.12	Corpus luteum cyst of left ovary ♀ ☑			
N83.291	Other ovarian cyst, right side ♀ ☑			
N83.292	Other ovarian cyst, left side ♀ ☑			
N83.6	Hematosalpinx ♀			
N83.8	Other noninflammatory disorders of ovary, fallopian tube and broad ligament ♀			
N84.0	Polyp of corpus uteri ♀			
N84.8	Polyp of other parts of female genital tract ♀			
N85.01	Benign endometrial hyperplasia ♀			
N85.02	Endometrial intraepithelial neoplasia [EIN] ♀			
N85.2	Hypertrophy of uterus ♀			
N85.7	Hematometra ♀			
N85.8	Other specified noninflammatory disorders of uterus ♀			
N87.0	Mild cervical dysplasia ♀			
N87.1	Moderate cervical dysplasia ♀			
N92.0	Excessive and frequent menstruation with regular cycle ♀			
N92.1	Excessive and frequent menstruation with irregular cycle ♀			
N92.5	Other specified irregular menstruation ♀			
N93.8	Other specified abnormal uterine and vaginal bleeding ♀			
N94.89	Other specified conditions associated with female genital organs and menstrual cycle ♀			
N95.0	Postmenopausal bleeding ♀			

AMA: **58262** 2019,Jul,6; 2014,Jan,11 **58263** 2019,Jul,6; 2014,Jan,11

Relative Value Units/Medicare Edits

Non-Facility RVU	Work	PE	MP	Total
58262	15.94	8.45	2.48	26.87
58263	17.23	8.93	2.71	28.87
Facility RVU	**Work**	**PE**	**MP**	**Total**
58262	15.94	8.45	2.48	26.87
58263	17.23	8.93	2.71	28.87

	FUD	Status	MUE	Modifiers				IOM Reference
58262	90	A	1(3)	51	N/A	62	80	None
58263	90	A	1(2)	51	N/A	62	80	

* with documentation

Terms To Know

enterocele. Intestinal herniation into the vaginal wall.

hysterectomy. Surgical removal of the uterus. A complete hysterectomy may also include removal of tubes and ovaries.

ligation. Tying off a blood vessel or duct with a suture or a soft, thin wire.

salpingo-oophorectomy. Surgical removal of both the fallopian tube and ovary.

58267

58267   Vaginal hysterectomy, for uterus 250 g or less; with colpo-urethrocystopexy (Marshall-Marchetti-Krantz type, Pereyra type) with or without endoscopic control

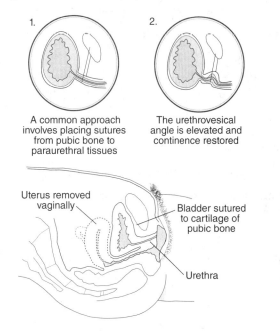

1.   A common approach involves placing sutures from pubic bone to paraurethral tissues

2.   The urethrovesical angle is elevated and continence restored

Uterus removed vaginally

Bladder sutured to cartilage of pubic bone

Urethra

Explanation

The physician performs a vaginal hysterectomy for a uterus 250 gm or less with colpo-urethrocystopexy, with or without endoscopic control. An incision is made around the cervix through the full thickness of the vaginal membrane. The cut vaginal edge is pulled toward the lower cervix and vaginal dissection is continued with countertraction. The posterior peritoneum is opened to admit a finger examination of the pelvis. The uterosacral ligaments are clamped and possibly shortened, cut from the uterus, and secured to the vagina. The vesicovaginal space is entered. The connective tissue fusing the bladder and vagina is dissected and the bladder is separated from the cervix. The bladder pillars are clamped, cut, and ligated near their cervical attachments, as well as the cardinal ligament tissue on each side of the cervix and the left and right uterine vessels. The physician clamps, cuts, and ligates the upper cardinal and lower broad ligament complex. Traction applied to the cervix moves the uterus down until the fundus is low in the pelvis. Hemostats are applied to the angle of the uterus on each side and the uterus is removed. Colpo-urethrocystopexy is done in cases of urinary incontinence to elevate the lower part of the bladder that connects to the urethra (bladder neck) and the urethra to a new position higher in the pelvis so the muscles of the pelvic floor can help control urination. After the uterus has been exteriorized and the bladder and urethra separated from surrounding structures, the physician lifts the vagina upward, suspends the bladder neck and urethra by placing sutures through the fibromuscular wall of the vagina lateral to the tissue surrounding the urethra, and sutures the tissue to the symphysis pubis (the midline junction of the pubic bones at the front). An endoscope may be placed to ensure no sutures pass through the lining of the bladder and to evaluate ureteral patency. The sutures are pulled tight to tack the structures to the pubic bone and provide support.

Coding Tips

This code does not include removal of tubes or ovaries. Colpo-urethrocystopexy is included and should not be identified separately. For colpo-urethrocystopexy without hysterectomy, see 51840 and 51841. Report 58270 when an enterocele is repaired at the same time. For other vaginal hysterectomy codes, see 58260–58263 and 58270–58294.

ICD-10-CM Diagnostic Codes

C53.0	Malignant neoplasm of endocervix ♀
C53.1	Malignant neoplasm of exocervix ♀
C53.8	Malignant neoplasm of overlapping sites of cervix uteri ♀
C54.0	Malignant neoplasm of isthmus uteri ♀
C54.1	Malignant neoplasm of endometrium ♀
C54.2	Malignant neoplasm of myometrium ♀
C54.3	Malignant neoplasm of fundus uteri ♀
C54.8	Malignant neoplasm of overlapping sites of corpus uteri ♀
C57.11	Malignant neoplasm of right broad ligament ♀ ☑
C57.12	Malignant neoplasm of left broad ligament ♀ ☑
C57.21	Malignant neoplasm of right round ligament ♀ ☑
C57.22	Malignant neoplasm of left round ligament ♀ ☑
C57.3	Malignant neoplasm of parametrium ♀
C57.7	Malignant neoplasm of other specified female genital organs ♀
C57.8	Malignant neoplasm of overlapping sites of female genital organs ♀
C79.82	Secondary malignant neoplasm of genital organs
D06.0	Carcinoma in situ of endocervix ♀
D06.1	Carcinoma in situ of exocervix ♀
D06.7	Carcinoma in situ of other parts of cervix ♀
D07.0	Carcinoma in situ of endometrium ♀
D07.39	Carcinoma in situ of other female genital organs ♀
D25.0	Submucous leiomyoma of uterus ♀
D25.1	Intramural leiomyoma of uterus ♀
D25.2	Subserosal leiomyoma of uterus ♀
D39.0	Neoplasm of uncertain behavior of uterus ♀
D39.2	Neoplasm of uncertain behavior of placenta Ⓜ ♀
D39.8	Neoplasm of uncertain behavior of other specified female genital organs ♀
D49.59	Neoplasm of unspecified behavior of other genitourinary organ
N39.3	Stress incontinence (female) (male)
N71.0	Acute inflammatory disease of uterus ♀
N71.1	Chronic inflammatory disease of uterus ♀
N72	Inflammatory disease of cervix uteri ♀
N73.0	Acute parametritis and pelvic cellulitis ♀
N73.1	Chronic parametritis and pelvic cellulitis ♀
N73.3	Female acute pelvic peritonitis ♀
N73.4	Female chronic pelvic peritonitis ♀
N73.6	Female pelvic peritoneal adhesions (postinfective) ♀
N73.8	Other specified female pelvic inflammatory diseases ♀
N80.0	Endometriosis of uterus ♀
N81.2	Incomplete uterovaginal prolapse ♀
N81.3	Complete uterovaginal prolapse ♀
N81.5	Vaginal enterocele ♀
N81.89	Other female genital prolapse ♀
N84.0	Polyp of corpus uteri ♀
N84.8	Polyp of other parts of female genital tract ♀
N85.01	Benign endometrial hyperplasia ♀
N85.02	Endometrial intraepithelial neoplasia [EIN] ♀

N85.2	Hypertrophy of uterus ♀
N85.7	Hematometra ♀
N85.8	Other specified noninflammatory disorders of uterus ♀
N87.0	Mild cervical dysplasia ♀
N87.1	Moderate cervical dysplasia ♀
N92.0	Excessive and frequent menstruation with regular cycle ♀
N92.1	Excessive and frequent menstruation with irregular cycle ♀
N92.5	Other specified irregular menstruation ♀
N93.8	Other specified abnormal uterine and vaginal bleeding ♀
N94.89	Other specified conditions associated with female genital organs and menstrual cycle ♀
N95.0	Postmenopausal bleeding ♀

AMA: 58267 2019,Jul,6; 2018,Jan,8; 2017,Jan,8; 2016,Jan,13; 2015,Jan,16; 2014,Jan,11

Relative Value Units/Medicare Edits

Non-Facility RVU	Work	PE	MP	Total
58267	18.36	9.69	2.86	30.91
Facility RVU	Work	PE	MP	Total
58267	18.36	9.69	2.86	30.91

	FUD	Status	MUE	Modifiers				IOM Reference
58267	90	A	1(2)	51	N/A	62*	80	None

* with documentation

Terms To Know

clamp. Tool used to grip, compress, join, or fasten body parts.

dissection. (dis. apart; -section, act of cutting) Separating by cutting tissue or body structures apart.

fundus uteri. Uterus.

ligation. Tying off a blood vessel or duct with a suture or a soft, thin wire.

Marshall-Marchetti-Krantz. Surgical procedure to correct urinary stress incontinence in which the bladder is suspended by placing several sutures through the tissue surrounding the urethra and into the vaginal wall. The sutures are pulled tight so that the tissues are tacked up to the symphysis pubis and the urethra is moved forward.

58270

| 58270 | Vaginal hysterectomy, for uterus 250 g or less; with repair of enterocele |

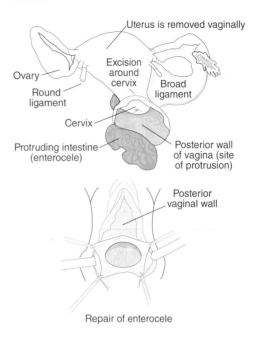

Repair of enterocele

Explanation

The physician performs a vaginal hysterectomy, for a uterus 250 gm or less with repair of an enterocele. An incision is made around the cervix through the full thickness of the vaginal membrane. The cut vaginal edge is pulled toward the lower cervix and vaginal dissection is continued with countertraction. The posterior peritoneum is opened to admit a finger examination of the pelvis. The uterosacral ligaments are clamped and possibly shortened, cut from the uterus, and secured to the vagina. The vesicovaginal space is entered. The connective tissue fusing the bladder and vagina is dissected and the bladder is separated from the cervix. The bladder pillars are clamped, cut, and ligated near their cervical attachments as well as the cardinal ligament tissue on each side of the cervix and the left and right uterine vessels. The anterior peritoneum is opened under direct vision to avoid damaging the bladder and admit finger exploration. The physician clamps, cuts, and ligates the upper cardinal and lower broad ligament complex now that the peritoneum is open both anterior and posterior to the uterine fundus. Hemostats are applied to the angle of the uterus on each side and the uterus is removed, usually posteriorly. The physician also repairs an enterocele, a herniation of intestine that protrudes against the vaginal wall, discovered during finger exploration. The hernia sac is bluntly and sharply dissected from the surrounding connective tissue, excised and ligated, and the surrounding tissues are strengthened and sutured. The peritoneum is closed with purse-string sutures that incorporate the proximal part of the uterosacral ligaments.

Coding Tips

Removal of the tubes and ovaries is not included in this procedure. However, the enterocele repair is included and should not be identified separately. For repair of an enterocele with removal of tubes and ovaries, report 58263. For other vaginal hysterectomy codes, see 58262–58267 and 58275–58294.

ICD-10-CM Diagnostic Codes

| C53.0 | Malignant neoplasm of endocervix ♀ |
| C53.1 | Malignant neoplasm of exocervix ♀ |

C53.8	Malignant neoplasm of overlapping sites of cervix uteri ♀	
C54.0	Malignant neoplasm of isthmus uteri ♀	
C54.1	Malignant neoplasm of endometrium ♀	
C54.2	Malignant neoplasm of myometrium ♀	
C54.3	Malignant neoplasm of fundus uteri ♀	
C54.8	Malignant neoplasm of overlapping sites of corpus uteri ♀	
C57.11	Malignant neoplasm of right broad ligament ♀ ☑	
C57.12	Malignant neoplasm of left broad ligament ♀ ☑	
C57.21	Malignant neoplasm of right round ligament ♀ ☑	
C57.22	Malignant neoplasm of left round ligament ♀ ☑	
C57.3	Malignant neoplasm of parametrium ♀	
C57.7	Malignant neoplasm of other specified female genital organs ♀	
C57.8	Malignant neoplasm of overlapping sites of female genital organs ♀	
C79.82	Secondary malignant neoplasm of genital organs	
D06.0	Carcinoma in situ of endocervix ♀	
D06.1	Carcinoma in situ of exocervix ♀	
D06.7	Carcinoma in situ of other parts of cervix ♀	
D07.0	Carcinoma in situ of endometrium ♀	
D07.39	Carcinoma in situ of other female genital organs ♀	
D25.0	Submucous leiomyoma of uterus ♀	
D25.1	Intramural leiomyoma of uterus ♀	
D25.2	Subserosal leiomyoma of uterus ♀	
D39.0	Neoplasm of uncertain behavior of uterus ♀	
D39.2	Neoplasm of uncertain behavior of placenta Ⓜ ♀	
D39.8	Neoplasm of uncertain behavior of other specified female genital organs ♀	
D49.59	Neoplasm of unspecified behavior of other genitourinary organ	
N71.0	Acute inflammatory disease of uterus ♀	
N71.1	Chronic inflammatory disease of uterus ♀	
N72	Inflammatory disease of cervix uteri ♀	
N73.0	Acute parametritis and pelvic cellulitis ♀	
N73.1	Chronic parametritis and pelvic cellulitis ♀	
N73.3	Female acute pelvic peritonitis ♀	
N73.4	Female chronic pelvic peritonitis ♀	
N73.6	Female pelvic peritoneal adhesions (postinfective) ♀	
N73.8	Other specified female pelvic inflammatory diseases ♀	
N80.0	Endometriosis of uterus ♀	
N81.2	Incomplete uterovaginal prolapse ♀	
N81.3	Complete uterovaginal prolapse ♀	
N81.5	Vaginal enterocele ♀	
N81.89	Other female genital prolapse ♀	
N84.0	Polyp of corpus uteri ♀	
N84.8	Polyp of other parts of female genital tract ♀	
N85.01	Benign endometrial hyperplasia ♀	
N85.02	Endometrial intraepithelial neoplasia [EIN] ♀	
N85.2	Hypertrophy of uterus ♀	
N85.7	Hematometra ♀	
N85.8	Other specified noninflammatory disorders of uterus ♀	
N87.0	Mild cervical dysplasia ♀	
N87.1	Moderate cervical dysplasia ♀	
N92.0	Excessive and frequent menstruation with regular cycle ♀	
N92.1	Excessive and frequent menstruation with irregular cycle ♀	

N92.5	Other specified irregular menstruation ♀	
N93.8	Other specified abnormal uterine and vaginal bleeding ♀	
N94.89	Other specified conditions associated with female genital organs and menstrual cycle ♀	
N95.0	Postmenopausal bleeding ♀	

AMA: **58270** 2019,Jul,6; 2014,Jan,11

Relative Value Units/Medicare Edits

Non-Facility RVU	Work	PE	MP	Total
58270	15.3	8.13	2.4	25.83
Facility RVU	**Work**	**PE**	**MP**	**Total**
58270	15.3	8.13	2.4	25.83

	FUD	Status	MUE	Modifiers				IOM Reference
58270	90	A	1(2)	51	N/A	62*	80	None

* with documentation

Terms To Know

anterior. Situated in the front area or toward the belly surface of the body.

blunt dissection. Surgical technique used to expose an underlying area by separating along natural cleavage lines of tissue, without cutting.

clamp. Tool used to grip, compress, join, or fasten body parts.

connective tissue. Body tissue made from fibroblasts, collagen, and elastic fibrils that connects, supports, and holds together other tissues and cells and includes cartilage, collagenous, fibrous, elastic, and osseous tissue.

enterocele. Intestinal herniation into the vaginal wall.

hemostat. Tool for clamping vessels and arresting hemorrhaging.

posterior. Located in the back part or caudal end of the body.

58275-58280

58275 Vaginal hysterectomy, with total or partial vaginectomy;
58280   with repair of enterocele

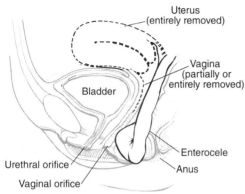

The uterus is removed.
The vagina is partially or entirely removed as well.

Explanation

The physician performs a vaginal hysterectomy with total or partial vaginectomy in 58275-58280 and with enterocele repair in 58280. An incision is made around the cervix through the full thickness of the vaginal membrane. The cut vaginal edge is pulled toward the lower cervix and vaginal dissection is continued with countertraction. The posterior peritoneum is opened to admit a finger examination of the pelvis. The uterosacral ligaments are clamped and possibly shortened, cut from the uterus, and secured to the vagina. The vesicovaginal space is entered. The connective tissue fusing the bladder and vagina is dissected and the bladder is separated from the cervix. The bladder pillars are clamped, cut, and ligated near their cervical attachments, as well as the cardinal ligament tissue on each side of the cervix and the left and right uterine vessels. The anterior peritoneum is opened under direct vision to avoid damaging the bladder and admit finger exploration. The physician clamps, cuts, and ligates the upper cardinal and lower broad ligament complex now that the peritoneum is open both anterior and posterior to the uterine fundus. Traction applied to the cervix moves the uterus down until the fundus is low in the pelvis. Hemostats are applied to the angle of the uterus on each side and the uterus is removed, usually posteriorly. The vagina is everted out through its opening and totally or partially removed in sections by blunt and sharp dissection. Any remaining vaginal tissue and the supporting tissues are inverted back into the resulting defect and are sutured in place with total vaginectomy obliterating the space. Report 58280 if the physician also repairs an enterocele, a herniation of intestine protruding through the vaginal wall. The hernia sac is bluntly and sharply dissected from the surrounding connective tissue, excised and ligated, and the surrounding tissues are strengthened and sutured. The peritoneum is closed with purse-string sutures that incorporate the proximal part of the uterosacral ligaments.

Coding Tips

Removing a narrow rim of vagina surrounding the cervix is standard with a vaginal hysterectomy; however, these codes include removing a significant amount of the vagina. For other vaginal hysterectomy codes, see 58262–58285 and 58550.

ICD-10-CM Diagnostic Codes

C52	Malignant neoplasm of vagina ♀
C53.0	Malignant neoplasm of endocervix ♀
C53.1	Malignant neoplasm of exocervix ♀
C53.8	Malignant neoplasm of overlapping sites of cervix uteri ♀
C54.0	Malignant neoplasm of isthmus uteri ♀
C54.1	Malignant neoplasm of endometrium ♀
C54.2	Malignant neoplasm of myometrium ♀
C54.3	Malignant neoplasm of fundus uteri ♀
C54.8	Malignant neoplasm of overlapping sites of corpus uteri ♀
C57.11	Malignant neoplasm of right broad ligament ♀ ☑
C57.12	Malignant neoplasm of left broad ligament ♀ ☑
C57.21	Malignant neoplasm of right round ligament ♀ ☑
C57.22	Malignant neoplasm of left round ligament ♀ ☑
C57.3	Malignant neoplasm of parametrium ♀
C57.7	Malignant neoplasm of other specified female genital organs ♀
C57.8	Malignant neoplasm of overlapping sites of female genital organs ♀
C79.82	Secondary malignant neoplasm of genital organs
D06.0	Carcinoma in situ of endocervix ♀
D06.1	Carcinoma in situ of exocervix ♀
D06.7	Carcinoma in situ of other parts of cervix ♀
D07.0	Carcinoma in situ of endometrium ♀
D07.2	Carcinoma in situ of vagina ♀
D07.39	Carcinoma in situ of other female genital organs ♀
D25.0	Submucous leiomyoma of uterus ♀
D25.1	Intramural leiomyoma of uterus ♀
D25.2	Subserosal leiomyoma of uterus ♀
D39.0	Neoplasm of uncertain behavior of uterus ♀
D39.2	Neoplasm of uncertain behavior of placenta Ⓜ ♀
D39.8	Neoplasm of uncertain behavior of other specified female genital organs ♀
D49.59	Neoplasm of unspecified behavior of other genitourinary organ
N71.0	Acute inflammatory disease of uterus ♀
N71.1	Chronic inflammatory disease of uterus ♀
N72	Inflammatory disease of cervix uteri ♀
N73.0	Acute parametritis and pelvic cellulitis ♀
N73.1	Chronic parametritis and pelvic cellulitis ♀
N73.3	Female acute pelvic peritonitis ♀
N73.4	Female chronic pelvic peritonitis ♀
N73.6	Female pelvic peritoneal adhesions (postinfective) ♀
N73.8	Other specified female pelvic inflammatory diseases ♀
N80.0	Endometriosis of uterus ♀
N81.2	Incomplete uterovaginal prolapse ♀
N81.3	Complete uterovaginal prolapse ♀
N81.5	Vaginal enterocele ♀
N81.89	Other female genital prolapse ♀
N84.0	Polyp of corpus uteri ♀
N84.8	Polyp of other parts of female genital tract ♀
N85.01	Benign endometrial hyperplasia ♀
N85.02	Endometrial intraepithelial neoplasia [EIN] ♀
N85.2	Hypertrophy of uterus ♀
N85.7	Hematometra ♀
N85.8	Other specified noninflammatory disorders of uterus ♀
N87.0	Mild cervical dysplasia ♀
N87.1	Moderate cervical dysplasia ♀

N92.0	Excessive and frequent menstruation with regular cycle ♀	
N92.1	Excessive and frequent menstruation with irregular cycle ♀	
N92.5	Other specified irregular menstruation ♀	
N93.8	Other specified abnormal uterine and vaginal bleeding ♀	
N94.89	Other specified conditions associated with female genital organs and menstrual cycle ♀	
N95.0	Postmenopausal bleeding ♀	

AMA: 58275 2019,Jul,6; 2014,Jan,11 **58280** 2019,Jul,6; 2014,Jan,11

Relative Value Units/Medicare Edits

Non-Facility RVU	Work	PE	MP	Total
58275	17.03	9.01	2.62	28.66
58280	18.33	9.5	2.89	30.72
Facility RVU	**Work**	**PE**	**MP**	**Total**
58275	17.03	9.01	2.62	28.66
58280	18.33	9.5	2.89	30.72

	FUD	Status	MUE	Modifiers				IOM Reference
58275	90	A	1(2)	51	N/A	62*	80	None
58280	90	A	1(2)	51	N/A	62*	80	

* with documentation

Terms To Know

connective tissue. Body tissue made from fibroblasts, collagen, and elastic fibrils that connects, supports, and holds together other tissues and cells and includes cartilage, collagenous, fibrous, elastic, and osseous tissue.

defect. Imperfection, flaw, or absence.

dissection. (dis. apart; -section, act of cutting) Separating by cutting tissue or body structures apart.

enterocele. Intestinal herniation into the vaginal wall.

full thickness. Consisting of skin and subcutaneous tissue.

incision. Act of cutting into tissue or an organ.

ligation. Tying off a blood vessel or duct with a suture or a soft, thin wire.

tissue. Group of similar cells with a similar function that form definite structures and organs. Tissue types include epithelial tissue, muscle tissue, connective tissue, and nervous tissue.

vaginectomy. Surgical excision of all or a portion of the vagina.

58285

58285 Vaginal hysterectomy, radical (Schauta type operation)

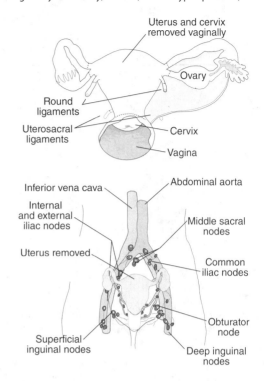

Explanation

The physician performs a radical vaginal hysterectomy. This includes the uterus, its surrounding tissues, and the pelvic lymph nodes. An incision is made around the cervix through the full thickness of the vaginal membrane. The cut vaginal edge is pulled toward the lower cervix and vaginal dissection is continued with countertraction. The posterior peritoneum is opened to admit a finger examination of the pelvis. The uterosacral ligaments are clamped and possibly shortened, cut from the uterus, and secured to the vagina. The vesicovaginal space is entered. The connective tissue fusing the bladder and vagina is dissected and the bladder is separated from the cervix. The bladder pillars are clamped, cut, and ligated near their cervical attachments, as well as the cardinal ligament tissue on each side of the cervix and the left and right uterine vessels. The anterior peritoneum is opened under direct vision to avoid damaging the bladder and admit finger exploration. The physician clamps, cuts, and ligates the upper cardinal and lower broad ligament complex now that the peritoneum is open both anterior and posterior to the uterine fundus. Traction applied to the cervix moves the uterus down until the fundus is low in the pelvis. Hemostats are applied to the angle of the uterus on each side and the uterus is removed, usually posteriorly. The physician also removes the surrounding tissues, including part or all of the vagina and the pelvic lymph nodes. Any incisions are closed by suturing.

Coding Tips

Removal of tubes and ovaries is not included in this code. Note that 58285 includes removal of more uterine adnexal tissue than 58275 or 58280. Several vaginal hysterectomy codes exist that include many different components and amounts of uterine and adnexal tissue dissection, see 58260–58280 and 58290–58294.

ICD-10-CM Diagnostic Codes

C53.0	Malignant neoplasm of endocervix ♀	
C53.1	Malignant neoplasm of exocervix ♀	

C53.8	Malignant neoplasm of overlapping sites of cervix uteri ♀	
C54.0	Malignant neoplasm of isthmus uteri ♀	
C54.1	Malignant neoplasm of endometrium ♀	
C54.2	Malignant neoplasm of myometrium ♀	
C54.3	Malignant neoplasm of fundus uteri ♀	
C54.8	Malignant neoplasm of overlapping sites of corpus uteri ♀	
C57.11	Malignant neoplasm of right broad ligament ♀ ☑	
C57.12	Malignant neoplasm of left broad ligament ♀ ☑	
C57.21	Malignant neoplasm of right round ligament ♀ ☑	
C57.22	Malignant neoplasm of left round ligament ♀ ☑	
C57.3	Malignant neoplasm of parametrium ♀	
C57.7	Malignant neoplasm of other specified female genital organs ♀	
C57.8	Malignant neoplasm of overlapping sites of female genital organs ♀	
C79.82	Secondary malignant neoplasm of genital organs	
D06.0	Carcinoma in situ of endocervix ♀	
D06.1	Carcinoma in situ of exocervix ♀	
D06.7	Carcinoma in situ of other parts of cervix ♀	
D07.0	Carcinoma in situ of endometrium ♀	
D07.39	Carcinoma in situ of other female genital organs ♀	
D25.0	Submucous leiomyoma of uterus ♀	
D25.1	Intramural leiomyoma of uterus ♀	
D25.2	Subserosal leiomyoma of uterus ♀	
D39.0	Neoplasm of uncertain behavior of uterus ♀	
D39.2	Neoplasm of uncertain behavior of placenta 🅜 ♀	
D39.8	Neoplasm of uncertain behavior of other specified female genital organs ♀	
D49.59	Neoplasm of unspecified behavior of other genitourinary organ	
N71.0	Acute inflammatory disease of uterus ♀	
N71.1	Chronic inflammatory disease of uterus ♀	
N72	Inflammatory disease of cervix uteri ♀	
N73.0	Acute parametritis and pelvic cellulitis ♀	
N73.1	Chronic parametritis and pelvic cellulitis ♀	
N73.3	Female acute pelvic peritonitis ♀	
N73.4	Female chronic pelvic peritonitis ♀	
N73.6	Female pelvic peritoneal adhesions (postinfective) ♀	
N73.8	Other specified female pelvic inflammatory diseases ♀	
N80.0	Endometriosis of uterus ♀	
N81.2	Incomplete uterovaginal prolapse ♀	
N81.3	Complete uterovaginal prolapse ♀	
N81.89	Other female genital prolapse ♀	
N84.0	Polyp of corpus uteri ♀	
N84.8	Polyp of other parts of female genital tract ♀	
N85.01	Benign endometrial hyperplasia ♀	
N85.02	Endometrial intraepithelial neoplasia [EIN] ♀	
N85.2	Hypertrophy of uterus ♀	
N85.7	Hematometra ♀	
N85.8	Other specified noninflammatory disorders of uterus ♀	
N87.0	Mild cervical dysplasia ♀	
N87.1	Moderate cervical dysplasia ♀	
N92.0	Excessive and frequent menstruation with regular cycle ♀	
N92.1	Excessive and frequent menstruation with irregular cycle ♀	
N92.5	Other specified irregular menstruation ♀	

N93.8	Other specified abnormal uterine and vaginal bleeding ♀
N94.89	Other specified conditions associated with female genital organs and menstrual cycle ♀
N95.0	Postmenopausal bleeding ♀

AMA: **58285** 2019,Jul,6; 2018,Jan,8; 2017,Jan,8; 2016,Jan,13; 2015,Jan,16; 2014,Jan,11

Relative Value Units/Medicare Edits

Non-Facility RVU	Work	PE	MP	Total
58285	23.38	13.39	3.7	40.47
Facility RVU	**Work**	**PE**	**MP**	**Total**
58285	23.38	13.39	3.7	40.47

	FUD	Status	MUE	Modifiers				IOM Reference
58285	90	A	1(3)	51	N/A	62*	80	None

* with documentation

Terms To Know

dissection. (dis. apart; -section, act of cutting) Separating by cutting tissue or body structures apart.

hysterectomy. Surgical removal of the uterus. A complete hysterectomy may also include removal of tubes and ovaries.

radical. Extensive surgery.

Schauta procedure. Surgical removal of the uterus, cervix, upper vagina, and parametrium through a vaginal approach.

58290

58290 Vaginal hysterectomy, for uterus greater than 250 g;

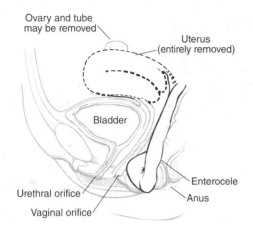

Ovary and tube may be removed

Uterus (entirely removed)

Bladder

Urethral orifice

Vaginal orifice

Enterocele

Anus

Explanation

The physician performs a vaginal hysterectomy, for a uterus greater than 250 gm. An incision is made around the cervix through the full thickness of the vaginal membrane. The cut vaginal edge is pulled toward the lower cervix and vaginal dissection is continued with countertraction. The posterior peritoneum is opened to admit a finger examination of the pelvis. The uterosacral ligaments are clamped and possibly shortened, cut from the uterus, and secured to the vagina. The vesicovaginal space is entered. The connective tissue fusing the bladder and vagina is dissected and the bladder is separated from the cervix. The bladder pillars are clamped, cut, and ligated near their cervical attachments as well as the cardinal ligament tissue on each side of the cervix and the left and right uterine vessels. The anterior peritoneum is opened under direct vision to avoid damaging the bladder and admit finger exploration. The physician clamps, cuts, and ligates the upper cardinal and lower broad ligament complex now that the peritoneum is open both anterior and posterior to the uterine fundus. Traction applied to the cervix moves the uterus down until the fundus is low in the pelvis. Hemostats are applied to the angle of the uterus on each side and the uterus is removed, usually posteriorly. When the uterus is too large to permit delivery through the anterior or posterior peritoneal opening, the myometrium may be incised circumferentially parallel to the uterine cavity axis and removed or the uterus can be dissected and removed one half at a time. The peritoneum is closed with purse-string sutures that incorporate the proximal part of the uterosacral ligaments. Colporrhaphy may be performed before the vaginal wall is closed by running or interrupted sutures placed side to side longitudinally.

Coding Tips

This code reports a hysterectomy for a uterus greater than 250 gm only. When tubes and ovaries are also removed, see 58291; and with repair of enterocele, see 58292. For other vaginal hysterectomy codes, see 58260–58285 and 58294. For laparoscopy with a vaginal hysterectomy only for a uterus greater than 250 gm, see 58553.

ICD-10-CM Diagnostic Codes

C53.0	Malignant neoplasm of endocervix ♀
C53.1	Malignant neoplasm of exocervix ♀
C53.8	Malignant neoplasm of overlapping sites of cervix uteri ♀
C54.0	Malignant neoplasm of isthmus uteri ♀
C54.1	Malignant neoplasm of endometrium ♀
C54.2	Malignant neoplasm of myometrium ♀
C54.3	Malignant neoplasm of fundus uteri ♀
C54.8	Malignant neoplasm of overlapping sites of corpus uteri ♀
C56.1	Malignant neoplasm of right ovary ♀ ☑
C56.2	Malignant neoplasm of left ovary ♀ ☑
C57.01	Malignant neoplasm of right fallopian tube ♀ ☑
C57.02	Malignant neoplasm of left fallopian tube ♀ ☑
C57.11	Malignant neoplasm of right broad ligament ♀ ☑
C57.12	Malignant neoplasm of left broad ligament ♀ ☑
C57.21	Malignant neoplasm of right round ligament ♀ ☑
C57.22	Malignant neoplasm of left round ligament ♀ ☑
C57.3	Malignant neoplasm of parametrium ♀
C57.7	Malignant neoplasm of other specified female genital organs ♀
C57.8	Malignant neoplasm of overlapping sites of female genital organs ♀
C79.61	Secondary malignant neoplasm of right ovary ♀ ☑
C79.62	Secondary malignant neoplasm of left ovary ♀ ☑
C79.82	Secondary malignant neoplasm of genital organs
D06.0	Carcinoma in situ of endocervix ♀
D06.1	Carcinoma in situ of exocervix ♀
D06.7	Carcinoma in situ of other parts of cervix ♀
D07.0	Carcinoma in situ of endometrium ♀
D07.39	Carcinoma in situ of other female genital organs ♀
D25.0	Submucous leiomyoma of uterus ♀
D25.1	Intramural leiomyoma of uterus ♀
D25.2	Subserosal leiomyoma of uterus ♀
D39.0	Neoplasm of uncertain behavior of uterus ♀
D39.11	Neoplasm of uncertain behavior of right ovary ♀ ☑
D39.12	Neoplasm of uncertain behavior of left ovary ♀ ☑
D39.2	Neoplasm of uncertain behavior of placenta Ⓜ ♀
D39.8	Neoplasm of uncertain behavior of other specified female genital organs ♀
D49.59	Neoplasm of unspecified behavior of other genitourinary organ
N70.01	Acute salpingitis ♀
N70.02	Acute oophoritis ♀
N70.03	Acute salpingitis and oophoritis ♀
N70.11	Chronic salpingitis ♀
N70.12	Chronic oophoritis ♀
N70.13	Chronic salpingitis and oophoritis ♀
N71.0	Acute inflammatory disease of uterus ♀
N71.1	Chronic inflammatory disease of uterus ♀
N72	Inflammatory disease of cervix uteri ♀
N73.0	Acute parametritis and pelvic cellulitis ♀
N73.1	Chronic parametritis and pelvic cellulitis ♀
N73.3	Female acute pelvic peritonitis ♀
N73.4	Female chronic pelvic peritonitis ♀
N73.6	Female pelvic peritoneal adhesions (postinfective) ♀
N73.8	Other specified female pelvic inflammatory diseases ♀
N80.0	Endometriosis of uterus ♀
N80.1	Endometriosis of ovary ♀
N80.2	Endometriosis of fallopian tube ♀
N81.2	Incomplete uterovaginal prolapse ♀
N81.3	Complete uterovaginal prolapse ♀
N81.5	Vaginal enterocele ♀

Ⓝ Newborn: 0 **Ⓟ Pediatric: 0-17** **Ⓜ Maternity: 9-64** **Ⓐ Adult: 15-124** ♂ **Male Only** ♀ **Female Only**

Coding Companion for Ob/Gyn

N81.89	Other female genital prolapse ♀
N83.01	Follicular cyst of right ovary ♀ ☑
N83.02	Follicular cyst of left ovary ♀ ☑
N83.11	Corpus luteum cyst of right ovary ♀ ☑
N83.12	Corpus luteum cyst of left ovary ♀ ☑
N83.291	Other ovarian cyst, right side ♀ ☑
N83.292	Other ovarian cyst, left side ♀ ☑
N83.6	Hematosalpinx ♀
N83.8	Other noninflammatory disorders of ovary, fallopian tube and broad ligament ♀
N84.0	Polyp of corpus uteri ♀
N84.8	Polyp of other parts of female genital tract ♀
N85.01	Benign endometrial hyperplasia ♀
N85.02	Endometrial intraepithelial neoplasia [EIN] ♀
N85.2	Hypertrophy of uterus ♀
N85.7	Hematometra ♀
N85.8	Other specified noninflammatory disorders of uterus ♀
N87.0	Mild cervical dysplasia ♀
N87.1	Moderate cervical dysplasia ♀
N92.0	Excessive and frequent menstruation with regular cycle ♀
N92.1	Excessive and frequent menstruation with irregular cycle ♀
N92.5	Other specified irregular menstruation ♀
N93.8	Other specified abnormal uterine and vaginal bleeding ♀
N94.89	Other specified conditions associated with female genital organs and menstrual cycle ♀
N95.0	Postmenopausal bleeding ♀

AMA: 58290 2019,Jul,6; 2014,Jan,11

Relative Value Units/Medicare Edits

Non-Facility RVU	Work	PE	MP	Total
58290	20.27	10.01	3.18	33.46
Facility RVU	**Work**	**PE**	**MP**	**Total**
58290	20.27	10.01	3.18	33.46

	FUD	Status	MUE	Modifiers				IOM Reference
58290	90	A	1(3)	51	N/A	62*	80	None

* with documentation

Terms To Know

connective tissue. Body tissue made from fibroblasts, collagen, and elastic fibrils that connects, supports, and holds together other tissues and cells and includes cartilage, collagenous, fibrous, elastic, and osseous tissue.

full thickness. Consisting of skin and subcutaneous tissue.

membrane. Thin, flexible tissue layer that covers or functions to separate or connect anatomic areas, structures, or organs. May also be described as having the characteristic of allowing certain substances to permeate or pass through but not others (semipermeable).

58291-58292

58291 Vaginal hysterectomy, for uterus greater than 250 g; with removal of tube(s) and/or ovary(s)

58292   with removal of tube(s) and/or ovary(s), with repair of enterocele

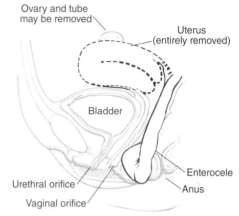

The uterus, tubes, and ovaries are removed vaginally in an open surgical session

Explanation

The physician performs a vaginal hysterectomy, for a uterus greater than 250 gm and removes the tubes and/or ovaries. An incision is made around the cervix through the full thickness of the vaginal membrane. The cut vaginal edge is pulled toward the lower cervix and vaginal dissection is continued with countertraction. The posterior peritoneum is opened to admit a finger examination of the pelvis. The uterosacral ligaments are clamped and possibly shortened, cut from the uterus, and secured to the vagina. The vesicovaginal space is entered. The connective tissue fusing the bladder and vagina is dissected and the bladder is separated from the cervix. The bladder pillars are clamped, cut, and ligated near their cervical attachments, as well as the cardinal ligament tissue on each side of the cervix and the left and right uterine vessels. The anterior peritoneum is opened under direct vision to avoid damaging the bladder and admit finger exploration. The physician clamps, cuts, and ligates the upper cardinal and lower broad ligament complex now that the peritoneum is open both anterior and posterior to the uterine fundus. Traction applied to the cervix moves the uterus down until the fundus is low in the pelvis. Hemostats are applied to the angle of the uterus on each side and the uterus is removed, usually posteriorly. After the uterus is exteriorized, care is taken to ensure ligation of the ovarian vessels. The ovary is excised under direct vision. For removal of both tubes and ovaries, the round ligament on one side at a time is clamped and divided. A tunnel is made through the layers of the uterine broad ligament that enclose the tube and the tube and ovary are clamped together. The structure is pulled forward, the two sheets of the broad ligament are each cut, and the broad ligament is opened completely. The whole specimen is separated from its attaching ligament, which is clamped, and the tube and ovary on that side are removed. Report 58292 if an enterocele is repaired in addition to removing the tube and/or ovary. An enterocele is a hernia of the intestine protruding against the vaginal wall. The hernia sac is bluntly and sharply dissected from the surrounding connective tissue, excised and ligated, and the surrounding tissues are strengthened and sutured. The peritoneal and vaginal wall incisions of the hysterectomy procedure are closed.

Coding Tips

For a vaginal hysterectomy only for a uterus greater than 250 gm, see 58290. For a vaginal hysterectomy for a uterus greater than 250 gm with repair of an enterocele without removal of tubes or ovaries, see 58294. For other vaginal

hysterectomy codes, see 58260–58285. For laparoscopic vaginal hysterectomy with removal of the tubes and/or ovaries for a uterus greater than 250 gm, see 58554.

ICD-10-CM Diagnostic Codes

C53.0	Malignant neoplasm of endocervix ♀
C53.1	Malignant neoplasm of exocervix ♀
C53.8	Malignant neoplasm of overlapping sites of cervix uteri ♀
C54.0	Malignant neoplasm of isthmus uteri ♀
C54.1	Malignant neoplasm of endometrium ♀
C54.2	Malignant neoplasm of myometrium ♀
C54.3	Malignant neoplasm of fundus uteri ♀
C54.8	Malignant neoplasm of overlapping sites of corpus uteri ♀
C56.1	Malignant neoplasm of right ovary ♀ ☑
C56.2	Malignant neoplasm of left ovary ♀ ☑
C57.01	Malignant neoplasm of right fallopian tube ♀ ☑
C57.02	Malignant neoplasm of left fallopian tube ♀ ☑
C57.11	Malignant neoplasm of right broad ligament ♀ ☑
C57.12	Malignant neoplasm of left broad ligament ♀ ☑
C57.21	Malignant neoplasm of right round ligament ♀ ☑
C57.22	Malignant neoplasm of left round ligament ♀ ☑
C57.3	Malignant neoplasm of parametrium ♀
C57.7	Malignant neoplasm of other specified female genital organs ♀
C57.8	Malignant neoplasm of overlapping sites of female genital organs ♀
C79.61	Secondary malignant neoplasm of right ovary ♀ ☑
C79.62	Secondary malignant neoplasm of left ovary ♀ ☑
C79.82	Secondary malignant neoplasm of genital organs
D06.0	Carcinoma in situ of endocervix ♀
D06.1	Carcinoma in situ of exocervix ♀
D06.7	Carcinoma in situ of other parts of cervix ♀
D07.0	Carcinoma in situ of endometrium ♀
D07.39	Carcinoma in situ of other female genital organs ♀
D25.0	Submucous leiomyoma of uterus ♀
D25.1	Intramural leiomyoma of uterus ♀
D25.2	Subserosal leiomyoma of uterus ♀
D39.0	Neoplasm of uncertain behavior of uterus ♀
D39.11	Neoplasm of uncertain behavior of right ovary ♀ ☑
D39.12	Neoplasm of uncertain behavior of left ovary ♀ ☑
D39.2	Neoplasm of uncertain behavior of placenta Ⓜ ♀
D39.8	Neoplasm of uncertain behavior of other specified female genital organs ♀
D49.59	Neoplasm of unspecified behavior of other genitourinary organ
N70.01	Acute salpingitis ♀
N70.02	Acute oophoritis ♀
N70.03	Acute salpingitis and oophoritis ♀
N70.11	Chronic salpingitis ♀
N70.12	Chronic oophoritis ♀
N70.13	Chronic salpingitis and oophoritis ♀
N71.0	Acute inflammatory disease of uterus ♀
N71.1	Chronic inflammatory disease of uterus ♀
N72	Inflammatory disease of cervix uteri ♀
N73.0	Acute parametritis and pelvic cellulitis ♀
N73.1	Chronic parametritis and pelvic cellulitis ♀
N73.3	Female acute pelvic peritonitis ♀
N73.4	Female chronic pelvic peritonitis ♀
N73.6	Female pelvic peritoneal adhesions (postinfective) ♀
N73.8	Other specified female pelvic inflammatory diseases ♀
N80.0	Endometriosis of uterus ♀
N80.1	Endometriosis of ovary ♀
N80.2	Endometriosis of fallopian tube ♀
N81.2	Incomplete uterovaginal prolapse ♀
N81.3	Complete uterovaginal prolapse ♀
N81.5	Vaginal enterocele ♀
N81.89	Other female genital prolapse ♀
N83.01	Follicular cyst of right ovary ♀ ☑
N83.02	Follicular cyst of left ovary ♀ ☑
N83.11	Corpus luteum cyst of right ovary ♀ ☑
N83.12	Corpus luteum cyst of left ovary ♀ ☑
N83.291	Other ovarian cyst, right side ♀ ☑
N83.292	Other ovarian cyst, left side ♀ ☑
N83.6	Hematosalpinx ♀
N83.8	Other noninflammatory disorders of ovary, fallopian tube and broad ligament ♀
N84.0	Polyp of corpus uteri ♀
N84.8	Polyp of other parts of female genital tract ♀
N85.01	Benign endometrial hyperplasia ♀
N85.02	Endometrial intraepithelial neoplasia [EIN] ♀
N85.2	Hypertrophy of uterus ♀
N85.7	Hematometra ♀
N85.8	Other specified noninflammatory disorders of uterus ♀
N87.0	Mild cervical dysplasia ♀
N87.1	Moderate cervical dysplasia ♀
N92.0	Excessive and frequent menstruation with regular cycle ♀
N92.1	Excessive and frequent menstruation with irregular cycle ♀
N92.5	Other specified irregular menstruation ♀
N93.8	Other specified abnormal uterine and vaginal bleeding ♀
N94.89	Other specified conditions associated with female genital organs and menstrual cycle ♀
N95.0	Postmenopausal bleeding ♀

AMA: **58291** 2019,Jul,6; 2014,Jan,11 **58292** 2019,Jul,6; 2014,Jan,11

Relative Value Units/Medicare Edits

Non-Facility RVU	Work	PE	MP	Total
58291	22.06	10.8	3.39	36.25
58292	23.35	11.18	3.68	38.21
Facility RVU	**Work**	**PE**	**MP**	**Total**
58291	22.06	10.8	3.39	36.25
58292	23.35	11.18	3.68	38.21

	FUD	Status	MUE	Modifiers				IOM Reference
58291	90	A	1(2)	51	N/A	62	80	None
58292	90	A	1(2)	51	N/A	62	80	

* with documentation

58294

58294   Vaginal hysterectomy, for uterus greater than 250 g; with repair of enterocele

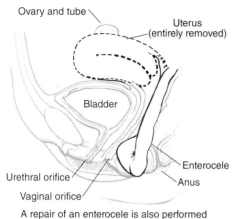

A uterus is removed vaginally

Ovary and tube

Uterus (entirely removed)

Bladder

Enterocele

Urethral orifice

Anus

Vaginal orifice

A repair of an enterocele is also performed

Explanation

The physician performs a vaginal hysterectomy, for a uterus greater than 250 gm, with repair of an enterocele. An incision is made around the cervix through the full thickness of the vaginal membrane. The cut vaginal edge is pulled toward the lower cervix and vaginal dissection is continued with countertraction. The posterior peritoneum is opened to admit a finger examination of the pelvis. The uterosacral ligaments are clamped and possibly shortened, cut from the uterus, and secured to the vagina. The vesicovaginal space is entered. The connective tissue fusing the bladder and vagina is dissected and the bladder is separated from the cervix. The bladder pillars are clamped, cut, and ligated near their cervical attachments, as well as the cardinal ligament tissue on each side of the cervix and the left and right uterine vessels. The anterior peritoneum is opened under direct vision. The physician clamps, cuts, and ligates the upper cardinal and lower broad ligament complex now that the peritoneum is open both anterior and posterior to the uterine fundus. Traction applied to the cervix moves the uterus down until the fundus is low in the pelvis. Hemostats are applied to the angle of the uterus on each side and the uterus is removed, usually posteriorly. The physician also repairs an enterocele, a herniation of intestine that protrudes against the vaginal wall, discovered during finger exploration. The hernia sac is bluntly and sharply dissected from the surrounding connective tissue, excised and ligated, and the surrounding tissues are strengthened and sutured. The peritoneum is closed with purse-string sutures that incorporate the proximal part of the uterosacral ligaments.

Coding Tips

This code does not include removal of tubes or ovaries. The enterocele repair is included and should not be identified separately. For repair of an enterocele with removal of tubes and ovaries, see 58292. For other vaginal hysterectomy codes, see 58260–58291.

ICD-10-CM Diagnostic Codes

C53.0	Malignant neoplasm of endocervix ♀
C53.1	Malignant neoplasm of exocervix ♀
C53.8	Malignant neoplasm of overlapping sites of cervix uteri ♀
C54.0	Malignant neoplasm of isthmus uteri ♀
C54.1	Malignant neoplasm of endometrium ♀
C54.2	Malignant neoplasm of myometrium ♀
C54.3	Malignant neoplasm of fundus uteri ♀
C54.8	Malignant neoplasm of overlapping sites of corpus uteri ♀
C57.11	Malignant neoplasm of right broad ligament ♀ ☑
C57.12	Malignant neoplasm of left broad ligament ♀ ☑
C57.21	Malignant neoplasm of right round ligament ♀ ☑
C57.22	Malignant neoplasm of left round ligament ♀ ☑
C57.3	Malignant neoplasm of parametrium ♀
C57.7	Malignant neoplasm of other specified female genital organs ♀
C57.8	Malignant neoplasm of overlapping sites of female genital organs ♀
C79.82	Secondary malignant neoplasm of genital organs
D06.0	Carcinoma in situ of endocervix ♀
D06.1	Carcinoma in situ of exocervix ♀
D06.7	Carcinoma in situ of other parts of cervix ♀
D07.0	Carcinoma in situ of endometrium ♀
D07.39	Carcinoma in situ of other female genital organs ♀
D25.0	Submucous leiomyoma of uterus ♀
D25.1	Intramural leiomyoma of uterus ♀
D25.2	Subserosal leiomyoma of uterus ♀
D39.0	Neoplasm of uncertain behavior of uterus ♀
D39.2	Neoplasm of uncertain behavior of placenta Ⓜ ♀
D39.8	Neoplasm of uncertain behavior of other specified female genital organs ♀
D49.59	Neoplasm of unspecified behavior of other genitourinary organ
N71.0	Acute inflammatory disease of uterus ♀
N71.1	Chronic inflammatory disease of uterus ♀
N72	Inflammatory disease of cervix uteri ♀
N73.0	Acute parametritis and pelvic cellulitis ♀
N73.1	Chronic parametritis and pelvic cellulitis ♀
N73.3	Female acute pelvic peritonitis ♀
N73.4	Female chronic pelvic peritonitis ♀
N73.6	Female pelvic peritoneal adhesions (postinfective) ♀
N73.8	Other specified female pelvic inflammatory diseases ♀
N80.0	Endometriosis of uterus ♀
N81.2	Incomplete uterovaginal prolapse ♀
N81.3	Complete uterovaginal prolapse ♀
N81.5	Vaginal enterocele ♀
N81.89	Other female genital prolapse ♀
N84.0	Polyp of corpus uteri ♀
N84.8	Polyp of other parts of female genital tract ♀
N85.01	Benign endometrial hyperplasia ♀
N85.02	Endometrial intraepithelial neoplasia [EIN] ♀
N85.2	Hypertrophy of uterus ♀
N85.7	Hematometra ♀
N85.8	Other specified noninflammatory disorders of uterus ♀
N87.0	Mild cervical dysplasia ♀
N87.1	Moderate cervical dysplasia ♀
N92.0	Excessive and frequent menstruation with regular cycle ♀
N92.1	Excessive and frequent menstruation with irregular cycle ♀
N92.5	Other specified irregular menstruation ♀
N93.8	Other specified abnormal uterine and vaginal bleeding ♀
N94.89	Other specified conditions associated with female genital organs and menstrual cycle ♀

N95.0   Postmenopausal bleeding ♀

AMA: **58294** 2019,Jul,6; 2014,Jan,11

Relative Value Units/Medicare Edits

Non-Facility RVU	Work	PE	MP	Total
58294	21.55	10.5	3.39	35.44
Facility RVU	Work	PE	MP	Total
58294	21.55	10.5	3.39	35.44

	FUD	Status	MUE	Modifiers				IOM Reference
58294	90	A	1(2)	51	N/A	62*	80	None

* with documentation

Terms To Know

clamp. Tool used to grip, compress, join, or fasten body parts.

enterocele. Intestinal herniation into the vaginal wall.

exploration. Examination for diagnostic purposes.

fundus uteri. Uterus.

hysterectomy. Surgical removal of the uterus. A complete hysterectomy may also include removal of tubes and ovaries.

repair. Surgical closure of a wound. The wound may be a result of injury/trauma or it may be a surgically created defect. Repairs are divided into three categories: simple, intermediate, and complex.

58300-58301

58300   Insertion of intrauterine device (IUD)
58301   Removal of intrauterine device (IUD)

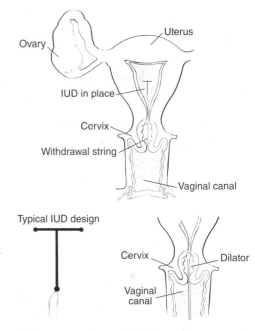

An intrauterine device (IUD) is inserted or removed

Explanation

The physician inserts a speculum into the vagina to visualize the cervix. A tool is used to gently pull down the cervix; it is dilated. In 58300, an intrauterine device (IUD), any of a variety of shapes (coil, loop, T, 7), is guided into the uterus through an insertion tube placed in the cervical os. In 58301, to remove a previously placed IUD from the uterus, a device is inserted through the cervical os and used to grasp and remove the IUD.

Coding Tips

These procedures may be performed by a registered nurse, physician assistant, nurse practitioner, or other trained paramedical person under a physician's supervision. For IUD removal and insertion of a new device during the same visit, report both the IUD removal (58301) and insertion (58300) codes separately. For insertion of a non-biodegradable drug delivery implant for contraception, see 11981; removal of implanted contraceptive capsules with subsequent reinsertion of the drug delivery implant, see 11976 with 11981. The cost of the IUD is not included in these codes and should be reported separately using the appropriate HCPCS Level II code (J7300). These procedures are usually not done out of medical necessity; therefore, the patient may be responsible for charges. Verify with the insurance carrier for coverage. Local anesthesia is included in these services. Report the HCPCS Level II code for Levonorgestrel-releasing intrauterine contraceptive system (Liletta), 52 mg (J7297) or Levonorgestrel-releasing intrauterine contraceptive system (Mirena), 52 mg (J7298). Surgical trays (A4550) are not separately reimbursed by Medicare; however, other third-party payers may cover them.

ICD-10-CM Diagnostic Codes

T83.31XA   Breakdown (mechanical) of intrauterine contraceptive device, initial encounter ♀

T83.32XA   Displacement of intrauterine contraceptive device, initial encounter ♀

T83.39XA	Other mechanical complication of intrauterine contraceptive device, initial encounter ♀	
T83.69XA	Infection and inflammatory reaction due to other prosthetic device, implant and graft in genital tract, initial encounter	
T83.81XA	Embolism due to genitourinary prosthetic devices, implants and grafts, initial encounter	
T83.82XA	Fibrosis due to genitourinary prosthetic devices, implants and grafts, initial encounter	
T83.83XA	Hemorrhage due to genitourinary prosthetic devices, implants and grafts, initial encounter	
T83.84XA	Pain due to genitourinary prosthetic devices, implants and grafts, initial encounter	
T83.85XA	Stenosis due to genitourinary prosthetic devices, implants and grafts, initial encounter	
T83.86XA	Thrombosis due to genitourinary prosthetic devices, implants and grafts, initial encounter	
T83.89XA	Other specified complication of genitourinary prosthetic devices, implants and grafts, initial encounter	
Z30.014	Encounter for initial prescription of intrauterine contraceptive device ♀	
Z30.430	Encounter for insertion of intrauterine contraceptive device ♀	
Z30.431	Encounter for routine checking of intrauterine contraceptive device ♀	
Z30.432	Encounter for removal of intrauterine contraceptive device ♀	
Z30.433	Encounter for removal and reinsertion of intrauterine contraceptive device ♀	

AMA: 58300 2019,Jul,6; 2018,Jan,8; 2017,Jan,8; 2016,Jan,13; 2015,Jan,16; 2014,Jan,11 **58301** 2019,Jul,6; 2018,Jan,8; 2017,Jan,8; 2016,Jan,13; 2015,Jan,16; 2014,Jan,11

Relative Value Units/Medicare Edits

Non-Facility RVU	Work	PE	MP	Total
58300	1.01	1.5	0.09	2.6
58301	1.27	1.45	0.19	2.91
Facility RVU	**Work**	**PE**	**MP**	**Total**
58300	1.01	0.39	0.09	1.49
58301	1.27	0.49	0.19	1.95

	FUD	Status	MUE	Modifiers				IOM Reference
58300	N/A	N	0(3)	N/A	N/A	N/A	N/A	None
58301	0	A	1(3)	51	N/A	N/A	80*	

* with documentation

Terms To Know

dilation. Artificial increase in the diameter of an opening or lumen made by medication or by instrumentation.

insertion. Placement or implantation into a body part.

IUD. Intrauterine device.

medical necessity. Medically appropriate and necessary to meet basic health needs; consistent with the diagnosis or condition and national medical practice guidelines regarding type, frequency, and duration of treatment; rendered in a cost-effective manner.

removal. Process of moving out of or away from, or the fact of being removed.

58321-58322

58321	Artificial insemination; intra-cervical
58322	intra-uterine

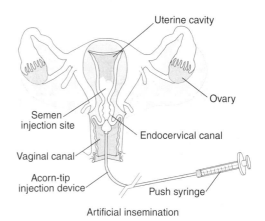

Artificial insemination

Explanation

In 58321, the physician performs artificial insemination by injecting semen into the endocervical canal by applying the blunt tip of a plastic syringe to the external os (opening) of the cervix. Sometimes a cervical cap is used to keep the semen in and around the cervix for eight to 16 hours. In 58322, the physician dilates the cervix and inserts a long flexible tube into the cavity of the uterus. Semen is injected into the uterus by a syringe connected to the tube.

Coding Tips

These procedures include only the semen injection and not the sperm preparation. For sperm preparation, see 58323. Because this procedure is usually not done out of medical necessity, the patient may be responsible for charges. Verify with the insurance carrier for coverage. For in vitro fertilization, see 58970–58976. Diagnostic coding should include male infertility in addition to the codes for female infertility. Surgical trays, A4550, are not separately reimbursed by Medicare; however, other third-party payers may cover them. Check with the specific payer to determine coverage.

ICD-10-CM Diagnostic Codes

N97.0	Female infertility associated with anovulation ♀	
N97.1	Female infertility of tubal origin ♀	
N97.2	Female infertility of uterine origin ♀	
N97.8	Female infertility of other origin ♀	
Z31.7	Encounter for procreative management and counseling for gestational carrier ♀	
Z31.83	Encounter for assisted reproductive fertility procedure cycle ♀	
Z31.89	Encounter for other procreative management	

AMA: 58321 2019,Jul,6; 2014,Jan,11 **58322** 2019,Jul,6; 2014,Jan,11

Relative Value Units/Medicare Edits

Non-Facility RVU	Work	PE	MP	Total
58321	0.92	1.21	0.13	2.26
58322	1.1	1.28	0.18	2.56
Facility RVU	Work	PE	MP	Total
58321	0.92	0.35	0.13	1.4
58322	1.1	0.42	0.18	1.7

	FUD	Status	MUE	Modifiers				IOM Reference
58321	0	A	1(2)	51	N/A	N/A	80*	None
58322	0	A	1(2)	51	N/A	N/A	80*	

* with documentation

Terms To Know

anovulation. Abnormal condition in which an ovum is not released each month. Anovulation is a prime factor in female infertility.

azoospermia. Failure of the development of sperm or the absence of sperm in semen; one of the most common factors in male infertility.

external os. Uterine opening through the cervix and into the vagina.

medical necessity. Medically appropriate and necessary to meet basic health needs; consistent with the diagnosis or condition and national medical practice guidelines regarding type, frequency, and duration of treatment; rendered in a cost-effective manner.

oligospermia. Insufficient production of sperm in semen, a common factor in male infertility.

stenosis. Narrowing or constriction of a passage.

stricture. Narrowing of an anatomical structure.

58323

58323   Sperm washing for artificial insemination

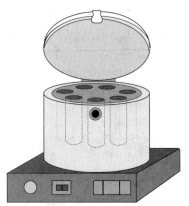

Spermatozoa are separated from seminal fluid by centrifuge

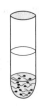

Washed sperm are resuspended in a solution in preparation for artificial insemination

Explanation

Sperm are spun in a centrifuge that removes the superficial antibodies on the sperm in order to facilitate fertilization. The sperm are first washed in a medium three times the volume of the collected semen. This mixture is spun in a centrifuge and the layer of liquid is discarded. The sperm are resuspended in a fresh medium. This method removes debris, bacteria, antibodies, and abnormal spermatozoa.

Coding Tips

Sperm washing is not routinely done with all sperm samples. Diagnostic coding should include codes for male infertility in addition to the codes for female infertility when applicable. Because this procedure is usually performed for the treatment of infertility, the patient may be responsible for charges. Verify with the insurance carrier for coverage. For artificial insemination, see 58321 and 58322. Surgical trays, A4550, are not separately reimbursed by Medicare; however, other third-party payers may cover them. Check with the specific payer to determine coverage.

ICD-10-CM Diagnostic Codes

N97.0	Female infertility associated with anovulation ♀
N97.1	Female infertility of tubal origin ♀
N97.2	Female infertility of uterine origin ♀
N97.8	Female infertility of other origin ♀
Z31.7	Encounter for procreative management and counseling for gestational carrier ♀
Z31.83	Encounter for assisted reproductive fertility procedure cycle ♀
Z31.89	Encounter for other procreative management

AMA: **58323** 2019,Jul,6; 2014,Jan,11

Relative Value Units/Medicare Edits

Non-Facility RVU	Work	PE	MP	Total
58323	0.23	0.17	0.05	0.45
Facility RVU	**Work**	**PE**	**MP**	**Total**
58323	0.23	0.09	0.05	0.37

	FUD	Status	MUE	Modifiers				IOM Reference
58323	0	A	1(3)	51	N/A	N/A	80*	None

* with documentation

Terms To Know

anovulation. Abnormal condition in which an ovum is not released each month. Anovulation is a prime factor in female infertility.

antibody. Protein that B cells of the immune system produce in response to the presence of a foreign antigen.

azoospermia. Failure of the development of sperm or the absence of sperm in semen; one of the most common factors in male infertility.

centrifuge. Machine used to simulate gravitational effects or centrifugal force to separate substances of different densities.

medical necessity. Medically appropriate and necessary to meet basic health needs; consistent with the diagnosis or condition and national medical practice guidelines regarding type, frequency, and duration of treatment; rendered in a cost-effective manner.

oligospermia. Insufficient production of sperm in semen, a common factor in male infertility.

stenosis. Narrowing or constriction of a passage.

stricture. Narrowing of an anatomical structure.

58340

58340 Catheterization and introduction of saline or contrast material for saline infusion sonohysterography (SIS) or hysterosalpingography

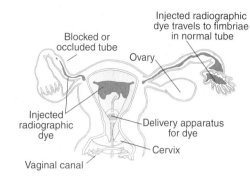

Explanation

A small catheter is introduced into the cervical opening and a saline solution (for saline infusion sonohysterography [SIS]) or liquid radiographic contrast material (for hysterosalpingography) is injected into the endometrial cavity with mild pressure to force the material into the fallopian tubes. The shadow of the contrast material appears on separately reported x-ray films, permitting examination of the uterus and fallopian tubes for any abnormalities or blockages. When sonohysterography is performed, a thin catheter is inserted into the uterus and one to two teaspoons of saline solution is injected into the uterine cavity. Separately reported, fluid enhanced endovaginal ultrasound is performed with the saline solution acting as a contrast medium to view any abnormal anatomic findings in the uterus.

Coding Tips

Report radiology services for this procedure separately. For hysterosonography, see 76831; hysterosalpingography, see 74740. For chromotubation of oviduct, see 58350. For transcervical introduction of fallopian tube catheter, see 58345.

ICD-10-CM Diagnostic Codes

A56.11	Chlamydial female pelvic inflammatory disease ♀
C54.1	Malignant neoplasm of endometrium ♀
C54.2	Malignant neoplasm of myometrium ♀
C54.3	Malignant neoplasm of fundus uteri ♀
C54.8	Malignant neoplasm of overlapping sites of corpus uteri ♀
C57.11	Malignant neoplasm of right broad ligament ♀ ☑
C57.12	Malignant neoplasm of left broad ligament ♀ ☑
C57.21	Malignant neoplasm of right round ligament ♀ ☑
C57.22	Malignant neoplasm of left round ligament ♀ ☑
C57.3	Malignant neoplasm of parametrium ♀
D06.0	Carcinoma in situ of endocervix ♀
D06.1	Carcinoma in situ of exocervix ♀
D06.7	Carcinoma in situ of other parts of cervix ♀
D25.0	Submucous leiomyoma of uterus ♀
D25.1	Intramural leiomyoma of uterus ♀
D25.2	Subserosal leiomyoma of uterus ♀
D26.0	Other benign neoplasm of cervix uteri ♀
D26.1	Other benign neoplasm of corpus uteri ♀
D26.7	Other benign neoplasm of other parts of uterus ♀
D28.2	Benign neoplasm of uterine tubes and ligaments ♀
D39.0	Neoplasm of uncertain behavior of uterus ♀

E28.2	Polycystic ovarian syndrome ♀	N93.8	Other specified abnormal uterine and vaginal bleeding ♀
E28.310	Symptomatic premature menopause 🅰 ♀	N94.4	Primary dysmenorrhea ♀
E28.319	Asymptomatic premature menopause 🅰 ♀	N94.5	Secondary dysmenorrhea ♀
E28.39	Other primary ovarian failure ♀	N94.89	Other specified conditions associated with female genital organs and menstrual cycle ♀
E28.8	Other ovarian dysfunction ♀	N95.0	Postmenopausal bleeding ♀
N70.11	Chronic salpingitis ♀	N97.0	Female infertility associated with anovulation ♀
N70.12	Chronic oophoritis ♀	N97.1	Female infertility of tubal origin ♀
N70.13	Chronic salpingitis and oophoritis ♀	N97.2	Female infertility of uterine origin ♀
N71.0	Acute inflammatory disease of uterus ♀	N97.8	Female infertility of other origin ♀
N71.1	Chronic inflammatory disease of uterus ♀	N99.83	Residual ovary syndrome ♀
N73.6	Female pelvic peritoneal adhesions (postinfective) ♀	N99.85	Post endometrial ablation syndrome ♀
N73.8	Other specified female pelvic inflammatory diseases ♀	Q50.4	Embryonic cyst of fallopian tube ♀
N80.0	Endometriosis of uterus ♀	Q50.5	Embryonic cyst of broad ligament ♀
N80.1	Endometriosis of ovary ♀	Q50.6	Other congenital malformations of fallopian tube and broad ligament ♀
N80.2	Endometriosis of fallopian tube ♀	Q51.0	Agenesis and aplasia of uterus ♀
N80.3	Endometriosis of pelvic peritoneum ♀	Q51.10	Doubling of uterus with doubling of cervix and vagina without obstruction ♀
N80.8	Other endometriosis ♀	Q51.11	Doubling of uterus with doubling of cervix and vagina with obstruction ♀
N83.291	Other ovarian cyst, right side ♀ ☑	Q51.21	Complete doubling of uterus ♀
N83.292	Other ovarian cyst, left side ♀ ☑	Q51.22	Partial doubling of uterus ♀
N83.41	Prolapse and hernia of right ovary and fallopian tube ♀ ☑	Q51.28	Other and unspecified doubling of uterus ♀
N83.42	Prolapse and hernia of left ovary and fallopian tube ♀ ☑	Q51.3	Bicornate uterus ♀
N83.511	Torsion of right ovary and ovarian pedicle ♀ ☑	Q51.4	Unicornate uterus ♀
N83.512	Torsion of left ovary and ovarian pedicle ♀ ☑	Q51.5	Agenesis and aplasia of cervix ♀
N83.521	Torsion of right fallopian tube ♀ ☑	Q51.810	Arcuate uterus ♀
N83.522	Torsion of left fallopian tube ♀ ☑	Q51.811	Hypoplasia of uterus ♀
N83.53	Torsion of ovary, ovarian pedicle and fallopian tube ♀	Q51.818	Other congenital malformations of uterus ♀
N83.6	Hematosalpinx ♀	Q51.820	Cervical duplication ♀
N83.8	Other noninflammatory disorders of ovary, fallopian tube and broad ligament ♀		
N84.0	Polyp of corpus uteri ♀		

AMA: **58340** 2019,Jul,6; 2018,Jan,8; 2017,Jan,8; 2016,Jan,13; 2015,Jan,16; 2014,Jan,11

N84.8	Polyp of other parts of female genital tract ♀	
N85.01	Benign endometrial hyperplasia ♀	
N85.02	Endometrial intraepithelial neoplasia [EIN] ♀	
N85.2	Hypertrophy of uterus ♀	
N85.3	Subinvolution of uterus ♀	
N85.4	Malposition of uterus ♀	
N85.5	Inversion of uterus ♀	
N85.6	Intrauterine synechiae ♀	
N85.7	Hematometra ♀	
N85.8	Other specified noninflammatory disorders of uterus ♀	
N89.7	Hematocolpos ♀	
N91.0	Primary amenorrhea ♀	
N91.1	Secondary amenorrhea ♀	
N91.3	Primary oligomenorrhea ♀	
N91.4	Secondary oligomenorrhea ♀	
N92.0	Excessive and frequent menstruation with regular cycle ♀	
N92.1	Excessive and frequent menstruation with irregular cycle ♀	
N92.2	Excessive menstruation at puberty 🅿 ♀	
N92.3	Ovulation bleeding ♀	
N92.4	Excessive bleeding in the premenopausal period ♀	
N92.5	Other specified irregular menstruation ♀	
N93.0	Postcoital and contact bleeding ♀	
N93.1	Pre-pubertal vaginal bleeding ♀	

Relative Value Units/Medicare Edits

Non-Facility RVU	Work	PE	MP	Total
58340	0.88	4.53	0.12	5.53
Facility RVU	**Work**	**PE**	**MP**	**Total**
58340	0.88	0.65	0.12	1.65

	FUD	Status	MUE	Modifiers				IOM Reference
58340	0	A	1(3)	51	N/A	N/A	N/A	None

* with documentation

Terms To Know

catheterization. Use or insertion of a tubular device into a duct, blood vessel, hollow organ, or body cavity for injecting or withdrawing fluids for diagnostic or therapeutic purposes.

hysterosalpingography. Radiographic pictures taken of the uterus and the fallopian tubes after the injection of a radiopaque dye.

58345

58345 Transcervical introduction of fallopian tube catheter for diagnosis and/or re-establishing patency (any method), with or without hysterosalpingography

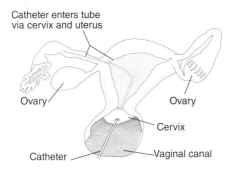

Catheter enters tube via cervix and uterus

Ovary

Ovary

Cervix

Catheter

Vaginal canal

Explanation

The physician introduces a catheter into the cervix, and takes it into the uterus and through the fallopian tube. The catheter must be made of a material that will show on x-ray film so that any blockages or abnormalities in the tube can be seen. The physician may inject radiographic contrast material into the endometrial cavity with mild pressure to force the material into the tubes. The shadow of this material on separately reported x-ray film permits examination of the uterus and tubes for any abnormalities or blockages.

Coding Tips

This procedure can be accomplished in a physician's office when radiology equipment is present or in a radiology facility. This code includes any method of re-establishing patency of the tube and a hysterosalpingography performed by the physician. For radiological supervision and interpretation of transcervical catheterization of a fallopian tube, see 74742. Because this procedure is usually performed for the treatment of infertility, the patient may be responsible for charges. Verify with the insurance carrier for coverage. For surgical treatment of an ectopic pregnancy, see 59120–59140. For laparoscopic treatment of an ectopic pregnancy, see 59150–59151.

ICD-10-CM Diagnostic Codes

E28.2	Polycystic ovarian syndrome ♀
E28.8	Other ovarian dysfunction ♀
N70.01	Acute salpingitis ♀
N70.02	Acute oophoritis ♀
N70.03	Acute salpingitis and oophoritis ♀
N70.11	Chronic salpingitis ♀
N70.12	Chronic oophoritis ♀
N70.13	Chronic salpingitis and oophoritis ♀
N73.6	Female pelvic peritoneal adhesions (postinfective) ♀
N80.2	Endometriosis of fallopian tube ♀
N83.321	Acquired atrophy of right fallopian tube ♀ ☑
N83.322	Acquired atrophy of left fallopian tube ♀ ☑
N83.331	Acquired atrophy of right ovary and fallopian tube ♀ ☑
N83.332	Acquired atrophy of left ovary and fallopian tube ♀ ☑
N83.41	Prolapse and hernia of right ovary and fallopian tube ♀ ☑
N83.42	Prolapse and hernia of left ovary and fallopian tube ♀ ☑
N83.521	Torsion of right fallopian tube ♀ ☑
N83.522	Torsion of left fallopian tube ♀ ☑
N83.53	Torsion of ovary, ovarian pedicle and fallopian tube ♀

N83.6	Hematosalpinx ♀
N83.8	Other noninflammatory disorders of ovary, fallopian tube and broad ligament ♀
N85.01	Benign endometrial hyperplasia ♀
N85.02	Endometrial intraepithelial neoplasia [EIN] ♀
N85.2	Hypertrophy of uterus ♀
N85.3	Subinvolution of uterus ♀
N85.5	Inversion of uterus ♀
N88.2	Stricture and stenosis of cervix uteri ♀
N88.8	Other specified noninflammatory disorders of cervix uteri ♀
N97.1	Female infertility of tubal origin ♀
N97.8	Female infertility of other origin ♀
N99.83	Residual ovary syndrome ♀
Q50.4	Embryonic cyst of fallopian tube ♀
Q50.6	Other congenital malformations of fallopian tube and broad ligament ♀
Z31.41	Encounter for fertility testing
Z31.42	Aftercare following sterilization reversal
Z31.49	Encounter for other procreative investigation and testing

AMA: **58345** 2019,Jul,6; 2018,Jan,8; 2017,Jan,8; 2016,Jan,13; 2015,Jan,16; 2014,Jan,11

Relative Value Units/Medicare Edits

Non-Facility RVU	Work	PE	MP	Total
58345	4.7	2.83	0.74	8.27
Facility RVU	**Work**	**PE**	**MP**	**Total**
58345	4.7	2.83	0.74	8.27

	FUD	Status	MUE	Modifiers				IOM Reference
58345	10	A	1(3)	51	50	62	80	None

* with documentation

Terms To Know

hysterosalpingography. Radiographic pictures taken of the uterus and the fallopian tubes after the injection of a radiopaque dye.

patency. State of a tube-like structure or conduit being open and unobstructed.

58346

58346 Insertion of Heyman capsules for clinical brachytherapy

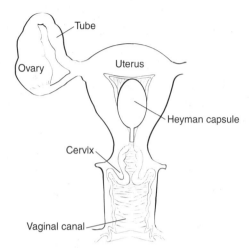

Heyman capsules are inserted into
the uterus for clinical brachytherapy

Explanation

The physician inserts radioactive Heyman capsules into the uterus to treat endometrial cancer. Radiotherapy is often the prescribed treatment for patients who are medically inoperable for endometrial carcinoma. Brachytherapy is administered via low dose radiation (LDR) or high dose radiation (HDR) technique, with the goal of achieving coverage of all uterine tissue. This is achieved with the placement of multiple Heyman capsules, inserted through the cervical os and placed in the uterus with consideration of appropriate radiation field. For low-dose treatment, Heyman capsules are used for patients with a large uterus to help expand the uterine cavity and cover the uterus. Heyman capsules also may be prescribed for patients with early-stage disease and low-grade histology, when radiation alone is the preferred therapy. Use this code once to report multiple capsules inserted during the same session.

Coding Tips

For insertion of intracavitary radioelement sources, see 77761–77763. For interstitial application of radioelement sources or ribbons, see 77770–77772. Placement of needles or catheters into pelvic organs and/or genitalia for the purposes of interstitial radioelement application is reported with 55920.

ICD-10-CM Diagnostic Codes

C53.0	Malignant neoplasm of endocervix ♀
C53.1	Malignant neoplasm of exocervix ♀
C53.8	Malignant neoplasm of overlapping sites of cervix uteri ♀
C54.0	Malignant neoplasm of isthmus uteri ♀
C54.1	Malignant neoplasm of endometrium ♀
C54.2	Malignant neoplasm of myometrium ♀
C54.3	Malignant neoplasm of fundus uteri ♀
C54.8	Malignant neoplasm of overlapping sites of corpus uteri ♀
C79.82	Secondary malignant neoplasm of genital organs
D06.0	Carcinoma in situ of endocervix ♀
D06.1	Carcinoma in situ of exocervix ♀
D06.7	Carcinoma in situ of other parts of cervix ♀
D07.0	Carcinoma in situ of endometrium ♀
D07.39	Carcinoma in situ of other female genital organs ♀
D39.0	Neoplasm of uncertain behavior of uterus ♀

D39.8	Neoplasm of uncertain behavior of other specified female genital organs ♀

AMA: 58346 2019,Jul,6; 2018,Jan,8; 2017,Jan,8; 2016,Jan,13; 2015,Jan,16; 2014,Jan,11

Relative Value Units/Medicare Edits

Non-Facility RVU	Work	PE	MP	Total
58346	7.56	5.55	0.54	13.65
Facility RVU	**Work**	**PE**	**MP**	**Total**
58346	7.56	5.55	0.54	13.65

	FUD	Status	MUE	Modifiers				IOM Reference
58346	90	A	1(2)	51	N/A	N/A	N/A	None

* with documentation

Terms To Know

brachytherapy. Form of radiation therapy in which radioactive pellets or seeds are implanted directly into the tissue being treated to deliver their dose of radiation in a more directed fashion. Brachytherapy provides radiation to the prescribed body area while minimizing exposure to normal tissue.

carcinoma in situ. Malignancy that arises from the cells of the vessel, gland, or organ of origin that remains confined to that site or has not invaded neighboring tissue.

endometrial carcinoma. Cancer of the inner lining of the uterine wall.

malignant. Any condition tending to progress toward death, specifically an invasive tumor with a loss of cellular differentiation that has the ability to spread or metastasize to other body areas.

secondary. Second in order of occurrence or importance, or appearing during the course of another disease or condition.

58350

58350 Chromotubation of oviduct, including materials

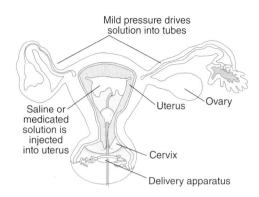

Mild pressure drives solution into tubes

Saline or medicated solution is injected into uterus

Uterus

Ovary

Cervix

Delivery apparatus

Explanation

The physician injects a liquid dye or solution into the uterine cavity or directly into the fallopian tubes. This procedure is frequently performed during a separately reported surgery, open or laparoscopic, to verify patency of tubes.

Coding Tips

When 58350 is performed with another separately identifiable procedure, the highest dollar value code is listed as the primary procedure and subsequent procedures are appended with modifier 51. Supply of materials should be reported separately with code 99070.

ICD-10-CM Diagnostic Codes

N70.01	Acute salpingitis ♀
N70.03	Acute salpingitis and oophoritis ♀
N70.11	Chronic salpingitis ♀
N70.13	Chronic salpingitis and oophoritis ♀
N80.2	Endometriosis of fallopian tube ♀
N83.321	Acquired atrophy of right fallopian tube ♀ ☑
N83.322	Acquired atrophy of left fallopian tube ♀ ☑
N83.331	Acquired atrophy of right ovary and fallopian tube ♀ ☑
N83.332	Acquired atrophy of left ovary and fallopian tube ♀ ☑
N83.521	Torsion of right fallopian tube ♀ ☑
N83.522	Torsion of left fallopian tube ♀ ☑
N83.53	Torsion of ovary, ovarian pedicle and fallopian tube ♀
N83.6	Hematosalpinx ♀
N83.8	Other noninflammatory disorders of ovary, fallopian tube and broad ligament ♀
N97.1	Female infertility of tubal origin ♀
Q50.4	Embryonic cyst of fallopian tube ♀
Q50.6	Other congenital malformations of fallopian tube and broad ligament ♀
Z31.41	Encounter for fertility testing
Z31.42	Aftercare following sterilization reversal

AMA: **58350** 2019,Jul,6; 2018,Jan,8; 2017,Jan,8; 2016,Jan,13; 2015,Jan,16; 2014,Jan,11

Corpus Uteri

Relative Value Units/Medicare Edits

Non-Facility RVU	Work	PE	MP	Total
58350	1.06	2.4	0.16	3.62
Facility RVU	**Work**	**PE**	**MP**	**Total**
58350	1.06	1.29	0.16	2.51

	FUD	Status	MUE	Modifiers				IOM Reference
58350	10	A	1(2)	51	50	N/A	N/A	None

* with documentation

Terms To Know

adhesion. Abnormal fibrous connection between two structures, soft tissue or bony structures, that may occur as the result of surgery, infection, or trauma.

chromotubation. Injection of a medication or saline solution into the uterine cavity and fallopian tubes to verify patency of the tubes.

endometriosis. Aberrant uterine mucosal tissue appearing in areas of the pelvic cavity outside of its normal location, lining the uterus, and inflaming surrounding tissues often resulting in infertility or spontaneous abortion.

follicular cyst. Common type of ovarian cyst related to the menstrual cycle that occurs when the follicle in which the ovum develops does not rupture and expel the egg. Follicular cysts normally disappear within two or three menstrual cycles and are usually benign.

oophoritis. Inflammation or infection of one or both ovaries that can cause chronic pelvic pain, ectopic pregnancy, or sterilization.

parametritis. Inflammation and infection of the tissue in the structures around the uterus.

patency. State of a tube-like structure or conduit being open and unobstructed.

salpingitis. Inflammation of the fallopian tubes, usually caused by a bacterial infection and occurring in conjunction with inflammation of the ovaries (oophoritis).

58353

58353 Endometrial ablation, thermal, without hysteroscopic guidance

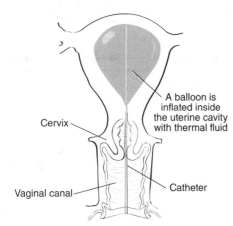

Cervix

A balloon is inflated inside the uterine cavity with thermal fluid

Vaginal canal

Catheter

Fluid in the balloon is heated to a scalding temperature, causing the lining to slough away

Explanation

The physician performs an endometrial ablation, using heat without hysteroscopic guidance. The physician inserts a soft, flexible balloon attached to a thin catheter into the vagina through the cervix and into the uterus. The balloon is inflated with fluid, which expands to fit the size and shape of the patient's uterus. The fluid in the balloon is heated to 87°C or 188°F and maintained for eight to nine minutes while the uterine lining is treated. When the treatment cycle is complete, all the fluid is withdrawn from the balloon and the balloon and catheter are removed.

Coding Tips

When 58353 is performed with another separately identifiable procedure, the highest dollar value code is listed as the primary procedure and subsequent procedures are appended with modifier 51. Local anesthesia is included in this service; however, this procedure may be performed under general anesthesia depending on the age and/or condition of the patient. For endometrial ablation with hysteroscopy, see 58563. Surgical trays, A4550, are not separately reimbursed by Medicare; however, other third-party payers may cover them. Check with the specific payer to determine coverage.

ICD-10-CM Diagnostic Codes

N80.0	Endometriosis of uterus ♀
N92.0	Excessive and frequent menstruation with regular cycle ♀
N92.1	Excessive and frequent menstruation with irregular cycle ♀
N92.3	Ovulation bleeding ♀
N92.4	Excessive bleeding in the premenopausal period ♀
N92.5	Other specified irregular menstruation ♀
N93.8	Other specified abnormal uterine and vaginal bleeding ♀
N95.0	Postmenopausal bleeding ♀
N95.8	Other specified menopausal and perimenopausal disorders ♀

AMA: 58353 2019,Jul,6; 2018,Jan,8; 2017,Jan,8; 2016,Jan,13; 2015,Jan,16; 2014,Jan,11

Relative Value Units/Medicare Edits

Non-Facility RVU	Work	PE	MP	Total
58353	3.6	24.35	0.56	28.51
Facility RVU	Work	PE	MP	Total
58353	3.6	2.38	0.56	6.54

	FUD	Status	MUE	Modifiers				IOM Reference
58353	10	A	1(3)	51	N/A	62	N/A	None

* with documentation

Terms To Know

ablation. Removal or destruction of a body part or tissue or its function. Ablation may be performed by surgical means, hormones, drugs, radiofrequency, heat, chemical application, or other methods.

catheter. Flexible tube inserted into an area of the body for introducing or withdrawing fluid.

endometriosis. Aberrant uterine mucosal tissue appearing in areas of the pelvic cavity outside of its normal location, lining the uterus, and inflaming surrounding tissues often resulting in infertility or spontaneous abortion.

metrorrhagia. Prolonged, irregular uterine bleeding of an inconsistent amount occurring in frequent bouts.

58356

58356   Endometrial cryoablation with ultrasonic guidance, including endometrial curettage, when performed

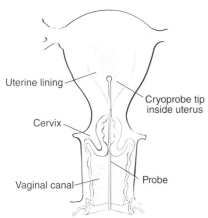

Uterine lining

Cryoprobe tip inside uterus

Cervix

Vaginal canal

Probe

Endometrial cryoablation is performed.
Dilation and curettage may also be performed.

Explanation

The physician performs endometrial cryoablation with any required endometrial curettage using ultrasound guidance. The physician inserts a speculum for visualization of the cervix. A numbing block is placed in the cervix. A thin cryoablation device is inserted through the cervix into the uterus. The cryoablation device freezes targeted uterine endometrial tissue. The instrument is withdrawn following completion of the procedure. Ultrasound provides visualization of probe placement and real-time monitoring of the ice ball growth. If endometrial curettage is required, the physician passes a curette into the uterus through the endocervical canal. The lining of the uterus is scraped.

Coding Tips

Biopsy of the endometrium, dilation and curettage, catheterization and contrast medium or saline infusion, and pelvic or abdominal ultrasound are included in 58356 and should not be reported separately. Do not report 58356 with 58100, 58120, 58340, 76700, or 76856. Surgical trays, A4550, are not separately reimbursed by Medicare; however, other third-party payers may cover them. Check with the specific payer to determine coverage.

ICD-10-CM Diagnostic Codes

N80.0	Endometriosis of uterus ♀
N92.0	Excessive and frequent menstruation with regular cycle ♀
N92.1	Excessive and frequent menstruation with irregular cycle ♀
N92.3	Ovulation bleeding ♀
N92.4	Excessive bleeding in the premenopausal period ♀
N92.5	Other specified irregular menstruation ♀
N93.8	Other specified abnormal uterine and vaginal bleeding ♀
N95.0	Postmenopausal bleeding ♀
N95.8	Other specified menopausal and perimenopausal disorders ♀

AMA: 58356 2019,Jul,6; 2014,Jan,11

Relative Value Units/Medicare Edits

Non-Facility RVU	Work	PE	MP	Total
58356	6.41	44.62	1.01	52.04
Facility RVU	**Work**	**PE**	**MP**	**Total**
58356	6.41	2.83	1.01	10.25

	FUD	Status	MUE	Modifiers				IOM Reference
58356	10	A	1(3)	51	N/A	62	80	None

* with documentation

Terms To Know

ablation. Removal or destruction of a body part or tissue or its function. Ablation may be performed by surgical means, hormones, drugs, radiofrequency, heat, chemical application, or other methods.

cryotherapy. Any surgical procedure that uses intense cold for treatment.

curettage. Removal of tissue by scraping.

curette. Spoon-shaped instrument used to scrape out abnormal tissue from a cavity or bone.

endometrium. Lining of the uterus, which thickens in preparation for fertilization. A fertilized ovum embeds into the thickened endometrium. When no fertilization takes place, the endometrial lining sheds during the process of menstruation.

speculum. Tool used to enlarge the opening of any canal or cavity.

ultrasound. Imaging using ultra-high sound frequency bounced off body structures.

58400

58400 Uterine suspension, with or without shortening of round ligaments, with or without shortening of sacrouterine ligaments; (separate procedure)

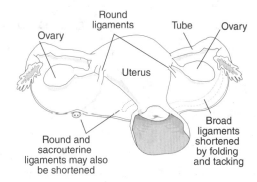

Round ligaments

Ovary

Tube Ovary

Uterus

Round and sacrouterine ligaments may also be shortened

Broad ligaments shortened by folding and tacking

Explanation

The physician plicates stretched uterine broad ligaments, bringing the uterus back into place. Plication shortens the ligament by folding and tacking it. The physician may elect to plicate the round and sacrouterine ligaments as well. This procedure may be done through a small abdominal incision or through an incision in the vagina.

Coding Tips

This separate procedure by definition is usually a component of a more complex service and is not identified separately. When performed alone or with other unrelated procedures/services it may be reported. If performed alone, list the code; if performed with other procedures/services, list the code and append modifier 59 or an X{EPSU} modifier. When 58400 is performed with another separately identifiable procedure, the highest dollar value code is listed as the primary procedure and subsequent procedures are appended with modifier 51. For uterine suspension, with or without shortening of round ligaments, with or without shortening of sacrouterine ligaments, with presacral sympathectomy, report 58410.

ICD-10-CM Diagnostic Codes

N81.2	Incomplete uterovaginal prolapse ♀
N81.3	Complete uterovaginal prolapse ♀
N85.4	Malposition of uterus ♀
N85.5	Inversion of uterus ♀

AMA: **58400** 2019,Jul,6; 2014,Jan,11

Relative Value Units/Medicare Edits

Non-Facility RVU	Work	PE	MP	Total
58400	7.14	4.96	1.04	13.14
Facility RVU	Work	PE	MP	Total
58400	7.14	4.96	1.04	13.14

	FUD	Status	MUE	Modifiers				IOM Reference
58400	90	A	1(3)	51	N/A	62*	80	None

* with documentation

58410

58410 Uterine suspension, with or without shortening of round ligaments, with or without shortening of sacrouterine ligaments; with presacral sympathectomy

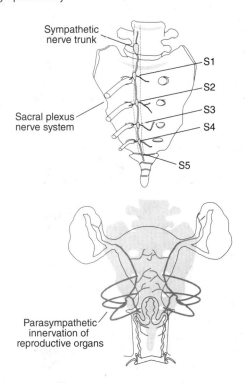

Sympathetic nerve trunk

S1
S2
S3
S4

Sacral plexus nerve system

S5

Parasympathetic innervation of reproductive organs

Explanation

The physician plicates stretched uterine broad ligaments, bringing the uterus back into place. Plication shortens the ligament by folding and tacking it. The physician may elect to plicate the round and sacrouterine ligaments as well. A portion of the presacral sympathetic nerve is removed or destroyed to alleviate pelvic pain. The procedure may be done through a small abdominal incision or through an incision in the vagina.

Coding Tips

When 58410 is performed with another separately identifiable procedure, the highest dollar value code is listed as the primary procedure and subsequent procedures are appended with modifier 51. For uterine suspension, with or without shortening of round ligaments, with or without shortening of sacrouterine ligaments, without presacral sympathectomy, report 58400.

ICD-10-CM Diagnostic Codes

N81.2	Incomplete uterovaginal prolapse ♀
N81.3	Complete uterovaginal prolapse ♀
N85.4	Malposition of uterus ♀
N85.5	Inversion of uterus ♀

AMA: **58410** 2019,Jul,6; 2018,Jan,8; 2017,Jan,8; 2016,Jan,13; 2015,Jan,16; 2014,Jan,11

Relative Value Units/Medicare Edits

Non-Facility RVU	Work	PE	MP	Total
58410	13.8	7.61	2.17	23.58
Facility RVU	Work	PE	MP	Total
58410	13.8	7.61	2.17	23.58

	FUD	Status	MUE	Modifiers				IOM Reference
58410	90	A	1(2)	51	N/A	62*	80	None

* with documentation

Terms To Know

chronic inversion of uterus. Persistent abnormality in which the uterus turns inside out.

female stress incontinence. Involuntary escape of urine at times of minor stress against the female bladder, such as coughing, sneezing, or laughing.

round ligament. Ligament between the uterus and the pelvic wall.

suspension. Fixation of an organ for support; temporary state of cessation of an activity, process, or experience.

uterovaginal prolapse. Uterus displaced downward and exposed in the external genitalia.

58520

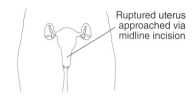

58520   Hysterorrhaphy, repair of ruptured uterus (nonobstetrical)

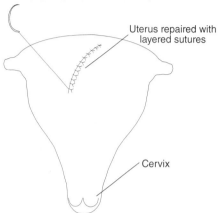

Ruptured uterus approached via midline incision

The injury may require additional procedures

Uterus repaired with layered sutures

Cervix

Explanation

The physician repairs a uterus that became lacerated or ruptured by nonobstetrical means. A large incision is made in the abdomen and the uterus is repaired with layered suturing of torn, crushed, or deeply lacerated tissue. The physician debrides the wound by removing foreign material or damaged tissue. Irrigation of the wound is performed and antimicrobial solutions are used to decontaminate and cleanse the wound. The physician may trim skin margins with a scalpel or scissors to allow for proper closure. The abdominal incision is closed.

Coding Tips

This code applies only to ruptures caused by injury or trauma, not by pregnancy. When 58520 is performed with another separately identifiable procedure, the highest dollar value code is listed as the primary procedure and subsequent procedures are appended with modifier 51. For repair of a ruptured uterus in an obstetrical setting, report 59350. When hysteroplasty is done to correct an anomaly present from birth, not an acquired condition due to trauma, age, or disease, see 58540.

ICD-10-CM Diagnostic Codes

S37.60XA	Unspecified injury of uterus, initial encounter ♀
S37.62XA	Contusion of uterus, initial encounter ♀
S37.63XA	Laceration of uterus, initial encounter ♀
S37.69XA	Other injury of uterus, initial encounter ♀

AMA: 58520 2019,Jul,6; 2014,Jan,11

Relative Value Units/Medicare Edits

Non-Facility RVU	Work	PE	MP	Total
58520	13.48	7.48	2.13	23.09
Facility RVU	Work	PE	MP	Total
58520	13.48	7.48	2.13	23.09

	FUD	Status	MUE	Modifiers				IOM Reference
58520	90	A	1(2)	51	N/A	62*	80	None

* with documentation

Terms To Know

debride. To remove all foreign objects and devitalized or infected tissue from a burn or wound to prevent infection and promote healing.

irrigation. To wash out or cleanse a body cavity, wound, or tissue with water or other fluid.

laceration. Tearing injury; a torn, ragged-edged wound.

margin. Boundary, edge, or border, as of a surface or structure.

repair. Surgical closure of a wound. The wound may be a result of injury/trauma or it may be a surgically created defect. Repairs are divided into three categories: simple, intermediate, and complex.

rupture. Tearing or breaking open of tissue.

suture. Numerous stitching techniques employed in wound closure.

wound. Injury to living tissue often involving a cut or break in the skin.

58540

58540 Hysteroplasty, repair of uterine anomaly (Strassman type)

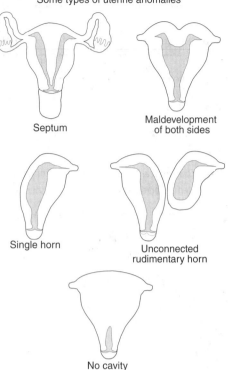

Some types of uterine anomalies

Septum

Maldevelopment of both sides

Single horn

Unconnected rudimentary horn

No cavity

Explanation

Through a small incision in the lower abdomen, the physician performs a plastic repair of a malformed uterus. This often is an extensive procedure that involves removing abnormal tissues, rearranging the uterine walls, and suturing.

Coding Tips

This code should be used when the hysteroplasty is done to correct an anomaly present from birth, not an acquired condition due to trauma, age, or disease. Use 58520 to report the repair of an acquired ruptured uterus. When 58540 is performed with another separately identifiable procedure, the highest dollar value code is listed as the primary procedure and subsequent procedures are appended with modifier 51. For repair of a ruptured uterus in an obstetrical setting, report 59350.

ICD-10-CM Diagnostic Codes

N85.8	Other specified noninflammatory disorders of uterus ♀
Q51.0	Agenesis and aplasia of uterus ♀
Q51.10	Doubling of uterus with doubling of cervix and vagina without obstruction ♀
Q51.11	Doubling of uterus with doubling of cervix and vagina with obstruction ♀
Q51.21	Complete doubling of uterus ♀
Q51.22	Partial doubling of uterus ♀
Q51.28	Other and unspecified doubling of uterus ♀
Q51.3	Bicornate uterus ♀
Q51.4	Unicornate uterus ♀
Q51.810	Arcuate uterus ♀

Q51.811 Hypoplasia of uterus ♀

Q51.818 Other congenital malformations of uterus ♀

AMA: 58540 2019,Jul,6; 2014,Jan,11

Relative Value Units/Medicare Edits

Non-Facility RVU	Work	PE	MP	Total
58540	15.71	8.38	2.47	26.56
Facility RVU	Work	PE	MP	Total
58540	15.71	8.38	2.47	26.56

	FUD	Status	MUE	Modifiers				IOM Reference
58540	90	A	1(3)	51	N/A	N/A	80	None

* with documentation

Terms To Know

agenesis. Absence of an organ due to developmental failure in the prenatal period.

anomaly. Irregularity in the structure or position of an organ or tissue.

aplasia. Incomplete development of an organ or tissue. Aplasia may be congenital (present at birth) or acquired.

congenital. Present at birth, occurring through heredity or an influence during gestation up to the moment of birth.

hypoplasia. Condition in which there is underdevelopment of an organ or tissue.

incision. Act of cutting into tissue or an organ.

suture. Numerous stitching techniques employed in wound closure.

[58674]

58674 Laparoscopy, surgical, ablation of uterine fibroid(s) including intraoperative ultrasound guidance and monitoring, radiofrequency

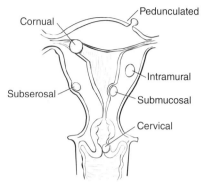

Types of uterine fibroids

Explanation

Radiofrequency ablation (RFA) of uterine fibroids is performed laparoscopically. The physician makes a small incision in the umbilicus through which the abdomen is insufflated and a fiberoptic laparoscope is inserted. Other incisions are made through which trocars can be passed into the abdominal cavity to deliver instruments, a video camera, and, when needed, an additional light source. The physician manipulates the tools so that the uterus and fibroids can be viewed through the laparoscope and/or video monitor. Using ultrasound guidance, the RFA catheter is inserted through the skin into a fibroid and electrical energy is delivered to the fibroid, heating the tissue and killing the tumor cells. The procedure is repeated as needed for additional fibroids. The catheter, laparoscope, and instruments are removed and the incisions are closed.

Coding Tips

Surgical laparoscopy always includes diagnostic laparoscopy. Do not report 58674 with 49320, 58541-58554, 58570-58573, or 76998.

ICD-10-CM Diagnostic Codes

D25.0 Submucous leiomyoma of uterus ♀

D25.1 Intramural leiomyoma of uterus ♀

D25.2 Subserosal leiomyoma of uterus ♀

AMA: 58674 2019,Jul,6; 2018,Jan,8; 2017,Feb,14; 2017,Apr,7

Relative Value Units/Medicare Edits

Non-Facility RVU	Work	PE	MP	Total
58674	14.08	7.39	2.21	23.68
Facility RVU	Work	PE	MP	Total
58674	14.08	7.39	2.21	23.68

	FUD	Status	MUE	Modifiers				IOM Reference
58674	90	A	1(2)	51	N/A	62	80	None

* with documentation

Terms To Know

leiomyoma. Benign tumor consisting of smooth muscle in the uterus.

radiofrequency ablation. To destroy by electromagnetic wave frequencies.

● New ▲ Revised + Add On ★ Telemedicine AMA: CPT Assist [Resequenced] ☑ Laterality © 2020 Optum360, LLC

58541-58542

58541 Laparoscopy, surgical, supracervical hysterectomy, for uterus 250 g or less;

58542 with removal of tube(s) and/or ovary(s)

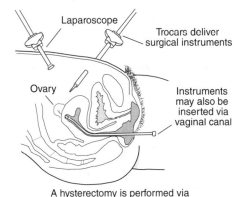

A hysterectomy is performed via laparoscopy and the cervix is preserved

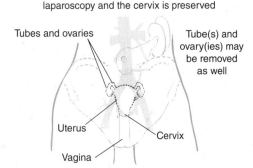

Tube(s) and ovary(ies) may be removed as well

Explanation

The physician performs a laparoscopic hysterectomy, removing a uterus with a total weight of 250 gm or less while preserving the cervix. The patient is placed in the dorsal lithotomy position. After the insertion of a speculum in the vagina, the physician grasps the cervix with an instrument to manipulate the uterus during the surgery. A trocar is inserted periumbilically and the abdomen is insufflated with gas. Additional trocars are placed in the right and left lower quadrants. The uterus is dissected free from the bladder and surrounding tissue and its body is separated from the cervix. Coagulation is achieved with the aid of electrocautery instruments. Alternatively, some vessels may be ligated. The uterus is morcellized and removed using endoscopic tools. In 58542, one or both ovaries and/or one or both fallopian tubes are removed in similar fashion. Once the excisions are complete, the abdominal cavity is deflated and instruments and trocars removed. The fascia and skin are closed with sutures.

Coding Tips

Surgical laparoscopy always includes diagnostic laparoscopy. For diagnostic laparoscopy, see 49320. For laparoscopic supracervical hysterectomy, for a uterus greater than 250 gm, see 58543; with removal of tubes and/or ovaries, see 58544. Do not report 58541-58542 with 49320, 57000, 57180, 57410, 58140–58146, 58545–58546, 58561, 58661, or 58670-58671.

ICD-10-CM Diagnostic Codes

C54.0	Malignant neoplasm of isthmus uteri ♀
C54.1	Malignant neoplasm of endometrium ♀
C54.2	Malignant neoplasm of myometrium ♀
C54.3	Malignant neoplasm of fundus uteri ♀
C54.8	Malignant neoplasm of overlapping sites of corpus uteri ♀
C56.1	Malignant neoplasm of right ovary ♀ ☑
C56.2	Malignant neoplasm of left ovary ♀ ☑
C57.01	Malignant neoplasm of right fallopian tube ♀ ☑
C57.02	Malignant neoplasm of left fallopian tube ♀ ☑
C57.11	Malignant neoplasm of right broad ligament ♀ ☑
C57.12	Malignant neoplasm of left broad ligament ♀ ☑
C57.21	Malignant neoplasm of right round ligament ♀ ☑
C57.22	Malignant neoplasm of left round ligament ♀ ☑
C57.3	Malignant neoplasm of parametrium ♀
C57.7	Malignant neoplasm of other specified female genital organs ♀
C57.8	Malignant neoplasm of overlapping sites of female genital organs ♀
C79.61	Secondary malignant neoplasm of right ovary ♀ ☑
C79.62	Secondary malignant neoplasm of left ovary ♀ ☑
C79.82	Secondary malignant neoplasm of genital organs ♀
D07.0	Carcinoma in situ of endometrium ♀
D07.39	Carcinoma in situ of other female genital organs ♀
D25.0	Submucous leiomyoma of uterus ♀
D25.1	Intramural leiomyoma of uterus ♀
D25.2	Subserosal leiomyoma of uterus ♀
D39.0	Neoplasm of uncertain behavior of uterus ♀
D39.11	Neoplasm of uncertain behavior of right ovary ♀ ☑
D39.12	Neoplasm of uncertain behavior of left ovary ♀ ☑
D39.2	Neoplasm of uncertain behavior of placenta Ⓜ ♀
D39.8	Neoplasm of uncertain behavior of other specified female genital organs ♀
D49.59	Neoplasm of unspecified behavior of other genitourinary organ
N39.3	Stress incontinence (female) (male)
N70.01	Acute salpingitis ♀
N70.02	Acute oophoritis ♀
N70.03	Acute salpingitis and oophoritis ♀
N70.11	Chronic salpingitis ♀
N70.12	Chronic oophoritis ♀
N70.13	Chronic salpingitis and oophoritis ♀
N71.0	Acute inflammatory disease of uterus ♀
N71.1	Chronic inflammatory disease of uterus ♀
N73.0	Acute parametritis and pelvic cellulitis ♀
N73.1	Chronic parametritis and pelvic cellulitis ♀
N73.3	Female acute pelvic peritonitis ♀
N73.4	Female chronic pelvic peritonitis ♀
N73.6	Female pelvic peritoneal adhesions (postinfective) ♀
N73.8	Other specified female pelvic inflammatory diseases ♀
N80.0	Endometriosis of uterus ♀
N80.1	Endometriosis of ovary ♀
N80.2	Endometriosis of fallopian tube ♀
N81.2	Incomplete uterovaginal prolapse ♀
N81.3	Complete uterovaginal prolapse ♀
N81.89	Other female genital prolapse ♀
N83.01	Follicular cyst of right ovary ♀ ☑
N83.02	Follicular cyst of left ovary ♀ ☑
N83.11	Corpus luteum cyst of right ovary ♀ ☑
N83.12	Corpus luteum cyst of left ovary ♀ ☑
N83.291	Other ovarian cyst, right side ♀ ☑

N83.292	Other ovarian cyst, left side ♀ ☑
N83.6	Hematosalpinx ♀
N83.8	Other noninflammatory disorders of ovary, fallopian tube and broad ligament ♀
N84.0	Polyp of corpus uteri ♀
N84.8	Polyp of other parts of female genital tract ♀
N85.01	Benign endometrial hyperplasia ♀
N85.02	Endometrial intraepithelial neoplasia [EIN] ♀
N85.2	Hypertrophy of uterus ♀
N85.7	Hematometra ♀
N85.8	Other specified noninflammatory disorders of uterus ♀
N87.0	Mild cervical dysplasia ♀
N87.1	Moderate cervical dysplasia ♀
N92.0	Excessive and frequent menstruation with regular cycle ♀
N92.1	Excessive and frequent menstruation with irregular cycle ♀
N92.5	Other specified irregular menstruation ♀
N93.8	Other specified abnormal uterine and vaginal bleeding ♀
N94.89	Other specified conditions associated with female genital organs and menstrual cycle ♀
N95.0	Postmenopausal bleeding ♀

AMA: **58541** 2019,Jul,6; 2018,Jan,8; 2017,Jan,8; 2017,Apr,7; 2016,Jan,13; 2015,Jan,16; 2014,Jan,11 **58542** 2019,Jul,6; 2018,Jan,8; 2017,Jan,8; 2017,Apr,7; 2016,Jan,13; 2015,Jan,16; 2014,Jan,11

Relative Value Units/Medicare Edits

Non-Facility RVU	Work	PE	MP	Total
58541	12.29	6.91	1.86	21.06
58542	14.16	7.64	2.17	23.97
Facility RVU	**Work**	**PE**	**MP**	**Total**
58541	12.29	6.91	1.86	21.06
58542	14.16	7.64	2.17	23.97

	FUD	Status	MUE	Modifiers				IOM Reference
58541	90	A	1(3)	51	N/A	62	80	100-03,230.3
58542	90	A	1(2)	51	N/A	62	80	

* with documentation

Terms To Know

dorsal. Pertaining to the back or posterior aspect.

lithotomy position. Common position patients may be placed in for some surgical procedures and examinations involving the pelvis and/or lower abdomen. The patient is placed supine (on their back), hips and knees flexed, thighs apart, with feet supported in raised stirrups.

trocar. Cannula or a sharp pointed instrument used to puncture and aspirate fluid from cavities.

58543-58544

58543   Laparoscopy, surgical, supracervical hysterectomy, for uterus greater than 250 g;
58544   with removal of tube(s) and/or ovary(s)

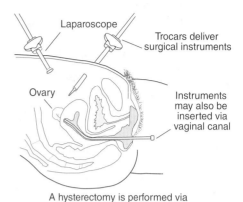

A hysterectomy is performed via laparoscopy and the cervix is preserved

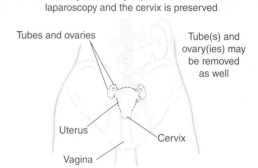

Explanation

The physician performs a laparoscopic hysterectomy, removing a uterus with a total weight of more than 250 gm while preserving the cervix. The patient is placed in the dorsal lithotomy position. After the insertion of a speculum in the vagina, the physician grasps the cervix with an instrument to manipulate the uterus during the surgery. A trocar is inserted periumbilically and the abdomen is insufflated with gas. Additional trocars are placed in the right and left lower quadrants. The uterus is dissected free from the bladder and surrounding tissue and its body is separated from the cervix. Coagulation is achieved with the aid of electrocautery instruments. Alternatively, some vessels may be ligated. The uterus is morcellized and removed using endoscopic tools. In 58544, one or both ovaries and/or one or both fallopian tubes are removed in similar fashion. Once the excisions are complete, the abdominal cavity is deflated and instruments and trocars removed. The fascia and skin are closed with sutures.

Coding Tips

Surgical laparoscopy always includes diagnostic laparoscopy. For diagnostic laparoscopy, see 49320. For laparoscopic supracervical hysterectomy, for a uterus 250 gm or less, see 58541; with removal of tubes and/or ovaries, see 58542. Do not report these codes with 49320, 57000, 57180, 57410, 58140–58146, 58545–58546, 58561, 58661, or 58670-58671.

ICD-10-CM Diagnostic Codes

C54.0	Malignant neoplasm of isthmus uteri ♀
C54.1	Malignant neoplasm of endometrium ♀
C54.2	Malignant neoplasm of myometrium ♀
C54.3	Malignant neoplasm of fundus uteri ♀
C54.8	Malignant neoplasm of overlapping sites of corpus uteri ♀

C56.1	Malignant neoplasm of right ovary ♀ ☑
C56.2	Malignant neoplasm of left ovary ♀ ☑
C57.01	Malignant neoplasm of right fallopian tube ♀ ☑
C57.02	Malignant neoplasm of left fallopian tube ♀ ☑
C57.11	Malignant neoplasm of right broad ligament ♀ ☑
C57.12	Malignant neoplasm of left broad ligament ♀ ☑
C57.21	Malignant neoplasm of right round ligament ♀ ☑
C57.22	Malignant neoplasm of left round ligament ♀ ☑
C57.3	Malignant neoplasm of parametrium ♀
C57.7	Malignant neoplasm of other specified female genital organs ♀
C57.8	Malignant neoplasm of overlapping sites of female genital organs ♀
C79.61	Secondary malignant neoplasm of right ovary ♀ ☑
C79.62	Secondary malignant neoplasm of left ovary ♀ ☑
C79.82	Secondary malignant neoplasm of genital organs
D07.0	Carcinoma in situ of endometrium ♀
D07.39	Carcinoma in situ of other female genital organs ♀
D25.0	Submucous leiomyoma of uterus ♀
D25.1	Intramural leiomyoma of uterus ♀
D25.2	Subserosal leiomyoma of uterus ♀
D39.0	Neoplasm of uncertain behavior of uterus ♀
D39.11	Neoplasm of uncertain behavior of right ovary ♀ ☑
D39.12	Neoplasm of uncertain behavior of left ovary ♀ ☑
D39.2	Neoplasm of uncertain behavior of placenta Ⓜ ♀
D39.8	Neoplasm of uncertain behavior of other specified female genital organs ♀
D49.59	Neoplasm of unspecified behavior of other genitourinary organ
N39.3	Stress incontinence (female) (male)
N70.01	Acute salpingitis ♀
N70.02	Acute oophoritis ♀
N70.03	Acute salpingitis and oophoritis ♀
N70.11	Chronic salpingitis ♀
N70.12	Chronic oophoritis ♀
N70.13	Chronic salpingitis and oophoritis ♀
N71.0	Acute inflammatory disease of uterus ♀
N71.1	Chronic inflammatory disease of uterus ♀
N73.0	Acute parametritis and pelvic cellulitis ♀
N73.1	Chronic parametritis and pelvic cellulitis ♀
N73.3	Female acute pelvic peritonitis ♀
N73.4	Female chronic pelvic peritonitis ♀
N73.6	Female pelvic peritoneal adhesions (postinfective) ♀
N73.8	Other specified female pelvic inflammatory diseases ♀
N80.0	Endometriosis of uterus ♀
N80.1	Endometriosis of ovary ♀
N80.2	Endometriosis of fallopian tube ♀
N81.2	Incomplete uterovaginal prolapse ♀
N81.3	Complete uterovaginal prolapse ♀
N81.89	Other female genital prolapse ♀
N83.01	Follicular cyst of right ovary ♀ ☑
N83.02	Follicular cyst of left ovary ♀ ☑
N83.11	Corpus luteum cyst of right ovary ♀ ☑
N83.12	Corpus luteum cyst of left ovary ♀ ☑
N83.291	Other ovarian cyst, right side ♀ ☑
N83.292	Other ovarian cyst, left side ♀ ☑
N83.6	Hematosalpinx ♀
N83.8	Other noninflammatory disorders of ovary, fallopian tube and broad ligament ♀
N84.0	Polyp of corpus uteri ♀
N84.8	Polyp of other parts of female genital tract ♀
N85.01	Benign endometrial hyperplasia ♀
N85.02	Endometrial intraepithelial neoplasia [EIN] ♀
N85.2	Hypertrophy of uterus ♀
N85.7	Hematometra ♀
N85.8	Other specified noninflammatory disorders of uterus ♀
N87.0	Mild cervical dysplasia ♀
N87.1	Moderate cervical dysplasia ♀
N92.0	Excessive and frequent menstruation with regular cycle ♀
N92.1	Excessive and frequent menstruation with irregular cycle ♀
N92.5	Other specified irregular menstruation ♀
N93.8	Other specified abnormal uterine and vaginal bleeding ♀
N94.89	Other specified conditions associated with female genital organs and menstrual cycle ♀
N95.0	Postmenopausal bleeding ♀

AMA: **58543** 2019,Jul,6; 2018,Jan,8; 2017,Jan,8; 2017,Apr,7; 2016,Jan,13; 2015,Jan,16; 2014,Jan,11 **58544** 2019,Jul,6; 2018,Jan,8; 2017,Jan,8; 2017,Apr,7; 2016,Jan,13; 2015,Jan,16; 2014,Jan,11

Relative Value Units/Medicare Edits

Non-Facility RVU	Work	PE	MP	Total
58543	14.39	7.7	2.27	24.36
58544	15.6	8.2	2.43	26.23
Facility RVU	**Work**	**PE**	**MP**	**Total**
58543	14.39	7.7	2.27	24.36
58544	15.6	8.2	2.43	26.23

	FUD	Status	MUE	Modifiers				IOM Reference
58543	90	A	1(3)	51	N/A	62	80	None
58544	90	A	1(2)	51	N/A	62	80	

* with documentation

58545

58545   Laparoscopy, surgical, myomectomy, excision; 1 to 4 intramural myomas with total weight of 250 g or less and/or removal of surface myomas

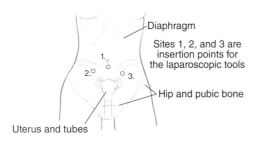

Sites 1, 2, and 3 are insertion points for the laparoscopic tools

Intramural myoma(s) are removed

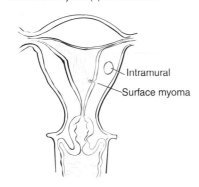

Explanation

The physician performs a laparoscopic myomectomy, removing one to four fibroid tumors from the wall of the uterus (intramural myomas) with a total weight of 250 gm or less and/or removes surface myomas. The patient is placed in the dorsal lithotomy position. A trocar is inserted periumbilically and the abdomen is insufflated with gas. Additional trocars are placed in the right and left lower quadrants. Electrocautery instruments and/or laser may be used to remove small surface myomas. Pedunculated myomas are removed by ligating, twisting, or snaring the stalk. The physician incises the uterus through the myometrium to expose the myoma, which is dissected free from the surrounding myometrium. The pedicle is isolated, clamped, and ligated and the myoma is dissected down to the pedicular blood supply. The adjacent myomas may be reached and removed by tunneling further through the initial incision. The uterine wall defects are sutured laparoscopically, the trocars are removed, and the wounds are closed.

Coding Tips

Surgical laparoscopy always includes diagnostic laparoscopy. For diagnostic laparoscopy, see 49320. Myomectomy performed via an abdominal (open) approach is reported with 58140 or 58146; vaginal approach, see 58145. Hysteroscopy with removal of leiomyomata should be reported with 58561.

ICD-10-CM Diagnostic Codes

D25.0	Submucous leiomyoma of uterus ♀
D25.1	Intramural leiomyoma of uterus ♀
D25.2	Subserosal leiomyoma of uterus ♀
D25.9	Leiomyoma of uterus, unspecified ♀

AMA: **58545** 2019,Jul,6; 2017,Apr,7; 2014,Jan,11

Relative Value Units/Medicare Edits

Non-Facility RVU	Work	PE	MP	Total
58545	15.55	8.04	2.48	26.07
Facility RVU	Work	PE	MP	Total
58545	15.55	8.04	2.48	26.07

	FUD	Status	MUE	Modifiers				IOM Reference
58545	90	A	1(2)	51	N/A	62	80	None

* with documentation

Terms To Know

dissect. Cut apart or separate tissue for surgical purposes or for visual or microscopic study.

electrocautery. Division or cutting of tissue using high-frequency electrical current to produce heat, which destroys cells.

insufflation. Blowing air or gas into a body cavity.

intramural uterine leiomyoma. Benign, smooth muscle tumor within the wall of the uterus.

laparoscopy. Direct visualization of the peritoneal cavity, outer fallopian tubes, uterus, and ovaries utilizing a laparoscope, a thin, flexible fiberoptic tube.

ligate. To tie off a blood vessel or duct with a suture or a soft, thin wire (ligature wire).

myometrium. Muscular middle layer of the uterine wall responsible for contractions associated with childbirth.

submucous uterine leiomyoma. Benign, smooth muscle tumor beneath the inner lining of the uterus.

subserous uterine leiomyoma. Benign, smooth muscle tumor beneath the serous membrane lining of the uterus.

trocar. Cannula or a sharp pointed instrument used to puncture and aspirate fluid from cavities.

58546

58546 Laparoscopy, surgical, myomectomy, excision; 5 or more intramural myomas and/or intramural myomas with total weight greater than 250 g

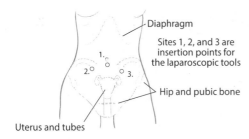

Sites 1, 2, and 3 are insertion points for the laparoscopic tools

Diaphragm

Hip and pubic bone

Uterus and tubes

Intramural myoma(s) are removed

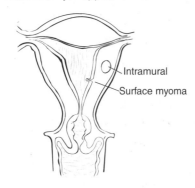

Intramural

Surface myoma

Explanation

The physician performs a laparoscopic myomectomy, removing five or more fibroid tumors from the wall of the uterus (intramural myomas) and/or intramural myomas with a total weight greater than 250 gm. The patient is placed in the dorsal lithotomy position. A trocar is inserted periumbilically and the abdomen is insufflated with gas. Additional trocars are placed in the right and left lower quadrants. The physician incises the uterus through the myometrium to expose the myoma, which is dissected free from the surrounding myometrium. The pedicle is isolated, clamped, and ligated and the myoma is dissected to the pedicular blood supply. The adjacent myomas may be reached and removed by tunneling further through the initial incision. After resecting large intramural myomas, removing them from the abdominal cavity may require making a culdotomy incision or using morcellation techniques. A minilaparotomy may be done with laparoscopic myomectomy as myomas are brought to the abdominal wall for removal and the uterus may be closed with some layered suturing. The laparoscopic instruments are removed and the wounds are closed.

Coding Tips

Surgical laparoscopy always includes diagnostic laparoscopy; the diagnostic laparoscopy should not be reported separately. For diagnostic laparoscopy, see 49320. For myomectomy performed via an abdominal approach, see 58140 and 58146; vaginal approach, see 58145. Hysteroscopy with removal of leiomyomata is reported with 58561.

ICD-10-CM Diagnostic Codes

D25.0	Submucous leiomyoma of uterus ♀
D25.1	Intramural leiomyoma of uterus ♀
D25.2	Subserosal leiomyoma of uterus ♀
D25.9	Leiomyoma of uterus, unspecified ♀

AMA: **58546** 2019,Jul,6; 2018,Jan,8; 2017,Jan,8; 2017,Apr,7; 2016,Jan,13; 2015,Jan,16; 2014,Jan,11

Relative Value Units/Medicare Edits

Non-Facility RVU	Work	PE	MP	Total
58546	19.94	9.46	3.11	32.51
Facility RVU	**Work**	**PE**	**MP**	**Total**
58546	19.94	9.46	3.11	32.51

	FUD	Status	MUE	Modifiers				IOM Reference
58546	90	A	1(2)	51	N/A	62	80	None

* with documentation

Terms To Know

blunt dissection. Surgical technique used to expose an underlying area by separating along natural cleavage lines of tissue, without cutting.

culdotomy/colpotomy. Incision through the vaginal wall into the cul-de-sac of Douglas (retro uterine pouch).

intramural uterine leiomyoma. Benign, smooth muscle tumor within the wall of the uterus.

laparoscopy. Direct visualization of the peritoneal cavity, outer fallopian tubes, uterus, and ovaries utilizing a laparoscope, a thin, flexible fiberoptic tube.

leiomyoma. Benign tumor consisting of smooth muscle in the uterus.

myometrium. Muscular middle layer of the uterine wall responsible for contractions associated with childbirth.

trocar. Cannula or a sharp pointed instrument used to puncture and aspirate fluid from cavities.

58548

58548 Laparoscopy, surgical, with radical hysterectomy, with bilateral total pelvic lymphadenectomy and para-aortic lymph node sampling (biopsy), with removal of tube(s) and ovary(s), if performed

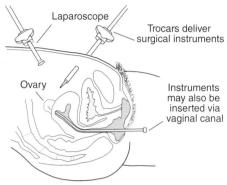

A radical hysterectomy is performed via laparoscope with removal of pelvic nodes and sampling of para-aortic nodes

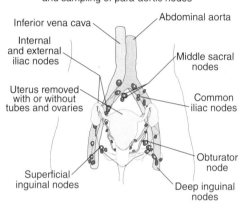

Explanation

The physician performs a laparoscopic hysterectomy, bilateral total pelvic lymphadenectomy, and para-aortic lymph node sampling, and may remove all or portions of the fallopian tubes and ovaries. The patient is placed in the dorsal lithotomy position. After the insertion of a speculum in the vagina, the physician grasps the cervix with an instrument to manipulate the uterus during the surgery. A trocar is inserted periumbilically and the abdomen is insufflated with gas. Additional trocars are placed in the right and left lower quadrants. The uterus is dissected free from the bladder and surrounding tissue and its body with the cervix is dissected from the vagina. Alternately, the vagina may also be excised. Coagulation is achieved with the aid of electrocautery instruments. Some vessels may be ligated. The uterus may be morcellized prior to being removed using endoscopic tools or it may be removed via the vagina. One or both ovaries and/or one or both fallopian tubes are removed in similar fashion. The physician removes the pelvic lymph nodes on both sides and takes samples or biopsies of the para-aortic lymph nodes. Once the excisions are complete, the abdominal cavity is deflated and instruments and trocars removed. The fascia and skin of the abdomen and vagina are closed with sutures.

Coding Tips

Surgical laparoscopy always includes a diagnostic laparoscopy; the diagnostic laparoscopy should not be reported separately. This code should not be reported with 38570–38572, 58210, 58285, or 58550–58554.

ICD-10-CM Diagnostic Codes

C51.8	Malignant neoplasm of overlapping sites of vulva ♀
C52	Malignant neoplasm of vagina ♀
C53.0	Malignant neoplasm of endocervix ♀
C53.1	Malignant neoplasm of exocervix ♀
C53.8	Malignant neoplasm of overlapping sites of cervix uteri ♀
C54.0	Malignant neoplasm of isthmus uteri ♀
C54.1	Malignant neoplasm of endometrium ♀
C54.2	Malignant neoplasm of myometrium ♀
C54.3	Malignant neoplasm of fundus uteri ♀
C54.8	Malignant neoplasm of overlapping sites of corpus uteri ♀
C56.1	Malignant neoplasm of right ovary ♀ ☑
C56.2	Malignant neoplasm of left ovary ♀ ☑
C57.01	Malignant neoplasm of right fallopian tube ♀ ☑
C57.02	Malignant neoplasm of left fallopian tube ♀ ☑
C57.11	Malignant neoplasm of right broad ligament ♀ ☑
C57.12	Malignant neoplasm of left broad ligament ♀ ☑
C57.21	Malignant neoplasm of right round ligament ♀ ☑
C57.22	Malignant neoplasm of left round ligament ♀ ☑
C57.3	Malignant neoplasm of parametrium ♀
C57.7	Malignant neoplasm of other specified female genital organs ♀
C57.8	Malignant neoplasm of overlapping sites of female genital organs ♀
C77.2	Secondary and unspecified malignant neoplasm of intra-abdominal lymph nodes
C77.5	Secondary and unspecified malignant neoplasm of intrapelvic lymph nodes
C79.61	Secondary malignant neoplasm of right ovary ♀ ☑
C79.62	Secondary malignant neoplasm of left ovary ♀ ☑
C79.82	Secondary malignant neoplasm of genital organs
D06.0	Carcinoma in situ of endocervix ♀
D06.1	Carcinoma in situ of exocervix ♀
D06.7	Carcinoma in situ of other parts of cervix ♀
D07.0	Carcinoma in situ of endometrium ♀
D07.39	Carcinoma in situ of other female genital organs ♀
D25.0	Submucous leiomyoma of uterus ♀
D25.1	Intramural leiomyoma of uterus ♀
D25.2	Subserosal leiomyoma of uterus ♀
D39.0	Neoplasm of uncertain behavior of uterus ♀
D39.11	Neoplasm of uncertain behavior of right ovary ♀ ☑
D39.12	Neoplasm of uncertain behavior of left ovary ♀ ☑
D39.2	Neoplasm of uncertain behavior of placenta Ⓜ ♀
D39.8	Neoplasm of uncertain behavior of other specified female genital organs ♀
D49.59	Neoplasm of unspecified behavior of other genitourinary organ
N70.01	Acute salpingitis ♀
N70.02	Acute oophoritis ♀
N70.03	Acute salpingitis and oophoritis ♀
N70.11	Chronic salpingitis ♀
N70.12	Chronic oophoritis ♀
N70.13	Chronic salpingitis and oophoritis ♀
N71.0	Acute inflammatory disease of uterus ♀
N71.1	Chronic inflammatory disease of uterus ♀

N72	Inflammatory disease of cervix uteri ♀	
N73.0	Acute parametritis and pelvic cellulitis ♀	
N73.1	Chronic parametritis and pelvic cellulitis ♀	
N73.3	Female acute pelvic peritonitis ♀	
N73.4	Female chronic pelvic peritonitis ♀	
N73.6	Female pelvic peritoneal adhesions (postinfective) ♀	
N73.8	Other specified female pelvic inflammatory diseases ♀	
N80.0	Endometriosis of uterus ♀	
N80.1	Endometriosis of ovary ♀	
N80.2	Endometriosis of fallopian tube ♀	
N81.2	Incomplete uterovaginal prolapse ♀	
N81.3	Complete uterovaginal prolapse ♀	
N81.89	Other female genital prolapse ♀	
N83.01	Follicular cyst of right ovary ♀ ☑	
N83.02	Follicular cyst of left ovary ♀ ☑	
N83.11	Corpus luteum cyst of right ovary ♀ ☑	
N83.12	Corpus luteum cyst of left ovary ♀ ☑	
N83.291	Other ovarian cyst, right side ♀ ☑	
N83.292	Other ovarian cyst, left side ♀ ☑	
N83.6	Hematosalpinx ♀	
N83.8	Other noninflammatory disorders of ovary, fallopian tube and broad ligament ♀	
N84.0	Polyp of corpus uteri ♀	
N84.8	Polyp of other parts of female genital tract ♀	
N85.01	Benign endometrial hyperplasia ♀	
N85.02	Endometrial intraepithelial neoplasia [EIN] ♀	
N85.2	Hypertrophy of uterus ♀	
N85.7	Hematometra ♀	
N85.8	Other specified noninflammatory disorders of uterus ♀	
N87.0	Mild cervical dysplasia ♀	
N87.1	Moderate cervical dysplasia ♀	
N92.0	Excessive and frequent menstruation with regular cycle ♀	
N92.1	Excessive and frequent menstruation with irregular cycle ♀	
N92.5	Other specified irregular menstruation ♀	
N93.8	Other specified abnormal uterine and vaginal bleeding ♀	
N94.89	Other specified conditions associated with female genital organs and menstrual cycle ♀	
N95.0	Postmenopausal bleeding ♀	

AMA: 58548 2019,Mar,5; 2019,Jul,6; 2018,Jan,8; 2017,Jan,8; 2017,Apr,7; 2016,Jan,13; 2015,Sep,12; 2015,Jan,16; 2014,Jan,11

Relative Value Units/Medicare Edits

Non-Facility RVU	Work	PE	MP	Total
58548	31.63	17.4	4.96	53.99
Facility RVU	**Work**	**PE**	**MP**	**Total**
58548	31.63	17.4	4.96	53.99

	FUD	Status	MUE	Modifiers				IOM Reference
58548	90	A	1(2)	51	N/A	62	80	None

* with documentation

58550-58552

58550 Laparoscopy, surgical, with vaginal hysterectomy, for uterus 250 g or less;

58552 with removal of tube(s) and/or ovary(s)

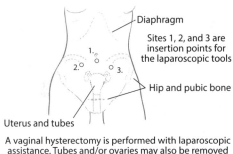

Diaphragm
Sites 1, 2, and 3 are insertion points for the laparoscopic tools
Hip and pubic bone
Uterus and tubes

A vaginal hysterectomy is performed with laparoscopic assistance. Tubes and/or ovaries may also be removed

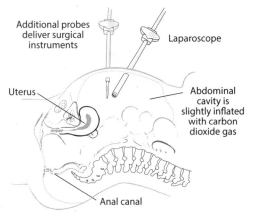

Additional probes deliver surgical instruments
Laparoscope
Uterus
Abdominal cavity is slightly inflated with carbon dioxide gas
Anal canal

Explanation

The physician performs surgical laparoscopy with vaginal hysterectomy for a uterus with a total weight of 250 gm or less. The laparoscope is used to perform the initial operative portion of the hysterectomy. The patient is placed in the dorsal lithotomy position for the endoscopic portion. For the vaginal portion, the patient is positioned in stirrups. A trocar is inserted periumbilically and the abdomen is insufflated with gas. Additional trocars are placed in the right and left lower quadrants. An intra-abdominal and pelvic survey is done and any adhesions are lysed. The round ligaments are ligated and incised. Starting on the left round ligament, the vesicouterine peritoneal fold is incised and the peritoneal vessels are dissected and desiccated. The physician continues the incision across the lower uterine segment to the round ligament on the other side and dissects the bladder off the uterus and cervix. Staples are inserted through one port on the side to be stapled or a bipolar coagulation unit is inserted for electrocautery. At this point, if tubes and/or ovaries are to be removed, the infundibulopelvic ligament is now ligated lateral to the ovary. If not, the ligation is done medial to the ovary. Staple ligation or electrodesiccation of the uterine vasculature is accomplished on both sides, followed by ligation or electrodesiccation of the cardinal ligaments. An anterior colpotomy incision is made to enter the vagina and the vaginal portion of the procedure is begun. The remaining supporting structures attached to the cervix and uterus are detached and the hysterectomy proceeds through a posterior cul-de-sac incision. The uterus is removed, the vaginal incision is closed, and hemostasis is confirmed before the trocars are removed and the skin incisions are closed. Report 58550 for removal of uterus or 58552 if uterus, tubes, and/or ovaries are removed.

Coding Tips

Surgical laparoscopy always includes a diagnostic laparoscopy; the diagnostic laparoscopy should not be reported separately. For a vaginal hysterectomy for a uterus 250 gm or less without laparoscopy, see 58260; with removal of the tubes and/or ovaries, see 58262; and with repair of enterocele, see 58263. For a vaginal hysterectomy for a uterus greater than 250 gm without laparoscopy, see 58290; with removal of the tubes and/or ovaries, see 58291; and with repair of enterocele, see 58292. For surgical laparoscopy with a vaginal hysterectomy for a uterus greater than 250 gm, see 58553; with removal of tubes and/or ovaries, see 58554.

ICD-10-CM Diagnostic Codes

C53.0	Malignant neoplasm of endocervix ♀
C53.1	Malignant neoplasm of exocervix ♀
C53.8	Malignant neoplasm of overlapping sites of cervix uteri ♀
C54.0	Malignant neoplasm of isthmus uteri ♀
C54.1	Malignant neoplasm of endometrium ♀
C54.2	Malignant neoplasm of myometrium ♀
C54.3	Malignant neoplasm of fundus uteri ♀
C54.8	Malignant neoplasm of overlapping sites of corpus uteri ♀
C56.1	Malignant neoplasm of right ovary ♀ ☑
C56.2	Malignant neoplasm of left ovary ♀ ☑
C57.01	Malignant neoplasm of right fallopian tube ♀ ☑
C57.02	Malignant neoplasm of left fallopian tube ♀ ☑
C57.11	Malignant neoplasm of right broad ligament ♀ ☑
C57.12	Malignant neoplasm of left broad ligament ♀ ☑
C57.21	Malignant neoplasm of right round ligament ♀ ☑
C57.22	Malignant neoplasm of left round ligament ♀ ☑
C57.3	Malignant neoplasm of parametrium ♀
C57.7	Malignant neoplasm of other specified female genital organs ♀
C57.8	Malignant neoplasm of overlapping sites of female genital organs ♀
C79.61	Secondary malignant neoplasm of right ovary ♀ ☑
C79.62	Secondary malignant neoplasm of left ovary ♀ ☑
C79.82	Secondary malignant neoplasm of genital organs
D06.0	Carcinoma in situ of endocervix ♀
D06.1	Carcinoma in situ of exocervix ♀
D06.7	Carcinoma in situ of other parts of cervix ♀
D07.0	Carcinoma in situ of endometrium ♀
D07.39	Carcinoma in situ of other female genital organs ♀
D25.0	Submucous leiomyoma of uterus ♀
D25.1	Intramural leiomyoma of uterus ♀
D25.2	Subserosal leiomyoma of uterus ♀
D39.0	Neoplasm of uncertain behavior of uterus ♀
D39.11	Neoplasm of uncertain behavior of right ovary ♀ ☑
D39.12	Neoplasm of uncertain behavior of left ovary ♀ ☑
D39.2	Neoplasm of uncertain behavior of placenta Ⓜ ♀
D39.8	Neoplasm of uncertain behavior of other specified female genital organs ♀
D49.59	Neoplasm of unspecified behavior of other genitourinary organ
N70.01	Acute salpingitis ♀
N70.02	Acute oophoritis ♀
N70.03	Acute salpingitis and oophoritis ♀
N70.11	Chronic salpingitis ♀
N70.12	Chronic oophoritis ♀
N70.13	Chronic salpingitis and oophoritis ♀
N71.0	Acute inflammatory disease of uterus ♀
N71.1	Chronic inflammatory disease of uterus ♀
N72	Inflammatory disease of cervix uteri ♀
N73.0	Acute parametritis and pelvic cellulitis ♀
N73.1	Chronic parametritis and pelvic cellulitis ♀
N73.3	Female acute pelvic peritonitis ♀
N73.4	Female chronic pelvic peritonitis ♀
N73.6	Female pelvic peritoneal adhesions (postinfective) ♀
N73.8	Other specified female pelvic inflammatory diseases ♀
N80.0	Endometriosis of uterus ♀
N80.1	Endometriosis of ovary ♀
N80.2	Endometriosis of fallopian tube ♀
N81.2	Incomplete uterovaginal prolapse ♀
N81.3	Complete uterovaginal prolapse ♀
N81.89	Other female genital prolapse ♀
N83.01	Follicular cyst of right ovary ♀ ☑
N83.02	Follicular cyst of left ovary ♀ ☑
N83.11	Corpus luteum cyst of right ovary ♀ ☑
N83.12	Corpus luteum cyst of left ovary ♀ ☑
N83.291	Other ovarian cyst, right side ♀ ☑
N83.292	Other ovarian cyst, left side ♀ ☑
N83.6	Hematosalpinx ♀
N83.8	Other noninflammatory disorders of ovary, fallopian tube and broad ligament ♀
N84.0	Polyp of corpus uteri ♀
N84.8	Polyp of other parts of female genital tract ♀
N85.01	Benign endometrial hyperplasia ♀
N85.02	Endometrial intraepithelial neoplasia [EIN] ♀
N85.2	Hypertrophy of uterus ♀
N85.7	Hematometra ♀
N85.8	Other specified noninflammatory disorders of uterus ♀
N87.0	Mild cervical dysplasia ♀
N87.1	Moderate cervical dysplasia ♀
N92.0	Excessive and frequent menstruation with regular cycle ♀
N92.1	Excessive and frequent menstruation with irregular cycle ♀
N92.5	Other specified irregular menstruation ♀
N93.8	Other specified abnormal uterine and vaginal bleeding ♀
N94.89	Other specified conditions associated with female genital organs and menstrual cycle ♀
N95.0	Postmenopausal bleeding ♀

AMA: **58550** 2019,Jul,6; 2018,Jan,8; 2017,Jan,8; 2017,Apr,7; 2016,Jan,13; 2015,Jan,16; 2014,Jan,11 **58552** 2019,Jul,6; 2018,Jan,8; 2017,Jan,8; 2017,Apr,7; 2016,Jan,13; 2015,Jan,16; 2014,Jan,11

Relative Value Units/Medicare Edits

Non-Facility RVU	Work	PE	MP	Total
58550	15.1	8.12	2.37	25.59
58552	16.91	8.94	2.67	28.52
Facility RVU	**Work**	**PE**	**MP**	**Total**
58550	15.1	8.12	2.37	25.59
58552	16.91	8.94	2.67	28.52

	FUD	Status	MUE	Modifiers				IOM Reference
58550	90	A	1(3)	51	N/A	62	80	None
58552	90	A	1(3)	51	N/A	62	80	

* with documentation

Terms To Know

hysterectomy. Surgical removal of the uterus. A complete hysterectomy may also include removal of tubes and ovaries.

laparoscopy. Direct visualization of the peritoneal cavity, outer fallopian tubes, uterus, and ovaries utilizing a laparoscope, a thin, flexible fiberoptic tube.

oophorectomy. Surgical removal of all or part of one or both ovaries, either as open procedure or laparoscopically. Menstruation and childbearing ability continues when one ovary is removed.

salpingectomy. Removal of all or part of one or both of the fallopian tubes. Indications include infection, ectopic pregnancy, sterilization, or cancer. This procedure is often performed in combination with other open or laparoscopic procedures.

salpingo-oophorectomy. Surgical removal of both the fallopian tube and ovary.

58553-58554

58553 Laparoscopy, surgical, with vaginal hysterectomy, for uterus greater than 250 g;

58554   with removal of tube(s) and/or ovary(s)

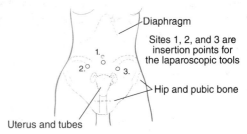

A vaginal hysterectomy is performed with laparoscopic assistance. Tubes and/or ovaries may also be removed

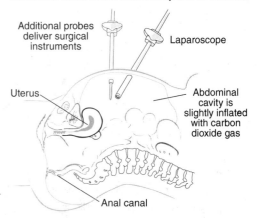

Explanation

The physician performs surgical laparoscopy with vaginal hysterectomy for a uterus with a total weight of more than 250 gm. The laparoscope is used to perform the initial operative portion of the hysterectomy. The patient is placed in the dorsal lithotomy position for the endoscopic portion. For the vaginal portion, the patient is positioned in stirrups. A trocar is inserted periumbilically and the abdomen is insufflated with gas. Additional trocars are placed in the right and left lower quadrants. An intra-abdominal and pelvic survey is done and any adhesions are lysed. The round ligaments are ligated and incised. Starting on the left round ligament, the vesicouterine peritoneal fold is incised and the peritoneal vessels are dissected and desiccated. The physician continues the incision across the lower uterine segment to the round ligament on the other side and dissects the bladder off the uterus and cervix. Staples are inserted through one port on the side to be stapled or a bipolar coagulation unit is inserted for electrocautery. At this point, if tubes and/or ovaries are to be removed, the infundibulopelvic ligament is now ligated lateral to the ovary. If not, the ligation is done medial to the ovary. Staple-ligation or electrodesiccation of the uterine vasculature is accomplished on both sides, followed by ligation or electrodesiccation of the cardinal ligaments. An anterior colpotomy incision is made to enter the vagina and the vaginal portion of the procedure is begun. The remaining supporting structures attached to the cervix and uterus are detached and the hysterectomy proceeds through a posterior cul-de-sac incision. The uterus is removed, the vaginal incision is closed, and hemostasis is confirmed before the trocars are removed and the skin incisions are closed. Report 58553 for removal of uterus or 58554 if uterus, tubes, and/or ovaries are removed.

Coding Tips

For surgical laparoscopy with a vaginal hysterectomy for a uterus weighing less than 250 gm, see 58550; with removal of tubes and/or ovaries, see 58552. For a vaginal hysterectomy for a uterus 250 gm or less without laparoscopy, see 58260; with removal of the tubes and/or ovaries, see 58262; and with repair of enterocele, see 58263. For a vaginal hysterectomy for a uterus greater than 250 gm without laparoscopy, see 58290; with removal of the tubes and/or ovaries, see 58291; and with repair of an enterocele, see 58292.

ICD-10-CM Diagnostic Codes

C53.0	Malignant neoplasm of endocervix ♀
C53.1	Malignant neoplasm of exocervix ♀
C53.8	Malignant neoplasm of overlapping sites of cervix uteri ♀
C54.0	Malignant neoplasm of isthmus uteri ♀
C54.1	Malignant neoplasm of endometrium ♀
C54.2	Malignant neoplasm of myometrium ♀
C54.3	Malignant neoplasm of fundus uteri ♀
C54.8	Malignant neoplasm of overlapping sites of corpus uteri ♀
C56.1	Malignant neoplasm of right ovary ♀ ☑
C56.2	Malignant neoplasm of left ovary ♀ ☑
C57.01	Malignant neoplasm of right fallopian tube ♀ ☑
C57.02	Malignant neoplasm of left fallopian tube ♀ ☑
C57.11	Malignant neoplasm of right broad ligament ♀ ☑
C57.12	Malignant neoplasm of left broad ligament ♀ ☑
C57.21	Malignant neoplasm of right round ligament ♀ ☑
C57.22	Malignant neoplasm of left round ligament ♀ ☑
C57.3	Malignant neoplasm of parametrium ♀
C57.7	Malignant neoplasm of other specified female genital organs ♀
C57.8	Malignant neoplasm of overlapping sites of female genital organs ♀
C79.61	Secondary malignant neoplasm of right ovary ♀ ☑
C79.62	Secondary malignant neoplasm of left ovary ♀ ☑
C79.82	Secondary malignant neoplasm of genital organs
D06.0	Carcinoma in situ of endocervix ♀
D06.1	Carcinoma in situ of exocervix ♀
D06.7	Carcinoma in situ of other parts of cervix ♀
D07.0	Carcinoma in situ of endometrium ♀
D07.39	Carcinoma in situ of other female genital organs ♀
D25.0	Submucous leiomyoma of uterus ♀
D25.1	Intramural leiomyoma of uterus ♀
D25.2	Subserosal leiomyoma of uterus ♀
D39.0	Neoplasm of uncertain behavior of uterus ♀
D39.11	Neoplasm of uncertain behavior of right ovary ♀ ☑
D39.12	Neoplasm of uncertain behavior of left ovary ♀ ☑
D39.2	Neoplasm of uncertain behavior of placenta Ⓜ ♀
D39.8	Neoplasm of uncertain behavior of other specified female genital organs ♀
D49.59	Neoplasm of unspecified behavior of other genitourinary organ
N70.01	Acute salpingitis ♀
N70.02	Acute oophoritis ♀
N70.03	Acute salpingitis and oophoritis ♀
N70.11	Chronic salpingitis ♀
N70.12	Chronic oophoritis ♀
N70.13	Chronic salpingitis and oophoritis ♀
N71.0	Acute inflammatory disease of uterus ♀
N71.1	Chronic inflammatory disease of uterus ♀
N72	Inflammatory disease of cervix uteri ♀
N73.0	Acute parametritis and pelvic cellulitis ♀
N73.1	Chronic parametritis and pelvic cellulitis ♀
N73.3	Female acute pelvic peritonitis ♀
N73.4	Female chronic pelvic peritonitis ♀
N73.6	Female pelvic peritoneal adhesions (postinfective) ♀
N73.8	Other specified female pelvic inflammatory diseases ♀
N80.0	Endometriosis of uterus ♀
N80.1	Endometriosis of ovary ♀
N80.2	Endometriosis of fallopian tube ♀
N81.2	Incomplete uterovaginal prolapse ♀
N81.3	Complete uterovaginal prolapse ♀
N81.89	Other female genital prolapse ♀
N83.01	Follicular cyst of right ovary ♀ ☑
N83.02	Follicular cyst of left ovary ♀ ☑
N83.11	Corpus luteum cyst of right ovary ♀ ☑
N83.12	Corpus luteum cyst of left ovary ♀ ☑
N83.291	Other ovarian cyst, right side ♀ ☑
N83.292	Other ovarian cyst, left side ♀ ☑
N83.6	Hematosalpinx ♀
N83.8	Other noninflammatory disorders of ovary, fallopian tube and broad ligament ♀
N84.0	Polyp of corpus uteri ♀
N84.8	Polyp of other parts of female genital tract ♀
N85.01	Benign endometrial hyperplasia ♀
N85.02	Endometrial intraepithelial neoplasia [EIN] ♀
N85.2	Hypertrophy of uterus ♀
N85.7	Hematometra ♀
N85.8	Other specified noninflammatory disorders of uterus ♀
N87.0	Mild cervical dysplasia ♀
N87.1	Moderate cervical dysplasia ♀
N92.0	Excessive and frequent menstruation with regular cycle ♀
N92.1	Excessive and frequent menstruation with irregular cycle ♀
N92.5	Other specified irregular menstruation ♀
N93.8	Other specified abnormal uterine and vaginal bleeding ♀
N94.89	Other specified conditions associated with female genital organs and menstrual cycle ♀
N95.0	Postmenopausal bleeding ♀

AMA: **58553** 2019,Jul,6; 2018,Jan,8; 2017,Apr,7; 2014,Jan,11 **58554** 2019,Jul,6; 2018,Jan,8; 2017,Apr,7; 2014,Jan,11

Relative Value Units/Medicare Edits

Non-Facility RVU	Work	PE	MP	Total
58553	20.06	9.51	3.13	32.7
58554	23.11	11.38	3.64	38.13
Facility RVU	**Work**	**PE**	**MP**	**Total**
58553	20.06	9.51	3.13	32.7
58554	23.11	11.38	3.64	38.13

	FUD	Status	MUE	Modifiers				IOM Reference
58553	90	A	1(3)	51	N/A	62	80	None
58554	90	A	1(2)	51	N/A	62	80	

* with documentation

Terms To Know

corpus luteum cyst. Common type of ovarian cyst that occurs when the corpus luteum fails to dissolve after the ovum is released and not fertilized. The cyst normally goes away in a few weeks but may enlarge to more than 10 cm and require surgical intervention.

dysplasia. Abnormality or alteration in the size, shape, and organization of cells from their normal pattern of development.

hematometra. Buildup of blood in the uterus, which causes uterine distention.

leiomyoma. Benign tumor consisting of smooth muscle in the uterus.

polyp. Small growth on a stalk-like attachment projecting from a mucous membrane.

postmenopause. Phase in a woman's life in which she has been free of menstrual periods for at least one year.

58555

58555   Hysteroscopy, diagnostic (separate procedure)

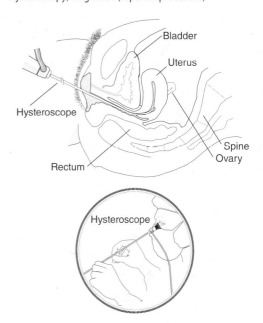

Explanation

The physician performs a diagnostic inspection of the uterus using a hysteroscope. The physician advances the hysteroscope through the vagina and into the cervical os to gain entry into the uterine cavity. The physician inspects the uterine cavity with the fiberoptic scope for diagnostic purposes.

Coding Tips

This separate procedure by definition is usually a component of a more complex service and is not identified separately. When performed alone or with other unrelated procedures/services it may be reported. If performed alone, list the code; if performed with other procedures/services, list the code and append modifier 59 or an X{EPSU} modifier. If biopsies or samples are taken from the endometrial surface, report 58558. If hysteroscopy is performed with lysis of intrauterine adhesions, report 58559. Local anesthesia is included in this service; however, this procedure may be performed under general anesthesia depending on the age and/or condition of the patient.

ICD-10-CM Diagnostic Codes

C53.0	Malignant neoplasm of endocervix ♀
C53.1	Malignant neoplasm of exocervix ♀
C53.8	Malignant neoplasm of overlapping sites of cervix uteri ♀
C54.0	Malignant neoplasm of isthmus uteri ♀
C54.1	Malignant neoplasm of endometrium ♀
C54.2	Malignant neoplasm of myometrium ♀
C54.3	Malignant neoplasm of fundus uteri ♀
C54.8	Malignant neoplasm of overlapping sites of corpus uteri ♀
C57.8	Malignant neoplasm of overlapping sites of female genital organs ♀
C79.82	Secondary malignant neoplasm of genital organs
D06.0	Carcinoma in situ of endocervix ♀
D06.1	Carcinoma in situ of exocervix ♀
D06.7	Carcinoma in situ of other parts of cervix ♀
D07.0	Carcinoma in situ of endometrium ♀

D07.39	Carcinoma in situ of other female genital organs ♀
D25.0	Submucous leiomyoma of uterus ♀
D25.1	Intramural leiomyoma of uterus ♀
D25.2	Subserosal leiomyoma of uterus ♀
D26.0	Other benign neoplasm of cervix uteri ♀
D26.1	Other benign neoplasm of corpus uteri ♀
D26.7	Other benign neoplasm of other parts of uterus ♀
D28.7	Benign neoplasm of other specified female genital organs ♀
D39.0	Neoplasm of uncertain behavior of uterus ♀
D39.8	Neoplasm of uncertain behavior of other specified female genital organs ♀
D49.59	Neoplasm of unspecified behavior of other genitourinary organ
N71.0	Acute inflammatory disease of uterus ♀
N71.1	Chronic inflammatory disease of uterus ♀
N72	Inflammatory disease of cervix uteri ♀
N73.1	Chronic parametritis and pelvic cellulitis ♀
N80.0	Endometriosis of uterus ♀
N81.2	Incomplete uterovaginal prolapse ♀
N81.3	Complete uterovaginal prolapse ♀
N81.89	Other female genital prolapse ♀
N84.0	Polyp of corpus uteri ♀
N84.1	Polyp of cervix uteri ♀
N84.8	Polyp of other parts of female genital tract ♀
N85.01	Benign endometrial hyperplasia ♀
N85.02	Endometrial intraepithelial neoplasia [EIN] ♀
N85.2	Hypertrophy of uterus ♀
N85.6	Intrauterine synechiae ♀
N85.7	Hematometra ♀
N85.8	Other specified noninflammatory disorders of uterus ♀
N86	Erosion and ectropion of cervix uteri ♀
N87.0	Mild cervical dysplasia ♀
N87.1	Moderate cervical dysplasia ♀
N88.0	Leukoplakia of cervix uteri ♀
N88.1	Old laceration of cervix uteri ♀
N88.2	Stricture and stenosis of cervix uteri ♀
N88.3	Incompetence of cervix uteri ♀
N88.4	Hypertrophic elongation of cervix uteri ♀
N88.8	Other specified noninflammatory disorders of cervix uteri ♀
N91.0	Primary amenorrhea ♀
N91.1	Secondary amenorrhea ♀
N92.0	Excessive and frequent menstruation with regular cycle ♀
N92.1	Excessive and frequent menstruation with irregular cycle ♀
N92.4	Excessive bleeding in the premenopausal period ♀
N92.5	Other specified irregular menstruation ♀
N93.8	Other specified abnormal uterine and vaginal bleeding ♀
N94.4	Primary dysmenorrhea ♀
N94.5	Secondary dysmenorrhea ♀
N94.89	Other specified conditions associated with female genital organs and menstrual cycle ♀
N95.0	Postmenopausal bleeding ♀
N96	Recurrent pregnancy loss ♀
N97.2	Female infertility of uterine origin ♀

Q51.10	Doubling of uterus with doubling of cervix and vagina without obstruction ♀
Q51.11	Doubling of uterus with doubling of cervix and vagina with obstruction ♀
Q51.21	Complete doubling of uterus ♀
Q51.22	Partial doubling of uterus ♀
Q51.28	Other and unspecified doubling of uterus ♀
Q51.3	Bicornate uterus ♀
Q51.4	Unicornate uterus ♀
Q51.6	Embryonic cyst of cervix ♀
Q51.7	Congenital fistulae between uterus and digestive and urinary tracts ♀
Q51.810	Arcuate uterus ♀
Q51.811	Hypoplasia of uterus ♀
Q51.818	Other congenital malformations of uterus ♀
Q51.820	Cervical duplication ♀
Q51.821	Hypoplasia of cervix ♀
Q51.828	Other congenital malformations of cervix ♀

AMA: **58555** 2019,Jul,6; 2018,Jan,8; 2017,Jan,8; 2016,Jan,13; 2015,Jan,16; 2014,Jan,11

Relative Value Units/Medicare Edits

Non-Facility RVU	Work	PE	MP	Total
58555	2.65	6.19	0.42	9.26
Facility RVU	**Work**	**PE**	**MP**	**Total**
58555	2.65	1.35	0.42	4.42

	FUD	Status	MUE	Modifiers				IOM Reference
58555	0	A	1(3)	51	N/A	62	80*	None

* with documentation

Terms To Know

hysteroscopy. Visualization and inspection of the uterus using a fiberoptic endoscope inserted through the vagina and cervical os into the uterine cavity. This may be done for diagnostic purposes alone or included with therapeutic procedures performed at the same time.

58558

58558 Hysteroscopy, surgical; with sampling (biopsy) of endometrium and/or polypectomy, with or without D & C

Numbers 1-4 show typical biopsy sites

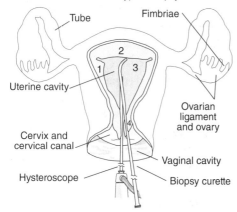

Explanation

The physician performs a diagnostic inspection of the uterus using a hysteroscope and removes a uterine polyp, removes uterine tissue for biopsy, and may perform cervical dilation and uterine curettage (D&C). The physician advances the hysteroscope through the vagina and into the cervical os to gain entry into the uterine cavity. The physician inspects the uterine cavity with the fiberoptic scope and removes a sample of the uterine lining and/or removes a growth (polypectomy) within the uterus and may perform a cervical dilation and uterine curettage, scraping (D&C) to take a complete sampling of the uterine lining.

Coding Tips

An excisional biopsy is not reported separately if a therapeutic excision is performed during the same surgical session. Surgical hysteroscopy always includes diagnostic hysteroscopy. For diagnostic hysteroscopy only, see 58555. When 58558 is performed with another separately identifiable procedure, the highest dollar value code is listed as the primary procedure and subsequent procedures are appended with modifier 51. If a hysteroscopy is performed with lysis of intrauterine adhesions, report 58559.

ICD-10-CM Diagnostic Codes

C53.0	Malignant neoplasm of endocervix ♀
C53.1	Malignant neoplasm of exocervix ♀
C53.8	Malignant neoplasm of overlapping sites of cervix uteri ♀
C54.0	Malignant neoplasm of isthmus uteri ♀
C54.1	Malignant neoplasm of endometrium ♀
C54.2	Malignant neoplasm of myometrium ♀
C54.3	Malignant neoplasm of fundus uteri ♀
C54.8	Malignant neoplasm of overlapping sites of corpus uteri ♀
C57.8	Malignant neoplasm of overlapping sites of female genital organs ♀
C79.82	Secondary malignant neoplasm of genital organs
D06.0	Carcinoma in situ of endocervix ♀
D06.1	Carcinoma in situ of exocervix ♀
D06.7	Carcinoma in situ of other parts of cervix ♀
D07.0	Carcinoma in situ of endometrium ♀
D07.39	Carcinoma in situ of other female genital organs ♀

D25.0	Submucous leiomyoma of uterus ♀
D25.1	Intramural leiomyoma of uterus ♀
D25.2	Subserosal leiomyoma of uterus ♀
D26.0	Other benign neoplasm of cervix uteri ♀
D26.1	Other benign neoplasm of corpus uteri ♀
D26.7	Other benign neoplasm of other parts of uterus ♀
D28.7	Benign neoplasm of other specified female genital organs ♀
D39.0	Neoplasm of uncertain behavior of uterus ♀
D39.8	Neoplasm of uncertain behavior of other specified female genital organs ♀
D49.59	Neoplasm of unspecified behavior of other genitourinary organ
N71.0	Acute inflammatory disease of uterus ♀
N71.1	Chronic inflammatory disease of uterus ♀
N72	Inflammatory disease of cervix uteri ♀
N73.1	Chronic parametritis and pelvic cellulitis ♀
N80.0	Endometriosis of uterus ♀
N81.2	Incomplete uterovaginal prolapse ♀
N81.3	Complete uterovaginal prolapse ♀
N81.89	Other female genital prolapse ♀
N84.0	Polyp of corpus uteri ♀
N84.1	Polyp of cervix uteri ♀
N84.8	Polyp of other parts of female genital tract ♀
N85.01	Benign endometrial hyperplasia ♀
N85.02	Endometrial intraepithelial neoplasia [EIN] ♀
N85.2	Hypertrophy of uterus ♀
N85.6	Intrauterine synechiae ♀
N85.7	Hematometra ♀
N85.8	Other specified noninflammatory disorders of uterus ♀
N86	Erosion and ectropion of cervix uteri ♀
N87.0	Mild cervical dysplasia ♀
N87.1	Moderate cervical dysplasia ♀
N88.0	Leukoplakia of cervix uteri ♀
N88.1	Old laceration of cervix uteri ♀
N88.2	Stricture and stenosis of cervix uteri ♀
N88.3	Incompetence of cervix uteri ♀
N88.4	Hypertrophic elongation of cervix uteri ♀
N88.8	Other specified noninflammatory disorders of cervix uteri ♀
N91.0	Primary amenorrhea ♀
N91.1	Secondary amenorrhea ♀
N92.0	Excessive and frequent menstruation with regular cycle ♀
N92.1	Excessive and frequent menstruation with irregular cycle ♀
N92.4	Excessive bleeding in the premenopausal period ♀
N92.5	Other specified irregular menstruation ♀
N93.8	Other specified abnormal uterine and vaginal bleeding ♀
N94.4	Primary dysmenorrhea ♀
N94.5	Secondary dysmenorrhea ♀
N94.89	Other specified conditions associated with female genital organs and menstrual cycle ♀
N95.0	Postmenopausal bleeding ♀
N96	Recurrent pregnancy loss ♀
N97.2	Female infertility of uterine origin ♀
Q51.6	Embryonic cyst of cervix ♀

AMA: **58558** 2019,Jul,6; 2018,Jan,8; 2017,Jan,8; 2016,Jan,13; 2015,Jan,16; 2014,Jan,11

Relative Value Units/Medicare Edits

Non-Facility RVU	Work	PE	MP	Total
58558	4.17	34.8	0.64	39.61
Facility RVU	**Work**	**PE**	**MP**	**Total**
58558	4.17	1.93	0.64	6.74

	FUD	Status	MUE	Modifiers				IOM Reference
58558	0	A	1(3)	51	N/A	62	N/A	None

* with documentation

Terms To Know

biopsy. Tissue or fluid removed for diagnostic purposes through analysis of the cells in the biopsy material.

curettage. Removal of tissue by scraping.

dilation. Artificial increase in the diameter of an opening or lumen made by medication or by instrumentation.

hysteroscopy. Visualization and inspection of the uterus using a fiberoptic endoscope inserted through the vagina and cervical os into the uterine cavity. This may be done for diagnostic purposes alone or included with therapeutic procedures performed at the same time.

polyp. Small growth on a stalk-like attachment projecting from a mucous membrane.

specimen. Tissue cells or sample of fluid taken for analysis, pathologic examination, and diagnosis.

tissue. Group of similar cells with a similar function that form definite structures and organs. Tissue types include epithelial tissue, muscle tissue, connective tissue, and nervous tissue.

58559-58560

58559   Hysteroscopy, surgical; with lysis of intrauterine adhesions (any method)

58560   with division or resection of intrauterine septum (any method)

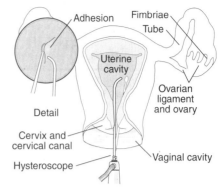

Adhesions separated under guidance of hysteroscope

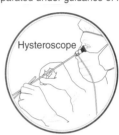

Explanation

The physician removes scar tissue (adhesions) from within the uterus using a fiberoptic hysteroscope. The physician advances the hysteroscope through the vagina and into the cervical os to gain entry into the uterine cavity. The physician inspects the uterine cavity with the fiberoptic scope and removes or divides adhesions (fibrous scar tissue) that are artificially connecting the walls of the uterus. In 58560, the physician divides or resects an intrauterine septum (tissue creating an abnormal partition in the uterus).

Coding Tips

An excisional biopsy is not reported separately if a therapeutic excision is performed during the same surgical session. Surgical hysteroscopy always includes diagnostic hysteroscopy. For diagnostic hysteroscopy only, see 58555. When either procedure is performed with another separately identifiable procedure, the highest dollar value code is listed as the primary procedure and subsequent procedures are appended with modifier 51. For excision of a vaginal septum, see 57130.

ICD-10-CM Diagnostic Codes

N85.6	Intrauterine synechiae ♀
Q51.21	Complete doubling of uterus ♀
Q51.22	Partial doubling of uterus ♀
Q51.28	Other and unspecified doubling of uterus ♀

AMA: **58559** 2019,Jul,6; 2018,Jan,8; 2017,Jan,8; 2016,Jan,13; 2015,Jan,16; 2014,Jan,11 **58560** 2019,Jul,6; 2018,Jan,8; 2017,Jan,8; 2016,Jan,13; 2015,Jan,16; 2014,Jan,11

Relative Value Units/Medicare Edits

Non-Facility RVU	Work	PE	MP	Total
58559	5.2	2.32	0.81	8.33
58560	5.75	2.51	0.9	9.16
Facility RVU	**Work**	**PE**	**MP**	**Total**
58559	5.2	2.32	0.81	8.33
58560	5.75	2.51	0.9	9.16

	FUD	Status	MUE	Modifiers				IOM Reference
58559	0	A	1(3)	51	N/A	62	N/A	None
58560	0	A	1(3)	51	N/A	62	80	

* with documentation

Terms To Know

adhesion. Abnormal fibrous connection between two structures, soft tissue or bony structures, that may occur as the result of surgery, infection, or trauma.

complication. Condition arising after the beginning of observation and treatment that modifies the course of the patient's illness or the medical care required, or an undesired result or misadventure in medical care.

congenital. Present at birth, occurring through heredity or an influence during gestation up to the moment of birth.

hysteroscopy. Visualization and inspection of the uterus using a fiberoptic endoscope inserted through the vagina and cervical os into the uterine cavity. This may be done for diagnostic purposes alone or included with therapeutic procedures performed at the same time.

intrauterine synechiae. Scarring and adhesions of the uterus, usually as a complication of a D&C.

lysis. Destruction, breakdown, dissolution, or decomposition of cells or substances by a specific catalyzing agent.

resection. Surgical removal of a part or all of an organ or body part.

scar tissue. Fibrous connective tissue that forms around a wounded area or injury, composed mainly of fibroblasts or collagenous fibers.

septum. Anatomical partition or dividing wall.

58561

58561   Hysteroscopy, surgical; with removal of leiomyomata

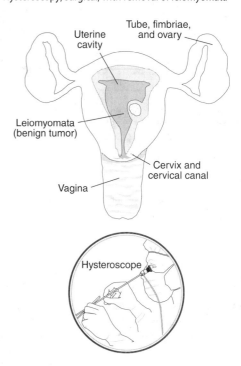

Explanation

The physician surgically removes a leiomyomata (uterine fibroid tumor) with the assistance of a fiberoptic hysteroscope. The physician advances the hysteroscope through the vagina and into the cervical os to gain entry into the uterine cavity. The physician inspects the uterine cavity with the fiberoptic scope and removes uterine leiomyomata with the assistance of the fiberoptic scope.

Coding Tips

An excisional biopsy is not reported separately if a therapeutic excision is performed during the same surgical session. Surgical hysteroscopy always includes diagnostic hysteroscopy. For diagnostic hysteroscopy only, see 58555. When 58561 is performed with another separately identifiable procedure, the highest dollar value code is listed as the primary procedure and subsequent procedures are appended with modifier 51. If hysteroscopy is performed with lysis of intrauterine adhesions, report 58559.

ICD-10-CM Diagnostic Codes

D25.0	Submucous leiomyoma of uterus ♀
D25.1	Intramural leiomyoma of uterus ♀
D25.2	Subserosal leiomyoma of uterus ♀
D25.9	Leiomyoma of uterus, unspecified ♀

AMA: 58561 2019,Jul,6; 2018,Jan,8; 2017,Jan,8; 2016,Jan,13; 2015,Jan,16; 2014,Jan,11

Relative Value Units/Medicare Edits

Non-Facility RVU	Work	PE	MP	Total
58561	6.6	2.84	1.04	10.48
Facility RVU	**Work**	**PE**	**MP**	**Total**
58561	6.6	2.84	1.04	10.48

	FUD	Status	MUE	Modifiers				IOM Reference
58561	0	A	1(3)	51	N/A	62	80*	None

* with documentation

Terms To Know

intramural uterine leiomyoma. Benign, smooth muscle tumor within the wall of the uterus.

leiomyoma. Benign tumor consisting of smooth muscle in the uterus.

metrorrhagia. Prolonged, irregular uterine bleeding of an inconsistent amount occurring in frequent bouts.

submucous uterine leiomyoma. Benign, smooth muscle tumor beneath the inner lining of the uterus.

subserous uterine leiomyoma. Benign, smooth muscle tumor beneath the serous membrane lining of the uterus.

58562

58562   Hysteroscopy, surgical; with removal of impacted foreign body

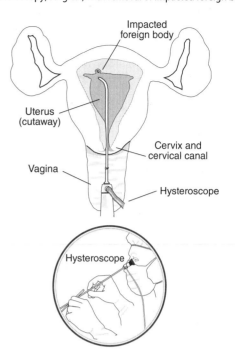

Explanation

The physician surgically removes an impacted foreign body with the assistance of a fiberoptic hysteroscope. The physician advances the hysteroscope through the vagina and into the cervical os to gain entry into the uterine cavity. The physician inspects the uterine cavity with the fiberoptic scope and removes an impacted foreign body from the uterine wall with the assistance of the hysteroscope.

Coding Tips

Surgical hysteroscopy always includes diagnostic hysteroscopy. For diagnostic hysteroscopy only, see 58555. When 58562 is performed with another separately identifiable procedure, the highest dollar value code is listed as the primary procedure and subsequent procedures are appended with modifier 51. For removal of an impacted vaginal foreign body under anesthesia, report 57415. If a laparoscopy is performed in conjunction with this procedure, report the appropriate laparoscopy code in addition to the hysteroscopy code.

ICD-10-CM Diagnostic Codes

T19.3XXA	Foreign body in uterus, initial encounter ♀
T83.31XA	Breakdown (mechanical) of intrauterine contraceptive device, initial encounter ♀
T83.32XA	Displacement of intrauterine contraceptive device, initial encounter ♀
T83.39XA	Other mechanical complication of intrauterine contraceptive device, initial encounter ♀
T83.69XA	Infection and inflammatory reaction due to other prosthetic device, implant and graft in genital tract, initial encounter

AMA: 58562 2019,Jul,6; 2018,Jan,8; 2017,Jan,8; 2016,Jan,13; 2015,Jan,16; 2014,Jan,11

Relative Value Units/Medicare Edits

Non-Facility RVU	Work	PE	MP	Total
58562	4.0	6.69	0.62	11.31
Facility RVU	Work	PE	MP	Total
58562	4.0	1.85	0.62	6.47

	FUD	Status	MUE	Modifiers				IOM Reference
58562	0	A	1(3)	51	N/A	62	N/A	None

* with documentation

Terms To Know

foreign body. Any object or substance found in an organ and tissue that does not belong under normal circumstances.

hysteroscopy. Visualization and inspection of the uterus using a fiberoptic endoscope inserted through the vagina and cervical os into the uterine cavity. This may be done for diagnostic purposes alone or included with therapeutic procedures performed at the same time.

impaction. State of being tightly wedged or lodged into or between something.

58563

58563   Hysteroscopy, surgical; with endometrial ablation (eg, endometrial resection, electrosurgical ablation, thermoablation)

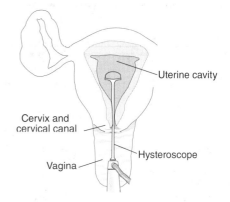

Explanation

The physician surgically removes (ablates) the inner lining of the uterus with the assistance of a fiberoptic hysteroscope. The physician advances the hysteroscope through the vagina and into the cervical os to gain entry into the uterine cavity. The physician inspects the uterine cavity with the fiberoptic scope and ablates the endometrium by various methods, such as resection, electrosurgical ablation, or thermoablation.

Coding Tips

Surgical hysteroscopy always includes diagnostic hysteroscopy. For diagnostic hysteroscopy only, see 58555. When 58563 is performed with another separately identifiable procedure, the highest dollar value code is listed as the primary procedure and subsequent procedures are appended with modifier 51. If a laparoscopy is performed in conjunction with this procedure, report the appropriate laparoscopy code in addition to the hysteroscopy code. For endometrial ablation without hysteroscopy, see 58353. Local anesthesia is included in this service; however, this procedure may be performed under general anesthesia depending on the age and/or condition of the patient.

ICD-10-CM Diagnostic Codes

N80.0	Endometriosis of uterus ♀
N92.0	Excessive and frequent menstruation with regular cycle ♀
N92.1	Excessive and frequent menstruation with irregular cycle ♀
N92.3	Ovulation bleeding ♀
N92.4	Excessive bleeding in the premenopausal period ♀
N92.5	Other specified irregular menstruation ♀
N93.8	Other specified abnormal uterine and vaginal bleeding ♀
N95.0	Postmenopausal bleeding ♀
N95.8	Other specified menopausal and perimenopausal disorders ♀

AMA: **58563** 2019,Jul,6; 2018,Jan,8; 2017,Jan,8; 2016,Jan,13; 2015,Jan,16; 2015,Jan,13; 2014,Jan,11

Relative Value Units/Medicare Edits

Non-Facility RVU	Work	PE	MP	Total
58563	4.47	50.46	0.68	55.61
Facility RVU	**Work**	**PE**	**MP**	**Total**
58563	4.47	2.03	0.68	7.18

	FUD	Status	MUE	Modifiers				IOM Reference
58563	0	A	1(3)	51	N/A	62	80*	None

* with documentation

Terms To Know

ablation. Removal or destruction of a body part or tissue or its function. Ablation may be performed by surgical means, hormones, drugs, radiofrequency, heat, chemical application, or other methods.

endometriosis. Aberrant uterine mucosal tissue appearing in areas of the pelvic cavity outside of its normal location, lining the uterus, and inflaming surrounding tissues often resulting in infertility or spontaneous abortion.

metrorrhagia. Prolonged, irregular uterine bleeding of an inconsistent amount occurring in frequent bouts.

58565

58565 Hysteroscopy, surgical; with bilateral fallopian tube cannulation to induce occlusion by placement of permanent implants

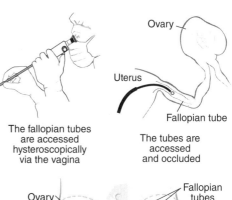

The fallopian tubes are accessed hysteroscopically via the vagina

The tubes are accessed and occluded

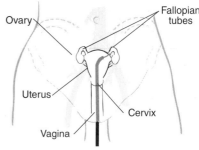

Explanation

The physician performs a hysteroscopy with bilateral fallopian tube cannulation and placement of permanent implants to occlude the fallopian tubes. The physician advances the hysteroscope through the vagina and into the cervical os to gain entry into the uterine cavity. The physician inserts a catheter into each fallopian tube. The catheter delivers a small metallic implant into each fallopian tube. The presence of the obstructive implant causes scar tissue to form, completely blocking the fallopian tube as a means of birth control.

Coding Tips

This is a bilateral procedure and as such is reported once even if the procedure is performed on both sides. If performed only on one side, append modifier 52. This procedure includes hysteroscopy and cervical dilation and should not be reported with 58555 or 57800.

ICD-10-CM Diagnostic Codes

Z30.2   Encounter for sterilization

AMA: 58565 2019,Jul,6; 2018,Jan,8; 2017,Jan,8; 2016,Jan,13; 2015,Jan,16; 2014,Jan,11

Relative Value Units/Medicare Edits

Non-Facility RVU	Work	PE	MP	Total
58565	7.12	43.4	1.13	51.65
Facility RVU	**Work**	**PE**	**MP**	**Total**
58565	7.12	4.72	1.13	12.97

	FUD	Status	MUE	Modifiers				IOM Reference
58565	90	A	1(2)	51	N/A	62	N/A	None

* with documentation

58570-58571

58570 Laparoscopy, surgical, with total hysterectomy, for uterus 250 g or less;

58571 with removal of tube(s) and/or ovary(s)

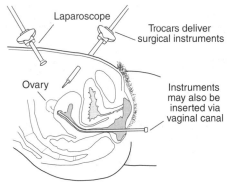

Laparoscope

Trocars deliver surgical instruments

Ovary

Instruments may also be inserted via vaginal canal

Laparoscopy assisted hysterectomy.
Tubes and ovaries may also be removed

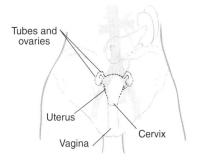

Tubes and ovaries

Uterus

Cervix

Vagina

Explanation

The physician performs a total laparoscopic hysterectomy (TLH), removing a uterus with a total weight of 250 gm or less. Following appropriate anesthesia, the patient is placed in the dorsal lithotomy position. A Foley catheter ensures that the bladder is emptied during the procedure. A trocar is inserted periumbilically and the abdomen is insufflated with gas. Ancillary trocars are also placed suprapubically. Following abdominal pelvic inspection and lysis of any adhesions present, the uterus is mobilized. The uterine ligaments are sectioned, and the uterus and cervix are dissected free from the bladder and surrounding tissues. Coagulation is achieved with the aid of electrocautery instruments. Alternately, some vessels may be ligated. The uterus and cervix are morcellized using endoscopic tools and removed through the abdominal incisions or the vagina. In 58571, one or both ovaries and/or one or both fallopian tubes are removed in similar fashion. Once the excisions are complete, the abdominal cavity is deflated and instruments and trocars are removed. The fascia and skin are closed with sutures.

Coding Tips

Surgical laparoscopy always includes a diagnostic laparoscopy; the diagnostic laparoscopy should not be reported separately. For a diagnostic laparoscopy, see 49320. For a laparoscopic supracervical hysterectomy for a uterus 250 gm or less, see 58541; with removal of tubes and/or ovaries, see 58542; greater than 250 gm, see 58543; with removal of tubes and/or ovaries, see 58544. Vaginal cuff closure is considered a component of a hysterectomy, regardless of approach.

ICD-10-CM Diagnostic Codes

C53.0	Malignant neoplasm of endocervix ♀
C53.1	Malignant neoplasm of exocervix ♀
C53.8	Malignant neoplasm of overlapping sites of cervix uteri ♀
C54.0	Malignant neoplasm of isthmus uteri ♀
C54.1	Malignant neoplasm of endometrium ♀
C54.2	Malignant neoplasm of myometrium ♀
C54.3	Malignant neoplasm of fundus uteri ♀
C54.8	Malignant neoplasm of overlapping sites of corpus uteri ♀
C56.1	Malignant neoplasm of right ovary ♀ ☑
C56.2	Malignant neoplasm of left ovary ♀ ☑
C57.01	Malignant neoplasm of right fallopian tube ♀ ☑
C57.02	Malignant neoplasm of left fallopian tube ♀ ☑
C57.11	Malignant neoplasm of right broad ligament ♀ ☑
C57.12	Malignant neoplasm of left broad ligament ♀ ☑
C57.21	Malignant neoplasm of right round ligament ♀ ☑
C57.22	Malignant neoplasm of left round ligament ♀ ☑
C57.3	Malignant neoplasm of parametrium ♀
C57.7	Malignant neoplasm of other specified female genital organs ♀
C57.8	Malignant neoplasm of overlapping sites of female genital organs ♀
C79.61	Secondary malignant neoplasm of right ovary ♀ ☑
C79.62	Secondary malignant neoplasm of left ovary ♀ ☑
C79.82	Secondary malignant neoplasm of genital organs
D06.0	Carcinoma in situ of endocervix ♀
D06.1	Carcinoma in situ of exocervix ♀
D06.7	Carcinoma in situ of other parts of cervix ♀
D07.0	Carcinoma in situ of endometrium ♀
D07.39	Carcinoma in situ of other female genital organs ♀
D25.0	Submucous leiomyoma of uterus ♀
D25.1	Intramural leiomyoma of uterus ♀
D25.2	Subserosal leiomyoma of uterus ♀
D39.0	Neoplasm of uncertain behavior of uterus ♀
D39.11	Neoplasm of uncertain behavior of right ovary ♀ ☑
D39.12	Neoplasm of uncertain behavior of left ovary ♀ ☑
D39.2	Neoplasm of uncertain behavior of placenta Ⓜ ♀
D39.8	Neoplasm of uncertain behavior of other specified female genital organs ♀
D49.59	Neoplasm of unspecified behavior of other genitourinary organ
N70.01	Acute salpingitis ♀
N70.02	Acute oophoritis ♀
N70.03	Acute salpingitis and oophoritis ♀
N70.11	Chronic salpingitis ♀
N70.12	Chronic oophoritis ♀
N70.13	Chronic salpingitis and oophoritis ♀
N71.0	Acute inflammatory disease of uterus ♀
N71.1	Chronic inflammatory disease of uterus ♀
N72	Inflammatory disease of cervix uteri ♀
N73.0	Acute parametritis and pelvic cellulitis ♀
N73.1	Chronic parametritis and pelvic cellulitis ♀
N73.3	Female acute pelvic peritonitis ♀
N73.4	Female chronic pelvic peritonitis ♀
N73.6	Female pelvic peritoneal adhesions (postinfective) ♀
N73.8	Other specified female pelvic inflammatory diseases ♀
N80.0	Endometriosis of uterus ♀
N80.1	Endometriosis of ovary ♀
N80.2	Endometriosis of fallopian tube ♀

N81.2	Incomplete uterovaginal prolapse ♀
N81.3	Complete uterovaginal prolapse ♀
N81.89	Other female genital prolapse ♀
N83.01	Follicular cyst of right ovary ♀ ☑
N83.02	Follicular cyst of left ovary ♀ ☑
N83.11	Corpus luteum cyst of right ovary ♀ ☑
N83.12	Corpus luteum cyst of left ovary ♀ ☑
N83.291	Other ovarian cyst, right side ♀ ☑
N83.292	Other ovarian cyst, left side ♀ ☑
N83.6	Hematosalpinx ♀
N83.8	Other noninflammatory disorders of ovary, fallopian tube and broad ligament ♀
N84.0	Polyp of corpus uteri ♀
N84.8	Polyp of other parts of female genital tract ♀
N85.01	Benign endometrial hyperplasia ♀
N85.02	Endometrial intraepithelial neoplasia [EIN] ♀
N85.2	Hypertrophy of uterus ♀
N85.7	Hematometra ♀
N85.8	Other specified noninflammatory disorders of uterus ♀
N87.0	Mild cervical dysplasia ♀
N87.1	Moderate cervical dysplasia ♀
N92.0	Excessive and frequent menstruation with regular cycle ♀
N92.1	Excessive and frequent menstruation with irregular cycle ♀
N92.5	Other specified irregular menstruation ♀
N93.8	Other specified abnormal uterine and vaginal bleeding ♀
N94.89	Other specified conditions associated with female genital organs and menstrual cycle ♀
N95.0	Postmenopausal bleeding ♀

AMA: 58570 2019,Jul,6; 2018,Jan,8; 2017,Apr,7; 2014,Jan,11 **58571** 2019,Jul,6; 2018,Jan,8; 2018,Feb,11; 2017,Jan,8; 2017,Apr,7; 2016,Jan,13; 2015,Jan,16; 2014,Jan,11

Relative Value Units/Medicare Edits

Non-Facility RVU	Work	PE	MP	Total
58570	13.36	7.55	2.08	22.99
58571	15.0	8.58	2.35	25.93
Facility RVU	**Work**	**PE**	**MP**	**Total**
58570	13.36	7.55	2.08	22.99
58571	15.0	8.58	2.35	25.93

	FUD	Status	MUE	Modifiers				IOM Reference
58570	90	A	1(3)	51	N/A	62	80	None
58571	90	A	1(2)	51	N/A	62	80	

* with documentation

58572-58573

58572 Laparoscopy, surgical, with total hysterectomy, for uterus greater than 250 g;

58573 with removal of tube(s) and/or ovary(s)

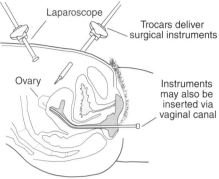

Laparoscopy assisted hysterectomy.
Tubes and ovaries may also be removed

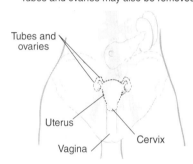

Explanation

The physician performs a total laparoscopic hysterectomy (TLH), removing a uterus with a total weight greater than 250 gm. Following appropriate anesthesia, the patient is placed in the dorsal lithotomy position. A Foley catheter ensures that the bladder is emptied during the procedure. A trocar is inserted periumbilically and the abdomen is insufflated with gas. Ancillary trocars are also placed suprapubically. Following abdominal pelvic inspection and lysis of any adhesions present, the uterus is mobilized. The uterine ligaments are sectioned, and the uterus and cervix are dissected free from the bladder and surrounding tissues. Coagulation is achieved with the aid of electrocautery instruments. Alternately, some vessels may be ligated. The uterus and cervix are morcellized using endoscopic tools and removed through the abdominal incisions or the vagina. In 58573, one or both ovaries and/or one or both fallopian tubes are removed in similar fashion. Once the excisions are complete, the abdominal cavity is deflated and instruments and trocars are removed. The fascia and skin are closed with sutures.

Coding Tips

Surgical laparoscopy always includes a diagnostic laparoscopy; the diagnostic laparoscopy should not be reported separately. For a diagnostic laparoscopy, see 49320. For a surgical laparoscopy, supracervical hysterectomy, for a uterus 250 gm or less, see 58541; with removal of tubes and/or ovaries, see 58542; for a uterus greater than 250 gm, see 58543; with removal of tubes and/or ovaries, see 58544.

ICD-10-CM Diagnostic Codes

C53.0	Malignant neoplasm of endocervix ♀
C53.1	Malignant neoplasm of exocervix ♀
C53.8	Malignant neoplasm of overlapping sites of cervix uteri ♀

C54.0	Malignant neoplasm of isthmus uteri ♀
C54.1	Malignant neoplasm of endometrium ♀
C54.2	Malignant neoplasm of myometrium ♀
C54.3	Malignant neoplasm of fundus uteri ♀
C54.8	Malignant neoplasm of overlapping sites of corpus uteri ♀
C56.1	Malignant neoplasm of right ovary ♀ ☑
C56.2	Malignant neoplasm of left ovary ♀ ☑
C57.01	Malignant neoplasm of right fallopian tube ♀ ☑
C57.02	Malignant neoplasm of left fallopian tube ♀ ☑
C57.11	Malignant neoplasm of right broad ligament ♀ ☑
C57.12	Malignant neoplasm of left broad ligament ♀ ☑
C57.21	Malignant neoplasm of right round ligament ♀ ☑
C57.22	Malignant neoplasm of left round ligament ♀ ☑
C57.3	Malignant neoplasm of parametrium ♀
C57.7	Malignant neoplasm of other specified female genital organs ♀
C57.8	Malignant neoplasm of overlapping sites of female genital organs ♀
C79.61	Secondary malignant neoplasm of right ovary ♀ ☑
C79.62	Secondary malignant neoplasm of left ovary ♀ ☑
C79.82	Secondary malignant neoplasm of genital organs
D06.0	Carcinoma in situ of endocervix ♀
D06.1	Carcinoma in situ of exocervix ♀
D06.7	Carcinoma in situ of other parts of cervix ♀
D07.0	Carcinoma in situ of endometrium ♀
D07.39	Carcinoma in situ of other female genital organs ♀
D25.0	Submucous leiomyoma of uterus ♀
D25.1	Intramural leiomyoma of uterus ♀
D25.2	Subserosal leiomyoma of uterus ♀
D39.0	Neoplasm of uncertain behavior of uterus ♀
D39.11	Neoplasm of uncertain behavior of right ovary ♀ ☑
D39.12	Neoplasm of uncertain behavior of left ovary ♀ ☑
D39.2	Neoplasm of uncertain behavior of placenta Ⓜ ♀
D39.8	Neoplasm of uncertain behavior of other specified female genital organs ♀
D49.59	Neoplasm of unspecified behavior of other genitourinary organ
N70.01	Acute salpingitis ♀
N70.02	Acute oophoritis ♀
N70.03	Acute salpingitis and oophoritis ♀
N70.11	Chronic salpingitis ♀
N70.12	Chronic oophoritis ♀
N70.13	Chronic salpingitis and oophoritis ♀
N71.0	Acute inflammatory disease of uterus ♀
N71.1	Chronic inflammatory disease of uterus ♀
N72	Inflammatory disease of cervix uteri ♀
N73.0	Acute parametritis and pelvic cellulitis ♀
N73.1	Chronic parametritis and pelvic cellulitis ♀
N73.3	Female acute pelvic peritonitis ♀
N73.4	Female chronic pelvic peritonitis ♀
N73.6	Female pelvic peritoneal adhesions (postinfective) ♀
N73.8	Other specified female pelvic inflammatory diseases ♀
N80.0	Endometriosis of uterus ♀
N80.1	Endometriosis of ovary ♀
N80.2	Endometriosis of fallopian tube ♀

N81.2	Incomplete uterovaginal prolapse ♀
N81.3	Complete uterovaginal prolapse ♀
N81.89	Other female genital prolapse ♀
N83.01	Follicular cyst of right ovary ♀ ☑
N83.02	Follicular cyst of left ovary ♀ ☑
N83.11	Corpus luteum cyst of right ovary ♀ ☑
N83.12	Corpus luteum cyst of left ovary ♀ ☑
N83.291	Other ovarian cyst, right side ♀ ☑
N83.292	Other ovarian cyst, left side ♀ ☑
N83.6	Hematosalpinx ♀
N83.8	Other noninflammatory disorders of ovary, fallopian tube and broad ligament ♀
N84.0	Polyp of corpus uteri ♀
N84.8	Polyp of other parts of female genital tract ♀
N85.01	Benign endometrial hyperplasia ♀
N85.02	Endometrial intraepithelial neoplasia [EIN] ♀
N85.2	Hypertrophy of uterus ♀
N85.7	Hematometra ♀
N85.8	Other specified noninflammatory disorders of uterus ♀
N87.0	Mild cervical dysplasia ♀
N87.1	Moderate cervical dysplasia ♀
N92.0	Excessive and frequent menstruation with regular cycle ♀
N92.1	Excessive and frequent menstruation with irregular cycle ♀
N92.5	Other specified irregular menstruation ♀
N93.8	Other specified abnormal uterine and vaginal bleeding ♀
N94.89	Other specified conditions associated with female genital organs and menstrual cycle ♀
N95.0	Postmenopausal bleeding ♀

AMA: **58572** 2019,Jul,6; 2018,Jan,8; 2017,Apr,7; 2014,Jan,11 **58573** 2019,Mar,5; 2019,Jul,6; 2018,Jan,8; 2018,Feb,11; 2018,Apr,10; 2017,Jan,8; 2017,Apr,7; 2016,Jan,13; 2015,Jan,16; 2014,Jan,11

Relative Value Units/Medicare Edits

Non-Facility RVU	Work	PE	MP	Total
58572	17.71	9.38	2.78	29.87
58573	20.79	10.98	3.26	35.03
Facility RVU	**Work**	**PE**	**MP**	**Total**
58572	17.71	9.38	2.78	29.87
58573	20.79	10.98	3.26	35.03

	FUD	Status	MUE	Modifiers				IOM Reference
58572	90	A	1(3)	51	N/A	62	80	None
58573	90	A	1(2)	51	N/A	62	80	

* with documentation

58575

58575 Laparoscopy, surgical, total hysterectomy for resection of malignancy (tumor debulking), with omentectomy including salpingo-oophorectomy, unilateral or bilateral, when performed

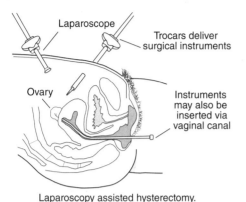

Laparoscopy assisted hysterectomy. Tubes and ovaries may also be removed

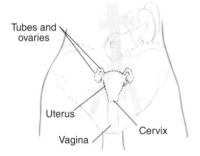

Explanation

Through small incisions made in the abdomen, the physician performs a total hysterectomy (removal the uterus and cervix) for an ovarian, fallopian, or peritoneal malignancy. After careful inspection of the abdomen and pelvis, aspiration of any pelvic ascites or peritoneal washings submitted for cytologic evaluation and tissue samples for frozen section may be performed to determine if malignant cells are still present and/or to determine if the cancer has metastasized. Tumor debulking is a procedure where a surgeon partially removes a surgically incurable malignant tumor to allow for subsequent therapies such as chemotherapy, radiation, or other adjunctive measures more effective with the goal of increasing the patient's survival rates. The physician also performs an omentectomy (removal of the membrane containing fat, lymph, and blood vessels that acts as a protective layer extending from the stomach to the transverse colon). Removal of one or both ovaries and/or fallopian tubes is included, when performed.

Coding Tips

Surgical laparoscopy always includes a diagnostic laparoscopy; the diagnostic laparoscopy should not be reported separately. Do not report 58575 with 49255, 49320-49321, 58570-58573, or 58661.

ICD-10-CM Diagnostic Codes

C48.1	Malignant neoplasm of specified parts of peritoneum
C48.8	Malignant neoplasm of overlapping sites of retroperitoneum and peritoneum
C53.0	Malignant neoplasm of endocervix ♀
C53.1	Malignant neoplasm of exocervix ♀
C53.8	Malignant neoplasm of overlapping sites of cervix uteri ♀
C54.0	Malignant neoplasm of isthmus uteri ♀
C54.1	Malignant neoplasm of endometrium ♀
C54.2	Malignant neoplasm of myometrium ♀
C54.3	Malignant neoplasm of fundus uteri ♀
C54.8	Malignant neoplasm of overlapping sites of corpus uteri ♀
C56.1	Malignant neoplasm of right ovary ♀ ☑
C56.2	Malignant neoplasm of left ovary ♀ ☑
C57.01	Malignant neoplasm of right fallopian tube ♀ ☑
C57.02	Malignant neoplasm of left fallopian tube ♀ ☑
C57.11	Malignant neoplasm of right broad ligament ♀ ☑
C57.12	Malignant neoplasm of left broad ligament ♀ ☑
C57.21	Malignant neoplasm of right round ligament ♀ ☑
C57.22	Malignant neoplasm of left round ligament ♀ ☑
C57.3	Malignant neoplasm of parametrium ♀
C57.7	Malignant neoplasm of other specified female genital organs ♀
C57.8	Malignant neoplasm of overlapping sites of female genital organs ♀
C78.6	Secondary malignant neoplasm of retroperitoneum and peritoneum
C79.61	Secondary malignant neoplasm of right ovary ♀ ☑
C79.62	Secondary malignant neoplasm of left ovary ♀ ☑
C79.82	Secondary malignant neoplasm of genital organs ♀
D06.0	Carcinoma in situ of endocervix ♀
D06.1	Carcinoma in situ of exocervix ♀
D06.7	Carcinoma in situ of other parts of cervix ♀
D07.0	Carcinoma in situ of endometrium ♀
D07.39	Carcinoma in situ of other female genital organs ♀
D25.0	Submucous leiomyoma of uterus ♀
D25.1	Intramural leiomyoma of uterus ♀
D25.2	Subserosal leiomyoma of uterus ♀
D39.0	Neoplasm of uncertain behavior of uterus ♀
D39.11	Neoplasm of uncertain behavior of right ovary ♀ ☑
D39.12	Neoplasm of uncertain behavior of left ovary ♀ ☑
D39.2	Neoplasm of uncertain behavior of placenta Ⓜ ♀
D39.8	Neoplasm of uncertain behavior of other specified female genital organs ♀
D49.59	Neoplasm of unspecified behavior of other genitourinary organ

AMA: **58575** 2019,Mar,5; 2019,Jul,6

Relative Value Units/Medicare Edits

Non-Facility RVU	Work	PE	MP	Total
58575	32.6	17.21	5.1	54.91
Facility RVU	**Work**	**PE**	**MP**	**Total**
58575	32.6	17.21	5.1	54.91

	FUD	Status	MUE	Modifiers				IOM Reference
58575	90	A	1(2)	51	N/A	62	80	None

* with documentation

58600-58605

58600 Ligation or transection of fallopian tube(s), abdominal or vaginal approach, unilateral or bilateral

58605 Ligation or transection of fallopian tube(s), abdominal or vaginal approach, postpartum, unilateral or bilateral, during same hospitalization (separate procedure)

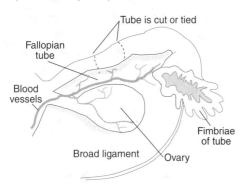

Explanation

The physician ties off the fallopian tube or removes a portion of it on one side or both. The procedure may be done through the vagina or through a small incision just above the pubic hairline. In 58605, the procedure is done during the same hospital stay as the delivery of a baby.

Coding Tips

Report 58605 only when a tubal ligation is completed while the patient is hospitalized following a delivery. Note that 58605, a separate procedure by definition, is usually a component of a more complex service and is not identified separately. When performed alone or with other unrelated procedures/services it may be reported. If performed alone, list the code; if performed with other procedures/services, list the code and append modifier 59 or an X{EPSU} modifier. When 58600 is performed with another separately identifiable procedure, the highest dollar value code is listed as the primary procedure and subsequent procedures are appended with modifier 51. For tubal ligation performed via laparoscopy, see 58670 and 58671.

ICD-10-CM Diagnostic Codes

Z30.2   Encounter for sterilization

AMA: 58600 2019,Jul,6; 2018,Jan,8; 2017,Jan,8; 2016,Jan,13; 2015,Jan,16; 2014,Jan,11 **58605** 2019,Jul,6; 2018,Jan,8; 2017,Jan,8; 2016,Jan,13; 2015,Jan,16; 2014,Jan,11

Relative Value Units/Medicare Edits

Non-Facility RVU	Work	PE	MP	Total
58600	5.91	3.83	0.92	10.66
58605	5.28	3.55	0.82	9.65
Facility RVU	Work	PE	MP	Total
58600	5.91	3.83	0.92	10.66
58605	5.28	3.55	0.82	9.65

	FUD	Status	MUE	Modifiers				IOM Reference
58600	90	A	1(2)	51	N/A	62*	80	100-03,230.3
58605	90	A	1(2)	51	N/A	N/A	80	

* with documentation

58611

+ 58611 Ligation or transection of fallopian tube(s) when done at the time of cesarean delivery or intra-abdominal surgery (not a separate procedure) (List separately in addition to code for primary procedure)

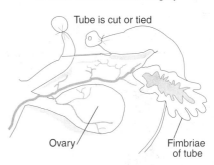

Performed in addition to C-section or other intra-abdominal surgery

Explanation

The physician ties off the fallopian tube or removes a portion of it on one side or both. This procedure is done at the time of a cesarean section or during intra-abdominal surgery.

Coding Tips

This code should only be used for a tubal ligation completed during a cesarean section or during intra-abdominal surgery. Unlike other minor procedures, 58611 is reported in conjunction with the primary procedure. No reimbursement reduction or modifier 51 is applied. To report a tubal ligation performed via laparoscopy, see 58670 and 58671.

ICD-10-CM Diagnostic Codes

Z30.2   Encounter for sterilization

AMA: 58611 2019,Jul,6; 2014,Jan,11

Relative Value Units/Medicare Edits

Non-Facility RVU	Work	PE	MP	Total
58611	1.45	0.55	0.24	2.24
Facility RVU	Work	PE	MP	Total
58611	1.45	0.55	0.24	2.24

	FUD	Status	MUE	Modifiers				IOM Reference
58611	N/A	A	1(2)	N/A	N/A	N/A	80	None

* with documentation

Terms To Know

fallopian tubes. Bilateral, paired tubes that extend from the uterus to the ovaries, through which an ovum released from the follicle travels to the uterus during ovulation.

intra. Within.

ligation. Tying off a blood vessel or duct with a suture or a soft, thin wire.

transection. Transverse dissection; to cut across a long axis; cross section.

Oviduct

58615

58615 Occlusion of fallopian tube(s) by device (eg, band, clip, Falope ring) vaginal or suprapubic approach

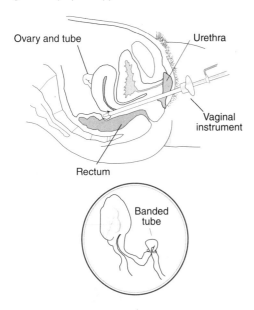

Ovary and tube

Urethra

Vaginal instrument

Rectum

Banded tube

Explanation

The physician blocks one or both of the fallopian tubes with a band, clip, or Falope ring. The physician may elect to do the procedure through the vagina or through a small incision just above the pubic hairline.

Coding Tips

This procedure is a reversible sterilization procedure. When 58615 is performed with another separately identifiable procedure, the highest dollar value code is listed as the primary procedure and subsequent procedures are appended with modifier 51. For a tubal occlusion performed via a laparoscopic approach, see 58671.

ICD-10-CM Diagnostic Codes

Z30.2   Encounter for sterilization

AMA: **58615** 2019,Jul,6; 2018,Jan,8; 2017,Jan,8; 2016,Jan,13; 2015,Jan,16; 2014,Jan,11

Relative Value Units/Medicare Edits

Non-Facility RVU	Work	PE	MP	Total
58615	3.94	2.68	0.62	7.24
Facility RVU	Work	PE	MP	Total
58615	3.94	2.68	0.62	7.24

	FUD	Status	MUE	Modifiers				IOM Reference
58615	10	A	1(2)	51	N/A	N/A	80	None

* with documentation

Terms To Know

approach. Method or anatomical location used to gain access to a body organ or specific area for procedures.

occlusion. Constriction, closure, or blockage of a passage.

58660

58660 Laparoscopy, surgical; with lysis of adhesions (salpingolysis, ovariolysis) (separate procedure)

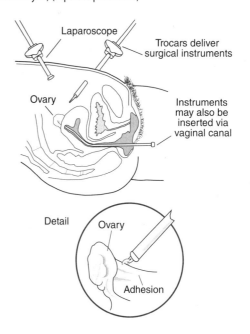

Laparoscope

Trocars deliver surgical instruments

Ovary

Instruments may also be inserted via vaginal canal

Detail

Ovary

Adhesion

Explanation

The physician performs a laparoscopic surgical cutting/releasing (lysis) of scar tissue (adhesions) surrounding the ovaries and/or fallopian tubes with the assistance of a fiberoptic laparoscope. The physician may first insert an instrument through the vagina to grasp the cervix and manipulate the uterus during surgery. Next, the physician makes a small incision just below the umbilicus through which a fiberoptic laparoscope is inserted. A second incision is made in the abdomen with additional instruments being placed through these incisions into the abdomen or pelvis. The physician manipulates the tools so that the pelvic organs can be observed, manipulated and lysis of adhesions can be performed. The abdomen is deflated, the trocars removed, and the incisions are closed with sutures.

Coding Tips

Surgical laparoscopy always includes diagnostic laparoscopy. For diagnostic laparoscopy only, see 49320. This separate procedure by definition is usually a component of a more complex service and is not identified separately. When performed alone or with other unrelated procedures/services it may be reported. If performed alone, list the code; if performed with other procedures/services, list the code and append modifier 59 or an X{EPSU} modifier. For hysteroscopic lysis of uterine adhesions, see 58559. For open lysis of adhesions (salpingolysis, ovariolysis), see 58740.

ICD-10-CM Diagnostic Codes

N73.6   Female pelvic peritoneal adhesions (postinfective) ♀
N99.4   Postprocedural pelvic peritoneal adhesions

AMA: **58660** 2019,Jul,6; 2018,Jan,8; 2017,Jan,8; 2016,Jan,13; 2015,Jan,16; 2014,Jan,11

Relative Value Units/Medicare Edits

Non-Facility RVU	Work	PE	MP	Total
58660	11.59	6.08	1.98	19.65
Facility RVU	**Work**	**PE**	**MP**	**Total**
58660	11.59	6.08	1.98	19.65

	FUD	Status	MUE	Modifiers				IOM Reference
58660	90	A	1(2)	51	N/A	62	80	100-03,230.3

* with documentation

Terms To Know

adhesion. Abnormal fibrous connection between two structures, soft tissue or bony structures, that may occur as the result of surgery, infection, or trauma.

lysis. Destruction, breakdown, dissolution, or decomposition of cells or substances by a specific catalyzing agent.

oophoritis. Inflammation or infection of one or both ovaries that can cause chronic pelvic pain, ectopic pregnancy, or sterilization.

salpingitis. Inflammation of the fallopian tubes, usually caused by a bacterial infection and occurring in conjunction with inflammation of the ovaries (oophoritis).

scar tissue. Fibrous connective tissue that forms around a wounded area or injury, composed mainly of fibroblasts or collagenous fibers.

separate procedures. Services commonly carried out as a fundamental part of a total service and, as such, do not usually warrant separate identification. These services are identified in CPT with the parenthetical phrase (separate procedure) at the end of the description and are payable only when performed alone.

58661

58661 Laparoscopy, surgical; with removal of adnexal structures (partial or total oophorectomy and/or salpingectomy)

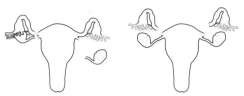

Removal of tubes and ovaries (salpingo-oophorectomy)

Removal of ovaries only   Removal of tubes only

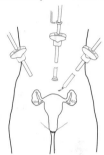

Explanation

The physician performs a laparoscopic surgical removal of one or both ovaries and their accompanying fallopian tubes with the assistance of a fiberoptic laparoscope. The physician may first insert an instrument through the vagina to grasp the cervix and manipulate the uterus during surgery. Next, the physician makes a small incision just below the umbilicus through which a fiberoptic laparoscope is inserted. A second incision is made on the left or right side of the abdomen with additional instruments being placed through these incisions into the abdomen or pelvis. The physician manipulates the tools so that the pelvic organs can be observed, manipulated and removal of one or both ovaries and fallopian tubes can be performed with the laparoscope. The abdomen is deflated, the trocars removed and the incisions are closed with sutures.

Coding Tips

This is a bilateral code and is reported once even if the procedure is performed on both sides according to CPT instructions. Surgical laparoscopy always includes diagnostic laparoscopy. For diagnostic laparoscopy only, see 49320. If the procedure is performed to treat an ectopic pregnancy, see 59151. When 58661 is performed with another separately identifiable procedure, the highest dollar value code is listed as the primary procedure and subsequent procedures are appended with modifier 51. Medicare instructions allow the reporting of modifier 50 when performed bilaterally. Check with individual payers for their instructions. To report open salpingectomy, see 58700; for open salpingo-oophorectomy, see 58720. If a hysteroscopy is performed in conjunction with this procedure, report the appropriate hysteroscopy code.

ICD-10-CM Diagnostic Codes

C56.1	Malignant neoplasm of right ovary ♀ ☑
C56.2	Malignant neoplasm of left ovary ♀ ☑
C57.01	Malignant neoplasm of right fallopian tube ♀ ☑
C57.02	Malignant neoplasm of left fallopian tube ♀ ☑
C79.61	Secondary malignant neoplasm of right ovary ♀ ☑
C79.62	Secondary malignant neoplasm of left ovary ♀ ☑

D07.39	Carcinoma in situ of other female genital organs ♀
D27.0	Benign neoplasm of right ovary ♀ ☑
D27.1	Benign neoplasm of left ovary ♀ ☑
D28.2	Benign neoplasm of uterine tubes and ligaments ♀
D28.7	Benign neoplasm of other specified female genital organs ♀
D39.11	Neoplasm of uncertain behavior of right ovary ♀ ☑
D39.12	Neoplasm of uncertain behavior of left ovary ♀ ☑
D39.8	Neoplasm of uncertain behavior of other specified female genital organs ♀
D49.59	Neoplasm of unspecified behavior of other genitourinary organ
E28.2	Polycystic ovarian syndrome ♀
E28.8	Other ovarian dysfunction ♀
N70.01	Acute salpingitis ♀
N70.02	Acute oophoritis ♀
N70.03	Acute salpingitis and oophoritis ♀
N70.11	Chronic salpingitis ♀
N70.12	Chronic oophoritis ♀
N70.13	Chronic salpingitis and oophoritis ♀
N73.6	Female pelvic peritoneal adhesions (postinfective) ♀
N80.1	Endometriosis of ovary ♀
N80.2	Endometriosis of fallopian tube ♀
N80.3	Endometriosis of pelvic peritoneum ♀
N83.01	Follicular cyst of right ovary ♀ ☑
N83.02	Follicular cyst of left ovary ♀ ☑
N83.11	Corpus luteum cyst of right ovary ♀ ☑
N83.12	Corpus luteum cyst of left ovary ♀ ☑
N83.291	Other ovarian cyst, right side ♀ ☑
N83.292	Other ovarian cyst, left side ♀ ☑
N83.321	Acquired atrophy of right fallopian tube ♀ ☑
N83.322	Acquired atrophy of left fallopian tube ♀ ☑
N83.511	Torsion of right ovary and ovarian pedicle ♀ ☑
N83.512	Torsion of left ovary and ovarian pedicle ♀ ☑
N83.521	Torsion of right fallopian tube ♀ ☑
N83.522	Torsion of left fallopian tube ♀ ☑
N83.53	Torsion of ovary, ovarian pedicle and fallopian tube ♀
N83.6	Hematosalpinx ♀
N83.8	Other noninflammatory disorders of ovary, fallopian tube and broad ligament ♀
N84.8	Polyp of other parts of female genital tract ♀
O00.101	Right tubal pregnancy without intrauterine pregnancy Ⓜ ♀
O00.102	Left tubal pregnancy without intrauterine pregnancy Ⓜ ♀
O00.111	Right tubal pregnancy with intrauterine pregnancy Ⓜ ♀
O00.112	Left tubal pregnancy with intrauterine pregnancy Ⓜ ♀
O00.201	Right ovarian pregnancy without intrauterine pregnancy Ⓜ ♀
O00.202	Left ovarian pregnancy without intrauterine pregnancy Ⓜ ♀
O00.211	Right ovarian pregnancy with intrauterine pregnancy Ⓜ ♀
O00.212	Left ovarian pregnancy with intrauterine pregnancy Ⓜ ♀
Q50.1	Developmental ovarian cyst ♀
Q50.2	Congenital torsion of ovary ♀

AMA: **58661** 2020,Jan,12; 2019,Jul,6; 2018,Jan,8; 2017,Jan,8; 2016,Jan,13; 2015,Jan,16; 2014,Jan,11

Relative Value Units/Medicare Edits

Non-Facility RVU	Work	PE	MP	Total
58661	11.35	5.71	1.8	18.86
Facility RVU	Work	PE	MP	Total
58661	11.35	5.71	1.8	18.86

	FUD	Status	MUE	Modifiers				IOM Reference
58661	10	A	1(2)	51	50	62	80	None

* with documentation

Terms To Know

adnexa. Appendages, adjunct parts, or connecting structures, related by functionality.

laparoscopy. Direct visualization of the peritoneal cavity, outer fallopian tubes, uterus, and ovaries utilizing a laparoscope, a thin, flexible fiberoptic tube.

oophorectomy. Surgical removal of all or part of one or both ovaries, either as open procedure or laparoscopically. Menstruation and childbearing ability continues when one ovary is removed.

salpingectomy. Removal of all or part of one or both of the fallopian tubes. Indications include infection, ectopic pregnancy, sterilization, or cancer. This procedure is often performed in combination with other open or laparoscopic procedures.

torsion of ovary or fallopian tube. Twisting or rotation of the ovary or fallopian tube upon itself, so as to compromise or cut off the blood supply.

58662

58662 Laparoscopy, surgical; with fulguration or excision of lesions of the ovary, pelvic viscera, or peritoneal surface by any method

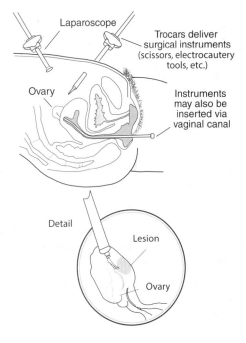

Laparoscope

Trocars deliver surgical instruments (scissors, electrocautery tools, etc.)

Ovary

Instruments may also be inserted via vaginal canal

Detail

Lesion

Ovary

Explanation

The physician performs a laparoscopic electrical cautery destruction of an ovarian, pelvic or peritoneal lesion with the assistance of a fiberoptic laparoscope. The physician may first insert an instrument through the vagina to grasp the cervix and manipulate the uterus during surgery. Next, the physician makes a small incision just below the umbilicus through which a fiberoptic laparoscope is inserted. A second incision is made on the left or right side of the abdomen with additional instruments being placed through these incisions into the abdomen or pelvis. The physician manipulates the tools so that the pelvic organs can be observed, manipulated and operated upon with the laparoscope. Once lesions are identified with the laparoscope, a third incision is typically made adjacent to the lesion through which an electric cautery tool, knife, or laser is inserted for lesion fulguration. The abdomen is deflated, the trocars removed and the incisions are closed with sutures.

Coding Tips

Surgical laparoscopy always includes diagnostic laparoscopy. For diagnostic laparoscopy only, see 49320. When 58662 is performed with another separately identifiable procedure, the highest dollar value code is listed as the primary procedure and subsequent procedures are appended with modifier 51. If a hysteroscopy is performed in conjunction with this procedure, report the appropriate hysteroscopy code. For laparotomy with excision or destruction of intra-abdominal or retroperitoneal tumors, cysts, or endometriomas, see 49203–49205. Report 58662 only once regardless of the number of lesions removed.

ICD-10-CM Diagnostic Codes

C48.1	Malignant neoplasm of specified parts of peritoneum
C48.8	Malignant neoplasm of overlapping sites of retroperitoneum and peritoneum
C56.1	Malignant neoplasm of right ovary ♀ ☑
C56.2	Malignant neoplasm of left ovary ♀ ☑

C78.6	Secondary malignant neoplasm of retroperitoneum and peritoneum
C79.61	Secondary malignant neoplasm of right ovary ♀ ☑
C79.62	Secondary malignant neoplasm of left ovary ♀ ☑
C7B.04	Secondary carcinoid tumors of peritoneum
D19.1	Benign neoplasm of mesothelial tissue of peritoneum
D27.0	Benign neoplasm of right ovary ♀ ☑
D27.1	Benign neoplasm of left ovary ♀ ☑
D39.11	Neoplasm of uncertain behavior of right ovary ♀ ☑
D39.12	Neoplasm of uncertain behavior of left ovary ♀ ☑
D48.4	Neoplasm of uncertain behavior of peritoneum
E28.2	Polycystic ovarian syndrome ♀
K66.8	Other specified disorders of peritoneum
N73.6	Female pelvic peritoneal adhesions (postinfective) ♀
N80.0	Endometriosis of uterus ♀
N80.1	Endometriosis of ovary ♀
N80.3	Endometriosis of pelvic peritoneum ♀
N80.8	Other endometriosis ♀
N83.01	Follicular cyst of right ovary ♀ ☑
N83.02	Follicular cyst of left ovary ♀ ☑
N83.11	Corpus luteum cyst of right ovary ♀ ☑
N83.12	Corpus luteum cyst of left ovary ♀ ☑
N83.291	Other ovarian cyst, right side ♀ ☑
N83.292	Other ovarian cyst, left side ♀ ☑
N83.8	Other noninflammatory disorders of ovary, fallopian tube and broad ligament ♀
N84.0	Polyp of corpus uteri ♀
N84.1	Polyp of cervix uteri ♀
N84.8	Polyp of other parts of female genital tract ♀
N85.01	Benign endometrial hyperplasia ♀
N85.02	Endometrial intraepithelial neoplasia [EIN] ♀
N94.4	Primary dysmenorrhea ♀
N94.5	Secondary dysmenorrhea ♀
N94.89	Other specified conditions associated with female genital organs and menstrual cycle ♀
N97.0	Female infertility associated with anovulation ♀
N97.1	Female infertility of tubal origin ♀
N97.2	Female infertility of uterine origin ♀
N97.8	Female infertility of other origin ♀
N99.83	Residual ovary syndrome ♀
Q50.4	Embryonic cyst of fallopian tube ♀
Q50.5	Embryonic cyst of broad ligament ♀

AMA: 58662 2019,Jul,6; 2018,Jan,8; 2017,Jan,8; 2017,Dec,14; 2016,Jan,13; 2015,Jan,16; 2014,Jan,11

Relative Value Units/Medicare Edits

Non-Facility RVU	Work	PE	MP	Total
58662	12.15	6.52	1.96	20.63
Facility RVU	**Work**	**PE**	**MP**	**Total**
58662	12.15	6.52	1.96	20.63

	FUD	Status	MUE	Modifiers				IOM Reference
58662	90	A	1(2)	51	N/A	62	80	None

* with documentation

Terms To Know

electrocautery. Division or cutting of tissue using high-frequency electrical current to produce heat, which destroys cells.

excision. Surgical removal of an organ or tissue.

fulguration. Destruction of living tissue by using sparks from a high-frequency electric current.

lesion. Area of damaged tissue that has lost continuity or function, due to disease or trauma.

peritoneal. Space between the lining of the abdominal wall, or parietal peritoneum, and the surface layer of the abdominal organs, or visceral peritoneum. It contains a thin, watery fluid that keeps the peritoneal surfaces moist.

viscera. Large interior organs enclosed within a cavity, generally referring to the abdominal organs.

58670-58671

58670   Laparoscopy, surgical; with fulguration of oviducts (with or without transection)

58671   with occlusion of oviducts by device (eg, band, clip, or Falope ring)

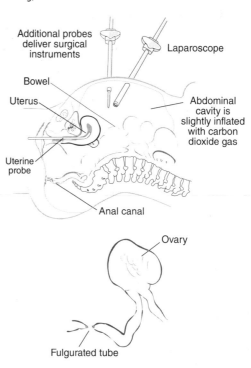

Additional probes deliver surgical instruments — Laparoscope — Bowel — Uterus — Abdominal cavity is slightly inflated with carbon dioxide gas — Uterine probe — Anal canal

Ovary — Fulgurated tube

Explanation

In both procedures, the physician uses a laparoscopic approach to perform electrical cautery destruction of an oviduct (the uterine tube), with or without complete cutting through the fallopian tubes (transection) or occlusion of the oviduct with the assistance of a fiberoptic laparoscope. The physician may insert an instrument through the vagina to grasp the cervix and manipulate the uterus during surgery. The physician makes a small incision just below the umbilicus through which a fiberoptic laparoscope is inserted. A second incision is made on the left or right side of the abdomen with additional instruments being placed through these incisions into the abdomen or pelvis. The physician manipulates the tools so that the pelvic organs can be observed, manipulated, and operated upon with the laparoscope. A third incision is typically made adjacent to the fallopian tubes. To fulgurate (58670) the fallopian tube, the physician inserts an electric cautery tool or a laser. The physician may cut the tubes and fulgurate or burn the ends. Additionally, the physician may transect (cut through) the fallopian tubes. To occlude (58671) the fallopian tubes, the physician places silicone rings or clips around the tubes through this incision. In both procedures, the abdomen is deflated, the trocars removed, and the incisions are closed with sutures.

Coding Tips

Surgical laparoscopy always includes diagnostic laparoscopy. For diagnostic laparoscopy only, see 49320. When either procedure is performed with another separately identifiable procedure, the highest dollar value code is listed as the primary procedure and subsequent procedures are appended with modifier 51. If a hysteroscopy is performed in conjunction with these procedures, report the appropriate hysteroscopy code. For occlusion of oviducts by vaginal or suprapubic approach, see 58615.

ICD-10-CM Diagnostic Codes

Z30.2   Encounter for sterilization

AMA: 58670 2019,Jul,6; 2018,Jan,8; 2017,Jan,8; 2016,Jan,13; 2015,Jan,16; 2014,Jan,11 **58671** 2019,Jul,6; 2018,Jan,8; 2017,Jan,8; 2016,Jan,13; 2015,Jan,16; 2014,Jan,11

Relative Value Units/Medicare Edits

Non-Facility RVU	Work	PE	MP	Total
58670	5.91	3.85	0.93	10.69
58671	5.91	3.84	0.92	10.67
Facility RVU	Work	PE	MP	Total
58670	5.91	3.85	0.93	10.69
58671	5.91	3.84	0.92	10.67

	FUD	Status	MUE	Modifiers				IOM Reference
58670	90	A	1(2)	51	N/A	62	N/A	None
58671	90	A	1(2)	51	N/A	62	N/A	

* with documentation

Terms To Know

electrocautery. Division or cutting of tissue using high-frequency electrical current to produce heat, which destroys cells.

fulguration. Destruction of living tissue by using sparks from a high-frequency electric current.

laparoscopy. Direct visualization of the peritoneal cavity, outer fallopian tubes, uterus, and ovaries utilizing a laparoscope, a thin, flexible fiberoptic tube.

multiparity. Condition of having had two or more pregnancies that resulted in viable fetuses; producing more than one fetus or offspring in the same gestation.

occlusion. Constriction, closure, or blockage of a passage.

transection. Transverse dissection; to cut across a long axis; cross section.

trocar. Cannula or a sharp pointed instrument used to puncture and aspirate fluid from cavities.

58672

58672   Laparoscopy, surgical; with fimbrioplasty

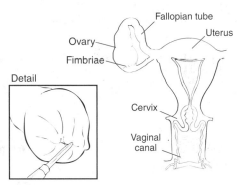

The occluded fimbriae are laparoscopically manipulated

Explanation

The physician performs a laparoscopic surgical repair of the ovarian fimbria (fingerlike processes on the distal part of the infundibulum of the uterine tube) with the assistance of a fiberoptic laparoscope. The physician may first insert an instrument through the vagina to grasp the cervix and manipulate the uterus during surgery. Next, the physician makes a small incision just below the umbilicus through which a fiberoptic laparoscope is inserted. A second incision is made on the left or right side of the abdomen with additional instruments being placed through these incisions into the abdomen or pelvis. The physician manipulates the tools so that the pelvic organs can be observed, manipulated and operated upon with the laparoscope. A third incision is typically made adjacent to the fallopian tubes. The physician performs surgical repair of the ovarian fimbria using instruments placed through the abdomen and pelvic trocars. The abdomen is deflated, the trocars removed and the incisions are closed with sutures.

Coding Tips

Report this code when the documentation specifies reconstruction of the fimbriae (hair-like projections) at the end of the tube. This code should not be used to report other tubal reconstruction. Surgical laparoscopy always includes diagnostic laparoscopy. For diagnostic laparoscopy only, see 49320. This is a unilateral procedure. If performed bilaterally, some payers require that the service be reported twice with modifier 50 appended to the second code while others require identification of the service only once with modifier 50 appended. Check with individual payers. Modifier 50 identifies a procedure performed identically on the opposite side of the body (mirror image). For open fimbrioplasty, see 58760. For tubotubal anastomosis, see 58750. For tubouterine implantation, see 58752. Because this procedure is usually not done out of medical necessity, the patient may be responsible for charges. Verify with the insurance carrier for coverage.

ICD-10-CM Diagnostic Codes

N70.11   Chronic salpingitis ♀

N70.13   Chronic salpingitis and oophoritis ♀

N97.1   Female infertility of tubal origin ♀

Q50.6   Other congenital malformations of fallopian tube and broad ligament ♀

AMA: 58672 2019,Jul,6; 2018,Jan,8; 2017,Jan,8; 2016,Jan,13; 2015,Jan,16; 2014,Jan,11

Oviduct

Relative Value Units/Medicare Edits

Non-Facility RVU	Work	PE	MP	Total
58672	12.91	6.38	2.02	21.31
Facility RVU	Work	PE	MP	Total
58672	12.91	6.38	2.02	21.31

	FUD	Status	MUE	Modifiers				IOM Reference
58672	90	A	1(2)	51	50	N/A	80	None

* with documentation

Terms To Know

-plasty. Indicates surgically formed or molded.

endometriosis. Aberrant uterine mucosal tissue appearing in areas of the pelvic cavity outside of its normal location, lining the uterus, and inflaming surrounding tissues often resulting in infertility or spontaneous abortion.

fimbria. Fringelike structure most often associated with the fallopian tube that helps move eggs toward the uterus.

laparoscopy. Direct visualization of the peritoneal cavity, outer fallopian tubes, uterus, and ovaries utilizing a laparoscope, a thin, flexible fiberoptic tube.

oophoritis. Inflammation or infection of one or both ovaries that can cause chronic pelvic pain, ectopic pregnancy, or sterilization.

salpingitis. Inflammation of the fallopian tubes, usually caused by a bacterial infection and occurring in conjunction with inflammation of the ovaries (oophoritis).

58673

58673 Laparoscopy, surgical; with salpingostomy (salpingoneostomy)

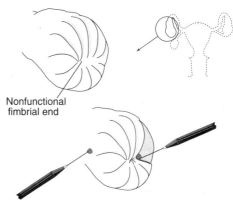

The physician uses laparoscopic microsurgery to remove mucosa, and expose tube opening, restoring patency

Nonfunctional fimbrial end

A new opening can be created in any location

Explanation

The physician performs a laparoscopic surgical restoration of the patency of the uterine tube damaged typically by infection, tumor or endometriosis. The physician may first insert an instrument through the vagina to grasp the cervix and manipulate the uterus during surgery. Next, the physician makes a small incision just below the umbilicus through which a fiberoptic laparoscope is inserted. A second incision is made on the left or right side of the abdomen with additional instruments being placed through these incisions into the abdomen or pelvis. The physician then manipulates the tools so that the pelvic organs can be observed, manipulated and operated upon with the laparoscope. A third incision is typically made adjacent to the fallopian tubes. The physician performs surgical restoration of the fallopian tube (salpingostomy) using instruments placed through the abdomen and pelvic trocars. The abdomen is then deflated, the trocars removed and the incisions are closed with sutures.

Coding Tips

Report 58673 for repair of the fimbrial end of the tube, not reconstruction of the fimbriae, which should be coded with 58672. Surgical laparoscopy always includes diagnostic laparoscopy. For diagnostic laparoscopy only, see 49320. This is a unilateral procedure. If performed bilaterally, some payers require that the service be reported twice with modifier 50 appended to the second code while others require identification of the service only once with modifier 50 appended. Check with individual payers. Modifier 50 identifies a procedure performed identically on the opposite side of the body (mirror image). For open salpingostomy, see 58770. Because this procedure is usually not done out of medical necessity, the patient may be responsible for charges. Verify with the insurance carrier for coverage.

ICD-10-CM Diagnostic Codes

N70.01	Acute salpingitis ♀
N70.03	Acute salpingitis and oophoritis ♀
N70.11	Chronic salpingitis ♀
N70.13	Chronic salpingitis and oophoritis ♀
N73.6	Female pelvic peritoneal adhesions (postinfective) ♀
N80.2	Endometriosis of fallopian tube ♀
N83.8	Other noninflammatory disorders of ovary, fallopian tube and broad ligament ♀

N97.1	Female infertility of tubal origin ♀
O00.101	Right tubal pregnancy without intrauterine pregnancy Ⓜ ♀
O00.102	Left tubal pregnancy without intrauterine pregnancy Ⓜ ♀
O00.111	Right tubal pregnancy with intrauterine pregnancy Ⓜ ♀
O00.112	Left tubal pregnancy with intrauterine pregnancy Ⓜ ♀
Q50.4	Embryonic cyst of fallopian tube ♀
S37.511A	Primary blast injury of fallopian tube, unilateral, initial encounter ♀
S37.512A	Primary blast injury of fallopian tube, bilateral, initial encounter ♀
S37.521A	Contusion of fallopian tube, unilateral, initial encounter ♀
S37.522A	Contusion of fallopian tube, bilateral, initial encounter ♀
S37.531A	Laceration of fallopian tube, unilateral, initial encounter ♀
S37.532A	Laceration of fallopian tube, bilateral, initial encounter ♀
S37.591A	Other injury of fallopian tube, unilateral, initial encounter ♀
S37.592A	Other injury of fallopian tube, bilateral, initial encounter ♀

AMA: **58673** 2019,Jul,6; 2018,Jan,8; 2017,Jan,8; 2016,Jan,13; 2015,Jan,16; 2014,Jan,11

Relative Value Units/Medicare Edits

Non-Facility RVU	Work	PE	MP	Total
58673	14.04	6.91	2.2	23.15
Facility RVU	**Work**	**PE**	**MP**	**Total**
58673	14.04	6.91	2.2	23.15

	FUD	Status	MUE	Modifiers				IOM Reference
58673	90	A	1(2)	51	50	N/A	80	None

* with documentation

Terms To Know

endometriosis. Aberrant uterine mucosal tissue appearing in areas of the pelvic cavity outside of its normal location, lining the uterus, and inflaming surrounding tissues often resulting in infertility or spontaneous abortion.

oophoritis. Inflammation or infection of one or both ovaries that can cause chronic pelvic pain, ectopic pregnancy, or sterilization.

patency. State of a tube-like structure or conduit being open and unobstructed.

salpingitis. Inflammation of the fallopian tubes, usually caused by a bacterial infection and occurring in conjunction with inflammation of the ovaries (oophoritis).

58700

58700   Salpingectomy, complete or partial, unilateral or bilateral (separate procedure)

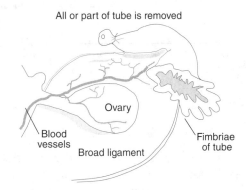

All or part of tube is removed

Ovary
Blood vessels
Broad ligament
Fimbriae of tube

Explanation

Through a small incision in the lower abdomen just above the pubic hairline, the physician removes part or all of the fallopian tube on one or both sides. The incision is closed by suturing.

Coding Tips

This separate procedure by definition is usually a component of a more complex service and is not identified separately. When performed alone or with other unrelated procedures/services it may be reported. If performed alone, list the code; if performed with other procedures/services, list the code and append modifier 59 or an X{EPSU} modifier. When 58700 is performed with another separately identifiable procedure, the highest dollar value code is listed as the primary procedure and subsequent procedures are appended with modifier 51. This code should only be used when completing an open invasive procedure, not when being performed through a laparoscopy; for laparoscopic salpingectomy, see 58661. If the ovary and fallopian tube are excised in an open approach, report 58720.

ICD-10-CM Diagnostic Codes

C57.01	Malignant neoplasm of right fallopian tube ♀ ☑
C57.02	Malignant neoplasm of left fallopian tube ♀ ☑
D07.39	Carcinoma in situ of other female genital organs ♀
D28.2	Benign neoplasm of uterine tubes and ligaments ♀
D39.8	Neoplasm of uncertain behavior of other specified female genital organs ♀
D49.59	Neoplasm of unspecified behavior of other genitourinary organ
N70.01	Acute salpingitis ♀
N70.03	Acute salpingitis and oophoritis ♀
N70.11	Chronic salpingitis ♀
N70.13	Chronic salpingitis and oophoritis ♀
N73.6	Female pelvic peritoneal adhesions (postinfective) ♀
N80.2	Endometriosis of fallopian tube ♀
N83.321	Acquired atrophy of right fallopian tube ♀ ☑
N83.322	Acquired atrophy of left fallopian tube ♀ ☑
N83.331	Acquired atrophy of right ovary and fallopian tube ♀ ☑
N83.332	Acquired atrophy of left ovary and fallopian tube ♀ ☑
N83.41	Prolapse and hernia of right ovary and fallopian tube ♀ ☑
N83.42	Prolapse and hernia of left ovary and fallopian tube ♀ ☑
N83.521	Torsion of right fallopian tube ♀ ☑
N83.522	Torsion of left fallopian tube ♀ ☑

N83.53	Torsion of ovary, ovarian pedicle and fallopian tube ♀
N83.6	Hematosalpinx ♀
N83.8	Other noninflammatory disorders of ovary, fallopian tube and broad ligament ♀
N84.8	Polyp of other parts of female genital tract ♀
O00.101	Right tubal pregnancy without intrauterine pregnancy Ⓜ ♀
O00.102	Left tubal pregnancy without intrauterine pregnancy Ⓜ ♀
O00.111	Right tubal pregnancy with intrauterine pregnancy Ⓜ ♀
O00.112	Left tubal pregnancy with intrauterine pregnancy Ⓜ ♀

AMA: 58700 2019,Jul,6; 2018,Sep,14; 2014,Jan,11

Relative Value Units/Medicare Edits

Non-Facility RVU	Work	PE	MP	Total
58700	12.95	7.7	2.25	22.9
Facility RVU	**Work**	**PE**	**MP**	**Total**
58700	12.95	7.7	2.25	22.9

	FUD	Status	MUE	Modifiers				IOM Reference
58700	90	A	1(2)	51	N/A	62*	80	None

* with documentation

Terms To Know

oophoritis. Inflammation or infection of one or both ovaries that can cause chronic pelvic pain, ectopic pregnancy, or sterilization.

prolapse. Falling, sliding, or sinking of an organ from its normal location in the body.

salpingitis. Inflammation of the fallopian tubes, usually caused by a bacterial infection and occurring in conjunction with inflammation of the ovaries (oophoritis).

torsion of ovary or fallopian tube. Twisting or rotation of the ovary or fallopian tube upon itself, so as to compromise or cut off the blood supply.

58720

58720	Salpingo-oophorectomy, complete or partial, unilateral or bilateral (separate procedure)

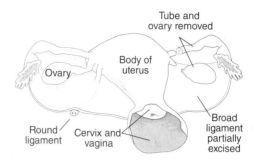

Tube and ovary removed
Body of uterus
Ovary
Round ligament
Cervix and vagina
Broad ligament partially excised

Oviduct

Explanation

Through a small incision in the abdomen just above the pubic hairline, the physician removes part or all of the ovary and part or all of its fallopian tube on one or both sides. The incision is closed by suturing.

Coding Tips

This code should only be used when completing an open invasive procedure, not when being performed through a laparoscopy; if performed through a laparoscopy, see 58661. This separate procedure by definition is usually a component of a more complex service and is not identified separately. When performed alone or with other unrelated procedures/services it may be reported. If performed alone, list the code; if performed with other procedures/services, list the code and append modifier 59 or an X{EPSU} modifier. When 58720 is performed with another separately identifiable procedure, the highest dollar value code is listed as the primary procedure and subsequent procedures are appended with modifier 51. If only the fallopian tubes are excised, report 58700.

ICD-10-CM Diagnostic Codes

C56.1	Malignant neoplasm of right ovary ♀ ☑
C56.2	Malignant neoplasm of left ovary ♀ ☑
C57.01	Malignant neoplasm of right fallopian tube ♀ ☑
C57.02	Malignant neoplasm of left fallopian tube ♀ ☑
C79.61	Secondary malignant neoplasm of right ovary ♀ ☑
C79.62	Secondary malignant neoplasm of left ovary ♀ ☑
D07.39	Carcinoma in situ of other female genital organs ♀
D27.0	Benign neoplasm of right ovary ♀ ☑
D27.1	Benign neoplasm of left ovary ♀ ☑
D28.2	Benign neoplasm of uterine tubes and ligaments ♀
D28.7	Benign neoplasm of other specified female genital organs ♀
D39.11	Neoplasm of uncertain behavior of right ovary ♀ ☑
D39.12	Neoplasm of uncertain behavior of left ovary ♀ ☑
D39.8	Neoplasm of uncertain behavior of other specified female genital organs ♀
D49.59	Neoplasm of unspecified behavior of other genitourinary organ
E28.2	Polycystic ovarian syndrome ♀
E28.8	Other ovarian dysfunction ♀
N70.01	Acute salpingitis ♀
N70.02	Acute oophoritis ♀
N70.03	Acute salpingitis and oophoritis ♀
N70.11	Chronic salpingitis ♀

N70.12	Chronic oophoritis ♀
N70.13	Chronic salpingitis and oophoritis ♀
N73.6	Female pelvic peritoneal adhesions (postinfective) ♀
N80.1	Endometriosis of ovary ♀
N80.2	Endometriosis of fallopian tube ♀
N80.3	Endometriosis of pelvic peritoneum ♀
N83.01	Follicular cyst of right ovary ♀ ☑
N83.02	Follicular cyst of left ovary ♀ ☑
N83.11	Corpus luteum cyst of right ovary ♀ ☑
N83.12	Corpus luteum cyst of left ovary ♀ ☑
N83.291	Other ovarian cyst, right side ♀ ☑
N83.292	Other ovarian cyst, left side ♀ ☑
N83.311	Acquired atrophy of right ovary ♀ ☑
N83.312	Acquired atrophy of left ovary ♀ ☑
N83.321	Acquired atrophy of right fallopian tube ♀ ☑
N83.322	Acquired atrophy of left fallopian tube ♀ ☑
N83.331	Acquired atrophy of right ovary and fallopian tube ♀ ☑
N83.332	Acquired atrophy of left ovary and fallopian tube ♀ ☑
N83.41	Prolapse and hernia of right ovary and fallopian tube ♀ ☑
N83.42	Prolapse and hernia of left ovary and fallopian tube ♀ ☑
N83.511	Torsion of right ovary and ovarian pedicle ♀ ☑
N83.512	Torsion of left ovary and ovarian pedicle ♀ ☑
N83.521	Torsion of right fallopian tube ♀ ☑
N83.522	Torsion of left fallopian tube ♀ ☑
N83.53	Torsion of ovary, ovarian pedicle and fallopian tube ♀
N83.6	Hematosalpinx ♀
N83.8	Other noninflammatory disorders of ovary, fallopian tube and broad ligament ♀
N84.8	Polyp of other parts of female genital tract ♀
O00.101	Right tubal pregnancy without intrauterine pregnancy Ⓜ ♀
O00.102	Left tubal pregnancy without intrauterine pregnancy Ⓜ ♀
O00.111	Right tubal pregnancy with intrauterine pregnancy Ⓜ ♀
O00.112	Left tubal pregnancy with intrauterine pregnancy Ⓜ ♀
O00.201	Right ovarian pregnancy without intrauterine pregnancy Ⓜ ♀
O00.202	Left ovarian pregnancy without intrauterine pregnancy Ⓜ ♀
O00.211	Right ovarian pregnancy with intrauterine pregnancy Ⓜ ♀
O00.212	Left ovarian pregnancy with intrauterine pregnancy Ⓜ ♀

AMA: **58720** 2019,Jul,6; 2018,Jan,8; 2017,Jan,8; 2016,Jan,13; 2015,Jan,16; 2014,Jan,11

Relative Value Units/Medicare Edits

Non-Facility RVU	Work	PE	MP	Total
58720	12.16	7.41	2.0	21.57
Facility RVU	Work	PE	MP	Total
58720	12.16	7.41	2.0	21.57

	FUD	Status	MUE	Modifiers				IOM Reference
58720	90	A	1(2)	51	N/A	62*	80	None

* with documentation

58740

58740   Lysis of adhesions (salpingolysis, ovariolysis)

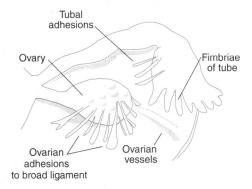

Explanation

The physician cuts free any fibrous tissue adhering to the ovaries or tubes through a small incision just above the pubic hairline.

Coding Tips

This procedure is performed to restore fertility and should not be coded for minor freeing of the tube and ovary as part of another procedure. For laparoscopic lysis of adhesions (salpingostomy, ovariolysis), see 58660. For laparoscopic fulguration or excision of lesions of the ovary, pelvic viscera, or peritoneal surface, see 58662. For excision or destruction of endometriomas via an open method, see 49203-49205 and 58957-58958.

ICD-10-CM Diagnostic Codes

N73.6	Female pelvic peritoneal adhesions (postinfective) ♀
N99.4	Postprocedural pelvic peritoneal adhesions
Q50.39	Other congenital malformation of ovary ♀

AMA: **58740** 2019,Jul,6; 2018,Jan,8; 2017,Jan,8; 2016,Jan,13; 2015,Jan,16; 2014,Jan,11

Relative Value Units/Medicare Edits

Non-Facility RVU	Work	PE	MP	Total
58740	14.9	8.48	2.58	25.96
Facility RVU	Work	PE	MP	Total
58740	14.9	8.48	2.58	25.96

	FUD	Status	MUE	Modifiers				IOM Reference
58740	90	A	1(2)	51	N/A	62*	80	None

* with documentation

Terms To Know

adhesion. Abnormal fibrous connection between two structures, soft tissue or bony structures, that may occur as the result of surgery, infection, or trauma.

fibrous tissue. Connective tissues.

lysis. Destruction, breakdown, dissolution, or decomposition of cells or substances by a specific catalyzing agent.

58750

58750 Tubotubal anastomosis

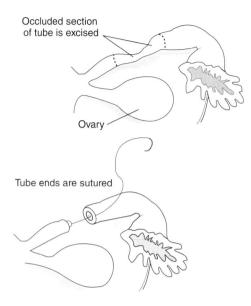

Occluded section
of tube is excised

Ovary

Tube ends are sutured

Explanation

Through a small incision just above the pubic hairline, the physician excises the closed or blocked portion of the tube and sutures the clean edges together. The procedure is generally performed microsurgically in order to do an accurate repair.

Coding Tips

This is usually an elective procedure to reverse prior sterilization. If performed to restore patency after a tubal pregnancy or after excision of a tubal lesion, submit a cover letter and operative report. This is a unilateral procedure. If performed bilaterally, some payers require that the service be reported twice with modifier 50 appended to the second code while others require identification of the service only once with modifier 50 appended. Check with individual payers. Modifier 50 identifies a procedure performed identically on the opposite side of the body (mirror image). Because this procedure is usually not done out of medical necessity, the patient may be responsible for charges. Verify with the insurance carrier for coverage.

ICD-10-CM Diagnostic Codes

N73.6	Female pelvic peritoneal adhesions (postinfective) ♀
N97.1	Female infertility of tubal origin ♀
Q50.6	Other congenital malformations of fallopian tube and broad ligament ♀
Z31.0	Encounter for reversal of previous sterilization

AMA: **58750** 2019,Jul,6; 2014,Jan,11

Relative Value Units/Medicare Edits

Non-Facility RVU	Work	PE	MP	Total
58750	15.64	8.26	2.46	26.36
Facility RVU	**Work**	**PE**	**MP**	**Total**
58750	15.64	8.26	2.46	26.36

	FUD	Status	MUE	Modifiers				IOM Reference
58750	90	A	1(2)	51	50	62*	80	None

* with documentation

Terms To Know

anastomosis. Surgically created connection between ducts, blood vessels, or bowel segments to allow flow from one to the other.

chronic. Persistent, continuing, or recurring.

occlusion. Constriction, closure, or blockage of a passage.

oophoritis. Inflammation or infection of one or both ovaries that can cause chronic pelvic pain, ectopic pregnancy, or sterilization.

peritonitis. Inflammation and infection within the peritoneal cavity, the space between the membrane lining the abdominopelvic walls and covering the internal organs.

salpingitis. Inflammation of the fallopian tubes, usually caused by a bacterial infection and occurring in conjunction with inflammation of the ovaries (oophoritis).

Oviduct

58752

58752   Tubouterine implantation

The physician excises a blocked section of
fallopian tube and reattaches the remaining
portion of the tube to the uterus

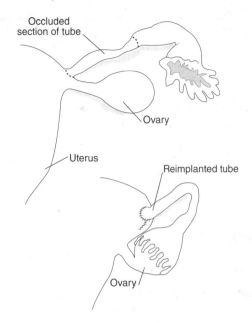

Explanation

Through a small incision just above the pubic hairline, the physician removes
a blocked portion of the tube near its junction with the uterus and reimplants
the tube into the uterus in the same place.

Coding Tips

This code should not be confused with 58750, tubotubal anastomosis, in which
a portion of the tube is excised and the two ends are sutured together. Report
this code when the procedure involves the tube and the uterus. This is a
unilateral procedure. If performed bilaterally, some payers require that the
service be reported twice with modifier 50 appended to the second code while
others require identification of the service only once with modifier 50
appended. Check with individual payers. Modifier 50 identifies a procedure
performed identically on the opposite side of the body (mirror image). Because
this procedure is usually not done out of medical necessity, the patient may
be responsible for charges. Verify with the insurance carrier for coverage.

ICD-10-CM Diagnostic Codes

D28.2	Benign neoplasm of uterine tubes and ligaments ♀
N70.01	Acute salpingitis ♀
N70.03	Acute salpingitis and oophoritis ♀
N70.11	Chronic salpingitis ♀
N70.13	Chronic salpingitis and oophoritis ♀
N73.6	Female pelvic peritoneal adhesions (postinfective) ♀
N83.8	Other noninflammatory disorders of ovary, fallopian tube and broad ligament ♀
N84.8	Polyp of other parts of female genital tract ♀
N97.1	Female infertility of tubal origin ♀
Q50.6	Other congenital malformations of fallopian tube and broad ligament ♀
Z31.0	Encounter for reversal of previous sterilization

AMA: **58752** 2019,Jul,6; 2014,Jan,11

Relative Value Units/Medicare Edits

Non-Facility RVU	Work	PE	MP	Total
58752	15.64	8.19	2.46	26.29
Facility RVU	**Work**	**PE**	**MP**	**Total**
58752	15.64	8.19	2.46	26.29

	FUD	Status	MUE	Modifiers				IOM Reference
58752	90	A	1(2)	51	50	N/A	80	None

* with documentation

Terms To Know

adhesion. Abnormal fibrous connection between two structures, soft tissue
or bony structures, that may occur as the result of surgery, infection, or trauma.

anomaly. Irregularity in the structure or position of an organ or tissue.

benign. Mild or nonmalignant in nature.

broad ligament. Fold of peritoneum extending from the side of the uterus
to the wall of the pelvis.

chronic. Persistent, continuing, or recurring.

congenital. Present at birth, occurring through heredity or an influence during
gestation up to the moment of birth.

neoplasm. New abnormal growth, tumor.

oophoritis. Inflammation or infection of one or both ovaries that can cause
chronic pelvic pain, ectopic pregnancy, or sterilization.

peritonitis. Inflammation and infection within the peritoneal cavity, the space
between the membrane lining the abdominopelvic walls and covering the
internal organs.

salpingitis. Inflammation of the fallopian tubes, usually caused by a bacterial
infection and occurring in conjunction with inflammation of the ovaries
(oophoritis).

58760

58760 Fimbrioplasty

The physician reconstructs
occluded fimbriae to restore patency

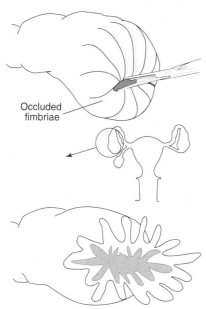

Occluded
fimbriae

Procedure may involve separating occluded fimbriae

Explanation

Through a small incision just above the pubic hairline, the physician reconstructs the existing fimbriae in a partially or totally obstructed (occluded) or closed off oviduct. Fimbriae are the hairlike fringes at the end of the fallopian tubes. Depending on the nature of the blockage, the physician may separate the fimbriae by gentle dilation or by electrosurgical dissection. The procedure is generally performed microsurgically in order to do an accurate repair.

Coding Tips

Report this code when the documentation specifies reconstruction of the fimbriae (hair-like projections) at the end of the tube. This code should not be used to report other tubal reconstruction. This is a unilateral procedure. If performed bilaterally, some payers require that the service be reported twice with modifier 50 appended to the second code while others require identification of the service only once with modifier 50 appended. Check with individual payers. Modifier 50 identifies a procedure performed identically on the opposite side of the body (mirror image). If significant additional time and effort is documented, append modifier 22 and submit a cover letter and operative report. For laparoscopic fimbrioplasty, see 58672. For tubotubal anastomosis, see 58750. For tubouterine implantation, see 58752. Because this procedure is usually not done out of medical necessity, the patient may be responsible for charges. Verify with the insurance carrier for coverage.

ICD-10-CM Diagnostic Codes

N70.11	Chronic salpingitis ♀
N70.13	Chronic salpingitis and oophoritis ♀
N97.1	Female infertility of tubal origin ♀
Q50.6	Other congenital malformations of fallopian tube and broad ligament ♀

AMA: 58760 2019,Jul,6; 2018,Jan,8; 2017,Jan,8; 2016,Jan,13; 2015,Jan,16; 2014,Jan,11

Relative Value Units/Medicare Edits

Non-Facility RVU	Work	PE	MP	Total
58760	13.93	7.62	2.19	23.74
Facility RVU	**Work**	**PE**	**MP**	**Total**
58760	13.93	7.62	2.19	23.74

	FUD	Status	MUE	Modifiers				IOM Reference
58760	90	A	1(2)	51	50	62*	80	None

* with documentation

Terms To Know

anomaly. Irregularity in the structure or position of an organ or tissue.

chronic. Persistent, continuing, or recurring.

congenital. Present at birth, occurring through heredity or an influence during gestation up to the moment of birth.

infertility. Inability to conceive for at least one year with regular intercourse.

oophoritis. Inflammation or infection of one or both ovaries that can cause chronic pelvic pain, ectopic pregnancy, or sterilization.

salpingitis. Inflammation of the fallopian tubes, usually caused by a bacterial infection and occurring in conjunction with inflammation of the ovaries (oophoritis).

58770

58770 Salpingostomy (salpingoneostomy)

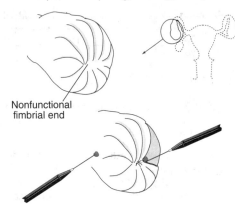

The physician uses laparoscopic microsurgery to remove mucosa, and expose tube opening, restoring patency

Nonfunctional fimbrial end

A new opening can be created in any location

Explanation

Through a small incision just above the pubic hairline, the physician creates a new opening in the fallopian tube where the fimbrial end has been closed by inflammation, infection, or injury. The procedure is generally performed microsurgically in order to do an accurate repair.

Coding Tips

Report 58770 for repair of the fimbrial end of the tube, not reconstruction of the fimbriae, which should be coded with 58760. This is a unilateral procedure. If performed bilaterally, some payers require that the service be reported twice with modifier 50 appended to the second code while others require identification of the service only once with modifier 50 appended. Check with individual payers. Modifier 50 identifies a procedure performed identically on the opposite side of the body (mirror image). For laparoscopic salpingostomy, see 58673. For tubotubal anastomosis, see 58750. For tubouterine implantation, see 58752. Because this procedure is usually not done out of medical necessity, the patient may be responsible for charges. Verify with the insurance carrier for coverage.

ICD-10-CM Diagnostic Codes

N70.01	Acute salpingitis ♀
N70.03	Acute salpingitis and oophoritis ♀
N70.11	Chronic salpingitis ♀
N70.13	Chronic salpingitis and oophoritis ♀
N73.6	Female pelvic peritoneal adhesions (postinfective) ♀
N80.2	Endometriosis of fallopian tube ♀
N83.8	Other noninflammatory disorders of ovary, fallopian tube and broad ligament ♀
N97.1	Female infertility of tubal origin ♀
O00.101	Right tubal pregnancy without intrauterine pregnancy Ⓜ ♀
O00.102	Left tubal pregnancy without intrauterine pregnancy Ⓜ ♀
O00.111	Right tubal pregnancy with intrauterine pregnancy Ⓜ ♀
O00.112	Left tubal pregnancy with intrauterine pregnancy Ⓜ ♀
Q50.4	Embryonic cyst of fallopian tube ♀
S37.511A	Primary blast injury of fallopian tube, unilateral, initial encounter ♀
S37.512A	Primary blast injury of fallopian tube, bilateral, initial encounter ♀
S37.521A	Contusion of fallopian tube, unilateral, initial encounter ♀
S37.522A	Contusion of fallopian tube, bilateral, initial encounter ♀
S37.531A	Laceration of fallopian tube, unilateral, initial encounter ♀
S37.532A	Laceration of fallopian tube, bilateral, initial encounter ♀
S37.591A	Other injury of fallopian tube, unilateral, initial encounter ♀
S37.592A	Other injury of fallopian tube, bilateral, initial encounter ♀

AMA: 58770 2019,Jul,6; 2018,Jan,8; 2017,Jan,8; 2016,Jan,13; 2015,Jan,16; 2014,Jan,11

Relative Value Units/Medicare Edits

Non-Facility RVU	Work	PE	MP	Total
58770	14.77	7.86˙	2.34	24.97
Facility RVU	**Work**	**PE**	**MP**	**Total**
58770	14.77	7.86	2.34	24.97

	FUD	Status	MUE	Modifiers				IOM Reference
58770	90	A	1(2)	51	50	N/A	80	None

* with documentation

Terms To Know

cellulitis. Infection of the skin and subcutaneous tissues, most often caused by Staphylococcus or Streptococcus bacteria secondary to a cutaneous lesion. Progression of the inflammation may lead to abscess and tissue death, or even systemic infection-like bacteremia.

endometriosis. Aberrant uterine mucosal tissue appearing in areas of the pelvic cavity outside of its normal location, lining the uterus, and inflaming surrounding tissues often resulting in infertility or spontaneous abortion.

oophoritis. Inflammation or infection of one or both ovaries that can cause chronic pelvic pain, ectopic pregnancy, or sterilization.

salpingitis. Inflammation of the fallopian tubes, usually caused by a bacterial infection and occurring in conjunction with inflammation of the ovaries (oophoritis).

Coding Companion for Ob/Gyn

58800-58805

58800 Drainage of ovarian cyst(s), unilateral or bilateral (separate procedure); vaginal approach

58805 abdominal approach

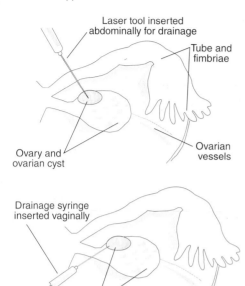

Laser tool inserted abdominally for drainage

Tube and fimbriae

Ovarian vessels

Ovary and ovarian cyst

Drainage syringe inserted vaginally

Ovary and ovarian cyst

Explanation

The physician drains a cyst or cysts on one or both ovaries through an incision in the vagina in 58800 and through an incision in the abdominal wall just above the pubic hairline in 58805. A cyst is a sac containing fluid or semisolid material. The cyst is ruptured with a surgical instrument, electrocautery, or a laser, and the fluid is removed.

Coding Tips

These separate procedures by definition are usually a component of a more complex service and are not identified separately. When performed alone or with other unrelated procedures/services they may be reported. If performed alone, list the code; if performed with other procedures/services, list the code and append modifier 59 or an X{EPSU} modifier. For drainage of an ovarian abscess vaginally, see 58820; abdominally, see 58822.

ICD-10-CM Diagnostic Codes

D27.0	Benign neoplasm of right ovary ♀ ☑
D27.1	Benign neoplasm of left ovary ♀ ☑
D39.11	Neoplasm of uncertain behavior of right ovary ♀ ☑
D39.12	Neoplasm of uncertain behavior of left ovary ♀ ☑
E28.2	Polycystic ovarian syndrome ♀
N83.01	Follicular cyst of right ovary ♀ ☑
N83.02	Follicular cyst of left ovary ♀ ☑
N83.11	Corpus luteum cyst of right ovary ♀ ☑
N83.12	Corpus luteum cyst of left ovary ♀ ☑
N83.291	Other ovarian cyst, right side ♀ ☑
N83.292	Other ovarian cyst, left side ♀ ☑
Q50.1	Developmental ovarian cyst ♀

AMA: **58800** 2019,Jul,6; 2014,Jan,11 **58805** 2019,Jul,6; 2014,Jan,11

Relative Value Units/Medicare Edits

Non-Facility RVU	Work	PE	MP	Total
58800	4.62	4.61	0.73	9.96
58805	6.42	4.68	1.01	12.11
Facility RVU	**Work**	**PE**	**MP**	**Total**
58800	4.62	3.57	0.73	8.92
58805	6.42	4.68	1.01	12.11

	FUD	Status	MUE	Modifiers			IOM Reference
58800	90	A	1(2)	51	N/A	N/A	N/A	None
58805	90	A	1(2)	51	N/A	62*	80	

* with documentation

Terms To Know

benign. Mild or nonmalignant in nature.

corpus luteum cyst or hematoma. Fluid-filled cyst or pocket of blood formed on the ovary at the site where a follicle has discharged its egg.

electrocautery. Division or cutting of tissue using high-frequency electrical current to produce heat, which destroys cells.

follicular cyst. Common type of ovarian cyst related to the menstrual cycle that occurs when the follicle in which the ovum develops does not rupture and expel the egg. Follicular cysts normally disappear within two or three menstrual cycles and are usually benign.

neoplasm. New abnormal growth, tumor.

polycystic. Multiple cysts.

Ovary

58820-58822

58820 Drainage of ovarian abscess; vaginal approach, open
58822   abdominal approach

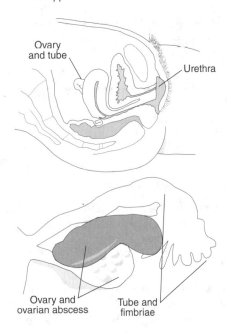

Ovary and tube

Urethra

Ovary and ovarian abscess

Tube and fimbriae

Explanation

The physician drains an abscess (infection) on the ovary through an incision in the vagina in 58820 and through a small abdominal incision just above the pubic hairline in 58822. The abscess is drained, cleaned out, and irrigated with antibiotics. Temporary catheters and tubes are often left in place to help drainage.

Coding Tips

These are unilateral procedures. If performed bilaterally, some payers require that the service be reported twice with modifier 50 appended to the second code while others require identification of the service only once with modifier 50 appended. Check with individual payers. Modifier 50 identifies a procedure performed identically on the opposite side of the body (mirror image). For drainage of an ovarian cyst, vaginal approach, see 58800; abdominal approach, see 58805. For transrectal or transvaginal image-guided drainage of a peritoneal or retroperitoneal fluid collection via catheter, see 49407.

ICD-10-CM Diagnostic Codes

N70.02	Acute oophoritis ♀
N70.03	Acute salpingitis and oophoritis ♀
N70.12	Chronic oophoritis ♀
N70.13	Chronic salpingitis and oophoritis ♀

AMA: **58820** 2019,Jul,6; 2014,Jan,11 **58822** 2019,Jul,6; 2014,Jan,11

Relative Value Units/Medicare Edits

Non-Facility RVU	Work	PE	MP	Total
58820	4.7	4.03	0.74	9.47
58822	11.81	6.91	1.86	20.58
Facility RVU	**Work**	**PE**	**MP**	**Total**
58820	4.7	4.03	0.74	9.47
58822	11.81	6.91	1.86	20.58

	FUD	Status	MUE	Modifiers				IOM Reference
58820	90	A	1(3)	51	50	N/A	80	None
58822	90	A	1(3)	51	50	62*	80	

* with documentation

Terms To Know

abscess. Circumscribed collection of pus resulting from bacteria, frequently associated with swelling and other signs of inflammation.

acute. Sudden, severe. Documentation and reporting of an acute condition is important to establishing medical necessity.

aspiration. Drawing fluid out by suction.

cellulitis. Infection of the skin and subcutaneous tissues, most often caused by Staphylococcus or Streptococcus bacteria secondary to a cutaneous lesion. Progression of the inflammation may lead to abscess and tissue death, or even systemic infection-like bacteremia.

chronic. Persistent, continuing, or recurring.

incision and drainage. Cutting open body tissue for the removal of tissue fluids or infected discharge from a wound or cavity.

irrigation. To wash out or cleanse a body cavity, wound, or tissue with water or other fluid.

oophoritis. Inflammation or infection of one or both ovaries that can cause chronic pelvic pain, ectopic pregnancy, or sterilization.

parametritis. Inflammation and infection of the tissue in the structures around the uterus.

salpingitis. Inflammation of the fallopian tubes, usually caused by a bacterial infection and occurring in conjunction with inflammation of the ovaries (oophoritis).

seroma. Swelling caused by the collection of serum, or clear fluid, in the tissues.

58825

58825 Transposition, ovary(s)

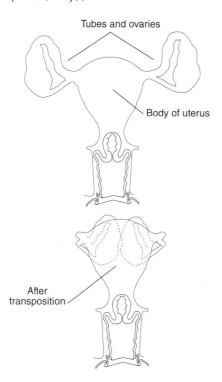

Tubes and ovaries

Body of uterus

After transposition

Explanation

The ovaries are placed behind the uterus and sutured in place prior to radiation therapy of the pelvis. The uterus acts as a shield protecting the ovaries from the radiation. The procedure is done through a small abdominal incision just above the pubic hairline.

Coding Tips

This is a bilateral code and is reported once even if the procedure is performed on both sides. When 58825 is performed with another separately identifiable procedure, the highest dollar value code is listed as the primary procedure and subsequent procedures are appended with modifier 51.

ICD-10-CM Diagnostic Codes

This code is associated with general malignancies and associated codes are too numerous to list here. Refer to the ICD-10-CM Neoplasm section.

AMA: **58825** 2019,Jul,6; 2014,Jan,11

Relative Value Units/Medicare Edits

Non-Facility RVU	Work	PE	MP	Total
58825	11.78	6.8	1.86	20.44
Facility RVU	Work	PE	MP	Total
58825	11.78	6.8	1.86	20.44

	FUD	Status	MUE	Modifiers				IOM Reference
58825	90	A	1(2)	51	N/A	62*	80	None

* with documentation

58900

58900 Biopsy of ovary, unilateral or bilateral (separate procedure)

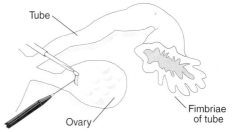

Tube

Fimbriae of tube

Ovary

Tissue sample removed for analysis

Explanation

The physician takes a tissue sample from one or both ovaries for diagnosis. This procedure may be done through the vagina or abdominally through a small incision just above the pubic hairline.

Coding Tips

This separate procedure by definition is usually a component of a more complex service and is not identified separately. When performed alone or with other unrelated procedures/services it may be reported. If performed alone, list the code; if performed with other procedures/services, list the code and append modifier 59 or an X{EPSU} modifier. Laparoscopic ovarian or fallopian tube biopsy is reported with 49321. For wedge resection or bisection of the ovary, see 58920. For an oophorectomy, partial or complete, see 58940.

ICD-10-CM Diagnostic Codes

C56.1	Malignant neoplasm of right ovary ♀ ☑
C56.2	Malignant neoplasm of left ovary ♀ ☑
C79.61	Secondary malignant neoplasm of right ovary ♀ ☑
C79.62	Secondary malignant neoplasm of left ovary ♀ ☑
D07.39	Carcinoma in situ of other female genital organs ♀
D27.0	Benign neoplasm of right ovary ♀ ☑
D27.1	Benign neoplasm of left ovary ♀ ☑
D39.11	Neoplasm of uncertain behavior of right ovary ♀ ☑
D39.12	Neoplasm of uncertain behavior of left ovary ♀ ☑
D49.59	Neoplasm of unspecified behavior of other genitourinary organ
E28.2	Polycystic ovarian syndrome ♀
E28.8	Other ovarian dysfunction ♀
E89.40	Asymptomatic postprocedural ovarian failure ♀
E89.41	Symptomatic postprocedural ovarian failure ♀
N80.1	Endometriosis of ovary ♀
N83.01	Follicular cyst of right ovary ♀ ☑
N83.02	Follicular cyst of left ovary ♀ ☑
N83.11	Corpus luteum cyst of right ovary ♀ ☑
N83.12	Corpus luteum cyst of left ovary ♀ ☑
N83.291	Other ovarian cyst, right side ♀ ☑
N83.292	Other ovarian cyst, left side ♀ ☑
N83.8	Other noninflammatory disorders of ovary, fallopian tube and broad ligament ♀
N99.83	Residual ovary syndrome ♀

AMA: **58900** 2019,Jul,6; 2018,Jan,8; 2017,Jan,8; 2016,Jan,13; 2015,Jan,16; 2014,Jan,11

Relative Value Units/Medicare Edits

Non-Facility RVU	Work	PE	MP	Total
58900	· 6.59	4.75	1.04	12.38
Facility RVU	Work	PE	MP	Total
58900	6.59	4.75	1.04	12.38

	FUD	Status	MUE	Modifiers				IOM Reference
58900	90	A	1(2)	51	N/A	62*	80	None

* with documentation

Terms To Know

biopsy. Tissue or fluid removed for diagnostic purposes through analysis of the cells in the biopsy material.

separate procedures. Services commonly carried out as a fundamental part of a total service and, as such, do not usually warrant separate identification. These services are identified in CPT with the parenthetical phrase (separate procedure) at the end of the description and are payable only when performed alone.

tissue. Group of similar cells with a similar function that form definite structures and organs. Tissue types include epithelial tissue, muscle tissue, connective tissue, and nervous tissue.

58920

58920   Wedge resection or bisection of ovary, unilateral or bilateral

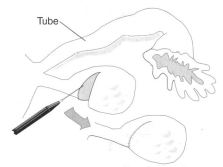

Tube

Section of ovary is removed and the excision sutured

Explanation

Through a small abdominal incision just above the pubic hairline, the physician takes a pie-shaped section or half of one or both of the ovaries to reduce the size and repairs each ovary with sutures.

Coding Tips

The documentation should reflect that a wedge or half of the ovary was removed, not simply a sample biopsy taken. This procedure can be performed unilaterally or bilaterally and is only reported once. For an open oophorectomy, partial or complete, see 58940. For laparoscopic oophorectomy, see 58661.

ICD-10-CM Diagnostic Codes

D27.0	Benign neoplasm of right ovary ♀ ☑
D27.1	Benign neoplasm of left ovary ♀ ☑
D39.11	Neoplasm of uncertain behavior of right ovary ♀ ☑
D39.12	Neoplasm of uncertain behavior of left ovary ♀ ☑
E28.2	Polycystic ovarian syndrome ♀
N83.01	Follicular cyst of right ovary ♀ ☑
N83.02	Follicular cyst of left ovary ♀ ☑
N83.11	Corpus luteum cyst of right ovary ♀ ☑
N83.12	Corpus luteum cyst of left ovary ♀ ☑
N83.291	Other ovarian cyst, right side ♀ ☑
N83.292	Other ovarian cyst, left side ♀ ☑

AMA: 58920 2019,Jul,6; 2014,Jan,11

Relative Value Units/Medicare Edits

Non-Facility RVU	Work	PE	MP	Total
58920	11.95	6.77	1.89	20.61
Facility RVU	Work	PE	MP	Total
58920	11.95	6.77	1.89	20.61

	FUD	Status	MUE	Modifiers				IOM Reference
58920	90	A	1(2)	51	N/A	62*	80	None

* with documentation

Terms To Know

wedge excision. Surgical removal of a section of tissue that is thick at one edge and tapers to a thin edge.

Ovary

58925

58925 Ovarian cystectomy, unilateral or bilateral

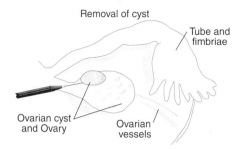

Removal of cyst

Tube and fimbriae

Ovarian cyst and Ovary

Ovarian vessels

Explanation

Through a small abdominal incision just above the pubic hairline, the physician removes a cyst or cysts on one or both of the ovaries.

Coding Tips

This procedure can be performed unilaterally or bilaterally and is only reported once. For an open oophorectomy, partial or complete, see 58940. For laparoscopic oophorectomy, see 58661. For drainage of an ovarian cyst via a vaginal approach, see 58800; abdominal approach, see 58805.

ICD-10-CM Diagnostic Codes

D27.0	Benign neoplasm of right ovary ♀ ☑
D27.1	Benign neoplasm of left ovary ♀ ☑
D39.11	Neoplasm of uncertain behavior of right ovary ♀ ☑
D39.12	Neoplasm of uncertain behavior of left ovary ♀ ☑
E28.2	Polycystic ovarian syndrome ♀
N83.01	Follicular cyst of right ovary ♀ ☑
N83.02	Follicular cyst of left ovary ♀ ☑
N83.11	Corpus luteum cyst of right ovary ♀ ☑
N83.12	Corpus luteum cyst of left ovary ♀ ☑
N83.291	Other ovarian cyst, right side ♀ ☑
N83.292	Other ovarian cyst, left side ♀ ☑
Q50.1	Developmental ovarian cyst ♀

AMA: 58925 2019,Jul,6; 2014,Jan,11

Relative Value Units/Medicare Edits

Non-Facility RVU	Work	PE	MP	Total
58925	12.43	7.38	2.17	21.98
Facility RVU	**Work**	**PE**	**MP**	**Total**
58925	12.43	7.38	2.17	21.98

	FUD	Status	MUE	Modifiers				IOM Reference
58925	90	A	1(3)	51	N/A	62*	80	None

* with documentation

Terms To Know

follicular cyst. Common type of ovarian cyst related to the menstrual cycle that occurs when the follicle in which the ovum develops does not rupture and expel the egg. Follicular cysts normally disappear within two or three menstrual cycles and are usually benign.

58940

58940 Oophorectomy, partial or total, unilateral or bilateral;

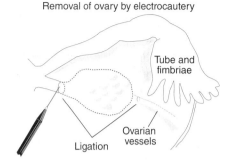

Removal of ovary by electrocautery

Tube and fimbriae

Ovarian vessels

Ligation

Explanation

Through a small abdominal incision just above the top of the pubic hairline, the physician removes part or all of one or both of the ovaries.

Coding Tips

This code should be used when completing an open invasive procedure. If performed through a laparoscope, see 58661. This can be performed unilaterally or bilaterally and is only reported once. When 58940 is performed with another separately identifiable procedure, the highest dollar value code is listed as the primary procedure and subsequent procedures are appended with modifier 51. For excision of the ovaries and fallopian tubes, see 58720. For an oophorectomy completed because of ovarian malignancy, with lymph node biopsies, see 58943.

ICD-10-CM Diagnostic Codes

C56.1	Malignant neoplasm of right ovary ♀ ☑
C56.2	Malignant neoplasm of left ovary ♀ ☑
C79.61	Secondary malignant neoplasm of right ovary ♀ ☑
C79.62	Secondary malignant neoplasm of left ovary ♀ ☑
D07.39	Carcinoma in situ of other female genital organs ♀
D27.0	Benign neoplasm of right ovary ♀ ☑
D27.1	Benign neoplasm of left ovary ♀ ☑
D39.11	Neoplasm of uncertain behavior of right ovary ♀ ☑
D39.12	Neoplasm of uncertain behavior of left ovary ♀ ☑
D49.59	Neoplasm of unspecified behavior of other genitourinary organ ♀
E28.2	Polycystic ovarian syndrome ♀
E28.8	Other ovarian dysfunction ♀
N70.02	Acute oophoritis ♀
N70.03	Acute salpingitis and oophoritis ♀
N70.12	Chronic oophoritis ♀
N70.13	Chronic salpingitis and oophoritis ♀
N73.6	Female pelvic peritoneal adhesions (postinfective) ♀
N80.1	Endometriosis of ovary ♀
N83.01	Follicular cyst of right ovary ♀ ☑
N83.02	Follicular cyst of left ovary ♀ ☑
N83.11	Corpus luteum cyst of right ovary ♀ ☑
N83.12	Corpus luteum cyst of left ovary ♀ ☑
N83.291	Other ovarian cyst, right side ♀ ☑
N83.292	Other ovarian cyst, left side ♀ ☑
N83.511	Torsion of right ovary and ovarian pedicle ♀ ☑
N83.512	Torsion of left ovary and ovarian pedicle ♀ ☑

N83.53	Torsion of ovary, ovarian pedicle and fallopian tube ♀
N83.8	Other noninflammatory disorders of ovary, fallopian tube and broad ligament ♀
N84.8	Polyp of other parts of female genital tract ♀
N99.83	Residual ovary syndrome ♀
O00.201	Right ovarian pregnancy without intrauterine pregnancy Ⓜ ♀
O00.202	Left ovarian pregnancy without intrauterine pregnancy Ⓜ ♀
O00.211	Right ovarian pregnancy with intrauterine pregnancy Ⓜ ♀
O00.212	Left ovarian pregnancy with intrauterine pregnancy Ⓜ ♀
Q50.1	Developmental ovarian cyst ♀
Q50.2	Congenital torsion of ovary ♀

AMA: 58940 2019,Jul,6; 2018,Jan,8; 2017,Jan,8; 2016,Jan,13; 2015,Jan,16; 2014,Jan,11

Relative Value Units/Medicare Edits

Non-Facility RVU	Work	PE	MP	Total
58940	8.22	5.96	1.47	15.65
Facility RVU	**Work**	**PE**	**MP**	**Total**
58940	8.22	5.96	1.47	15.65

	FUD	Status	MUE	Modifiers				IOM Reference
58940	90	A	1(2)	51	N/A	62*	80	100-03,230.3

* with documentation

Terms To Know

benign. Mild or nonmalignant in nature.

corpus luteum cyst. Common type of ovarian cyst that occurs when the corpus luteum fails to dissolve after the ovum is released and not fertilized. The cyst normally goes away in a few weeks but may enlarge to more than 10 cm and require surgical intervention.

malignant. Any condition tending to progress toward death, specifically an invasive tumor with a loss of cellular differentiation that has the ability to spread or metastasize to other body areas.

oophorectomy. Surgical removal of all or part of one or both ovaries, either as open procedure or laparoscopically. Menstruation and childbearing ability continues when one ovary is removed.

polycystic ovarian syndrome. Common hormonal disorder among women of reproductive age that involves enlarged ovaries with numerous small cysts located along the outer ovarian edge.

torsion of ovary or fallopian tube. Twisting or rotation of the ovary or fallopian tube upon itself, so as to compromise or cut off the blood supply.

58943

58943	Oophorectomy, partial or total, unilateral or bilateral; for ovarian, tubal or primary peritoneal malignancy, with para-aortic and pelvic lymph node biopsies, peritoneal washings, peritoneal biopsies, diaphragmatic assessments, with or without salpingectomy(s), with or without omentectomy

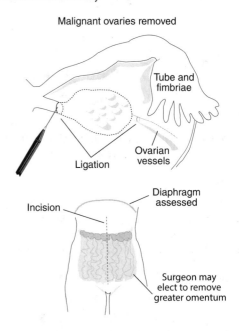

Malignant ovaries removed

Explanation

Through an abdominal incision extending from the top of the pubic hairline to the rib cage, the physician removes part or all of one or both ovaries depending on the extent of the malignancy. The physician takes a sampling of the lymph nodes surrounding the lower aorta within the pelvis and flushes the peritoneum, which is the lining of the abdominal cavity, with saline. The saline solution is suctioned from the peritoneum for separately reportable examination. Multiple tissue samples are excised. The physician also examines and takes tissue samples of the diaphragm. The physician may elect to remove one or both fallopian tubes and the omentum. The abdominal incision is closed with layered sutures.

Coding Tips

For a radical resection of ovarian malignancy with bilateral salpingo-oophorectomy and omentectomy, see 58950. When 58943 is performed with another separately identifiable procedure, the highest dollar value code is listed as the primary procedure and subsequent procedures are appended with modifier 51.

ICD-10-CM Diagnostic Codes

C48.1	Malignant neoplasm of specified parts of peritoneum
C48.8	Malignant neoplasm of overlapping sites of retroperitoneum and peritoneum
C56.1	Malignant neoplasm of right ovary ♀ ☑
C56.2	Malignant neoplasm of left ovary ♀ ☑
C57.01	Malignant neoplasm of right fallopian tube ♀ ☑
C57.02	Malignant neoplasm of left fallopian tube ♀ ☑
C77.2	Secondary and unspecified malignant neoplasm of intra-abdominal lymph nodes

C77.5	Secondary and unspecified malignant neoplasm of intrapelvic lymph nodes
C79.61	Secondary malignant neoplasm of right ovary ♀ ☑
C79.62	Secondary malignant neoplasm of left ovary ♀ ☑
C79.82	Secondary malignant neoplasm of genital organs

AMA: 58943 2019,Jul,6; 2014,Jan,11

Relative Value Units/Medicare Edits

Non-Facility RVU	Work	PE	MP	Total
58943	19.52	11.06	3.1	33.68
Facility RVU	**Work**	**PE**	**MP**	**Total**
58943	19.52	11.06	3.1	33.68

	FUD	Status	MUE	Modifiers				IOM Reference
58943	90	A	1(2)	51	N/A	62*	80	None

* with documentation

Terms To Know

biopsy. Tissue or fluid removed for diagnostic purposes through analysis of the cells in the biopsy material.

lymph nodes. Bean-shaped structures along the lymphatic vessels that intercept and destroy foreign materials in the tissue and bloodstream.

malignant neoplasm. Any cancerous tumor or lesion exhibiting uncontrolled tissue growth that can progressively invade other parts of the body with its disease-generating cells.

omentum. Fold of peritoneal tissue suspended between the stomach and neighboring visceral organs of the abdominal cavity.

secondary. Second in order of occurrence or importance, or appearing during the course of another disease or condition.

58950

| 58950 | Resection (initial) of ovarian, tubal or primary peritoneal malignancy with bilateral salpingo-oophorectomy and omentectomy; |

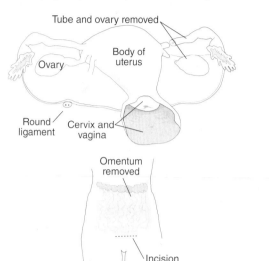

An ovarian, tubal, or primary peritoneal malignancy is removed with bilateral salpingo-oophorectomy and omentectomy

Explanation

The physician performs the initial resection of an ovarian, tubal, or primary peritoneal malignancy. Through a full abdominal incision, the physician removes both tubes, both ovaries, and the omentum, which is a membrane of lymph nodes, blood vessels, and fat that forms a protective layer extending from the stomach to the transverse colon. The abdominal incision is closed with layered sutures.

Coding Tips

The documentation or pathology report should verify a total removal of both tubes, ovaries, and the omentum due to malignancy. This is a bilateral code and is reported once even if the procedure is performed on both sides. If performed with a total abdominal hysterectomy, see 58951. If performed with radical dissection and debulking, see 58952.

ICD-10-CM Diagnostic Codes

C48.1	Malignant neoplasm of specified parts of peritoneum
C48.8	Malignant neoplasm of overlapping sites of retroperitoneum and peritoneum
C56.1	Malignant neoplasm of right ovary ♀ ☑
C56.2	Malignant neoplasm of left ovary ♀ ☑
C57.01	Malignant neoplasm of right fallopian tube ♀ ☑
C57.02	Malignant neoplasm of left fallopian tube ♀ ☑
C78.6	Secondary malignant neoplasm of retroperitoneum and peritoneum
C79.61	Secondary malignant neoplasm of right ovary ♀ ☑
C79.62	Secondary malignant neoplasm of left ovary ♀ ☑
C79.82	Secondary malignant neoplasm of genital organs

AMA: 58950 2019,Jul,6; 2014,Jan,11

Relative Value Units/Medicare Edits

Non-Facility RVU	Work	PE	MP	Total
58950	18.37	11.38	2.93	32.68
Facility RVU	Work	PE	MP	Total
58950	18.37	11.38	2.93	32.68

	FUD	Status	MUE	Modifiers				IOM Reference
58950	90	A	1(2)	51	N/A	62*	80	None

* with documentation

Terms To Know

lymph nodes. Bean-shaped structures along the lymphatic vessels that intercept and destroy foreign materials in the tissue and bloodstream.

malignant. Any condition tending to progress toward death, specifically an invasive tumor with a loss of cellular differentiation that has the ability to spread or metastasize to other body areas.

omentum. Fold of peritoneal tissue suspended between the stomach and neighboring visceral organs of the abdominal cavity.

peritoneal. Space between the lining of the abdominal wall, or parietal peritoneum, and the surface layer of the abdominal organs, or visceral peritoneum. It contains a thin, watery fluid that keeps the peritoneal surfaces moist.

resection. Surgical removal of a part or all of an organ or body part.

secondary. Second in order of occurrence or importance, or appearing during the course of another disease or condition.

58951

58951 Resection (initial) of ovarian, tubal or primary peritoneal malignancy with bilateral salpingo-oophorectomy and omentectomy; with total abdominal hysterectomy, pelvic and limited para-aortic lymphadenectomy

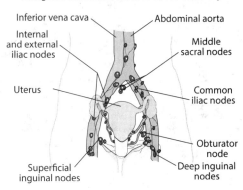

Malignant ovaries and tubes removed bilaterally

Pelvic lymph nodes and some aortic nodes removed. The uterus is also removed

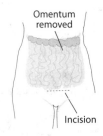

Explanation

Through a full abdominal incision extending from just above the pubic hairline to the rib cage, the physician treats an ovarian, tubal, or peritoneal malignancy by taking out both tubes, both ovaries, and the omentum, which is a membrane of lymph nodes, blood vessels, and fat that forms a protective layer extending from the stomach to the transverse colon. The physician also removes the uterus, the pelvic lymph nodes, and a portion of the lymph nodes surrounding the lower aorta. The abdominal incision is closed with layered sutures. This code is to be used only for the initial surgical resection of the malignancy.

Coding Tips

The documentation or pathology report should verify a total removal of both tubes, ovaries, and the omentum with a total hysterectomy due to malignancy. The pelvic or limited para-aortic lymphadenectomies are not identified separately. If this procedure is performed with radical dissection and debulking, report 58952. If completing the hysterectomy for reasons other than malignancy, see 58150–58285 for the most appropriate choice.

ICD-10-CM Diagnostic Codes

C48.1	Malignant neoplasm of specified parts of peritoneum
C48.8	Malignant neoplasm of overlapping sites of retroperitoneum and peritoneum
C56.1	Malignant neoplasm of right ovary ♀ ☑
C56.2	Malignant neoplasm of left ovary ♀ ☑
C57.01	Malignant neoplasm of right fallopian tube ♀ ☑
C57.02	Malignant neoplasm of left fallopian tube ♀ ☑
C77.2	Secondary and unspecified malignant neoplasm of intra-abdominal lymph nodes

Ovary

C77.5	Secondary and unspecified malignant neoplasm of intrapelvic lymph nodes
C78.6	Secondary malignant neoplasm of retroperitoneum and peritoneum
C79.61	Secondary malignant neoplasm of right ovary ♀ ☑
C79.62	Secondary malignant neoplasm of left ovary ♀ ☑
C79.82	Secondary malignant neoplasm of genital organs

AMA: 58951 2019,Jul,6; 2018,Jan,8; 2017,Jan,8; 2016,Jan,13; 2015,Jan,16; 2014,Jan,11

Relative Value Units/Medicare Edits

Non-Facility RVU	Work	PE	MP	Total
58951	24.26	13.27	3.83	41.36
Facility RVU	Work	PE	MP	Total
58951	24.26	13.27	3.83	41.36

	FUD	Status	MUE	Modifiers				IOM Reference
58951	90	A	1(2)	51	N/A	62*	80	None

* with documentation

Terms To Know

hysterectomy. Surgical removal of the uterus. A complete hysterectomy may also include removal of tubes and ovaries.

lymph nodes. Bean-shaped structures along the lymphatic vessels that intercept and destroy foreign materials in the tissue and bloodstream.

malignant neoplasm. Any cancerous tumor or lesion exhibiting uncontrolled tissue growth that can progressively invade other parts of the body with its disease-generating cells.

omentum. Fold of peritoneal tissue suspended between the stomach and neighboring visceral organs of the abdominal cavity.

resection. Surgical removal of a part or all of an organ or body part.

58952

58952	Resection (initial) of ovarian, tubal or primary peritoneal malignancy with bilateral salpingo-oophorectomy and omentectomy; with radical dissection for debulking (ie, radical excision or destruction, intra-abdominal or retroperitoneal tumors)

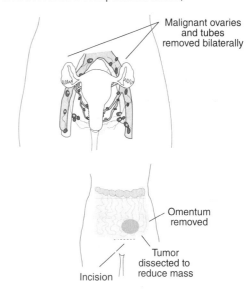

Malignant ovaries and tubes removed bilaterally

Omentum removed

Tumor dissected to reduce mass

Incision

Ovary

Explanation

Through a full abdominal incision extending from just above the pubic hairline to the rib cage, the physician treats an ovarian, tubal, or peritoneal malignancy by excising both tubes, both ovaries, and the omentum, which is a membrane containing fat, lymph, and blood vessels that acts as a protective layer extending from the stomach to the transverse colon. The physician also reduces the size of a tumor that has grown large enough to cause discomfort or problems. Due to the size and location, it may not be possible to remove the tumor. The abdominal incision is closed with layered sutures. This code is to be used only for the initial surgical resection of the malignancy.

Coding Tips

The documentation or pathology report should verify a total removal of both tubes, ovaries, and the omentum with radical excision of an intra-abdominal or retroperitoneal tumor due to malignancy. This procedure involves an extensive amount of work debulking the surrounding tissues and there is a large amount of clean up involved, which is not identified separately. If performed with total abdominal hysterectomy and lymphadenectomies, see 58951. For resection of a recurrent ovarian, tubal, primary peritoneal, or uterine malignancy, see 58957-58958.

ICD-10-CM Diagnostic Codes

C48.1	Malignant neoplasm of specified parts of peritoneum
C48.8	Malignant neoplasm of overlapping sites of retroperitoneum and peritoneum
C56.1	Malignant neoplasm of right ovary ♀ ☑
C56.2	Malignant neoplasm of left ovary ♀ ☑
C57.01	Malignant neoplasm of right fallopian tube ♀ ☑
C57.02	Malignant neoplasm of left fallopian tube ♀ ☑
C78.6	Secondary malignant neoplasm of retroperitoneum and peritoneum
C79.61	Secondary malignant neoplasm of right ovary ♀ ☑
C79.62	Secondary malignant neoplasm of left ovary ♀ ☑

C79.82   Secondary malignant neoplasm of genital organs

AMA: 58952 2019,Jul,6; 2018,Jan,8; 2017,Jan,8; 2016,Jan,13; 2015,Jan,16; 2014,Jan,11

Relative Value Units/Medicare Edits

Non-Facility RVU	Work	PE	MP	Total
58952	27.29	15.35	4.33	46.97
Facility RVU	**Work**	**PE**	**MP**	**Total**
58952	27.29	15.35	4.33	46.97

	FUD	Status	MUE	Modifiers				IOM Reference
58952	90	A	1(2)	51	N/A	62*	80	None

* with documentation

Terms To Know

dissection. Separating by cutting tissue or body structures apart.

intra. Within.

malignant neoplasm. Any cancerous tumor or lesion exhibiting uncontrolled tissue growth that can progressively invade other parts of the body with its disease-generating cells.

radical resection. Removal of an entire tumor (e.g., malignant neoplasm) along with a large area of surrounding tissue, including adjacent lymph nodes that may have been infiltrated.

tumor. Pathological swelling or enlargement; a neoplastic growth of uncontrolled, abnormal multiplication of cells.

58953

58953   Bilateral salpingo-oophorectomy with omentectomy, total abdominal hysterectomy and radical dissection for debulking;

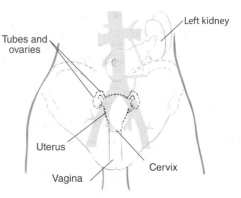

The tubes, ovaries, and the uterus are removed along with the omentum

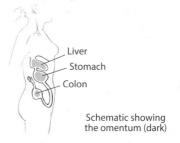

Schematic showing the omentum (dark)

Explanation

Through a full abdominal incision extending from just above the pubic hairline to the rib cage, the physician treats an ovarian malignancy. The physician makes a full abdominal incision and carries dissection down to the abdominal cavity. The physician excises the fallopian tubes, both ovaries, the uterus, and the omentum, which is a membrane containing lymph, blood vessels, and fat in a protective layer that extends from the stomach to the transverse colon. The physician removes or reduces metastatic ovarian cancer implants from the abdominal cavity. The abdominal incision is closed with layered sutures.

Coding Tips

For bilateral salpingo-oophorectomy with omentectomy, total abdominal hysterectomy and radical dissection for debulking, with pelvic lymphadenectomy and limited para-aortic lymphadenectomy, see 58954. For resection of ovarian, tubal, or primary peritoneal malignancy with bilateral salpingo-oophorectomy and omentectomy alone, see 58950; with radical dissection for debulking, without total abdominal hysterectomy, see 58952. For resection of ovarian, tubal, or primary peritoneal malignancy with bilateral salpingo-oophorectomy and omentectomy, with total abdominal hysterectomy, pelvic and limited para-aortic lymphadenectomy, without radical dissection for debulking, see 58951.

ICD-10-CM Diagnostic Codes

C56.1	Malignant neoplasm of right ovary ♀ ☑
C56.2	Malignant neoplasm of left ovary ♀ ☑
C57.01	Malignant neoplasm of right fallopian tube ♀ ☑
C57.02	Malignant neoplasm of left fallopian tube ♀ ☑
C79.61	Secondary malignant neoplasm of right ovary ♀ ☑
C79.62	Secondary malignant neoplasm of left ovary ♀ ☑
C79.82	Secondary malignant neoplasm of genital organs

Ovary

AMA: **58953** 2019,Jul,6; 2018,Jan,8; 2017,Jan,8; 2016,Jan,13; 2015,Jan,16; 2014,May,10; 2014,Jan,11

Relative Value Units/Medicare Edits

Non-Facility RVU	Work	PE	MP	Total
58953	34.13	18.09	5.39	57.61
Facility RVU	Work	PE	MP	Total
58953	34.13	18.09	5.39	57.61

	FUD	Status	MUE	Modifiers				IOM Reference
58953	90	A	1(2)	51	N/A	62*	80	None

* with documentation

Terms To Know

dissection. Separating by cutting tissue or body structures apart.

hysterectomy. Surgical removal of the uterus. A complete hysterectomy may also include removal of tubes and ovaries.

malignant. Any condition tending to progress toward death, specifically an invasive tumor with a loss of cellular differentiation that has the ability to spread or metastasize to other body areas.

metastasize. Spread, invade, or extend to a new location.

omentum. Fold of peritoneal tissue suspended between the stomach and neighboring visceral organs of the abdominal cavity.

radical. Extensive surgery.

salpingo-oophorectomy. Surgical removal of both the fallopian tube and ovary.

58954

58954 Bilateral salpingo-oophorectomy with omentectomy, total abdominal hysterectomy and radical dissection for debulking; with pelvic lymphadenectomy and limited para-aortic lymphadenectomy

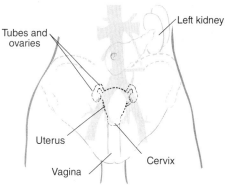

The tubes, ovaries, and the uterus are removed along with the omentum, pelvic, and para-aortic lymph nodes

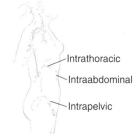

Schematic showing lymph nodes

Explanation

Through a full abdominal incision extending from just above the pubic hairline to the rib cage, the physician treats an ovarian malignancy. Additionally, the physician excises pelvic lymph nodes and partially removes para-aortic lymph nodes. The physician makes a full abdominal incision and carries dissection down to the abdominal cavity. The physician excises the fallopian tubes, both ovaries, the uterus, and the omentum, which is a membrane containing lymph, blood vessels, and fat in a protective layer that extends from the stomach to the transverse colon. The physician removes or reduces metastatic ovarian cancer implants from the abdominal cavity. The physician additionally removes pelvic lymph nodes and a portion of the lymph nodes that surrounds the lower aorta within the pelvis. The abdominal incision is closed with layered sutures.

Coding Tips

For bilateral salpingo-oophorectomy with omentectomy, total abdominal hysterectomy and radical dissection for debulking, see 58953. For resection of ovarian, tubal, or primary peritoneal malignancy with bilateral salpingo-oophorectomy and omentectomy alone, see 58950; with radical dissection for debulking without total abdominal hysterectomy, see 58952. For resection of ovarian, tubal, or primary peritoneal malignancy with bilateral salpingo-oophorectomy and omentectomy, with total abdominal hysterectomy, pelvic and limited para-aortic lymphadenectomy, without radical dissection for debulking, see 58951.

ICD-10-CM Diagnostic Codes

C56.1	Malignant neoplasm of right ovary ♀ ☑
C56.2	Malignant neoplasm of left ovary ♀ ☑
C57.01	Malignant neoplasm of right fallopian tube ♀ ☑
C57.02	Malignant neoplasm of left fallopian tube ♀ ☑

Ovary

C77.2	Secondary and unspecified malignant neoplasm of intra-abdominal lymph nodes
C77.5	Secondary and unspecified malignant neoplasm of intrapelvic lymph nodes
C79.61	Secondary malignant neoplasm of right ovary ♀ ☑
C79.62	Secondary malignant neoplasm of left ovary ♀ ☑
C79.82	Secondary malignant neoplasm of genital organs

AMA: 58954 2019,Jul,6; 2018,Jan,8; 2017,Jan,8; 2016,Jan,13; 2015,Jan,16; 2014,Jan,11

Relative Value Units/Medicare Edits

Non-Facility RVU	Work	PE	MP	Total
58954	37.13	19.43	5.87	62.43
Facility RVU	**Work**	**PE**	**MP**	**Total**
58954	37.13	19.43	5.87	62.43

	FUD	Status	MUE	Modifiers				IOM Reference
58954	90	A	1(2)	51	N/A	62*	80	None

* with documentation

Terms To Know

dissection. Separating by cutting tissue or body structures apart.

lymph nodes. Bean-shaped structures along the lymphatic vessels that intercept and destroy foreign materials in the tissue and bloodstream.

lymphadenectomy. Dissection of lymph nodes free from the vessels and removal for examination by frozen section in a separate procedure to detect early-stage metastases.

malignant neoplasm. Any cancerous tumor or lesion exhibiting uncontrolled tissue growth that can progressively invade other parts of the body with its disease-generating cells.

radical. Extensive surgery.

salpingo-oophorectomy. Surgical removal of both the fallopian tube and ovary.

58956

| 58956 | Bilateral salpingo-oophorectomy with total omentectomy, total abdominal hysterectomy for malignancy |

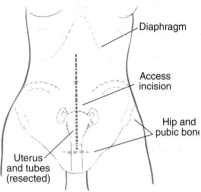

The uterus, tubes, and ovaries are removed along with the omentum

Explanation

The physician performs a bilateral salpingo-oophorectomy with total omentectomy and total abdominal hysterectomy to treat a malignancy. A full abdominal incision is made extending from just above the pubic hairline to the rib cage. Dissection is carried down to the abdominal cavity. The physician excises the fallopian tubes, ovaries, the uterus, and the omentum. The supporting pedicles containing the tubes, ligaments, and arteries are clamped and cut free. The uterus and cervix are removed along with a narrow rim or cuff of the vaginal lining. The vaginal defect is often left open for drainage. Attention is directed to the omentum, a membrane of lymph, blood vessels, and fat that forms a protective layer that extends from the stomach to the transverse colon. The omentum is mobilized from the stomach and colon, divided from its blood supply, and removed. The physician inspects the abdominal cavity and removes any metastatic lesions. The abdominal incision is closed with layered sutures.

Coding Tips

This is a bilateral procedure. If salpingo-oophorectomy is performed only on one side, append modifier 52. This procedure should not be reported with the following codes: 49255, 58150, 58180, 58262, 58263, 58550, 58661, 58700, 58720, 58900, 58925, 58940, 58957, or 58958.

ICD-10-CM Diagnostic Codes

C48.1	Malignant neoplasm of specified parts of peritoneum
C48.8	Malignant neoplasm of overlapping sites of retroperitoneum and peritoneum
C52	Malignant neoplasm of vagina ♀
C53.0	Malignant neoplasm of endocervix ♀
C53.1	Malignant neoplasm of exocervix ♀
C53.8	Malignant neoplasm of overlapping sites of cervix uteri ♀
C54.0	Malignant neoplasm of isthmus uteri ♀
C54.1	Malignant neoplasm of endometrium ♀
C54.2	Malignant neoplasm of myometrium ♀
C54.3	Malignant neoplasm of fundus uteri ♀
C54.8	Malignant neoplasm of overlapping sites of corpus uteri ♀
C56.1	Malignant neoplasm of right ovary ♀ ☑
C56.2	Malignant neoplasm of left ovary ♀ ☑
C57.01	Malignant neoplasm of right fallopian tube ♀ ☑

Coding Companion for Ob/Gyn

Ovary

C57.02	Malignant neoplasm of left fallopian tube ♀ ☑	
C57.11	Malignant neoplasm of right broad ligament ♀ ☑	
C57.12	Malignant neoplasm of left broad ligament ♀ ☑	
C57.21	Malignant neoplasm of right round ligament ♀ ☑	
C57.22	Malignant neoplasm of left round ligament ♀ ☑	
C57.3	Malignant neoplasm of parametrium ♀	
C57.7	Malignant neoplasm of other specified female genital organs ♀	
C57.8	Malignant neoplasm of overlapping sites of female genital organs ♀	
C78.5	Secondary malignant neoplasm of large intestine and rectum	
C78.6	Secondary malignant neoplasm of retroperitoneum and peritoneum	
C79.11	Secondary malignant neoplasm of bladder	
C79.19	Secondary malignant neoplasm of other urinary organs	
C79.61	Secondary malignant neoplasm of right ovary ♀ ☑	
C79.62	Secondary malignant neoplasm of left ovary ♀ ☑	
C79.82	Secondary malignant neoplasm of genital organs	

AMA: 58956 2019,Jul,6; 2018,Jan,8; 2017,Jan,8; 2016,Jan,13; 2015,Jan,16; 2014,May,10; 2014,Jan,11

Relative Value Units/Medicare Edits

Non-Facility RVU	Work	PE	MP	Total
58956	22.8	12.72	3.63	39.15
Facility RVU	Work	PE	MP	Total
58956	22.8	12.72	3.63	39.15

	FUD	Status	MUE	Modifiers				IOM Reference
58956	90	A	1(2)	51	N/A	62*	80	None

* with documentation

Terms To Know

dissection. (dis. apart; -section, act of cutting) Separating by cutting tissue or body structures apart.

malignant neoplasm. Any cancerous tumor or lesion exhibiting uncontrolled tissue growth that can progressively invade other parts of the body with its disease-generating cells.

omentum. Fold of peritoneal tissue suspended between the stomach and neighboring visceral organs of the abdominal cavity.

salpingo-oophorectomy. Surgical removal of both the fallopian tube and ovary.

secondary. Second in order of occurrence or importance, or appearing during the course of another disease or condition.

58957-58958

58957 Resection (tumor debulking) of recurrent ovarian, tubal, primary peritoneal, uterine malignancy (intra-abdominal, retroperitoneal tumors), with omentectomy, if performed;

58958   with pelvic lymphadenectomy and limited para-aortic lymphadenectomy

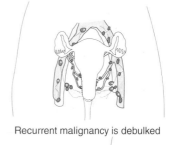

Pelvic and limited para-aortic lymphadenectomy may also be performed

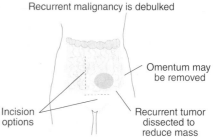

Recurrent malignancy is debulked

Omentum may be removed

Incision options

Recurrent tumor dissected to reduce mass

Explanation

These codes report tumor debulking in recurrent ovarian, uterine, tubal, or peritoneal malignancies. Through a full abdominal incision extending from just above the pubic hairline to the rib cage, the physician explores the abdomen, pelvis, and viscera. In addition to debulking recurrent malignancy, the physician releases intestinal adhesions or excises all or portions of the omentum, ovaries, or fallopian tubes. The physician may remove all visible tumors or only reduce their size, depending on the nature of the malignancy and the structures involved. The abdominal incision is closed with layered sutures. Report 58958 when pelvic and para-aortic lymph nodes are also removed.

Coding Tips

If significant additional time and effort is documented, append modifier 22 and submit a cover letter and operative report. This is a bilateral procedure and as such is reported once even if the procedure is performed on both sides. Code 58958 includes any lymphadenectomy or omentectomy the physician may perform. For initial malignancy of the ovaries, uterus, tubes, or primary peritoneal structures, see 58900–58952. For staging of tubal, ovarian, or primary peritoneal malignancy, see 58960.

ICD-10-CM Diagnostic Codes

C48.1	Malignant neoplasm of specified parts of peritoneum	
C48.8	Malignant neoplasm of overlapping sites of retroperitoneum and peritoneum	
C54.0	Malignant neoplasm of isthmus uteri ♀	
C54.1	Malignant neoplasm of endometrium ♀	
C54.2	Malignant neoplasm of myometrium ♀	
C54.3	Malignant neoplasm of fundus uteri ♀	
C54.8	Malignant neoplasm of overlapping sites of corpus uteri ♀	
C56.1	Malignant neoplasm of right ovary ♀ ☑	

C56.2	Malignant neoplasm of left ovary ♀ ☑
C57.01	Malignant neoplasm of right fallopian tube ♀ ☑
C57.02	Malignant neoplasm of left fallopian tube ♀ ☑
C77.2	Secondary and unspecified malignant neoplasm of intra-abdominal lymph nodes
C77.5	Secondary and unspecified malignant neoplasm of intrapelvic lymph nodes
C78.6	Secondary malignant neoplasm of retroperitoneum and peritoneum
C79.61	Secondary malignant neoplasm of right ovary ♀ ☑
C79.62	Secondary malignant neoplasm of left ovary ♀ ☑
C79.82	Secondary malignant neoplasm of genital organs

AMA: 58957 2019,Jul,6; 2014,Jan,11 **58958** 2019,Jul,6; 2014,Jan,11

Relative Value Units/Medicare Edits

Non-Facility RVU	Work	PE	MP	Total
58957	26.22	14.99	4.25	45.46
58958	29.22	16.29	4.82	50.33
Facility RVU	Work	PE	MP	Total
58957	26.22	14.99	4.25	45.46
58958	29.22	16.29	4.82	50.33

	FUD	Status	MUE	Modifiers				IOM Reference
58957	90	A	1(2)	51	N/A	62*	80	None
58958	90	A	1(2)	51	N/A	62*	80	

* with documentation

Terms To Know

intra. Within.

lymphadenectomy. Dissection of lymph nodes free from the vessels and removal for examination by frozen section in a separate procedure to detect early-stage metastases.

omentum. Fold of peritoneal tissue suspended between the stomach and neighboring visceral organs of the abdominal cavity.

peritoneal. Space between the lining of the abdominal wall, or parietal peritoneum, and the surface layer of the abdominal organs, or visceral peritoneum. It contains a thin, watery fluid that keeps the peritoneal surfaces moist.

resection. Surgical removal of a part or all of an organ or body part.

retroperitoneal. Located behind the peritoneum, the membrane that lines the abdominopelvic walls and forms a covering for the internal organs.

58960

58960 Laparotomy, for staging or restaging of ovarian, tubal, or primary peritoneal malignancy (second look), with or without omentectomy, peritoneal washing, biopsy of abdominal and pelvic peritoneum, diaphragmatic assessment with pelvic and limited para-aortic lymphadenectomy

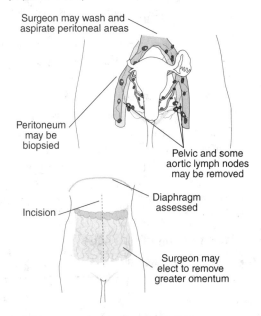

Surgeon may wash and aspirate peritoneal areas

Peritoneum may be biopsied

Pelvic and some aortic lymph nodes may be removed

Incision

Diaphragm assessed

Surgeon may elect to remove greater omentum

Explanation

This procedure is the second operation to check for a recurrence of the ovarian malignancy. Through a full abdominal incision extending from just above the pubic hairline to the rib cage, the physician may elect to remove the omentum, a membrane of lymph, blood vessels, and fat that forms a protective layer that extends from the stomach to the transverse colon. The physician may flush the lining of the abdominal cavity (peritoneum) and remove the liquid to check for cancerous cells. A tissue sample of the abdominal and pelvic peritoneum may be taken. The physician also may examine and take tissue samples of the diaphragm. The pelvic lymph nodes are removed and a portion of the lymph nodes that surrounds the lower aorta within the pelvis is removed. The abdominal incision is closed with layered sutures.

Coding Tips

A prior surgery for ovarian malignancy should be documented. For initial treatment and guidelines, see 58950–58952. Do not report 58960 with 58957-58958.

ICD-10-CM Diagnostic Codes

C48.1	Malignant neoplasm of specified parts of peritoneum
C48.8	Malignant neoplasm of overlapping sites of retroperitoneum and peritoneum
C56.1	Malignant neoplasm of right ovary ♀ ☑
C56.2	Malignant neoplasm of left ovary ♀ ☑
C57.01	Malignant neoplasm of right fallopian tube ♀ ☑
C57.02	Malignant neoplasm of left fallopian tube ♀ ☑
C78.6	Secondary malignant neoplasm of retroperitoneum and peritoneum
C79.61	Secondary malignant neoplasm of right ovary ♀ ☑
C79.62	Secondary malignant neoplasm of left ovary ♀ ☑
C79.82	Secondary malignant neoplasm of genital organs

Ovary

AMA: **58960** 2019,Jul,6; 2014,Jan,11

Relative Value Units/Medicare Edits

Non-Facility RVU	Work	PE	MP	Total
58960	15.79	9.58	2.62	27.99
Facility RVU	Work	PE	MP	Total
58960	15.79	9.58	2.62	27.99

	FUD	Status	MUE	Modifiers				IOM Reference
58960	90	A	1(2)	51	N/A	62*	80	None

* with documentation

Terms To Know

lymphadenectomy. Dissection of lymph nodes free from the vessels and removal for examination by frozen section in a separate procedure to detect early-stage metastases.

malignant. Any condition tending to progress toward death, specifically an invasive tumor with a loss of cellular differentiation that has the ability to spread or metastasize to other body areas.

omentum. Fold of peritoneal tissue suspended between the stomach and neighboring visceral organs of the abdominal cavity.

peritoneum. Strong, continuous membrane that forms the lining of the abdominal and pelvic cavity. The parietal peritoneum, or outer layer, is attached to the abdominopelvic walls and the visceral peritoneum, or inner layer, surrounds the organs inside the abdominal cavity.

Ovary

58970

58970 Follicle puncture for oocyte retrieval, any method

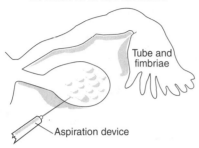

The physician aspirates an egg from the follicle for in vitro fertilization

Tube and fimbriae

Aspiration device

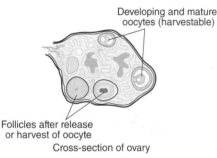

Developing and mature oocytes (harvestable)

Follicles after release or harvest of oocyte

Cross-section of ovary

Explanation

The physician aspirates a mature or nearly mature egg from its follicle for in vitro fertilization. Visualization of the aspiration may be done laparoscopically or by ultrasound. The laparoscopic method uses three puncture sites in the lower abdomen: one for the laparoscope, one for the holding forceps, and one for the aspirating needle. The ultrasound guided technique involves using a transabdominal ultrasound transducer for guidance. The aspirating needle is passed through the bladder wall to the ovary or through the urethra and into the pelvic cavity. Another ultrasound method uses transvaginal ultrasound and transvaginal needle aspiration of the ovary. In all methods, the ovary and preovulatory follicle are visualized and punctured with a needle to withdraw the follicular fluid containing the egg.

Coding Tips

This procedure only reports the retrieval of an oocyte. This code includes any method of retrieval performed by the physician. For culture and fertilization of an oocyte, see 89250. For assisted oocyte fertilization by microtechnique, see 89280–89281. For subsequent intrauterine embryo transfer, see 58974. For gamete, zygote, or embryo intrafallopian transfer, see 58976. When 58970 is performed with another separately identifiable procedure, the highest dollar value code is listed as the primary procedure and subsequent procedures are appended with modifier 51. For ultrasonic guidance (supervision and interpretation), see 76948.

ICD-10-CM Diagnostic Codes

N97.0	Female infertility associated with anovulation ♀
N97.1	Female infertility of tubal origin ♀
N97.2	Female infertility of uterine origin ♀
N97.8	Female infertility of other origin ♀
Z31.7	Encounter for procreative management and counseling for gestational carrier ♀
Z31.83	Encounter for assisted reproductive fertility procedure cycle ♀
Z31.84	Encounter for fertility preservation procedure
Z31.89	Encounter for other procreative management
Z52.810	Egg (Oocyte) donor under age 35, anonymous recipient ♀
Z52.811	Egg (Oocyte) donor under age 35, designated recipient ♀
Z52.812	Egg (Oocyte) donor age 35 and over, anonymous recipient ♀
Z52.813	Egg (Oocyte) donor age 35 and over, designated recipient ♀

AMA: **58970** 2019,Jul,6; 2014,Jan,11

Relative Value Units/Medicare Edits

Non-Facility RVU	Work	PE	MP	Total
58970	3.52	2.67	0.56	6.75
Facility RVU	**Work**	**PE**	**MP**	**Total**
58970	3.52	1.66	0.56	5.74

	FUD	Status	MUE	Modifiers				IOM Reference
58970	0	A	1(3)	51	N/A	N/A	80*	None

* with documentation

Terms To Know

aspirate. To withdraw fluid or air from a body cavity by suction.

infertility. Inability to conceive for at least one year with regular intercourse.

laparoscopy. Direct visualization of the peritoneal cavity, outer fallopian tubes, uterus, and ovaries utilizing a laparoscope, a thin, flexible fiberoptic tube.

oocyte. Female gametocyte or germ cell involved in reproduction. It is an immature ovum or egg cell.

polycystic. Multiple cysts.

puncture. Creating a hole.

trans. *1)* Across, through. *2)* Transverse.

ultrasound. Imaging using ultra-high sound frequency bounced off body structures.

In Vitro

58974

58974　Embryo transfer, intrauterine

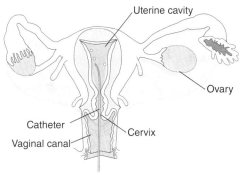

The physician injects fertilized eggs into the uterus

Explanation

The physician places fertilized eggs in the uterus after the eggs have undergone 48 to 72 hours of laboratory culture. The embryos are aspirated into a small catheter. The catheter is passed through the cervical os and into the uterus. The eggs are injected into the uterus.

Coding Tips

This code includes only intrauterine transfer. For gamete, zygote, or embryo intrafallopian transfer, any method, see 58976. For preparation of embryo for transfer, see 89255. For follicle puncture for oocyte retrieval, any method, see 58970. Because this procedure is usually not done out of medical necessity, the patient may be responsible for charges. Verify with the insurance carrier for coverage.

ICD-10-CM Diagnostic Codes

N97.0　Female infertility associated with anovulation ♀

N97.1　Female infertility of tubal origin ♀

N97.2　Female infertility of uterine origin ♀

N97.8　Female infertility of other origin ♀

Z31.81　Encounter for male factor infertility in female patient ♀

Z31.83　Encounter for assisted reproductive fertility procedure cycle ♀

AMA: 58974 2019,Jul,6; 2014,Jan,11

Relative Value Units/Medicare Edits

Non-Facility RVU	Work	PE	MP	Total
58974	0.0	0.0	0.0	0.0
Facility RVU	**Work**	**PE**	**MP**	**Total**
58974	0.0	0.0	0.0	0.0

	FUD	Status	MUE	Modifiers				IOM Reference
58974	0	C	1(3)	51	N/A	62*	80	None

* with documentation

Terms To Know

embryo. Developing cells of a new organism that will become a fetus; the period defined from the fourth day after fertilization to the end of the eighth week.

58976

58976　Gamete, zygote, or embryo intrafallopian transfer, any method

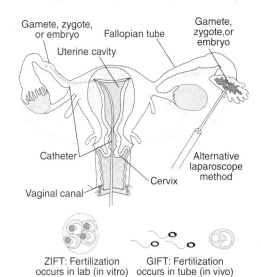

ZIFT: Fertilization occurs in lab (in vitro)　　GIFT: Fertilization occurs in tube (in vivo)

In Vitro

Explanation

In gamete intrafallopian transfer (GIFT), the physician mixes previously captured eggs with sperm and draws the mixture into a catheter. The catheter is passed through the cervix and uterus and into the tubes or passed through an abdominal incision and directly into the fimbrial end of the fallopian tube. The physician deposits the eggs and sperm in the tubes, permitting fertilization. In a zygote intrafallopian transfer (ZIFT), a physician draws an already fertilized egg into a catheter. The catheter is passed through the cervix and uterus and into the tube where the egg is deposited. GIFT is a one-step procedure while ZIFT is a two-step process. In ZIFT, the egg is collected and fertilized and transferred to the fallopian tube at a later time. GIFT and ZIFT can be done laparoscopically or hysteroscopically.

Coding Tips

For follicle puncture for oocyte retrieval, any method, see 58970. For culture and fertilization of an oocyte, see 89250. For embryo transfer, intrauterine, see 58974. For adnexa procedures via laparoscopy, see 58660-58673. This code can be reported more than once to reflect additional transfers. When 58976 is performed with another separately identifiable procedure, the highest dollar value code is listed as the primary procedure and subsequent procedures are appended with modifier 51.

ICD-10-CM Diagnostic Codes

N97.0　Female infertility associated with anovulation ♀

N97.1　Female infertility of tubal origin ♀

N97.2　Female infertility of uterine origin ♀

N97.8　Female infertility of other origin ♀

Z31.81　Encounter for male factor infertility in female patient ♀

Z31.83　Encounter for assisted reproductive fertility procedure cycle ♀

AMA: 58976 2019,Jul,6; 2018,Jan,8; 2017,Jan,8; 2016,Jan,13; 2015,Jan,16; 2014,Jan,11

Relative Value Units/Medicare Edits

Non-Facility RVU	Work	PE	MP	Total
58976	3.82	2.91	0.6	7.33
Facility RVU	Work	PE	MP	Total
58976	3.82	1.78	0.6	6.2

	FUD	Status	MUE	Modifiers				IOM Reference
58976	0	A	2(3)	51	N/A	62*	80	None

* with documentation

Terms To Know

anovulation. Abnormal condition in which an ovum is not released each month. Anovulation is a prime factor in female infertility.

catheter. Flexible tube inserted into an area of the body for introducing or withdrawing fluid.

cyst. Elevated encapsulated mass containing fluid, semisolid, or solid material with a membranous lining.

embryo. Developing cells of a new organism that will become a fetus; the period defined from the fourth day after fertilization to the end of the eighth week.

endometriosis. Aberrant uterine mucosal tissue appearing in areas of the pelvic cavity outside of its normal location, lining the uterus, and inflaming surrounding tissues often resulting in infertility or spontaneous abortion.

fallopian tubes. Bilateral, paired tubes that extend from the uterus to the ovaries, through which an ovum released from the follicle travels to the uterus during ovulation.

gamete. Unfertilized male or female reproductive cell; an ovum or a spermatozoon.

GIFT. Gamete intrafallopian transfer.

infertility. Inability to conceive for at least one year with regular intercourse.

intra. Within.

polycystic. Multiple cysts.

ZIFT. Zygote intrafallopian transfer.

zygote. Fertilized ovum or the cell created after the union of a male and female gamete.

59000

59000 Amniocentesis; diagnostic

The physician aspirates amniotic fluid from the pregnant uterus for analysis

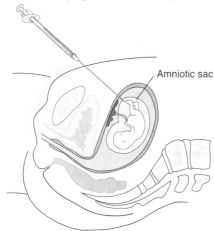

Amniotic sac

Explanation

The physician aspirates fluid from the amniotic sac for diagnostic purposes. Using separately reportable ultrasonic guidance, the physician inserts an amniocentesis needle through the abdominal wall into the interior of the pregnant uterus and directly into the amniotic sac to collect amniotic fluid for separately reportable analysis.

Coding Tips

For radiological supervision and interpretation, see 76946. For fetal lung maturity assessment, lecithin sphingomyelin (L/S) ratio testing, see 83661. For chromosome analysis, see 88267 and 88269. For alpha-fetoprotein by amniotic fluid specimen, see 82106. For amniotic fluid scan (spectrophotometric), see 82143.

ICD-10-CM Diagnostic Codes

O09.12	Supervision of pregnancy with history of ectopic pregnancy, second trimester ⓜ ♀
O09.13	Supervision of pregnancy with history of ectopic pregnancy, third trimester ⓜ ♀
O09.291	Supervision of pregnancy with other poor reproductive or obstetric history, first trimester ⓜ ♀
O09.292	Supervision of pregnancy with other poor reproductive or obstetric history, second trimester ⓜ ♀
O09.293	Supervision of pregnancy with other poor reproductive or obstetric history, third trimester ⓜ ♀
O09.511	Supervision of elderly primigravida, first trimester ⓜ ♀
O09.512	Supervision of elderly primigravida, second trimester ⓜ ♀
O09.513	Supervision of elderly primigravida, third trimester ⓜ ♀
O09.521	Supervision of elderly multigravida, first trimester ⓜ ♀
O09.522	Supervision of elderly multigravida, second trimester ⓜ ♀
O09.523	Supervision of elderly multigravida, third trimester ⓜ ♀
O09.621	Supervision of young multigravida, first trimester ⓜ ♀
O09.622	Supervision of young multigravida, second trimester ⓜ ♀
O09.623	Supervision of young multigravida, third trimester ⓜ ♀
O09.71	Supervision of high risk pregnancy due to social problems, first trimester ⓜ ♀
O09.72	Supervision of high risk pregnancy due to social problems, second trimester ⓜ ♀
O09.73	Supervision of high risk pregnancy due to social problems, third trimester ⓜ ♀
O09.811	Supervision of pregnancy resulting from assisted reproductive technology, first trimester ⓜ ♀
O09.812	Supervision of pregnancy resulting from assisted reproductive technology, second trimester ⓜ ♀
O09.813	Supervision of pregnancy resulting from assisted reproductive technology, third trimester ⓜ ♀
O09.821	Supervision of pregnancy with history of in utero procedure during previous pregnancy, first trimester ⓜ ♀
O09.822	Supervision of pregnancy with history of in utero procedure during previous pregnancy, second trimester ⓜ ♀
O09.823	Supervision of pregnancy with history of in utero procedure during previous pregnancy, third trimester ⓜ ♀
O09.891	Supervision of other high risk pregnancies, first trimester ⓜ ♀
O09.892	Supervision of other high risk pregnancies, second trimester ⓜ ♀
O09.893	Supervision of other high risk pregnancies, third trimester ⓜ ♀
O09.A1	Supervision of pregnancy with history of molar pregnancy, first trimester ⓜ ♀
O09.A2	Supervision of pregnancy with history of molar pregnancy, second trimester ⓜ ♀
O09.A3	Supervision of pregnancy with history of molar pregnancy, third trimester ⓜ ♀
O28.0	Abnormal hematological finding on antenatal screening of mother ⓜ ♀
O28.1	Abnormal biochemical finding on antenatal screening of mother ⓜ ♀
O28.2	Abnormal cytological finding on antenatal screening of mother ⓜ ♀
O28.3	Abnormal ultrasonic finding on antenatal screening of mother ⓜ ♀
O28.4	Abnormal radiological finding on antenatal screening of mother ⓜ ♀
O28.5	Abnormal chromosomal and genetic finding on antenatal screening of mother ⓜ ♀
O28.8	Other abnormal findings on antenatal screening of mother ⓜ ♀
O35.0XX1	Maternal care for (suspected) central nervous system malformation in fetus, fetus 1 ⓜ ♀
O35.0XX2	Maternal care for (suspected) central nervous system malformation in fetus, fetus 2 ⓜ ♀
O35.0XX3	Maternal care for (suspected) central nervous system malformation in fetus, fetus 3 ⓜ ♀
O35.1XX1	Maternal care for (suspected) chromosomal abnormality in fetus, fetus 1 ⓜ ♀
O35.1XX2	Maternal care for (suspected) chromosomal abnormality in fetus, fetus 2 ⓜ ♀
O35.1XX3	Maternal care for (suspected) chromosomal abnormality in fetus, fetus 3 ⓜ ♀
O35.2XX1	Maternal care for (suspected) hereditary disease in fetus, fetus 1 ⓜ ♀
O35.2XX2	Maternal care for (suspected) hereditary disease in fetus, fetus 2 ⓜ ♀
O35.2XX3	Maternal care for (suspected) hereditary disease in fetus, fetus 3 ⓜ ♀

Maternity Care

O35.3XX1	Maternal care for (suspected) damage to fetus from viral disease in mother, fetus 1 Ⓜ ♀
O35.3XX2	Maternal care for (suspected) damage to fetus from viral disease in mother, fetus 2 Ⓜ ♀
O35.3XX3	Maternal care for (suspected) damage to fetus from viral disease in mother, fetus 3 Ⓜ ♀
O35.4XX1	Maternal care for (suspected) damage to fetus from alcohol, fetus 1 Ⓜ ♀
O35.4XX2	Maternal care for (suspected) damage to fetus from alcohol, fetus 2 Ⓜ ♀
O35.4XX3	Maternal care for (suspected) damage to fetus from alcohol, fetus 3 Ⓜ ♀
O35.8XX1	Maternal care for other (suspected) fetal abnormality and damage, fetus 1 Ⓜ ♀
O35.8XX2	Maternal care for other (suspected) fetal abnormality and damage, fetus 2 Ⓜ ♀
O35.8XX3	Maternal care for other (suspected) fetal abnormality and damage, fetus 3 Ⓜ ♀
O36.0111	Maternal care for anti-D [Rh] antibodies, first trimester, fetus 1 Ⓜ ♀
O36.0112	Maternal care for anti-D [Rh] antibodies, first trimester, fetus 2 Ⓜ ♀
O36.0113	Maternal care for anti-D [Rh] antibodies, first trimester, fetus 3 Ⓜ ♀
O36.0121	Maternal care for anti-D [Rh] antibodies, second trimester, fetus 1 Ⓜ ♀
O36.0122	Maternal care for anti-D [Rh] antibodies, second trimester, fetus 2 Ⓜ ♀
O36.0123	Maternal care for anti-D [Rh] antibodies, second trimester, fetus 3 Ⓜ ♀
O36.0131	Maternal care for anti-D [Rh] antibodies, third trimester, fetus 1 Ⓜ ♀
O36.0132	Maternal care for anti-D [Rh] antibodies, third trimester, fetus 2 Ⓜ ♀
O36.0133	Maternal care for anti-D [Rh] antibodies, third trimester, fetus 3 Ⓜ ♀
O36.21X1	Maternal care for hydrops fetalis, first trimester, fetus 1 Ⓜ ♀
O36.21X2	Maternal care for hydrops fetalis, first trimester, fetus 2 Ⓜ ♀
O36.21X3	Maternal care for hydrops fetalis, first trimester, fetus 3 Ⓜ ♀
O36.22X1	Maternal care for hydrops fetalis, second trimester, fetus 1 Ⓜ ♀
O36.22X2	Maternal care for hydrops fetalis, second trimester, fetus 2 Ⓜ ♀
O36.22X3	Maternal care for hydrops fetalis, second trimester, fetus 3 Ⓜ ♀
O36.23X1	Maternal care for hydrops fetalis, third trimester, fetus 1 Ⓜ ♀
O36.23X2	Maternal care for hydrops fetalis, third trimester, fetus 2 Ⓜ ♀
O36.23X3	Maternal care for hydrops fetalis, third trimester, fetus 3 Ⓜ ♀
O40.1XX1	Polyhydramnios, first trimester, fetus 1 Ⓜ ♀
O40.1XX2	Polyhydramnios, first trimester, fetus 2 Ⓜ ♀
O40.1XX3	Polyhydramnios, first trimester, fetus 3 Ⓜ ♀
O40.2XX1	Polyhydramnios, second trimester, fetus 1 Ⓜ ♀
O40.2XX2	Polyhydramnios, second trimester, fetus 2 Ⓜ ♀
O40.2XX3	Polyhydramnios, second trimester, fetus 3 Ⓜ ♀
O40.3XX1	Polyhydramnios, third trimester, fetus 1 Ⓜ ♀
O40.3XX2	Polyhydramnios, third trimester, fetus 2 Ⓜ ♀
O40.3XX3	Polyhydramnios, third trimester, fetus 3 Ⓜ ♀
O40.3XX4	Polyhydramnios, third trimester, fetus 4 Ⓜ ♀
O40.3XX5	Polyhydramnios, third trimester, fetus 5 Ⓜ ♀
O40.3XX9	Polyhydramnios, third trimester, other fetus Ⓜ ♀
O41.01X1	Oligohydramnios, first trimester, fetus 1 Ⓜ ♀
O41.01X2	Oligohydramnios, first trimester, fetus 2 Ⓜ ♀
O41.01X3	Oligohydramnios, first trimester, fetus 3 Ⓜ ♀
O41.02X1	Oligohydramnios, second trimester, fetus 1 Ⓜ ♀
O41.02X2	Oligohydramnios, second trimester, fetus 2 Ⓜ ♀
O41.02X3	Oligohydramnios, second trimester, fetus 3 Ⓜ ♀
O41.03X1	Oligohydramnios, third trimester, fetus 1 Ⓜ ♀
O41.03X2	Oligohydramnios, third trimester, fetus 2 Ⓜ ♀
O41.03X3	Oligohydramnios, third trimester, fetus 3 Ⓜ ♀
Z03.71	Encounter for suspected problem with amniotic cavity and membrane ruled out Ⓜ ♀
Z13.71	Encounter for nonprocreative screening for genetic disease carrier status
Z13.79	Encounter for other screening for genetic and chromosomal anomalies

AMA: **59000** 2019,Jul,6; 2018,Jan,8; 2017,Jan,8; 2016,Jan,13; 2015,Jan,16; 2014,Jan,11

Relative Value Units/Medicare Edits

Non-Facility RVU	Work	PE	MP	Total
59000	1.3	1.82	0.35	3.47
Facility RVU	**Work**	**PE**	**MP**	**Total**
59000	1.3	0.68	0.35	2.33

	FUD	Status	MUE	Modifiers				IOM Reference
59000	0	A	2(3)	51	N/A	N/A	N/A	None

* with documentation

Terms To Know

amniocentesis. Surgical puncture through the abdominal wall, with a specialized needle and under ultrasonic guidance, into the interior of the pregnant uterus and directly into the amniotic sac to collect fluid for diagnostic analysis or therapeutic reduction of fluid levels.

amniotic sac. Commonly referred to as the "bag of waters," the amniotic sac is created from the amnion, which is the inner one of two fetal membranes containing amniotic fluid that surrounds the fetus during pregnancy.

analysis. Study of body fluid, tissue, section, or parts.

aspirate. To withdraw fluid or air from a body cavity by suction.

diagnostic. Examination or procedure to which the patient is subjected, or which is performed on materials derived from a hospital outpatient, to obtain information to aid in the assessment of a medical condition or the identification of a disease. Among these examinations and tests are diagnostic laboratory services such as hematology and chemistry, diagnostic x-rays, isotope studies, EKGs, pulmonary function studies, thyroid function tests, psychological tests, and other tests given to determine the nature and severity of an ailment or injury.

59001

59001 Amniocentesis; therapeutic amniotic fluid reduction (includes ultrasound guidance)

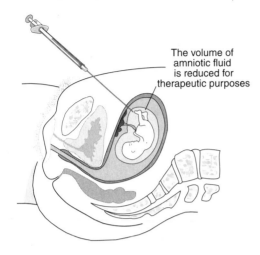

The volume of amniotic fluid is reduced for therapeutic purposes

Explanation

The physician performs a therapeutic amniotic fluid reduction. Using ultrasonic guidance, the physician inserts an 18- or 20-gauge amniocentesis needle through the abdominal wall into the interior of the pregnant uterus and directly into the amniotic sac to remove excess levels of amniotic fluid (amnioreduction). Serial amniotic fluid volume reduction may be accomplished on an ongoing basis by repeating the procedure.

Coding Tips

Note that this amniocentesis procedure is for the therapeutic purpose of reducing excess amniotic fluid only. For an amniocentesis for diagnostic purposes, see 59000.

ICD-10-CM Diagnostic Codes

O40.1XX0	Polyhydramnios, first trimester, not applicable or unspecified Ⓜ ♀
O40.1XX1	Polyhydramnios, first trimester, fetus 1 Ⓜ ♀
O40.1XX2	Polyhydramnios, first trimester, fetus 2 Ⓜ ♀
O40.1XX3	Polyhydramnios, first trimester, fetus 3 Ⓜ ♀
O40.1XX4	Polyhydramnios, first trimester, fetus 4 Ⓜ ♀
O40.1XX5	Polyhydramnios, first trimester, fetus 5 Ⓜ ♀
O40.1XX9	Polyhydramnios, first trimester, other fetus Ⓜ ♀
O40.2XX0	Polyhydramnios, second trimester, not applicable or unspecified Ⓜ ♀
O40.2XX1	Polyhydramnios, second trimester, fetus 1 Ⓜ ♀
O40.2XX2	Polyhydramnios, second trimester, fetus 2 Ⓜ ♀
O40.2XX3	Polyhydramnios, second trimester, fetus 3 Ⓜ ♀
O40.2XX4	Polyhydramnios, second trimester, fetus 4 Ⓜ ♀
O40.2XX5	Polyhydramnios, second trimester, fetus 5 Ⓜ ♀
O40.2XX9	Polyhydramnios, second trimester, other fetus Ⓜ ♀
O40.3XX0	Polyhydramnios, third trimester, not applicable or unspecified Ⓜ ♀
O40.3XX1	Polyhydramnios, third trimester, fetus 1 Ⓜ ♀
O40.3XX2	Polyhydramnios, third trimester, fetus 2 Ⓜ ♀
O40.3XX3	Polyhydramnios, third trimester, fetus 3 Ⓜ ♀
O40.3XX4	Polyhydramnios, third trimester, fetus 4 Ⓜ ♀
O40.3XX5	Polyhydramnios, third trimester, fetus 5 Ⓜ ♀
O40.3XX9	Polyhydramnios, third trimester, other fetus Ⓜ ♀

AMA: 59001 2019,Jul,6; 2018,Jan,8; 2017,Jan,8; 2016,Jan,13; 2015,Jan,16; 2014,Jan,11

Relative Value Units/Medicare Edits

Non-Facility RVU	Work	PE	MP	Total
59001	3.0	1.36	0.82	5.18
Facility RVU	**Work**	**PE**	**MP**	**Total**
59001	3.0	1.36	0.82	5.18

	FUD	Status	MUE	Modifiers			IOM Reference
59001	0	A	2(3)	51	N/A	N/A	N/A	None

* with documentation

Terms To Know

amniocentesis. Surgical puncture through the abdominal wall, with a specialized needle and under ultrasonic guidance, into the interior of the pregnant uterus and directly into the amniotic sac to collect fluid for diagnostic analysis or therapeutic reduction of fluid levels.

polyhydramnios. Excess amniotic fluid surrounding the fetus, typically defined as a total fluid volume of greater than 24.0 cc.

therapeutic. Act meant to alleviate a medical or mental condition.

ultrasound. Imaging using ultra-high sound frequency bounced off body structures.

59012

59012   Cordocentesis (intrauterine), any method

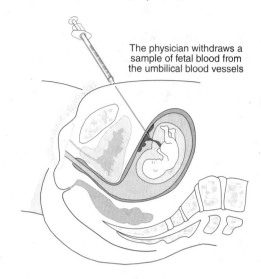

The physician withdraws a sample of fetal blood from the umbilical blood vessels

Explanation

The physician removes blood from the fetal umbilical cord for diagnostic purposes. Using separately reportable ultrasonic guidance, the physician inserts an amniocentesis needle through the abdominal wall into the cavity of the pregnant uterus and into the umbilical vessels to obtain fetal blood. This may be accomplished with a transplacental or transamniotic approach.

Coding Tips

For radiological supervision and interpretation, see 76941. For diagnostic amniocentesis, see 59000. For chorionic villus sampling, see 59015. For fetal hemoglobin test, see 83030 and 83033. For fetal hemoglobin or RBCs for fetomaternal hemorrhage, see 85460–85461.

ICD-10-CM Diagnostic Codes

O09.891	Supervision of other high risk pregnancies, first trimester Ⓜ ♀
O09.892	Supervision of other high risk pregnancies, second trimester Ⓜ ♀
O09.893	Supervision of other high risk pregnancies, third trimester Ⓜ ♀
O28.0	Abnormal hematological finding on antenatal screening of mother Ⓜ ♀
O28.1	Abnormal biochemical finding on antenatal screening of mother Ⓜ ♀
O28.2	Abnormal cytological finding on antenatal screening of mother Ⓜ ♀
O28.3	Abnormal ultrasonic finding on antenatal screening of mother Ⓜ ♀
O28.4	Abnormal radiological finding on antenatal screening of mother Ⓜ ♀
O28.5	Abnormal chromosomal and genetic finding on antenatal screening of mother Ⓜ ♀
O28.8	Other abnormal findings on antenatal screening of mother Ⓜ ♀
O35.1XX1	Maternal care for (suspected) chromosomal abnormality in fetus, fetus 1 Ⓜ ♀
O35.1XX2	Maternal care for (suspected) chromosomal abnormality in fetus, fetus 2 Ⓜ ♀
O35.1XX3	Maternal care for (suspected) chromosomal abnormality in fetus, fetus 3 Ⓜ ♀

O35.2XX1	Maternal care for (suspected) hereditary disease in fetus, fetus 1 Ⓜ ♀
O35.2XX2	Maternal care for (suspected) hereditary disease in fetus, fetus 2 Ⓜ ♀
O35.2XX3	Maternal care for (suspected) hereditary disease in fetus, fetus 3 Ⓜ ♀
O35.3XX1	Maternal care for (suspected) damage to fetus from viral disease in mother, fetus 1 Ⓜ ♀
O35.3XX2	Maternal care for (suspected) damage to fetus from viral disease in mother, fetus 2 Ⓜ ♀
O35.3XX3	Maternal care for (suspected) damage to fetus from viral disease in mother, fetus 3 Ⓜ ♀
O35.4XX1	Maternal care for (suspected) damage to fetus from alcohol, fetus 1 Ⓜ ♀
O35.4XX2	Maternal care for (suspected) damage to fetus from alcohol, fetus 2 Ⓜ ♀
O35.4XX3	Maternal care for (suspected) damage to fetus from alcohol, fetus 3 Ⓜ ♀
O35.8XX1	Maternal care for other (suspected) fetal abnormality and damage, fetus 1 Ⓜ ♀
O35.8XX2	Maternal care for other (suspected) fetal abnormality and damage, fetus 2 Ⓜ ♀
O35.8XX3	Maternal care for other (suspected) fetal abnormality and damage, fetus 3 Ⓜ ♀
O36.0111	Maternal care for anti-D [Rh] antibodies, first trimester, fetus 1 Ⓜ ♀
O36.0112	Maternal care for anti-D [Rh] antibodies, first trimester, fetus 2 Ⓜ ♀
O36.0113	Maternal care for anti-D [Rh] antibodies, first trimester, fetus 3 Ⓜ ♀
O36.0121	Maternal care for anti-D [Rh] antibodies, second trimester, fetus 1 Ⓜ ♀
O36.0122	Maternal care for anti-D [Rh] antibodies, second trimester, fetus 2 Ⓜ ♀
O36.0123	Maternal care for anti-D [Rh] antibodies, second trimester, fetus 3 Ⓜ ♀
O36.0131	Maternal care for anti-D [Rh] antibodies, third trimester, fetus 1 Ⓜ ♀
O36.0132	Maternal care for anti-D [Rh] antibodies, third trimester, fetus 2 Ⓜ ♀
O36.0133	Maternal care for anti-D [Rh] antibodies, third trimester, fetus 3 Ⓜ ♀
O36.0911	Maternal care for other rhesus isoimmunization, first trimester, fetus 1 Ⓜ ♀
O36.0912	Maternal care for other rhesus isoimmunization, first trimester, fetus 2 Ⓜ ♀
O36.0913	Maternal care for other rhesus isoimmunization, first trimester, fetus 3 Ⓜ ♀
O36.0921	Maternal care for other rhesus isoimmunization, second trimester, fetus 1 Ⓜ ♀
O36.0922	Maternal care for other rhesus isoimmunization, second trimester, fetus 2 Ⓜ ♀
O36.0923	Maternal care for other rhesus isoimmunization, second trimester, fetus 3 Ⓜ ♀
O36.0931	Maternal care for other rhesus isoimmunization, third trimester, fetus 1 Ⓜ ♀

O36.0932	Maternal care for other rhesus isoimmunization, third trimester, fetus 2 Ⓜ ♀
O36.0933	Maternal care for other rhesus isoimmunization, third trimester, fetus 3 Ⓜ ♀
O36.1111	Maternal care for Anti-A sensitization, first trimester, fetus 1 Ⓜ ♀
O36.1112	Maternal care for Anti-A sensitization, first trimester, fetus 2 Ⓜ ♀
O36.1113	Maternal care for Anti-A sensitization, first trimester, fetus 3 Ⓜ ♀
O36.1121	Maternal care for Anti-A sensitization, second trimester, fetus 1 Ⓜ ♀
O36.1122	Maternal care for Anti-A sensitization, second trimester, fetus 2 Ⓜ ♀
O36.1123	Maternal care for Anti-A sensitization, second trimester, fetus 3 Ⓜ ♀
O36.1131	Maternal care for Anti-A sensitization, third trimester, fetus 1 Ⓜ ♀
O36.1132	Maternal care for Anti-A sensitization, third trimester, fetus 2 Ⓜ ♀
O36.1133	Maternal care for Anti-A sensitization, third trimester, fetus 3 Ⓜ ♀
O36.1911	Maternal care for other isoimmunization, first trimester, fetus 1 Ⓜ ♀
O36.1912	Maternal care for other isoimmunization, first trimester, fetus 2 Ⓜ ♀
O36.1913	Maternal care for other isoimmunization, first trimester, fetus 3 Ⓜ ♀
O36.1921	Maternal care for other isoimmunization, second trimester, fetus 1 Ⓜ ♀
O36.1922	Maternal care for other isoimmunization, second trimester, fetus 2 Ⓜ ♀
O36.1923	Maternal care for other isoimmunization, second trimester, fetus 3 Ⓜ ♀
O36.1931	Maternal care for other isoimmunization, third trimester, fetus 1 Ⓜ ♀
O36.1932	Maternal care for other isoimmunization, third trimester, fetus 2 Ⓜ ♀
O36.1933	Maternal care for other isoimmunization, third trimester, fetus 3 Ⓜ ♀
O36.21X1	Maternal care for hydrops fetalis, first trimester, fetus 1 Ⓜ ♀
O36.21X2	Maternal care for hydrops fetalis, first trimester, fetus 2 Ⓜ ♀
O36.21X3	Maternal care for hydrops fetalis, first trimester, fetus 3 Ⓜ ♀
O36.22X1	Maternal care for hydrops fetalis, second trimester, fetus 1 Ⓜ ♀
O36.22X2	Maternal care for hydrops fetalis, second trimester, fetus 2 Ⓜ ♀
O36.22X3	Maternal care for hydrops fetalis, second trimester, fetus 3 Ⓜ ♀
O36.23X1	Maternal care for hydrops fetalis, third trimester, fetus 1 Ⓜ ♀
O36.23X2	Maternal care for hydrops fetalis, third trimester, fetus 2 Ⓜ ♀
O36.23X3	Maternal care for hydrops fetalis, third trimester, fetus 3 Ⓜ ♀
O36.61X1	Maternal care for excessive fetal growth, first trimester, fetus 1 Ⓜ ♀
O36.61X2	Maternal care for excessive fetal growth, first trimester, fetus 2 Ⓜ ♀
O36.61X3	Maternal care for excessive fetal growth, first trimester, fetus 3 Ⓜ ♀
O36.62X1	Maternal care for excessive fetal growth, second trimester, fetus 1 Ⓜ ♀
O36.62X2	Maternal care for excessive fetal growth, second trimester, fetus 2 Ⓜ ♀
O36.62X3	Maternal care for excessive fetal growth, second trimester, fetus 3 Ⓜ ♀

O36.63X1	Maternal care for excessive fetal growth, third trimester, fetus 1 Ⓜ ♀
O36.63X2	Maternal care for excessive fetal growth, third trimester, fetus 2 Ⓜ ♀
O36.63X3	Maternal care for excessive fetal growth, third trimester, fetus 3 Ⓜ ♀
O36.8211	Fetal anemia and thrombocytopenia, first trimester, fetus 1 Ⓜ ♀
O36.8212	Fetal anemia and thrombocytopenia, first trimester, fetus 2 Ⓜ ♀
O36.8213	Fetal anemia and thrombocytopenia, first trimester, fetus 3 Ⓜ ♀
O36.8221	Fetal anemia and thrombocytopenia, second trimester, fetus 1 Ⓜ ♀
O36.8222	Fetal anemia and thrombocytopenia, second trimester, fetus 2 Ⓜ ♀
O36.8223	Fetal anemia and thrombocytopenia, second trimester, fetus 3 Ⓜ ♀
O36.8231	Fetal anemia and thrombocytopenia, third trimester, fetus 1 Ⓜ ♀
O36.8232	Fetal anemia and thrombocytopenia, third trimester, fetus 2 Ⓜ ♀
O36.8233	Fetal anemia and thrombocytopenia, third trimester, fetus 3 Ⓜ ♀
Z13.71	Encounter for nonprocreative screening for genetic disease carrier status
Z13.79	Encounter for other screening for genetic and chromosomal anomalies
Z36.0	Encounter for antenatal screening for chromosomal anomalies Ⓜ ♀
Z36.3	Encounter for antenatal screening for malformations Ⓜ ♀
Z36.5	Encounter for antenatal screening for isoimmunization Ⓜ ♀
Z36.89	Encounter for other specified antenatal screening Ⓜ ♀
Z36.8A	Encounter for antenatal screening for other genetic defects Ⓜ ♀

AMA: **59012** 2019,Jul,6; 2014,Jan,11

Relative Value Units/Medicare Edits

Non-Facility RVU	Work	PE	MP	Total
59012	3.44	1.48	0.95	5.87
Facility RVU	Work	PE	MP	Total
59012	3.44	1.48	0.95	5.87

	FUD	Status	MUE	Modifiers				IOM Reference
59012	0	A	2(3)	51	N/A	N/A	80*	None

* with documentation

Terms To Know

approach. Method or anatomical location used to gain access to a body organ or specific area for procedures.

cordocentesis. Aspiration of a sample of fetal blood from the umbilical vein under ultrasonic guidance. The specialized amniocentesis needle is placed into the cavity of the pregnant uterus and into the umbilical vessels. This procedure is done in the second or third trimester and is used for rapid chromosome analysis for fetal genetic information to help diagnose defects.

59015

59015 Chorionic villus sampling, any method

The physician aspirates placental tissue into a catheter

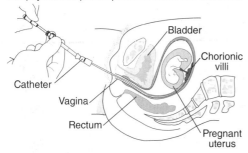

Labels: Bladder; Chorionic villi; Catheter; Vagina; Rectum; Pregnant uterus

Explanation

The physician samples tissue from the placenta for diagnostic purposes. This procedure uses ultrasonic guidance and can be done by any one of three methods. In the transcervical method, the physician inserts a catheter through the cervix and into the uterine cavity toward the placental site. A sample of the placenta (chorionic villus) is aspirated to obtain placental cells for analysis for chromosomal abnormalities. The procedure may also be performed transvaginally or transabdominally.

Coding Tips

For radiological supervision and interpretation, see 76945. For diagnostic amniocentesis, see 59000. For cordocentesis (intrauterine), see 59012. For chromosome analysis, see 88267.

ICD-10-CM Diagnostic Codes

O09.12	Supervision of pregnancy with history of ectopic pregnancy, second trimester ⓜ ♀
O09.13	Supervision of pregnancy with history of ectopic pregnancy, third trimester ⓜ ♀
O09.291	Supervision of pregnancy with other poor reproductive or obstetric history, first trimester ⓜ ♀
O09.292	Supervision of pregnancy with other poor reproductive or obstetric history, second trimester ⓜ ♀
O09.293	Supervision of pregnancy with other poor reproductive or obstetric history, third trimester ⓜ ♀
O09.511	Supervision of elderly primigravida, first trimester ⓜ ♀
O09.512	Supervision of elderly primigravida, second trimester ⓜ ♀
O09.513	Supervision of elderly primigravida, third trimester ⓜ ♀
O09.521	Supervision of elderly multigravida, first trimester ⓜ ♀
O09.522	Supervision of elderly multigravida, second trimester ⓜ ♀
O09.523	Supervision of elderly multigravida, third trimester ⓜ ♀
O09.621	Supervision of young multigravida, first trimester ⓜ ♀
O09.622	Supervision of young multigravida, second trimester ⓜ ♀
O09.623	Supervision of young multigravida, third trimester ⓜ ♀
O09.71	Supervision of high risk pregnancy due to social problems, first trimester ⓜ ♀
O09.72	Supervision of high risk pregnancy due to social problems, second trimester ⓜ ♀
O09.73	Supervision of high risk pregnancy due to social problems, third trimester ⓜ ♀
O09.811	Supervision of pregnancy resulting from assisted reproductive technology, first trimester ⓜ ♀
O09.812	Supervision of pregnancy resulting from assisted reproductive technology, second trimester ⓜ ♀
O09.813	Supervision of pregnancy resulting from assisted reproductive technology, third trimester ⓜ ♀
O09.821	Supervision of pregnancy with history of in utero procedure during previous pregnancy, first trimester ⓜ ♀
O09.822	Supervision of pregnancy with history of in utero procedure during previous pregnancy, second trimester ⓜ ♀
O09.823	Supervision of pregnancy with history of in utero procedure during previous pregnancy, third trimester ⓜ ♀
O09.891	Supervision of other high risk pregnancies, first trimester ⓜ ♀
O09.892	Supervision of other high risk pregnancies, second trimester ⓜ ♀
O09.893	Supervision of other high risk pregnancies, third trimester ⓜ ♀
O09.A1	Supervision of pregnancy with history of molar pregnancy, first trimester ⓜ ♀
O09.A2	Supervision of pregnancy with history of molar pregnancy, second trimester ⓜ ♀
O09.A3	Supervision of pregnancy with history of molar pregnancy, third trimester ⓜ ♀
O28.0	Abnormal hematological finding on antenatal screening of mother ⓜ ♀
O28.1	Abnormal biochemical finding on antenatal screening of mother ⓜ ♀
O28.2	Abnormal cytological finding on antenatal screening of mother ⓜ ♀
O28.3	Abnormal ultrasonic finding on antenatal screening of mother ⓜ ♀
O28.4	Abnormal radiological finding on antenatal screening of mother ⓜ ♀
O28.5	Abnormal chromosomal and genetic finding on antenatal screening of mother ⓜ ♀
O28.8	Other abnormal findings on antenatal screening of mother ⓜ ♀
O35.0XX1	Maternal care for (suspected) central nervous system malformation in fetus, fetus 1 ⓜ ♀
O35.0XX2	Maternal care for (suspected) central nervous system malformation in fetus, fetus 2 ⓜ ♀
O35.0XX3	Maternal care for (suspected) central nervous system malformation in fetus, fetus 3 ⓜ ♀
O35.1XX1	Maternal care for (suspected) chromosomal abnormality in fetus, fetus 1 ⓜ ♀
O35.1XX2	Maternal care for (suspected) chromosomal abnormality in fetus, fetus 2 ⓜ ♀
O35.1XX3	Maternal care for (suspected) chromosomal abnormality in fetus, fetus 3 ⓜ ♀
O35.2XX1	Maternal care for (suspected) hereditary disease in fetus, fetus 1 ⓜ ♀
O35.2XX2	Maternal care for (suspected) hereditary disease in fetus, fetus 2 ⓜ ♀
O35.2XX3	Maternal care for (suspected) hereditary disease in fetus, fetus 3 ⓜ ♀
O35.3XX1	Maternal care for (suspected) damage to fetus from viral disease in mother, fetus 1 ⓜ ♀
O35.3XX2	Maternal care for (suspected) damage to fetus from viral disease in mother, fetus 2 ⓜ ♀
O35.3XX3	Maternal care for (suspected) damage to fetus from viral disease in mother, fetus 3 ⓜ ♀

Maternity Care

O35.4XX1	Maternal care for (suspected) damage to fetus from alcohol, fetus 1 🔟 ♀
O35.4XX2	Maternal care for (suspected) damage to fetus from alcohol, fetus 2 🔟 ♀
O35.4XX3	Maternal care for (suspected) damage to fetus from alcohol, fetus 3 🔟 ♀
O35.8XX1	Maternal care for other (suspected) fetal abnormality and damage, fetus 1 🔟 ♀
O35.8XX2	Maternal care for other (suspected) fetal abnormality and damage, fetus 2 🔟 ♀
O35.8XX3	Maternal care for other (suspected) fetal abnormality and damage, fetus 3 🔟 ♀
O36.80X1	Pregnancy with inconclusive fetal viability, fetus 1 🔟 ♀
O36.80X2	Pregnancy with inconclusive fetal viability, fetus 2 🔟 ♀
O36.80X3	Pregnancy with inconclusive fetal viability, fetus 3 🔟 ♀
Z03.71	Encounter for suspected problem with amniotic cavity and membrane ruled out 🔟 ♀
Z03.72	Encounter for suspected placental problem ruled out 🔟 ♀
Z03.73	Encounter for suspected fetal anomaly ruled out 🔟 ♀
Z03.79	Encounter for other suspected maternal and fetal conditions ruled out 🔟 ♀
Z13.71	Encounter for nonprocreative screening for genetic disease carrier status
Z13.79	Encounter for other screening for genetic and chromosomal anomalies
Z36.0	Encounter for antenatal screening for chromosomal anomalies 🔟 ♀
Z36.3	Encounter for antenatal screening for malformations 🔟 ♀
Z36.89	Encounter for other specified antenatal screening 🔟 ♀
Z36.8A	Encounter for antenatal screening for other genetic defects 🔟 ♀

AMA: 59015 2019,Jul,6; 2018,Jan,8; 2017,Jan,8; 2016,Jan,13; 2015,Jan,16; 2014,Jan,11

Relative Value Units/Medicare Edits

Non-Facility RVU	Work	PE	MP	Total
59015	2.2	1.71	0.6	4.51
Facility RVU	Work	PE	MP	Total
59015	2.2	1.02	0.6	3.82

	FUD	Status	MUE	Modifiers				IOM Reference
59015	0	A	2(3)	51	N/A	N/A	80*	None

* with documentation

59020

59020 Fetal contraction stress test

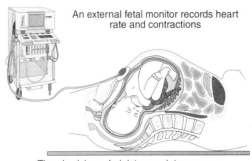

An external fetal monitor records heart rate and contractions

The physician administers an intravenous injection to induce contractions (stress)

Explanation

The physician evaluates fetal response to induced contractions in the mother. The physician applies external fetal monitors to the maternal abdominal wall. Pitocin is given intravenously to the mother to cause uterine contractions. The fetal heart rate and uterine contractions are monitored and recorded for 20 minutes to determine the effect of contractions on the fetus. This procedure is usually performed during the third trimester.

Coding Tips

For a fetal non-stress test, see 59025; fetal scalp blood sampling, see 59030.

ICD-10-CM Diagnostic Codes

O09.03	Supervision of pregnancy with history of infertility, third trimester 🔟 ♀
O12.03	Gestational edema, third trimester 🔟 ♀
O12.13	Gestational proteinuria, third trimester 🔟 ♀
O12.23	Gestational edema with proteinuria, third trimester 🔟 ♀
O14.12	Severe pre-eclampsia, second trimester 🔟 ♀
O14.13	Severe pre-eclampsia, third trimester 🔟 ♀
O14.22	HELLP syndrome (HELLP), second trimester 🔟 ♀
O14.23	HELLP syndrome (HELLP), third trimester 🔟 ♀
O15.02	Eclampsia complicating pregnancy, second trimester 🔟 ♀
O15.03	Eclampsia complicating pregnancy, third trimester 🔟 ♀
O15.1	Eclampsia complicating labor 🔟 ♀
O20.0	Threatened abortion 🔟 ♀
O30.013	Twin pregnancy, monochorionic/monoamniotic, third trimester 🔟 ♀
O30.033	Twin pregnancy, monochorionic/diamniotic, third trimester 🔟 ♀
O30.043	Twin pregnancy, dichorionic/diamniotic, third trimester 🔟 ♀
O30.113	Triplet pregnancy with two or more monochorionic fetuses, third trimester 🔟 ♀
O30.123	Triplet pregnancy with two or more monoamniotic fetuses, third trimester 🔟 ♀
O35.1XX1	Maternal care for (suspected) chromosomal abnormality in fetus, fetus 1 🔟 ♀
O35.1XX2	Maternal care for (suspected) chromosomal abnormality in fetus, fetus 2 🔟 ♀
O35.1XX3	Maternal care for (suspected) chromosomal abnormality in fetus, fetus 3 🔟 ♀

O35.2XX1	Maternal care for (suspected) hereditary disease in fetus, fetus 1 Ⓜ ♀	
O35.2XX2	Maternal care for (suspected) hereditary disease in fetus, fetus 2 Ⓜ ♀	
O35.2XX3	Maternal care for (suspected) hereditary disease in fetus, fetus 3 Ⓜ ♀	
O36.80X1	Pregnancy with inconclusive fetal viability, fetus 1 Ⓜ ♀	
O36.80X2	Pregnancy with inconclusive fetal viability, fetus 2 Ⓜ ♀	
O36.80X3	Pregnancy with inconclusive fetal viability, fetus 3 Ⓜ ♀	
O40.1XX1	Polyhydramnios, first trimester, fetus 1 Ⓜ ♀	
O40.1XX2	Polyhydramnios, first trimester, fetus 2 Ⓜ ♀	
O40.1XX3	Polyhydramnios, first trimester, fetus 3 Ⓜ ♀	
O40.2XX1	Polyhydramnios, second trimester, fetus 1 Ⓜ ♀	
O40.2XX2	Polyhydramnios, second trimester, fetus 2 Ⓜ ♀	
O40.2XX3	Polyhydramnios, second trimester, fetus 3 Ⓜ ♀	
O40.3XX1	Polyhydramnios, third trimester, fetus 1 Ⓜ ♀	
O40.3XX2	Polyhydramnios, third trimester, fetus 2 Ⓜ ♀	
O40.3XX3	Polyhydramnios, third trimester, fetus 3 Ⓜ ♀	
O41.01X1	Oligohydramnios, first trimester, fetus 1 Ⓜ ♀	
O41.01X2	Oligohydramnios, first trimester, fetus 2 Ⓜ ♀	
O41.01X3	Oligohydramnios, first trimester, fetus 3 Ⓜ ♀	
O41.02X1	Oligohydramnios, second trimester, fetus 1 Ⓜ ♀	
O41.02X2	Oligohydramnios, second trimester, fetus 2 Ⓜ ♀	
O41.02X3	Oligohydramnios, second trimester, fetus 3 Ⓜ ♀	
O41.03X1	Oligohydramnios, third trimester, fetus 1 Ⓜ ♀	
O41.03X2	Oligohydramnios, third trimester, fetus 2 Ⓜ ♀	
O41.03X3	Oligohydramnios, third trimester, fetus 3 Ⓜ ♀	
O44.03	Complete placenta previa NOS or without hemorrhage, third trimester Ⓜ ♀	
O44.13	Complete placenta previa with hemorrhage, third trimester Ⓜ ♀	
O45.012	Premature separation of placenta with afibrinogenemia, second trimester Ⓜ ♀	
O45.013	Premature separation of placenta with afibrinogenemia, third trimester Ⓜ ♀	
O45.023	Premature separation of placenta with disseminated intravascular coagulation, third trimester Ⓜ ♀	
O46.013	Antepartum hemorrhage with afibrinogenemia, third trimester Ⓜ ♀	
O46.023	Antepartum hemorrhage with disseminated intravascular coagulation, third trimester Ⓜ ♀	
O61.0	Failed medical induction of labor Ⓜ ♀	
O61.1	Failed instrumental induction of labor Ⓜ ♀	
O62.4	Hypertonic, incoordinate, and prolonged uterine contractions Ⓜ ♀	
O63.0	Prolonged first stage (of labor) Ⓜ ♀	
O63.1	Prolonged second stage (of labor) Ⓜ ♀	
O68	Labor and delivery complicated by abnormality of fetal acid-base balance Ⓜ ♀	
O75.5	Delayed delivery after artificial rupture of membranes Ⓜ ♀	
O76	Abnormality in fetal heart rate and rhythm complicating labor and delivery Ⓜ ♀	
O77.0	Labor and delivery complicated by meconium in amniotic fluid Ⓜ ♀	
O77.1	Fetal stress in labor or delivery due to drug administration Ⓜ ♀	

AMA: **59020** 2019,Jul,6; 2018,Jan,8; 2017,Jan,8; 2016,Jan,13; 2015,Jan,16; 2014,Jan,11

Relative Value Units/Medicare Edits

Non-Facility RVU	Work	PE	MP	Total
59020	0.66	1.17	0.17	2.0
Facility RVU	**Work**	**PE**	**MP**	**Total**
59020	0.66	1.17	0.17	2.0

	FUD	Status	MUE	Modifiers				IOM Reference
59020	0	A	2(3)	N/A	N/A	N/A	80*	None

* with documentation

Terms To Know

eclampsia. Tetany and toxemia producing seizure activity or coma in a pregnant patient who most often has presented with prior preeclampsia (i.e., hypertension, albuminuria, and edema).

gestation. Carrying of offspring in the womb throughout the period of development of the fetus(es) during pregnancy.

oligohydramnios. Low amniotic fluid, occurring most frequently in the last trimester.

polyhydramnios. Excess amniotic fluid surrounding the fetus, typically defined as a total fluid volume of greater than 24.0 cc.

59025

59025 Fetal non-stress test

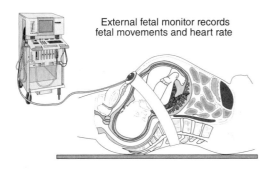

External fetal monitor records fetal movements and heart rate

Explanation

The physician evaluates fetal heart rate response to its own activity. The patient reports fetal movements as an external monitor records fetal heart rate changes. The procedure is noninvasive and takes 20 to 40 minutes to perform. If the fetus is not active, an acoustic device may be used to stimulate activity.

Coding Tips

Check with third-party payers to see if one fetal non-stress test is included in the total obstetrical package. For patients with conditions complicating pregnancy, 59025 is typically performed weekly for the last six weeks of gestation. The non-stress test is usually the primary means of surveillance for most conditions that place the fetus at high risk for placental insufficiency. Procedure 59025 has both a technical and professional component. To claim only the professional component, append modifier 26. To claim only the technical component, append modifier TC. To claim the complete procedure (i.e., both the professional and technical components), submit without a modifier. For fetal contraction stress test, see 59020.

ICD-10-CM Diagnostic Codes

O09.01	Supervision of pregnancy with history of infertility, first trimester ⓜ ♀
O09.02	Supervision of pregnancy with history of infertility, second trimester ⓜ ♀
O09.03	Supervision of pregnancy with history of infertility, third trimester ⓜ ♀
O09.11	Supervision of pregnancy with history of ectopic pregnancy, first trimester ⓜ ♀
O09.12	Supervision of pregnancy with history of ectopic pregnancy, second trimester ⓜ ♀
O09.13	Supervision of pregnancy with history of ectopic pregnancy, third trimester ⓜ ♀
O09.211	Supervision of pregnancy with history of pre-term labor, first trimester ⓜ ♀
O09.212	Supervision of pregnancy with history of pre-term labor, second trimester ⓜ ♀
O09.213	Supervision of pregnancy with history of pre-term labor, third trimester ⓜ ♀
O09.511	Supervision of elderly primigravida, first trimester ⓜ ♀
O09.512	Supervision of elderly primigravida, second trimester ⓜ ♀
O09.513	Supervision of elderly primigravida, third trimester ⓜ ♀
O09.611	Supervision of young primigravida, first trimester ⓜ ♀
O09.612	Supervision of young primigravida, second trimester ⓜ ♀
O09.613	Supervision of young primigravida, third trimester ⓜ ♀

O12.01	Gestational edema, first trimester ⓜ ♀
O12.02	Gestational edema, second trimester ⓜ ♀
O12.03	Gestational edema, third trimester ⓜ ♀
O12.11	Gestational proteinuria, first trimester ⓜ ♀
O12.12	Gestational proteinuria, second trimester ⓜ ♀
O12.13	Gestational proteinuria, third trimester ⓜ ♀
O12.21	Gestational edema with proteinuria, first trimester ⓜ ♀
O12.22	Gestational edema with proteinuria, second trimester ⓜ ♀
O12.23	Gestational edema with proteinuria, third trimester ⓜ ♀
O13.1	Gestational [pregnancy-induced] hypertension without significant proteinuria, first trimester ⓜ ♀
O13.2	Gestational [pregnancy-induced] hypertension without significant proteinuria, second trimester ⓜ ♀
O13.3	Gestational [pregnancy-induced] hypertension without significant proteinuria, third trimester ⓜ ♀
O14.12	Severe pre-eclampsia, second trimester ⓜ ♀
O14.13	Severe pre-eclampsia, third trimester ⓜ ♀
O14.22	HELLP syndrome (HELLP), second trimester ⓜ ♀
O14.23	HELLP syndrome (HELLP), third trimester ⓜ ♀
O15.02	Eclampsia complicating pregnancy, second trimester ⓜ ♀
O15.03	Eclampsia complicating pregnancy, third trimester ⓜ ♀
O15.1	Eclampsia complicating labor ⓜ ♀
O20.0	Threatened abortion ⓜ ♀
O21.1	Hyperemesis gravidarum with metabolic disturbance ⓜ ♀
O21.2	Late vomiting of pregnancy ⓜ ♀
O24.410	Gestational diabetes mellitus in pregnancy, diet controlled ⓜ ♀
O24.414	Gestational diabetes mellitus in pregnancy, insulin controlled ⓜ ♀
O30.011	Twin pregnancy, monochorionic/monoamniotic, first trimester ⓜ ♀
O30.012	Twin pregnancy, monochorionic/monoamniotic, second trimester ⓜ ♀
O30.013	Twin pregnancy, monochorionic/monoamniotic, third trimester ⓜ ♀
O30.031	Twin pregnancy, monochorionic/diamniotic, first trimester ⓜ ♀
O30.032	Twin pregnancy, monochorionic/diamniotic, second trimester ⓜ ♀
O30.033	Twin pregnancy, monochorionic/diamniotic, third trimester ⓜ ♀
O30.041	Twin pregnancy, dichorionic/diamniotic, first trimester ⓜ ♀
O30.042	Twin pregnancy, dichorionic/diamniotic, second trimester ⓜ ♀
O30.043	Twin pregnancy, dichorionic/diamniotic, third trimester ⓜ ♀
O30.111	Triplet pregnancy with two or more monochorionic fetuses, first trimester ⓜ ♀
O30.112	Triplet pregnancy with two or more monochorionic fetuses, second trimester ⓜ ♀
O30.113	Triplet pregnancy with two or more monochorionic fetuses, third trimester ⓜ ♀
O30.121	Triplet pregnancy with two or more monoamniotic fetuses, first trimester ⓜ ♀
O30.122	Triplet pregnancy with two or more monoamniotic fetuses, second trimester ⓜ ♀
O30.123	Triplet pregnancy with two or more monoamniotic fetuses, third trimester ⓜ ♀
O36.80X1	Pregnancy with inconclusive fetal viability, fetus 1 ⓜ ♀
O36.80X2	Pregnancy with inconclusive fetal viability, fetus 2 ⓜ ♀

O36.80X3	Pregnancy with inconclusive fetal viability, fetus 3 Ⓜ ♀
O40.1XX1	Polyhydramnios, first trimester, fetus 1 Ⓜ ♀
O40.1XX2	Polyhydramnios, first trimester, fetus 2 Ⓜ ♀
O40.1XX3	Polyhydramnios, first trimester, fetus 3 Ⓜ ♀
O40.2XX1	Polyhydramnios, second trimester, fetus 1 Ⓜ ♀
O40.2XX2	Polyhydramnios, second trimester, fetus 2 Ⓜ ♀
O40.2XX3	Polyhydramnios, second trimester, fetus 3 Ⓜ ♀
O40.3XX1	Polyhydramnios, third trimester, fetus 1 Ⓜ ♀
O40.3XX2	Polyhydramnios, third trimester, fetus 2 Ⓜ ♀
O40.3XX3	Polyhydramnios, third trimester, fetus 3 Ⓜ ♀
O41.01X1	Oligohydramnios, first trimester, fetus 1 Ⓜ ♀
O41.01X2	Oligohydramnios, first trimester, fetus 2 Ⓜ ♀
O41.01X3	Oligohydramnios, first trimester, fetus 3 Ⓜ ♀
O41.02X1	Oligohydramnios, second trimester, fetus 1 Ⓜ ♀
O41.02X2	Oligohydramnios, second trimester, fetus 2 Ⓜ ♀
O41.02X3	Oligohydramnios, second trimester, fetus 3 Ⓜ ♀
O41.03X1	Oligohydramnios, third trimester, fetus 1 Ⓜ ♀
O41.03X2	Oligohydramnios, third trimester, fetus 2 Ⓜ ♀
O41.03X3	Oligohydramnios, third trimester, fetus 3 Ⓜ ♀
O44.01	Complete placenta previa NOS or without hemorrhage, first trimester Ⓜ ♀
O44.02	Complete placenta previa NOS or without hemorrhage, second trimester Ⓜ ♀
O44.03	Complete placenta previa NOS or without hemorrhage, third trimester Ⓜ ♀
O44.11	Complete placenta previa with hemorrhage, first trimester Ⓜ ♀
O44.12	Complete placenta previa with hemorrhage, second trimester Ⓜ ♀
O44.13	Complete placenta previa with hemorrhage, third trimester Ⓜ ♀
O45.012	Premature separation of placenta with afibrinogenemia, second trimester Ⓜ ♀
O45.013	Premature separation of placenta with afibrinogenemia, third trimester Ⓜ ♀
O45.021	Premature separation of placenta with disseminated intravascular coagulation, first trimester Ⓜ ♀
O45.022	Premature separation of placenta with disseminated intravascular coagulation, second trimester Ⓜ ♀
O45.023	Premature separation of placenta with disseminated intravascular coagulation, third trimester Ⓜ ♀
O46.011	Antepartum hemorrhage with afibrinogenemia, first trimester Ⓜ ♀
O46.012	Antepartum hemorrhage with afibrinogenemia, second trimester Ⓜ ♀
O46.013	Antepartum hemorrhage with afibrinogenemia, third trimester Ⓜ ♀
O46.021	Antepartum hemorrhage with disseminated intravascular coagulation, first trimester Ⓜ ♀
O46.022	Antepartum hemorrhage with disseminated intravascular coagulation, second trimester Ⓜ ♀
O46.023	Antepartum hemorrhage with disseminated intravascular coagulation, third trimester Ⓜ ♀
O48.0	Post-term pregnancy Ⓜ ♀
O48.1	Prolonged pregnancy Ⓜ ♀
O67.0	Intrapartum hemorrhage with coagulation defect Ⓜ ♀
O67.8	Other intrapartum hemorrhage Ⓜ ♀
O68	Labor and delivery complicated by abnormality of fetal acid-base balance Ⓜ ♀
O76	Abnormality in fetal heart rate and rhythm complicating labor and delivery Ⓜ ♀

Associated HCPCS Codes

A4649	Surgical supply; miscellaneous

AMA: **59025** 2019,Jul,6; 2018,Jan,8; 2017,Jan,8; 2016,Jan,13; 2015,Jan,16; 2014,Jan,11

Relative Value Units/Medicare Edits

Non-Facility RVU	Work	PE	MP	Total
59025	0.53	0.72	0.12	1.37
Facility RVU	**Work**	**PE**	**MP**	**Total**
59025	0.53	0.72	0.12	1.37

	FUD	Status	MUE	Modifiers				IOM Reference
59025	0	A	2(3)	N/A	N/A	N/A	80*	None

* with documentation

Terms To Know

antepartum. Period of pregnancy between conception and the onset of labor.

eclampsia. Tetany and toxemia producing seizure activity or coma in a pregnant patient who most often has presented with prior preeclampsia (i.e., hypertension, albuminuria, and edema).

fetal nonstress test. Noninvasive procedure in which the patient reports fetal movements as an external monitor records fetal heart rate changes. Electrodes that measure both the fetal heart rate as well as the ability of the uterus to contract are placed on the maternal abdomen over a conducting jelly and the accelerations of the fetal heart rate with normal movement are gauged.

gestation. Carrying of offspring in the womb throughout the period of development of the fetus(es) during pregnancy.

HELLP syndrome. Group of symptoms occurring in pregnancy, including hemolysis, elevated liver enzymes, and a low platelet count. These symptoms may occur simultaneously with preeclampsia or may be present prior to the patient becoming preeclamptic.

monitoring. Recording of events; keep track, regulate, or control patient activities and record findings.

oligohydramnios. Low amniotic fluid, occurring most frequently in the last trimester.

polyhydramnios. Excess amniotic fluid surrounding the fetus, typically defined as a total fluid volume of greater than 24.0 cc.

59030

59030   Fetal scalp blood sampling

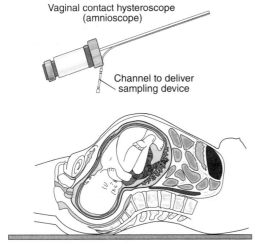

Vaginal contact hysteroscope
(amnioscope)

Channel to deliver
sampling device

The physician removes a sample of fetal scalp blood

Explanation

The physician samples fetal scalp blood during active labor for diagnostic purposes. This test, which assesses fetal distress during labor, must be done when the cervix is dilated more than 2 cm and the fetal vertex is low in the pelvis. The physician breaks the amniotic sac in patients whose water has not broken spontaneously and inserts an amnioscope through the vagina. An incision is made in the scalp with a narrow blade that penetrates no more than 2 mm. Blood is aspirated into a tube.

Coding Tips

For repeat fetal scalp blood sampling by the same physician or other qualified health care professional, report 59030 and append modifier 76; by a different clinician, append modifier 77. Note that 59030 can be reported in addition to the maternity package.

ICD-10-CM Diagnostic Codes

O11.1	Pre-existing hypertension with pre-eclampsia, first trimester ⋓ ♀
O11.2	Pre-existing hypertension with pre-eclampsia, second trimester ⋓ ♀
O11.3	Pre-existing hypertension with pre-eclampsia, third trimester ⋓ ♀
O11.4	Pre-existing hypertension with pre-eclampsia, complicating childbirth ⋓ ♀
O14.02	Mild to moderate pre-eclampsia, second trimester ⋓ ♀
O14.03	Mild to moderate pre-eclampsia, third trimester ⋓ ♀
O14.04	Mild to moderate pre-eclampsia, complicating childbirth ⋓ ♀
O14.12	Severe pre-eclampsia, second trimester ⋓ ♀
O14.13	Severe pre-eclampsia, third trimester ⋓ ♀
O14.14	Severe pre-eclampsia complicating childbirth ⋓ ♀
O14.22	HELLP syndrome (HELLP), second trimester ⋓ ♀
O14.23	HELLP syndrome (HELLP), third trimester ⋓ ♀
O14.24	HELLP syndrome, complicating childbirth ⋓ ♀
O15.02	Eclampsia complicating pregnancy, second trimester ⋓ ♀

O15.03	Eclampsia complicating pregnancy, third trimester ⋓ ♀
O15.1	Eclampsia complicating labor ⋓ ♀
O63.0	Prolonged first stage (of labor) ⋓ ♀
O63.1	Prolonged second stage (of labor) ⋓ ♀
O68	Labor and delivery complicated by abnormality of fetal acid-base balance ⋓ ♀
O75.5	Delayed delivery after artificial rupture of membranes ⋓ ♀
O76	Abnormality in fetal heart rate and rhythm complicating labor and delivery ⋓ ♀
O77.8	Labor and delivery complicated by other evidence of fetal stress ⋓ ♀

AMA: 59030 2019,Jul,6; 2014,Jan,11

Relative Value Units/Medicare Edits

Non-Facility RVU	Work	PE	MP	Total
59030	1.99	0.75	0.54	3.28
Facility RVU	**Work**	**PE**	**MP**	**Total**
59030	1.99	0.75	0.54	3.28

	FUD	Status	MUE	Modifiers				IOM Reference
59030	0	A	2(3)	51	N/A	N/A	80*	None

* with documentation

Terms To Know

complication. Condition arising after the beginning of observation and treatment that modifies the course of the patient's illness or the medical care required, or an undesired result or misadventure in medical care.

diagnostic. Examination or procedure to which the patient is subjected, or which is performed on materials derived from a hospital outpatient, to obtain information to aid in the assessment of a medical condition or the identification of a disease. Among these examinations and tests are diagnostic laboratory services such as hematology and chemistry, diagnostic x-rays, isotope studies, EKGs, pulmonary function studies, thyroid function tests, psychological tests, and other tests given to determine the nature and severity of an ailment or injury.

HELLP syndrome. Group of symptoms occurring in pregnancy, including hemolysis, elevated liver enzymes, and a low platelet count. These symptoms may occur simultaneously with preeclampsia or may be present prior to the patient becoming preeclamptic.

preeclampsia. Complication of pregnancy manifesting in the development of borderline hypertension, protein in the urine, and unresponsive swelling between the 20th week of pregnancy and the end of the first week following birth in mild to moderate cases. Severe preeclampsia presents with hypertension, associated with marked swelling, proteinuria, abdominal pain, and/or visual changes.

59050-59051

59050 Fetal monitoring during labor by consulting physician (ie, non-attending physician) with written report; supervision and interpretation
59051   interpretation only

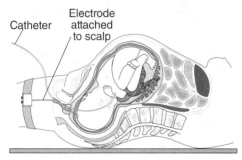
Internal fetal monitoring

Explanation

In 59050, a consultant other than the attending physician attaches an electrode directly to the presenting fetus' scalp via the cervix. The electrocardiographic impulses are transmitted to a cardiotachometer which converts the fetal electrocardiographic pattern into recorded electronic impulses. A catheter is inserted through the dilated cervix into the amniotic sac to measure and record the intervals between contractions. The procedure is supervised during labor until delivery. The recordings are analyzed and accompanied by an interpretive written report. In 59051, the consultant initiates the monitoring, provides the analysis and interpretive report, but does not supervise the patient during labor.

Coding Tips

These codes are to be used by the consulting (non-attending) physician only. They are part of the maternity package when performed by the attending physician.

ICD-10-CM Diagnostic Codes

O10.011	Pre-existing essential hypertension complicating pregnancy, first trimester ⓜ ♀
O10.012	Pre-existing essential hypertension complicating pregnancy, second trimester ⓜ ♀
O10.013	Pre-existing essential hypertension complicating pregnancy, third trimester ⓜ ♀
O10.111	Pre-existing hypertensive heart disease complicating pregnancy, first trimester ⓜ ♀
O10.112	Pre-existing hypertensive heart disease complicating pregnancy, second trimester ⓜ ♀
O10.113	Pre-existing hypertensive heart disease complicating pregnancy, third trimester ⓜ ♀
O10.12	Pre-existing hypertensive heart disease complicating childbirth ⓜ ♀
O10.22	Pre-existing hypertensive chronic kidney disease complicating childbirth ⓜ ♀
O10.32	Pre-existing hypertensive heart and chronic kidney disease complicating childbirth ⓜ ♀
O10.42	Pre-existing secondary hypertension complicating childbirth ⓜ ♀
O11.1	Pre-existing hypertension with pre-eclampsia, first trimester ⓜ ♀
O11.2	Pre-existing hypertension with pre-eclampsia, second trimester ⓜ ♀
O11.3	Pre-existing hypertension with pre-eclampsia, third trimester ⓜ ♀
O11.4	Pre-existing hypertension with pre-eclampsia, complicating childbirth ⓜ ♀
O12.04	Gestational edema, complicating childbirth ⓜ ♀
O12.14	Gestational proteinuria, complicating childbirth ⓜ ♀
O12.24	Gestational edema with proteinuria, complicating childbirth ⓜ ♀
O13.4	Gestational [pregnancy-induced] hypertension without significant proteinuria, complicating childbirth ⓜ ♀
O14.04	Mild to moderate pre-eclampsia, complicating childbirth ⓜ ♀
O14.14	Severe pre-eclampsia complicating childbirth ⓜ ♀
O14.24	HELLP syndrome, complicating childbirth ⓜ ♀
O15.1	Eclampsia complicating labor ⓜ ♀
O76	Abnormality in fetal heart rate and rhythm complicating labor and delivery ⓜ ♀

AMA: 59050 2019,Jul,6; 2014,Jan,11 **59051** 2019,Jul,6; 2014,Jan,11

Relative Value Units/Medicare Edits

Non-Facility RVU	Work	PE	MP	Total
59050	0.89	0.34	0.26	1.49
59051	0.74	0.28	0.21	1.23
Facility RVU	**Work**	**PE**	**MP**	**Total**
59050	0.89	0.34	0.26	1.49
59051	0.74	0.28	0.21	1.23

	FUD	Status	MUE	Modifiers				IOM Reference
59050	N/A	A	2(3)	N/A	N/A	N/A	80*	None
59051	N/A	A	2(3)	N/A	N/A	N/A	80*	

* with documentation

Terms To Know

eclampsia. Tetany and toxemia producing seizure activity or coma in a pregnant patient who most often has presented with prior preeclampsia (i.e., hypertension, albuminuria, and edema).

internal os. Opening through the cervix into the uterus.

placenta previa. Implantation of the placenta in the lower segment of the uterus, over or near the internal cervical os. In total previa, the cervical os is completely covered by the placenta; in partial previa, only a portion is covered.

preeclampsia. Complication of pregnancy manifesting in the development of borderline hypertension, protein in the urine, and unresponsive swelling between the 20th week of pregnancy and the end of the first week following birth in mild to moderate cases. Severe preeclampsia presents with hypertension, associated with marked swelling, proteinuria, abdominal pain, and/or visual changes.

Maternity Care

59070

59070 Transabdominal amnioinfusion, including ultrasound guidance

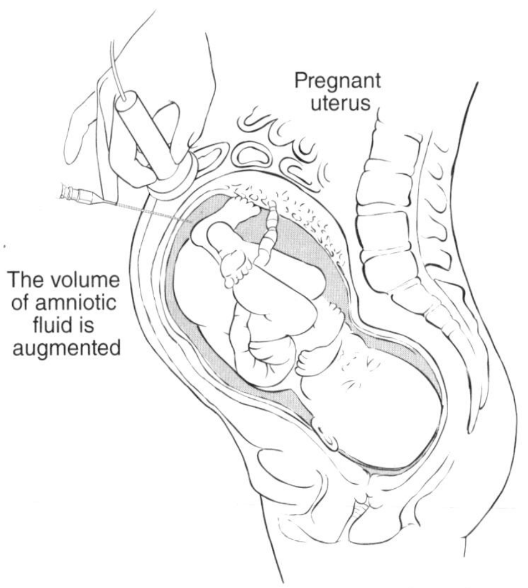
Pregnant uterus
The volume of amniotic fluid is augmented

Amniotic fluid (saline, or Ringer's solution) is infused into the pregnant uterus under ultrasound guidance

Explanation

The physician infuses an abnormally underhydrated amniotic sac with fluid. This may be done as a prophylactic measure for the fetus or to enhance sonographic imaging. An amniocentesis needle is placed through the mother's abdomen and advanced between extremities of the fetus under separately reportable ultrasound guidance. Normal sterile saline is infused into the uterus until the fetal anatomy is adequately visualized. The needle is removed and a detailed ultrasound is carried out.

Coding Tips

This procedure includes the radiology services of ultrasound guidance. This procedure may be necessary before more invasive procedures, such as fetal shunt placement, can be done. For fetal shunt placement, see 59076.

ICD-10-CM Diagnostic Codes

O36.21X1	Maternal care for hydrops fetalis, first trimester, fetus 1 M ♀
O36.21X2	Maternal care for hydrops fetalis, first trimester, fetus 2 M ♀
O36.21X3	Maternal care for hydrops fetalis, first trimester, fetus 3 M ♀
O36.22X1	Maternal care for hydrops fetalis, second trimester, fetus 1 M ♀
O36.22X2	Maternal care for hydrops fetalis, second trimester, fetus 2 M ♀
O36.22X3	Maternal care for hydrops fetalis, second trimester, fetus 3 M ♀
O36.23X1	Maternal care for hydrops fetalis, third trimester, fetus 1 M ♀
O36.23X2	Maternal care for hydrops fetalis, third trimester, fetus 2 M ♀
O36.23X3	Maternal care for hydrops fetalis, third trimester, fetus 3 M ♀
O36.71X1	Maternal care for viable fetus in abdominal pregnancy, first trimester, fetus 1 M ♀
O36.71X2	Maternal care for viable fetus in abdominal pregnancy, first trimester, fetus 2 M ♀
O36.71X3	Maternal care for viable fetus in abdominal pregnancy, first trimester, fetus 3 M ♀
O36.72X1	Maternal care for viable fetus in abdominal pregnancy, second trimester, fetus 1 M ♀
O36.72X2	Maternal care for viable fetus in abdominal pregnancy, second trimester, fetus 2 M ♀
O36.72X3	Maternal care for viable fetus in abdominal pregnancy, second trimester, fetus 3 M ♀
O36.73X1	Maternal care for viable fetus in abdominal pregnancy, third trimester, fetus 1 M ♀
O36.73X2	Maternal care for viable fetus in abdominal pregnancy, third trimester, fetus 2 M ♀
O36.73X3	Maternal care for viable fetus in abdominal pregnancy, third trimester, fetus 3 M ♀
O36.8911	Maternal care for other specified fetal problems, first trimester, fetus 1 M ♀
O36.8912	Maternal care for other specified fetal problems, first trimester, fetus 2 M ♀
O36.8913	Maternal care for other specified fetal problems, first trimester, fetus 3 M ♀
O36.8921	Maternal care for other specified fetal problems, second trimester, fetus 1 M ♀
O36.8922	Maternal care for other specified fetal problems, second trimester, fetus 2 M ♀
O36.8923	Maternal care for other specified fetal problems, second trimester, fetus 3 M ♀
O36.8931	Maternal care for other specified fetal problems, third trimester, fetus 1 M ♀
O36.8932	Maternal care for other specified fetal problems, third trimester, fetus 2 M ♀
O36.8933	Maternal care for other specified fetal problems, third trimester, fetus 3 M ♀
O41.01X1	Oligohydramnios, first trimester, fetus 1 M ♀
O41.01X2	Oligohydramnios, first trimester, fetus 2 M ♀
O41.01X3	Oligohydramnios, first trimester, fetus 3 M ♀
O41.02X1	Oligohydramnios, second trimester, fetus 1 M ♀
O41.02X2	Oligohydramnios, second trimester, fetus 2 M ♀
O41.02X3	Oligohydramnios, second trimester, fetus 3 M ♀
O41.03X1	Oligohydramnios, third trimester, fetus 1 M ♀
O41.03X2	Oligohydramnios, third trimester, fetus 2 M ♀
O41.03X3	Oligohydramnios, third trimester, fetus 3 M ♀
O42.011	Preterm premature rupture of membranes, onset of labor within 24 hours of rupture, first trimester M ♀
O42.012	Preterm premature rupture of membranes, onset of labor within 24 hours of rupture, second trimester M ♀
O42.013	Preterm premature rupture of membranes, onset of labor within 24 hours of rupture, third trimester M ♀
O42.02	Full-term premature rupture of membranes, onset of labor within 24 hours of rupture M ♀
O42.111	Preterm premature rupture of membranes, onset of labor more than 24 hours following rupture, first trimester M ♀
O42.112	Preterm premature rupture of membranes, onset of labor more than 24 hours following rupture, second trimester M ♀
O42.113	Preterm premature rupture of membranes, onset of labor more than 24 hours following rupture, third trimester M ♀
O43.891	Other placental disorders, first trimester M ♀
O43.892	Other placental disorders, second trimester M ♀
O43.893	Other placental disorders, third trimester M ♀
O68	Labor and delivery complicated by abnormality of fetal acid-base balance M ♀
O69.0XX0	Labor and delivery complicated by prolapse of cord, not applicable or unspecified M ♀

O69.1XX0	Labor and delivery complicated by cord around neck, with compression, not applicable or unspecified ⓜ ♀
O69.2XX0	Labor and delivery complicated by other cord entanglement, with compression, not applicable or unspecified ⓜ ♀
O76	Abnormality in fetal heart rate and rhythm complicating labor and delivery ⓜ ♀
O77.0	Labor and delivery complicated by meconium in amniotic fluid ⓜ ♀
O77.1	Fetal stress in labor or delivery due to drug administration ⓜ ♀
O77.8	Labor and delivery complicated by other evidence of fetal stress ⓜ ♀

AMA: 59070 2019,Jul,6; 2018,Jan,8; 2017,Jan,8; 2016,Jan,13; 2015,Jan,16; 2014,Jan,11

Relative Value Units/Medicare Edits

Non-Facility RVU	Work	PE	MP	Total
59070	5.24	4.94	1.44	11.62
Facility RVU	Work	PE	MP	Total
59070	5.24	2.31	1.44	8.99

	FUD	Status	MUE	Modifiers				IOM Reference
59070	0	A	2(3)	51	N/A	N/A	80	None

* with documentation

Terms To Know

hypoplasia. Condition in which there is underdevelopment of an organ or tissue.

meconium. First stool passed by a fetus, sometimes while still in the uterus. In this event, the meconium combines with the maternal amniotic fluid. Complications may occur if meconium is aspirated by the fetus while in utero or at the time of birth.

oligohydramnios. Low amniotic fluid, occurring most frequently in the last trimester.

prolapse. Falling, sliding, or sinking of an organ from its normal location in the body.

ultrasound. Imaging using ultra-high sound frequency bounced off body structures.

59072

59072 Fetal umbilical cord occlusion, including ultrasound guidance

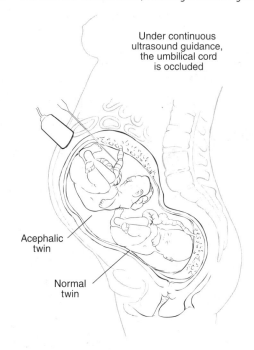

Under continuous ultrasound guidance, the umbilical cord is occluded

Acephalic twin

Normal twin

Explanation

Fetal umbilical cord occlusion is carried out in cases of complicated monochorionic multiple gestation pregnancies or in cases to terminate a pregnancy due to a birth defect. Ultrasound is used to locate access to the umbilical cord, avoiding the placenta. Using ultrasound guidance, small forceps are advanced into the uterus and the cord of the affected fetus is identified and grasped. The umbilical cord may be ligated, occluded, or compressed. Complete absence of flow through the cord is confirmed and the instruments are removed.

Coding Tips

This procedure includes ultrasound guidance.

ICD-10-CM Diagnostic Codes

O30.011	Twin pregnancy, monochorionic/monoamniotic, first trimester ⓜ ♀
O30.012	Twin pregnancy, monochorionic/monoamniotic, second trimester ⓜ ♀
O30.013	Twin pregnancy, monochorionic/monoamniotic, third trimester ⓜ ♀
O30.021	Conjoined twin pregnancy, first trimester ⓜ ♀
O30.022	Conjoined twin pregnancy, second trimester ⓜ ♀
O30.023	Conjoined twin pregnancy, third trimester ⓜ ♀
O30.031	Twin pregnancy, monochorionic/diamniotic, first trimester ⓜ ♀
O30.032	Twin pregnancy, monochorionic/diamniotic, second trimester ⓜ ♀
O30.033	Twin pregnancy, monochorionic/diamniotic, third trimester ⓜ ♀
O30.041	Twin pregnancy, dichorionic/diamniotic, first trimester ⓜ ♀
O30.042	Twin pregnancy, dichorionic/diamniotic, second trimester ⓜ ♀
O30.043	Twin pregnancy, dichorionic/diamniotic, third trimester ⓜ ♀
O30.111	Triplet pregnancy with two or more monochorionic fetuses, first trimester ⓜ ♀

Maternity Care

O30.112	Triplet pregnancy with two or more monochorionic fetuses, second trimester ⓜ ♀
O30.113	Triplet pregnancy with two or more monochorionic fetuses, third trimester ⓜ ♀
O30.121	Triplet pregnancy with two or more monoamniotic fetuses, first trimester ⓜ ♀
O30.122	Triplet pregnancy with two or more monoamniotic fetuses, second trimester ⓜ ♀
O30.123	Triplet pregnancy with two or more monoamniotic fetuses, third trimester ⓜ ♀
O30.131	Triplet pregnancy, trichorionic/triamniotic, first trimester ⓜ ♀
O30.132	Triplet pregnancy, trichorionic/triamniotic, second trimester ⓜ ♀
O30.133	Triplet pregnancy, trichorionic/triamniotic, third trimester ⓜ ♀
O30.811	Other specified multiple gestation with two or more monochorionic fetuses, first trimester ⓜ ♀
O30.812	Other specified multiple gestation with two or more monochorionic fetuses, second trimester ⓜ ♀
O30.813	Other specified multiple gestation with two or more monochorionic fetuses, third trimester ⓜ ♀
O30.821	Other specified multiple gestation with two or more monoamniotic fetuses, first trimester ⓜ ♀
O30.822	Other specified multiple gestation with two or more monoamniotic fetuses, second trimester ⓜ ♀
O30.823	Other specified multiple gestation with two or more monoamniotic fetuses, third trimester ⓜ ♀
O31.31X1	Continuing pregnancy after elective fetal reduction of one fetus or more, first trimester, fetus 1 ⓜ ♀
O31.31X2	Continuing pregnancy after elective fetal reduction of one fetus or more, first trimester, fetus 2 ⓜ ♀
O31.31X3	Continuing pregnancy after elective fetal reduction of one fetus or more, first trimester, fetus 3 ⓜ ♀
O31.32X1	Continuing pregnancy after elective fetal reduction of one fetus or more, second trimester, fetus 1 ⓜ ♀
O31.32X2	Continuing pregnancy after elective fetal reduction of one fetus or more, second trimester, fetus 2 ⓜ ♀
O31.32X3	Continuing pregnancy after elective fetal reduction of one fetus or more, second trimester, fetus 3 ⓜ ♀
O31.33X1	Continuing pregnancy after elective fetal reduction of one fetus or more, third trimester, fetus 1 ⓜ ♀
O31.33X2	Continuing pregnancy after elective fetal reduction of one fetus or more, third trimester, fetus 2 ⓜ ♀
O31.33X3	Continuing pregnancy after elective fetal reduction of one fetus or more, third trimester, fetus 3 ⓜ ♀
O31.8X11	Other complications specific to multiple gestation, first trimester, fetus 1 ⓜ ♀
O31.8X12	Other complications specific to multiple gestation, first trimester, fetus 2 ⓜ ♀
O31.8X13	Other complications specific to multiple gestation, first trimester, fetus 3 ⓜ ♀
O31.8X21	Other complications specific to multiple gestation, second trimester, fetus 1 ⓜ ♀
O31.8X22	Other complications specific to multiple gestation, second trimester, fetus 2 ⓜ ♀
O31.8X23	Other complications specific to multiple gestation, second trimester, fetus 3 ⓜ ♀
O31.8X31	Other complications specific to multiple gestation, third trimester, fetus 1 ⓜ ♀
O31.8X32	Other complications specific to multiple gestation, third trimester, fetus 2 ⓜ ♀
O31.8X33	Other complications specific to multiple gestation, third trimester, fetus 3 ⓜ ♀

AMA: **59072** 2019,Jul,6; 2018,Jan,8; 2017,Jan,8; 2016,Jan,13; 2015,Jan,16; 2014,Jan,11

Relative Value Units/Medicare Edits

Non-Facility RVU	Work	PE	MP	Total
59072	8.99	3.73	2.48	15.2
Facility RVU	**Work**	**PE**	**MP**	**Total**
59072	8.99	3.73	2.48	15.2

	FUD	Status	MUE	Modifiers				IOM Reference
59072	0	A	2(3)	51	N/A	N/A	N/A	None

* with documentation

Terms To Know

fetus. Unborn offspring past the embryonic stage that has developed major structures. It is the period defined from nine weeks after fertilization until birth.

ligation. Tying off a blood vessel or duct with a suture or a soft, thin wire.

occlusion. Constriction, closure, or blockage of a passage.

oligohydramnios. Low amniotic fluid, occurring most frequently in the last trimester.

polyhydramnios. Excess amniotic fluid surrounding the fetus, typically defined as a total fluid volume of greater than 24.0 cc.

ultrasound. Imaging using ultra-high sound frequency bounced off body structures.

Maternity Care

59074

59074 Fetal fluid drainage (eg, vesicocentesis, thoracocentesis, paracentesis), including ultrasound guidance

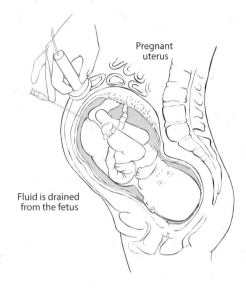

Pregnant uterus

Fluid is drained from the fetus

Explanation

Fetal fluid drainage is done in cases of pleural effusions or pulmonary cysts, and especially in fetal megavesica, a rare syndrome caused by functional obstruction of the fetal urethra. The fetus' bladder is enlarged due to the megavesica. Oligohydramnios, dilation of the lower and upper urinary tract, and hydronephrosis may also be present. Pulmonary hypoplasia can result and lead to hypoplastic abdominal musculature, urinary tract anomalies, and cryptorchidism. The fetal urinary bladder is emptied by transabdominal intrauterine vesicocentesis. Under continual ultrasound guidance, a 20 to 22 gauge needle is inserted through the mother's abdomen and advanced into the fetus' bladder. Fetal urine is aspirated and sent to the lab for analysis of urinary electrolytes and to determine renal function. The needle is removed and the patient kept for monitoring for up to another hour to check for refilling in the bladder. Similar fluid drainage is done by transabdominal intrauterine thoracocentesis for fetal pleural effusion.

Coding Tips

This procedure includes ultrasound guidance.

ICD-10-CM Diagnostic Codes

O35.8XX1	Maternal care for other (suspected) fetal abnormality and damage, fetus 1 **M** ♀
O35.8XX2	Maternal care for other (suspected) fetal abnormality and damage, fetus 2 **M** ♀
O35.8XX3	Maternal care for other (suspected) fetal abnormality and damage, fetus 3 **M** ♀
O36.21X1	Maternal care for hydrops fetalis, first trimester, fetus 1 **M** ♀
O36.21X2	Maternal care for hydrops fetalis, first trimester, fetus 2 **M** ♀
O36.21X3	Maternal care for hydrops fetalis, first trimester, fetus 3 **M** ♀
O36.22X1	Maternal care for hydrops fetalis, second trimester, fetus 1 **M** ♀
O36.22X2	Maternal care for hydrops fetalis, second trimester, fetus 2 **M** ♀
O36.22X3	Maternal care for hydrops fetalis, second trimester, fetus 3 **M** ♀
O36.23X1	Maternal care for hydrops fetalis, third trimester, fetus 1 **M** ♀
O36.23X2	Maternal care for hydrops fetalis, third trimester, fetus 2 **M** ♀
O36.23X3	Maternal care for hydrops fetalis, third trimester, fetus 3 **M** ♀

O41.01X1	Oligohydramnios, first trimester, fetus 1 **M** ♀
O41.01X2	Oligohydramnios, first trimester, fetus 2 **M** ♀
O41.01X3	Oligohydramnios, first trimester, fetus 3 **M** ♀
O41.02X1	Oligohydramnios, second trimester, fetus 1 **M** ♀
O41.02X2	Oligohydramnios, second trimester, fetus 2 **M** ♀
O41.02X3	Oligohydramnios, second trimester, fetus 3 **M** ♀
O41.03X1	Oligohydramnios, third trimester, fetus 1 **M** ♀
O41.03X2	Oligohydramnios, third trimester, fetus 2 **M** ♀
O41.03X3	Oligohydramnios, third trimester, fetus 3 **M** ♀

AMA: **59074** 2019,Jul,6; 2018,Jan,8; 2017,Jan,8; 2016,Jan,13; 2015,Jan,16; 2014,Jan,11

Relative Value Units/Medicare Edits

Non-Facility RVU	Work	PE	MP	Total
59074	5.24	4.49	1.44	11.17
Facility RVU	**Work**	**PE**	**MP**	**Total**
59074	5.24	2.31	1.44	8.99

	FUD	Status	MUE	Modifiers				IOM Reference
59074	0	A	2(3)	51	N/A	N/A	80	None

* with documentation

Terms To Know

aspirate. To withdraw fluid or air from a body cavity by suction.

centesis. Puncture, as with a needle, trocar, or aspirator, often done for withdrawing fluid from a cavity.

fetus. Unborn offspring past the embryonic stage that has developed major structures. It is the period defined from nine weeks after fertilization until birth.

hydronephrosis. Distension of the kidney caused by an accumulation of urine that cannot flow out due to an obstruction that may be caused by conditions such as kidney stones or vesicoureteral reflux.

oligohydramnios. Low amniotic fluid, occurring most frequently in the last trimester.

polyhydramnios. Excess amniotic fluid surrounding the fetus, typically defined as a total fluid volume of greater than 24.0 cc.

ultrasound. Imaging using ultra-high sound frequency bounced off body structures.

Maternity Care

59076

59076 Fetal shunt placement, including ultrasound guidance

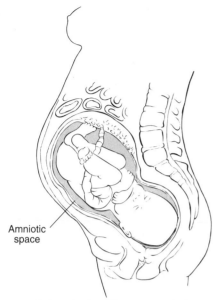

A shunt is placed from an area in the fetus that requires drainage (e.g., bladder) to the amniotic space surrounding the fetus

Explanation

Fetal shunt placement is performed for pleural or vesical amniotic shunting in cases of pleural effusion, pulmonary cysts, or fetal megavesica, where the bladder is enlarged because of urethra blockage. Shunting is done to supply continuous drainage when reaccumulation of fluid is not successfully treated by isolated vesicocentesis or thoracocentesis. Fluids can be drained into the amniotic cavity through a double pigtailed catheter. The entry site on the mother's abdomen is cleaned with antiseptic solution and local anesthetic is infiltrated down to the myometrium. Under ultrasound guidance, a metal cannula with a trocar is introduced transabdominally into the amniotic cavity and inserted through the fetal chest wall in the midthoracic region, into the effusion or cyst (if megavesical fluid accumulation is the problem, the shunt is placed into the bladder). The trocar is removed and the catheter is inserted into the cannula. A short introducer rod is used to place the proximal half of the catheter into the effusion or cyst. The cannula is gradually removed into the amniotic cavity where the other half of the catheter is pushed by a longer introducer. There is now a conduit for fluid drainage into the amniotic space. Placement of the shunt is confirmed, the instruments are removed, and the patient is monitored for one to two hours. Follow-up ultrasound scans are performed at weekly intervals to check drainage and determine if the effusions reaccumulate, in which case another shunt may be inserted. The drains are immediately clamped and removed after delivery.

Coding Tips

This procedure includes ultrasound guidance.

ICD-10-CM Diagnostic Codes

O35.8XX1	Maternal care for other (suspected) fetal abnormality and damage, fetus 1 🖪 ♀
O35.8XX2	Maternal care for other (suspected) fetal abnormality and damage, fetus 2 🖪 ♀
O35.8XX3	Maternal care for other (suspected) fetal abnormality and damage, fetus 3 🖪 ♀

O36.21X1	Maternal care for hydrops fetalis, first trimester, fetus 1 🖪 ♀
O36.21X2	Maternal care for hydrops fetalis, first trimester, fetus 2 🖪 ♀
O36.21X3	Maternal care for hydrops fetalis, first trimester, fetus 3 🖪 ♀
O36.22X1	Maternal care for hydrops fetalis, second trimester, fetus 1 🖪 ♀
O36.22X2	Maternal care for hydrops fetalis, second trimester, fetus 2 🖪 ♀
O36.22X3	Maternal care for hydrops fetalis, second trimester, fetus 3 🖪 ♀
O36.23X1	Maternal care for hydrops fetalis, third trimester, fetus 1 🖪 ♀
O36.23X2	Maternal care for hydrops fetalis, third trimester, fetus 2 🖪 ♀
O36.23X3	Maternal care for hydrops fetalis, third trimester, fetus 3 🖪 ♀
O41.01X1	Oligohydramnios, first trimester, fetus 1 🖪 ♀
O41.01X2	Oligohydramnios, first trimester, fetus 2 🖪 ♀
O41.01X3	Oligohydramnios, first trimester, fetus 3 🖪 ♀
O41.02X1	Oligohydramnios, second trimester, fetus 1 🖪 ♀
O41.02X2	Oligohydramnios, second trimester, fetus 2 🖪 ♀
O41.02X3	Oligohydramnios, second trimester, fetus 3 🖪 ♀
O41.03X1	Oligohydramnios, third trimester, fetus 1 🖪 ♀
O41.03X2	Oligohydramnios, third trimester, fetus 2 🖪 ♀
O41.03X3	Oligohydramnios, third trimester, fetus 3 🖪 ♀

AMA: 59076 2019,Jul,6; 2018,Jan,8; 2017,Jan,8; 2016,Jan,13; 2015,Jan,16; 2014,Jan,11

Relative Value Units/Medicare Edits

Non-Facility RVU	Work	PE	MP	Total
59076	8.99	3.73	2.48	15.2
Facility RVU	**Work**	**PE**	**MP**	**Total**
59076	8.99	3.73	2.48	15.2

	FUD	Status	MUE	Modifiers				IOM Reference
59076	0	A	2(3)	51	N/A	N/A	80	None

* with documentation

Terms To Know

cannula. Tube inserted into a blood vessel, duct, or body cavity to facilitate passage.

catheter. Flexible tube inserted into an area of the body for introducing or withdrawing fluid.

centesis. Puncture, as with a needle, trocar, or aspirator, often done for withdrawing fluid from a cavity.

shunt. Surgically created passage between blood vessels or other natural passages, such as an arteriovenous anastomosis, to divert or bypass blood flow from the normal channel.

Maternity Care

59100

59100   Hysterotomy, abdominal (eg, for hydatidiform mole, abortion)

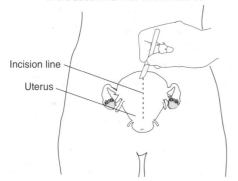

The physician removes an embryo or hydatidiform mole through an incision in the abdominal wall and the uterus

Incision line

Uterus

Explanation

The physician removes an embryo or hydatidiform mole through an incision in the abdominal wall and uterus. The surgery is similar to a cesarean section but the abdominal and uterine incisions are smaller. The lower abdominal wall is opened with a vertical or horizontal incision and the uterus is entered through the lower uterine segment. The physician removes the embryo or hydatidiform mole and may also remove any remaining membranes and placenta from the uterine cavity. Curettage of the uterine cavity may also be performed. The abdominal and uterine incisions are closed by suturing.

Coding Tips

Hysterotomy for abortion or for hydatidiform molar pregnancy is rarely performed. Suction curettage has replaced hysterotomy as the method of choice in the treatment of hydatidiform mole. For treatment of hydatidiform mole by suction curettage, see 59870. When tubal ligation is performed at the same time as hysterotomy, report 58611 with 59100. Because 58611 is a subsidiary or "in addition to" code, reimbursement reduction and modifier 51 do not apply.

ICD-10-CM Diagnostic Codes

O01.0	Classical hydatidiform mole	Ⓜ ♀
O01.1	Incomplete and partial hydatidiform mole	Ⓜ ♀
O02.0	Blighted ovum and nonhydatidiform mole	Ⓜ ♀
O02.1	Missed abortion	Ⓜ ♀
O02.89	Other abnormal products of conception	Ⓜ ♀

AMA: 59100 2019,Jul,6; 2014,Jan,11

Relative Value Units/Medicare Edits

Non-Facility RVU	Work	PE	MP	Total
59100	13.37	7.59	3.7	24.66
Facility RVU	Work	PE	MP	Total
59100	13.37	7.59	3.7	24.66

	FUD	Status	MUE	Modifiers				IOM Reference
59100	90	A	1(2)	51	N/A	62*	80	100-03,230.3

* with documentation

59120-59121

59120   Surgical treatment of ectopic pregnancy; tubal or ovarian, requiring salpingectomy and/or oophorectomy, abdominal or vaginal approach

59121   tubal or ovarian, without salpingectomy and/or oophorectomy

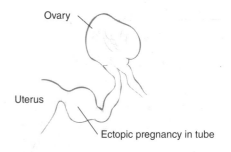

Ovary

Uterus

Ectopic pregnancy in tube

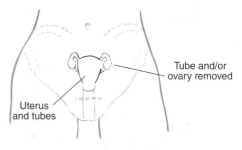

Tube and/or ovary removed

Uterus and tubes

Explanation

The physician treats a tubal or ovarian ectopic pregnancy by removing the fallopian tube and/or ovary. Through the vagina or through an incision in the lower abdomen, the physician explores the pelvic cavity, inspects the gestation site for bleeding, and removes all products of conception, clots, and free blood. If the tube is affected, it may be excised by cutting a small wedge of the uterine wall at the junction of the fallopian tube and body of the uterus. If the ovary is affected, it may be removed. Lysis of adhesions may be indicated and the pelvis lavaged with saline solution. If an abdominal approach is used, the incision is closed with sutures. In 59121, the physician removes an embryo from the tube or ovary. If the embryo is implanted in the fallopian tube, the physician may do one of the following: manually remove the embryo from the tube, make an incision to remove the embryo, or excise the section of the tube containing the embryo. If the embryo is implanted in the ovary, the physician resects the ovary to remove the embryo. Lysis of adhesions may be indicated and the pelvis lavaged with saline solution. The incision is closed with sutures.

Coding Tips

For surgical treatment of interstitial uterine ectopic pregnancy requiring total hysterectomy, see 59135; with partial resection, see 59136; cervical with evacuation, see 59140. For laparoscopic treatment of an ectopic pregnancy without removal of fallopian tubes and/or ovaries, see 59150; with removal of fallopian tubes, see 59151. Complications such as control of hemorrhage resulting from the ectopic pregnancy are not included and are reported separately.

ICD-10-CM Diagnostic Codes

O00.101	Right tubal pregnancy without intrauterine pregnancy	Ⓜ ♀
O00.102	Left tubal pregnancy without intrauterine pregnancy	Ⓜ ♀
O00.111	Right tubal pregnancy with intrauterine pregnancy	Ⓜ ♀
O00.112	Left tubal pregnancy with intrauterine pregnancy	Ⓜ ♀
O00.201	Right ovarian pregnancy without intrauterine pregnancy	Ⓜ ♀

Maternity Care

O00.202	Left ovarian pregnancy without intrauterine pregnancy Ⓜ ♀
O00.211	Right ovarian pregnancy with intrauterine pregnancy Ⓜ ♀
O00.212	Left ovarian pregnancy with intrauterine pregnancy Ⓜ ♀

AMA: **59120** 2019,Jul,6; 2014,Jan,11 **59121** 2019,Jul,6; 2014,Jan,11

Relative Value Units/Medicare Edits

Non-Facility RVU	Work	PE	MP	Total
59120	12.67	7.33	3.49	23.49
59121	12.74	7.27	3.51	23.52
Facility RVU	**Work**	**PE**	**MP**	**Total**
59120	12.67	7.33	3.49	23.49
59121	12.74	7.27	3.51	23.52

	FUD	Status	MUE	Modifiers				IOM Reference
59120	90	A	1(3)	51	N/A	62*	80	None
59121	90	A	1(3)	51	N/A	62*	80	

* with documentation

Terms To Know

approach. Method or anatomical location used to gain access to a body organ or specific area for procedures.

ectopic pregnancy. Fertilized ovum that implants and develops outside the uterus. The ovum may implant itself in different sites, such as the fallopian tube, the ovary, the abdomen, or the cervix.

embryo. Developing cells of a new organism that will become a fetus; the period defined from the fourth day after fertilization to the end of the eighth week.

oophorectomy. Surgical removal of all or part of one or both ovaries, either as open procedure or laparoscopically. Menstruation and childbearing ability continues when one ovary is removed.

salpingectomy. Removal of all or part of one or both of the fallopian tubes. Indications include infection, ectopic pregnancy, sterilization, or cancer. This procedure is often performed in combination with other open or laparoscopic procedures.

59130

| 59130 | Surgical treatment of ectopic pregnancy; abdominal pregnancy |

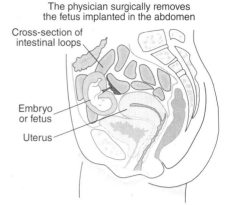

The physician surgically removes the fetus implanted in the abdomen

Cross-section of intestinal loops

Embryo or fetus

Uterus

Explanation

The physician removes an embryo or fetus implanted in the abdomen. The fertilized ovum may have implanted directly in the abdomen (primary) or it may have implanted after escaping from the tube through a rupture or through the fimbriated end (secondary). After making an abdominal incision, the physician surgically removes the fetus from the abdomen. The membranes are also removed and the cord is ligated near the placenta. The placenta is usually not removed unless attached to the fallopian tube, ovary, or uterine broad ligament. Abdominal lavage may also be indicated. The abdominal incision is closed with sutures. Although this procedure is rare, it can be done any time during gestation, even at or near term.

Coding Tips

For surgical treatment of an ectopic pregnancy with removal of fallopian tubes and/or ovaries, abdominal or vaginal approach, see 59120; without removal of fallopian tubes and/or ovaries, see 59121; interstitial uterine ectopic pregnancy requiring total hysterectomy, see 59135; with partial resection, see 59136; cervical with evacuation, see 59140. For laparoscopic treatment of an ectopic pregnancy without removal of fallopian tubes and/or ovaries, see 59150; with removal of fallopian tubes, see 59151. Complications such as control of hemorrhage resulting from the ectopic pregnancy are not included and are reported separately.

ICD-10-CM Diagnostic Codes

| O00.00 | Abdominal pregnancy without intrauterine pregnancy Ⓜ ♀ |
| O00.01 | Abdominal pregnancy with intrauterine pregnancy Ⓜ ♀ |

AMA: **59130** 2019,Jul,6; 2014,Jan,11

Relative Value Units/Medicare Edits

Non-Facility RVU	Work	PE	MP	Total
59130	15.08	8.14	4.16	27.38
Facility RVU	**Work**	**PE**	**MP**	**Total**
59130	15.08	8.14	4.16	27.38

	FUD	Status	MUE	Modifiers			IOM Reference
59130	90	A	1(3)	51	N/A	N/A	80*	None

* with documentation

59135

59135   Surgical treatment of ectopic pregnancy; interstitial, uterine pregnancy requiring total hysterectomy

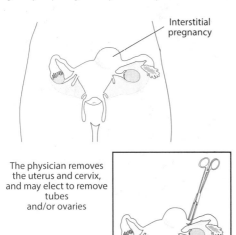

The physician removes the uterus and cervix, and may elect to remove tubes and/or ovaries

Explanation

The physician treats an interstitial pregnancy where the fertilized ovum has implanted in the portion of the tube that transverses the uterine wall by removing the uterus and cervix. Through an incision extending from just above the pubic hairline to the rib cage, the physician clamps and cuts free the supporting pedicles containing the tubes, ligaments, and arteries. The physician removes the uterus and cervix and may elect to remove the tubes and/or ovaries. Abdominal or pelvic lavage may also be indicated. The abdominal incision is closed with sutures.

Coding Tips

For surgical treatment of an ectopic pregnancy with removal of fallopian tubes and/or ovaries, abdominal or vaginal approach, see 59120; without removal of fallopian tubes and/or ovaries, see 59121; interstitial uterine ectopic pregnancy with partial resection, see 59136; cervical with evacuation, see 59140. For laparoscopic treatment of an ectopic pregnancy without removal of fallopian tubes and/or ovaries, see 59150; with removal of fallopian tubes, see 59151. Complications such as control of hemorrhage resulting from the ectopic pregnancy are not included and are reported separately.

ICD-10-CM Diagnostic Codes

O00.80	Other ectopic pregnancy without intrauterine pregnancy Ⓜ ♀
O00.81	Other ectopic pregnancy with intrauterine pregnancy Ⓜ ♀

AMA: 59135 2019,Jul,6; 2014,Jan,11

Relative Value Units/Medicare Edits

Non-Facility RVU	Work	PE	MP	Total
59135	14.92	8.02	4.13	27.07
Facility RVU	Work	PE	MP	Total
59135	14.92	8.02	4.13	27.07

	FUD	Status	MUE	Modifiers				IOM Reference
59135	90	A	1(3)	51	N/A	N/A	80*	None

* with documentation

59136

59136   Surgical treatment of ectopic pregnancy; interstitial, uterine pregnancy with partial resection of uterus

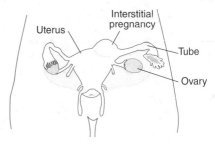

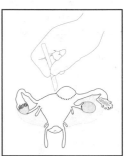

The physician resects the uterus to remove an interstitial ectopic pregnancy

Explanation

The physician treats an interstitial ectopic pregnancy where the fertilized ovum has implanted in the portion of the tube that transverses the uterine wall by partially resecting the uterus. Through an incision extending from just above the pubic hairline to the rib cage, the physician resects and reconstructs the uterine wall. The physician may also remove a portion or all of the fallopian tube. Abdominal or pelvic lavage may be indicated. The abdominal incision is closed with sutures.

Coding Tips

For surgical treatment of an ectopic pregnancy with removal of fallopian tubes and/or ovaries, abdominal or vaginal approach, see 59120; without removal of fallopian tubes and/or ovaries, see 59121; interstitial uterine ectopic pregnancy requiring total hysterectomy, see 59135; cervical with evacuation, see 59140. For laparoscopic treatment of an ectopic pregnancy without removal of fallopian tubes and/or ovaries, see 59150; with removal of fallopian tubes, see 59151. Complications such as control of hemorrhage resulting from the ectopic pregnancy are not included and are reported separately.

ICD-10-CM Diagnostic Codes

O00.80	Other ectopic pregnancy without intrauterine pregnancy Ⓜ ♀
O00.81	Other ectopic pregnancy with intrauterine pregnancy Ⓜ ♀

AMA: 59136 2019,Jul,6; 2014,Jan,11

Maternity Care

Relative Value Units/Medicare Edits

Non-Facility RVU	Work	PE	MP	Total
59136	14.25	7.77	3.94	25.96
Facility RVU	Work	PE	MP	Total
59136	14.25	7.77	3.94	25.96

	FUD	Status	MUE	Modifiers				IOM Reference
59136	90	A	1(3)	51	N/A	N/A	80	None

* with documentation

Terms To Know

cornua. Paired superior lateral extremities of the uterus that mark the entrance to the uterine tube.

ectopic pregnancy. Fertilized ovum that implants and develops outside the uterus. The ovum may implant itself in different sites, such as the fallopian tube, the ovary, the abdomen, or the cervix.

interstitial. Within the small spaces or gaps occurring in tissue or organs.

59140

59140   Surgical treatment of ectopic pregnancy; cervical, with evacuation

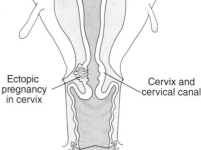

The physician removes a cervical ectopic pregnancy vaginally or abdominally

Ectopic pregnancy in cervix

Cervix and cervical canal

Explanation

The physician treats an ectopic pregnancy where the embryo has implanted in the cervix. If the pregnancy is less than 12 weeks gestation, the physician usually removes the embryo through the vagina. The physician ligates the hypogastric arteries or the cervical branches of the uterus to control bleeding. Curettage of the endocervix and endometrium may stop heavy bleeding. Sutures and gauze packing may also be necessary. If later than 12 weeks gestation, the physician may treat the cervical pregnancy by performing an abdominal hysterectomy. Through a horizontal incision just within the pubic hairline, the physician clamps and cuts free the supporting pedicles containing the tubes, ligaments, and arteries. The uterus is removed above the cervix, and the incision is closed by suturing.

Coding Tips

For surgical treatment of an ectopic pregnancy with removal of fallopian tubes and/or ovaries, abdominal or vaginal approach, see 59120; without removal of fallopian tubes and/or ovaries, see 59121; interstitial uterine ectopic pregnancy requiring total hysterectomy, see 59135; with partial resection, see 59136. For laparoscopic treatment of an ectopic pregnancy without removal of fallopian tubes and/or ovaries, see 59150; with removal of fallopian tubes, see 59151. Complications such as control of hemorrhage resulting from the ectopic pregnancy are not included and are reported separately.

ICD-10-CM Diagnostic Codes

O00.80	Other ectopic pregnancy without intrauterine pregnancy 🅼 ♀
O00.81	Other ectopic pregnancy with intrauterine pregnancy 🅼 ♀

AMA: 59140 2019,Jul,6; 2014,Jan,11

Relative Value Units/Medicare Edits

Non-Facility RVU	Work	PE	MP	Total
59140	5.94	4.35	1.64	11.93
Facility RVU	Work	PE	MP	Total
59140	5.94	4.35	1.64	11.93

	FUD	Status	MUE	Modifiers				IOM Reference
59140	90	A	1(2)	51	N/A	N/A	80	None

* with documentation

Maternity Care

59150

59150 Laparoscopic treatment of ectopic pregnancy; without salpingectomy and/or oophorectomy

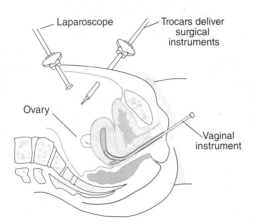

The physician removes a tubal ectopic pregnancy by laparoscopy

Laparoscope

Trocars deliver surgical instruments

Ovary

Vaginal instrument

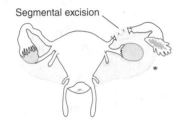

Segmental excision

Explanation

The physician treats an ectopic pregnancy by laparoscopy without salpingectomy and/or oophorectomy. The physician inserts an instrument through the vagina to grasp the cervix while passing another instrument through the cervix and into the uterus to manipulate the uterus. Next, the physician makes a 1 cm incision in the umbilicus through which the abdomen is inflated and a fiberoptic laparoscope is inserted. A second incision is made on the left or right side of the abdomen. After locating the site of the gestation, another small incision is made above the site. Instruments are passed into the abdomen through the incisions. The physician removes the ectopic pregnancy by making an incision in the tube or ovary or by segmental excision. The abdominal incisions are closed with sutures.

Coding Tips

If significant additional time and effort is documented, append modifier 22 and submit a cover letter and operative report. This code includes diagnostic laparoscopy performed by the physician. This code is appropriate for reporting this procedure when performed with any technique or combination of techniques (e.g., laser, hot cautery). For failed laparoscopic procedures followed by an open procedure, code the open procedure as the primary procedure and a diagnostic laparoscopy as a secondary procedure with modifier 51. For laparoscopic treatment of an ectopic pregnancy, with salpingectomy and/or oophorectomy, see 59151.

ICD-10-CM Diagnostic Codes

O00.00	Abdominal pregnancy without intrauterine pregnancy Ⓜ ♀
O00.01	Abdominal pregnancy with intrauterine pregnancy Ⓜ ♀
O00.101	Right tubal pregnancy without intrauterine pregnancy Ⓜ ♀
O00.102	Left tubal pregnancy without intrauterine pregnancy Ⓜ ♀
O00.111	Right tubal pregnancy with intrauterine pregnancy Ⓜ ♀
O00.112	Left tubal pregnancy with intrauterine pregnancy Ⓜ ♀
O00.201	Right ovarian pregnancy without intrauterine pregnancy Ⓜ ♀
O00.202	Left ovarian pregnancy without intrauterine pregnancy Ⓜ ♀
O00.211	Right ovarian pregnancy with intrauterine pregnancy Ⓜ ♀
O00.212	Left ovarian pregnancy with intrauterine pregnancy Ⓜ ♀
O00.80	Other ectopic pregnancy without intrauterine pregnancy Ⓜ ♀
O00.81	Other ectopic pregnancy with intrauterine pregnancy Ⓜ ♀

AMA: **59150** 2019,Jul,6; 2018,Jan,8; 2017,Jan,8; 2016,Jan,13; 2015,Jan,16; 2014,Jan,11

Relative Value Units/Medicare Edits

Non-Facility RVU	Work	PE	MP	Total
59150	12.29	7.11	3.39	22.79
Facility RVU	**Work**	**PE**	**MP**	**Total**
59150	12.29	7.11	3.39	22.79

	FUD	Status	MUE	Modifiers				IOM Reference
59150	90	A	1(3)	51	N/A	N/A	80	None

* with documentation

Terms To Know

ectopic pregnancy. Fertilized ovum that implants and develops outside the uterus. The ovum may implant itself in different sites, such as the fallopian tube, the ovary, the abdomen, or the cervix.

gestation. Carrying of offspring in the womb throughout the period of development of the fetus(es) during pregnancy.

laparoscopy. Direct visualization of the peritoneal cavity, outer fallopian tubes, uterus, and ovaries utilizing a laparoscope, a thin, flexible fiberoptic tube.

Maternity Care

59151

59151 Laparoscopic treatment of ectopic pregnancy; with salpingectomy and/or oophorectomy

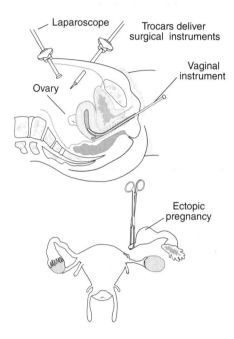

The physician removes a fallopian tube to treat ectopic pregnancy; ovary may also be removed

Laparoscope

Trocars deliver surgical instruments

Vaginal instrument

Ovary

Ectopic pregnancy

Explanation

The physician treats an ectopic pregnancy by laparoscopy with salpingectomy and/or oophorectomy. The physician inserts an instrument through the vagina to grasp the cervix while passing another instrument through the cervix and into the uterus to manipulate the uterus. Next, the physician makes a 1 cm incision in the umbilicus through which the abdomen is inflated and a fiberoptic laparoscope is inserted. A second incision is made on the left or right side of the abdomen. After locating the site of the gestation, another small incision is made above the site. Instruments are passed into the abdomen through the incisions. The physician removes the tube and/or ovary containing the embryo and closes the abdominal incisions with sutures.

Coding Tips

A diagnostic laparoscopy is included in this procedure and should not be reported separately. This code is appropriate for reporting this procedure when performed with any technique or combination of techniques (e.g., laser, hot cautery). If significant additional time and effort is documented, append modifier 22 and submit a cover letter and operative report. For laparoscopic treatment of an ectopic pregnancy, without salpingectomy and/or oophorectomy, see 59150.

ICD-10-CM Diagnostic Codes

O00.00	Abdominal pregnancy without intrauterine pregnancy Ⓜ ♀
O00.01	Abdominal pregnancy with intrauterine pregnancy Ⓜ ♀
O00.101	Right tubal pregnancy without intrauterine pregnancy Ⓜ ♀
O00.102	Left tubal pregnancy without intrauterine pregnancy Ⓜ ♀
O00.111	Right tubal pregnancy with intrauterine pregnancy Ⓜ ♀
O00.112	Left tubal pregnancy with intrauterine pregnancy Ⓜ ♀
O00.201	Right ovarian pregnancy without intrauterine pregnancy Ⓜ ♀
O00.202	Left ovarian pregnancy without intrauterine pregnancy Ⓜ ♀
O00.211	Right ovarian pregnancy with intrauterine pregnancy Ⓜ ♀
O00.212	Left ovarian pregnancy with intrauterine pregnancy Ⓜ ♀
O00.80	Other ectopic pregnancy without intrauterine pregnancy Ⓜ ♀
O00.81	Other ectopic pregnancy with intrauterine pregnancy Ⓜ ♀

AMA: 59151 2019,Jul,6; 2014,Jan,11

Relative Value Units/Medicare Edits

Non-Facility RVU	Work	PE	MP	Total
59151	12.11	6.8	3.34	22.25
Facility RVU	**Work**	**PE**	**MP**	**Total**
59151	12.11	6.8	3.34	22.25

	FUD	Status	MUE	Modifiers				IOM Reference
59151	90	A	1(3)	51	N/A	N/A	80	None

* with documentation

Terms To Know

ectopic pregnancy. Fertilized ovum that implants and develops outside the uterus. The ovum may implant itself in different sites, such as the fallopian tube, the ovary, the abdomen, or the cervix.

oophorectomy. Surgical removal of all or part of one or both ovaries, either as open procedure or laparoscopically. Menstruation and childbearing ability continues when one ovary is removed.

salpingectomy. Removal of all or part of one or both of the fallopian tubes. Indications include infection, ectopic pregnancy, sterilization, or cancer. This procedure is often performed in combination with other open or laparoscopic procedures.

Maternity Care

59160

59160 Curettage, postpartum

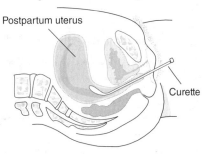

The physician scrapes the endometrial lining of the uterus following childbirth

Postpartum uterus

Curette

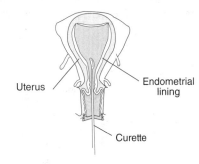

Uterus

Endometrial lining

Curette

Explanation

The physician scrapes the endometrial lining of the uterus following childbirth. The physician passes a curette through the cervix and endocervical canal, and into the uterus. Due to the large, soft postpartum uterus that is especially susceptible to perforation, a large blunt curette, also known as a "banjo" curette, is preferable to the suction curette. The physician gently scrapes the endometrial lining of the uterus to control bleeding, treat obstetric lacerations, or remove any remaining placental tissue.

Coding Tips

Because the postpartum uterus has been previously dilated during delivery of the newborn, dilation is not required for this surgery. This code is only to be used for postpartum curettage. For dilation and curettage, diagnostic and/or therapeutic (nonobstetrical), see 58120.

ICD-10-CM Diagnostic Codes

O43.211	Placenta accreta, first trimester 🅼 ♀
O43.212	Placenta accreta, second trimester 🅼 ♀
O43.213	Placenta accreta, third trimester 🅼 ♀
O43.221	Placenta increta, first trimester 🅼 ♀
O43.222	Placenta increta, second trimester 🅼 ♀
O43.223	Placenta increta, third trimester 🅼 ♀
O43.231	Placenta percreta, first trimester 🅼 ♀
O43.232	Placenta percreta, second trimester 🅼 ♀
O43.233	Placenta percreta, third trimester 🅼 ♀
O72.0	Third-stage hemorrhage 🅼 ♀
O72.1	Other immediate postpartum hemorrhage 🅼 ♀
O72.2	Delayed and secondary postpartum hemorrhage 🅼 ♀
O72.3	Postpartum coagulation defects 🅼 ♀
O73.0	Retained placenta without hemorrhage 🅼 ♀
O73.1	Retained portions of placenta and membranes, without hemorrhage 🅼 ♀

AMA: 59160 2019,Jul,6; 2018,Jan,8; 2017,Jan,8; 2016,Jan,13; 2015,Jan,16; 2014,Jan,11

Relative Value Units/Medicare Edits

Non-Facility RVU	Work	PE	MP	Total
59160	2.76	3.42	0.74	6.92
Facility RVU	**Work**	**PE**	**MP**	**Total**
59160	2.76	1.79	0.74	5.29

	FUD	Status	MUE	Modifiers				IOM Reference
59160	10	A	1(2)	51	N/A	N/A	80*	None

* with documentation

Terms To Know

curettage. Removal of tissue by scraping.

curette. Spoon-shaped instrument used to scrape out abnormal tissue from a cavity or bone.

hemorrhage syndrome. Fulminating meningococcal septicemia occurring in children younger than 10 years of age with vomiting, cyanosis, diarrhea, purpura, convulsions, circulatory collapse, meningitis, and hemorrhaging into adrenal glands.

laceration. Tearing injury; a torn, ragged-edged wound.

placenta. Temporary organ within the uterus during pregnancy, joining the mother and fetus. Attached to the fetus via the umbilical cord, it provides oxygen and nutrients and helps to eliminate carbon dioxide and waste through the selective exchange of soluble substances carried via the blood. The placenta is expelled from the uterus after the baby is delivered, and is then termed the afterbirth.

placenta accreta. Condition where the placenta adheres too deeply to the uterine wall; often associated with placenta previa and results in premature delivery, retention of all or a portion of the placenta, or postpartum bleeding.

placenta increta. Condition where the placenta adheres too deeply to the uterine wall and penetrates the muscle; often associated with placenta previa and results in premature delivery, retention of all or a portion of the placenta, or postpartum bleeding.

placenta previa. Placenta implanted in the lower segment of the uterus, which commonly causes hemorrhage in the last trimester of pregnancy.

postpartum. Period of time following childbirth.

Maternity Care

59200

59200 Insertion of cervical dilator (eg, laminaria, prostaglandin) (separate procedure)

The physician inserts a cervical dilator to expand cervical opening

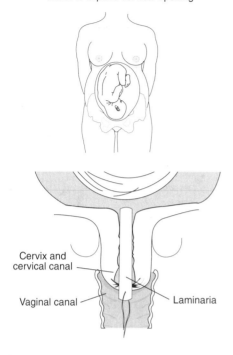

Cervix and cervical canal

Vaginal canal

Laminaria

Explanation

The physician inserts a cervical dilator, such as a laminaria or prostaglandin, into the endocervix to chemically stimulate and dilate the cervical canal. Using a speculum, the physician views the cervix and uses a tool to grasp it and pull it down. A laminaria, which is a sterile applicator made of kelp or synthetic material, may be placed in the cervical canal where it absorbs moisture, swells, and gradually dilates the cervix prior to inducing labor. Or the physician may insert prostaglandin in the form of gel or suppositories into the cervix in order to prime it six to 12 hours before induction.

Coding Tips

Code 59200 does not require the use of laminaria or prostaglandin in order to report this service as these represent only one method of dilation. Mechanical dilation such as the use of a Foley catheter to induce labor for a patient delivering on another day may be reported using this code. Cervical dilation of a pregnant patient on the same day as a subsequent delivery is not reported as it is included in the obstetric package. This separate procedure by definition is usually a component of a more complex service and is not identified separately. When performed alone or with other unrelated procedures/services it may be reported. If performed alone, list the code; if performed with other procedures/services, list the code and append modifier 59 or an X{EPSU} modifier. For introduction of a hypertonic solution and/or prostaglandin to initiate labor, see 59850–59857. Report intrauterine fetal transfusion with 36460.

ICD-10-CM Diagnostic Codes

O36.4XX0	Maternal care for intrauterine death, not applicable or unspecified ⓜ ♀
O36.4XX1	Maternal care for intrauterine death, fetus 1 ⓜ ♀
O36.4XX2	Maternal care for intrauterine death, fetus 2 ⓜ ♀
O36.4XX3	Maternal care for intrauterine death, fetus 3 ⓜ ♀
O36.4XX4	Maternal care for intrauterine death, fetus 4 ⓜ ♀
O36.4XX5	Maternal care for intrauterine death, fetus 5 ⓜ ♀
O36.4XX9	Maternal care for intrauterine death, other fetus ⓜ ♀
O42.011	Preterm premature rupture of membranes, onset of labor within 24 hours of rupture, first trimester ⓜ ♀
O42.012	Preterm premature rupture of membranes, onset of labor within 24 hours of rupture, second trimester ⓜ ♀
O42.013	Preterm premature rupture of membranes, onset of labor within 24 hours of rupture, third trimester ⓜ ♀
O42.02	Full-term premature rupture of membranes, onset of labor within 24 hours of rupture ⓜ ♀
O42.111	Preterm premature rupture of membranes, onset of labor more than 24 hours following rupture, first trimester ⓜ ♀
O42.112	Preterm premature rupture of membranes, onset of labor more than 24 hours following rupture, second trimester ⓜ ♀
O42.113	Preterm premature rupture of membranes, onset of labor more than 24 hours following rupture, third trimester ⓜ ♀
O42.12	Full-term premature rupture of membranes, onset of labor more than 24 hours following rupture ⓜ ♀
O48.0	Post-term pregnancy ⓜ ♀
O48.1	Prolonged pregnancy ⓜ ♀
O61.0	Failed medical induction of labor ⓜ ♀
O61.8	Other failed induction of labor ⓜ ♀
O62.0	Primary inadequate contractions ⓜ ♀
O62.1	Secondary uterine inertia ⓜ ♀
O62.2	Other uterine inertia ⓜ ♀
O62.4	Hypertonic, incoordinate, and prolonged uterine contractions ⓜ ♀
O62.8	Other abnormalities of forces of labor ⓜ ♀
O63.0	Prolonged first stage (of labor) ⓜ ♀
O75.5	Delayed delivery after artificial rupture of membranes ⓜ ♀

AMA: **59200** 2019,Jul,6; 2018,Jan,8; 2017,Jan,8; 2017,Dec,14; 2016,Jan,13; 2015,Jan,16; 2014,Jan,11

Relative Value Units/Medicare Edits

Non-Facility RVU	Work	PE	MP	Total
59200	0.79	1.56	0.21	2.56
Facility RVU	**Work**	**PE**	**MP**	**Total**
59200	0.79	0.3	0.21	1.3

	FUD	Status	MUE	Modifiers				IOM Reference
59200	0	A	1(3)	51	N/A	N/A	N/A	None

* with documentation

59300

59300　Episiotomy or vaginal repair, by other than attending

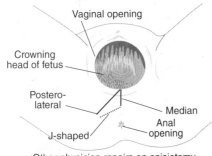

Other physician repairs an episiotomy
or vaginal tear incurred during delivery

Explanation

A qualified health care provider, other than the provider who performed the delivery, repairs an episiotomy, vaginal tear, or laceration using sutures.

Coding Tips

This code is for use by the non-attending provider only. For tracheloplasty, see 57700. Local anesthesia is included in this service. However, this procedure may be performed under general anesthesia, depending on the age and/or condition of the patient. Surgical trays, A4550, are not separately reimbursed by Medicare; however, other third-party payers may cover them. Check with the specific payer to determine coverage.

ICD-10-CM Diagnostic Codes

O70.0	First degree perineal laceration during delivery Ⓜ ♀
O70.1	Second degree perineal laceration during delivery Ⓜ ♀
O70.21	Third degree perineal laceration during delivery, IIIa Ⓜ ♀
O70.22	Third degree perineal laceration during delivery, IIIb Ⓜ ♀
O70.23	Third degree perineal laceration during delivery, IIIc Ⓜ ♀
O70.3	Fourth degree perineal laceration during delivery Ⓜ ♀
O71.4	Obstetric high vaginal laceration alone Ⓜ ♀

AMA: 59300 2019,Jul,6; 2014,Jan,11

Relative Value Units/Medicare Edits

Non-Facility RVU	Work	PE	MP	Total
59300	2.41	3.1	0.64	6.15
Facility RVU	**Work**	**PE**	**MP**	**Total**
59300	2.41	1.21	0.64	4.26

	FUD	Status	MUE	Modifiers				IOM Reference
59300	0	A	1(2)	51	N/A	N/A	80*	None

* with documentation

Terms To Know

episiotomy. Deliberate incision in the perineal tissue to facilitate delivery of the fetus and avoid traumatic tearing. In a midline or median episiotomy, the incision is made from the vagina straight down toward the anus. In a mediolateral episiotomy, the incision slants to one side.

laceration. Tearing injury; a torn, ragged-edged wound.

59320

59320　Cerclage of cervix, during pregnancy; vaginal

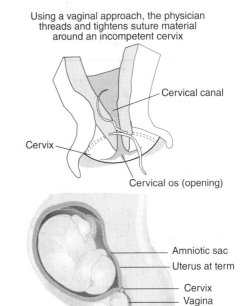

Using a vaginal approach, the physician threads and tightens suture material around an incompetent cervix

Explanation

The physician threads suture material or wraps banding around the cervix to close an incompetent cervix. An incompetent cervix is one that dilates during the second trimester and will eventually allow the pregnancy to fall out. After inserting a speculum into the vagina to view the cervix, heavy suture material or wire is threaded around the cervix using purse-string sutures. The sutures are pulled tight to make the opening smaller and prevent spontaneous abortion.

Coding Tips

For cerclage of cervix, during pregnancy, abdominal, see 59325. For nonobstetric cerclage, see 57700.

ICD-10-CM Diagnostic Codes

O34.31	Maternal care for cervical incompetence, first trimester Ⓜ ♀
O34.32	Maternal care for cervical incompetence, second trimester Ⓜ ♀
O34.33	Maternal care for cervical incompetence, third trimester Ⓜ ♀

AMA: 59320 2019,Jul,6; 2018,Jan,8; 2017,Jan,8; 2016,Jan,13; 2015,Jan,16; 2014,Jan,11

Relative Value Units/Medicare Edits

Non-Facility RVU	Work	PE	MP	Total
59320	2.48	1.24	0.66	4.38
Facility RVU	**Work**	**PE**	**MP**	**Total**
59320	2.48	1.24	0.66	4.38

	FUD	Status	MUE	Modifiers				IOM Reference
59320	0	A	1(2)	51	N/A	N/A	80*	None

* with documentation

Coding Companion for Ob/Gyn

59325

59325 Cerclage of cervix, during pregnancy; abdominal

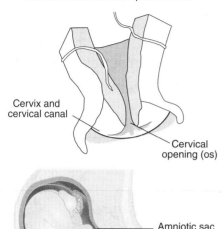

Using an abdominal surgical approach, the physician wraps and tightens banding material around an incompetent cervix

Cervix and cervical canal

Cervical opening (os)

Amniotic sac
Uterus at term
Cervix
Vagina
Pubic bone

Explanation

Through a small abdominal incision just above the pubic hairline, the physician places a band around the cervix at the level of the internal os (opening) to make the cervical opening smaller and prevent spontaneous abortion from an incompetent cervix. An incompetent cervix is one that dilates during the second trimester and will eventually allow the pregnancy to fall out. The abdominal incision is then closed with sutures.

Coding Tips

Intra-abdominal cerclage is rare and only indicated in such instances as traumatic cervical laceration, congenital shortening of the cervix, previous failed vaginal cerclage, and advanced cervical effacement. For vaginal cerclage of the cervix during pregnancy, see 59320. For nonobstetric cerclage, see 57700.

ICD-10-CM Diagnostic Codes

O34.31 Maternal care for cervical incompetence, first trimester Ⓜ ♀
O34.32 Maternal care for cervical incompetence, second trimester Ⓜ ♀
O34.33 Maternal care for cervical incompetence, third trimester Ⓜ ♀

AMA: 59325 2019,Jul,6; 2018,Jan,8; 2017,Jan,8; 2016,Jan,13; 2015,Jan,16; 2014,Jan,11

Relative Value Units/Medicare Edits

Non-Facility RVU	Work	PE	MP	Total
59325	4.06	1.84	1.13	7.03
Facility RVU	Work	PE	MP	Total
59325	4.06	1.84	1.13	7.03

	FUD	Status	MUE	Modifiers				IOM Reference
59325	0	A	1(2)	51	N/A	N/A	80*	None

* with documentation

Terms To Know

cerclage. Looping or encircling an organ or tissue with wire or ligature for positional support.

incompetent cervix. Narrow end of the uterus opening into the birth canal that abnormally dilates during the second trimester of the pregnancy and can lead to a miscarriage or premature delivery.

internal os. Opening through the cervix into the uterus.

spontaneous abortion. Early expulsion of the products of conception from the uterus that occurs naturally, without chemical intervention or instrumentation, before completion of 20 weeks of gestation. Spontaneous abortion may be complete, in which all of the products of conception are expelled; or incomplete, in which parts of the placental material or fetus are retained.

trimester. Normal pregnancy has a duration of approximately 40 weeks and is grouped into three-month periods consisting of three trimesters. ICD-10-CM counts trimesters from the first day of the last menstrual period as follows: 1st trimester less than 14 weeks and 0 days; 2nd trimester 14 weeks, 0 days to less than 28 weeks and 0 days; and 3rd trimester 28 weeks and 0 days until delivery.

Maternity Care

59350

59350   Hysterorrhaphy of ruptured uterus

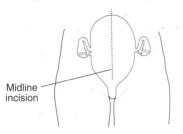

Layered sutures are used to repair a uterus
ruptured or lacerated during pregnancy

Midline
incision

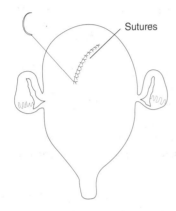

Sutures

Explanation

The physician repairs a uterus that is lacerated or ruptured during pregnancy. A large incision is made in the abdomen and the uterus is sutured in layers. The abdominal incision is closed with sutures.

Coding Tips

For nonobstetric hysterorrhaphy, see 58520. For hysteroplasty, repair of uterine anomaly, see 58540.

ICD-10-CM Diagnostic Codes

O34.29	Maternal care due to uterine scar from other previous surgery 🅜 ♀
O71.02	Rupture of uterus before onset of labor, second trimester 🅜 ♀
O71.03	Rupture of uterus before onset of labor, third trimester 🅜 ♀
O71.1	Rupture of uterus during labor 🅜 ♀
O71.81	Laceration of uterus, not elsewhere classified 🅜 ♀

AMA: 59350 2019,Jul,6; 2014,Jan,11

Relative Value Units/Medicare Edits

Non-Facility RVU	Work	PE	MP	Total
59350	4.94	1.86	1.36	8.16
Facility RVU	**Work**	**PE**	**MP**	**Total**
59350	4.94	1.86	1.36	8.16

	FUD	Status	MUE	Modifiers				IOM Reference
59350	0	A	1(2)	51	N/A	N/A	80	None

* with documentation

59400

59400   Routine obstetric care including antepartum care, vaginal delivery (with or without episiotomy, and/or forceps) and postpartum care

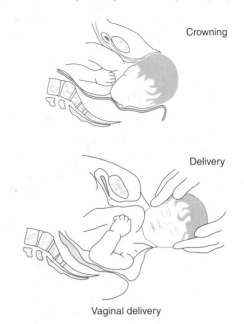

Crowning

Delivery

Vaginal delivery

Explanation

The physician delivers an infant and placenta through the uterus and vagina. The physician may elect to assist the delivery with the use of forceps, vacuum extraction, or rupture of membranes. The physician may also elect to do an episiotomy, which is an incision in the perineum to widen the external opening. Episiotomy and laceration repair are included as well. This procedure covers both antepartum and postpartum care. Antepartum or prenatal care includes the initial and subsequent histories, physical examinations, recording of weight, blood pressures, fetal heart tones, and routine chemical urinalysis. It includes monthly visits up to 28 weeks gestation, biweekly visits to 36 weeks gestation, and weekly visits until delivery. Postpartum care includes hospital and office visits following delivery.

Coding Tips

Note that 59400 includes total OB care; if services provided do not match the code description of total OB care, use the appropriate stand-alone code (e.g., antepartum care, 59425–59426). If care rendered was less than the listed service (i.e., the one that most closely describes the service performed), append modifier 52 and reduce the cost of the service. See notes in CPT for directions in the use of the maternity care and delivery codes. For vaginal delivery only, without antepartum or postpartum care, see 59409. For vaginal delivery only, including postpartum care, see 59410. For cesarean delivery, including antepartum and postpartum care, see 59510.

ICD-10-CM Diagnostic Codes

O11.5	Pre-existing hypertension with pre-eclampsia, complicating the puerperium 🅜 ♀
O12.05	Gestational edema, complicating the puerperium 🅜 ♀
O12.15	Gestational proteinuria, complicating the puerperium 🅜 ♀
O12.25	Gestational edema with proteinuria, complicating the puerperium 🅜 ♀
O13.5	Gestational [pregnancy-induced] hypertension without significant proteinuria, complicating the puerperium 🅜 ♀

Maternity Care

O14.05	Mild to moderate pre-eclampsia, complicating the puerperium ⓜ ♀
O14.15	Severe pre-eclampsia, complicating the puerperium ⓜ ♀
O14.25	HELLP syndrome, complicating the puerperium ⓜ ♀
O24.435	Gestational diabetes mellitus in puerperium, controlled by oral hypoglycemic drugs ⓜ ♀
O30.013	Twin pregnancy, monochorionic/monoamniotic, third trimester ⓜ ♀
O30.033	Twin pregnancy, monochorionic/diamniotic, third trimester ⓜ ♀
O30.043	Twin pregnancy, dichorionic/diamniotic, third trimester ⓜ ♀
O42.013	Preterm premature rupture of membranes, onset of labor within 24 hours of rupture, third trimester ⓜ ♀
O70.0	First degree perineal laceration during delivery ⓜ ♀
O70.1	Second degree perineal laceration during delivery ⓜ ♀
O70.21	Third degree perineal laceration during delivery, IIIa ⓜ ♀
O70.22	Third degree perineal laceration during delivery, IIIb ⓜ ♀
O70.23	Third degree perineal laceration during delivery, IIIc ⓜ ♀
O70.3	Fourth degree perineal laceration during delivery ⓜ ♀
O80	Encounter for full-term uncomplicated delivery ⓜ ♀
Z33.3	Pregnant state, gestational carrier ⓜ ♀
Z34.01	Encounter for supervision of normal first pregnancy, first trimester ⓜ ♀
Z34.02	Encounter for supervision of normal first pregnancy, second trimester ⓜ ♀
Z34.03	Encounter for supervision of normal first pregnancy, third trimester ⓜ ♀
Z34.81	Encounter for supervision of other normal pregnancy, first trimester ⓜ ♀
Z34.82	Encounter for supervision of other normal pregnancy, second trimester ⓜ ♀
Z34.83	Encounter for supervision of other normal pregnancy, third trimester ⓜ ♀
Z36.0	Encounter for antenatal screening for chromosomal anomalies ⓜ ♀
Z36.1	Encounter for antenatal screening for raised alphafetoprotein level ⓜ ♀
Z36.2	Encounter for other antenatal screening follow-up ⓜ ♀
Z36.3	Encounter for antenatal screening for malformations ⓜ ♀
Z36.4	Encounter for antenatal screening for fetal growth retardation ⓜ ♀
Z36.5	Encounter for antenatal screening for isoimmunization ⓜ ♀
Z36.81	Encounter for antenatal screening for hydrops fetalis ⓜ ♀
Z36.82	Encounter for antenatal screening for nuchal translucency ⓜ ♀
Z36.83	Encounter for fetal screening for congenital cardiac abnormalities ⓜ ♀
Z36.84	Encounter for antenatal screening for fetal lung maturity ⓜ ♀
Z36.85	Encounter for antenatal screening for Streptococcus B ⓜ ♀
Z36.86	Encounter for antenatal screening for cervical length ⓜ ♀
Z36.87	Encounter for antenatal screening for uncertain dates ⓜ ♀
Z36.88	Encounter for antenatal screening for fetal macrosomia ⓜ ♀
Z36.89	Encounter for other specified antenatal screening ⓜ ♀
Z36.8A	Encounter for antenatal screening for other genetic defects ⓜ ♀
Z39.0	Encounter for care and examination of mother immediately after delivery ⓜ ♀
Z39.1	Encounter for care and examination of lactating mother ⓜ ♀
Z39.2	Encounter for routine postpartum follow-up ⓜ ♀

AMA: **59400** 2019,Jul,6; 2018,Jan,8; 2017,Jan,8; 2016,Jan,13; 2015,Jan,16; 2014,Jan,11

Relative Value Units/Medicare Edits

Non-Facility RVU	Work	PE	MP	Total
59400	32.16	21.24	8.13	61.53
Facility RVU	Work	PE	MP	Total
59400	32.16	21.24	8.13	61.53

	FUD	Status	MUE	Modifiers				IOM Reference
59400	N/A	A	1(2)	51	N/A	N/A	N/A	100-02,15,20.1; 100-02,15,180

* with documentation

Terms To Know

antepartum. Period of pregnancy between conception and the onset of labor.

delivery. Expulsion or extraction of a newborn and the afterbirth.

episiotomy. Deliberate incision in the perineal tissue to facilitate delivery of the fetus and avoid traumatic tearing. In a midline or median episiotomy, the incision is made from the vagina straight down toward the anus. In a mediolateral episiotomy, the incision slants to one side.

forceps. Tool used for grasping or compressing tissue.

placenta. Temporary organ within the uterus during pregnancy, joining the mother and fetus. Attached to the fetus via the umbilical cord, it provides oxygen and nutrients and helps to eliminate carbon dioxide and waste through the selective exchange of soluble substances carried via the blood. The placenta is expelled from the uterus after the baby is delivered, and is then termed the afterbirth.

rupture. Tearing or breaking open of tissue.

59409-59410

59409 Vaginal delivery only (with or without episiotomy and/or forceps);
59410   including postpartum care

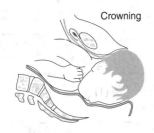

Crowning

The physician delivers the infant through the vagina

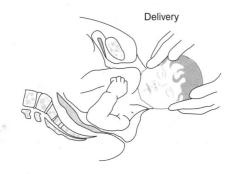

Delivery

Explanation

The physician delivers an infant and placenta through the uterus and vagina. The physician may elect to assist the delivery with the use of forceps, vacuum extraction, or rupture of membranes. The physician may also elect to do an episiotomy, which is an incision in the perineum to widen the external opening. Episiotomy and laceration repair are included as well. Code 59409 represents the vaginal delivery only and does not include antepartum or postpartum care. Code 59410 covers the vaginal delivery with postpartum care, which includes hospital and office visits following delivery.

Coding Tips

If services provided do not match the code description of vaginal delivery only (59409) or vaginal delivery with postpartum care (59410), use the appropriate stand-alone code (e.g., postpartum care only, 59430, or total OB care, 59400). If care rendered was less than the listed service (i.e., the one that most closely describes the service performed), append modifier 52 and reduce the cost of the service. See notes in CPT for directions on the use of the maternity care and delivery codes. For a vaginal delivery with routine obstetric care including antepartum and postpartum care, see 59400. For cesarean delivery only, see 59514. For cesarean delivery including postpartum care, see 59515. For vaginal delivery after previous cesarean section, see 59610–59614.

ICD-10-CM Diagnostic Codes

O11.5	Pre-existing hypertension with pre-eclampsia, complicating the puerperium 🅼 ♀
O12.05	Gestational edema, complicating the puerperium 🅼 ♀
O12.15	Gestational proteinuria, complicating the puerperium 🅼 ♀
O12.25	Gestational edema with proteinuria, complicating the puerperium 🅼 ♀
O13.5	Gestational [pregnancy-induced] hypertension without significant proteinuria, complicating the puerperium 🅼 ♀
O14.05	Mild to moderate pre-eclampsia, complicating the puerperium 🅼 ♀
O14.15	Severe pre-eclampsia, complicating the puerperium 🅼 ♀
O14.25	HELLP syndrome, complicating the puerperium 🅼 ♀
O24.435	Gestational diabetes mellitus in puerperium, controlled by oral hypoglycemic drugs 🅼 ♀
O36.0930	Maternal care for other rhesus isoimmunization, third trimester, not applicable or unspecified 🅼 ♀
O36.1130	Maternal care for Anti-A sensitization, third trimester, not applicable or unspecified 🅼 ♀
O36.1930	Maternal care for other isoimmunization, third trimester, not applicable or unspecified 🅼 ♀
O36.4XX0	Maternal care for intrauterine death, not applicable or unspecified 🅼 ♀
O36.5130	Maternal care for known or suspected placental insufficiency, third trimester, not applicable or unspecified 🅼 ♀
O36.5930	Maternal care for other known or suspected poor fetal growth, third trimester, not applicable or unspecified 🅼 ♀
O36.63X0	Maternal care for excessive fetal growth, third trimester, not applicable or unspecified 🅼 ♀
O36.8130	Decreased fetal movements, third trimester, not applicable or unspecified 🅼 ♀
O36.8230	Fetal anemia and thrombocytopenia, third trimester, not applicable or unspecified 🅼 ♀
O36.8930	Maternal care for other specified fetal problems, third trimester, not applicable or unspecified 🅼 ♀
O70.0	First degree perineal laceration during delivery 🅼 ♀
O80	Encounter for full-term uncomplicated delivery 🅼 ♀
Z39.0	Encounter for care and examination of mother immediately after delivery 🅼 ♀
Z39.2	Encounter for routine postpartum follow-up 🅼 ♀

AMA: **59409** 2019,Jul,6; 2018,Jan,8; 2017,Jan,8; 2016,Jan,13; 2015,Jan,16; 2014,Jan,11 **59410** 2019,Jul,6; 2014,Jan,11

Relative Value Units/Medicare Edits

Non-Facility RVU	Work	PE	MP	Total
59409	14.37	5.57	3.59	23.53
59410	18.01	7.77	4.51	30.29
Facility RVU	**Work**	**PE**	**MP**	**Total**
59409	14.37	5.57	3.59	23.53
59410	18.01	7.77	4.51	30.29

	FUD	Status	MUE	Modifiers				IOM Reference
59409	N/A	A	2(3)	51	N/A	N/A	80*	None
59410	N/A	A	1(2)	51	N/A	N/A	N/A	

* with documentation

Maternity Care

59412

59412   External cephalic version, with or without tocolysis

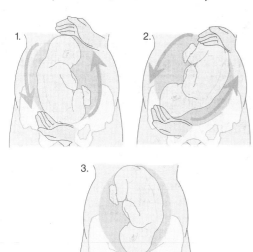

The baby is in breech presentation (1), the physician
feels for the baby's head and bottom externally.
By applying pressure the baby is turned (2)
to a cephalic presentation for delivery (3)

Explanation

The physician turns the fetus from a breech presenting position to a cephalic presenting position. External cephalic version is performed by manipulating the fetus from the outside of the abdominal wall. The physician places both hands on the patient's abdomen and locates each pole of the fetus by palpation. The fetus is shifted so that the breech or rear end of the fetus is moved upward and the head downward. The physician may elect to use tocolytic drug therapy to suppress uterine contractions during the manipulation.

Coding Tips

This code may be used for manipulation prior to or during delivery. It may be reported in addition to any of the delivery codes (59400–59622). Procedure 59412 has not been designated in CPT as an "add-on" code or exempt from modifier 51. However, this procedure is not billed as a stand-alone service and it is recommended that it be reported using "add-on" reporting guidelines when the same physician performs the service/procedure on the same date of service as other related services/procedures.

ICD-10-CM Diagnostic Codes

O32.1XX0	Maternal care for breech presentation, not applicable or unspecified ⓜ ♀
O32.1XX1	Maternal care for breech presentation, fetus 1 ⓜ ♀
O32.1XX2	Maternal care for breech presentation, fetus 2 ⓜ ♀
O32.1XX3	Maternal care for breech presentation, fetus 3 ⓜ ♀
O32.1XX4	Maternal care for breech presentation, fetus 4 ⓜ ♀
O32.1XX5	Maternal care for breech presentation, fetus 5 ⓜ ♀
O32.1XX9	Maternal care for breech presentation, other fetus ⓜ ♀
O64.1XX0	Obstructed labor due to breech presentation, not applicable or unspecified ⓜ ♀
O64.1XX1	Obstructed labor due to breech presentation, fetus 1 ⓜ ♀
O64.1XX2	Obstructed labor due to breech presentation, fetus 2 ⓜ ♀
O64.1XX3	Obstructed labor due to breech presentation, fetus 3 ⓜ ♀
O64.1XX4	Obstructed labor due to breech presentation, fetus 4 ⓜ ♀
O64.1XX5	Obstructed labor due to breech presentation, fetus 5 ⓜ ♀
O64.1XX9	Obstructed labor due to breech presentation, other fetus ⓜ ♀

AMA: 59412 2019,Jul,6; 2014,Jan,11

Relative Value Units/Medicare Edits

Non-Facility RVU	Work	PE	MP	Total
59412	1.71	0.81	0.48	3.0
Facility RVU	**Work**	**PE**	**MP**	**Total**
59412	1.71	0.81	0.48	3.0

	FUD	Status	MUE	Modifiers				IOM Reference
59412	N/A	A	1(3)	N/A	N/A	N/A	80*	100-02,15,20.1; 100-02,15,180

* with documentation

Terms To Know

breech presentation. Abnormal condition in which the fetal buttocks present first. In frank breech, the legs of the fetus extend over the abdomen and thorax so that the feet lie beside the face. In complete breech, the legs are flexed and crossed, while incomplete breech presents with one or both lower legs and feet prolapsed into the vagina.

cephalad. Toward the head.

tocolytic. Drug administered during pregnancy in order to relax the uterus and reduce or halt contractions, administered primarily to stop premature labor.

Maternity Care

59414

59414   Delivery of placenta (separate procedure)

The physician delivers the placenta through the vagina

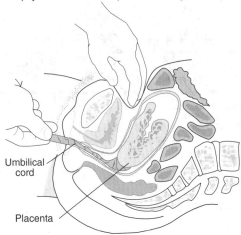

Umbilical cord

Placenta

Explanation

The physician removes a retained placenta following delivery of the fetus, usually unattended, and after separation of the placenta from its intrauterine attachment. The physician places abdominal pressure just above the symphysis to elevate the uterus into the abdomen and prevent inversion of the uterus. This also helps move the placenta downward into the vagina. The umbilical cord is very gently pulled to help guide the placenta out of the birth canal. If the placenta cannot be removed by this technique or there is brisk bleeding, manual removal of the placenta may be indicated. Manual removal requires adequate analgesia or anesthesia. It is accomplished by grasping the fundus of the uterus with a hand on the abdomen. The other hand, wearing an elbow-length glove, is passed through the vagina into the uterus to separate the placenta and remove it.

Coding Tips

This separate procedure by definition is usually a component of a more complex service and is not identified separately. When performed alone or with other unrelated procedures/services it may be reported. If performed alone, list the code; if performed with other procedures/services, list the code and append modifier 59 or an X{EPSU} modifier. Complications (e.g., control of hemorrhage) are not included in 59414 and are reported separately. For postpartum curettage, see 59160.

ICD-10-CM Diagnostic Codes

O73.0	Retained placenta without hemorrhage Ⓜ ♀
O73.1	Retained portions of placenta and membranes, without hemorrhage Ⓜ ♀

AMA: **59414** 2019,Jul,6; 2018,Jan,8; 2017,Jan,8; 2016,Jan,13; 2015,Jan,16; 2014,Jan,11

Relative Value Units/Medicare Edits

Non-Facility RVU	Work	PE	MP	Total
59414	1.61	0.61	0.44	2.66
Facility RVU	**Work**	**PE**	**MP**	**Total**
59414	1.61	0.61	0.44	2.66

	FUD	Status	MUE	Modifiers				IOM Reference
59414	N/A	A	1(3)	51	N/A	N/A	80*	None

* with documentation

Terms To Know

placenta. Temporary organ within the uterus during pregnancy, joining the mother and fetus. Attached to the fetus via the umbilical cord, it provides oxygen and nutrients and helps to eliminate carbon dioxide and waste through the selective exchange of soluble substances carried via the blood. The placenta is expelled from the uterus after the baby is delivered, and is then termed the afterbirth.

secundines. Placenta and membranes; the afterbirth.

separate procedures. Services commonly carried out as a fundamental part of a total service and, as such, do not usually warrant separate identification. These services are identified in CPT with the parenthetical phrase (separate procedure) at the end of the description and are payable only when performed alone.

59425-59426

59425 Antepartum care only; 4-6 visits
59426   7 or more visits

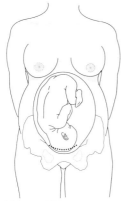

The physician provides antepartum care only

Explanation

Antepartum or prenatal care includes the initial and subsequent histories, physical examinations, recording of weight, blood pressures, fetal heart tones, and routine chemical urinalysis. It includes monthly visits up to 28 weeks gestation, biweekly visits to 36 weeks gestation, and weekly visits until delivery. 59425 includes four to six visits. 59426 covers seven or more visits.

Coding Tips

For one to three antepartum care visits, see the appropriate E/M code. Medical visits not related to maternity care, but within the antepartum time, may be reported separately.

ICD-10-CM Diagnostic Codes

Z33.3	Pregnant state, gestational carrier 🅼 ♀
Z34.01	Encounter for supervision of normal first pregnancy, first trimester 🅼 ♀
Z34.02	Encounter for supervision of normal first pregnancy, second trimester 🅼 ♀
Z34.03	Encounter for supervision of normal first pregnancy, third trimester 🅼 ♀
Z34.81	Encounter for supervision of other normal pregnancy, first trimester 🅼 ♀
Z34.82	Encounter for supervision of other normal pregnancy, second trimester 🅼 ♀
Z34.83	Encounter for supervision of other normal pregnancy, third trimester 🅼 ♀

AMA: 59425 2019,Jul,6; 2018,Jan,8; 2017,Jan,8; 2016,Jan,13; 2015,Jan,16; 2014,Jan,11 **59426** 2019,Jul,6; 2018,Jan,8; 2017,Jan,8; 2016,Jan,13; 2015,Jan,16; 2014,Jan,11

Relative Value Units/Medicare Edits

Non-Facility RVU	Work	PE	MP	Total
59425	6.31	5.62	1.59	13.52
59426	11.16	10.16	2.74	24.06
Facility RVU	**Work**	**PE**	**MP**	**Total**
59425	6.31	2.43	1.59	10.33
59426	11.16	4.31	2.74	18.21

	FUD	Status	MUE	Modifiers				IOM Reference
59425	N/A	A	1(2)	N/A	N/A	N/A	80*	100-02,15,20.1;
59426	N/A	A	1(2)	N/A	N/A	N/A	80*	100-02,15,180

* with documentation

Terms To Know

eclampsia. Tetany and toxemia producing seizure activity or coma in a pregnant patient who most often has presented with prior preeclampsia (i.e., hypertension, albuminuria, and edema).

elderly primigravida. Female in her first pregnancy who will be 35 years or older at her expected date of delivery. Women in this category are considered to be at high risk during pregnancy.

multigravida. Female who has had two or more pregnancies. Women in this category are considered to be at high risk during pregnancy.

oligohydramnios. Low amniotic fluid, occurring most frequently in the last trimester.

placenta previa. Implantation of the placenta in the lower segment of the uterus, over or near the internal cervical os. In total previa, the cervical os is completely covered by the placenta; in partial previa, only a portion is covered.

polyhydramnios. Excess amniotic fluid surrounding the fetus, typically defined as a total fluid volume of greater than 24.0 cc.

preeclampsia. Complication of pregnancy manifesting in the development of borderline hypertension, protein in the urine, and unresponsive swelling between the 20th week of pregnancy and the end of the first week following birth in mild to moderate cases. Severe preeclampsia presents with hypertension, associated with marked swelling, proteinuria, abdominal pain, and/or visual changes.

59430

59430   Postpartum care only (separate procedure)

Explanation

Postpartum care includes hospital and office visits following vaginal or cesarean section delivery.

Coding Tips

This separate procedure by definition is usually a component of a more complex service and is not identified separately. When performed alone or with other unrelated procedures/services it may be reported. If performed alone, list the code; if performed with other procedures/services, list the code and append modifier 59 or an X{EPSU} modifier. Office or other outpatient encounters following a vaginal or cesarean delivery are included in the description of this service. If services provided do not match the code description of postpartum care only, use the appropriate stand-alone code (e.g., vaginal delivery with postpartum care, 59410, or total OB care, 59400). If care rendered was less than the listed service (i.e., the one that most closely describes the service performed), append modifier 52 and reduce the cost of the service. See notes in CPT for directions in the use of the maternity care and delivery codes. For antepartum care, four or more visits, see 59425 and 59426.

ICD-10-CM Diagnostic Codes

O11.5	Pre-existing hypertension with pre-eclampsia, complicating the puerperium Ⓜ ♀
O12.05	Gestational edema, complicating the puerperium Ⓜ ♀
O12.15	Gestational proteinuria, complicating the puerperium Ⓜ ♀
O12.25	Gestational edema with proteinuria, complicating the puerperium Ⓜ ♀
O13.5	Gestational [pregnancy-induced] hypertension without significant proteinuria, complicating the puerperium Ⓜ ♀
O14.05	Mild to moderate pre-eclampsia, complicating the puerperium Ⓜ ♀
O14.15	Severe pre-eclampsia, complicating the puerperium Ⓜ ♀
O14.25	HELLP syndrome, complicating the puerperium Ⓜ ♀
O24.435	Gestational diabetes mellitus in puerperium, controlled by oral hypoglycemic drugs Ⓜ ♀
Z39.0	Encounter for care and examination of mother immediately after delivery Ⓜ ♀
Z39.1	Encounter for care and examination of lactating mother Ⓜ ♀
Z39.2	Encounter for routine postpartum follow-up Ⓜ ♀

AMA: 59430 2019,Jul,6; 2018,Jan,8; 2017,Jan,8; 2016,Jan,13; 2015,Jan,16; 2014,Jan,11

Relative Value Units/Medicare Edits

Non-Facility RVU	Work	PE	MP	Total
59430	2.47	2.87	0.62	5.96
Facility RVU	**Work**	**PE**	**MP**	**Total**
59430	2.47	0.96	0.62	4.05

	FUD	Status	MUE	Modifiers				IOM Reference
59430	N/A	A	1(2)	51	N/A	N/A	N/A	None

* with documentation

59510

59510   Routine obstetric care including antepartum care, cesarean delivery, and postpartum care

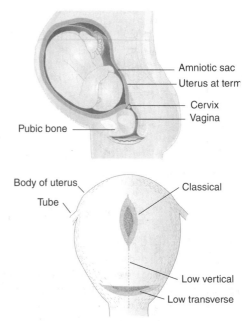

The physician delivers the infant through an abdominal incision

Explanation

The physician delivers an infant through a horizontal or vertical incision in the abdomen and uterus. Once the incisions are made, the infant is delivered and the placenta separated and removed. The uterine and abdominal incisions are closed with sutures. This procedure includes both antepartum and postpartum care. Antepartum or prenatal care includes the initial and subsequent histories, physical examinations, recording of weight, blood pressures, fetal heart tones, and routine chemical urinalysis. It includes monthly visits up to 28 weeks gestation, biweekly visits to 36 weeks gestation, and weekly visits until delivery. Postpartum care includes hospital and office visits following delivery.

Coding Tips

If services provided do not match the code description of cesarean delivery, including antepartum and postpartum care, use the appropriate stand-alone code (e.g., antepartum care, 59425–59426, or cesarean delivery only, 59514). If care rendered was less than the listed service (i.e., the one that most closely describes the service performed), append modifier 52 and reduce the cost of the service. See notes in CPT for directions in the use of the maternity care and delivery codes. For standby attendance for infant, see 99360. For cesarean delivery only, see 59514. For cesarean delivery including postpartum care, see 59515. Note that codes 59618–59622 report a cesarean delivery following attempted vaginal delivery after a previous cesarean section.

ICD-10-CM Diagnostic Codes

O30.013	Twin pregnancy, monochorionic/monoamniotic, third trimester Ⓜ ♀
O30.033	Twin pregnancy, monochorionic/diamniotic, third trimester Ⓜ ♀
O30.043	Twin pregnancy, dichorionic/diamniotic, third trimester Ⓜ ♀
O30.113	Triplet pregnancy with two or more monochorionic fetuses, third trimester Ⓜ ♀

O30.123	Triplet pregnancy with two or more monoamniotic fetuses, third trimester Ⓜ ♀
O32.0XX1	Maternal care for unstable lie, fetus 1 Ⓜ ♀
O32.0XX2	Maternal care for unstable lie, fetus 2 Ⓜ ♀
O32.0XX3	Maternal care for unstable lie, fetus 3 Ⓜ ♀
O32.1XX1	Maternal care for breech presentation, fetus 1 Ⓜ ♀
O32.1XX2	Maternal care for breech presentation, fetus 2 Ⓜ ♀
O32.1XX3	Maternal care for breech presentation, fetus 3 Ⓜ ♀
O32.2XX1	Maternal care for transverse and oblique lie, fetus 1 Ⓜ ♀
O32.2XX2	Maternal care for transverse and oblique lie, fetus 2 Ⓜ ♀
O32.2XX3	Maternal care for transverse and oblique lie, fetus 3 Ⓜ ♀
O32.3XX1	Maternal care for face, brow and chin presentation, fetus 1 Ⓜ ♀
O32.3XX2	Maternal care for face, brow and chin presentation, fetus 2 Ⓜ ♀
O32.3XX3	Maternal care for face, brow and chin presentation, fetus 3 Ⓜ ♀
O32.4XX1	Maternal care for high head at term, fetus 1 Ⓜ ♀
O32.4XX2	Maternal care for high head at term, fetus 2 Ⓜ ♀
O32.4XX3	Maternal care for high head at term, fetus 3 Ⓜ ♀
O32.6XX1	Maternal care for compound presentation, fetus 1 Ⓜ ♀
O32.6XX2	Maternal care for compound presentation, fetus 2 Ⓜ ♀
O32.6XX3	Maternal care for compound presentation, fetus 3 Ⓜ ♀
O32.8XX1	Maternal care for other malpresentation of fetus, fetus 1 Ⓜ ♀
O32.8XX2	Maternal care for other malpresentation of fetus, fetus 2 Ⓜ ♀
O32.8XX3	Maternal care for other malpresentation of fetus, fetus 3 Ⓜ ♀
O34.29	Maternal care due to uterine scar from other previous surgery Ⓜ ♀
O34.33	Maternal care for cervical incompetence, third trimester Ⓜ ♀
O34.43	Maternal care for other abnormalities of cervix, third trimester Ⓜ ♀
O61.0	Failed medical induction of labor Ⓜ ♀
O61.1	Failed instrumental induction of labor Ⓜ ♀
O61.8	Other failed induction of labor Ⓜ ♀
O64.0XX1	Obstructed labor due to incomplete rotation of fetal head, fetus 1 Ⓜ ♀
O64.0XX2	Obstructed labor due to incomplete rotation of fetal head, fetus 2 Ⓜ ♀
O64.0XX3	Obstructed labor due to incomplete rotation of fetal head, fetus 3 Ⓜ ♀
O64.1XX1	Obstructed labor due to breech presentation, fetus 1 Ⓜ ♀
O64.1XX2	Obstructed labor due to breech presentation, fetus 2 Ⓜ ♀
O64.1XX3	Obstructed labor due to breech presentation, fetus 3 Ⓜ ♀
O64.2XX1	Obstructed labor due to face presentation, fetus 1 Ⓜ ♀
O64.2XX2	Obstructed labor due to face presentation, fetus 2 Ⓜ ♀
O64.2XX3	Obstructed labor due to face presentation, fetus 3 Ⓜ ♀
O64.3XX1	Obstructed labor due to brow presentation, fetus 1 Ⓜ ♀
O64.3XX2	Obstructed labor due to brow presentation, fetus 2 Ⓜ ♀
O64.3XX3	Obstructed labor due to brow presentation, fetus 3 Ⓜ ♀
O64.4XX1	Obstructed labor due to shoulder presentation, fetus 1 Ⓜ ♀
O64.4XX2	Obstructed labor due to shoulder presentation, fetus 2 Ⓜ ♀
O64.4XX3	Obstructed labor due to shoulder presentation, fetus 3 Ⓜ ♀
O64.5XX1	Obstructed labor due to compound presentation, fetus 1 Ⓜ ♀
O64.5XX2	Obstructed labor due to compound presentation, fetus 2 Ⓜ ♀
O64.5XX3	Obstructed labor due to compound presentation, fetus 3 Ⓜ ♀
O64.8XX1	Obstructed labor due to other malposition and malpresentation, fetus 1 Ⓜ ♀
O64.8XX2	Obstructed labor due to other malposition and malpresentation, fetus 2 Ⓜ ♀
O64.8XX3	Obstructed labor due to other malposition and malpresentation, fetus 3 Ⓜ ♀
O65.0	Obstructed labor due to deformed pelvis Ⓜ ♀
O65.1	Obstructed labor due to generally contracted pelvis Ⓜ ♀
O65.2	Obstructed labor due to pelvic inlet contraction Ⓜ ♀
O65.3	Obstructed labor due to pelvic outlet and mid-cavity contraction Ⓜ ♀
O65.5	Obstructed labor due to abnormality of maternal pelvic organs Ⓜ ♀
O65.8	Obstructed labor due to other maternal pelvic abnormalities Ⓜ ♀
O66.0	Obstructed labor due to shoulder dystocia Ⓜ ♀
O66.1	Obstructed labor due to locked twins Ⓜ ♀
O66.2	Obstructed labor due to unusually large fetus Ⓜ ♀
O66.3	Obstructed labor due to other abnormalities of fetus Ⓜ ♀
O66.41	Failed attempted vaginal birth after previous cesarean delivery Ⓜ ♀
O66.5	Attempted application of vacuum extractor and forceps Ⓜ ♀
O66.6	Obstructed labor due to other multiple fetuses Ⓜ ♀
O66.8	Other specified obstructed labor Ⓜ ♀
O68	Labor and delivery complicated by abnormality of fetal acid-base balance Ⓜ ♀
O69.0XX1	Labor and delivery complicated by prolapse of cord, fetus 1 Ⓜ ♀
O69.0XX2	Labor and delivery complicated by prolapse of cord, fetus 2 Ⓜ ♀
O69.0XX3	Labor and delivery complicated by prolapse of cord, fetus 3 Ⓜ ♀
O69.3XX1	Labor and delivery complicated by short cord, fetus 1 Ⓜ ♀
O69.3XX2	Labor and delivery complicated by short cord, fetus 2 Ⓜ ♀
O69.3XX3	Labor and delivery complicated by short cord, fetus 3 Ⓜ ♀
O69.4XX1	Labor and delivery complicated by vasa previa, fetus 1 Ⓜ ♀
O69.4XX2	Labor and delivery complicated by vasa previa, fetus 2 Ⓜ ♀
O69.4XX3	Labor and delivery complicated by vasa previa, fetus 3 Ⓜ ♀
O69.81X1	Labor and delivery complicated by cord around neck, without compression, fetus 1 Ⓜ ♀
O69.81X2	Labor and delivery complicated by cord around neck, without compression, fetus 2 Ⓜ ♀
O69.81X3	Labor and delivery complicated by cord around neck, without compression, fetus 3 Ⓜ ♀
O69.82X1	Labor and delivery complicated by other cord entanglement, without compression, fetus 1 Ⓜ ♀
O69.82X2	Labor and delivery complicated by other cord entanglement, without compression, fetus 2 Ⓜ ♀
O69.82X3	Labor and delivery complicated by other cord entanglement, without compression, fetus 3 Ⓜ ♀
O69.89X1	Labor and delivery complicated by other cord complications, fetus 1 Ⓜ ♀
O69.89X2	Labor and delivery complicated by other cord complications, fetus 2 Ⓜ ♀
O69.89X3	Labor and delivery complicated by other cord complications, fetus 3 Ⓜ ♀
O77.0	Labor and delivery complicated by meconium in amniotic fluid Ⓜ ♀
O77.1	Fetal stress in labor or delivery due to drug administration Ⓜ ♀
O77.8	Labor and delivery complicated by other evidence of fetal stress Ⓜ ♀

O82	Encounter for cesarean delivery without indication ⓜ ♀
O99.213	Obesity complicating pregnancy, third trimester ⓜ ♀
O99.214	Obesity complicating childbirth ⓜ ♀
Z36.0	Encounter for antenatal screening for chromosomal anomalies ⓜ ♀
Z36.1	Encounter for antenatal screening for raised alphafetoprotein level ⓜ ♀
Z36.2	Encounter for other antenatal screening follow-up ⓜ ♀
Z36.3	Encounter for antenatal screening for malformations ⓜ ♀
Z36.4	Encounter for antenatal screening for fetal growth retardation ⓜ ♀
Z36.5	Encounter for antenatal screening for isoimmunization ⓜ ♀
Z36.81	Encounter for antenatal screening for hydrops fetalis ⓜ ♀
Z36.82	Encounter for antenatal screening for nuchal translucency ⓜ ♀
Z36.83	Encounter for fetal screening for congenital cardiac abnormalities ⓜ ♀
Z36.84	Encounter for antenatal screening for fetal lung maturity ⓜ ♀
Z36.85	Encounter for antenatal screening for Streptococcus B ⓜ ♀
Z36.86	Encounter for antenatal screening for cervical length ⓜ ♀
Z36.87	Encounter for antenatal screening for uncertain dates ⓜ ♀
Z36.88	Encounter for antenatal screening for fetal macrosomia ⓜ ♀
Z39.0	Encounter for care and examination of mother immediately after delivery ⓜ ♀

AMA: 59510 2019,Jul,6; 2018,Jan,8; 2017,Jan,8; 2016,Jan,13; 2015,Jan,16; 2014,Jan,11

Relative Value Units/Medicare Edits

Non-Facility RVU	Work	PE	MP	Total
59510	35.64	22.86	9.74	68.24
Facility RVU	**Work**	**PE**	**MP**	**Total**
59510	35.64	22.86	9.74	68.24

	FUD	Status	MUE	Modifiers			IOM Reference
59510	N/A	A	1(2)	51	N/A	N/A	N/A	None

* with documentation

Terms To Know

elderly primigravida. Female in her first pregnancy who will be 35 years or older at her expected date of delivery. Women in this category are considered to be at high risk during pregnancy.

placenta previa. Implantation of the placenta in the lower segment of the uterus, over or near the internal cervical os. In total previa, the cervical os is completely covered by the placenta; in partial previa, only a portion is covered.

preeclampsia. Complication of pregnancy manifesting in the development of borderline hypertension, protein in the urine, and unresponsive swelling between the 20th week of pregnancy and the end of the first week following birth in mild to moderate cases. Severe preeclampsia presents with hypertension, associated with marked swelling, proteinuria, abdominal pain, and/or visual changes.

59514-59515

| 59514 | Cesarean delivery only; |
| 59515 | including postpartum care |

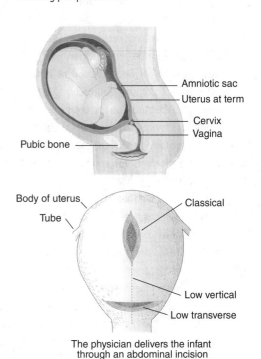

The physician delivers the infant through an abdominal incision

Explanation

The physician delivers an infant through a horizontal or vertical incision in the abdomen and uterus. Once the incisions are made, the infant is delivered and the placenta separated and removed. The uterine and abdominal incisions are closed with sutures. Code 59514 represents the cesarean delivery only and does not include antepartum or postpartum care. Code 59515 covers the cesarean delivery with postpartum care, which includes hospital and office visits following delivery.

Coding Tips

If services provided do not match the code description of cesarean delivery only (59514) or cesarean delivery with postpartum care (59515), use the appropriate stand-alone code (e.g., antepartum care, 59425–59426, or total cesarean care, 59510). If care rendered was less than the listed service (i.e., the one that most closely describes the service performed), append modifier 52 and reduce the cost of the service. See notes in CPT for directions in the use of the maternity care and delivery codes. For cesarean delivery including antepartum and postpartum care, see 59510. For cesarean delivery following attempted vaginal delivery after a previous cesarean section, see 59618–59622.

ICD-10-CM Diagnostic Codes

O30.013	Twin pregnancy, monochorionic/monoamniotic, third trimester ⓜ ♀
O30.033	Twin pregnancy, monochorionic/diamniotic, third trimester ⓜ ♀
O30.043	Twin pregnancy, dichorionic/diamniotic, third trimester ⓜ ♀
O30.113	Triplet pregnancy with two or more monochorionic fetuses, third trimester ⓜ ♀
O30.123	Triplet pregnancy with two or more monoamniotic fetuses, third trimester ⓜ ♀
O32.0XX1	Maternal care for unstable lie, fetus 1 ⓜ ♀

O32.0XX2	Maternal care for unstable lie, fetus 2 ⬚ ♀
O32.0XX3	Maternal care for unstable lie, fetus 3 ⬚ ♀
O32.1XX1	Maternal care for breech presentation, fetus 1 ⬚ ♀
O32.1XX2	Maternal care for breech presentation, fetus 2 ⬚ ♀
O32.1XX3	Maternal care for breech presentation, fetus 3 ⬚ ♀
O32.2XX1	Maternal care for transverse and oblique lie, fetus 1 ⬚ ♀
O32.2XX2	Maternal care for transverse and oblique lie, fetus 2 ⬚ ♀
O32.2XX3	Maternal care for transverse and oblique lie, fetus 3 ⬚ ♀
O32.3XX1	Maternal care for face, brow and chin presentation, fetus 1 ⬚ ♀
O32.3XX2	Maternal care for face, brow and chin presentation, fetus 2 ⬚ ♀
O32.3XX3	Maternal care for face, brow and chin presentation, fetus 3 ⬚ ♀
O32.4XX1	Maternal care for high head at term, fetus 1 ⬚ ♀
O32.4XX2	Maternal care for high head at term, fetus 2 ⬚ ♀
O32.4XX3	Maternal care for high head at term, fetus 3 ⬚ ♀
O32.6XX1	Maternal care for compound presentation, fetus 1 ⬚ ♀
O32.6XX2	Maternal care for compound presentation, fetus 2 ⬚ ♀
O32.6XX3	Maternal care for compound presentation, fetus 3 ⬚ ♀
O32.8XX1	Maternal care for other malpresentation of fetus, fetus 1 ⬚ ♀
O32.8XX2	Maternal care for other malpresentation of fetus, fetus 2 ⬚ ♀
O32.8XX3	Maternal care for other malpresentation of fetus, fetus 3 ⬚ ♀
O34.29	Maternal care due to uterine scar from other previous surgery ⬚ ♀
O34.33	Maternal care for cervical incompetence, third trimester ⬚ ♀
O34.43	Maternal care for other abnormalities of cervix, third trimester ⬚ ♀
O61.0	Failed medical induction of labor ⬚ ♀
O61.1	Failed instrumental induction of labor ⬚ ♀
O61.8	Other failed induction of labor ⬚ ♀
O64.0XX1	Obstructed labor due to incomplete rotation of fetal head, fetus 1 ⬚ ♀
O64.0XX2	Obstructed labor due to incomplete rotation of fetal head, fetus 2 ⬚ ♀
O64.0XX3	Obstructed labor due to incomplete rotation of fetal head, fetus 3 ⬚ ♀
O64.1XX1	Obstructed labor due to breech presentation, fetus 1 ⬚ ♀
O64.1XX2	Obstructed labor due to breech presentation, fetus 2 ⬚ ♀
O64.1XX3	Obstructed labor due to breech presentation, fetus 3 ⬚ ♀
O64.2XX1	Obstructed labor due to face presentation, fetus 1 ⬚ ♀
O64.2XX2	Obstructed labor due to face presentation, fetus 2 ⬚ ♀
O64.2XX3	Obstructed labor due to face presentation, fetus 3 ⬚ ♀
O64.3XX1	Obstructed labor due to brow presentation, fetus 1 ⬚ ♀
O64.3XX2	Obstructed labor due to brow presentation, fetus 2 ⬚ ♀
O64.3XX3	Obstructed labor due to brow presentation, fetus 3 ⬚ ♀
O64.4XX1	Obstructed labor due to shoulder presentation, fetus 1 ⬚ ♀
O64.4XX2	Obstructed labor due to shoulder presentation, fetus 2 ⬚ ♀
O64.4XX3	Obstructed labor due to shoulder presentation, fetus 3 ⬚ ♀
O64.5XX1	Obstructed labor due to compound presentation, fetus 1 ⬚ ♀
O64.5XX2	Obstructed labor due to compound presentation, fetus 2 ⬚ ♀
O64.5XX3	Obstructed labor due to compound presentation, fetus 3 ⬚ ♀
O64.8XX1	Obstructed labor due to other malposition and malpresentation, fetus 1 ⬚ ♀
O64.8XX2	Obstructed labor due to other malposition and malpresentation, fetus 2 ⬚ ♀

O64.8XX3	Obstructed labor due to other malposition and malpresentation, fetus 3 ⬚ ♀
O65.0	Obstructed labor due to deformed pelvis ⬚ ♀
O65.1	Obstructed labor due to generally contracted pelvis ⬚ ♀
O65.2	Obstructed labor due to pelvic inlet contraction ⬚ ♀
O65.3	Obstructed labor due to pelvic outlet and mid-cavity contraction ⬚ ♀
O65.5	Obstructed labor due to abnormality of maternal pelvic organs ⬚ ♀
O65.8	Obstructed labor due to other maternal pelvic abnormalities ⬚ ♀
O66.0	Obstructed labor due to shoulder dystocia ⬚ ♀
O66.1	Obstructed labor due to locked twins ⬚ ♀
O66.2	Obstructed labor due to unusually large fetus ⬚ ♀
O66.3	Obstructed labor due to other abnormalities of fetus ⬚ ♀
O66.41	Failed attempted vaginal birth after previous cesarean delivery ⬚ ♀
O66.5	Attempted application of vacuum extractor and forceps ⬚ ♀
O66.6	Obstructed labor due to other multiple fetuses ⬚ ♀
O66.8	Other specified obstructed labor ⬚ ♀
O68	Labor and delivery complicated by abnormality of fetal acid-base balance ⬚ ♀
O69.0XX1	Labor and delivery complicated by prolapse of cord, fetus 1 ⬚ ♀
O69.0XX2	Labor and delivery complicated by prolapse of cord, fetus 2 ⬚ ♀
O69.0XX3	Labor and delivery complicated by prolapse of cord, fetus 3 ⬚ ♀
O69.3XX1	Labor and delivery complicated by short cord, fetus 1 ⬚ ♀
O69.3XX2	Labor and delivery complicated by short cord, fetus 2 ⬚ ♀
O69.3XX3	Labor and delivery complicated by short cord, fetus 3 ⬚ ♀
O69.4XX1	Labor and delivery complicated by vasa previa, fetus 1 ⬚ ♀
O69.4XX2	Labor and delivery complicated by vasa previa, fetus 2 ⬚ ♀
O69.4XX3	Labor and delivery complicated by vasa previa, fetus 3 ⬚ ♀
O69.81X1	Labor and delivery complicated by cord around neck, without compression, fetus 1 ⬚ ♀
O69.81X2	Labor and delivery complicated by cord around neck, without compression, fetus 2 ⬚ ♀
O69.81X3	Labor and delivery complicated by cord around neck, without compression, fetus 3 ⬚ ♀
O69.82X1	Labor and delivery complicated by other cord entanglement, without compression, fetus 1 ⬚ ♀
O69.82X2	Labor and delivery complicated by other cord entanglement, without compression, fetus 2 ⬚ ♀
O69.82X3	Labor and delivery complicated by other cord entanglement, without compression, fetus 3 ⬚ ♀
O69.89X1	Labor and delivery complicated by other cord complications, fetus 1 ⬚ ♀
O69.89X2	Labor and delivery complicated by other cord complications, fetus 2 ⬚ ♀
O69.89X3	Labor and delivery complicated by other cord complications, fetus 3 ⬚ ♀
O77.0	Labor and delivery complicated by meconium in amniotic fluid ⬚ ♀
O77.1	Fetal stress in labor or delivery due to drug administration ⬚ ♀
O77.8	Labor and delivery complicated by other evidence of fetal stress ⬚ ♀
O82	Encounter for cesarean delivery without indication ⬚ ♀
O99.213	Obesity complicating pregnancy, third trimester ⬚ ♀

| O99.214 | Obesity complicating childbirth Ⓜ ♀ |
| Z39.0 | Encounter for care and examination of mother immediately after delivery Ⓜ ♀ |

AMA: **59514** 2019,Jul,6; 2018,Jan,8; 2017,Jan,8; 2016,Jan,13; 2015,Jan,16; 2014,Jan,11 **59515** 2019,Jul,6; 2018,Jan,8; 2017,Jan,8; 2016,Jan,13; 2015,Jan,16; 2014,Jan,11

Relative Value Units/Medicare Edits

Non-Facility RVU	Work	PE	MP	Total
59514	16.13	6.16	4.3	26.59
59515	21.47	9.58	5.84	36.89
Facility RVU	**Work**	**PE**	**MP**	**Total**
59514	16.13	6.16	4.3	26.59
59515	21.47	9.58	5.84	36.89

	FUD	Status	MUE	Modifiers				IOM Reference
59514	N/A	A	1(3)	51	N/A	62*	80	None
59515	N/A	A	1(2)	51	N/A	N/A	N/A	

* with documentation

Terms To Know

eclampsia. Tetany and toxemia producing seizure activity or coma in a pregnant patient who most often has presented with prior preeclampsia (i.e., hypertension, albuminuria, and edema).

multiparity. Condition of having had two or more pregnancies that resulted in viable fetuses; producing more than one fetus or offspring in the same gestation.

preeclampsia. Complication of pregnancy manifesting in the development of borderline hypertension, protein in the urine, and unresponsive swelling between the 20th week of pregnancy and the end of the first week following birth in mild to moderate cases. Severe preeclampsia presents with hypertension, associated with marked swelling, proteinuria, abdominal pain, and/or visual changes.

secundines. Placenta and membranes; the afterbirth.

59525

+ **59525** Subtotal or total hysterectomy after cesarean delivery (List separately in addition to code for primary procedure)

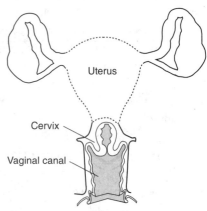

The physician removes the uterus, with or without removing the cervix, and leaving any combination of tubes and ovaries

Explanation

The physician performs a hysterectomy immediately following cesarean delivery. Through the abdominal incision, the physician clamps and cuts free the supporting pedicles containing the tubes, ligaments, and arteries. The uterus is removed and the physician may elect to remove the cervix as well. In a subtotal hysterectomy, just the uterus is removed. In a total hysterectomy, both the uterus and cervix are removed. The abdominal incision is closed with sutures.

Coding Tips

Report 59525 in addition to 59510, 59514, 59515, 59618, 59620, and 59622. For extraperitoneal cesarean section or C-section with a subtotal or total hysterectomy, see 59510, 59515, and 59525. For physician standby attendance for cesarean/high-risk delivery for newborn care, see 99360.

ICD-10-CM Diagnostic Codes

This/these CPT code(s) are add-on code(s). See the primary procedure code that this code is performed with for your ICD-10-CM code selections. Diagnostic code(s) would be the same as the actual procedure performed.

AMA: **59525** 2019,Jul,6; 2014,Jan,11

Relative Value Units/Medicare Edits

Non-Facility RVU	Work	PE	MP	Total
59525	8.53	3.22	2.35	14.1
Facility RVU	**Work**	**PE**	**MP**	**Total**
59525	8.53	3.22	2.35	14.1

	FUD	Status	MUE	Modifiers			IOM Reference
59525	N/A	A	1(2)	N/A	N/A	62*	80	None

* with documentation

Maternity Care

59610

59610 Routine obstetric care including antepartum care, vaginal delivery (with or without episiotomy, and/or forceps) and postpartum care, after previous cesarean delivery

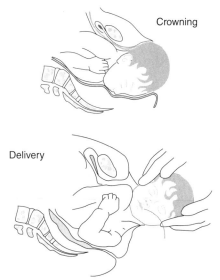

Crowning

Delivery

The physician provides successfully delivers the infant through the vagina

Explanation

The physician delivers an infant and placenta through the vagina. The patient has previously delivered by cesarean section. The physician may elect to assist the delivery with the use of forceps, vacuum extraction, or rupture of membranes. The physician may also elect to do an episiotomy, which is an incision in the perineum to widen the external opening. Episiotomy and laceration repair are included as well. This procedure covers both antepartum and postpartum care. Antepartum or prenatal care includes the initial and subsequent histories, physical examinations, recording of weight, blood pressures, fetal heart tones, and routine chemical urinalysis. It includes monthly visits up to 28 weeks gestation, biweekly visits to 36 weeks gestation, and weekly visits until delivery (approximately 12-15 visits). Because of the previous cesarean delivery, the physician monitors the patient during labor and delivery. Postpartum care includes hospital and office visits following delivery.

Coding Tips

Code 59610 includes total OB care; if services provided do not match the code description of vaginal delivery, including antepartum and postpartum care, following a previous cesarean delivery, use the appropriate stand-alone code. If care rendered was less than the listed service (i.e., the one that most closely describes the service performed), append modifier 52 and reduce the cost of the service. See notes in CPT for directions on the use of maternity care and delivery codes. For vaginal delivery only, after previous cesarean, without antepartum or postpartum care, see 59612. For vaginal delivery including postpartum care, after previous cesarean, see 59614.

ICD-10-CM Diagnostic Codes

O11.5	Pre-existing hypertension with pre-eclampsia, complicating the puerperium ♀ ♀
O12.05	Gestational edema, complicating the puerperium ♀ ♀
O12.15	Gestational proteinuria, complicating the puerperium ♀ ♀
O12.25	Gestational edema with proteinuria, complicating the puerperium ♀ ♀
O13.5	Gestational [pregnancy-induced] hypertension without significant proteinuria, complicating the puerperium ♀ ♀
O14.05	Mild to moderate pre-eclampsia, complicating the puerperium ♀ ♀
O14.15	Severe pre-eclampsia, complicating the puerperium ♀ ♀
O14.25	HELLP syndrome, complicating the puerperium ♀ ♀
O24.435	Gestational diabetes mellitus in puerperium, controlled by oral hypoglycemic drugs ♀ ♀
O34.211	Maternal care for low transverse scar from previous cesarean delivery ♀ ♀
O34.212	Maternal care for vertical scar from previous cesarean delivery ♀ ♀
O34.218	Maternal care for other type scar from previous cesarean delivery ♀ ♀
O34.22	Maternal care for cesarean scar defect (isthmocele) ♀ ♀
O70.0	First degree perineal laceration during delivery ♀ ♀
O70.1	Second degree perineal laceration during delivery ♀ ♀
O70.21	Third degree perineal laceration during delivery, IIIa ♀ ♀
O70.22	Third degree perineal laceration during delivery, IIIb ♀ ♀
O70.23	Third degree perineal laceration during delivery, IIIc ♀ ♀
O70.3	Fourth degree perineal laceration during delivery ♀ ♀
O80	Encounter for full-term uncomplicated delivery ♀ ♀
Z34.01	Encounter for supervision of normal first pregnancy, first trimester ♀ ♀
Z34.02	Encounter for supervision of normal first pregnancy, second trimester ♀ ♀
Z34.03	Encounter for supervision of normal first pregnancy, third trimester ♀ ♀
Z34.81	Encounter for supervision of other normal pregnancy, first trimester ♀ ♀
Z34.82	Encounter for supervision of other normal pregnancy, second trimester ♀ ♀
Z34.83	Encounter for supervision of other normal pregnancy, third trimester ♀ ♀
Z36.0	Encounter for antenatal screening for chromosomal anomalies ♀ ♀
Z36.1	Encounter for antenatal screening for raised alphafetoprotein level ♀ ♀
Z36.2	Encounter for other antenatal screening follow-up ♀ ♀
Z36.3	Encounter for antenatal screening for malformations ♀ ♀
Z36.4	Encounter for antenatal screening for fetal growth retardation ♀ ♀
Z36.5	Encounter for antenatal screening for isoimmunization ♀ ♀
Z36.81	Encounter for antenatal screening for hydrops fetalis ♀ ♀
Z36.82	Encounter for antenatal screening for nuchal translucency ♀ ♀
Z36.83	Encounter for fetal screening for congenital cardiac abnormalities ♀ ♀
Z36.84	Encounter for antenatal screening for fetal lung maturity ♀ ♀
Z36.85	Encounter for antenatal screening for Streptococcus B ♀ ♀
Z36.86	Encounter for antenatal screening for cervical length ♀ ♀
Z36.87	Encounter for antenatal screening for uncertain dates ♀ ♀
Z36.88	Encounter for antenatal screening for fetal macrosomia ♀ ♀
Z36.89	Encounter for other specified antenatal screening ♀ ♀
Z36.8A	Encounter for antenatal screening for other genetic defects ♀ ♀

Z39.0	Encounter for care and examination of mother immediately after delivery Ⓜ ♀
Z39.1	Encounter for care and examination of lactating mother Ⓜ ♀
Z39.2	Encounter for routine postpartum follow-up Ⓜ ♀

AMA: 59610 2019,Jul,6; 2018,Jan,8; 2017,Jan,8; 2016,Jan,13; 2015,Jan,16; 2014,Jan,11

Relative Value Units/Medicare Edits

Non-Facility RVU	Work	PE	MP	Total
59610	33.87	21.51	9.36	64.74
Facility RVU	Work	PE	MP	Total
59610	33.87	21.51	9.36	64.74

	FUD	Status	MUE	Modifiers				IOM Reference
59610	N/A	A	1(2)	51	N/A	N/A	80*	100-02,15,20.1; 100-02,15,180

* with documentation

Terms To Know

elderly primigravida. Female in her first pregnancy who will be 35 years or older at her expected date of delivery. Women in this category are considered to be at high risk during pregnancy.

episiotomy. Deliberate incision in the perineal tissue to facilitate delivery of the fetus and avoid traumatic tearing. In a midline or median episiotomy, the incision is made from the vagina straight down toward the anus. In a mediolateral episiotomy, the incision slants to one side.

multigravida. Female who has had two or more pregnancies. Women in this category are considered to be at high risk during pregnancy.

multiparity. Condition of having had two or more pregnancies that resulted in viable fetuses; producing more than one fetus or offspring in the same gestation.

placenta previa. Implantation of the placenta in the lower segment of the uterus, over or near the internal cervical os. In total previa, the cervical os is completely covered by the placenta; in partial previa, only a portion is covered.

preeclampsia. Complication of pregnancy manifesting in the development of borderline hypertension, protein in the urine, and unresponsive swelling between the 20th week of pregnancy and the end of the first week following birth in mild to moderate cases. Severe preeclampsia presents with hypertension, associated with marked swelling, proteinuria, abdominal pain, and/or visual changes.

59612-59614

| 59612 | Vaginal delivery only, after previous cesarean delivery (with or without episiotomy and/or forceps); |
| 59614 | including postpartum care |

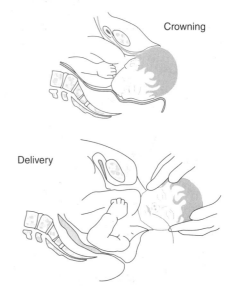

Crowning

Delivery

The physician provides successfully delivers the infant through the vagina

Explanation

The physician delivers an infant and placenta through the vagina. The patient has previously delivered by cesarean section. The physician may elect to assist the delivery with the use of forceps. The physician may also elect to do an episiotomy, which is an incision in the perineum to widen the external opening. Episiotomy and laceration repair are included. Because of the previous cesarean delivery, the physician monitors the patient during labor and delivery. Code 59614 includes postpartum care, hospital office visits following delivery.

Coding Tips

If services provided do not match the code description of vaginal delivery only after previous cesarean (59612) or vaginal delivery including postpartum care, following a previous cesarean delivery (59614), use the appropriate stand-alone code. If care rendered was less than the listed service (i.e., the one that most closely describes the service performed), append modifier 52 and reduce the cost of the service. See notes in CPT for directions on the use of maternity care and delivery codes. For vaginal delivery, after previous cesarean delivery, with antepartum and postpartum care, see 59610.

ICD-10-CM Diagnostic Codes

O11.5	Pre-existing hypertension with pre-eclampsia, complicating the puerperium Ⓜ ♀
O12.05	Gestational edema, complicating the puerperium Ⓜ ♀
O12.15	Gestational proteinuria, complicating the puerperium Ⓜ ♀
O12.25	Gestational edema with proteinuria, complicating the puerperium Ⓜ ♀
O13.5	Gestational [pregnancy-induced] hypertension without significant proteinuria, complicating the puerperium Ⓜ ♀
O14.05	Mild to moderate pre-eclampsia, complicating the puerperium Ⓜ ♀
O14.15	Severe pre-eclampsia, complicating the puerperium Ⓜ ♀
O14.25	HELLP syndrome, complicating the puerperium Ⓜ ♀

Coding Companion for Ob/Gyn

O24.435	Gestational diabetes mellitus in puerperium, controlled by oral hypoglycemic drugs Ⓜ ♀
O34.211	Maternal care for low transverse scar from previous cesarean delivery Ⓜ ♀
O34.212	Maternal care for vertical scar from previous cesarean delivery Ⓜ ♀
O34.218	Maternal care for other type scar from previous cesarean delivery Ⓜ ♀
O34.22	Maternal care for cesarean scar defect (isthmocele) Ⓜ ♀
O70.0	First degree perineal laceration during delivery Ⓜ ♀
O70.1	Second degree perineal laceration during delivery Ⓜ ♀
O70.21	Third degree perineal laceration during delivery, IIIa Ⓜ ♀
O70.22	Third degree perineal laceration during delivery, IIIb Ⓜ ♀
O70.23	Third degree perineal laceration during delivery, IIIc Ⓜ ♀
O70.3	Fourth degree perineal laceration during delivery Ⓜ ♀
Z39.0	Encounter for care and examination of mother immediately after delivery Ⓜ ♀
Z39.1	Encounter for care and examination of lactating mother Ⓜ ♀
Z39.2	Encounter for routine postpartum follow-up Ⓜ ♀

AMA: **59612** 2019,Jul,6; 2018,Jan,8; 2017,Jan,8; 2016,Jan,13; 2015,Jan,16; 2014,Jan,11 **59614** 2019,Jul,6; 2018,Jan,8; 2017,Jan,8; 2016,Jan,13; 2015,Jan,16; 2014,Jan,11

Relative Value Units/Medicare Edits

Non-Facility RVU	Work	PE	MP	Total
59612	16.09	6.07	4.43	26.59
59614	19.73	7.87	5.45	33.05
Facility RVU	Work	PE	MP	Total
59612	16.09	6.07	4.43	26.59
59614	19.73	7.87	5.45	33.05

	FUD	Status	MUE	Modifiers				IOM Reference
59612	N/A	A	2(3)	51	N/A	N/A	80*	None
59614	N/A	A	1(2)	51	N/A	N/A	80*	

* with documentation

Terms To Know

eclampsia. Tetany and toxemia producing seizure activity or coma in a pregnant patient who most often has presented with prior preeclampsia (i.e., hypertension, albuminuria, and edema).

elderly primigravida. Female in her first pregnancy who will be 35 years or older at her expected date of delivery. Women in this category are considered to be at high risk during pregnancy.

episiotomy. Deliberate incision in the perineal tissue to facilitate delivery of the fetus and avoid traumatic tearing. In a midline or median episiotomy, the incision is made from the vagina straight down toward the anus. In a mediolateral episiotomy, the incision slants to one side.

multiparity. Condition of having had two or more pregnancies that resulted in viable fetuses; producing more than one fetus or offspring in the same gestation.

59618

59618	Routine obstetric care including antepartum care, cesarean delivery, and postpartum care, following attempted vaginal delivery after previous cesarean delivery

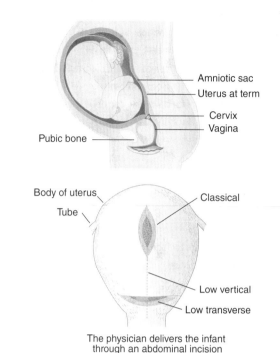

The physician delivers the infant through an abdominal incision

Explanation

After first attempting a vaginal delivery, the physician delivers an infant through a horizontal or vertical incision in the abdomen and uterus. The patient has previously delivered by cesarean section. Once the incisions are made, the infant is delivered and the placenta separated and removed. The uterine and abdominal incisions are closed with layered sutures. This procedure includes both antepartum and postpartum care. Antepartum or prenatal care includes the initial and subsequent histories, physical examinations, recording of weight, blood pressures, fetal heart tones, and routine chemical urinalysis. It includes monthly visits up to 28 weeks gestation, biweekly visits to 36 weeks gestation, and weekly visits until delivery (approximately 13-15 visits). Because of the previous cesarean delivery and the attempted vaginal delivery, the physician monitors the patient during labor and delivery. Postpartum care includes hospital and office visits following delivery.

Coding Tips

Code 59618 includes total OB care; if services provided do not match the code description of cesarean delivery, including antepartum and postpartum care, after attempted vaginal delivery, following a previous cesarean, use the appropriate stand-alone code. If care rendered was less than the listed service (i.e., the one that most closely describes the service performed), append modifier 52 and reduce the cost of the service. See notes in CPT for directions on the use of the maternity care and delivery codes. For cesarean delivery only, following attempted vaginal delivery after previous cesarean, see 59620. For cesarean delivery, following attempted vaginal delivery after previous cesarean, including postpartum care, see 59622.

ICD-10-CM Diagnostic Codes

O30.013	Twin pregnancy, monochorionic/monoamniotic, third trimester Ⓜ ♀

O30.033	Twin pregnancy, monochorionic/diamniotic, third trimester Ⓜ ♀
O30.113	Triplet pregnancy with two or more monochorionic fetuses, third trimester Ⓜ ♀
O30.123	Triplet pregnancy with two or more monoamniotic fetuses, third trimester Ⓜ ♀
O32.0XX1	Maternal care for unstable lie, fetus 1 Ⓜ ♀
O32.0XX2	Maternal care for unstable lie, fetus 2 Ⓜ ♀
O32.0XX3	Maternal care for unstable lie, fetus 3 Ⓜ ♀
O32.1XX1	Maternal care for breech presentation, fetus 1 Ⓜ ♀
O32.1XX2	Maternal care for breech presentation, fetus 2 Ⓜ ♀
O32.1XX3	Maternal care for breech presentation, fetus 3 Ⓜ ♀
O32.2XX1	Maternal care for transverse and oblique lie, fetus 1 Ⓜ ♀
O32.2XX2	Maternal care for transverse and oblique lie, fetus 2 Ⓜ ♀
O32.2XX3	Maternal care for transverse and oblique lie, fetus 3 Ⓜ ♀
O32.3XX1	Maternal care for face, brow and chin presentation, fetus 1 Ⓜ ♀
O32.3XX2	Maternal care for face, brow and chin presentation, fetus 2 Ⓜ ♀
O32.3XX3	Maternal care for face, brow and chin presentation, fetus 3 Ⓜ ♀
O32.4XX1	Maternal care for high head at term, fetus 1 Ⓜ ♀
O32.4XX2	Maternal care for high head at term, fetus 2 Ⓜ ♀
O32.4XX3	Maternal care for high head at term, fetus 3 Ⓜ ♀
O32.6XX1	Maternal care for compound presentation, fetus 1 Ⓜ ♀
O32.6XX2	Maternal care for compound presentation, fetus 2 Ⓜ ♀
O32.6XX3	Maternal care for compound presentation, fetus 3 Ⓜ ♀
O32.8XX1	Maternal care for other malpresentation of fetus, fetus 1 Ⓜ ♀
O32.8XX2	Maternal care for other malpresentation of fetus, fetus 2 Ⓜ ♀
O32.8XX3	Maternal care for other malpresentation of fetus, fetus 3 Ⓜ ♀
O34.211	Maternal care for low transverse scar from previous cesarean delivery Ⓜ ♀
O34.212	Maternal care for vertical scar from previous cesarean delivery Ⓜ ♀
O34.218	Maternal care for other type scar from previous cesarean delivery Ⓜ ♀
O34.22	Maternal care for cesarean scar defect (isthmocele) Ⓜ ♀
O34.29	Maternal care due to uterine scar from other previous surgery Ⓜ ♀
O34.33	Maternal care for cervical incompetence, third trimester Ⓜ ♀
O34.43	Maternal care for other abnormalities of cervix, third trimester Ⓜ ♀
O61.0	Failed medical induction of labor Ⓜ ♀
O61.1	Failed instrumental induction of labor Ⓜ ♀
O61.8	Other failed induction of labor Ⓜ ♀
O64.0XX1	Obstructed labor due to incomplete rotation of fetal head, fetus 1 Ⓜ ♀
O64.0XX2	Obstructed labor due to incomplete rotation of fetal head, fetus 2 Ⓜ ♀
O64.0XX3	Obstructed labor due to incomplete rotation of fetal head, fetus 3 Ⓜ ♀
O64.1XX1	Obstructed labor due to breech presentation, fetus 1 Ⓜ ♀
O64.1XX2	Obstructed labor due to breech presentation, fetus 2 Ⓜ ♀
O64.1XX3	Obstructed labor due to breech presentation, fetus 3 Ⓜ ♀
O64.2XX1	Obstructed labor due to face presentation, fetus 1 Ⓜ ♀
O64.2XX2	Obstructed labor due to face presentation, fetus 2 Ⓜ ♀
O64.2XX3	Obstructed labor due to face presentation, fetus 3 Ⓜ ♀
O64.3XX1	Obstructed labor due to brow presentation, fetus 1 Ⓜ ♀
O64.3XX2	Obstructed labor due to brow presentation, fetus 2 Ⓜ ♀
O64.3XX3	Obstructed labor due to brow presentation, fetus 3 Ⓜ ♀
O64.4XX1	Obstructed labor due to shoulder presentation, fetus 1 Ⓜ ♀
O64.4XX2	Obstructed labor due to shoulder presentation, fetus 2 Ⓜ ♀
O64.4XX3	Obstructed labor due to shoulder presentation, fetus 3 Ⓜ ♀
O64.5XX1	Obstructed labor due to compound presentation, fetus 1 Ⓜ ♀
O64.5XX2	Obstructed labor due to compound presentation, fetus 2 Ⓜ ♀
O64.5XX3	Obstructed labor due to compound presentation, fetus 3 Ⓜ ♀
O64.8XX1	Obstructed labor due to other malposition and malpresentation, fetus 1 Ⓜ ♀
O64.8XX2	Obstructed labor due to other malposition and malpresentation, fetus 2 Ⓜ ♀
O64.8XX3	Obstructed labor due to other malposition and malpresentation, fetus 3 Ⓜ ♀
O65.0	Obstructed labor due to deformed pelvis Ⓜ ♀
O65.1	Obstructed labor due to generally contracted pelvis Ⓜ ♀
O65.2	Obstructed labor due to pelvic inlet contraction Ⓜ ♀
O65.3	Obstructed labor due to pelvic outlet and mid-cavity contraction Ⓜ ♀
O65.5	Obstructed labor due to abnormality of maternal pelvic organs Ⓜ ♀
O65.8	Obstructed labor due to other maternal pelvic abnormalities Ⓜ ♀
O66.0	Obstructed labor due to shoulder dystocia Ⓜ ♀
O66.1	Obstructed labor due to locked twins Ⓜ ♀
O66.2	Obstructed labor due to unusually large fetus Ⓜ ♀
O66.3	Obstructed labor due to other abnormalities of fetus Ⓜ ♀
O66.41	Failed attempted vaginal birth after previous cesarean delivery Ⓜ ♀
O66.5	Attempted application of vacuum extractor and forceps Ⓜ ♀
O66.6	Obstructed labor due to other multiple fetuses Ⓜ ♀
O66.8	Other specified obstructed labor Ⓜ ♀
O68	Labor and delivery complicated by abnormality of fetal acid-base balance Ⓜ ♀
O69.0XX1	Labor and delivery complicated by prolapse of cord, fetus 1 Ⓜ ♀
O69.0XX2	Labor and delivery complicated by prolapse of cord, fetus 2 Ⓜ ♀
O69.0XX3	Labor and delivery complicated by prolapse of cord, fetus 3 Ⓜ ♀
O69.3XX1	Labor and delivery complicated by short cord, fetus 1 Ⓜ ♀
O69.3XX2	Labor and delivery complicated by short cord, fetus 2 Ⓜ ♀
O69.3XX3	Labor and delivery complicated by short cord, fetus 3 Ⓜ ♀
O69.4XX1	Labor and delivery complicated by vasa previa, fetus 1 Ⓜ ♀
O69.4XX2	Labor and delivery complicated by vasa previa, fetus 2 Ⓜ ♀
O69.4XX3	Labor and delivery complicated by vasa previa, fetus 3 Ⓜ ♀
O69.81X1	Labor and delivery complicated by cord around neck, without compression, fetus 1 Ⓜ ♀
O69.81X2	Labor and delivery complicated by cord around neck, without compression, fetus 2 Ⓜ ♀
O69.81X3	Labor and delivery complicated by cord around neck, without compression, fetus 3 Ⓜ ♀
O69.82X1	Labor and delivery complicated by other cord entanglement, without compression, fetus 1 Ⓜ ♀
O69.82X2	Labor and delivery complicated by other cord entanglement, without compression, fetus 2 Ⓜ ♀
O69.82X3	Labor and delivery complicated by other cord entanglement, without compression, fetus 3 Ⓜ ♀

O69.89X1	Labor and delivery complicated by other cord complications, fetus 1 ▥ ♀
O69.89X2	Labor and delivery complicated by other cord complications, fetus 2 ▥ ♀
O69.89X3	Labor and delivery complicated by other cord complications, fetus 3 ▥ ♀
O77.0	Labor and delivery complicated by meconium in amniotic fluid ▥ ♀
O77.1	Fetal stress in labor or delivery due to drug administration ▥ ♀
O77.8	Labor and delivery complicated by other evidence of fetal stress ▥ ♀
O99.213	Obesity complicating pregnancy, third trimester ▥ ♀
O99.214	Obesity complicating childbirth ▥ ♀
Z36.0	Encounter for antenatal screening for chromosomal anomalies ▥ ♀
Z36.1	Encounter for antenatal screening for raised alphafetoprotein level ▥ ♀
Z36.2	Encounter for other antenatal screening follow-up ▥ ♀
Z36.3	Encounter for antenatal screening for malformations ▥ ♀
Z36.4	Encounter for antenatal screening for fetal growth retardation ▥ ♀
Z36.5	Encounter for antenatal screening for isoimmunization ▥ ♀
Z36.81	Encounter for antenatal screening for hydrops fetalis ▥ ♀
Z36.82	Encounter for antenatal screening for nuchal translucency ▥ ♀
Z36.83	Encounter for fetal screening for congenital cardiac abnormalities ▥ ♀
Z36.84	Encounter for antenatal screening for fetal lung maturity ▥ ♀
Z36.85	Encounter for antenatal screening for Streptococcus B ▥ ♀
Z36.86	Encounter for antenatal screening for cervical length ▥ ♀
Z36.87	Encounter for antenatal screening for uncertain dates ▥ ♀
Z36.88	Encounter for antenatal screening for fetal macrosomia ▥ ♀
Z39.0	Encounter for care and examination of mother immediately after delivery ▥ ♀

AMA: **59618** 2019,Jul,6; 2018,Jan,8; 2017,Jan,8; 2016,Jan,13; 2015,Jan,16; 2014,Jan,11

Relative Value Units/Medicare Edits

Non-Facility RVU	Work	PE	MP	Total
59618	36.16	22.95	10.01	69.12
Facility RVU	**Work**	**PE**	**MP**	**Total**
59618	36.16	22.95	10.01	69.12

	FUD	Status	MUE	Modifiers				IOM Reference
59618	N/A	A	1(2)	51	N/A	N/A	80*	None

* with documentation

59620-59622

| 59620 | Cesarean delivery only, following attempted vaginal delivery after previous cesarean delivery; |
| 59622 | including postpartum care |

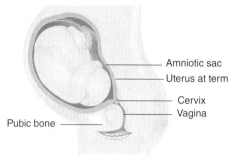

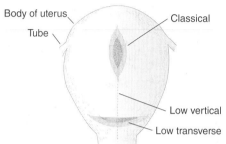

The physician delivers the infant through an abdominal incision

Explanation

After first attempting a vaginal delivery, the physician delivers an infant through a horizontal or vertical incision in the abdomen and uterus. The patient has previously delivered by cesarean section. Once the incisions are made, the infant is delivered and the placenta separated and removed. The uterine and abdominal incisions are closed with layered sutures because of the previous cesarean delivery and the attempted vaginal delivery, the physician monitors the patient during labor and delivery. Only delivery is included in 59620. Postpartum care is included in 59622. Postpartum care includes hospital and office visits following delivery.

Coding Tips

Code 59620 represents a cesarean delivery following attempted vaginal delivery after previous cesarean delivery only and does not include postpartum care. Code 59622 represents a cesarean delivery including postpartum care, following attempted vaginal delivery, after previous cesarean delivery. See notes in CPT for directions on the use of the maternity care and delivery codes. For cesarean delivery including antepartum and postpartum care, following attempted vaginal delivery after previous cesarean delivery, see 59618.

ICD-10-CM Diagnostic Codes

O11.5	Pre-existing hypertension with pre-eclampsia, complicating the puerperium ▥ ♀
O12.05	Gestational edema, complicating the puerperium ▥ ♀
O12.15	Gestational proteinuria, complicating the puerperium ▥ ♀
O12.25	Gestational edema with proteinuria, complicating the puerperium ▥ ♀
O13.5	Gestational [pregnancy-induced] hypertension without significant proteinuria, complicating the puerperium ▥ ♀

Maternity Care

O30.013	Twin pregnancy, monochorionic/monoamniotic, third trimester Ⓜ ♀
O30.023	Conjoined twin pregnancy, third trimester Ⓜ ♀
O30.033	Twin pregnancy, monochorionic/diamniotic, third trimester Ⓜ ♀
O30.043	Twin pregnancy, dichorionic/diamniotic, third trimester Ⓜ ♀
O30.113	Triplet pregnancy with two or more monochorionic fetuses, third trimester Ⓜ ♀
O30.123	Triplet pregnancy with two or more monoamniotic fetuses, third trimester Ⓜ ♀
O32.0XX1	Maternal care for unstable lie, fetus 1 Ⓜ ♀
O32.0XX2	Maternal care for unstable lie, fetus 2 Ⓜ ♀
O32.0XX3	Maternal care for unstable lie, fetus 3 Ⓜ ♀
O32.1XX1	Maternal care for breech presentation, fetus 1 Ⓜ ♀
O32.1XX2	Maternal care for breech presentation, fetus 2 Ⓜ ♀
O32.1XX3	Maternal care for breech presentation, fetus 3 Ⓜ ♀
O32.2XX1	Maternal care for transverse and oblique lie, fetus 1 Ⓜ ♀
O32.2XX2	Maternal care for transverse and oblique lie, fetus 2 Ⓜ ♀
O32.2XX3	Maternal care for transverse and oblique lie, fetus 3 Ⓜ ♀
O32.3XX1	Maternal care for face, brow and chin presentation, fetus 1 Ⓜ ♀
O32.3XX2	Maternal care for face, brow and chin presentation, fetus 2 Ⓜ ♀
O32.3XX3	Maternal care for face, brow and chin presentation, fetus 3 Ⓜ ♀
O32.4XX1	Maternal care for high head at term, fetus 1 Ⓜ ♀
O32.4XX2	Maternal care for high head at term, fetus 2 Ⓜ ♀
O32.4XX3	Maternal care for high head at term, fetus 3 Ⓜ ♀
O32.6XX1	Maternal care for compound presentation, fetus 1 Ⓜ ♀
O32.6XX2	Maternal care for compound presentation, fetus 2 Ⓜ ♀
O32.6XX3	Maternal care for compound presentation, fetus 3 Ⓜ ♀
O32.8XX1	Maternal care for other malpresentation of fetus, fetus 1 Ⓜ ♀
O32.8XX2	Maternal care for other malpresentation of fetus, fetus 2 Ⓜ ♀
O32.8XX3	Maternal care for other malpresentation of fetus, fetus 3 Ⓜ ♀
O34.211	Maternal care for low transverse scar from previous cesarean delivery Ⓜ ♀
O34.212	Maternal care for vertical scar from previous cesarean delivery Ⓜ ♀
O34.29	Maternal care due to uterine scar from other previous surgery ♀
O34.33	Maternal care for cervical incompetence, third trimester Ⓜ ♀
O34.43	Maternal care for other abnormalities of cervix, third trimester Ⓜ ♀
O61.0	Failed medical induction of labor Ⓜ ♀
O61.1	Failed instrumental induction of labor Ⓜ ♀
O61.8	Other failed induction of labor Ⓜ ♀
O64.0XX1	Obstructed labor due to incomplete rotation of fetal head, fetus 1 Ⓜ ♀
O64.0XX2	Obstructed labor due to incomplete rotation of fetal head, fetus 2 Ⓜ ♀
O64.0XX3	Obstructed labor due to incomplete rotation of fetal head, fetus 3 Ⓜ ♀
O64.1XX1	Obstructed labor due to breech presentation, fetus 1 Ⓜ ♀
O64.1XX2	Obstructed labor due to breech presentation, fetus 2 Ⓜ ♀
O64.1XX3	Obstructed labor due to breech presentation, fetus 3 Ⓜ ♀
O64.2XX1	Obstructed labor due to face presentation, fetus 1 Ⓜ ♀
O64.2XX2	Obstructed labor due to face presentation, fetus 2 Ⓜ ♀
O64.2XX3	Obstructed labor due to face presentation, fetus 3 Ⓜ ♀

O64.3XX1	Obstructed labor due to brow presentation, fetus 1 Ⓜ ♀
O64.3XX2	Obstructed labor due to brow presentation, fetus 2 Ⓜ ♀
O64.3XX3	Obstructed labor due to brow presentation, fetus 3 Ⓜ ♀
O64.4XX1	Obstructed labor due to shoulder presentation, fetus 1 Ⓜ ♀
O64.4XX2	Obstructed labor due to shoulder presentation, fetus 2 Ⓜ ♀
O64.4XX3	Obstructed labor due to shoulder presentation, fetus 3 Ⓜ ♀
O64.5XX1	Obstructed labor due to compound presentation, fetus 1 Ⓜ ♀
O64.5XX2	Obstructed labor due to compound presentation, fetus 2 Ⓜ ♀
O64.5XX3	Obstructed labor due to compound presentation, fetus 3 Ⓜ ♀
O64.8XX1	Obstructed labor due to other malposition and malpresentation, fetus 1 Ⓜ ♀
O64.8XX2	Obstructed labor due to other malposition and malpresentation, fetus 2 Ⓜ ♀
O64.8XX3	Obstructed labor due to other malposition and malpresentation, fetus 3 Ⓜ ♀
O65.0	Obstructed labor due to deformed pelvis Ⓜ ♀
O65.1	Obstructed labor due to generally contracted pelvis Ⓜ ♀
O65.2	Obstructed labor due to pelvic inlet contraction Ⓜ ♀
O65.3	Obstructed labor due to pelvic outlet and mid-cavity contraction Ⓜ ♀
O65.5	Obstructed labor due to abnormality of maternal pelvic organs Ⓜ ♀
O65.8	Obstructed labor due to other maternal pelvic abnormalities Ⓜ ♀
O66.0	Obstructed labor due to shoulder dystocia Ⓜ ♀
O66.1	Obstructed labor due to locked twins Ⓜ ♀
O66.2	Obstructed labor due to unusually large fetus Ⓜ ♀
O66.3	Obstructed labor due to other abnormalities of fetus Ⓜ ♀
O66.41	Failed attempted vaginal birth after previous cesarean delivery Ⓜ ♀
O66.5	Attempted application of vacuum extractor and forceps Ⓜ ♀
O66.6	Obstructed labor due to other multiple fetuses Ⓜ ♀
O66.8	Other specified obstructed labor Ⓜ ♀
O68	Labor and delivery complicated by abnormality of fetal acid-base balance Ⓜ ♀
O69.0XX1	Labor and delivery complicated by prolapse of cord, fetus 1 Ⓜ ♀
O69.0XX2	Labor and delivery complicated by prolapse of cord, fetus 2 Ⓜ ♀
O69.0XX3	Labor and delivery complicated by prolapse of cord, fetus 3 Ⓜ ♀
O69.0XX9	Labor and delivery complicated by prolapse of cord, other fetus Ⓜ ♀
O69.3XX1	Labor and delivery complicated by short cord, fetus 1 Ⓜ ♀
O69.3XX2	Labor and delivery complicated by short cord, fetus 2 Ⓜ ♀
O69.3XX3	Labor and delivery complicated by short cord, fetus 3 Ⓜ ♀
O69.4XX1	Labor and delivery complicated by vasa previa, fetus 1 Ⓜ ♀
O69.4XX2	Labor and delivery complicated by vasa previa, fetus 2 Ⓜ ♀
O69.4XX3	Labor and delivery complicated by vasa previa, fetus 3 Ⓜ ♀
O69.81X1	Labor and delivery complicated by cord around neck, without compression, fetus 1 Ⓜ ♀
O69.81X2	Labor and delivery complicated by cord around neck, without compression, fetus 2 Ⓜ ♀
O69.81X3	Labor and delivery complicated by cord around neck, without compression, fetus 3 Ⓜ ♀
O69.82X1	Labor and delivery complicated by other cord entanglement, without compression, fetus 1 Ⓜ ♀
O69.82X2	Labor and delivery complicated by other cord entanglement, without compression, fetus 2 Ⓜ ♀

Maternity Care

O69.82X3	Labor and delivery complicated by other cord entanglement, without compression, fetus 3 ▥ ♀
O69.89X1	Labor and delivery complicated by other cord complications, fetus 1 ▥ ♀
O69.89X2	Labor and delivery complicated by other cord complications, fetus 2 ▥ ♀
O69.89X3	Labor and delivery complicated by other cord complications, fetus 3 ▥ ♀
O77.0	Labor and delivery complicated by meconium in amniotic fluid ▥ ♀
O77.1	Fetal stress in labor or delivery due to drug administration ▥ ♀
O77.8	Labor and delivery complicated by other evidence of fetal stress ▥ ♀
O99.213	Obesity complicating pregnancy, third trimester ▥ ♀
O99.214	Obesity complicating childbirth ▥ ♀

AMA: **59620** 2019,Jul,6; 2018,Jan,8; 2017,Jan,8; 2016,Jan,13; 2015,Jan,16; 2014,Jan,11 **59622** 2019,Jul,6; 2018,Jan,8; 2017,Jan,8; 2016,Jan,13; 2015,Jan,16; 2014,Jan,11

Relative Value Units/Medicare Edits

Non-Facility RVU	Work	PE	MP	Total
59620	16.66	6.28	4.61	27.55
59622	22.0	10.05	6.07	38.12
Facility RVU	**Work**	**PE**	**MP**	**Total**
59620	16.66	6.28	4.61	27.55
59622	22.0	10.05	6.07	38.12

	FUD	Status	MUE	Modifiers				IOM Reference
59620	N/A	A	1(2)	51	N/A	N/A	80	None
59622	N/A	A	1(2)	51	N/A	N/A	80*	

* with documentation

Terms To Know

eclampsia. Tetany and toxemia producing seizure activity or coma in a pregnant patient who most often has presented with prior preeclampsia (i.e., hypertension, albuminuria, and edema).

elderly primigravida. Female in her first pregnancy who will be 35 years or older at her expected date of delivery. Women in this category are considered to be at high risk during pregnancy.

multiparity. Condition of having had two or more pregnancies that resulted in viable fetuses; producing more than one fetus or offspring in the same gestation.

placenta previa. Implantation of the placenta in the lower segment of the uterus, over or near the internal cervical os. In total previa, the cervical os is completely covered by the placenta; in partial previa, only a portion is covered.

preeclampsia. Complication of pregnancy manifesting in the development of borderline hypertension, protein in the urine, and unresponsive swelling between the 20th week of pregnancy and the end of the first week following birth in mild to moderate cases. Severe preeclampsia presents with hypertension, associated with marked swelling, proteinuria, abdominal pain, and/or visual changes.

secundines. Placenta and membranes; the afterbirth.

59812

| 59812 | Treatment of incomplete abortion, any trimester, completed surgically |

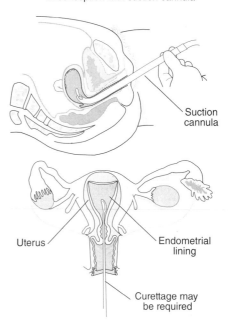

The physician removes remaining products of conception with suction cannula

Suction cannula

Uterus

Endometrial lining

Curettage may be required

Explanation

The physician removes the products of conception remaining after an incomplete abortion in any trimester. To evacuate the uterus, the physician performs a dilation and suction curettage. The physician inserts a speculum into the vagina to view the cervix. A tenaculum is used to grasp the cervix, pull it down, and exert traction. If the cervix is not sufficiently dilated, a dilator is inserted into the endocervix and through the cervical canal to enlarge the opening. The physician places a cannula in the endocervical canal and passes it into the uterus. The suction machine is activated and the uterine contents are evacuated by rotation of the cannula. After suction curettage, a sharp curette may be used to gently scrape the uterus to ensure that it is empty.

Coding Tips

For medical treatment of a spontaneous complete abortion, any trimester, see 99202–99233. For treatment of a missed abortion completed surgically, first trimester, see 59820; second trimester, see 59821. For induced abortion, see 59840-59857.

ICD-10-CM Diagnostic Codes

O03.0	Genital tract and pelvic infection following incomplete spontaneous abortion ▥ ♀
O03.1	Delayed or excessive hemorrhage following incomplete spontaneous abortion ▥ ♀
O03.2	Embolism following incomplete spontaneous abortion ▥ ♀
O03.31	Shock following incomplete spontaneous abortion ▥ ♀
O03.32	Renal failure following incomplete spontaneous abortion ▥ ♀
O03.33	Metabolic disorder following incomplete spontaneous abortion ▥ ♀
O03.34	Damage to pelvic organs following incomplete spontaneous abortion ▥ ♀
O03.35	Other venous complications following incomplete spontaneous abortion ▥ ♀

Maternity Care

O03.36	Cardiac arrest following incomplete spontaneous abortion Ⓜ ♀
O03.37	Sepsis following incomplete spontaneous abortion Ⓜ ♀
O03.38	Urinary tract infection following incomplete spontaneous abortion Ⓜ ♀
O03.39	Incomplete spontaneous abortion with other complications Ⓜ ♀
O03.4	Incomplete spontaneous abortion without complication Ⓜ ♀

AMA: **59812** 2019,Jul,6; 2018,Jan,8; 2017,Jan,8; 2016,Jan,13; 2015,Jan,16; 2014,Jan,11

Relative Value Units/Medicare Edits

Non-Facility RVU	Work	PE	MP	Total
59812	4.44	4.23	1.22	9.89
Facility RVU	**Work**	**PE**	**MP**	**Total**
59812	4.44	3.13	1.22	8.79

	FUD	Status	MUE	Modifiers			IOM Reference
59812	90	A	1(2)	51	N/A	N/A	N/A	100-02,15,20.1

* with documentation

Terms To Know

abortion. Premature expulsion or extraction of the products of conception.

cannula. Tube inserted into a blood vessel, duct, or body cavity to facilitate passage.

curettage. Removal of tissue by scraping.

dilation. Artificial increase in the diameter of an opening or lumen made by medication or by instrumentation.

suction. Vacuum evacuation of fluid or tissue.

trimester. Normal pregnancy has a duration of approximately 40 weeks and is grouped into three-month periods consisting of three trimesters. ICD-10-CM counts trimesters from the first day of the last menstrual period as follows: 1st trimester less than 14 weeks and 0 days; 2nd trimester 14 weeks, 0 days to less than 28 weeks and 0 days; and 3rd trimester 28 weeks and 0 days until delivery.

59820-59821

| 59820 | Treatment of missed abortion, completed surgically; first trimester |
| 59821 | second trimester |

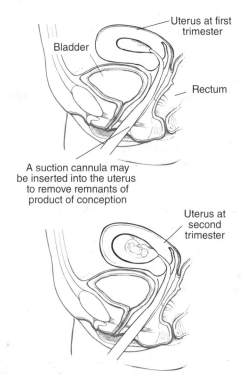

Bladder
Uterus at first trimester
Rectum

A suction cannula may be inserted into the uterus to remove remnants of product of conception

Uterus at second trimester

Explanation

The physician treats a missed abortion by suction curettage in the first trimester for 59820, and in the second trimester for 59821. In missed abortion, the fetus remains in the uterus four to eight weeks following its death. Ultrasonography may be needed to determine the size of the fetus prior to the procedure. The physician inserts a speculum into the vagina to view the cervix. A tenaculum is used to grasp the cervix, pull it down, and exert traction. A dilator is inserted into the endocervix and through the cervical canal to enlarge the opening. The physician places a cannula in the endocervical canal and passes it into the uterus. The suction machine is activated and the uterine contents are evacuated by rotation of the cannula. After suction curettage, a sharp curette may be used to gently scrape the uterus to ensure that it is empty.

Coding Tips

For surgical treatment of an incomplete abortion, any trimester, see 59812. For medical treatment of a spontaneous complete abortion, any trimester, see 99202–99233. For induced abortion, see 59840–59857.

ICD-10-CM Diagnostic Codes

| O02.1 | Missed abortion Ⓜ ♀ |

AMA: **59820** 2019,Jul,6; 2018,Jan,8; 2017,Jan,8; 2016,Jan,13; 2015,Jan,16; 2014,Jan,11 **59821** 2019,Jul,6; 2018,Jan,8; 2017,Jan,8; 2016,Jan,13; 2015,Jan,16; 2014,Jan,11

Maternity Care

Relative Value Units/Medicare Edits

Non-Facility RVU	Work	PE	MP	Total
59820	4.84	5.7	1.32	11.86
59821	5.09	5.32	1.41	11.82
Facility RVU	Work	PE	MP	Total
59820	4.84	4.6	1.32	10.76
59821	5.09	4.16	1.41	10.66

	FUD	Status	MUE	Modifiers				IOM Reference
59820	90	A	1(2)	51	N/A	N/A	N/A	None
59821	90	A	1(2)	51	N/A	N/A	80*	

* with documentation

Terms To Know

abortion. Premature expulsion or extraction of the products of conception.

curettage. Removal of tissue by scraping.

curette. Spoon-shaped instrument used to scrape out abnormal tissue from a cavity or bone.

dilation. Artificial increase in the diameter of an opening or lumen made by medication or by instrumentation.

fetus. Unborn offspring past the embryonic stage that has developed major structures. It is the period defined from nine weeks after fertilization until birth.

missed abortion. Retention of a dead fetus within the uterus in cases where fetal demise occurred before 20 weeks gestation. Abortion in this context refers to retained products of conception from the death of a normal fetus that does not result in spontaneous or induced abortion, or missed delivery.

secundines. Placenta and membranes; the afterbirth.

speculum. Tool used to enlarge the opening of any canal or cavity.

suction. Vacuum evacuation of fluid or tissue.

59830

59830   Treatment of septic abortion, completed surgically

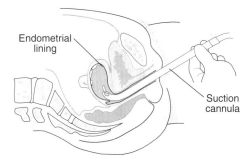

The physician removes remaining matter using a suction cannula; intravenous antibiotics and fluids may be required

Endometrial lining

Suction cannula

Explanation

The physician treats a septic abortion with prompt evacuation of the uterus and vigorous medical treatment of the patient. A septic abortion is one complicated by generalized fever and infection. There is also inflammation and infection of the endometrium and in the cellular tissue around the uterus. The physician treats the infection with intravenous antibiotics and blood transfusions as necessary. To evacuate the uterus, the physician inserts a speculum into the vagina to view the cervix. A tenaculum is used to grasp the cervix, pull it down, and exert traction. A dilator is inserted into the endocervix and through the cervical canal to enlarge the opening. The physician places a cannula in the endocervical canal and passes it into the uterus. The suction machine is activated and the uterine contents are evacuated by rotation of the cannula. After suction curettage, a sharp curette may be used to gently scrape the uterus to ensure that it is empty.

Coding Tips

To report surgical treatment of an incomplete abortion, any trimester, see 59812. For medical treatment of a spontaneous complete abortion, any trimester, see 99202–99233. For treatment of a missed abortion, completed surgically, see 59820–59821. For induced abortion, see 59840–59857.

ICD-10-CM Diagnostic Codes

O03.37	Sepsis following incomplete spontaneous abortion 🄼 ♀
O03.87	Sepsis following complete or unspecified spontaneous abortion 🄼 ♀
O04.87	Sepsis following (induced) termination of pregnancy 🄼 ♀

AMA: 59830 2019,Jul,6; 2018,Jan,8; 2017,Jan,8; 2016,Jan,13; 2015,Jan,16; 2014,Jan,11

Relative Value Units/Medicare Edits

Non-Facility RVU	Work	PE	MP	Total
59830	6.59	4.72	1.81	13.12
Facility RVU	Work	PE	MP	Total
59830	6.59	4.72	1.81	13.12

	FUD	Status	MUE	Modifiers				IOM Reference
59830	90	A	1(2)	51	N/A	N/A	80*	None

* with documentation

59840

59840 Induced abortion, by dilation and curettage

The physician dilates the cervix, then uses a curette to scrape the uterine wall

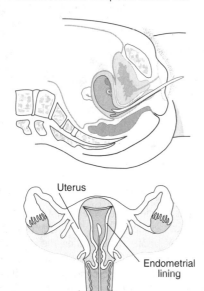

Uterus

Endometrial lining

Curette

Explanation

The physician terminates a pregnancy by dilation and curettage. The physician inserts a speculum into the vagina to view the cervix. A tenaculum is used to grasp the cervix, pull it down, and exert traction. A dilator is inserted into the endocervix and through the cervical canal to enlarge the opening. The physician places a curette in the endocervical canal and passes it into the uterus. The uterine contents are removed by rotating the curette and gently scraping the uterus until all the products of conception are removed.

Coding Tips

For induced abortion by dilation and evacuation, see 59841. For other induced abortion, see 59850–59857. For medical treatment of a spontaneous complete abortion, any trimester, see 99202–99233. For surgical treatment of an incomplete abortion, any trimester, see 59812. For treatment of a missed abortion, completed surgically, first trimester, see 59820; second trimester, see 59821. Because this procedure may not be done out of medical necessity, the patient may be responsible for charges. Verify with the insurance carrier for coverage.

ICD-10-CM Diagnostic Codes

O02.89	Other abnormal products of conception ⓜ ♀
O10.211	Pre-existing hypertensive chronic kidney disease complicating pregnancy, first trimester ⓜ ♀
O10.311	Pre-existing hypertensive heart and chronic kidney disease complicating pregnancy, first trimester ⓜ ♀
O35.0XX0	Maternal care for (suspected) central nervous system malformation in fetus, not applicable or unspecified ⓜ ♀
O35.1XX0	Maternal care for (suspected) chromosomal abnormality in fetus, not applicable or unspecified ⓜ ♀
O35.2XX0	Maternal care for (suspected) hereditary disease in fetus, not applicable or unspecified ⓜ ♀

O35.3XX0	Maternal care for (suspected) damage to fetus from viral disease in mother, not applicable or unspecified ⓜ ♀
O35.4XX0	Maternal care for (suspected) damage to fetus from alcohol, not applicable or unspecified ⓜ ♀
O35.5XX0	Maternal care for (suspected) damage to fetus by drugs, not applicable or unspecified ⓜ ♀
O35.6XX0	Maternal care for (suspected) damage to fetus by radiation, not applicable or unspecified ⓜ ♀
O35.7XX0	Maternal care for (suspected) damage to fetus by other medical procedures, not applicable or unspecified ⓜ ♀
O35.8XX0	Maternal care for other (suspected) fetal abnormality and damage, not applicable or unspecified ⓜ ♀
O35.9XX0	Maternal care for (suspected) fetal abnormality and damage, unspecified, not applicable or unspecified ⓜ ♀
O36.0110	Maternal care for anti-D [Rh] antibodies, first trimester, not applicable or unspecified ⓜ ♀
O36.0910	Maternal care for other rhesus isoimmunization, first trimester, not applicable or unspecified ⓜ ♀
O36.1110	Maternal care for Anti-A sensitization, first trimester, not applicable or unspecified ⓜ ♀
O36.1910	Maternal care for other isoimmunization, first trimester, not applicable or unspecified ⓜ ♀
O36.21X0	Maternal care for hydrops fetalis, first trimester, not applicable or unspecified ⓜ ♀
O36.4XX0	Maternal care for intrauterine death, not applicable or unspecified ⓜ ♀
O36.5110	Maternal care for known or suspected placental insufficiency, first trimester, not applicable or unspecified ⓜ ♀
O36.5910	Maternal care for other known or suspected poor fetal growth, first trimester, not applicable or unspecified ⓜ ♀
O36.8910	Maternal care for other specified fetal problems, first trimester, not applicable or unspecified ⓜ ♀
O99.111	Other diseases of the blood and blood-forming organs and certain disorders involving the immune mechanism complicating pregnancy, first trimester ⓜ ♀
O99.411	Diseases of the circulatory system complicating pregnancy, first trimester ⓜ ♀
Z33.2	Encounter for elective termination of pregnancy ⓜ ♀

AMA: 59840 2019,Jul,6; 2018,Jan,8; 2017,Jan,8; 2016,Jan,13; 2015,Jan,16; 2014,Jan,11

Relative Value Units/Medicare Edits

Non-Facility RVU	Work	PE	MP	Total
59840	3.01	2.99	0.84	6.84
Facility RVU	**Work**	**PE**	**MP**	**Total**
59840	3.01	2.42	0.84	6.27

	FUD	Status	MUE	Modifiers				IOM Reference
59840	10	R	1(2)	51	N/A	N/A	80*	100-02,1,90; 100-03,140.1; 100-04,3,100.1

* with documentation

Maternity Care

59841

59841 Induced abortion, by dilation and evacuation

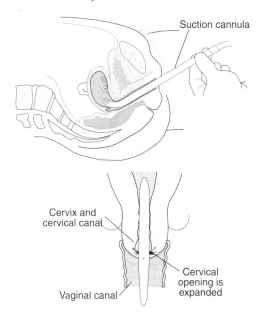

Suction cannula

Cervix and cervical canal

Cervical opening is expanded

Vaginal canal

Explanation

The physician terminates a pregnancy by dilation and evacuation (D&E). Because D&E requires wider cervical dilation than curettage, the physician may dilate the cervix with a laminaria several hours to several days before the procedure. At the time of the procedure, the physician inserts a speculum into the vagina to view the cervix. A tenaculum is used to grasp the cervix, pull it down, and exert traction. The physician places a cannula in the dilated endocervical canal and passes it into the uterus. The suction machine is activated and the uterine contents are evacuated by rotation of the cannula. For pregnancies through 16 weeks, the cannula will usually evacuate the pregnancy. For later pregnancies, the cannula is used to drain amniotic fluid and to draw tissue into the lower uterus for extraction by forceps. In either case, a sharp curette may be used to gently scrape the uterus to ensure that it is empty.

Coding Tips

For induced abortion by dilation and curettage, see 59840. For other induced abortion, see 59850–59857. For medical treatment of a spontaneous complete abortion, any trimester, see 99202–99233. For surgical treatment of an incomplete abortion, any trimester, see 59812. For treatment of a missed abortion, completed surgically, first trimester, see 59820; second trimester, see 59821. Because this procedure may not be done out of medical necessity, the patient may be responsible for charges. Verify with the insurance carrier for coverage.

ICD-10-CM Diagnostic Codes

O02.89	Other abnormal products of conception ⓜ ♀
O10.211	Pre-existing hypertensive chronic kidney disease complicating pregnancy, first trimester ⓜ ♀
O10.212	Pre-existing hypertensive chronic kidney disease complicating pregnancy, second trimester ⓜ ♀
O10.311	Pre-existing hypertensive heart and chronic kidney disease complicating pregnancy, first trimester ⓜ ♀
O10.312	Pre-existing hypertensive heart and chronic kidney disease complicating pregnancy, second trimester ⓜ ♀

O35.0XX0	Maternal care for (suspected) central nervous system malformation in fetus, not applicable or unspecified ⓜ ♀
O35.1XX0	Maternal care for (suspected) chromosomal abnormality in fetus, not applicable or unspecified ⓜ ♀
O35.2XX0	Maternal care for (suspected) hereditary disease in fetus, not applicable or unspecified ⓜ ♀
O35.3XX0	Maternal care for (suspected) damage to fetus from viral disease in mother, not applicable or unspecified ⓜ ♀
O35.4XX0	Maternal care for (suspected) damage to fetus from alcohol, not applicable or unspecified ⓜ ♀
O35.5XX0	Maternal care for (suspected) damage to fetus by drugs, not applicable or unspecified ⓜ ♀
O35.6XX0	Maternal care for (suspected) damage to fetus by radiation, not applicable or unspecified ⓜ ♀
O35.7XX0	Maternal care for (suspected) damage to fetus by other medical procedures, not applicable or unspecified ⓜ ♀
O35.8XX0	Maternal care for other (suspected) fetal abnormality and damage, not applicable or unspecified ⓜ ♀
O35.9XX0	Maternal care for (suspected) fetal abnormality and damage, unspecified, not applicable or unspecified ⓜ ♀
O36.0110	Maternal care for anti-D [Rh] antibodies, first trimester, not applicable or unspecified ⓜ ♀
O36.0120	Maternal care for anti-D [Rh] antibodies, second trimester, not applicable or unspecified ⓜ ♀
O36.0910	Maternal care for other rhesus isoimmunization, first trimester, not applicable or unspecified ⓜ ♀
O36.0920	Maternal care for other rhesus isoimmunization, second trimester, not applicable or unspecified ⓜ ♀
O36.1110	Maternal care for Anti-A sensitization, first trimester, not applicable or unspecified ⓜ ♀
O36.1120	Maternal care for Anti-A sensitization, second trimester, not applicable or unspecified ⓜ ♀
O36.1910	Maternal care for other isoimmunization, first trimester, not applicable or unspecified ⓜ ♀
O36.1920	Maternal care for other isoimmunization, second trimester, not applicable or unspecified ⓜ ♀
O36.21X0	Maternal care for hydrops fetalis, first trimester, not applicable or unspecified ⓜ ♀
O36.22X0	Maternal care for hydrops fetalis, second trimester, not applicable or unspecified ⓜ ♀
O36.4XX0	Maternal care for intrauterine death, not applicable or unspecified ⓜ ♀
O36.5110	Maternal care for known or suspected placental insufficiency, first trimester, not applicable or unspecified ⓜ ♀
O36.5120	Maternal care for known or suspected placental insufficiency, second trimester, not applicable or unspecified ⓜ ♀
O36.5910	Maternal care for other known or suspected poor fetal growth, first trimester, not applicable or unspecified ⓜ ♀
O36.5920	Maternal care for other known or suspected poor fetal growth, second trimester, not applicable or unspecified ⓜ ♀
O36.8910	Maternal care for other specified fetal problems, first trimester, not applicable or unspecified ⓜ ♀
O36.8920	Maternal care for other specified fetal problems, second trimester, not applicable or unspecified ⓜ ♀
O99.111	Other diseases of the blood and blood-forming organs and certain disorders involving the immune mechanism complicating pregnancy, first trimester ⓜ ♀

O99.112	Other diseases of the blood and blood-forming organs and certain disorders involving the immune mechanism complicating pregnancy, second trimester 🅼 ♀
O99.411	Diseases of the circulatory system complicating pregnancy, first trimester 🅼 ♀
O99.412	Diseases of the circulatory system complicating pregnancy, second trimester 🅼 ♀
Z33.2	Encounter for elective termination of pregnancy 🅼 ♀

AMA: 59841 2019,Jul,6; 2018,Jan,8; 2017,Jan,8; 2016,Jan,13; 2015,Jan,16; 2014,Jan,11

Relative Value Units/Medicare Edits

Non-Facility RVU	Work	PE	MP	Total
59841	5.65	4.56	1.56	11.77
Facility RVU	**Work**	**PE**	**MP**	**Total**
59841	5.65	3.47	1.56	10.68

	FUD	Status	MUE	Modifiers				IOM Reference
59841	10	R	1(2)	51	N/A	N/A	80*	None

* with documentation

Terms To Know

fetus. Unborn offspring past the embryonic stage that has developed major structures. It is the period defined from nine weeks after fertilization until birth.

legally induced abortion. Elective or therapeutic termination of pregnancy performed within legal parameters by a licensed physician or other qualified medical professionals.

59850

| 59850 | Induced abortion, by 1 or more intra-amniotic injections (amniocentesis-injections), including hospital admission and visits, delivery of fetus and secundines; |

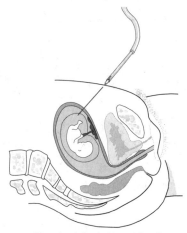

The physician induces abortion using an intra-amniotic injection

Explanation

The physician terminates a pregnancy by inducing labor with amniocentesis and intra-amniotic injections. This method is usually used after the first trimester (13 weeks or more). The physician inserts an amniocentesis needle into the abdomen to obtain a free flow of clear amniotic fluid. A hypertonic solution is administered by gravity drip. The hypertonic solution results in fetal death and labor usually results. The fetus and placenta are delivered through the vagina.

Coding Tips

For induced abortion by one or more intra-amniotic injections, with dilation and curettage and/or evacuation, see 59851; with hysterotomy, see 59852; by other methods, see 59855–59857. For medical treatment of a spontaneous complete abortion, any trimester, see 99202–99233. For surgical treatment of an incomplete abortion, any trimester, see 59812. For treatment of a missed abortion, completed surgically, first trimester, see 59820; second trimester, see 59821.

ICD-10-CM Diagnostic Codes

O02.89	Other abnormal products of conception 🅼 ♀
O10.211	Pre-existing hypertensive chronic kidney disease complicating pregnancy, first trimester 🅼 ♀
O10.212	Pre-existing hypertensive chronic kidney disease complicating pregnancy, second trimester 🅼 ♀
O10.213	Pre-existing hypertensive chronic kidney disease complicating pregnancy, third trimester 🅼 ♀
O10.311	Pre-existing hypertensive heart and chronic kidney disease complicating pregnancy, first trimester 🅼 ♀
O10.312	Pre-existing hypertensive heart and chronic kidney disease complicating pregnancy, second trimester 🅼 ♀
O10.313	Pre-existing hypertensive heart and chronic kidney disease complicating pregnancy, third trimester 🅼 ♀
O35.0XX0	Maternal care for (suspected) central nervous system malformation in fetus, not applicable or unspecified 🅼 ♀

O35.1XX0 Maternal care for (suspected) chromosomal abnormality in fetus, not applicable or unspecified Ⓜ ♀

O35.2XX0 Maternal care for (suspected) hereditary disease in fetus, not applicable or unspecified Ⓜ ♀

O35.3XX0 Maternal care for (suspected) damage to fetus from viral disease in mother, not applicable or unspecified Ⓜ ♀

O35.4XX0 Maternal care for (suspected) damage to fetus from alcohol, not applicable or unspecified Ⓜ ♀

O35.5XX0 Maternal care for (suspected) damage to fetus by drugs, not applicable or unspecified Ⓜ ♀

O35.6XX0 Maternal care for (suspected) damage to fetus by radiation, not applicable or unspecified Ⓜ ♀

O35.7XX0 Maternal care for (suspected) damage to fetus by other medical procedures, not applicable or unspecified Ⓜ ♀

O35.8XX0 Maternal care for other (suspected) fetal abnormality and damage, not applicable or unspecified Ⓜ ♀

O35.9XX0 Maternal care for (suspected) fetal abnormality and damage, unspecified, not applicable or unspecified Ⓜ ♀

O36.0110 Maternal care for anti-D [Rh] antibodies, first trimester, not applicable or unspecified Ⓜ ♀

O36.0120 Maternal care for anti-D [Rh] antibodies, second trimester, not applicable or unspecified Ⓜ ♀

O36.0130 Maternal care for anti-D [Rh] antibodies, third trimester, not applicable or unspecified Ⓜ ♀

O36.0910 Maternal care for other rhesus isoimmunization, first trimester, not applicable or unspecified Ⓜ ♀

O36.0920 Maternal care for other rhesus isoimmunization, second trimester, not applicable or unspecified Ⓜ ♀

O36.0930 Maternal care for other rhesus isoimmunization, third trimester, not applicable or unspecified Ⓜ ♀

O36.1110 Maternal care for Anti-A sensitization, first trimester, not applicable or unspecified Ⓜ ♀

O36.1120 Maternal care for Anti-A sensitization, second trimester, not applicable or unspecified Ⓜ ♀

O36.1130 Maternal care for Anti-A sensitization, third trimester, not applicable or unspecified Ⓜ ♀

O36.1910 Maternal care for other isoimmunization, first trimester, not applicable or unspecified Ⓜ ♀

O36.1920 Maternal care for other isoimmunization, second trimester, not applicable or unspecified Ⓜ ♀

O36.1930 Maternal care for other isoimmunization, third trimester, not applicable or unspecified Ⓜ ♀

O36.21X0 Maternal care for hydrops fetalis, first trimester, not applicable or unspecified Ⓜ ♀

O36.22X0 Maternal care for hydrops fetalis, second trimester, not applicable or unspecified Ⓜ ♀

O36.23X0 Maternal care for hydrops fetalis, third trimester, not applicable or unspecified Ⓜ ♀

O36.4XX0 Maternal care for intrauterine death, not applicable or unspecified Ⓜ ♀

O36.5110 Maternal care for known or suspected placental insufficiency, first trimester, not applicable or unspecified Ⓜ ♀

O36.5120 Maternal care for known or suspected placental insufficiency, second trimester, not applicable or unspecified Ⓜ ♀

O36.5130 Maternal care for known or suspected placental insufficiency, third trimester, not applicable or unspecified Ⓜ ♀

O36.5910 Maternal care for other known or suspected poor fetal growth, first trimester, not applicable or unspecified Ⓜ ♀

O36.5920 Maternal care for other known or suspected poor fetal growth, second trimester, not applicable or unspecified Ⓜ ♀

O36.5930 Maternal care for other known or suspected poor fetal growth, third trimester, not applicable or unspecified Ⓜ ♀

O36.8910 Maternal care for other specified fetal problems, first trimester, not applicable or unspecified Ⓜ ♀

O36.8920 Maternal care for other specified fetal problems, second trimester, not applicable or unspecified Ⓜ ♀

O36.8930 Maternal care for other specified fetal problems, third trimester, not applicable or unspecified Ⓜ ♀

O99.111 Other diseases of the blood and blood-forming organs and certain disorders involving the immune mechanism complicating pregnancy, first trimester Ⓜ ♀

O99.112 Other diseases of the blood and blood-forming organs and certain disorders involving the immune mechanism complicating pregnancy, second trimester Ⓜ ♀

O99.113 Other diseases of the blood and blood-forming organs and certain disorders involving the immune mechanism complicating pregnancy, third trimester Ⓜ ♀

O99.411 Diseases of the circulatory system complicating pregnancy, first trimester Ⓜ ♀

O99.412 Diseases of the circulatory system complicating pregnancy, second trimester Ⓜ ♀

O99.413 Diseases of the circulatory system complicating pregnancy, third trimester Ⓜ ♀

Z33.2 Encounter for elective termination of pregnancy Ⓜ ♀

AMA: 59850 2019,Jul,6; 2018,Jan,8; 2017,Jan,8; 2016,Jan,13; 2015,Jan,16; 2014,Jan,11

Relative Value Units/Medicare Edits

Non-Facility RVU	Work	PE	MP	Total
59850	5.9	3.7	1.63	11.23
Facility RVU	**Work**	**PE**	**MP**	**Total**
59850	5.9	3.7	1.63	11.23

	FUD	Status	MUE	Modifiers				IOM Reference
59850	90	R	1(2)	51	N/A	N/A	80*	None

* with documentation

CPT © 2020 American Medical Association. All Rights Reserved.   ● New   ▲ Revised   + Add On   ★ Telemedicine   AMA: CPT Assist   [Resequenced]   ☑ Laterality   © 2020 Optum360, LLC

Maternity Care

59851

59851   Induced abortion, by 1 or more intra-amniotic injections (amniocentesis-injections), including hospital admission and visits, delivery of fetus and secundines; with dilation and curettage and/or evacuation

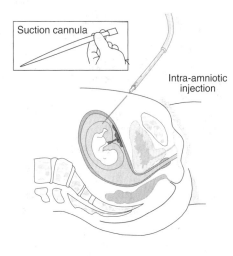

Suction cannula

Intra-amniotic injection

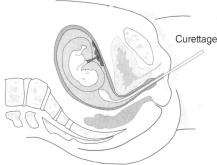

Curettage

The physician induces abortion with Intra-amniotic injections and uses dilation and curettage and/or evacuation when all products of conception are not expelled

Explanation

The physician begins the termination of a pregnancy by inducing labor with amniocentesis and intra-amniotic injections. This method is usually used after the first trimester (13 weeks or more). The physician inserts an amniocentesis needle into the abdomen to obtain a free flow of clear amniotic fluid. A hypertonic solution is administered by gravity drip. The hypertonic solution results in fetal death and labor usually results. Code 59851 is used when this method fails to expel all products of conception, and a dilation and curettage and/or evacuation is used to remove the remaining tissue.

Coding Tips

For induced abortion, by one or more intra-amniotic injections, see 59850; with hysterotomy, see 59852; by other methods, see 59855–59857. For medical treatment of a spontaneous complete abortion, any trimester, see 99202–99233. For surgical treatment of an incomplete abortion, any trimester, see 59812. For treatment of a missed abortion, completed surgically, first trimester, see 59820; second trimester, see 59821.

ICD-10-CM Diagnostic Codes

O02.89   Other abnormal products of conception ⓜ ♀
O10.211   Pre-existing hypertensive chronic kidney disease complicating pregnancy, first trimester ⓜ ♀

O10.212   Pre-existing hypertensive chronic kidney disease complicating pregnancy, second trimester ⓜ ♀
O10.213   Pre-existing hypertensive chronic kidney disease complicating pregnancy, third trimester ⓜ ♀
O10.311   Pre-existing hypertensive heart and chronic kidney disease complicating pregnancy, first trimester ⓜ ♀
O10.312   Pre-existing hypertensive heart and chronic kidney disease complicating pregnancy, second trimester ⓜ ♀
O10.313   Pre-existing hypertensive heart and chronic kidney disease complicating pregnancy, third trimester ⓜ ♀
O35.0XX0 Maternal care for (suspected) central nervous system malformation in fetus, not applicable or unspecified ⓜ ♀
O35.1XX0 Maternal care for (suspected) chromosomal abnormality in fetus, not applicable or unspecified ⓜ ♀
O35.2XX0 Maternal care for (suspected) hereditary disease in fetus, not applicable or unspecified ⓜ ♀
O35.3XX0 Maternal care for (suspected) damage to fetus from viral disease in mother, not applicable or unspecified ⓜ ♀
O35.4XX0 Maternal care for (suspected) damage to fetus from alcohol, not applicable or unspecified ⓜ ♀
O35.5XX0 Maternal care for (suspected) damage to fetus by drugs, not applicable or unspecified ⓜ ♀
O35.6XX0 Maternal care for (suspected) damage to fetus by radiation, not applicable or unspecified ⓜ ♀
O35.7XX0 Maternal care for (suspected) damage to fetus by other medical procedures, not applicable or unspecified ⓜ ♀
O35.8XX0 Maternal care for other (suspected) fetal abnormality and damage, not applicable or unspecified ⓜ ♀
O35.9XX0 Maternal care for (suspected) fetal abnormality and damage, unspecified, not applicable or unspecified ⓜ ♀
O36.0110 Maternal care for anti-D [Rh] antibodies, first trimester, not applicable or unspecified ⓜ ♀
O36.0120 Maternal care for anti-D [Rh] antibodies, second trimester, not applicable or unspecified ⓜ ♀
O36.0130 Maternal care for anti-D [Rh] antibodies, third trimester, not applicable or unspecified ⓜ ♀
O36.0910 Maternal care for other rhesus isoimmunization, first trimester, not applicable or unspecified ⓜ ♀
O36.0920 Maternal care for other rhesus isoimmunization, second trimester, not applicable or unspecified ⓜ ♀
O36.0930 Maternal care for other rhesus isoimmunization, third trimester, not applicable or unspecified ⓜ ♀
O36.1110 Maternal care for Anti-A sensitization, first trimester, not applicable or unspecified ⓜ ♀
O36.1120 Maternal care for Anti-A sensitization, second trimester, not applicable or unspecified ⓜ ♀
O36.1130 Maternal care for Anti-A sensitization, third trimester, not applicable or unspecified ⓜ ♀
O36.1910 Maternal care for other isoimmunization, first trimester, not applicable or unspecified ⓜ ♀
O36.1920 Maternal care for other isoimmunization, second trimester, not applicable or unspecified ⓜ ♀
O36.1930 Maternal care for other isoimmunization, third trimester, not applicable or unspecified ⓜ ♀
O36.21X0 Maternal care for hydrops fetalis, first trimester, not applicable or unspecified ⓜ ♀

Maternity Care

O36.22X0	Maternal care for hydrops fetalis, second trimester, not applicable or unspecified 🅜 ♀
O36.23X0	Maternal care for hydrops fetalis, third trimester, not applicable or unspecified 🅜 ♀
O36.4XX0	Maternal care for intrauterine death, not applicable or unspecified 🅜 ♀
O36.5110	Maternal care for known or suspected placental insufficiency, first trimester, not applicable or unspecified 🅜 ♀
O36.5120	Maternal care for known or suspected placental insufficiency, second trimester, not applicable or unspecified 🅜 ♀
O36.5130	Maternal care for known or suspected placental insufficiency, third trimester, not applicable or unspecified 🅜 ♀
O36.5910	Maternal care for other known or suspected poor fetal growth, first trimester, not applicable or unspecified 🅜 ♀
O36.5920	Maternal care for other known or suspected poor fetal growth, second trimester, not applicable or unspecified 🅜 ♀
O36.5930	Maternal care for other known or suspected poor fetal growth, third trimester, not applicable or unspecified 🅜 ♀
O36.8910	Maternal care for other specified fetal problems, first trimester, not applicable or unspecified 🅜 ♀
O36.8920	Maternal care for other specified fetal problems, second trimester, not applicable or unspecified 🅜 ♀
O36.8930	Maternal care for other specified fetal problems, third trimester, not applicable or unspecified 🅜 ♀
O99.111	Other diseases of the blood and blood-forming organs and certain disorders involving the immune mechanism complicating pregnancy, first trimester 🅜 ♀
O99.112	Other diseases of the blood and blood-forming organs and certain disorders involving the immune mechanism complicating pregnancy, second trimester 🅜 ♀
O99.113	Other diseases of the blood and blood-forming organs and certain disorders involving the immune mechanism complicating pregnancy, third trimester 🅜 ♀
O99.411	Diseases of the circulatory system complicating pregnancy, first trimester 🅜 ♀
O99.412	Diseases of the circulatory system complicating pregnancy, second trimester 🅜 ♀
O99.413	Diseases of the circulatory system complicating pregnancy, third trimester 🅜 ♀
Z33.2	Encounter for elective termination of pregnancy 🅜 ♀

AMA: 59851 2019,Jul,6; 2018,Jan,8; 2017,Jan,8; 2016,Jan,13; 2015,Jan,16; 2014,Jan,11

Relative Value Units/Medicare Edits

Non-Facility RVU	Work	PE	MP	Total
59851	5.92	4.49	1.63	12.04
Facility RVU	**Work**	**PE**	**MP**	**Total**
59851	5.92	4.49	1.63	12.04

	FUD	Status	MUE	Modifiers				IOM Reference
59851	90	R	1(2)	51	N/A	N/A	80*	None

* with documentation

59852

59852	Induced abortion, by 1 or more intra-amniotic injections (amniocentesis-injections), including hospital admission and visits, delivery of fetus and secundines; with hysterotomy (failed intra-amniotic injection)

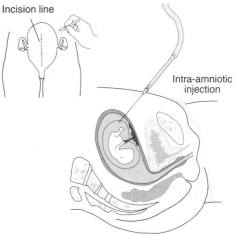

Incision line

Intra-amniotic injection

Intra-amniotic injections are performed and when all products of conception are not expelled, a hysterotomy is performed

Explanation

The physician begins the termination of a pregnancy by inducing labor with amniocentesis and intra-amniotic injections. This method is usually used after the first trimester (13 weeks or more). The physician inserts an amniocentesis needle into the abdomen to obtain a free flow of clear amniotic fluid. A hypertonic solution is administered by gravity drip. The hypertonic solution results in fetal death and labor usually results. Code 59852 is used when this method fails to expel all products of conception, and a hysterotomy, through an incision in the abdominal wall and uterus, is used to remove the remaining tissue. Following removal, the incision is closed with sutures.

Coding Tips

For induced abortion, by one or more intra-amniotic injections, see 59850; with dilation and curettage and/or evacuation, see 59851; by other methods, see 59855–59857. For medical treatment of a spontaneous complete abortion, any trimester, see 99202–99233. For surgical treatment of an incomplete abortion, any trimester, see 59812. For treatment of a missed abortion, completed surgically, first trimester, see 59820; second trimester, see 59821. For insertion of a cervical dilator only, see 59200.

ICD-10-CM Diagnostic Codes

O02.89	Other abnormal products of conception 🅜 ♀
O10.211	Pre-existing hypertensive chronic kidney disease complicating pregnancy, first trimester 🅜 ♀
O10.212	Pre-existing hypertensive chronic kidney disease complicating pregnancy, second trimester 🅜 ♀
O10.213	Pre-existing hypertensive chronic kidney disease complicating pregnancy, third trimester 🅜 ♀
O10.311	Pre-existing hypertensive heart and chronic kidney disease complicating pregnancy, first trimester 🅜 ♀
O35.5XX0	Maternal care for (suspected) damage to fetus by drugs, not applicable or unspecified 🅜 ♀
O35.6XX0	Maternal care for (suspected) damage to fetus by radiation, not applicable or unspecified 🅜 ♀

Maternity Care

O35.7XX0   Maternal care for (suspected) damage to fetus by other medical procedures, not applicable or unspecified ▯ ♀

O35.8XX0   Maternal care for other (suspected) fetal abnormality and damage, not applicable or unspecified ▯ ♀

O35.9XX0   Maternal care for (suspected) fetal abnormality and damage, unspecified, not applicable or unspecified ▯ ♀

O36.0110   Maternal care for anti-D [Rh] antibodies, first trimester, not applicable or unspecified ▯ ♀

O36.0120   Maternal care for anti-D [Rh] antibodies, second trimester, not applicable or unspecified ▯ ♀

O36.0130   Maternal care for anti-D [Rh] antibodies, third trimester, not applicable or unspecified ▯ ♀

O36.0910   Maternal care for other rhesus isoimmunization, first trimester, not applicable or unspecified ▯ ♀

O36.0920   Maternal care for other rhesus isoimmunization, second trimester, not applicable or unspecified ▯ ♀

O36.0930   Maternal care for other rhesus isoimmunization, third trimester, not applicable or unspecified ▯ ♀

O36.1110   Maternal care for Anti-A sensitization, first trimester, not applicable or unspecified ▯ ♀

O36.1120   Maternal care for Anti-A sensitization, second trimester, not applicable or unspecified ▯ ♀

O36.1130   Maternal care for Anti-A sensitization, third trimester, not applicable or unspecified ▯ ♀

O36.1910   Maternal care for other isoimmunization, first trimester, not applicable or unspecified ▯ ♀

O36.1920   Maternal care for other isoimmunization, second trimester, not applicable or unspecified ▯ ♀

O36.1930   Maternal care for other isoimmunization, third trimester, not applicable or unspecified ▯ ♀

O36.21X0   Maternal care for hydrops fetalis, first trimester, not applicable or unspecified ▯ ♀

O36.22X0   Maternal care for hydrops fetalis, second trimester, not applicable or unspecified ▯ ♀

O36.23X0   Maternal care for hydrops fetalis, third trimester, not applicable or unspecified ▯ ♀

O36.4XX0   Maternal care for intrauterine death, not applicable or unspecified ▯ ♀

O36.5110   Maternal care for known or suspected placental insufficiency, first trimester, not applicable or unspecified ▯ ♀

O36.5120   Maternal care for known or suspected placental insufficiency, second trimester, not applicable or unspecified ▯ ♀

O36.5130   Maternal care for known or suspected placental insufficiency, third trimester, not applicable or unspecified ▯ ♀

O36.5910   Maternal care for other known or suspected poor fetal growth, first trimester, not applicable or unspecified ▯ ♀

O36.5920   Maternal care for other known or suspected poor fetal growth, second trimester, not applicable or unspecified ▯ ♀

O36.5930   Maternal care for other known or suspected poor fetal growth, third trimester, not applicable or unspecified ▯ ♀

O36.8910   Maternal care for other specified fetal problems, first trimester, not applicable or unspecified ▯ ♀

O36.8920   Maternal care for other specified fetal problems, second trimester, not applicable or unspecified ▯ ♀

O36.8930   Maternal care for other specified fetal problems, third trimester, not applicable or unspecified ▯ ♀

O99.111   Other diseases of the blood and blood-forming organs and certain disorders involving the immune mechanism complicating pregnancy, first trimester ▯ ♀

O99.112   Other diseases of the blood and blood-forming organs and certain disorders involving the immune mechanism complicating pregnancy, second trimester ▯ ♀

O99.113   Other diseases of the blood and blood-forming organs and certain disorders involving the immune mechanism complicating pregnancy, third trimester ▯ ♀

O99.411   Diseases of the circulatory system complicating pregnancy, first trimester ▯ ♀

O99.412   Diseases of the circulatory system complicating pregnancy, second trimester ▯ ♀

O99.413   Diseases of the circulatory system complicating pregnancy, third trimester ▯ ♀

Z33.2   Encounter for elective termination of pregnancy ▯ ♀

AMA: **59852** 2019,Jul,6; 2018,Jan,8; 2017,Jan,8; 2016,Jan,13; 2015,Jan,16; 2014,Jan,11

Relative Value Units/Medicare Edits

Non-Facility RVU	Work	PE	MP	Total
59852	8.23	6.07	2.28	16.58
Facility RVU	**Work**	**PE**	**MP**	**Total**
59852	8.23	6.07	2.28	16.58

	FUD	Status	MUE	Modifiers				IOM Reference
59852	90	R	1(2)	51	N/A	N/A	80*	None

* with documentation

59855

59855 Induced abortion, by 1 or more vaginal suppositories (eg, prostaglandin) with or without cervical dilation (eg, laminaria), including hospital admission and visits, delivery of fetus and secundines;

A laminaria may be inserted first to soften the cervix

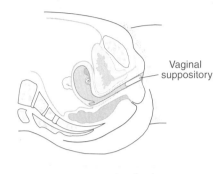

Vaginal suppository

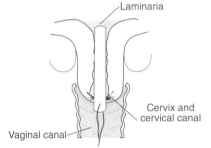

Laminaria

Cervix and cervical canal

Vaginal canal

Explanation

The physician terminates a pregnancy by inducing labor with vaginal suppositories. Before using the suppositories, a laminaria, which is an applicator made of kelp or synthetic material, may be inserted in the cervix to soften and expand the cervical canal. Once the cervix is ready, the physician inserts the vaginal suppositories and labor usually results. The fetus and placenta are delivered through the vagina.

Coding Tips

For induced abortion with dilation and curettage and/or evacuation, see 59856; with a hysterotomy, see 59857. For induced abortion, by one or more intra-amniotic injections, see 59850; with dilation and curettage and/or evacuation, see 59851; with hysterotomy, see 59852. For medical treatment of a spontaneous complete abortion, any trimester, see 99202–99233. For surgical treatment of an incomplete abortion, any trimester, see 59812. For treatment of a missed abortion, completed surgically, first trimester, see 59820; second trimester, see 59821. For insertion of a cervical dilator only, see 59200.

ICD-10-CM Diagnostic Codes

O02.89	Other abnormal products of conception ⚥ ♀
O10.211	Pre-existing hypertensive chronic kidney disease complicating pregnancy, first trimester ⚥ ♀
O10.212	Pre-existing hypertensive chronic kidney disease complicating pregnancy, second trimester ⚥ ♀
O10.213	Pre-existing hypertensive chronic kidney disease complicating pregnancy, third trimester ⚥ ♀
O10.311	Pre-existing hypertensive heart and chronic kidney disease complicating pregnancy, first trimester ⚥ ♀
O35.5XX0	Maternal care for (suspected) damage to fetus by drugs, not applicable or unspecified ⚥ ♀

O35.6XX0	Maternal care for (suspected) damage to fetus by radiation, not applicable or unspecified ⚥ ♀
O35.7XX0	Maternal care for (suspected) damage to fetus by other medical procedures, not applicable or unspecified ⚥ ♀
O35.8XX0	Maternal care for other (suspected) fetal abnormality and damage, not applicable or unspecified ⚥ ♀
O35.9XX0	Maternal care for (suspected) fetal abnormality and damage, unspecified, not applicable or unspecified ⚥ ♀
O36.0110	Maternal care for anti-D [Rh] antibodies, first trimester, not applicable or unspecified ⚥ ♀
O36.0120	Maternal care for anti-D [Rh] antibodies, second trimester, not applicable or unspecified ⚥ ♀
O36.0130	Maternal care for anti-D [Rh] antibodies, third trimester, not applicable or unspecified ⚥ ♀
O36.0910	Maternal care for other rhesus isoimmunization, first trimester, not applicable or unspecified ⚥ ♀
O36.0920	Maternal care for other rhesus isoimmunization, second trimester, not applicable or unspecified ⚥ ♀
O36.0930	Maternal care for other rhesus isoimmunization, third trimester, not applicable or unspecified ⚥ ♀
O36.1110	Maternal care for Anti-A sensitization, first trimester, not applicable or unspecified ⚥ ♀
O36.1120	Maternal care for Anti-A sensitization, second trimester, not applicable or unspecified ⚥ ♀
O36.1130	Maternal care for Anti-A sensitization, third trimester, not applicable or unspecified ⚥ ♀
O36.1910	Maternal care for other isoimmunization, first trimester, not applicable or unspecified ⚥ ♀
O36.1920	Maternal care for other isoimmunization, second trimester, not applicable or unspecified ⚥ ♀
O36.1930	Maternal care for other isoimmunization, third trimester, not applicable or unspecified ⚥ ♀
O36.21X0	Maternal care for hydrops fetalis, first trimester, not applicable or unspecified ⚥ ♀
O36.22X0	Maternal care for hydrops fetalis, second trimester, not applicable or unspecified ⚥ ♀
O36.23X0	Maternal care for hydrops fetalis, third trimester, not applicable or unspecified ⚥ ♀
O36.4XX0	Maternal care for intrauterine death, not applicable or unspecified ⚥ ♀
O36.5110	Maternal care for known or suspected placental insufficiency, first trimester, not applicable or unspecified ⚥ ♀
O36.5120	Maternal care for known or suspected placental insufficiency, second trimester, not applicable or unspecified ⚥ ♀
O36.5130	Maternal care for known or suspected placental insufficiency, third trimester, not applicable or unspecified ⚥ ♀
O36.5910	Maternal care for other known or suspected poor fetal growth, first trimester, not applicable or unspecified ⚥ ♀
O36.5920	Maternal care for other known or suspected poor fetal growth, second trimester, not applicable or unspecified ⚥ ♀
O36.5930	Maternal care for other known or suspected poor fetal growth, third trimester, not applicable or unspecified ⚥ ♀
O36.8910	Maternal care for other specified fetal problems, first trimester, not applicable or unspecified ⚥ ♀
O36.8920	Maternal care for other specified fetal problems, second trimester, not applicable or unspecified ⚥ ♀

O36.8930	Maternal care for other specified fetal problems, third trimester, not applicable or unspecified Ⓜ ♀
O99.111	Other diseases of the blood and blood-forming organs and certain disorders involving the immune mechanism complicating pregnancy, first trimester Ⓜ ♀
O99.112	Other diseases of the blood and blood-forming organs and certain disorders involving the immune mechanism complicating pregnancy, second trimester Ⓜ ♀
O99.113	Other diseases of the blood and blood-forming organs and certain disorders involving the immune mechanism complicating pregnancy, third trimester Ⓜ ♀
O99.411	Diseases of the circulatory system complicating pregnancy, first trimester Ⓜ ♀
O99.412	Diseases of the circulatory system complicating pregnancy, second trimester Ⓜ ♀
O99.413	Diseases of the circulatory system complicating pregnancy, third trimester Ⓜ ♀
Z33.2	Encounter for elective termination of pregnancy Ⓜ ♀

AMA: 59855 2019,Jul,6; 2014,Jan,11

Relative Value Units/Medicare Edits

Non-Facility RVU	Work	PE	MP	Total
59855	6.43	4.02	1.78	12.23
Facility RVU	**Work**	**PE**	**MP**	**Total**
59855	6.43	4.02	1.78	12.23

	FUD	Status	MUE	Modifiers				IOM Reference
59855	90	R	1(2)	51	N/A	N/A	80*	None

* with documentation

59856

| 59856 | Induced abortion, by 1 or more vaginal suppositories (eg, prostaglandin) with or without cervical dilation (eg, laminaria), including hospital admission and visits, delivery of fetus and secundines; with dilation and curettage and/or evacuation |

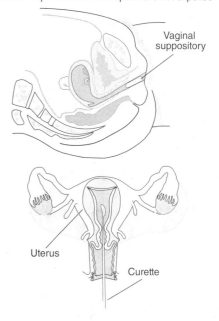

A laminaria may be inserted to soften the cervix. The physician uses dilation and curettage and/or evacuation when all products of conception are not expelled

Explanation

The physician begins the termination of a pregnancy by inducing labor with vaginal suppositories. Before using the suppositories, a laminaria, which is an applicator made of kelp or synthetic material, may be inserted in the cervix to soften and expand the cervical canal. Once the cervix is ready, the physician inserts the vaginal suppositories and labor usually results. 59856 is used when this method fails to expel all products of conception, and a dilation and curettage and/or evacuation is used to remove the remaining tissue.

Coding Tips

For induced abortion with one or more vaginal suppositories, with or without cervical dilation, with all hospital care, see 59855; with a hysterotomy, see 59857. For induced abortion, by one or more intra-amniotic injections, see 59850; with dilation and curettage and/or evacuation, see 59851; with hysterotomy, see 59852. For medical treatment of a spontaneous complete abortion, any trimester, see 99202–99233. For surgical treatment of an incomplete abortion, any trimester, see 59812. For treatment of a missed abortion, completed surgically, first trimester, see 59820; second trimester, see 59821. For insertion of a cervical dilator only, see 59200.

ICD-10-CM Diagnostic Codes

O02.89	Other abnormal products of conception Ⓜ ♀
O10.211	Pre-existing hypertensive chronic kidney disease complicating pregnancy, first trimester Ⓜ ♀
O10.212	Pre-existing hypertensive chronic kidney disease complicating pregnancy, second trimester Ⓜ ♀
O10.213	Pre-existing hypertensive chronic kidney disease complicating pregnancy, third trimester Ⓜ ♀

O10.311	Pre-existing hypertensive heart and chronic kidney disease complicating pregnancy, first trimester ⓜ ♀
O35.5XX0	Maternal care for (suspected) damage to fetus by drugs, not applicable or unspecified ⓜ ♀
O35.6XX0	Maternal care for (suspected) damage to fetus by radiation, not applicable or unspecified ⓜ ♀
O35.7XX0	Maternal care for (suspected) damage to fetus by other medical procedures, not applicable or unspecified ⓜ ♀
O35.8XX0	Maternal care for other (suspected) fetal abnormality and damage, not applicable or unspecified ⓜ ♀
O35.9XX0	Maternal care for (suspected) fetal abnormality and damage, unspecified, not applicable or unspecified ⓜ ♀
O36.0110	Maternal care for anti-D [Rh] antibodies, first trimester, not applicable or unspecified ⓜ ♀
O36.0120	Maternal care for anti-D [Rh] antibodies, second trimester, not applicable or unspecified ⓜ ♀
O36.0130	Maternal care for anti-D [Rh] antibodies, third trimester, not applicable or unspecified ⓜ ♀
O36.0910	Maternal care for other rhesus isoimmunization, first trimester, not applicable or unspecified ⓜ ♀
O36.0920	Maternal care for other rhesus isoimmunization, second trimester, not applicable or unspecified ⓜ ♀
O36.0930	Maternal care for other rhesus isoimmunization, third trimester, not applicable or unspecified ⓜ ♀
O36.1110	Maternal care for Anti-A sensitization, first trimester, not applicable or unspecified ⓜ ♀
O36.1120	Maternal care for Anti-A sensitization, second trimester, not applicable or unspecified ⓜ ♀
O36.1130	Maternal care for Anti-A sensitization, third trimester, not applicable or unspecified ⓜ ♀
O36.1910	Maternal care for other isoimmunization, first trimester, not applicable or unspecified ⓜ ♀
O36.1920	Maternal care for other isoimmunization, second trimester, not applicable or unspecified ⓜ ♀
O36.1930	Maternal care for other isoimmunization, third trimester, not applicable or unspecified ⓜ ♀
O36.21X0	Maternal care for hydrops fetalis, first trimester, not applicable or unspecified ⓜ ♀
O36.22X0	Maternal care for hydrops fetalis, second trimester, not applicable or unspecified ⓜ ♀
O36.23X0	Maternal care for hydrops fetalis, third trimester, not applicable or unspecified ⓜ ♀
O36.4XX0	Maternal care for intrauterine death, not applicable or unspecified ⓜ ♀
O36.5110	Maternal care for known or suspected placental insufficiency, first trimester, not applicable or unspecified ⓜ ♀
O36.5120	Maternal care for known or suspected placental insufficiency, second trimester, not applicable or unspecified ⓜ ♀
O36.5130	Maternal care for known or suspected placental insufficiency, third trimester, not applicable or unspecified ⓜ ♀
O36.5910	Maternal care for other known or suspected poor fetal growth, first trimester, not applicable or unspecified ⓜ ♀
O36.5920	Maternal care for other known or suspected poor fetal growth, second trimester, not applicable or unspecified ⓜ ♀
O36.5930	Maternal care for other known or suspected poor fetal growth, third trimester, not applicable or unspecified ⓜ ♀

O36.8910	Maternal care for other specified fetal problems, first trimester, not applicable or unspecified ⓜ ♀
O36.8920	Maternal care for other specified fetal problems, second trimester, not applicable or unspecified ⓜ ♀
O36.8930	Maternal care for other specified fetal problems, third trimester, not applicable or unspecified ⓜ ♀
O99.111	Other diseases of the blood and blood-forming organs and certain disorders involving the immune mechanism complicating pregnancy, first trimester ⓜ ♀
O99.112	Other diseases of the blood and blood-forming organs and certain disorders involving the immune mechanism complicating pregnancy, second trimester ⓜ ♀
O99.113	Other diseases of the blood and blood-forming organs and certain disorders involving the immune mechanism complicating pregnancy, third trimester ⓜ ♀
O99.411	Diseases of the circulatory system complicating pregnancy, first trimester ⓜ ♀
O99.412	Diseases of the circulatory system complicating pregnancy, second trimester ⓜ ♀
O99.413	Diseases of the circulatory system complicating pregnancy, third trimester ⓜ ♀
Z33.2	Encounter for elective termination of pregnancy ⓜ ♀

AMA: **59856** 2019,Jul,6; 2014,Jan,11

Relative Value Units/Medicare Edits

Non-Facility RVU	Work	PE	MP	Total
59856	7.79	4.41	2.16	14.36
Facility RVU	**Work**	**PE**	**MP**	**Total**
59856	7.79	4.41	2.16	14.36

	FUD	Status	MUE	Modifiers				IOM Reference
59856	90	R	1(2)	51	N/A	N/A	80*	None

* with documentation

Maternity Care

59857

59857 Induced abortion, by 1 or more vaginal suppositories (eg, prostaglandin) with or without cervical dilation (eg, laminaria), including hospital admission and visits, delivery of fetus and secundines; with hysterotomy (failed medical evacuation)

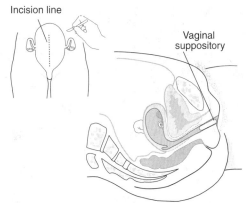

Incision line

Vaginal suppository

The physician induces abortion with vaginal suppositories and when all products of conception are not expelled, performs a hysterotomy.

Explanation

The physician begins the termination of a pregnancy by inducing labor with vaginal suppositories. Before using the suppositories, a laminaria, which is an applicator made of kelp or synthetic material, may be inserted in the cervix to soften and expand the cervical canal. Once the cervix is ready, the physician inserts the vaginal suppositories and labor usually results. 59857 is used when this method fails to expel all products of conception, and a hysterotomy, through an incision in the abdominal wall and uterus, is used to remove the remaining tissue. Following removal, the incision is closed with sutures.

Coding Tips

For induced abortion with one or more vaginal suppositories, with or without cervical dilation, with all hospital care, see 59855; with dilation and curettage and/or evacuation, see 59856. For induced abortion, by one or more intra-amniotic injections, see 59850; with dilation and curettage and/or evacuation, see 59851; with hysterotomy, see 59852. For medical treatment of a spontaneous complete abortion, any trimester, see 99202–99233. For surgical treatment of an incomplete abortion, any trimester, see 59812. For treatment of a missed abortion, completed surgically, first trimester, see 59820; second trimester, see 59821. For insertion of a cervical dilator only, see 59200.

ICD-10-CM Diagnostic Codes

O02.89	Other abnormal products of conception 🅜 ♀
O10.211	Pre-existing hypertensive chronic kidney disease complicating pregnancy, first trimester 🅜 ♀
O10.212	Pre-existing hypertensive chronic kidney disease complicating pregnancy, second trimester 🅜 ♀
O10.213	Pre-existing hypertensive chronic kidney disease complicating pregnancy, third trimester 🅜 ♀
O10.311	Pre-existing hypertensive heart and chronic kidney disease complicating pregnancy, first trimester 🅜 ♀
O35.5XX0	Maternal care for (suspected) damage to fetus by drugs, not applicable or unspecified 🅜 ♀
O35.6XX0	Maternal care for (suspected) damage to fetus by radiation, not applicable or unspecified 🅜 ♀
O35.7XX0	Maternal care for (suspected) damage to fetus by other medical procedures, not applicable or unspecified 🅜 ♀
O35.8XX0	Maternal care for other (suspected) fetal abnormality and damage, not applicable or unspecified 🅜 ♀
O35.9XX0	Maternal care for (suspected) fetal abnormality and damage, unspecified, not applicable or unspecified 🅜 ♀
O36.0110	Maternal care for anti-D [Rh] antibodies, first trimester, not applicable or unspecified 🅜 ♀
O36.0120	Maternal care for anti-D [Rh] antibodies, second trimester, not applicable or unspecified 🅜 ♀
O36.0130	Maternal care for anti-D [Rh] antibodies, third trimester, not applicable or unspecified 🅜 ♀
O36.0910	Maternal care for other rhesus isoimmunization, first trimester, not applicable or unspecified 🅜 ♀
O36.0920	Maternal care for other rhesus isoimmunization, second trimester, not applicable or unspecified 🅜 ♀
O36.0930	Maternal care for other rhesus isoimmunization, third trimester, not applicable or unspecified 🅜 ♀
O36.1110	Maternal care for Anti-A sensitization, first trimester, not applicable or unspecified 🅜 ♀
O36.1120	Maternal care for Anti-A sensitization, second trimester, not applicable or unspecified 🅜 ♀
O36.1130	Maternal care for Anti-A sensitization, third trimester, not applicable or unspecified 🅜 ♀
O36.1910	Maternal care for other isoimmunization, first trimester, not applicable or unspecified 🅜 ♀
O36.1920	Maternal care for other isoimmunization, second trimester, not applicable or unspecified 🅜 ♀
O36.1930	Maternal care for other isoimmunization, third trimester, not applicable or unspecified 🅜 ♀
O36.21X0	Maternal care for hydrops fetalis, first trimester, not applicable or unspecified 🅜 ♀
O36.22X0	Maternal care for hydrops fetalis, second trimester, not applicable or unspecified 🅜 ♀
O36.23X0	Maternal care for hydrops fetalis, third trimester, not applicable or unspecified 🅜 ♀
O36.4XX0	Maternal care for intrauterine death, not applicable or unspecified 🅜 ♀
O36.5110	Maternal care for known or suspected placental insufficiency, first trimester, not applicable or unspecified 🅜 ♀
O36.5120	Maternal care for known or suspected placental insufficiency, second trimester, not applicable or unspecified 🅜 ♀
O36.5130	Maternal care for known or suspected placental insufficiency, third trimester, not applicable or unspecified 🅜 ♀
O36.5910	Maternal care for other known or suspected poor fetal growth, first trimester, not applicable or unspecified 🅜 ♀
O36.5920	Maternal care for other known or suspected poor fetal growth, second trimester, not applicable or unspecified 🅜 ♀
O36.5930	Maternal care for other known or suspected poor fetal growth, third trimester, not applicable or unspecified 🅜 ♀
O36.8910	Maternal care for other specified fetal problems, first trimester, not applicable or unspecified 🅜 ♀
O36.8920	Maternal care for other specified fetal problems, second trimester, not applicable or unspecified 🅜 ♀
O36.8930	Maternal care for other specified fetal problems, third trimester, not applicable or unspecified 🅜 ♀

Maternity Care

O99.111	Other diseases of the blood and blood-forming organs and certain disorders involving the immune mechanism complicating pregnancy, first trimester ℳ ♀
O99.112	Other diseases of the blood and blood-forming organs and certain disorders involving the immune mechanism complicating pregnancy, second trimester ℳ ♀
O99.113	Other diseases of the blood and blood-forming organs and certain disorders involving the immune mechanism complicating pregnancy, third trimester ℳ ♀
O99.411	Diseases of the circulatory system complicating pregnancy, first trimester ℳ ♀
O99.412	Diseases of the circulatory system complicating pregnancy, second trimester ℳ ♀
O99.413	Diseases of the circulatory system complicating pregnancy, third trimester ℳ ♀
Z33.2	Encounter for elective termination of pregnancy ℳ ♀

AMA: 59857 2019,Jul,6; 2014,Jan,11

Relative Value Units/Medicare Edits

Non-Facility RVU	Work	PE	MP	Total
59857	9.33	4.9	2.58	16.81
Facility RVU	**Work**	**PE**	**MP**	**Total**
59857	9.33	4.9	2.58	16.81

	FUD	Status	MUE	Modifiers				IOM Reference
59857	90	R	1(2)	51	N/A	N/A	80*	None

* with documentation

59866

59866   Multifetal pregnancy reduction(s) (MPR)

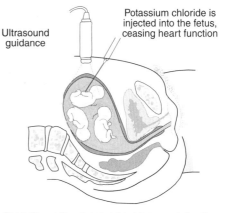

Typically, under ultrasound guidance, a potassium chloride solution is injected into the fetal thorax

Explanation

Selective reduction is performed to eliminate one or more fetuses of a multiple pregnancy in an attempt to increase the viability of the remaining fetuses. Fetuses are usually eliminated in this procedure until only a twin or triplet pregnancy remains. Physicians most often use ultrasound guided intracardiac injection of potassium chloride to reduce the number of fetuses, although injection of potassium chloride in any part of the fetal body accomplishes the same result. When an intracardiac injection is performed, a 22 gauge spinal needle is advanced through the abdominal and uterine walls toward a cardiac echo using high-resolution ultrasound as a guide. With the needle position in the heart, a solution of potassium chloride is injected at intervals until prolonged cardiac standstill is observed. The physician withdraws the needle and redirects it into another gestational sac, as needed. The embryo(s) or fetus(es) that have been injected shrivel and decompose, leaving the remaining fetuses in utero an increased chance of surviving to term. Any sacs that remain intact are removed during delivery of the surviving fetus(es).

Coding Tips

For induced abortion, see 59840–59857. For medical treatment of a spontaneous complete abortion, any trimester, see 99202–99233.

ICD-10-CM Diagnostic Codes

O30.011	Twin pregnancy, monochorionic/monoamniotic, first trimester ℳ ♀
O30.012	Twin pregnancy, monochorionic/monoamniotic, second trimester ℳ ♀
O30.031	Twin pregnancy, monochorionic/diamniotic, first trimester ℳ ♀
O30.032	Twin pregnancy, monochorionic/diamniotic, second trimester ℳ ♀
O30.041	Twin pregnancy, dichorionic/diamniotic, first trimester ℳ ♀
O30.042	Twin pregnancy, dichorionic/diamniotic, second trimester ℳ ♀
O30.091	Twin pregnancy, unable to determine number of placenta and number of amniotic sacs, first trimester ℳ ♀
O30.092	Twin pregnancy, unable to determine number of placenta and number of amniotic sacs, second trimester ℳ ♀
O30.111	Triplet pregnancy with two or more monochorionic fetuses, first trimester ℳ ♀

O30.112 Triplet pregnancy with two or more monochorionic fetuses, second trimester Ⓜ ♀

O30.121 Triplet pregnancy with two or more monoamniotic fetuses, first trimester Ⓜ ♀

O30.122 Triplet pregnancy with two or more monoamniotic fetuses, second trimester Ⓜ ♀

O30.131 Triplet pregnancy, trichorionic/triamniotic, first trimester Ⓜ ♀

O30.132 Triplet pregnancy, trichorionic/triamniotic, second trimester Ⓜ ♀

O30.191 Triplet pregnancy, unable to determine number of placenta and number of amniotic sacs, first trimester Ⓜ ♀

O30.192 Triplet pregnancy, unable to determine number of placenta and number of amniotic sacs, second trimester Ⓜ ♀

O30.211 Quadruplet pregnancy with two or more monochorionic fetuses, first trimester Ⓜ ♀

O30.212 Quadruplet pregnancy with two or more monochorionic fetuses, second trimester Ⓜ ♀

O30.221 Quadruplet pregnancy with two or more monoamniotic fetuses, first trimester Ⓜ ♀

O30.222 Quadruplet pregnancy with two or more monoamniotic fetuses, second trimester Ⓜ ♀

O30.231 Quadruplet pregnancy, quadrachorionic/quadra-amniotic, first trimester Ⓜ ♀

O30.232 Quadruplet pregnancy, quadrachorionic/quadra-amniotic, second trimester Ⓜ ♀

O30.291 Quadruplet pregnancy, unable to determine number of placenta and number of amniotic sacs, first trimester Ⓜ ♀

O30.292 Quadruplet pregnancy, unable to determine number of placenta and number of amniotic sacs, second trimester Ⓜ ♀

O30.811 Other specified multiple gestation with two or more monochorionic fetuses, first trimester Ⓜ ♀

O30.812 Other specified multiple gestation with two or more monochorionic fetuses, second trimester Ⓜ ♀

O30.821 Other specified multiple gestation with two or more monoamniotic fetuses, first trimester Ⓜ ♀

O30.822 Other specified multiple gestation with two or more monoamniotic fetuses, second trimester Ⓜ ♀

O30.831 Other specified multiple gestation, number of chorions and amnions are both equal to the number of fetuses, first trimester Ⓜ ♀

O30.832 Other specified multiple gestation, number of chorions and amnions are both equal to the number of fetuses, second trimester Ⓜ ♀

O30.891 Other specified multiple gestation, unable to determine number of placenta and number of amniotic sacs, first trimester Ⓜ ♀

O30.892 Other specified multiple gestation, unable to determine number of placenta and number of amniotic sacs, second trimester Ⓜ ♀

O31.8X10 Other complications specific to multiple gestation, first trimester, not applicable or unspecified Ⓜ ♀

O31.8X11 Other complications specific to multiple gestation, first trimester, fetus 1 Ⓜ ♀

O31.8X12 Other complications specific to multiple gestation, first trimester, fetus 2 Ⓜ ♀

O31.8X13 Other complications specific to multiple gestation, first trimester, fetus 3 Ⓜ ♀

O31.8X14 Other complications specific to multiple gestation, first trimester, fetus 4 Ⓜ ♀

O31.8X15 Other complications specific to multiple gestation, first trimester, fetus 5 Ⓜ ♀

O31.8X19 Other complications specific to multiple gestation, first trimester, other fetus Ⓜ ♀

O31.8X20 Other complications specific to multiple gestation, second trimester, not applicable or unspecified Ⓜ ♀

O31.8X21 Other complications specific to multiple gestation, second trimester, fetus 1 Ⓜ ♀

O31.8X22 Other complications specific to multiple gestation, second trimester, fetus 2 Ⓜ ♀

O31.8X23 Other complications specific to multiple gestation, second trimester, fetus 3 Ⓜ ♀

O31.8X24 Other complications specific to multiple gestation, second trimester, fetus 4 Ⓜ ♀

O31.8X25 Other complications specific to multiple gestation, second trimester, fetus 5 Ⓜ ♀

O31.8X29 Other complications specific to multiple gestation, second trimester, other fetus Ⓜ ♀

AMA: **59866** 2019,Jul,6; 2014,Jan,11

Relative Value Units/Medicare Edits

Non-Facility RVU	Work	PE	MP	Total
59866	3.99	1.84	1.11	6.94
Facility RVU	**Work**	**PE**	**MP**	**Total**
59866	3.99	1.84	1.11	6.94

	FUD	Status	MUE	Modifiers				IOM Reference
59866	0	R	1(2)	51	N/A	62*	80	None

* with documentation

Terms To Know

fetus. Unborn offspring past the embryonic stage that has developed major structures. It is the period defined from nine weeks after fertilization until birth.

multifetal pregnancy reduction. Selective reduction, most often using potassium chloride injections, performed to eliminate one or more fetuses of a multiple pregnancy in an attempt to increase the viability of the remaining fetuses. Fetuses are usually eliminated in this procedure until only a twin or triplet pregnancy remains. *Synonym(s): MPR, selective abortion.*

viability. Ability to live, develop, grow, or survive after birth.

59870

59870 Uterine evacuation and curettage for hydatidiform mole

The physician removes a molar pregnancy by curettage

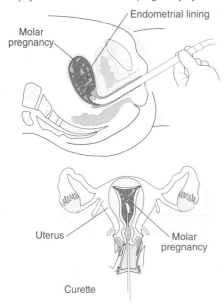

Explanation

The physician treats a hydatidiform mole (molar pregnancy) by evacuation and curettage of the uterus. The physician inserts a speculum into the vagina to view the cervix. A tenaculum is used to grasp the cervix, pull it down, and exert traction. A dilator is inserted into the endocervix and through the cervical canal to enlarge the opening. The physician places a cannula in the endocervical canal and passes it into the uterus. The suction machine is activated and the hydatidiform mole is evacuated by rotation of the cannula. After suction curettage, a sharp curette may be used to scrape the uterus and confirm that it is empty.

Coding Tips

For treatment of a hydatidiform mole by hysterotomy, see 59100. For insertion of a cervical dilator, see 59200. For induced abortion, see 59840–59857.

ICD-10-CM Diagnostic Codes

O01.0	Classical hydatidiform mole ▥ ♀
O01.1	Incomplete and partial hydatidiform mole ▥ ♀

AMA: **59870** 2019,Jul,6; 2018,Jan,8; 2017,Jan,8; 2016,Jan,13; 2015,Jan,16; 2014,Jan,11

Relative Value Units/Medicare Edits

Non-Facility RVU	Work	PE	MP	Total
59870	6.57	6.33	1.81	14.71
Facility RVU	**Work**	**PE**	**MP**	**Total**
59870	6.57	6.33	1.81	14.71

	FUD	Status	MUE	Modifiers				IOM Reference
59870	90	A	1(2)	51	N/A	N/A	80	None

* with documentation

59871

59871 Removal of cerclage suture under anesthesia (other than local)

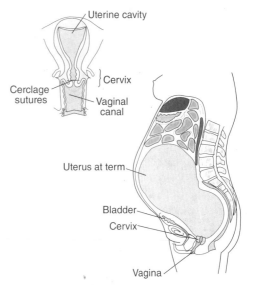

Cerclage sutures encircle the cervical opening, keeping it from premature dilation

Explanation

The physician removes a cervical cerclage, a suture that had been placed to hold the cervix closed. A cerclage is most often placed when a cervix dilates too early during pregnancy and risks a miscarriage. The physician severs the sutures and removes them. This code includes anesthesia other than local.

Coding Tips

For cerclage of cervix, during pregnancy, vaginal, see 59320; abdominal, see 59325. For non-obstetrical cerclage, see 57700.

ICD-10-CM Diagnostic Codes

Z48.02	Encounter for removal of sutures

AMA: **59871** 2019,Jul,6; 2018,Jan,8; 2017,Jan,8; 2016,Jan,13; 2015,Jan,16; 2014,Jan,11

Relative Value Units/Medicare Edits

Non-Facility RVU	Work	PE	MP	Total
59871	2.13	1.14	0.58	3.85
Facility RVU	**Work**	**PE**	**MP**	**Total**
59871	2.13	1.14	0.58	3.85

	FUD	Status	MUE	Modifiers				IOM Reference
59871	0	A	1(2)	51	N/A	N/A	80*	None

* with documentation

64430-64435

64430 Injection(s), anesthetic agent(s) and/or steroid; pudendal nerve
64435 paracervical (uterine) nerve

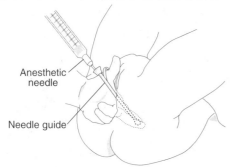

An anesthetic agent is injected to block the pudendal nerve or the paracervical (uterine) nerve

Anesthetic needle

Needle guide

A needle guide may be used to direct the injection using anatomical landmarks

Explanation

The physician anesthetizes the pudendal nerve for anesthesia of the perineum, rectum, and parts of the bladder and genitals. In 64430, the pudendal nerve is blocked, typically for perineal pain control, for example, during vaginal delivery. Code 64435 is a female-only procedure in which the area around the cervix is injected with a local anesthetic to supply pain control for the first stage of labor.

Coding Tips

For anesthetic injection into the superior hypogastric plexus, see 64517. Surgical trays, A4550, are not separately reimbursed by Medicare; however, other third-party payers may cover them. Check with the specific payer to determine coverage.

ICD-10-CM Diagnostic Codes

N73.8	Other specified female pelvic inflammatory diseases ♀
N76.0	Acute vaginitis ♀
N76.1	Subacute and chronic vaginitis ♀
N76.2	Acute vulvitis ♀
N76.3	Subacute and chronic vulvitis ♀
N76.4	Abscess of vulva ♀
N76.5	Ulceration of vagina ♀
N76.6	Ulceration of vulva ♀
N76.81	Mucositis (ulcerative) of vagina and vulva ♀
N76.89	Other specified inflammation of vagina and vulva ♀
N88.2	Stricture and stenosis of cervix uteri ♀
N88.3	Incompetence of cervix uteri ♀
N89.0	Mild vaginal dysplasia ♀
N89.1	Moderate vaginal dysplasia ♀
N89.5	Stricture and atresia of vagina ♀
N89.6	Tight hymenal ring ♀
N89.7	Hematocolpos ♀
N89.8	Other specified noninflammatory disorders of vagina ♀
N94.11	Superficial (introital) dyspareunia ♀
N94.12	Deep dyspareunia ♀
N94.19	Other specified dyspareunia ♀
N94.818	Other vulvodynia ♀

O02.1	Missed abortion Ⓜ ♀
O02.89	Other abnormal products of conception Ⓜ ♀
O34.31	Maternal care for cervical incompetence, first trimester Ⓜ ♀
O34.32	Maternal care for cervical incompetence, second trimester Ⓜ ♀
O34.33	Maternal care for cervical incompetence, third trimester Ⓜ ♀
O70.0	First degree perineal laceration during delivery Ⓜ ♀
O70.1	Second degree perineal laceration during delivery Ⓜ ♀
O70.21	Third degree perineal laceration during delivery, IIIa Ⓜ ♀
O70.22	Third degree perineal laceration during delivery, IIIb Ⓜ ♀
O70.23	Third degree perineal laceration during delivery, IIIc Ⓜ ♀
O70.3	Fourth degree perineal laceration during delivery Ⓜ ♀
O70.4	Anal sphincter tear complicating delivery, not associated with third degree laceration Ⓜ ♀
O71.82	Other specified trauma to perineum and vulva Ⓜ ♀
O80	Encounter for full-term uncomplicated delivery Ⓜ ♀
R10.2	Pelvic and perineal pain
S30.814A	Abrasion of vagina and vulva, initial encounter ♀

AMA: 64430 2018,Jan,8; 2017,Jan,8; 2016,Jan,13; 2015,Jan,16; 2014,Jan,11
64435 2018,Jan,8; 2017,Jan,8; 2016,Jan,13; 2015,Jan,16; 2014,Jan,11

Relative Value Units/Medicare Edits

Non-Facility RVU	Work	PE	MP	Total
64430	1.0	1.46	0.11	2.57
64435	0.75	1.23	0.11	2.09
Facility RVU	**Work**	**PE**	**MP**	**Total**
64430	1.0	0.48	0.11	1.59
64435	0.75	0.4	0.11	1.26

	FUD	Status	MUE	Modifiers				IOM Reference
64430	0	A	1(3)	51	50	N/A	N/A	None
64435	0	A	1(3)	51	50	N/A	N/A	

* with documentation

Terms To Know

anesthesia. Loss of feeling or sensation, usually induced to permit the performance of surgery or other painful procedures.

injection. Forcing a liquid substance into a body part such as a joint or muscle.

paracervical nerve. Nerve close to the cervix that the pain from uterine contractions travels through.

pudendal nerve. Nerve that serves most of the perineum and the external anal sphincter and provides sensation to the external genitalia.

Nervous

64486-64489

64486 Transversus abdominis plane (TAP) block (abdominal plane block, rectus sheath block) unilateral; by injection(s) (includes imaging guidance, when performed)

64487 by continuous infusion(s) (includes imaging guidance, when performed)

64488 Transversus abdominis plane (TAP) block (abdominal plane block, rectus sheath block) bilateral; by injections (includes imaging guidance, when performed)

64489 by continuous infusions (includes imaging guidance, when performed)

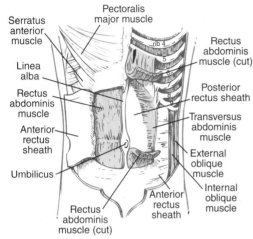

Anterior Abdominal Wall Muscles

Explanation

The transversus abdominis plane (TAP) block is a relatively new regional anesthesia technique with a high margin of safety and is technically simple to perform. The physician injects a local anesthetic in the space between the aponeurosis of the internal oblique and transversus abdominis muscles to anesthetize the nerves that supply the anterior abdominal wall (T6–L1) for postoperative pain control in a wide variety of abdominal procedures, including large bowel resection, open/laparoscopic appendectomy, cesarean section, total abdominal hysterectomy, laparoscopic cholecystectomy, open prostatectomy, renal transplant surgery, abdominoplasty with/without flank liposuction, iliac crest bone graft, and inguinal hernia repairs. This technique is also useful for procedures in which epidural analgesia is contraindicated (e.g., anticoagulated patients). For prolonged analgesia, continuous infusions via a catheter may also be performed. Imaging guidance, when performed, is included in these services. Report 64486 for a unilateral TAP, by injection; 64487 for a unilateral TAP, continuous infusion; 64488 for a bilateral TAP, by injection; and 64489 for a bilateral TAP, continuous infusion.

Coding Tips

For injection of an anesthetic agent or steroid, transforaminal epidural, with imaging guidance (CT or fluoroscopy), see 64479–64480 and 64483–64484.

ICD-10-CM Diagnostic Codes

G89.18 Other acute postprocedural pain
G89.28 Other chronic postprocedural pain

AMA: 64486 2018,Jan,8; 2017,Jan,8; 2016,Jan,13; 2015,Jun,3 **64487** 2018,Jan,8; 2017,Jan,8; 2016,Jan,13; 2015,Jun,3 **64488** 2018,Jan,8; 2017,Jan,8; 2016,Jan,13; 2015,Jun,3 **64489** 2018,Jan,8; 2017,Jan,8; 2016,Jan,13; 2015,Jun,3

Relative Value Units/Medicare Edits

Non-Facility RVU	Work	PE	MP	Total
64486	1.27	1.79	0.11	3.17
64487	1.48	3.57	0.11	5.16
64488	1.6	2.17	0.12	3.89
64489	1.8	6.06	0.13	7.99
Facility RVU	**Work**	**PE**	**MP**	**Total**
64486	1.27	0.24	0.11	1.62
64487	1.48	0.26	0.11	1.85
64488	1.6	0.28	0.12	2.0
64489	1.8	0.32	0.13	2.25

	FUD	Status	MUE		Modifiers			IOM Reference
64486	0	A	1(3)	51	50	N/A	N/A	None
64487	0	A	1(2)	51	50	N/A	N/A	
64488	0	A	1(3)	51	N/A	N/A	N/A	
64489	0	A	1(2)	51	N/A	N/A	N/A	

* with documentation

Terms To Know

analgesia. Absence of a normal sense of pain without loss of consciousness.

bilateral. Consisting of or affecting two sides.

epidural. Anesthesia commonly used during labor and delivery achieved by the injection of an anesthetic agent between the vertebrae into the extradural space.

imaging. Radiologic means of producing pictures for clinical study of the internal structures and functions of the body, such as x-ray, ultrasound, magnetic resonance, or positron emission tomography.

infusion. Introduction of a therapeutic fluid, other than blood, into the bloodstream.

injection. Forcing a liquid substance into a body part such as a joint or muscle.

unilateral. Located on or affecting one side.

Nervous

64517

64517   Injection, anesthetic agent; superior hypogastric plexus

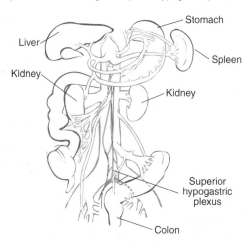

The plexus lies near the bifurcation of the
aorta just anterior to the sacrum

Explanation

The physician performs a nerve block on the superior hypogastric plexus by injecting an anesthetic agent through a needle inserted in the L5/S1 interspace. The superior hypogastric plexus, also called the presacral nerve, is located in front of the upper part of the sacrum and is formed by lower lumbar nerves responsible for pain sensation in the pelvic area. This nerve block is done in such cases as severe, intractable menstrual pain and pain due to pelvic area metastases from cancer. The patient is placed in the prone position and prepped. A 6-inch needle is guided under radiological imaging, such as fluoroscopy (reported separately), into the ventral lateral spine and through the L5/S1 interspace. Needle position is checked by injecting contrast material and aspirating for the return of any blood, urine, or cerebral spinal fluid. With negative aspiration results and imaging verifying that the needle position is in the prevertebral space and not within a blood vessel, a ureter, or spinal nerves, local anesthetic is injected on both sides.

Coding Tips

Local anesthesia is included in this service. Fluoroscopic guidance is reported separately. Surgical trays, A4550, are not separately reimbursed by Medicare; however, other third-party payers may cover them. Check with the specific payer to determine coverage.

ICD-10-CM Diagnostic Codes

C41.4	Malignant neoplasm of pelvic bones, sacrum and coccyx
C79.82	Secondary malignant neoplasm of genital organs
C79.89	Secondary malignant neoplasm of other specified sites
G89.18	Other acute postprocedural pain
G89.28	Other chronic postprocedural pain
G89.29	Other chronic pain
G89.3	Neoplasm related pain (acute) (chronic)
N94.4	Primary dysmenorrhea ♀
N94.5	Secondary dysmenorrhea ♀
R10.2	Pelvic and perineal pain

AMA: **64517** 2018,Jan,8; 2017,Jan,8; 2016,Jan,13; 2015,Jan,16; 2014,Jan,11

Relative Value Units/Medicare Edits

Non-Facility RVU	Work	PE	MP	Total
64517	2.2	3.08	0.19	5.47
Facility RVU	**Work**	**PE**	**MP**	**Total**
64517	2.2	1.21	0.19	3.6

	FUD	Status	MUE	Modifiers				IOM Reference
64517	0	A	1(3)	51	N/A	N/A	N/A	None

* with documentation

Terms To Know

anesthesia. Loss of feeling or sensation, usually induced to permit the performance of surgery or other painful procedures.

dysmenorrhea. Painful menstruation that may be primary, or essential, due to prostaglandin production and the onset of menstruation; secondary due to uterine, tubal, or ovarian abnormality or disease; spasmodic arising uterine contractions; or obstructive due to some mechanical blockage or interference with the menstrual flow.

fluoroscopy. Radiology technique that allows visual examination of part of the body or a function of an organ using a device that projects an x-ray image on a fluorescent screen.

imaging. Radiologic means of producing pictures for clinical study of the internal structures and functions of the body, such as x-ray, ultrasound, magnetic resonance, or positron emission tomography.

injection. Forcing a liquid substance into a body part such as a joint or muscle.

nerve block. Regional anesthesia/analgesia administered by injection that prevents sensory nerve impulses from reaching the central nervous system.

plexus. Bundle of nerves that serve a particular region of the body that lies relatively deep in the body as opposed to superficial nerves, which are close to the surface of the skin.

prone. Lying face downward.

sacrum. Lower portion of the spine composed of five fused vertebrae designated as S1-S5.

superior hypogastric plexus. Part of the autonomic nervous system, the superior hypogastric plexus is formed of parasympathetic fibers that are a continuation of the intermesenteric plexus. It divides into the left and right hypogastric nerves.

Nervous

64681

64681 Destruction by neurolytic agent, with or without radiologic monitoring; superior hypogastric plexus

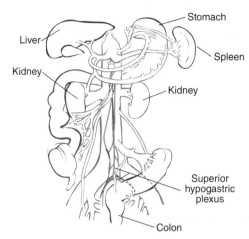

The nerve is injected with a neurolytic agent.
This plexus lies near the bifurcation of
the aorta just anterior to the sacrum

Explanation

The physician performs a neurolysis on the superior hypogastric plexus by injecting a chemical, thermal, or electrical agent through a needle inserted in the L5/S1 interspace. The superior hypogastric plexus, also called the presacral nerve, is located in front of the upper part of the sacrum and is formed by lower lumbar nerves responsible for pain sensation in the pelvic area. Nerve destruction is done in such cases as severe, intractable menstrual pain and pain due to pelvic area metastases from cancer such as prostatic malignancy when an anesthetic nerve block does not offer sufficient relief. The patient is placed in the prone position and prepped. A 6-inch needle is guided under radiological imaging, such as fluoroscopy (reported separately), into the ventral lateral spine and through the L5/S1 interspace. Needle position is checked by injecting contrast material and aspirating for the return of any blood, urine, or cerebral spinal fluid. With negative aspiration results and imaging verifying that the needle position is in the prevertebral space and not within a blood vessel, a ureter, or spinal nerves, the neurolytic agent is injected, or delivered, to both sides.

Coding Tips

Code 64681 includes the injection of other therapeutic agents (e.g., corticosteroids). For destruction by neurolytic agent, with or without radiologic monitoring, celiac plexus, see 64680.

ICD-10-CM Diagnostic Codes ·

C18.6	Malignant neoplasm of descending colon
C19	Malignant neoplasm of rectosigmoid junction
C20	Malignant neoplasm of rectum
C41.4	Malignant neoplasm of pelvic bones, sacrum and coccyx
C49.5	Malignant neoplasm of connective and soft tissue of pelvis
C51.0	Malignant neoplasm of labium majus ♀
C51.1	Malignant neoplasm of labium minus ♀
C51.2	Malignant neoplasm of clitoris ♀
C51.8	Malignant neoplasm of overlapping sites of vulva ♀
C52	Malignant neoplasm of vagina ♀
C53.0	Malignant neoplasm of endocervix ♀
C53.1	Malignant neoplasm of exocervix ♀
C53.8	Malignant neoplasm of overlapping sites of cervix uteri ♀
C54.0	Malignant neoplasm of isthmus uteri ♀
C54.1	Malignant neoplasm of endometrium ♀
C54.2	Malignant neoplasm of myometrium ♀
C54.3	Malignant neoplasm of fundus uteri ♀
C54.8	Malignant neoplasm of overlapping sites of corpus uteri ♀
C67.0	Malignant neoplasm of trigone of bladder
C67.1	Malignant neoplasm of dome of bladder
C67.2	Malignant neoplasm of lateral wall of bladder
C67.3	Malignant neoplasm of anterior wall of bladder
C67.4	Malignant neoplasm of posterior wall of bladder
C67.5	Malignant neoplasm of bladder neck
C67.6	Malignant neoplasm of ureteric orifice
C67.7	Malignant neoplasm of urachus
C67.8	Malignant neoplasm of overlapping sites of bladder
C68.0	Malignant neoplasm of urethra
C68.1	Malignant neoplasm of paraurethral glands
C68.8	Malignant neoplasm of overlapping sites of urinary organs
G89.3	Neoplasm related pain (acute) (chronic)
N80.0	Endometriosis of uterus ♀
N80.1	Endometriosis of ovary ♀
N80.2	Endometriosis of fallopian tube ♀
N80.3	Endometriosis of pelvic peritoneum ♀
N80.4	Endometriosis of rectovaginal septum and vagina ♀
N80.5	Endometriosis of intestine ♀
N80.8	Other endometriosis ♀

AMA: **64681** 2019,Apr,9; 2018,Jan,8; 2017,Jan,8; 2016,Jan,13; 2015,Jan,16; 2014,Jan,11

Relative Value Units/Medicare Edits

Non-Facility RVU	Work	PE	MP	Total
64681	3.78	11.47	0.87	16.12
Facility RVU	**Work**	**PE**	**MP**	**Total**
64681	3.78	2.85	0.87	7.5

	FUD	Status	MUE	Modifiers				IOM Reference
64681	10	A	1(2)	51	N/A	N/A	N/A	None

* with documentation

Terms To Know

destruction. Ablation or eradication of a structure or tissue.

interspace. Space between two similar objects.

neurolysis. Dissection of a nerve.

neurolytic. Destruction of nerve tissue.

sacrum. Lower portion of the spine composed of five fused vertebrae designated as S1-S5.

superior hypogastric plexus. Part of the autonomic nervous system, the superior hypogastric plexus is formed of parasympathetic fibers that are a continuation of the intermesenteric plexus. It divides into the left and right hypogastric nerves.

Nervous

69990

+ 69990 Microsurgical techniques, requiring use of operating microscope (List separately in addition to code for primary procedure)

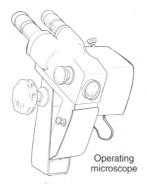

Operating microscope

Explanation

The physician uses a surgical microscope when the services are performed using the techniques of microsurgery, except when the microscopy is part of the procedure (such as in 15756). This code is reported in addition to the primary procedure.

Coding Tips

Report 69990 in addition to the code for the primary procedure performed. A surgical microscope is employed when surgical services are performed using techniques of microsurgery. It should not be used for visualization with magnifying loupes or corrected vision. It should not be reported with procedures where use of an operating microscope is an inclusive component: 15756-15758, 15842, 19364, 19368, 20955-20962, 20969-20973, 22551-22552, 22856-22861, 26551-26554, 26556, 31526, 31531, 31536, 31541, 31545-31546, 31561, 31571, 43116, 43180, 43496, 46601, 46607, 49906, 61548, 63075-63078, 64727, 64820-64823, 64912, 64913, 65091-68850, 0184T, 0308T, 0402T, and 0583T.

ICD-10-CM Diagnostic Codes

The application of this code is too broad to adequately present ICD-10-CM diagnostic code links here. Refer to your ICD-10-CM book.

AMA: 69990 2018,Jan,8; 2018,Feb,11; 2017,Jan,8; 2017,Dec,12; 2017,Dec,13; 2017,Dec,14; 2016,Jan,13; 2016,Feb,12; 2015,Jan,16; 2014,Sep,13; 2014,Jan,8; 2014,Jan,11; 2014,Apr,10

Relative Value Units/Medicare Edits

Non-Facility RVU	Work	PE	MP	Total
69990	3.46	1.59	1.25	6.3
Facility RVU	Work	PE	MP	Total
69990	3.46	1.59	1.25	6.3

	FUD	Status	MUE	Modifiers				IOM Reference
69990	N/A	R	1(3)	N/A	N/A	N/A	80	None

* with documentation

Terms To Know

microsurgery. Surgical procedures performed under magnification using a surgical microscope.

76801-76802

76801 Ultrasound, pregnant uterus, real time with image documentation, fetal and maternal evaluation, first trimester (< 14 weeks 0 days), transabdominal approach; single or first gestation

+ 76802 each additional gestation (List separately in addition to code for primary procedure)

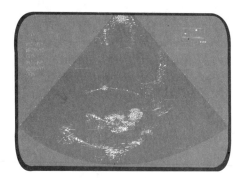

A real time ultrasound is taken of a pregnant uterus in the first trimester.

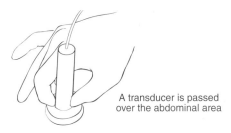

A transducer is passed over the abdominal area

Explanation

Diagnostic ultrasound is an imaging technique bouncing sound waves far above the level of human perception through interior body structures. The sound waves pass through different densities of tissue and reflect back to a receiving unit at varying speeds. The unit converts the waves to electrical pulses that are immediately displayed in picture form on screen. Real time scanning displays both two-dimensional structure images and movement with time. Use 76801 to report real time ultrasound, transabdominal, with image documentation on a pregnant uterus for fetal and maternal evaluation in the first trimester of a single or first gestation. This includes determining the number of fetuses and gestational sacs and taking their measurements, surveying the visible fetal and placental structure, assessing amniotic fluid volume and sac shape, and examining the maternal uterus and adnexa. Report 76802 for each additional gestation evaluation.

Coding Tips

Report 76802 in addition to 76801. Report first trimester fetal nuchal translucency measurement with 76813-76814. Results must be documented in the report for each of the elements described in the code description. It is appropriate to code an obstetrical ultrasound for a patient who has an established diagnosis of pregnancy, who presents with indications necessitating the exam that may be pregnancy related, even when the outcome shows that the patient is no longer currently pregnant.

ICD-10-CM Diagnostic Codes

O09.521	Supervision of elderly multigravida, first trimester ⚕ ♀
O09.522	Supervision of elderly multigravida, second trimester ⚕ ♀
O09.523	Supervision of elderly multigravida, third trimester ⚕ ♀
O09.891	Supervision of other high risk pregnancies, first trimester ⚕ ♀

O10.011	Pre-existing essential hypertension complicating pregnancy, first trimester ⚕ ♀
O10.111	Pre-existing hypertensive heart disease complicating pregnancy, first trimester ⚕ ♀
O10.211	Pre-existing hypertensive chronic kidney disease complicating pregnancy, first trimester ⚕ ♀
O10.311	Pre-existing hypertensive heart and chronic kidney disease complicating pregnancy, first trimester ⚕ ♀
O10.411	Pre-existing secondary hypertension complicating pregnancy, first trimester ⚕ ♀
O11.1	Pre-existing hypertension with pre-eclampsia, first trimester ⚕ ♀
O13.1	Gestational [pregnancy-induced] hypertension without significant proteinuria, first trimester ⚕ ♀
O20.0	Threatened abortion ⚕ ♀
O25.11	Malnutrition in pregnancy, first trimester ⚕ ♀
O26.11	Low weight gain in pregnancy, first trimester ⚕ ♀
O26.21	Pregnancy care for patient with recurrent pregnancy loss, first trimester ⚕ ♀
O26.31	Retained intrauterine contraceptive device in pregnancy, first trimester ⚕ ♀
O26.711	Subluxation of symphysis (pubis) in pregnancy, first trimester ⚕ ♀
O26.841	Uterine size-date discrepancy, first trimester ⚕ ♀
O26.851	Spotting complicating pregnancy, first trimester ⚕ ♀
O29.011	Aspiration pneumonitis due to anesthesia during pregnancy, first trimester ⚕ ♀
O29.021	Pressure collapse of lung due to anesthesia during pregnancy, first trimester ⚕ ♀
O29.091	Other pulmonary complications of anesthesia during pregnancy, first trimester ⚕ ♀
O29.111	Cardiac arrest due to anesthesia during pregnancy, first trimester ⚕ ♀
O29.121	Cardiac failure due to anesthesia during pregnancy, first trimester ⚕ ♀
O29.211	Cerebral anoxia due to anesthesia during pregnancy, first trimester ⚕ ♀
O29.291	Other central nervous system complications of anesthesia during pregnancy, first trimester ⚕ ♀
O29.3X1	Toxic reaction to local anesthesia during pregnancy, first trimester ⚕ ♀
O29.8X1	Other complications of anesthesia during pregnancy, first trimester ⚕ ♀
O33.0	Maternal care for disproportion due to deformity of maternal pelvic bones ⚕ ♀
O34.11	Maternal care for benign tumor of corpus uteri, first trimester ⚕ ♀
O34.41	Maternal care for other abnormalities of cervix, first trimester ⚕ ♀
O34.511	Maternal care for incarceration of gravid uterus, first trimester ⚕ ♀
O34.521	Maternal care for prolapse of gravid uterus, first trimester ⚕ ♀
O34.531	Maternal care for retroversion of gravid uterus, first trimester ⚕ ♀
O34.61	Maternal care for abnormality of vagina, first trimester ⚕ ♀
O34.71	Maternal care for abnormality of vulva and perineum, first trimester ⚕ ♀
O35.0XX1	Maternal care for (suspected) central nervous system malformation in fetus, fetus 1 ⚕ ♀

Radiology

O35.1XX1 Maternal care for (suspected) chromosomal abnormality in fetus, fetus 1 M ♀

O35.2XX1 Maternal care for (suspected) hereditary disease in fetus, fetus 1 M ♀

O35.3XX1 Maternal care for (suspected) damage to fetus from viral disease in mother, fetus 1 M ♀

O35.4XX1 Maternal care for (suspected) damage to fetus from alcohol, fetus 1 M ♀

O35.5XX1 Maternal care for (suspected) damage to fetus by drugs, fetus 1 M ♀

O35.6XX1 Maternal care for (suspected) damage to fetus by radiation, fetus 1 M ♀

O35.8XX1 Maternal care for other (suspected) fetal abnormality and damage, fetus 1 M ♀

O36.0111 Maternal care for anti-D [Rh] antibodies, first trimester, fetus 1 M ♀

O36.0911 Maternal care for other rhesus isoimmunization, first trimester, fetus 1 M ♀

O36.1111 Maternal care for Anti-A sensitization, first trimester, fetus 1 M ♀

O36.1911 Maternal care for other isoimmunization, first trimester, fetus 1 M ♀

O36.4XX1 Maternal care for intrauterine death, fetus 1 M ♀

O36.5110 Maternal care for known or suspected placental insufficiency, first trimester, not applicable or unspecified M ♀

O36.5111 Maternal care for known or suspected placental insufficiency, first trimester, fetus 1 M ♀

O36.5112 Maternal care for known or suspected placental insufficiency, first trimester, fetus 2 M ♀

O36.5911 Maternal care for other known or suspected poor fetal growth, first trimester, fetus 1 M ♀

O36.80X1 Pregnancy with inconclusive fetal viability, fetus 1 M ♀

O36.8911 Maternal care for other specified fetal problems, first trimester, fetus 1 M ♀

O40.1XX1 Polyhydramnios, first trimester, fetus 1 M ♀

O41.01X1 Oligohydramnios, first trimester, fetus 1 M ♀

O41.1211 Chorioamnionitis, first trimester, fetus 1 M ♀

O41.1411 Placentitis, first trimester, fetus 1 M ♀

O41.8X11 Other specified disorders of amniotic fluid and membranes, first trimester, fetus 1 M ♀

O42.011 Preterm premature rupture of membranes, onset of labor within 24 hours of rupture, first trimester M ♀

O43.011 Fetomaternal placental transfusion syndrome, first trimester M ♀

O43.111 Circumvallate placenta, first trimester M ♀

O43.191 Other malformation of placenta, first trimester M ♀

O43.811 Placental infarction, first trimester M ♀

O43.891 Other placental disorders, first trimester M ♀

O44.01 Complete placenta previa NOS or without hemorrhage, first trimester M ♀

O44.11 Complete placenta previa with hemorrhage, first trimester M ♀

O45.011 Premature separation of placenta with afibrinogenemia, first trimester M ♀

O45.021 Premature separation of placenta with disseminated intravascular coagulation, first trimester M ♀

O45.091 Premature separation of placenta with other coagulation defect, first trimester M ♀

O45.8X1 Other premature separation of placenta, first trimester M ♀

O46.011 Antepartum hemorrhage with afibrinogenemia, first trimester M ♀

O46.021 Antepartum hemorrhage with disseminated intravascular coagulation, first trimester M ♀

O46.091 Antepartum hemorrhage with other coagulation defect, first trimester M ♀

O46.8X1 Other antepartum hemorrhage, first trimester M ♀

O99.211 Obesity complicating pregnancy, first trimester M ♀

O99.311 Alcohol use complicating pregnancy, first trimester M ♀

O99.321 Drug use complicating pregnancy, first trimester M ♀

O99.331 Smoking (tobacco) complicating pregnancy, first trimester M ♀

O9A.211 Injury, poisoning and certain other consequences of external causes complicating pregnancy, first trimester M ♀

Z33.3 Pregnant state, gestational carrier M ♀

Z36.0 Encounter for antenatal screening for chromosomal anomalies M ♀

Z36.2 Encounter for other antenatal screening follow-up M ♀

Z36.3 Encounter for antenatal screening for malformations M ♀

Z36.4 Encounter for antenatal screening for fetal growth retardation M ♀

Z36.5 Encounter for antenatal screening for isoimmunization M ♀

Z36.81 Encounter for antenatal screening for hydrops fetalis M ♀

Z36.83 Encounter for fetal screening for congenital cardiac abnormalities M ♀

Z36.84 Encounter for antenatal screening for fetal lung maturity M ♀

Z36.86 Encounter for antenatal screening for cervical length M ♀

Z36.87 Encounter for antenatal screening for uncertain dates M ♀

Z36.88 Encounter for antenatal screening for fetal macrosomia M ♀

Z36.8A Encounter for antenatal screening for other genetic defects M ♀

AMA: 76801 2018,Jan,8; 2017,Jan,8; 2016,Jan,13; 2015,Jan,16; 2014,Jan,11
76802 2018,Jan,8; 2017,Jan,8; 2016,Jan,13; 2015,Jan,16; 2014,Jan,11

Relative Value Units/Medicare Edits

Non-Facility RVU	Work	PE	MP	Total
76801	0.99	2.4	0.06	3.45
76802	0.83	0.92	0.03	1.78
Facility RVU	Work	PE	MP	Total
76801	0.99	2.4	0.06	3.45
76802	0.83	0.92	0.03	1.78

	FUD	Status	MUE	Modifiers				IOM Reference
76801	N/A	A	1(2)	N/A	N/A	N/A	80*	None
76802	N/A	A	2(3)	N/A	N/A	N/A	80*	

* with documentation

Terms To Know

fetus. Unborn offspring past the embryonic stage that has developed major structures. It is the period defined from nine weeks after fertilization until birth.

real-time. Immediate imaging, with movement as it happens.

ultrasound. Imaging using ultra-high sound frequency bounced off body structures.

76805-76810

76805 Ultrasound, pregnant uterus, real time with image documentation, fetal and maternal evaluation, after first trimester (> or = 14 weeks 0 days), transabdominal approach; single or first gestation

+ 76810 each additional gestation (List separately in addition to code for primary procedure)

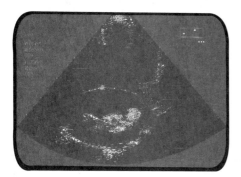

A real time ultrasound is taken of a pregnant uterus in the first trimester.

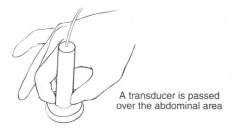

A transducer is passed over the abdominal area

Explanation

Diagnostic ultrasound is an imaging technique bouncing sound waves far above the level of human perception through interior body structures. The sound waves pass through different densities of tissue and reflect back to a receiving unit at varying speeds. The unit converts the waves to electrical pulses that are immediately displayed in picture form on screen. Real time scanning displays both two-dimensional structure images and movement with time. Use 76805 to report real time ultrasound, transabdominal, with image documentation on a pregnant uterus for fetal and maternal evaluation after the first trimester of a single or first gestation. This includes determining the number of fetuses and amniotic/chorionic sacs, taking measurements appropriate for gestational age, surveying intracranial, spinal, abdominal, and heart chamber anatomy as well as the insertion site of the umbilical cord and the location of the placenta, and assessing amniotic fluid and maternal adnexa. Report 76810 for each additional gestation evaluation.

Coding Tips

Report 76810 in addition to 76805. Results must be documented in the report for each of the elements described in the code description. It is appropriate to code an obstetrical ultrasound for a patient who has an established diagnosis of pregnancy, who presents with indications necessitating the exam that may be pregnancy related, even when the outcome shows that the patient is no longer currently pregnant.

ICD-10-CM Diagnostic Codes

O12.02	Gestational edema, second trimester Ⓜ ♀
O12.03	Gestational edema, third trimester Ⓜ ♀
O14.22	HELLP syndrome (HELLP), second trimester Ⓜ ♀
O14.23	HELLP syndrome (HELLP), third trimester Ⓜ ♀

O15.02	Eclampsia complicating pregnancy, second trimester Ⓜ ♀
O15.03	Eclampsia complicating pregnancy, third trimester Ⓜ ♀
O20.0	Threatened abortion Ⓜ ♀
O26.712	Subluxation of symphysis (pubis) in pregnancy, second trimester Ⓜ ♀
O26.713	Subluxation of symphysis (pubis) in pregnancy, third trimester Ⓜ ♀
O26.842	Uterine size-date discrepancy, second trimester Ⓜ ♀
O26.843	Uterine size-date discrepancy, third trimester Ⓜ ♀
O26.852	Spotting complicating pregnancy, second trimester Ⓜ ♀
O26.853	Spotting complicating pregnancy, third trimester Ⓜ ♀
O32.0XX1	Maternal care for unstable lie, fetus 1 Ⓜ ♀
O32.1XX1	Maternal care for breech presentation, fetus 1 Ⓜ ♀
O32.2XX1	Maternal care for transverse and oblique lie, fetus 1 Ⓜ ♀
O32.3XX1	Maternal care for face, brow and chin presentation, fetus 1 Ⓜ ♀
O32.4XX1	Maternal care for high head at term, fetus 1 Ⓜ ♀
O32.6XX1	Maternal care for compound presentation, fetus 1 Ⓜ ♀
O33.3XX1	Maternal care for disproportion due to outlet contraction of pelvis, fetus 1 Ⓜ ♀
O33.4XX1	Maternal care for disproportion of mixed maternal and fetal origin, fetus 1 Ⓜ ♀
O33.5XX1	Maternal care for disproportion due to unusually large fetus, fetus 1 Ⓜ ♀
O33.6XX1	Maternal care for disproportion due to hydrocephalic fetus, fetus 1 Ⓜ ♀
O33.7XX1	Maternal care for disproportion due to other fetal deformities, fetus 1 Ⓜ ♀
O33.7XX2	Maternal care for disproportion due to other fetal deformities, fetus 2 Ⓜ ♀
O33.7XX3	Maternal care for disproportion due to other fetal deformities, fetus 3 Ⓜ ♀
O34.512	Maternal care for incarceration of gravid uterus, second trimester Ⓜ ♀
O34.513	Maternal care for incarceration of gravid uterus, third trimester Ⓜ ♀
O34.522	Maternal care for prolapse of gravid uterus, second trimester Ⓜ ♀
O34.523	Maternal care for prolapse of gravid uterus, third trimester Ⓜ ♀
O34.532	Maternal care for retroversion of gravid uterus, second trimester Ⓜ ♀
O34.533	Maternal care for retroversion of gravid uterus, third trimester Ⓜ ♀
O35.0XX1	Maternal care for (suspected) central nervous system malformation in fetus, fetus 1 Ⓜ ♀
O35.1XX1	Maternal care for (suspected) chromosomal abnormality in fetus, fetus 1 Ⓜ ♀
O35.2XX1	Maternal care for (suspected) hereditary disease in fetus, fetus 1 Ⓜ ♀
O36.0121	Maternal care for anti-D [Rh] antibodies, second trimester, fetus 1 Ⓜ ♀
O36.0131	Maternal care for anti-D [Rh] antibodies, third trimester, fetus 1 Ⓜ ♀
O36.0921	Maternal care for other rhesus isoimmunization, second trimester, fetus 1 Ⓜ ♀
O36.0931	Maternal care for other rhesus isoimmunization, third trimester, fetus 1 Ⓜ ♀

Radiology

O36.1121 Maternal care for Anti-A sensitization, second trimester, fetus 1 Ⓜ ♀

O36.1131 Maternal care for Anti-A sensitization, third trimester, fetus 1 Ⓜ ♀

O36.1921 Maternal care for other isoimmunization, second trimester, fetus 1 Ⓜ ♀

O36.1931 Maternal care for other isoimmunization, third trimester, fetus 1 Ⓜ ♀

O36.22X1 Maternal care for hydrops fetalis, second trimester, fetus 1 Ⓜ ♀

O36.23X1 Maternal care for hydrops fetalis, third trimester, fetus 1 Ⓜ ♀

O36.5121 Maternal care for known or suspected placental insufficiency, second trimester, fetus 1 Ⓜ ♀

O36.5131 Maternal care for known or suspected placental insufficiency, third trimester, fetus 1 Ⓜ ♀

O36.5921 Maternal care for other known or suspected poor fetal growth, second trimester, fetus 1 Ⓜ ♀

O36.5931 Maternal care for other known or suspected poor fetal growth, third trimester, fetus 1 Ⓜ ♀

O36.62X1 Maternal care for excessive fetal growth, second trimester, fetus 1 Ⓜ ♀

O36.63X1 Maternal care for excessive fetal growth, third trimester, fetus 1 Ⓜ ♀

O36.8121 Decreased fetal movements, second trimester, fetus 1 Ⓜ ♀

O36.8131 Decreased fetal movements, third trimester, fetus 1 Ⓜ ♀

O36.8221 Fetal anemia and thrombocytopenia, second trimester, fetus 1 Ⓜ ♀

O36.8231 Fetal anemia and thrombocytopenia, third trimester, fetus 1 Ⓜ ♀

O36.8921 Maternal care for other specified fetal problems, second trimester, fetus 1 Ⓜ ♀

O40.2XX1 Polyhydramnios, second trimester, fetus 1 Ⓜ ♀

O40.3XX1 Polyhydramnios, third trimester, fetus 1 Ⓜ ♀

O41.02X1 Oligohydramnios, second trimester, fetus 1 Ⓜ ♀

O41.03X1 Oligohydramnios, third trimester, fetus 1 Ⓜ ♀

O41.1221 Chorioamnionitis, second trimester, fetus 1 Ⓜ ♀

O41.1231 Chorioamnionitis, third trimester, fetus 1 Ⓜ ♀

O41.1421 Placentitis, second trimester, fetus 1 Ⓜ ♀

O41.1431 Placentitis, third trimester, fetus 1 Ⓜ ♀

O42.012 Preterm premature rupture of membranes, onset of labor within 24 hours of rupture, second trimester Ⓜ ♀

O42.013 Preterm premature rupture of membranes, onset of labor within 24 hours of rupture, third trimester Ⓜ ♀

O42.112 Preterm premature rupture of membranes, onset of labor more than 24 hours following rupture, second trimester Ⓜ ♀

O42.113 Preterm premature rupture of membranes, onset of labor more than 24 hours following rupture, third trimester Ⓜ ♀

O43.012 Fetomaternal placental transfusion syndrome, second trimester Ⓜ ♀

O43.013 Fetomaternal placental transfusion syndrome, third trimester Ⓜ ♀

O43.022 Fetus-to-fetus placental transfusion syndrome, second trimester Ⓜ ♀

O43.023 Fetus-to-fetus placental transfusion syndrome, third trimester Ⓜ ♀

O43.112 Circumvallate placenta, second trimester Ⓜ ♀

O43.113 Circumvallate placenta, third trimester Ⓜ ♀

O43.812 Placental infarction, second trimester Ⓜ ♀

O43.813 Placental infarction, third trimester Ⓜ ♀

O44.02 Complete placenta previa NOS or without hemorrhage, second trimester Ⓜ ♀

O44.03 Complete placenta previa NOS or without hemorrhage, third trimester Ⓜ ♀

O44.12 Complete placenta previa with hemorrhage, second trimester Ⓜ ♀

O44.13 Complete placenta previa with hemorrhage, third trimester Ⓜ ♀

O45.012 Premature separation of placenta with afibrinogenemia, second trimester Ⓜ ♀

O45.013 Premature separation of placenta with afibrinogenemia, third trimester Ⓜ ♀

O45.022 Premature separation of placenta with disseminated intravascular coagulation, second trimester Ⓜ ♀

O45.023 Premature separation of placenta with disseminated intravascular coagulation, third trimester Ⓜ ♀

O45.092 Premature separation of placenta with other coagulation defect, second trimester Ⓜ ♀

O45.093 Premature separation of placenta with other coagulation defect, third trimester Ⓜ ♀

O46.012 Antepartum hemorrhage with afibrinogenemia, second trimester Ⓜ ♀

O46.013 Antepartum hemorrhage with afibrinogenemia, third trimester Ⓜ ♀

O46.022 Antepartum hemorrhage with disseminated intravascular coagulation, second trimester Ⓜ ♀

O46.023 Antepartum hemorrhage with disseminated intravascular coagulation, third trimester Ⓜ ♀

O46.092 Antepartum hemorrhage with other coagulation defect, second trimester Ⓜ ♀

O46.093 Antepartum hemorrhage with other coagulation defect, third trimester Ⓜ ♀

Z34.02 Encounter for supervision of normal first pregnancy, second trimester Ⓜ ♀

Z34.03 Encounter for supervision of normal first pregnancy, third trimester Ⓜ ♀

AMA: **76805** 2018,Jan,8; 2017,Jan,8; 2016,Jan,13; 2015,Jan,16; 2014,Jan,11 **76810** 2018,Jan,8; 2017,Jan,8; 2016,Jan,13; 2015,Jan,16; 2014,Jan,11

Relative Value Units/Medicare Edits

Non-Facility RVU	Work	PE	MP	Total
76805	0.99	2.9	0.06	3.95
76810	0.98	1.55	0.06	2.59
Facility RVU	Work	PE	MP	Total
76805	0.99	2.9	0.06	3.95
76810	0.98	1.55	0.06	2.59

	FUD	Status	MUE	Modifiers				IOM Reference
76805	N/A	A	1(2)	N/A	N/A	N/A	80*	None
76810	N/A	A	2(3)	N/A	N/A	N/A	80*	

* with documentation

76811-76812

76811 Ultrasound, pregnant uterus, real time with image documentation, fetal and maternal evaluation plus detailed fetal anatomic examination, transabdominal approach; single or first gestation

+ 76812 each additional gestation (List separately in addition to code for primary procedure)

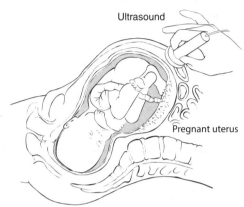

Ultrasound

Pregnant uterus

Ultrasound is performed on a pregnant uterus, real time with documentation

Explanation

Diagnostic ultrasound is an imaging technique bouncing sound waves far above the level of human perception through interior body structures. The sound waves pass through different densities of tissue and reflect back to a receiving unit at varying speeds. The unit converts the waves to electrical pulses that are immediately displayed in picture form on screen. Real time scanning displays both two-dimensional structure images and movement with time. Use 76811 to report real time ultrasound, transabdominal, with image documentation on a pregnant uterus for fetal and maternal evaluation plus detailed fetal anatomic examination of a single or first gestation. This includes determining the number of fetuses and amniotic/chorionic sacs, taking measurements appropriate for gestational age, and surveying intracranial, spinal, abdominal, and heart chamber anatomy plus a detailed evaluation of the brain and ventricles, face, heart and outflow tracts, chest, abdominal organs, and number, length, and structure of the limbs. Assessing amniotic fluid, maternal adnexa, and any other fetal anatomy is also done with a detailed evaluation of the umbilical cord and the placenta. Report 76812 for each additional gestation evaluation.

Coding Tips

Report 76812 in addition to 76811. Results must be documented in the report for each of the elements described in the code description. It is appropriate to code an obstetrical ultrasound for a patient who has an established diagnosis of pregnancy, who presents with indications necessitating the exam that may be pregnancy related, even when the outcome shows that the patient is no longer currently pregnant.

ICD-10-CM Diagnostic Codes

O12.02	Gestational edema, second trimester ⓜ ♀
O12.03	Gestational edema, third trimester ⓜ ♀
O14.22	HELLP syndrome (HELLP), second trimester ⓜ ♀
O14.23	HELLP syndrome (HELLP), third trimester ⓜ ♀
O15.02	Eclampsia complicating pregnancy, second trimester ⓜ ♀
O15.03	Eclampsia complicating pregnancy, third trimester ⓜ ♀
O20.0	Threatened abortion ⓜ ♀

O26.712	Subluxation of symphysis (pubis) in pregnancy, second trimester ⓜ ♀
O26.713	Subluxation of symphysis (pubis) in pregnancy, third trimester ⓜ ♀
O26.842	Uterine size-date discrepancy, second trimester ⓜ ♀
O26.843	Uterine size-date discrepancy, third trimester ⓜ ♀
O26.852	Spotting complicating pregnancy, second trimester ⓜ ♀
O26.853	Spotting complicating pregnancy, third trimester ⓜ ♀
O26.872	Cervical shortening, second trimester ⓜ ♀
O26.873	Cervical shortening, third trimester ⓜ ♀
O32.0XX1	Maternal care for unstable lie, fetus 1 ⓜ ♀
O32.1XX1	Maternal care for breech presentation, fetus 1 ⓜ ♀
O32.2XX1	Maternal care for transverse and oblique lie, fetus 1 ⓜ ♀
O32.3XX1	Maternal care for face, brow and chin presentation, fetus 1 ⓜ ♀
O32.4XX1	Maternal care for high head at term, fetus 1 ⓜ ♀
O32.6XX1	Maternal care for compound presentation, fetus 1 ⓜ ♀
O32.8XX1	Maternal care for other malpresentation of fetus, fetus 1 ⓜ ♀
O33.3XX1	Maternal care for disproportion due to outlet contraction of pelvis, fetus 1 ⓜ ♀
O33.4XX1	Maternal care for disproportion of mixed maternal and fetal origin, fetus 1 ⓜ ♀
O33.5XX1	Maternal care for disproportion due to unusually large fetus, fetus 1 ⓜ ♀
O33.6XX1	Maternal care for disproportion due to hydrocephalic fetus, fetus 1 ⓜ ♀
O33.7XX1	Maternal care for disproportion due to other fetal deformities, fetus 1 ⓜ ♀
O33.7XX2	Maternal care for disproportion due to other fetal deformities, fetus 2 ⓜ ♀
O33.7XX3	Maternal care for disproportion due to other fetal deformities, fetus 3 ⓜ ♀
O34.512	Maternal care for incarceration of gravid uterus, second trimester ⓜ ♀
O34.513	Maternal care for incarceration of gravid uterus, third trimester ⓜ ♀
O34.522	Maternal care for prolapse of gravid uterus, second trimester ⓜ ♀
O34.523	Maternal care for prolapse of gravid uterus, third trimester ⓜ ♀
O34.532	Maternal care for retroversion of gravid uterus, second trimester ⓜ ♀
O34.533	Maternal care for retroversion of gravid uterus, third trimester ⓜ ♀
O35.1XX1	Maternal care for (suspected) chromosomal abnormality in fetus, fetus 1 ⓜ ♀
O35.2XX1	Maternal care for (suspected) hereditary disease in fetus, fetus 1 ⓜ ♀
O36.0121	Maternal care for anti-D [Rh] antibodies, second trimester, fetus 1 ⓜ ♀
O36.0131	Maternal care for anti-D [Rh] antibodies, third trimester, fetus 1 ⓜ ♀
O36.0921	Maternal care for other rhesus isoimmunization, second trimester, fetus 1 ⓜ ♀
O36.0931	Maternal care for other rhesus isoimmunization, third trimester, fetus 1 ⓜ ♀
O36.1121	Maternal care for Anti-A sensitization, second trimester, fetus 1 ⓜ ♀
O36.1131	Maternal care for Anti-A sensitization, third trimester, fetus 1 ⓜ ♀

Radiology

O36.1911	Maternal care for other isoimmunization, first trimester, fetus 1 Ⓜ ♀
O36.1921	Maternal care for other isoimmunization, second trimester, fetus 1 Ⓜ ♀
O36.1931	Maternal care for other isoimmunization, third trimester, fetus 1 Ⓜ ♀
O36.22X1	Maternal care for hydrops fetalis, second trimester, fetus 1 Ⓜ ♀
O36.23X1	Maternal care for hydrops fetalis, third trimester, fetus 1 Ⓜ ♀
O36.5121	Maternal care for known or suspected placental insufficiency, second trimester, fetus 1 Ⓜ ♀
O36.5131	Maternal care for known or suspected placental insufficiency, third trimester, fetus 1 Ⓜ ♀
O36.5921	Maternal care for other known or suspected poor fetal growth, second trimester, fetus 1 Ⓜ ♀
O36.5931	Maternal care for other known or suspected poor fetal growth, third trimester, fetus 1 Ⓜ ♀
O36.62X1	Maternal care for excessive fetal growth, second trimester, fetus 1 Ⓜ ♀
O36.63X1	Maternal care for excessive fetal growth, third trimester, fetus 1 Ⓜ ♀
O36.8121	Decreased fetal movements, second trimester, fetus 1 Ⓜ ♀
O36.8131	Decreased fetal movements, third trimester, fetus 1 Ⓜ ♀
O40.2XX1	Polyhydramnios, second trimester, fetus 1 Ⓜ ♀
O40.3XX1	Polyhydramnios, third trimester, fetus 1 Ⓜ ♀
O41.02X1	Oligohydramnios, second trimester, fetus 1 Ⓜ ♀
O41.03X1	Oligohydramnios, third trimester, fetus 1 Ⓜ ♀
O41.1221	Chorioamnionitis, second trimester, fetus 1 Ⓜ ♀
O41.1231	Chorioamnionitis, third trimester, fetus 1 Ⓜ ♀
O41.1421	Placentitis, second trimester, fetus 1 Ⓜ ♀
O41.1431	Placentitis, third trimester, fetus 1 Ⓜ ♀
O43.112	Circumvallate placenta, second trimester Ⓜ ♀
O43.113	Circumvallate placenta, third trimester Ⓜ ♀
O43.192	Other malformation of placenta, second trimester Ⓜ ♀
O43.193	Other malformation of placenta, third trimester Ⓜ ♀
O43.812	Placental infarction, second trimester Ⓜ ♀
O43.813	Placental infarction, third trimester Ⓜ ♀
O43.892	Other placental disorders, second trimester Ⓜ ♀
O43.893	Other placental disorders, third trimester Ⓜ ♀
O44.02	Complete placenta previa NOS or without hemorrhage, second trimester Ⓜ ♀
O44.03	Complete placenta previa NOS or without hemorrhage, third trimester Ⓜ ♀
O44.12	Complete placenta previa with hemorrhage, second trimester Ⓜ ♀
O44.13	Complete placenta previa with hemorrhage, third trimester Ⓜ ♀
O45.012	Premature separation of placenta with afibrinogenemia, second trimester Ⓜ ♀
O45.013	Premature separation of placenta with afibrinogenemia, third trimester Ⓜ ♀
O45.022	Premature separation of placenta with disseminated intravascular coagulation, second trimester Ⓜ ♀
O45.023	Premature separation of placenta with disseminated intravascular coagulation, third trimester Ⓜ ♀
O45.092	Premature separation of placenta with other coagulation defect, second trimester Ⓜ ♀
O45.093	Premature separation of placenta with other coagulation defect, third trimester Ⓜ ♀
O45.8X2	Other premature separation of placenta, second trimester Ⓜ ♀
O45.8X3	Other premature separation of placenta, third trimester Ⓜ ♀
O46.012	Antepartum hemorrhage with afibrinogenemia, second trimester Ⓜ ♀
O46.013	Antepartum hemorrhage with afibrinogenemia, third trimester Ⓜ ♀
O46.022	Antepartum hemorrhage with disseminated intravascular coagulation, second trimester Ⓜ ♀
O46.023	Antepartum hemorrhage with disseminated intravascular coagulation, third trimester Ⓜ ♀
O46.092	Antepartum hemorrhage with other coagulation defect, second trimester Ⓜ ♀
O46.093	Antepartum hemorrhage with other coagulation defect, third trimester Ⓜ ♀
O47.02	False labor before 37 completed weeks of gestation, second trimester Ⓜ ♀
O47.03	False labor before 37 completed weeks of gestation, third trimester Ⓜ ♀
O68	Labor and delivery complicated by abnormality of fetal acid-base balance Ⓜ ♀
O76	Abnormality in fetal heart rate and rhythm complicating labor and delivery Ⓜ ♀
Z33.3	Pregnant state, gestational carrier Ⓜ ♀
Z34.02	Encounter for supervision of normal first pregnancy, second trimester Ⓜ ♀
Z34.03	Encounter for supervision of normal first pregnancy, third trimester Ⓜ ♀

AMA: **76811** 2018,Jan,8; 2017,Jan,8; 2016,Jan,13; 2015,Jan,16; 2014,Jan,11
76812 2018,Jan,8; 2017,Jan,8; 2016,Jan,13; 2015,Jan,16; 2014,Jan,11

Relative Value Units/Medicare Edits

Non-Facility RVU	Work	PE	MP	Total
76811	1.9	3.03	0.08	5.01
76812	1.78	3.75	0.08	5.61
Facility RVU	**Work**	**PE**	**MP**	**Total**
76811	1.9	3.03	0.08	5.01
76812	1.78	3.75	0.08	5.61

	FUD	Status	MUE	Modifiers				IOM Reference
76811	N/A	A	1(2)	N/A	N/A	N/A	80*	None
76812	N/A	A	2(3)	N/A	N/A	N/A	80*	

* with documentation

76813-76814

76813 Ultrasound, pregnant uterus, real time with image documentation, first trimester fetal nuchal translucency measurement, transabdominal or transvaginal approach; single or first gestation

+ 76814 each additional gestation (List separately in addition to code for primary procedure)

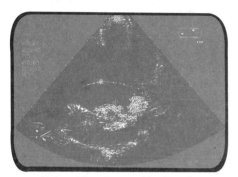

A real time ultrasound is taken of a pregnant uterus to exam nuchal translucency measurement of transabdominal or transvaginal approach

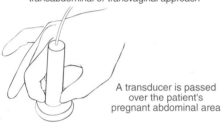

A transducer is passed over the patient's pregnant abdominal area

Explanation

Fetal nuchal translucency provides a noninvasive method to screen for chromosomal abnormalities or heart defects in the first trimester. Nuchal pertains to the back of the neck. Until the lymphatic system of the fetus develops, the back of the neck is a good predictor of fetal health, because the fetus will lie on its back and edema will form in the neck if circulatory problems are present. In a fetal nuchal translucency test, ultrasound transducers on the maternal abdomen or vagina focus on the fetal neck, and the depth of tissue there is measured. The examination includes a calculation of fetal length, and the two measurements are correlated. Fetal nuchal edema does not provide a definitive diagnosis, but would warrant further testing (e.g., chorionic villus sampling). Report 76813 for fetal nuchal translucency testing of one fetus and 76814 for each additional fetus.

Coding Tips

Report 76814 in addition to 76813. For fetal and maternal evaluation performed with detailed fetal anatomic examination, see 76811–76812.

ICD-10-CM Diagnostic Codes

O09.511	Supervision of elderly primigravida, first trimester ⚕ ♀
O35.1XX0	Maternal care for (suspected) chromosomal abnormality in fetus, not applicable or unspecified ⚕ ♀
O35.1XX1	Maternal care for (suspected) chromosomal abnormality in fetus, fetus 1 ⚕ ♀
O35.1XX2	Maternal care for (suspected) chromosomal abnormality in fetus, fetus 2 ⚕ ♀
O35.1XX3	Maternal care for (suspected) chromosomal abnormality in fetus, fetus 3 ⚕ ♀
O35.1XX4	Maternal care for (suspected) chromosomal abnormality in fetus, fetus 4 ⚕ ♀
O35.1XX5	Maternal care for (suspected) chromosomal abnormality in fetus, fetus 5 ⚕ ♀
O35.1XX9	Maternal care for (suspected) chromosomal abnormality in fetus, other fetus ⚕ ♀
Z03.73	Encounter for suspected fetal anomaly ruled out ⚕ ♀
Z36.82	Encounter for antenatal screening for nuchal translucency ⚕ ♀

AMA: **76813** 2018,Jan,8; 2017,Jan,8; 2016,Jan,13; 2015,Jan,16; 2014,Jan,11 **76814** 2018,Jan,8; 2017,Jan,8; 2016,Jan,13; 2015,Jan,16; 2014,Jan,11

Relative Value Units/Medicare Edits

Non-Facility RVU	Work	PE	MP	Total
76813	1.18	2.18	0.06	3.42
76814	0.99	1.19	0.04	2.22
Facility RVU	**Work**	**PE**	**MP**	**Total**
76813	1.18	2.18	0.06	3.42
76814	0.99	1.19	0.04	2.22

	FUD	Status	MUE	Modifiers				IOM Reference
76813	N/A	A	1(2)	N/A	N/A	N/A	80*	None
76814	N/A	A	2(3)	N/A	N/A	N/A	80*	

* with documentation

Terms To Know

approach. Method or anatomical location used to gain access to a body organ or specific area for procedures.

fetal nuchal translucency. Fluid collection residing behind the neck of the fetus that occurs, in part, due to the fetus position, primarily on its' back, as well as the laxity of the neck skin. Fluid collection in the nuchal or neck area in the fetus, like fluid collection in the ankle (edema), can point to a number of pathological processes, such as heart failure. The process of fluid collecting behind the fetal neck may be identified and measured on ultrasound as nuchal translucency with more fluid present representing a higher risk for abnormalities.

fetus. Unborn offspring past the embryonic stage that has developed major structures. It is the period defined from nine weeks after fertilization until birth.

gestation. Carrying of offspring in the womb throughout the period of development of the fetus(es) during pregnancy.

real-time. Immediate imaging, with movement as it happens.

trimester. Normal pregnancy has a duration of approximately 40 weeks and is grouped into three-month periods consisting of three trimesters. ICD-10-CM counts trimesters from the first day of the last menstrual period as follows: 1st trimester less than 14 weeks and 0 days; 2nd trimester 14 weeks, 0 days to less than 28 weeks and 0 days; and 3rd trimester 28 weeks and 0 days until delivery.

ultrasound. Imaging using ultra-high sound frequency bounced off body structures.

Radiology

76815-76816

76815 Ultrasound, pregnant uterus, real time with image documentation, limited (eg, fetal heart beat, placental location, fetal position and/or qualitative amniotic fluid volume), 1 or more fetuses

76816 Ultrasound, pregnant uterus, real time with image documentation, follow-up (eg, re-evaluation of fetal size by measuring standard growth parameters and amniotic fluid volume, re-evaluation of organ system(s) suspected or confirmed to be abnormal on a previous scan), transabdominal approach, per fetus

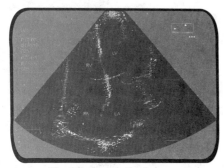

The fetus is visualized on-screen and recordings taken for later analysis

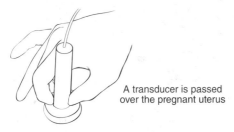

A transducer is passed over the pregnant uterus

Explanation

Diagnostic ultrasound is an imaging technique bouncing sound waves far above the level of human perception through interior body structures. The sound waves pass through different densities of tissue and reflect back to a receiving unit at varying speeds. The unit converts the waves to electrical pulses that are immediately displayed in picture form on screen. Real time scanning displays both two-dimensional structure images and movement with time. Use 76815 to report real time ultrasound with image documentation on a pregnant uterus for a limited evaluation focused on the assessment of one or more of the following: fetal heartbeat, placental location, fetal position, and/or qualitative amniotic fluid volume for one or more fetuses. Use 76816 to report real time ultrasound, transabdominal, with image documentation on a pregnant uterus for a follow-up to reassess fetal size by measuring standard growth parameters and amniotic fluid volume, and to re-evaluate an organ system suspected or confirmed to be abnormal on a previous scan. Report 76816 per fetus evaluated.

Coding Tips

Code 76815 is an exam focused only on evaluating one or more of the elements listed in the code descriptor based on certain clinical indications that necessitate a quick look assessment by ultrasound. It may only be reported per exam and not per element evaluated. Append modifier 59 or an X{EPSU} modifier to code 76816 for each additional fetus evaluated for patients with a multiple pregnancy. It is appropriate to code an obstetrical ultrasound for a patient who has an established diagnosis of pregnancy, who presents with indications necessitating the exam that may be pregnancy related, even when

the outcome shows that the patient is no longer currently pregnant. For fetal nuchal translucency measurement, first trimester, see 76813 and 76814.

ICD-10-CM Diagnostic Codes

O09.891	Supervision of other high risk pregnancies, first trimester ⓜ ♀
O09.892	Supervision of other high risk pregnancies, second trimester ⓜ ♀
O09.893	Supervision of other high risk pregnancies, third trimester ⓜ ♀
O26.711	Subluxation of symphysis (pubis) in pregnancy, first trimester ⓜ ♀
O26.712	Subluxation of symphysis (pubis) in pregnancy, second trimester ⓜ ♀
O26.713	Subluxation of symphysis (pubis) in pregnancy, third trimester ⓜ ♀
O26.841	Uterine size-date discrepancy, first trimester ⓜ ♀
O26.842	Uterine size-date discrepancy, second trimester ⓜ ♀
O26.843	Uterine size-date discrepancy, third trimester ⓜ ♀
O30.011	Twin pregnancy, monochorionic/monoamniotic, first trimester ⓜ ♀
O30.012	Twin pregnancy, monochorionic/monoamniotic, second trimester ⓜ ♀
O30.013	Twin pregnancy, monochorionic/monoamniotic, third trimester ⓜ ♀
O30.031	Twin pregnancy, monochorionic/diamniotic, first trimester ⓜ ♀
O30.032	Twin pregnancy, monochorionic/diamniotic, second trimester ⓜ ♀
O30.033	Twin pregnancy, monochorionic/diamniotic, third trimester ⓜ ♀
O30.041	Twin pregnancy, dichorionic/diamniotic, first trimester ⓜ ♀
O30.042	Twin pregnancy, dichorionic/diamniotic, second trimester ⓜ ♀
O30.043	Twin pregnancy, dichorionic/diamniotic, third trimester ⓜ ♀
O30.111	Triplet pregnancy with two or more monochorionic fetuses, first trimester ⓜ ♀
O30.112	Triplet pregnancy with two or more monochorionic fetuses, second trimester ⓜ ♀
O30.113	Triplet pregnancy with two or more monochorionic fetuses, third trimester ⓜ ♀
O30.121	Triplet pregnancy with two or more monoamniotic fetuses, first trimester ⓜ ♀
O30.122	Triplet pregnancy with two or more monoamniotic fetuses, second trimester ⓜ ♀
O30.123	Triplet pregnancy with two or more monoamniotic fetuses, third trimester ⓜ ♀
O32.0XX1	Maternal care for unstable lie, fetus 1 ⓜ ♀
O32.0XX2	Maternal care for unstable lie, fetus 2 ⓜ ♀
O32.0XX3	Maternal care for unstable lie, fetus 3 ⓜ ♀
O32.1XX1	Maternal care for breech presentation, fetus 1 ⓜ ♀
O32.1XX2	Maternal care for breech presentation, fetus 2 ⓜ ♀
O32.1XX3	Maternal care for breech presentation, fetus 3 ⓜ ♀
O32.2XX1	Maternal care for transverse and oblique lie, fetus 1 ⓜ ♀
O32.2XX2	Maternal care for transverse and oblique lie, fetus 2 ⓜ ♀
O32.2XX3	Maternal care for transverse and oblique lie, fetus 3 ⓜ ♀
O32.3XX1	Maternal care for face, brow and chin presentation, fetus 1 ⓜ ♀
O32.3XX2	Maternal care for face, brow and chin presentation, fetus 2 ⓜ ♀
O32.3XX3	Maternal care for face, brow and chin presentation, fetus 3 ⓜ ♀
O32.4XX1	Maternal care for high head at term, fetus 1 ⓜ ♀
O32.4XX2	Maternal care for high head at term, fetus 2 ⓜ ♀

Radiology

O32.4XX3 Maternal care for high head at term, fetus 3 Ⓜ ♀
O32.6XX1 Maternal care for compound presentation, fetus 1 Ⓜ ♀
O32.6XX2 Maternal care for compound presentation, fetus 2 Ⓜ ♀
O32.6XX3 Maternal care for compound presentation, fetus 3 Ⓜ ♀
O33.4XX1 Maternal care for disproportion of mixed maternal and fetal origin, fetus 1 Ⓜ ♀
O33.4XX2 Maternal care for disproportion of mixed maternal and fetal origin, fetus 2 Ⓜ ♀
O33.4XX3 Maternal care for disproportion of mixed maternal and fetal origin, fetus 3 Ⓜ ♀
O33.5XX1 Maternal care for disproportion due to unusually large fetus, fetus 1 Ⓜ ♀
O33.5XX2 Maternal care for disproportion due to unusually large fetus, fetus 2 Ⓜ ♀
O33.5XX3 Maternal care for disproportion due to unusually large fetus, fetus 3 Ⓜ ♀
O33.6XX1 Maternal care for disproportion due to hydrocephalic fetus, fetus 1 Ⓜ ♀
O33.6XX2 Maternal care for disproportion due to hydrocephalic fetus, fetus 2 Ⓜ ♀
O33.6XX3 Maternal care for disproportion due to hydrocephalic fetus, fetus 3 Ⓜ ♀
O35.2XX1 Maternal care for (suspected) hereditary disease in fetus, fetus 1 Ⓜ ♀
O35.2XX2 Maternal care for (suspected) hereditary disease in fetus, fetus 2 Ⓜ ♀
O35.2XX3 Maternal care for (suspected) hereditary disease in fetus, fetus 3 Ⓜ ♀
O36.21X1 Maternal care for hydrops fetalis, first trimester, fetus 1 Ⓜ ♀
O36.21X2 Maternal care for hydrops fetalis, first trimester, fetus 2 Ⓜ ♀
O36.21X3 Maternal care for hydrops fetalis, first trimester, fetus 3 Ⓜ ♀
O36.22X1 Maternal care for hydrops fetalis, second trimester, fetus 1 Ⓜ ♀
O36.22X2 Maternal care for hydrops fetalis, second trimester, fetus 2 Ⓜ ♀
O36.22X3 Maternal care for hydrops fetalis, second trimester, fetus 3 Ⓜ ♀
O36.23X1 Maternal care for hydrops fetalis, third trimester, fetus 1 Ⓜ ♀
O36.23X2 Maternal care for hydrops fetalis, third trimester, fetus 2 Ⓜ ♀
O36.23X3 Maternal care for hydrops fetalis, third trimester, fetus 3 Ⓜ ♀
O36.71X1 Maternal care for viable fetus in abdominal pregnancy, first trimester, fetus 1 Ⓜ ♀
O36.71X2 Maternal care for viable fetus in abdominal pregnancy, first trimester, fetus 2 Ⓜ ♀
O36.71X3 Maternal care for viable fetus in abdominal pregnancy, first trimester, fetus 3 Ⓜ ♀
O36.72X1 Maternal care for viable fetus in abdominal pregnancy, second trimester, fetus 1 Ⓜ ♀
O36.72X2 Maternal care for viable fetus in abdominal pregnancy, second trimester, fetus 2 Ⓜ ♀
O36.72X3 Maternal care for viable fetus in abdominal pregnancy, second trimester, fetus 3 Ⓜ ♀
O36.73X1 Maternal care for viable fetus in abdominal pregnancy, third trimester, fetus 1 Ⓜ ♀
O36.73X2 Maternal care for viable fetus in abdominal pregnancy, third trimester, fetus 2 Ⓜ ♀
O36.73X3 Maternal care for viable fetus in abdominal pregnancy, third trimester, fetus 3 Ⓜ ♀
O40.1XX1 Polyhydramnios, first trimester, fetus 1 Ⓜ ♀
O40.1XX2 Polyhydramnios, first trimester, fetus 2 Ⓜ ♀
O40.1XX3 Polyhydramnios, first trimester, fetus 3 Ⓜ ♀
O40.2XX1 Polyhydramnios, second trimester, fetus 1 Ⓜ ♀
O40.2XX2 Polyhydramnios, second trimester, fetus 2 Ⓜ ♀
O40.2XX3 Polyhydramnios, second trimester, fetus 3 Ⓜ ♀
O40.3XX1 Polyhydramnios, third trimester, fetus 1 Ⓜ ♀
O40.3XX2 Polyhydramnios, third trimester, fetus 2 Ⓜ ♀
O40.3XX3 Polyhydramnios, third trimester, fetus 3 Ⓜ ♀
O41.01X1 Oligohydramnios, first trimester, fetus 1 Ⓜ ♀
O41.01X2 Oligohydramnios, first trimester, fetus 2 Ⓜ ♀
O41.01X3 Oligohydramnios, first trimester, fetus 3 Ⓜ ♀
O41.02X1 Oligohydramnios, second trimester, fetus 1 Ⓜ ♀
O41.02X2 Oligohydramnios, second trimester, fetus 2 Ⓜ ♀
O41.02X3 Oligohydramnios, second trimester, fetus 3 Ⓜ ♀
O41.03X1 Oligohydramnios, third trimester, fetus 1 Ⓜ ♀
O41.03X2 Oligohydramnios, third trimester, fetus 2 Ⓜ ♀
O41.03X3 Oligohydramnios, third trimester, fetus 3 Ⓜ ♀
O41.1433 Placentitis, third trimester, fetus 3 Ⓜ ♀
O43.111 Circumvallate placenta, first trimester Ⓜ ♀
O43.112 Circumvallate placenta, second trimester Ⓜ ♀
O43.113 Circumvallate placenta, third trimester Ⓜ ♀
O43.811 Placental infarction, first trimester Ⓜ ♀
O43.812 Placental infarction, second trimester Ⓜ ♀
O43.813 Placental infarction, third trimester Ⓜ ♀
O44.01 Complete placenta previa NOS or without hemorrhage, first trimester Ⓜ ♀
O44.02 Complete placenta previa NOS or without hemorrhage, second trimester Ⓜ ♀
O44.03 Complete placenta previa NOS or without hemorrhage, third trimester Ⓜ ♀
O44.11 Complete placenta previa with hemorrhage, first trimester Ⓜ ♀
O44.12 Complete placenta previa with hemorrhage, second trimester Ⓜ ♀
O44.13 Complete placenta previa with hemorrhage, third trimester Ⓜ ♀

AMA: **76815** 2018,Jan,8; 2017,Jan,8; 2016,Jan,13; 2015,Jan,16; 2014,Jan,11
76816 2018,Jan,8; 2017,Jan,8; 2016,Jan,13; 2015,Jan,16; 2014,Jan,11

Relative Value Units/Medicare Edits

Non-Facility RVU	Work	PE	MP	Total
76815	0.65	1.68	0.04	2.37
76816	0.85	2.3	0.04	3.19
Facility RVU	Work	PE	MP	Total
76815	0.65	1.68	0.04	2.37
76816	0.85	2.3	0.04	3.19

	FUD	Status	MUE	Modifiers				IOM Reference
76815	N/A	A	1(2)	N/A	N/A	N/A	80*	None
76816	N/A	A	2(3)	N/A	N/A	N/A	80*	

* with documentation

Radiology

76817

76817   Ultrasound, pregnant uterus, real time with image documentation, transvaginal

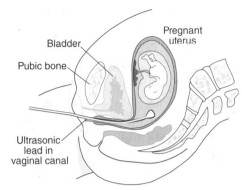

Ultrasound is performed in real time with image documentation by a transvaginal approach

Explanation

Diagnostic ultrasound is an imaging technique bouncing sound waves far above the level of human perception through interior body structures. The sound waves pass through different densities of tissue and reflect back to a receiving unit at varying speeds. The unit converts the waves to electrical pulses that are immediately displayed in picture form on screen. Real time scanning displays both two-dimensional structure images and movement with time. Use 76817 to report real time ultrasound on a pregnant uterus done transvaginally, with image documentation.

Coding Tips

A transvaginal ultrasound may be performed separately or in addition to a transabdominal ultrasound. When this procedure is done in addition to a transabdominal obstetrical ultrasound examination, report this code and the appropriate transabdominal exam code. See 76830 for a non-obstetrical transvaginal ultrasound. It is appropriate to code an obstetrical ultrasound for a patient who has an established diagnosis of pregnancy, who presents with indications necessitating the exam that may be pregnancy related, even when the outcome shows that the patient is no longer currently pregnant.

ICD-10-CM Diagnostic Codes

O26.712	Subluxation of symphysis (pubis) in pregnancy, second trimester ♀
O26.713	Subluxation of symphysis (pubis) in pregnancy, third trimester ♀
O26.841	Uterine size-date discrepancy, first trimester ♀
O26.842	Uterine size-date discrepancy, second trimester ♀
O26.843	Uterine size-date discrepancy, third trimester ♀
O30.011	Twin pregnancy, monochorionic/monoamniotic, first trimester ♀
O30.012	Twin pregnancy, monochorionic/monoamniotic, second trimester ♀
O30.013	Twin pregnancy, monochorionic/monoamniotic, third trimester ♀
O30.031	Twin pregnancy, monochorionic/diamniotic, first trimester ♀
O30.032	Twin pregnancy, monochorionic/diamniotic, second trimester ♀
O30.033	Twin pregnancy, monochorionic/diamniotic, third trimester ♀
O30.041	Twin pregnancy, dichorionic/diamniotic, first trimester ♀
O30.042	Twin pregnancy, dichorionic/diamniotic, second trimester ♀
O30.043	Twin pregnancy, dichorionic/diamniotic, third trimester ♀
O30.111	Triplet pregnancy with two or more monochorionic fetuses, first trimester ♀
O30.112	Triplet pregnancy with two or more monochorionic fetuses, second trimester ♀
O30.113	Triplet pregnancy with two or more monochorionic fetuses, third trimester ♀
O30.121	Triplet pregnancy with two or more monoamniotic fetuses, first trimester ♀
O30.122	Triplet pregnancy with two or more monoamniotic fetuses, second trimester ♀
O30.123	Triplet pregnancy with two or more monoamniotic fetuses, third trimester ♀
O32.0XX1	Maternal care for unstable lie, fetus 1 ♀
O32.0XX2	Maternal care for unstable lie, fetus 2 ♀
O32.0XX3	Maternal care for unstable lie, fetus 3 ♀
O32.1XX1	Maternal care for breech presentation, fetus 1 ♀
O32.1XX2	Maternal care for breech presentation, fetus 2 ♀
O32.1XX3	Maternal care for breech presentation, fetus 3 ♀
O32.2XX1	Maternal care for transverse and oblique lie, fetus 1 ♀
O32.2XX2	Maternal care for transverse and oblique lie, fetus 2 ♀
O32.2XX3	Maternal care for transverse and oblique lie, fetus 3 ♀
O32.3XX1	Maternal care for face, brow and chin presentation, fetus 1 ♀
O32.3XX2	Maternal care for face, brow and chin presentation, fetus 2 ♀
O32.3XX3	Maternal care for face, brow and chin presentation, fetus 3 ♀
O32.4XX1	Maternal care for high head at term, fetus 1 ♀
O32.4XX2	Maternal care for high head at term, fetus 2 ♀
O32.4XX3	Maternal care for high head at term, fetus 3 ♀
O32.6XX1	Maternal care for compound presentation, fetus 1 ♀
O32.6XX2	Maternal care for compound presentation, fetus 2 ♀
O32.6XX3	Maternal care for compound presentation, fetus 3 ♀
O33.4XX1	Maternal care for disproportion of mixed maternal and fetal origin, fetus 1 ♀
O33.4XX2	Maternal care for disproportion of mixed maternal and fetal origin, fetus 2 ♀
O33.4XX3	Maternal care for disproportion of mixed maternal and fetal origin, fetus 3 ♀
O33.5XX1	Maternal care for disproportion due to unusually large fetus, fetus 1 ♀
O33.5XX2	Maternal care for disproportion due to unusually large fetus, fetus 2 ♀
O33.5XX3	Maternal care for disproportion due to unusually large fetus, fetus 3 ♀
O33.6XX1	Maternal care for disproportion due to hydrocephalic fetus, fetus 1 ♀
O33.6XX2	Maternal care for disproportion due to hydrocephalic fetus, fetus 2 ♀
O33.6XX3	Maternal care for disproportion due to hydrocephalic fetus, fetus 3 ♀
O35.2XX1	Maternal care for (suspected) hereditary disease in fetus, fetus 1 ♀
O35.2XX2	Maternal care for (suspected) hereditary disease in fetus, fetus 2 ♀

Radiology

O35.2XX3	Maternal care for (suspected) hereditary disease in fetus, fetus 3 Ⓜ ♀
O36.21X1	Maternal care for hydrops fetalis, first trimester, fetus 1 Ⓜ ♀
O36.21X2	Maternal care for hydrops fetalis, first trimester, fetus 2 Ⓜ ♀
O36.21X3	Maternal care for hydrops fetalis, first trimester, fetus 3 Ⓜ ♀
O36.22X1	Maternal care for hydrops fetalis, second trimester, fetus 1 Ⓜ ♀
O36.22X2	Maternal care for hydrops fetalis, second trimester, fetus 2 Ⓜ ♀
O36.22X3	Maternal care for hydrops fetalis, second trimester, fetus 3 Ⓜ ♀
O36.23X1	Maternal care for hydrops fetalis, third trimester, fetus 1 Ⓜ ♀
O36.23X2	Maternal care for hydrops fetalis, third trimester, fetus 2 Ⓜ ♀
O36.23X3	Maternal care for hydrops fetalis, third trimester, fetus 3 Ⓜ ♀
O36.71X1	Maternal care for viable fetus in abdominal pregnancy, first trimester, fetus 1 Ⓜ ♀
O36.71X2	Maternal care for viable fetus in abdominal pregnancy, first trimester, fetus 2 Ⓜ ♀
O36.71X3	Maternal care for viable fetus in abdominal pregnancy, first trimester, fetus 3 Ⓜ ♀
O36.72X1	Maternal care for viable fetus in abdominal pregnancy, second trimester, fetus 1 Ⓜ ♀
O36.72X2	Maternal care for viable fetus in abdominal pregnancy, second trimester, fetus 2 Ⓜ ♀
O36.72X3	Maternal care for viable fetus in abdominal pregnancy, second trimester, fetus 3 Ⓜ ♀
O36.73X1	Maternal care for viable fetus in abdominal pregnancy, third trimester, fetus 1 Ⓜ ♀
O36.73X2	Maternal care for viable fetus in abdominal pregnancy, third trimester, fetus 2 Ⓜ ♀
O36.73X3	Maternal care for viable fetus in abdominal pregnancy, third trimester, fetus 3 Ⓜ ♀
O36.80X1	Pregnancy with inconclusive fetal viability, fetus 1 Ⓜ ♀
O36.80X2	Pregnancy with inconclusive fetal viability, fetus 2 Ⓜ ♀
O36.80X3	Pregnancy with inconclusive fetal viability, fetus 3 Ⓜ ♀
O40.1XX1	Polyhydramnios, first trimester, fetus 1 Ⓜ ♀
O40.1XX2	Polyhydramnios, first trimester, fetus 2 Ⓜ ♀
O40.1XX3	Polyhydramnios, first trimester, fetus 3 Ⓜ ♀
O40.2XX1	Polyhydramnios, second trimester, fetus 1 Ⓜ ♀
O40.2XX2	Polyhydramnios, second trimester, fetus 2 Ⓜ ♀
O40.2XX3	Polyhydramnios, second trimester, fetus 3 Ⓜ ♀
O40.3XX1	Polyhydramnios, third trimester, fetus 1 Ⓜ ♀
O40.3XX2	Polyhydramnios, third trimester, fetus 2 Ⓜ ♀
O40.3XX3	Polyhydramnios, third trimester, fetus 3 Ⓜ ♀
O41.01X1	Oligohydramnios, first trimester, fetus 1 Ⓜ ♀
O41.01X2	Oligohydramnios, first trimester, fetus 2 Ⓜ ♀
O41.01X3	Oligohydramnios, first trimester, fetus 3 Ⓜ ♀
O41.02X1	Oligohydramnios, second trimester, fetus 1 Ⓜ ♀
O41.02X2	Oligohydramnios, second trimester, fetus 2 Ⓜ ♀
O41.02X3	Oligohydramnios, second trimester, fetus 3 Ⓜ ♀
O41.03X1	Oligohydramnios, third trimester, fetus 1 Ⓜ ♀
O41.03X2	Oligohydramnios, third trimester, fetus 2 Ⓜ ♀
O41.03X3	Oligohydramnios, third trimester, fetus 3 Ⓜ ♀
O41.1433	Placentitis, third trimester, fetus 3 Ⓜ ♀
O43.111	Circumvallate placenta, first trimester Ⓜ ♀
O43.112	Circumvallate placenta, second trimester Ⓜ ♀
O43.811	Placental infarction, first trimester Ⓜ ♀

O43.812	Placental infarction, second trimester Ⓜ ♀
O44.01	Complete placenta previa NOS or without hemorrhage, first trimester Ⓜ ♀
O44.02	Complete placenta previa NOS or without hemorrhage, second trimester Ⓜ ♀
O44.11	Complete placenta previa with hemorrhage, first trimester Ⓜ ♀
O44.12	Complete placenta previa with hemorrhage, second trimester Ⓜ ♀
O46.011	Antepartum hemorrhage with afibrinogenemia, first trimester Ⓜ ♀
O46.012	Antepartum hemorrhage with afibrinogenemia, second trimester Ⓜ ♀
O46.013	Antepartum hemorrhage with afibrinogenemia, third trimester Ⓜ ♀
Z36.0	Encounter for antenatal screening for chromosomal anomalies Ⓜ ♀
Z36.2	Encounter for other antenatal screening follow-up Ⓜ ♀
Z36.3	Encounter for antenatal screening for malformations Ⓜ ♀
Z36.4	Encounter for antenatal screening for fetal growth retardation Ⓜ ♀
Z36.81	Encounter for antenatal screening for hydrops fetalis Ⓜ ♀
Z36.82	Encounter for antenatal screening for nuchal translucency Ⓜ ♀
Z36.83	Encounter for fetal screening for congenital cardiac abnormalities Ⓜ ♀
Z36.84	Encounter for antenatal screening for fetal lung maturity Ⓜ ♀
Z36.86	Encounter for antenatal screening for cervical length Ⓜ ♀
Z36.87	Encounter for antenatal screening for uncertain dates Ⓜ ♀
Z36.88	Encounter for antenatal screening for fetal macrosomia Ⓜ ♀

AMA: 76817 2018,Jan,8; 2017,Jan,8; 2016,Jan,13; 2015,Jan,16; 2014,Jan,11

Relative Value Units/Medicare Edits

Non-Facility RVU	Work	PE	MP	Total
76817	0.75	1.91	0.04	2.7
Facility RVU	Work	PE	MP	Total
76817	0.75	1.91	0.04	2.7

	FUD	Status	MUE	Modifiers				IOM Reference
76817	N/A	A	1(3)	N/A	N/A	N/A	80*	None

* with documentation

Terms To Know

fetus. Unborn offspring past the embryonic stage that has developed major structures. It is the period defined from nine weeks after fertilization until birth.

real-time. Immediate imaging, with movement as it happens.

trans. *1)* Across, through. *2)* Transverse.

ultrasound. Imaging using ultra-high sound frequency bounced off body structures.

Radiology

76818-76819

76818 Fetal biophysical profile; with non-stress testing
76819   without non-stress testing

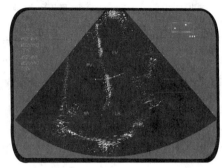

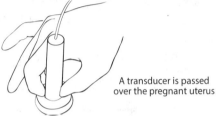

A transducer is passed over the pregnant uterus

Explanation

The health of a term or near-term fetus is assessed using ultrasound to monitor the fetus' movements, tone, and breathing, as well as to check amniotic fluid volume. The fetal heart rate is also monitored electronically in a biophysical profile. The physician conducts a non-stress test which monitors the baby's heart rate over a period of 20 minutes or more to look for accelerations with the baby's movement. Report 76819 if the fetal profile is done without non-stress testing.

Coding Tips

If biophysical profile assessments are done on multiple fetuses, report 76818 or 76819 separately, as appropriate, for each fetus after the first and append modifier 59 or an X{EPSU} modifier. For qualitative amniotic fluid volume assessment, see 76815.

ICD-10-CM Diagnostic Codes

O12.01	Gestational edema, first trimester Ⓜ ♀
O12.02	Gestational edema, second trimester Ⓜ ♀
O12.03	Gestational edema, third trimester Ⓜ ♀
O12.21	Gestational edema with proteinuria, first trimester Ⓜ ♀
O12.22	Gestational edema with proteinuria, second trimester Ⓜ ♀
O12.23	Gestational edema with proteinuria, third trimester Ⓜ ♀
O30.011	Twin pregnancy, monochorionic/monoamniotic, first trimester Ⓜ ♀
O30.012	Twin pregnancy, monochorionic/monoamniotic, second trimester Ⓜ ♀
O30.013	Twin pregnancy, monochorionic/monoamniotic, third trimester Ⓜ ♀
O30.031	Twin pregnancy, monochorionic/diamniotic, first trimester Ⓜ ♀
O30.032	Twin pregnancy, monochorionic/diamniotic, second trimester Ⓜ ♀
O30.033	Twin pregnancy, monochorionic/diamniotic, third trimester Ⓜ ♀
O30.041	Twin pregnancy, dichorionic/diamniotic, first trimester Ⓜ ♀
O30.042	Twin pregnancy, dichorionic/diamniotic, second trimester Ⓜ ♀
O30.043	Twin pregnancy, dichorionic/diamniotic, third trimester Ⓜ ♀
O30.111	Triplet pregnancy with two or more monochorionic fetuses, first trimester Ⓜ ♀
O30.112	Triplet pregnancy with two or more monochorionic fetuses, second trimester Ⓜ ♀
O30.113	Triplet pregnancy with two or more monochorionic fetuses, third trimester Ⓜ ♀
O30.121	Triplet pregnancy with two or more monoamniotic fetuses, first trimester Ⓜ ♀
O30.122	Triplet pregnancy with two or more monoamniotic fetuses, second trimester Ⓜ ♀
O30.123	Triplet pregnancy with two or more monoamniotic fetuses, third trimester Ⓜ ♀
O36.8131	Decreased fetal movements, third trimester, fetus 1 Ⓜ ♀
O36.8132	Decreased fetal movements, third trimester, fetus 2 Ⓜ ♀
O36.8133	Decreased fetal movements, third trimester, fetus 3 Ⓜ ♀
O40.1XX1	Polyhydramnios, first trimester, fetus 1 Ⓜ ♀
O40.1XX2	Polyhydramnios, first trimester, fetus 2 Ⓜ ♀
O40.1XX3	Polyhydramnios, first trimester, fetus 3 Ⓜ ♀
O40.2XX1	Polyhydramnios, second trimester, fetus 1 Ⓜ ♀
O40.2XX2	Polyhydramnios, second trimester, fetus 2 Ⓜ ♀
O40.2XX3	Polyhydramnios, second trimester, fetus 3 Ⓜ ♀
O40.3XX1	Polyhydramnios, third trimester, fetus 1 Ⓜ ♀
O40.3XX2	Polyhydramnios, third trimester, fetus 2 Ⓜ ♀
O40.3XX3	Polyhydramnios, third trimester, fetus 3 Ⓜ ♀
O41.01X1	Oligohydramnios, first trimester, fetus 1 Ⓜ ♀
O41.01X2	Oligohydramnios, first trimester, fetus 2 Ⓜ ♀
O41.01X3	Oligohydramnios, first trimester, fetus 3 Ⓜ ♀
O41.02X1	Oligohydramnios, second trimester, fetus 1 Ⓜ ♀
O41.02X2	Oligohydramnios, second trimester, fetus 2 Ⓜ ♀
O41.02X3	Oligohydramnios, second trimester, fetus 3 Ⓜ ♀
O41.03X1	Oligohydramnios, third trimester, fetus 1 Ⓜ ♀
O41.03X2	Oligohydramnios, third trimester, fetus 2 Ⓜ ♀
O41.03X3	Oligohydramnios, third trimester, fetus 3 Ⓜ ♀
O41.1211	Chorioamnionitis, first trimester, fetus 1 Ⓜ ♀
O41.1212	Chorioamnionitis, first trimester, fetus 2 Ⓜ ♀
O41.1213	Chorioamnionitis, first trimester, fetus 3 Ⓜ ♀
O41.1221	Chorioamnionitis, second trimester, fetus 1 Ⓜ ♀
O41.1222	Chorioamnionitis, second trimester, fetus 2 Ⓜ ♀
O41.1223	Chorioamnionitis, second trimester, fetus 3 Ⓜ ♀
O41.1231	Chorioamnionitis, third trimester, fetus 1 Ⓜ ♀
O41.1232	Chorioamnionitis, third trimester, fetus 2 Ⓜ ♀
O41.1233	Chorioamnionitis, third trimester, fetus 3 Ⓜ ♀
O41.1411	Placentitis, first trimester, fetus 1 Ⓜ ♀
O41.1412	Placentitis, first trimester, fetus 2 Ⓜ ♀
O41.1413	Placentitis, first trimester, fetus 3 Ⓜ ♀
O41.1421	Placentitis, second trimester, fetus 1 Ⓜ ♀
O41.1422	Placentitis, second trimester, fetus 2 Ⓜ ♀
O41.1423	Placentitis, second trimester, fetus 3 Ⓜ ♀
O41.1431	Placentitis, third trimester, fetus 1 Ⓜ ♀
O41.1432	Placentitis, third trimester, fetus 2 Ⓜ ♀
O41.1433	Placentitis, third trimester, fetus 3 Ⓜ ♀

Radiology

O42.011	Preterm premature rupture of membranes, onset of labor within 24 hours of rupture, first trimester ⬛ ♀
O42.012	Preterm premature rupture of membranes, onset of labor within 24 hours of rupture, second trimester ⬛ ♀
O42.013	Preterm premature rupture of membranes, onset of labor within 24 hours of rupture, third trimester ⬛ ♀
O43.011	Fetomaternal placental transfusion syndrome, first trimester ⬛ ♀
O43.012	Fetomaternal placental transfusion syndrome, second trimester ⬛ ♀
O43.013	Fetomaternal placental transfusion syndrome, third trimester ⬛ ♀
O44.01	Complete placenta previa NOS or without hemorrhage, first trimester ⬛ ♀
O44.02	Complete placenta previa NOS or without hemorrhage, second trimester ⬛ ♀
O44.03	Complete placenta previa NOS or without hemorrhage, third trimester ⬛ ♀
O44.11	Complete placenta previa with hemorrhage, first trimester ⬛ ♀
O44.12	Complete placenta previa with hemorrhage, second trimester ⬛ ♀
O44.13	Complete placenta previa with hemorrhage, third trimester ⬛ ♀
O45.011	Premature separation of placenta with afibrinogenemia, first trimester ⬛ ♀
O45.012	Premature separation of placenta with afibrinogenemia, second trimester ⬛ ♀
O45.013	Premature separation of placenta with afibrinogenemia, third trimester ⬛ ♀
O45.021	Premature separation of placenta with disseminated intravascular coagulation, first trimester ⬛ ♀
O45.022	Premature separation of placenta with disseminated intravascular coagulation, second trimester ⬛ ♀
O45.023	Premature separation of placenta with disseminated intravascular coagulation, third trimester ⬛ ♀
O45.091	Premature separation of placenta with other coagulation defect, first trimester ⬛ ♀
O45.092	Premature separation of placenta with other coagulation defect, second trimester ⬛ ♀
O45.093	Premature separation of placenta with other coagulation defect, third trimester ⬛ ♀
O45.8X1	Other premature separation of placenta, first trimester ⬛ ♀
O45.8X2	Other premature separation of placenta, second trimester ⬛ ♀
O45.8X3	Other premature separation of placenta, third trimester ⬛ ♀
O46.011	Antepartum hemorrhage with afibrinogenemia, first trimester ⬛ ♀
O46.012	Antepartum hemorrhage with afibrinogenemia, second trimester ⬛ ♀
O46.013	Antepartum hemorrhage with afibrinogenemia, third trimester ⬛ ♀
O46.021	Antepartum hemorrhage with disseminated intravascular coagulation, first trimester ⬛ ♀
O46.022	Antepartum hemorrhage with disseminated intravascular coagulation, second trimester ⬛ ♀
O46.023	Antepartum hemorrhage with disseminated intravascular coagulation, third trimester ⬛ ♀
O46.091	Antepartum hemorrhage with other coagulation defect, first trimester ⬛ ♀
O46.092	Antepartum hemorrhage with other coagulation defect, second trimester ⬛ ♀
O46.093	Antepartum hemorrhage with other coagulation defect, third trimester ⬛ ♀
O76	Abnormality in fetal heart rate and rhythm complicating labor and delivery ⬛ ♀
Z03.71	Encounter for suspected problem with amniotic cavity and membrane ruled out ⬛ ♀
Z03.72	Encounter for suspected placental problem ruled out ⬛ ♀
Z03.73	Encounter for suspected fetal anomaly ruled out ⬛ ♀
Z03.74	Encounter for suspected problem with fetal growth ruled out ⬛ ♀
Z03.79	Encounter for other suspected maternal and fetal conditions ruled out ⬛ ♀

AMA: **76818** 2018,Jan,8; 2017,Jan,8; 2016,Jan,13; 2015,Jan,16; 2014,Jan,11 **76819** 2018,Jan,8; 2017,Jan,8; 2016,Jan,13; 2015,Jan,16; 2014,Jan,11

Relative Value Units/Medicare Edits

Non-Facility RVU	Work	PE	MP	Total
76818	1.05	2.23	0.05	3.33
76819	0.77	1.64	0.04	2.45
Facility RVU	**Work**	**PE**	**MP**	**Total**
76818	1.05	2.23	0.05	3.33
76819	0.77	1.64	0.04	2.45

	FUD	Status	MUE	Modifiers				IOM Reference
76818	N/A	A	2(3)	N/A	N/A	N/A	80*	None
76819	N/A	A	2(3)	N/A	N/A	N/A	80*	

* with documentation

Terms To Know

fetal biophysical profile. Monitoring by ultrasound the health of a term or near-term fetus by assessing fetal breathing movements, body movements, tone, and amniotic fluid volume. Fetal biophysical profiles are excluded from the maternity care global package. *Synonym(s): BPP.*

fetus. Unborn offspring past the embryonic stage that has developed major structures. It is the period defined from nine weeks after fertilization until birth.

ultrasound. Imaging using ultra-high sound frequency bounced off body structures.

Radiology

76820-76821

76820 Doppler velocimetry, fetal; umbilical artery
76821 middle cerebral artery

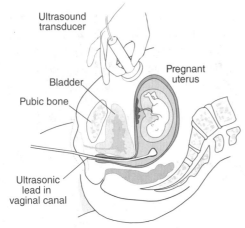

Ultrasound transducer
Pregnant uterus
Bladder
Pubic bone
Ultrasonic lead in vaginal canal

Ultrasonography or echography is performed

Explanation

Doppler ultrasonography, or echography, is performed for fetal surveillance to determine the velocity of blood flow through the umbilical artery (76820) or the middle cerebral artery (76821). Doppler works off the principle that when emitted sound waves reflect back off a moving object, the frequency of the reflected waves will vary in relation to the speed of the moving object. The frequency of sound waves bouncing back off moving blood cells is converted to the velocity of blood flow through the vessel and is seen on screen as a wave with peak, systole, and diastole. Velocity waveforms through the umbilical artery of a normally growing fetus are different from those of a growth-retarded fetus. The peak systolic velocity through the middle cerebral artery is inversely related to the amount of hematocrit in fetal blood. These tests determine the timing of labor induction and when fetal anemia is severe enough to require a transfusion. The ultrasound is carried out transabdominally or endovaginally.

Coding Tips

For fetal Doppler echocardiography, see 76827–76828.

ICD-10-CM Diagnostic Codes

O35.0XX1	Maternal care for (suspected) central nervous system malformation in fetus, fetus 1 Ⓜ ♀
O35.0XX2	Maternal care for (suspected) central nervous system malformation in fetus, fetus 2 Ⓜ ♀
O35.0XX3	Maternal care for (suspected) central nervous system malformation in fetus, fetus 3 Ⓜ ♀
O35.1XX1	Maternal care for (suspected) chromosomal abnormality in fetus, fetus 1 Ⓜ ♀
O35.1XX2	Maternal care for (suspected) chromosomal abnormality in fetus, fetus 2 Ⓜ ♀
O35.1XX3	Maternal care for (suspected) chromosomal abnormality in fetus, fetus 3 Ⓜ ♀
O35.2XX1	Maternal care for (suspected) hereditary disease in fetus, fetus 1 Ⓜ ♀
O35.2XX2	Maternal care for (suspected) hereditary disease in fetus, fetus 2 Ⓜ ♀

O35.3XX2	Maternal care for (suspected) damage to fetus from viral disease in mother, fetus 2 Ⓜ ♀
O35.3XX3	Maternal care for (suspected) damage to fetus from viral disease in mother, fetus 3 ♀
O35.4XX1	Maternal care for (suspected) damage to fetus from alcohol, fetus 1 Ⓜ ♀
O35.5XX1	Maternal care for (suspected) damage to fetus by drugs, fetus 1 Ⓜ ♀
O35.5XX2	Maternal care for (suspected) damage to fetus by drugs, fetus 2 Ⓜ ♀
O35.5XX3	Maternal care for (suspected) damage to fetus by drugs, fetus 3 Ⓜ ♀
O35.6XX1	Maternal care for (suspected) damage to fetus by radiation, fetus 1 Ⓜ ♀
O35.6XX2	Maternal care for (suspected) damage to fetus by radiation, fetus 2 Ⓜ ♀
O35.6XX3	Maternal care for (suspected) damage to fetus by radiation, fetus 3 Ⓜ ♀
O35.8XX1	Maternal care for other (suspected) fetal abnormality and damage, fetus 1 Ⓜ ♀
O35.8XX2	Maternal care for other (suspected) fetal abnormality and damage, fetus 2 Ⓜ ♀
O35.8XX3	Maternal care for other (suspected) fetal abnormality and damage, fetus 3 Ⓜ ♀
O36.8211	Fetal anemia and thrombocytopenia, first trimester, fetus 1 Ⓜ ♀
O36.8212	Fetal anemia and thrombocytopenia, first trimester, fetus 2 Ⓜ ♀
O36.8213	Fetal anemia and thrombocytopenia, first trimester, fetus 3 Ⓜ ♀
O36.8221	Fetal anemia and thrombocytopenia, second trimester, fetus 1 Ⓜ ♀
O36.8222	Fetal anemia and thrombocytopenia, second trimester, fetus 2 Ⓜ ♀
O36.8223	Fetal anemia and thrombocytopenia, second trimester, fetus 3 Ⓜ ♀
O36.8231	Fetal anemia and thrombocytopenia, third trimester, fetus 1 Ⓜ ♀
O36.8232	Fetal anemia and thrombocytopenia, third trimester, fetus 2 Ⓜ ♀
O36.8233	Fetal anemia and thrombocytopenia, third trimester, fetus 3 Ⓜ ♀
O43.112	Circumvallate placenta, second trimester Ⓜ ♀
O43.113	Circumvallate placenta, third trimester Ⓜ ♀
O43.812	Placental infarction, second trimester Ⓜ ♀
O43.813	Placental infarction, third trimester Ⓜ ♀
O44.02	Complete placenta previa NOS or without hemorrhage, second trimester Ⓜ ♀
O44.03	Complete placenta previa NOS or without hemorrhage, third trimester Ⓜ ♀
O44.12	Complete placenta previa with hemorrhage, second trimester Ⓜ ♀
O44.13	Complete placenta previa with hemorrhage, third trimester Ⓜ ♀
O45.012	Premature separation of placenta with afibrinogenemia, second trimester Ⓜ ♀
O45.013	Premature separation of placenta with afibrinogenemia, third trimester Ⓜ ♀
O45.022	Premature separation of placenta with disseminated intravascular coagulation, second trimester Ⓜ ♀
O45.023	Premature separation of placenta with disseminated intravascular coagulation, third trimester Ⓜ ♀

Radiology

O45.092	Premature separation of placenta with other coagulation defect, second trimester ⓜ ♀
O45.093	Premature separation of placenta with other coagulation defect, third trimester ⓜ ♀
O46.012	Antepartum hemorrhage with afibrinogenemia, second trimester ⓜ ♀
O46.013	Antepartum hemorrhage with afibrinogenemia, third trimester ⓜ ♀
O46.022	Antepartum hemorrhage with disseminated intravascular coagulation, second trimester ⓜ ♀
O46.023	Antepartum hemorrhage with disseminated intravascular coagulation, third trimester ⓜ ♀
O46.092	Antepartum hemorrhage with other coagulation defect, second trimester ⓜ ♀
O76	Abnormality in fetal heart rate and rhythm complicating labor and delivery ⓜ ♀

AMA: 76820 2018,Jan,8; 2017,Jan,8; 2016,Jul,8; 2016,Jan,13; 2015,Jan,16; 2014,Jan,11 **76821** 2018,Jan,8; 2017,Jan,8; 2016,Jan,13; 2015,Jan,16; 2014,Jan,11

Relative Value Units/Medicare Edits

Non-Facility RVU	Work	PE	MP	Total
76820	0.5	0.79	0.03	1.32
76821	0.7	1.82	0.03	2.55
Facility RVU	**Work**	**PE**	**MP**	**Total**
76820	0.5	0.79	0.03	1.32
76821	0.7	1.82	0.03	2.55

	FUD	Status	MUE	Modifiers				IOM Reference
76820	N/A	A	3(3)	N/A	N/A	N/A	80*	None
76821	N/A	A	2(3)	N/A	N/A	N/A	80*	

* with documentation

Terms To Know

doppler. Ultrasonography used to augment two-dimensional images by registering velocity. When emitted sound waves reflect back off a moving object, the frequency of the reflected sound waves varies in relation to the speed of the moving object and may be used in many different procedures.

echography. Radiographic imaging that uses sound waves reflected off the different densities of anatomic structures to create images.

fetus. Unborn offspring past the embryonic stage that has developed major structures. It is the period defined from nine weeks after fertilization until birth.

ultrasound. Imaging using ultra-high sound frequency bounced off body structures.

76825-76826

76825	Echocardiography, fetal, cardiovascular system, real time with image documentation (2D), with or without M-mode recording;
76826	follow-up or repeat study

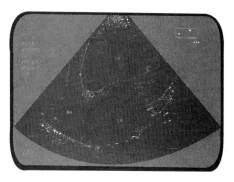

An echocardiogram study is performed on a fetus

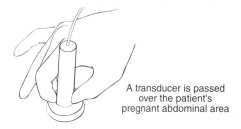

A transducer is passed over the patient's pregnant abdominal area

Explanation

Diagnostic ultrasound is an imaging technique bouncing sound waves far above the level of human perception through interior body structures. The sound waves pass through different densities of tissue and reflect back to a receiving unit at varying speeds. The unit converts the waves to electrical pulses that are immediately displayed in picture form on screen. These codes report fetal echocardiography, real time, with or without M-mode recording. Real time scanning displays both two-dimensional structure images and movement with time. M-mode is a single dimension method of recording amplitude and velocity of a moving structure producing the echoes being studied. Report 76825 for a complete evaluation of a fetal cardiovascular system and 76826 for a follow-up or repeat study.

Coding Tips

Procedures 76825 and 76826 have both a technical and professional component. To claim only the professional component, append modifier 26. To claim only the technical component, append modifier TC. To claim the complete procedure (i.e., both the professional and technical components), submit without a modifier. When 76825 or 76826 is performed with another separately identifiable procedure, the highest dollar value code is listed as the primary procedure and subsequent procedures are appended with modifier 51. For fetal Doppler echocardiography, see 76827-76828.

ICD-10-CM Diagnostic Codes

O35.0XX1	Maternal care for (suspected) central nervous system malformation in fetus, fetus 1 ⓜ ♀
O35.0XX2	Maternal care for (suspected) central nervous system malformation in fetus, fetus 2 ♀
O35.0XX3	Maternal care for (suspected) central nervous system malformation in fetus, fetus 3 ⓜ ♀
O35.1XX1	Maternal care for (suspected) chromosomal abnormality in fetus, fetus 1 ⓜ ♀

Radiology

O35.1XX2	Maternal care for (suspected) chromosomal abnormality in fetus, fetus 2 Ⓜ ♀
O35.1XX3	Maternal care for (suspected) chromosomal abnormality in fetus, fetus 3 Ⓜ ♀
O35.2XX1	Maternal care for (suspected) hereditary disease in fetus, fetus 1 Ⓜ ♀
O35.2XX2	Maternal care for (suspected) hereditary disease in fetus, fetus 2 Ⓜ ♀
O35.3XX1	Maternal care for (suspected) damage to fetus from viral disease in mother, fetus 1 Ⓜ ♀
O35.3XX2	Maternal care for (suspected) damage to fetus from viral disease in mother, fetus 2 Ⓜ ♀
O35.3XX3	Maternal care for (suspected) damage to fetus from viral disease in mother, fetus 3 Ⓜ ♀
O35.4XX1	Maternal care for (suspected) damage to fetus from alcohol, fetus 1 Ⓜ ♀
O35.4XX2	Maternal care for (suspected) damage to fetus from alcohol, fetus 2 Ⓜ ♀
O35.4XX3	Maternal care for (suspected) damage to fetus from alcohol, fetus 3 Ⓜ ♀
O35.5XX1	Maternal care for (suspected) damage to fetus by drugs, fetus 1 Ⓜ ♀
O35.5XX2	Maternal care for (suspected) damage to fetus by drugs, fetus 2 Ⓜ ♀
O35.5XX3	Maternal care for (suspected) damage to fetus by drugs, fetus 3 Ⓜ ♀
O35.6XX1	Maternal care for (suspected) damage to fetus by radiation, fetus 1 Ⓜ ♀
O35.6XX2	Maternal care for (suspected) damage to fetus by radiation, fetus 2 Ⓜ ♀
O35.6XX3	Maternal care for (suspected) damage to fetus by radiation, fetus 3 Ⓜ ♀
O35.8XX1	Maternal care for other (suspected) fetal abnormality and damage, fetus 1 Ⓜ ♀
O35.8XX2	Maternal care for other (suspected) fetal abnormality and damage, fetus 2 Ⓜ ♀
O35.8XX3	Maternal care for other (suspected) fetal abnormality and damage, fetus 3 Ⓜ ♀
Z03.73	Encounter for suspected fetal anomaly ruled out Ⓜ ♀
Z03.79	Encounter for other suspected maternal and fetal conditions ruled out Ⓜ ♀

AMA: 76825 2018,Jan,8; 2017,Sep,14; 2017,Jan,8; 2016,Jan,13; 2015,Jan,16; 2014,Jan,11 **76826** 2018,Jan,8; 2017,Sep,14

Relative Value Units/Medicare Edits

Non-Facility RVU	Work	PE	MP	Total
76825	1.67	5.97	0.07	7.71
76826	0.83	3.7	0.05	4.58
Facility RVU	**Work**	**PE**	**MP**	**Total**
76825	1.67	5.97	0.07	7.71
76826	0.83	3.7	0.05	4.58

	FUD	Status	MUE	Modifiers				IOM Reference
76825	N/A	A	2(3)	N/A	N/A	N/A	80*	None
76826	N/A	A	2(3)	N/A	N/A	N/A	80*	

* with documentation

Terms To Know

professional component. Portion of a charge for health care services that represents the physician's (or other practitioner's) work in providing the service, including interpretation and report of the procedure. This component of the service usually is charged for and billed separately from the inpatient hospital charges.

spectral display. Visual display mode in Doppler ultrasonography that shows the blood-flow velocity range present. The most common form of spectral display indicates blood flow velocity shifts.

technical component. Portion of a health care service that identifies the provision of the equipment, supplies, technical personnel, and costs attendant to the performance of the procedure other than the professional services.

transducer. Apparatus that transfers or translates one type of energy into another, such as converting pressure to an electrical signal.

ultrasound. Imaging using ultra-high sound frequency bounced off body structures.

Radiology

76827-76828

76827 Doppler echocardiography, fetal, pulsed wave and/or continuous wave with spectral display; complete
76828   follow-up or repeat study

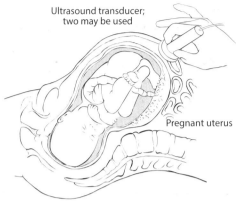

Ultrasound transducer; two may be used

Pregnant uterus

Doppler echocardiography is performed on a fetus

Explanation

Diagnostic ultrasound is an imaging technique bouncing sound waves far above the level of human perception through interior body structures. The sound waves pass through different densities of tissue and reflect back to a receiving unit at varying speeds. The unit converts the waves to electrical pulses that are immediately displayed in picture form on screen. These codes report fetal doppler echocardiography by pulsed or continuous sound wave. Fetal echocardiography is done to study the unborn baby's heart in much greater detail than is possible with a routine pregnancy ultrasound when the mother is at risk for giving birth to a baby with heart defects. Doppler echography uses the frequency shifts of the emitted waves against their echoes to measure velocity, such as for blood flow through the heart. Pulsed wave transmits and records from a single source to determine a precise site of signal origin but not high velocity. Continuous wave uses two transducers: one to continually transmit and the other to record. This scan determines high velocities. Report 76827 for a complete fetal echocardiographic evaluation and 76828 for a follow-up or repeat study.

Coding Tips

Procedures 76827 and 76828 have both a technical and professional component. To claim only the professional component, append modifier 26. To claim only the technical component, append modifier TC. To claim the complete procedure (i.e., both the professional and technical components), submit without a modifier. When 76827 or 76828 is performed with another separately identifiable procedure, the highest dollar value code is listed as the primary procedure and subsequent procedures are appended with modifier 51. For color flow velocity mapping for Doppler echocardiography, use 93325.

ICD-10-CM Diagnostic Codes

O35.0XX1	Maternal care for (suspected) central nervous system malformation in fetus, fetus 1 Ⓜ ♀
O35.0XX2	Maternal care for (suspected) central nervous system malformation in fetus, fetus 2 Ⓜ ♀
O35.0XX3	Maternal care for (suspected) central nervous system malformation in fetus, fetus 3 Ⓜ ♀
O35.1XX1	Maternal care for (suspected) chromosomal abnormality in fetus, fetus 1 Ⓜ ♀
O35.1XX2	Maternal care for (suspected) chromosomal abnormality in fetus, fetus 2 Ⓜ ♀
O35.1XX3	Maternal care for (suspected) chromosomal abnormality in fetus, fetus 3 Ⓜ ♀
O35.2XX1	Maternal care for (suspected) hereditary disease in fetus, fetus 1 Ⓜ ♀
O35.2XX2	Maternal care for (suspected) hereditary disease in fetus, fetus 2 Ⓜ ♀
O35.2XX3	Maternal care for (suspected) hereditary disease in fetus, fetus 3 Ⓜ ♀
O35.3XX1	Maternal care for (suspected) damage to fetus from viral disease in mother, fetus 1 Ⓜ ♀
O35.3XX2	Maternal care for (suspected) damage to fetus from viral disease in mother, fetus 2 Ⓜ ♀
O35.3XX3	Maternal care for (suspected) damage to fetus from viral disease in mother, fetus 3 Ⓜ ♀
O35.4XX1	Maternal care for (suspected) damage to fetus from alcohol, fetus 1 Ⓜ ♀
O35.4XX2	Maternal care for (suspected) damage to fetus from alcohol, fetus 2 Ⓜ ♀
O35.4XX3	Maternal care for (suspected) damage to fetus from alcohol, fetus 3 Ⓜ ♀
O35.5XX1	Maternal care for (suspected) damage to fetus by drugs, fetus 1 Ⓜ ♀
O35.5XX2	Maternal care for (suspected) damage to fetus by drugs, fetus 2 Ⓜ ♀
O35.5XX3	Maternal care for (suspected) damage to fetus by drugs, fetus 3 Ⓜ ♀
O35.6XX1	Maternal care for (suspected) damage to fetus by radiation, fetus 1 Ⓜ ♀
O35.6XX2	Maternal care for (suspected) damage to fetus by radiation, fetus 2 Ⓜ ♀
O35.6XX3	Maternal care for (suspected) damage to fetus by radiation, fetus 3 Ⓜ ♀
O35.8XX1	Maternal care for other (suspected) fetal abnormality and damage, fetus 1 Ⓜ ♀
O35.8XX2	Maternal care for other (suspected) fetal abnormality and damage, fetus 2 Ⓜ ♀
O35.8XX3	Maternal care for other (suspected) fetal abnormality and damage, fetus 3 Ⓜ ♀

AMA: **76827** 2018,Jan,8; 2017,Jan,8; 2016,Jan,13; 2015,Jan,16; 2014,Jan,11
76828 2018,Jan,8; 2017,Jan,8; 2016,Jan,13; 2015,Jan,16; 2014,Jan,11

Relative Value Units/Medicare Edits

Non-Facility RVU	Work	PE	MP	Total
76827	0.58	1.46	0.03	2.07
76828	0.56	0.88	0.03	1.47
Facility RVU	**Work**	**PE**	**MP**	**Total**
76827	0.58	1.46	0.03	2.07
76828	0.56	0.88	0.03	1.47

	FUD	Status	MUE	Modifiers				IOM Reference
76827	N/A	A	2(3)	N/A	N/A	N/A	80*	None
76828	N/A	A	2(3)	N/A	N/A	N/A	80*	

* with documentation

Radiology

76830

76830 Ultrasound, transvaginal

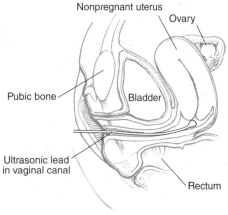

Nonpregnant uterus
Ovary
Pubic bone
Bladder
Ultrasonic lead
in vaginal canal
Rectum

Ultrasound is performed in real time with image
documentation by a transvaginal approach

Explanation

Diagnostic ultrasound is an imaging technique bouncing sound waves far
above the level of human perception through interior body structures. The
sound waves pass through different densities of tissue and reflect back to a
receiving unit at varying speeds. The unit converts the waves to electrical
pulses that are immediately displayed in picture form on screen. This code
reports transvaginal ultrasonography.

Coding Tips

When 76830 is performed with another separately identifiable procedure, the
highest dollar value code is listed as the primary procedure and subsequent
procedures are appended with modifier 51. If transvaginal ultrasound
(nonobstetric) is done in addition to a transabdominal ultrasound exam, report
76830 in addition to the appropriate code for the transabdominal ultrasound.
For transvaginal ultrasound on a gravid uterus, see 76817.

ICD-10-CM Diagnostic Codes

D25.0	Submucous leiomyoma of uterus ♀
D25.1	Intramural leiomyoma of uterus ♀
D25.2	Subserosal leiomyoma of uterus ♀
E28.2	Polycystic ovarian syndrome ♀
E28.310	Symptomatic premature menopause 🅐 ♀
E89.40	Asymptomatic postprocedural ovarian failure ♀
E89.41	Symptomatic postprocedural ovarian failure ♀
N70.01	Acute salpingitis ♀
N70.02	Acute oophoritis ♀
N70.03	Acute salpingitis and oophoritis ♀
N70.11	Chronic salpingitis ♀
N70.12	Chronic oophoritis ♀
N70.13	Chronic salpingitis and oophoritis ♀
N71.0	Acute inflammatory disease of uterus ♀
N71.1	Chronic inflammatory disease of uterus ♀
N76.0	Acute vaginitis ♀
N76.1	Subacute and chronic vaginitis ♀
N76.2	Acute vulvitis ♀
N76.3	Subacute and chronic vulvitis ♀

N80.0	Endometriosis of uterus ♀
N80.1	Endometriosis of ovary ♀
N80.2	Endometriosis of fallopian tube ♀
N80.4	Endometriosis of rectovaginal septum and vagina ♀
N81.0	Urethrocele ♀
N81.6	Rectocele ♀
N81.81	Perineocele ♀
N81.82	Incompetence or weakening of pubocervical tissue ♀
N81.83	Incompetence or weakening of rectovaginal tissue ♀
N83.01	Follicular cyst of right ovary ♀ ☑
N83.02	Follicular cyst of left ovary ♀ ☑
N83.11	Corpus luteum cyst of right ovary ♀ ☑
N83.12	Corpus luteum cyst of left ovary ♀ ☑
N83.291	Other ovarian cyst, right side ♀ ☑
N83.292	Other ovarian cyst, left side ♀ ☑
N83.311	Acquired atrophy of right ovary ♀ ☑
N83.312	Acquired atrophy of left ovary ♀ ☑
N83.321	Acquired atrophy of right fallopian tube ♀ ☑
N83.322	Acquired atrophy of left fallopian tube ♀ ☑
N83.331	Acquired atrophy of right ovary and fallopian tube ♀ ☑
N83.332	Acquired atrophy of left ovary and fallopian tube ♀ ☑
N83.41	Prolapse and hernia of right ovary and fallopian tube ♀ ☑
N83.42	Prolapse and hernia of left ovary and fallopian tube ♀ ☑
N83.511	Torsion of right ovary and ovarian pedicle ♀ ☑
N83.512	Torsion of left ovary and ovarian pedicle ♀ ☑
N83.521	Torsion of right fallopian tube ♀ ☑
N83.522	Torsion of left fallopian tube ♀ ☑
N83.53	Torsion of ovary, ovarian pedicle and fallopian tube ♀
N83.6	Hematosalpinx ♀
N83.7	Hematoma of broad ligament ♀
N84.0	Polyp of corpus uteri ♀
N85.01	Benign endometrial hyperplasia ♀
N85.02	Endometrial intraepithelial neoplasia [EIN] ♀
N85.2	Hypertrophy of uterus ♀
N85.3	Subinvolution of uterus ♀
N85.4	Malposition of uterus ♀
N85.5	Inversion of uterus ♀
N85.6	Intrauterine synechiae ♀
N85.7	Hematometra ♀
N87.0	Mild cervical dysplasia ♀
N87.1	Moderate cervical dysplasia ♀
N89.7	Hematocolpos ♀
N91.0	Primary amenorrhea ♀
N91.1	Secondary amenorrhea ♀
N91.3	Primary oligomenorrhea ♀
N91.4	Secondary oligomenorrhea ♀
N92.0	Excessive and frequent menstruation with regular cycle ♀
N92.1	Excessive and frequent menstruation with irregular cycle ♀
N92.2	Excessive menstruation at puberty 🅟 ♀
N92.3	Ovulation bleeding ♀
N92.4	Excessive bleeding in the premenopausal period ♀
N92.5	Other specified irregular menstruation ♀
N93.0	Postcoital and contact bleeding ♀

Radiology

N94.0	Mittelschmerz ♀
N94.2	Vaginismus ♀
N94.4	Primary dysmenorrhea ♀
N94.5	Secondary dysmenorrhea ♀
N95.0	Postmenopausal bleeding ♀
N95.1	Menopausal and female climacteric states ♀
N96	Recurrent pregnancy loss ♀
N97.0	Female infertility associated with anovulation ♀
N97.1	Female infertility of tubal origin ♀
N98.1	Hyperstimulation of ovaries ♀
N99.83	Residual ovary syndrome ♀
N99.85	Post endometrial ablation syndrome ♀
Q50.01	Congenital absence of ovary, unilateral ♀
Q50.02	Congenital absence of ovary, bilateral ♀
Q50.1	Developmental ovarian cyst ♀
Q50.2	Congenital torsion of ovary ♀
Q50.31	Accessory ovary ♀
Q50.32	Ovarian streak ♀
Q50.4	Embryonic cyst of fallopian tube ♀
Q50.5	Embryonic cyst of broad ligament ♀
Q51.0	Agenesis and aplasia of uterus ♀
Q51.10	Doubling of uterus with doubling of cervix and vagina without obstruction ♀
Q51.11	Doubling of uterus with doubling of cervix and vagina with obstruction ♀
Q51.21	Complete doubling of uterus ♀
Q51.22	Partial doubling of uterus ♀
Q51.3	Bicornate uterus ♀
Q51.4	Unicornate uterus ♀
Q51.5	Agenesis and aplasia of cervix ♀
Q51.6	Embryonic cyst of cervix ♀
Q51.7	Congenital fistulae between uterus and digestive and urinary tracts ♀
Q51.810	Arcuate uterus ♀
Q51.811	Hypoplasia of uterus ♀
Q51.820	Cervical duplication ♀
Q51.821	Hypoplasia of cervix ♀
Q52.0	Congenital absence of vagina ♀
Q52.11	Transverse vaginal septum ♀
Q52.2	Congenital rectovaginal fistula ♀

AMA: **76830** 2018,Jan,8; 2017,Oct,9; 2017,Jan,8; 2016,Jan,13; 2015,Jan,16; 2014,Jan,11

Relative Value Units/Medicare Edits

Non-Facility RVU	Work	PE	MP	Total
76830	0.69	2.74	0.04	3.47
Facility RVU	**Work**	**PE**	**MP**	**Total**
76830	0.69	2.74	0.04	3.47

	FUD	Status	MUE	Modifiers				IOM Reference
76830	N/A	A	1(3)	N/A	N/A	N/A	80*	None

* with documentation

76856-76857

76856 Ultrasound, pelvic (nonobstetric), real time with image documentation; complete
76857 limited or follow-up (eg, for follicles)

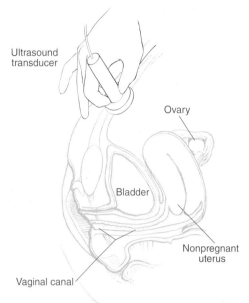

Nonobstetric ultrasound is performed

Explanation

Diagnostic ultrasound is an imaging technique bouncing sound waves far above the level of human perception through interior body structures. The sound waves pass through different densities of tissue and reflect back to a receiving unit at varying speeds. The unit converts the waves to electrical pulses that are immediately displayed in picture form on screen. Real time scanning displays both structure images and movement with time. Report 76856 for a complete pelvic evaluation in a patient who is not pregnant and 76857 for a limited or follow-up pelvic evaluation, for example, to monitor real time follicle development on the ovary to evaluate gonadotrophin therapy.

Coding Tips

It is appropriate to code a nonobstetrical pelvic ultrasound in cases where a patient, without an established diagnosis of pregnancy, has gynecological signs and symptoms that would necessitate an ultrasound even when the outcome results in a diagnosis of pregnancy or a complication of a pregnancy.

ICD-10-CM Diagnostic Codes

C54.1	Malignant neoplasm of endometrium ♀
C54.2	Malignant neoplasm of myometrium ♀
C54.3	Malignant neoplasm of fundus uteri ♀
C56.1	Malignant neoplasm of right ovary ♀ ☑
C56.2	Malignant neoplasm of left ovary ♀ ☑
C57.01	Malignant neoplasm of right fallopian tube ♀ ☑
C57.02	Malignant neoplasm of left fallopian tube ♀ ☑
C57.11	Malignant neoplasm of right broad ligament ♀ ☑
C57.12	Malignant neoplasm of left broad ligament ♀ ☑
C57.21	Malignant neoplasm of right round ligament ♀ ☑
C57.22	Malignant neoplasm of left round ligament ♀ ☑
C57.3	Malignant neoplasm of parametrium ♀

Radiology

D25.0	Submucous leiomyoma of uterus ♀	N83.332	Acquired atrophy of left ovary and fallopian tube ♀ ☑
D25.1	Intramural leiomyoma of uterus ♀	N83.41	Prolapse and hernia of right ovary and fallopian tube ♀ ☑
D25.2	Subserosal leiomyoma of uterus ♀	N83.42	Prolapse and hernia of left ovary and fallopian tube ♀ ☑
D27.0	Benign neoplasm of right ovary ♀ ☑	N83.511	Torsion of right ovary and ovarian pedicle ♀ ☑
D27.1	Benign neoplasm of left ovary ♀ ☑	N83.512	Torsion of left ovary and ovarian pedicle ♀ ☑
D28.2	Benign neoplasm of uterine tubes and ligaments ♀	N83.521	Torsion of right fallopian tube ♀ ☑
D39.0	Neoplasm of uncertain behavior of uterus ♀	N83.522	Torsion of left fallopian tube ♀ ☑
D39.11	Neoplasm of uncertain behavior of right ovary ♀ ☑	N83.53	Torsion of ovary, ovarian pedicle and fallopian tube ♀
D39.12	Neoplasm of uncertain behavior of left ovary ♀ ☑	N84.0	Polyp of corpus uteri ♀
E28.2	Polycystic ovarian syndrome ♀	N84.8	Polyp of other parts of female genital tract ♀
E28.310	Symptomatic premature menopause 🅰 ♀	N85.01	Benign endometrial hyperplasia ♀
E28.319	Asymptomatic premature menopause 🅰 ♀	N85.02	Endometrial intraepithelial neoplasia [EIN] ♀
E30.0	Delayed puberty	N85.2	Hypertrophy of uterus ♀
E30.1	Precocious puberty 🅿	N85.3	Subinvolution of uterus ♀
E89.40	Asymptomatic postprocedural ovarian failure ♀	N85.4	Malposition of uterus ♀
E89.41	Symptomatic postprocedural ovarian failure ♀	N85.5	Inversion of uterus ♀
F32.81	Premenstrual dysphoric disorder ♀	N85.6	Intrauterine synechiae ♀
N39.3	Stress incontinence (female) (male)	N85.7	Hematometra ♀
N70.01	Acute salpingitis ♀	N89.7	Hematocolpos ♀
N70.02	Acute oophoritis ♀	N91.0	Primary amenorrhea ♀
N70.03	Acute salpingitis and oophoritis ♀	N91.1	Secondary amenorrhea ♀
N70.11	Chronic salpingitis ♀	N91.3	Primary oligomenorrhea ♀
N70.12	Chronic oophoritis ♀	N91.4	Secondary oligomenorrhea ♀
N70.13	Chronic salpingitis and oophoritis ♀	N92.0	Excessive and frequent menstruation with regular cycle ♀
N71.0	Acute inflammatory disease of uterus ♀	N92.1	Excessive and frequent menstruation with irregular cycle ♀
N71.1	Chronic inflammatory disease of uterus ♀	N92.2	Excessive menstruation at puberty 🅿 ♀
N73.0	Acute parametritis and pelvic cellulitis ♀	N92.3	Ovulation bleeding ♀
N73.6	Female pelvic peritoneal adhesions (postinfective) ♀	N92.4	Excessive bleeding in the premenopausal period ♀
N80.0	Endometriosis of uterus ♀	N93.0	Postcoital and contact bleeding ♀
N80.1	Endometriosis of ovary ♀	N94.0	Mittelschmerz ♀
N80.2	Endometriosis of fallopian tube ♀	N94.11	Superficial (introital) dyspareunia ♀
N80.3	Endometriosis of pelvic peritoneum ♀	N94.12	Deep dyspareunia ♀
N81.11	Cystocele, midline ♀	N94.3	Premenstrual tension syndrome ♀
N81.12	Cystocele, lateral ♀	N94.4	Primary dysmenorrhea ♀
N81.2	Incomplete uterovaginal prolapse ♀	N94.5	Secondary dysmenorrhea ♀
N81.3	Complete uterovaginal prolapse ♀	N95.0	Postmenopausal bleeding ♀
N81.6	Rectocele ♀	N95.1	Menopausal and female climacteric states ♀
N81.81	Perineocele ♀	N96	Recurrent pregnancy loss ♀
N81.84	Pelvic muscle wasting ♀	N97.0	Female infertility associated with anovulation ♀
N82.0	Vesicovaginal fistula ♀	N97.2	Female infertility of uterine origin ♀
N82.2	Fistula of vagina to small intestine ♀	N98.1	Hyperstimulation of ovaries ♀
N82.3	Fistula of vagina to large intestine ♀	N99.510	Cystostomy hemorrhage
N83.01	Follicular cyst of right ovary ♀ ☑	N99.511	Cystostomy infection
N83.02	Follicular cyst of left ovary ♀ ☑	N99.512	Cystostomy malfunction
N83.11	Corpus luteum cyst of right ovary ♀ ☑	N99.83	Residual ovary syndrome ♀
N83.12	Corpus luteum cyst of left ovary ♀ ☑	N99.85	Post endometrial ablation syndrome ♀
N83.291	Other ovarian cyst, right side ♀ ☑	Q50.01	Congenital absence of ovary, unilateral ♀
N83.292	Other ovarian cyst, left side ♀ ☑	Q50.02	Congenital absence of ovary, bilateral ♀
N83.311	Acquired atrophy of right ovary ♀ ☑	Q50.1	Developmental ovarian cyst ♀
N83.312	Acquired atrophy of left ovary ♀ ☑	Q50.2	Congenital torsion of ovary ♀
N83.321	Acquired atrophy of right fallopian tube ♀ ☑	Q50.31	Accessory ovary ♀
N83.322	Acquired atrophy of left fallopian tube ♀ ☑	Q50.32	Ovarian streak ♀
N83.331	Acquired atrophy of right ovary and fallopian tube ♀ ☑	Q50.4	Embryonic cyst of fallopian tube ♀

Radiology

Q50.5	Embryonic cyst of broad ligament ♀
Q51.0	Agenesis and aplasia of uterus ♀
Q51.10	Doubling of uterus with doubling of cervix and vagina without obstruction ♀
Q51.11	Doubling of uterus with doubling of cervix and vagina with obstruction ♀
Q51.21	Complete doubling of uterus ♀
Q51.22	Partial doubling of uterus ♀
Q51.28	Other and unspecified doubling of uterus ♀
Q51.3	Bicornate uterus ♀
Q51.4	Unicornate uterus ♀
Q51.5	Agenesis and aplasia of cervix ♀
Q51.810	Arcuate uterus ♀
Q51.811	Hypoplasia of uterus ♀
Q51.820	Cervical duplication ♀
Q52.0	Congenital absence of vagina ♀
Q52.11	Transverse vaginal septum ♀
Q52.120	Longitudinal vaginal septum, nonobstructing ♀
Q52.121	Longitudinal vaginal septum, obstructing, right side ♀ ☑
Q52.122	Longitudinal vaginal septum, obstructing, left side ♀ ☑
Q52.123	Longitudinal vaginal septum, microperforate, right side ♀ ☑
Q52.124	Longitudinal vaginal septum, microperforate, left side ♀ ☑
T83.31XA	Breakdown (mechanical) of intrauterine contraceptive device, initial encounter ♀
T83.32XA	Displacement of intrauterine contraceptive device, initial encounter ♀
T83.711A	Erosion of implanted vaginal mesh to surrounding organ or tissue, initial encounter ♀
T83.721A	Exposure of implanted vaginal mesh into vagina, initial encounter ♀
Z30.431	Encounter for routine checking of intrauterine contraceptive device ♀

AMA: **76856** 2018,Jan,8; 2017,Oct,9; 2017,Jan,8; 2016,Jan,13; 2016,Aug,9; 2015,Jan,16; 2014,Jan,11 **76857** 2018,Jan,8; 2017,Oct,9; 2017,Jan,8; 2016,Jan,13; 2015,Jan,16; 2014,Jan,11

Relative Value Units/Medicare Edits

Non-Facility RVU	Work	PE	MP	Total
76856	0.69	2.36	0.04	3.09
76857	0.5	0.84	0.03	1.37
Facility RVU	**Work**	**PE**	**MP**	**Total**
76856	0.69	2.36	0.04	3.09
76857	0.5	0.84	0.03	1.37

	FUD	Status	MUE	Modifiers				IOM Reference
76856	N/A	A	1(3)	51	N/A	N/A	80*	None
76857	N/A	A	1(3)	51	N/A	N/A	80*	

* with documentation

● New ▲ Revised + Add On ★ Telemedicine AMA: CPT Assist [Resequenced] ☑ Laterality © 2020 Optum360, LLC

90384-90386

90384 Rho(D) immune globulin (RhIg), human, full-dose, for intramuscular use

90385 Rho(D) immune globulin (RhIg), human, mini-dose, for intramuscular use

90386 Rho(D) immune globulin (RhIgIV), human, for intravenous use

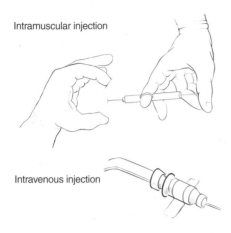

Intramuscular injection

Intravenous injection

Explanation

Code 90384 identifies the human Rho(D) immune globulin (RhIg) for intramuscular use, full-dose; 90385 is for a mini-dose. Code 90386 identifies the human Rho(D) immune globulin (RhIgIV) for intravenous use. This immune globulin is a passive immunization agent that gives protection against reactions between blood that is negative for the presence of Rh antigens on the surface of red blood cells to blood that is positive for the presence of Rh antigens on the RBC. Report these codes with the appropriate administration code.

Coding Tips

Modifier 51 should not be reported with the immune globulin codes when performed with another procedure. Report with the appropriate administration code. Assign the appropriate E/M service code when a significant and separately identifiable service is performed in addition to the administration of the vaccine/toxoid. Supplies used when providing this procedure may be reported with the appropriate HCPCS Level II code. Check with the specific payer to determine coverage.

ICD-10-CM Diagnostic Codes

O36.0110	Maternal care for anti-D [Rh] antibodies, first trimester, not applicable or unspecified 🅼 ♀
O36.0111	Maternal care for anti-D [Rh] antibodies, first trimester, fetus 1 🅼 ♀
O36.0112	Maternal care for anti-D [Rh] antibodies, first trimester, fetus 2 🅼 ♀
O36.0113	Maternal care for anti-D [Rh] antibodies, first trimester, fetus 3 🅼 ♀
O36.0114	Maternal care for anti-D [Rh] antibodies, first trimester, fetus 4 🅼 ♀
O36.0115	Maternal care for anti-D [Rh] antibodies, first trimester, fetus 5 🅼 ♀
O36.0119	Maternal care for anti-D [Rh] antibodies, first trimester, other fetus 🅼 ♀
O36.0120	Maternal care for anti-D [Rh] antibodies, second trimester, not applicable or unspecified 🅼 ♀
O36.0121	Maternal care for anti-D [Rh] antibodies, second trimester, fetus 1 🅼 ♀
O36.0122	Maternal care for anti-D [Rh] antibodies, second trimester, fetus 2 🅼 ♀
O36.0123	Maternal care for anti-D [Rh] antibodies, second trimester, fetus 3 🅼 ♀
O36.0124	Maternal care for anti-D [Rh] antibodies, second trimester, fetus 4 🅼 ♀
O36.0125	Maternal care for anti-D [Rh] antibodies, second trimester, fetus 5 🅼 ♀
O36.0129	Maternal care for anti-D [Rh] antibodies, second trimester, other fetus 🅼 ♀
O36.0130	Maternal care for anti-D [Rh] antibodies, third trimester, not applicable or unspecified 🅼 ♀
O36.0131	Maternal care for anti-D [Rh] antibodies, third trimester, fetus 1 🅼 ♀
O36.0132	Maternal care for anti-D [Rh] antibodies, third trimester, fetus 2 🅼 ♀
O36.0133	Maternal care for anti-D [Rh] antibodies, third trimester, fetus 3 🅼 ♀
O36.0134	Maternal care for anti-D [Rh] antibodies, third trimester, fetus 4 🅼 ♀
O36.0135	Maternal care for anti-D [Rh] antibodies, third trimester, fetus 5 🅼 ♀
O36.0139	Maternal care for anti-D [Rh] antibodies, third trimester, other fetus 🅼 ♀
O36.0910	Maternal care for other rhesus isoimmunization, first trimester, not applicable or unspecified 🅼 ♀
O36.0911	Maternal care for other rhesus isoimmunization, first trimester, fetus 1 🅼 ♀
O36.0912	Maternal care for other rhesus isoimmunization, first trimester, fetus 2 🅼 ♀
O36.0913	Maternal care for other rhesus isoimmunization, first trimester, fetus 3 🅼 ♀
O36.0914	Maternal care for other rhesus isoimmunization, first trimester, fetus 4 🅼 ♀
O36.0915	Maternal care for other rhesus isoimmunization, first trimester, fetus 5 🅼 ♀
O36.0919	Maternal care for other rhesus isoimmunization, first trimester, other fetus 🅼 ♀
O36.0920	Maternal care for other rhesus isoimmunization, second trimester, not applicable or unspecified 🅼 ♀
O36.0921	Maternal care for other rhesus isoimmunization, second trimester, fetus 1 🅼 ♀
O36.0922	Maternal care for other rhesus isoimmunization, second trimester, fetus 2 🅼 ♀
O36.0923	Maternal care for other rhesus isoimmunization, second trimester, fetus 3 🅼 ♀
O36.0924	Maternal care for other rhesus isoimmunization, second trimester, fetus 4 🅼 ♀
O36.0925	Maternal care for other rhesus isoimmunization, second trimester, fetus 5 🅼 ♀
O36.0929	Maternal care for other rhesus isoimmunization, second trimester, other fetus 🅼 ♀
O36.0930	Maternal care for other rhesus isoimmunization, third trimester, not applicable or unspecified 🅼 ♀
O36.0931	Maternal care for other rhesus isoimmunization, third trimester, fetus 1 🅼 ♀
O36.0932	Maternal care for other rhesus isoimmunization, third trimester, fetus 2 🅼 ♀

Medicine

O36.0933	Maternal care for other rhesus isoimmunization, third trimester, fetus 3 ▣ ♀
O36.0934	Maternal care for other rhesus isoimmunization, third trimester, fetus 4 ▣ ♀
O36.0935	Maternal care for other rhesus isoimmunization, third trimester, fetus 5 ▣ ♀
O36.0939	Maternal care for other rhesus isoimmunization, third trimester, other fetus ▣ ♀
Z41.8	Encounter for other procedures for purposes other than remedying health state

Associated HCPCS Codes

J2790	Injection, Rho D immune globulin, human, full dose, 300 mcg (1500 IU)

AMA: 90384 2020,Jan,11; 2018,Jan,8; 2017,Jan,8; 2016,Jan,13; 2015,Jan,16; 2014,Jan,11 **90385** 2020,Jan,11; 2018,Jan,8; 2017,Jan,8; 2016,Jan,13; 2015,Jan,16; 2014,Jan,11 **90386** 2020,Jan,11; 2018,Jan,8; 2017,Jan,8; 2016,Jan,13; 2015,Jan,16; 2014,Jan,11

Relative Value Units/Medicare Edits

Non-Facility RVU	Work	PE	MP	Total
90384	0.0	0.0	0.0	0.0
90385	0.0	0.0	0.0	0.0
90386	0.0	0.0	0.0	0.0
Facility RVU	**Work**	**PE**	**MP**	**Total**
90384	0.0	0.0	0.0	0.0
90385	0.0	0.0	0.0	0.0
90386	0.0	0.0	0.0	0.0

	FUD	Status	MUE	Modifiers				IOM Reference
90384	N/A	I	0(3)	N/A	N/A	N/A	N/A	None
90385	N/A	E	1(2)	N/A	N/A	N/A	N/A	
90386	N/A	I	0(3)	N/A	N/A	N/A	N/A	

* with documentation

Terms To Know

immune globulin. Serum immunoglobulins, glycoproteins that function as antibodies, are injected to provide passive immunity by increasing the amount of circulating antibodies. It is used to help prevent infections in patients exposed to certain pathogens and to boost immune systems in patients who suffer primary humoral immunodeficiency. Correct code assignment is dependent upon dosage. May be sold under the brand names Flebogamma, Gammagard, Gamunex, Hepagam B, Octagam, Privigen, and Vivaglobin.

intramuscular. Within a muscle.

intravenous. Within a vein or veins.

99500-99501

99500	Home visit for prenatal monitoring and assessment to include fetal heart rate, non-stress test, uterine monitoring, and gestational diabetes monitoring
99501	Home visit for postnatal assessment and follow-up care

Explanation

The home health provider may visit patients with prenatal complications from the first month until the birth of the baby in 99500. The home nurse may obtain vaginal-anorectal/cervical cultures, perform a non-stress test and uterine and fetal heart rate monitoring, draw blood for serology (including offering of AFP/HIV testing), and other tests such as glucose screening to check for gestational diabetes. In 99501, the home visit for postnatal assessment may include a review of plans for future health maintenance and care, including routine infant immunizations, identification of illness and periodic health evaluations, and linking the family with other sources of support such as social services, parenting classes, and lactation consultants as necessary.

Coding Tips

Home visits take place at the patient's place of residence and may include assisted living residences, group homes, non-traditional private homes, and custodial care facilities. Services are reported by non-physician health care professionals. Home visits performed by a physician should be reported with the appropriate E/M home visit codes (99341–99350) with any other appropriate codes other than those in the 99500–99602 range for any additional procedures or services provided by the physician in the patient's home. Health care professionals who report E/M home visit codes (99341–99350) may also report these codes when both services are performed.

ICD-10-CM Diagnostic Codes

O10.012	Pre-existing essential hypertension complicating pregnancy, second trimester ▣ ♀
O10.013	Pre-existing essential hypertension complicating pregnancy, third trimester ▣ ♀
O10.111	Pre-existing hypertensive heart disease complicating pregnancy, first trimester ▣ ♀
O10.112	Pre-existing hypertensive heart disease complicating pregnancy, second trimester ▣ ♀
O10.113	Pre-existing hypertensive heart disease complicating pregnancy, third trimester ▣ ♀
O10.211	Pre-existing hypertensive chronic kidney disease complicating pregnancy, first trimester ▣ ♀
O10.212	Pre-existing hypertensive chronic kidney disease complicating pregnancy, second trimester ▣ ♀
O10.213	Pre-existing hypertensive chronic kidney disease complicating pregnancy, third trimester ▣ ♀
O10.311	Pre-existing hypertensive heart and chronic kidney disease complicating pregnancy, first trimester ▣ ♀
O10.312	Pre-existing hypertensive heart and chronic kidney disease complicating pregnancy, second trimester ▣ ♀
O10.313	Pre-existing hypertensive heart and chronic kidney disease complicating pregnancy, third trimester ▣ ♀
O10.411	Pre-existing secondary hypertension complicating pregnancy, first trimester ▣ ♀
O10.412	Pre-existing secondary hypertension complicating pregnancy, second trimester ▣ ♀

Medicine

O10.413	Pre-existing secondary hypertension complicating pregnancy, third trimester Ⓜ ♀
O11.1	Pre-existing hypertension with pre-eclampsia, first trimester Ⓜ ♀
O11.2	Pre-existing hypertension with pre-eclampsia, second trimester Ⓜ ♀
O11.3	Pre-existing hypertension with pre-eclampsia, third trimester Ⓜ ♀
O14.02	Mild to moderate pre-eclampsia, second trimester Ⓜ ♀
O14.03	Mild to moderate pre-eclampsia, third trimester Ⓜ ♀
O21.0	Mild hyperemesis gravidarum Ⓜ ♀
O21.1	Hyperemesis gravidarum with metabolic disturbance Ⓜ ♀
O24.011	Pre-existing type 1 diabetes mellitus, in pregnancy, first trimester Ⓜ ♀
O24.012	Pre-existing type 1 diabetes mellitus, in pregnancy, second trimester Ⓜ ♀
O24.013	Pre-existing type 1 diabetes mellitus, in pregnancy, third trimester Ⓜ ♀
O24.03	Pre-existing type 1 diabetes mellitus, in the puerperium Ⓜ ♀
O24.111	Pre-existing type 2 diabetes mellitus, in pregnancy, first trimester Ⓜ ♀
O24.112	Pre-existing type 2 diabetes mellitus, in pregnancy, second trimester Ⓜ ♀
O24.113	Pre-existing type 2 diabetes mellitus, in pregnancy, third trimester Ⓜ ♀
O24.13	Pre-existing type 2 diabetes mellitus, in the puerperium Ⓜ ♀
O24.410	Gestational diabetes mellitus in pregnancy, diet controlled Ⓜ ♀
O24.414	Gestational diabetes mellitus in pregnancy, insulin controlled Ⓜ ♀
O24.415	Gestational diabetes mellitus in pregnancy, controlled by oral hypoglycemic drugs Ⓜ ♀
O24.430	Gestational diabetes mellitus in the puerperium, diet controlled Ⓜ ♀
O24.434	Gestational diabetes mellitus in the puerperium, insulin controlled Ⓜ ♀
O24.811	Other pre-existing diabetes mellitus in pregnancy, first trimester Ⓜ ♀
O24.812	Other pre-existing diabetes mellitus in pregnancy, second trimester Ⓜ ♀
O24.813	Other pre-existing diabetes mellitus in pregnancy, third trimester Ⓜ ♀
O24.83	Other pre-existing diabetes mellitus in the puerperium Ⓜ ♀
O44.01	Complete placenta previa NOS or without hemorrhage, first trimester Ⓜ ♀
O44.02	Complete placenta previa NOS or without hemorrhage, second trimester Ⓜ ♀
O44.03	Complete placenta previa NOS or without hemorrhage, third trimester Ⓜ ♀
O44.21	Partial placenta previa NOS or without hemorrhage, first trimester Ⓜ ♀
O44.22	Partial placenta previa NOS or without hemorrhage, second trimester Ⓜ ♀
O44.23	Partial placenta previa NOS or without hemorrhage, third trimester Ⓜ ♀
O44.31	Partial placenta previa with hemorrhage, first trimester Ⓜ ♀
O44.32	Partial placenta previa with hemorrhage, second trimester Ⓜ ♀
O44.33	Partial placenta previa with hemorrhage, third trimester Ⓜ ♀

O44.41	Low lying placenta NOS or without hemorrhage, first trimester Ⓜ ♀
O44.42	Low lying placenta NOS or without hemorrhage, second trimester Ⓜ ♀
O44.43	Low lying placenta NOS or without hemorrhage, third trimester Ⓜ ♀
O44.51	Low lying placenta with hemorrhage, first trimester Ⓜ ♀
O44.52	Low lying placenta with hemorrhage, second trimester Ⓜ ♀
O44.53	Low lying placenta with hemorrhage, third trimester Ⓜ ♀
O47.02	False labor before 37 completed weeks of gestation, second trimester Ⓜ ♀
O47.03	False labor before 37 completed weeks of gestation, third trimester Ⓜ ♀
O47.1	False labor at or after 37 completed weeks of gestation Ⓜ ♀
O60.02	Preterm labor without delivery, second trimester Ⓜ ♀
O60.03	Preterm labor without delivery, third trimester Ⓜ ♀
O99.810	Abnormal glucose complicating pregnancy Ⓜ ♀
O99.815	Abnormal glucose complicating the puerperium Ⓜ ♀
Z33.3	Pregnant state, gestational carrier Ⓜ ♀
Z34.01	Encounter for supervision of normal first pregnancy, first trimester Ⓜ ♀
Z34.02	Encounter for supervision of normal first pregnancy, second trimester Ⓜ ♀
Z34.03	Encounter for supervision of normal first pregnancy, third trimester Ⓜ ♀
Z34.81	Encounter for supervision of other normal pregnancy, first trimester Ⓜ ♀
Z34.82	Encounter for supervision of other normal pregnancy, second trimester Ⓜ ♀
Z34.83	Encounter for supervision of other normal pregnancy, third trimester Ⓜ ♀

AMA: **99500** 2018,Jan,8; 2017,Jan,8; 2016,Jan,13; 2015,Jan,16; 2014,Jan,11
99501 2018,Jan,8; 2017,Jan,8; 2016,Jan,13; 2015,Jan,16; 2014,Jan,11

Relative Value Units/Medicare Edits

Non-Facility RVU	Work	PE	MP	Total
99500	0.0	0.0	0.0	0.0
99501	0.0	0.0	0.0	0.0
Facility RVU	**Work**	**PE**	**MP**	**Total**
99500	0.0	0.0	0.0	0.0
99501	0.0	0.0	0.0	0.0

	FUD	Status	MUE	Modifiers				IOM Reference
99500	N/A	I	0(3)	N/A	N/A	N/A	N/A	None
99501	N/A	I	0(3)	N/A	N/A	N/A	N/A	

* with documentation

Medicine

G0101

G0101   Cervical or vaginal cancer screening; pelvic and clinical breast examination

Explanation

This code reports a cervical or vaginal cancer screening and a pelvic and clinical breast examination. The specimen for cancer screening is collected by cervical, endocervical, or vaginal scrapings or by aspiration of vaginal fluid and cells. The pelvic and breast exams are done manually by the physician to check for abnormalities, pain, and/or any palpable lumps or masses.

Coding Tips

If a separately identifiable service is performed in addition to this procedure, an E/M service may be reported with modifier 25 appended. Some payers may require this service to be reported using CPT preventive medicine service codes, new patient, see 99384-99387; established patient, see 99394-99397. Check with specific payers to determine coverage.

ICD-10-CM Diagnostic Codes

Z01.411	Encounter for gynecological examination (general) (routine) with abnormal findings ♀
Z01.419	Encounter for gynecological examination (general) (routine) without abnormal findings ♀
Z12.39	Encounter for other screening for malignant neoplasm of breast
Z12.4	Encounter for screening for malignant neoplasm of cervix ♀
Z12.72	Encounter for screening for malignant neoplasm of vagina ♀

Relative Value Units/Medicare Edits

Non-Facility RVU	Work	PE	MP	Total
G0101	0.45	0.6	0.08	1.13
Facility RVU	**Work**	**PE**	**MP**	**Total**
G0101	0.45	0.28	0.08	0.81

	FUD	Status	MUE	Modifiers				IOM Reference
G0101	N/A	A	1(2)	N/A	N/A	N/A	80*	None

* with documentation

Terms To Know

endocervical canal. Opening between the uterus and the vagina, through the cervix, lined with mucous membrane.

examination. Comprehensive visual and tactile screening and specific testing leading to diagnosis or, as appropriate, to a referral to another practitioner.

malignant. Any condition tending to progress toward death, specifically an invasive tumor with a loss of cellular differentiation that has the ability to spread or metastasize to other body areas.

screening pap smear. Diagnostic laboratory test consisting of a routine exfoliative cytology test (Papanicolaou test) provided to a woman for the early detection of cervical or vaginal cancer. The exam includes a clinical breast examination and a physician's interpretation of the results.

specimen. Tissue cells or sample of fluid taken for analysis, pathologic examination, and diagnosis.

G0130

G0130   Single energy x-ray absorptiometry (SEXA) bone density study, one or more sites; appendicular skeleton (peripheral) (e.g., radius, wrist, heel)

Explanation

Bone mineral density studies are used to evaluate diseases of bone and/or the responses of bone disease to treatment. Densities are measured at the wrist, radius, hip, pelvis, spine, or heel. The studies assess bone mass or density associated with such diseases as osteoporosis, osteomalacia, and renal osteodystrophy. Single energy x-ray absorptiometry (SEXA) utilizes an x-ray tube as the radiation source that is pulsed at a certain energy level. SEXA is used to scan bone that is in a superficial location with little adjacent soft tissue, such as the wrist or heel. There is a differential attenuation between bone and soft tissue for the energy beam. Excessive soft tissue renders the measurement incorrect. An attenuation profile of the bony components is calculated and the results are given in two scores, which are reported as standard deviations from the normal bone density of a person the same sex, 30 years old, which is the age of peak bone mass, and from the normal bone density of an "age matched" that compares the patient's bone density to what is expected in someone the same age, sex, and size.

Coding Tips

When medically necessary, Medicare may cover a bone mass measurement for a patient once every two years or more for specific conditions. For non-Medicare patients, check with the specific payer to determine coverage.

ICD-10-CM Diagnostic Codes

E83.31	Familial hypophosphatemia
E83.32	Hereditary vitamin D-dependent rickets (type 1) (type 2)
M80.011A	Age-related osteoporosis with current pathological fracture, right shoulder, initial encounter for fracture 🅰 ☑
M80.021A	Age-related osteoporosis with current pathological fracture, right humerus, initial encounter for fracture 🅰 ☑
M80.031A	Age-related osteoporosis with current pathological fracture, right forearm, initial encounter for fracture 🅰 ☑
M80.041A	Age-related osteoporosis with current pathological fracture, right hand, initial encounter for fracture 🅰 ☑
M80.051A	Age-related osteoporosis with current pathological fracture, right femur, initial encounter for fracture 🅰 ☑
M80.061A	Age-related osteoporosis with current pathological fracture, right lower leg, initial encounter for fracture 🅰 ☑
M80.071A	Age-related osteoporosis with current pathological fracture, right ankle and foot, initial encounter for fracture 🅰 ☑
M80.0AXA	Age-related osteoporosis with current pathological fracture, other site, initial encounter for fracture 🅰
M80.811A	Other osteoporosis with current pathological fracture, right shoulder, initial encounter for fracture ☑
M80.821A	Other osteoporosis with current pathological fracture, right humerus, initial encounter for fracture ☑
M80.831A	Other osteoporosis with current pathological fracture, right forearm, initial encounter for fracture ☑
M80.841A	Other osteoporosis with current pathological fracture, right hand, initial encounter for fracture ☑
M80.851A	Other osteoporosis with current pathological fracture, right femur, initial encounter for fracture ☑
M80.861A	Other osteoporosis with current pathological fracture, right lower leg, initial encounter for fracture ☑

M80.871A Other osteoporosis with current pathological fracture, right ankle and foot, initial encounter for fracture ☑

M80.88XA Other osteoporosis with current pathological fracture, vertebra(e), initial encounter for fracture

M80.8AXA Other osteoporosis with current pathological fracture, other site, initial encounter for fracture

M81.0 Age-related osteoporosis without current pathological fracture ▲

M81.6 Localized osteoporosis [Lequesne]

M81.8 Other osteoporosis without current pathological fracture

M83.0 Puerperal osteomalacia Ⓜ ♀

M83.1 Senile osteomalacia ▲

M83.2 Adult osteomalacia due to malabsorption ▲

M83.3 Adult osteomalacia due to malnutrition ▲

M83.4 Aluminum bone disease

M83.5 Other drug-induced osteomalacia in adults ▲

M83.8 Other adult osteomalacia ▲

N25.0 Renal osteodystrophy

Relative Value Units/Medicare Edits

Non-Facility RVU	Work	PE	MP	Total
G0130	0.22	0.75	0.02	0.99
Facility RVU	Work	PE	MP	Total
G0130	0.22	0.75	0.02	0.99

	FUD	Status	MUE	Modifiers				IOM Reference
G0130	N/A	A	1(2)	N/A	N/A	N/A	80*	None

* with documentation

Terms To Know

appendicular. Appendage, referring to the limbs and not the axis.

osteomalacia. Bones softened by a deficiency of calcium, characterized by bone pain, muscle weakness, and weight loss.

osteoporosis. Bone degeneration caused by the breakdown of the bony matrix without equivalent regeneration, resulting in a weak, porous, fragile bone structure.

SEXA. Single energy x-ray absorptiometry.

G0168

G0168 Wound closure utilizing tissue adhesive(s) only

Explanation

Wound closure done by using tissue adhesive only, not any kind of suturing or stapling, is reported with this code. Tissue adhesives, such as Dermabond, are materials that are applied directly to the skin or tissue of an open wound to hold the margins closed for healing.

Coding Tips

Code G0168 is reported when a Medicare patient undergoes a superficial repair or closure using a tissue adhesive only. This also includes those instances where sutures have been used for the repair of deeper layers and tissue adhesive is used to close the superficial layer. Payment for this service is at the discretion of the carrier.

ICD-10-CM Diagnostic Codes

S21.011A Laceration without foreign body of right breast, initial encounter ☑

S21.012A Laceration without foreign body of left breast, initial encounter ☑

S21.031A Puncture wound without foreign body of right breast, initial encounter ☑

S21.032A Puncture wound without foreign body of left breast, initial encounter ☑

S21.051A Open bite of right breast, initial encounter ☑

S21.052A Open bite of left breast, initial encounter ☑

S30.810A Abrasion of lower back and pelvis, initial encounter

S30.811A Abrasion of abdominal wall, initial encounter

S30.814A Abrasion of vagina and vulva, initial encounter ♀

S30.817A Abrasion of anus, initial encounter

S31.010A Laceration without foreign body of lower back and pelvis without penetration into retroperitoneum, initial encounter

S31.030A Puncture wound without foreign body of lower back and pelvis without penetration into retroperitoneum, initial encounter

S31.050A Open bite of lower back and pelvis without penetration into retroperitoneum, initial encounter

S31.110A Laceration without foreign body of abdominal wall, right upper quadrant without penetration into peritoneal cavity, initial encounter ☑

S31.111A Laceration without foreign body of abdominal wall, left upper quadrant without penetration into peritoneal cavity, initial encounter ☑

S31.112A Laceration without foreign body of abdominal wall, epigastric region without penetration into peritoneal cavity, initial encounter

S31.113A Laceration without foreign body of abdominal wall, right lower quadrant without penetration into peritoneal cavity, initial encounter ☑

S31.114A Laceration without foreign body of abdominal wall, left lower quadrant without penetration into peritoneal cavity, initial encounter ☑

S31.115A Laceration without foreign body of abdominal wall, periumbilic region without penetration into peritoneal cavity, initial encounter

S31.130A	Puncture wound of abdominal wall without foreign body, right upper quadrant without penetration into peritoneal cavity, initial encounter ☑	
S31.131A	Puncture wound of abdominal wall without foreign body, left upper quadrant without penetration into peritoneal cavity, initial encounter ☑	
S31.132A	Puncture wound of abdominal wall without foreign body, epigastric region without penetration into peritoneal cavity, initial encounter	
S31.133A	Puncture wound of abdominal wall without foreign body, right lower quadrant without penetration into peritoneal cavity, initial encounter ☑	
S31.134A	Puncture wound of abdominal wall without foreign body, left lower quadrant without penetration into peritoneal cavity, initial encounter ☑	
S31.135A	Puncture wound of abdominal wall without foreign body, periumbilic region without penetration into peritoneal cavity, initial encounter	
S31.150A	Open bite of abdominal wall, right upper quadrant without penetration into peritoneal cavity, initial encounter ☑	
S31.151A	Open bite of abdominal wall, left upper quadrant without penetration into peritoneal cavity, initial encounter ☑	
S31.152A	Open bite of abdominal wall, epigastric region without penetration into peritoneal cavity, initial encounter	
S31.153A	Open bite of abdominal wall, right lower quadrant without penetration into peritoneal cavity, initial encounter ☑	
S31.154A	Open bite of abdominal wall, left lower quadrant without penetration into peritoneal cavity, initial encounter ☑	
S31.155A	Open bite of abdominal wall, periumbilic region without penetration into peritoneal cavity, initial encounter	
S31.41XA	Laceration without foreign body of vagina and vulva, initial encounter ♀	
S31.43XA	Puncture wound without foreign body of vagina and vulva, initial encounter ♀	
S31.45XA	Open bite of vagina and vulva, initial encounter ♀	
S31.831A	Laceration without foreign body of anus, initial encounter	
S31.833A	Puncture wound without foreign body of anus, initial encounter	
S31.835A	Open bite of anus, initial encounter	
S71.111A	Laceration without foreign body, right thigh, initial encounter ☑	
S71.112A	Laceration without foreign body, left thigh, initial encounter ☑	
S71.131A	Puncture wound without foreign body, right thigh, initial encounter ☑	
S71.132A	Puncture wound without foreign body, left thigh, initial encounter ☑	
S71.151A	Open bite, right thigh, initial encounter ☑	
S71.152A	Open bite, left thigh, initial encounter ☑	

Relative Value Units/Medicare Edits

Non-Facility RVU	Work	PE	MP	Total
G0168	0.31	2.66	0.06	3.03
Facility RVU	**Work**	**PE**	**MP**	**Total**
G0168	0.31	0.17	0.06	0.54

	FUD	Status	MUE	Modifiers				IOM Reference
G0168	0	A	2(3)	51	N/A	N/A	N/A	None

* with documentation

G0124

G0124 Screening cytopathology, cervical or vaginal (any reporting system), collected in preservative fluid, automated thin layer preparation, requiring interpretation by physician

Explanation

These cervical or vaginal cytopathology screenings (any reporting system) of specimens collected in preservative fluid may be identified as "thin prep." The specimen is collected by cervical, endocervical, or vaginal scrapings or by aspiration of vaginal fluid and cells. This method saves time by eliminating the need for the physician to prepare a smear; the specimen is placed in a preservative suspension instead. At the laboratory, special instruments take the cells in the preservative suspension and "plate-out" a monolayer for screening, which will carefully review the specimen for abnormal cells.

Relative Value Units/Medicare Edits

Non-Facility RVU	Work	PE	MP	Total
G0124	0.26	0.46	0.01	0.73
Facility RVU	**Work**	**PE**	**MP**	**Total**
G0124	0.26	0.46	0.01	0.73

G0141

G0141 Screening cytopathology smears, cervical or vaginal, performed by automated system, with manual rescreening, requiring interpretation by physician

Explanation

This cervical or vaginal cytopathology screening is done on specimens prepared in a smear. The specimen is collected by cervical, endocervical, or vaginal scrapings or by aspiration of vaginal fluid and cells. The screening method is microscopy examination of a spray or liquid fixated smear prepared by the physician collecting the specimen. Screening, defined as the careful review of the specimen for abnormal cells, may then be accomplished by different methods that involve the use of automated systems.

Relative Value Units/Medicare Edits

Non-Facility RVU	Work	PE	MP	Total
G0141	0.26	0.46	0.01	0.73
Facility RVU	**Work**	**PE**	**MP**	**Total**
G0141	0.26	0.46	0.01	0.73

G0425-G0427

G0425 Telehealth consultation, emergency department or initial inpatient, typically 30 minutes communicating with the patient via telehealth

G0426 Telehealth consultation, emergency department or initial inpatient, typically 50 minutes communicating with the patient via telehealth

G0427 Telehealth consultation, emergency department or initial inpatient, typically 70 minutes or more communicating with the patient via telehealth

Explanation

These codes are used to report an initial inpatient or emergency department consultative visit or consultations that are furnished via telehealth in response to a request by the attending physician. Telehealth is the delivery of health-related services via telecommunications equipment. These services include counseling and coordination of patient care with the other providers.

Relative Value Units/Medicare Edits

Non-Facility RVU	Work	PE	MP	Total
G0425	1.92	0.77	0.13	2.82
G0426	2.61	1.06	0.16	3.83
G0427	3.86	1.57	0.25	5.68
Facility RVU	**Work**	**PE**	**MP**	**Total**
G0425	1.92	0.77	0.13	2.82
G0426	2.61	1.06	0.16	3.83
G0427	3.86	1.57	0.25	5.68

G0438-G0439

G0438 Annual wellness visit; includes a personalized prevention plan of service (PPS), initial visit

G0439 Annual wellness visit, includes a personalized prevention plan of service (PPS), subsequent visit

Explanation

The initial annual wellness visit (AWV) includes taking the patient's history; compiling a list of the patient's current providers; taking the patient's vital signs, including height and weight; reviewing the patient's risk factor for depression; identifying any cognitive impairment; reviewing the patient's functional ability and level of safety (based on observation or screening questions); setting up a written patient screening schedule; compiling a list of risk factors, and furnishing personalized health services and referrals, as necessary. Subsequent annual wellness visits (AWV) include updating the patient's medical and family history, updating the current provider list, obtaining the patient's vital signs and weight, identifying cognitive impairment, updating the screening schedule, updating the risk factors list, and providing personalized health advice to the patient.

Relative Value Units/Medicare Edits

Non-Facility RVU	Work	PE	MP	Total
G0438	2.43	2.23	0.13	4.79
G0439	1.5	1.66	0.09	3.25
Facility RVU	**Work**	**PE**	**MP**	**Total**
G0438	2.43	2.23	0.13	4.79
G0439	1.5	1.66	0.09	3.25

P3001

P3001 Screening Papanicolaou smear, cervical or vaginal, up to three smears, requiring interpretation by physician

Explanation

A screening Papanicolaou (commonly referred to as Pap) smear, cervical or vaginal, is a microscopic examination of cells scraped from the cervix or vaginal wall. The smears are examined for any cells that appear to be abnormal. It is a screening procedure when no known disease process exists.

Relative Value Units/Medicare Edits

Non-Facility RVU	Work	PE	MP	Total
P3001	0.26	0.46	0.01	0.73
Facility RVU	**Work**	**PE**	**MP**	**Total**
P3001	0.26	0.46	0.01	0.73

Q0091

Q0091 Screening Papanicolaou smear; obtaining, preparing and conveyance of cervical or vaginal smear to laboratory

Explanation

A screening Papanicolaou (commonly referred to as Pap) smear, cervical or vaginal, is a microscopic examination of cells scraped from the cervix or vaginal wall. The smears are examined for any abnormal appearing cells. It is a screening procedure when no known disease process currently exists and the test is looking for any possible abnormalities. This code reports the collection and preparation of a screening vaginal or cervical Pap smear and includes the conveyance or transportation of the smear to the laboratory.

Relative Value Units/Medicare Edits

Non-Facility RVU	Work	PE	MP	Total
Q0091	0.37	0.81	0.03	1.21
Facility RVU	**Work**	**PE**	**MP**	**Total**
Q0091	0.37	0.14	0.03	0.54

76641-76642

76641 Ultrasound, breast, unilateral, real time with image documentation, including axilla when performed; complete

76642 limited

Explanation

Breast ultrasound is a noninvasive diagnostic imaging technique that produces images used to assess breast tissues. Ultrasound uses a transducer that sends out ultrasound waves at a frequency too high to be heard. The ultrasound transducer is placed on the skin, and the ultrasound waves move through different densities of breast tissue. The sound waves bounce off the tissues like an echo and return to the transducer. The transducer processes the reflected waves, which are then converted by a computer into an image of the breast tissues being examined. Real time scanning displays structure images and movement with time. Report 76641 for a complete ultrasound, which includes examination of all four quadrants of the breast, as well as the retroareolar region. Report 76642 for a limited ultrasound, which pays particular attention to one or more, but not all, of the elements described by 76641. Examination of the axilla is included in both codes, when performed.

Relative Value Units/Medicare Edits

Non-Facility RVU	Work	PE	MP	Total
76641	0.73	2.25	0.04	3.02
76642	0.68	1.75	0.04	2.47
Facility RVU	**Work**	**PE**	**MP**	**Total**
76641	0.73	2.25	0.04	3.02
76642	0.68	1.75	0.04	2.47

76700-76705

76700 Ultrasound, abdominal, real time with image documentation; complete

76705 limited (eg, single organ, quadrant, follow-up)

Explanation

Diagnostic ultrasound is an imaging technique bouncing sound waves far above the level of human perception through interior body structures. The sound waves pass through different densities of tissue and reflect back to a receiving unit at varying speeds. The unit converts the waves to electrical pulses that are immediately displayed in picture form on screen. Real time scanning displays structure images and movement with time. Report 76700 for ultrasound and real time of the entire abdomen and 76705 for a single quadrant or organ of the abdomen.

Relative Value Units/Medicare Edits

Non-Facility RVU	Work	PE	MP	Total
76700	0.81	2.6	0.06	3.47
76705	0.59	1.94	0.04	2.57
Facility RVU	**Work**	**PE**	**MP**	**Total**
76700	0.81	2.6	0.06	3.47
76705	0.59	1.94	0.04	2.57

76945

76945 Ultrasonic guidance for chorionic villus sampling, imaging supervision and interpretation

Explanation

The physician aspirates cells from the chorionic villus (early stage of the placenta) under ultrasonic guidance. Ultrasound is an imaging technique bouncing sound waves far above the level of human perception through interior body structures. The sound waves pass through different densities of tissue and reflect back to a receiving unit, which converts the waves to electrical pulses that are immediately displayed in picture form on screen. In the transcervical method, a catheter is inserted through the cervix and into the uterine cavity toward the chorionic villus or early placenta. Aspirated cells are obtained for abnormal chromosome analysis. The procedure may also be done transvaginally or transabdominally. The transabdominal approach can be done throughout pregnancy while the other approaches are usually done between 9 and 12 weeks gestation. This code reports the imaging supervision and interpretation only for this procedure.

Relative Value Units/Medicare Edits

Non-Facility RVU	Work	PE	MP	Total
76945	0.0	0.0	0.0	0.0
Facility RVU	**Work**	**PE**	**MP**	**Total**
76945	0.0	0.0	0.0	0.0

76946

76946 Ultrasonic guidance for amniocentesis, imaging supervision and interpretation

Explanation

The physician withdraws fluid from the amniotic sac under ultrasonic guidance. Ultrasound is an imaging technique bouncing sound waves far above the level of human perception through interior body structures. The sound waves pass through different densities of tissue and reflect back to a receiving unit, which converts the waves to electrical pulses that are immediately displayed in picture form on screen. Following preparation of the skin and administration of a local anesthetic, a small gauge needle is introduced into the amniotic sac and fluid aspirated. This code reports the imaging supervision and interpretation only for this procedure.

Relative Value Units/Medicare Edits

Non-Facility RVU	Work	PE	MP	Total
76946	0.38	0.51	0.02	0.91
Facility RVU	**Work**	**PE**	**MP**	**Total**
76946	0.38	0.51	0.02	0.91

76948

76948 Ultrasonic guidance for aspiration of ova, imaging supervision and interpretation

Explanation

The physician aspirates ova under ultrasonic guidance. Ultrasound is an imaging technique bouncing sound waves far above the level of human perception through interior body structures. The sound waves pass through different densities of tissue and reflect back to a receiving unit, which converts the waves to electrical pulses that are immediately displayed in picture form on screen. Following preparation of the skin and administration of a local anesthetic, a small gauge needle is introduced into the ovary and the ova are aspirated. This code reports the imaging supervision and interpretation only for this procedure.

Relative Value Units/Medicare Edits

Non-Facility RVU	Work	PE	MP	Total
76948	0.67	1.45	0.03	2.15
Facility RVU	**Work**	**PE**	**MP**	**Total**
76948	0.67	1.45	0.03	2.15

80050

80050   General health panel This panel must include the following: Comprehensive metabolic panel (80053) Blood count, complete (CBC), automated and automated differential WBC count (85025 or 85027 and 85004) OR Blood count, complete (CBC), automated (85027) and appropriate manual differential WBC count (85007 or 85009) Thyroid stimulating hormone (TSH) (84443)

Explanation

A general health panel includes the following tests: albumin (82040), total bilirubin (82247), calcium (82310), carbon dioxide (bicarbonate) (82374), chloride (82435), creatinine (82565), glucose (82947), alkaline phosphatase (84075), potassium (84132), total protein (84155), sodium (84295), alanine amino transferase (ALT) (SGPT) (84460), aspartate amino transferase (AST) (SGOT) (84450), urea nitrogen (BUN) (84520), and thyroid stimulating hormone (84443). In addition, this panel includes a hemogram with automated differential (85025 or 85027 and 85004) or hemogram (85027) with manual differential (85007 or 85009). Blood specimen is obtained by venipuncture. See specific codes for additional information about the listed tests.

Relative Value Units/Medicare Edits

Non-Facility RVU	Work	PE	MP	Total
80050	0.0	0.0	0.0	0.0
Facility RVU	**Work**	**PE**	**MP**	**Total**
80050	0.0	0.0	0.0	0.0

80051

80051   Electrolyte panel This panel must include the following: Carbon dioxide (bicarbonate) (82374) Chloride (82435) Potassium (84132) Sodium (84295)

Explanation

An electrolyte panel includes the following tests: carbon dioxide (82374), chloride (82435), potassium (84132), and sodium (84295). Blood specimen is obtained by venipuncture. See specific codes for additional information about the listed tests.

Relative Value Units/Medicare Edits

Non-Facility RVU	Work	PE	MP	Total
80051	0.0	0.0	0.0	0.0
Facility RVU	**Work**	**PE**	**MP**	**Total**
80051	0.0	0.0	0.0	0.0

80055 [80081]

80055   Obstetric panel This panel must include the following: Blood count, complete (CBC), automated and automated differential WBC count (85025 or 85027 and 85004) OR Blood count, complete (CBC), automated (85027) and appropriate manual differential WBC count (85007 or 85009) Hepatitis B surface antigen (HBsAg) (87340) Antibody, rubella (86762) Syphilis test, non-treponemal antibody; qualitative (eg, VDRL, RPR, ART) (86592) Antibody screen, RBC, each serum technique (86850) Blood typing, ABO (86900) AND Blood typing, Rh (D) (86901)

80081   Obstetric panel (includes HIV testing)

Explanation

An obstetric panel (80055) includes the following tests: hepatitis B surface antigen (HBsAg) (87340), rubella antibody (86762), qualitative non-treponemal antibody syphilis test (VDRL, RPR, ART) (86592), RBC antibody screen (86850), ABO blood typing (86900), and Rh (D) blood typing (86901). In addition, this panel includes an automated complete blood count (CBC) and automated differential white blood count (WBC) as described by 85025 or 85027 and 85004 OR automated CBC (85027) and appropriate manual differential WBC count (85007 or 85009). Blood specimen is obtained by venipuncture. See specific codes for additional information about the listed tests. Report 80081 when the obstetric panel also includes HIV-1 antigen(s) with HIV-1 and HIV-2 antibodies reported as a single result (87389).

Relative Value Units/Medicare Edits

Non-Facility RVU	Work	PE	MP	Total
80055	0.0	0.0	0.0	0.0
80081	0.0	0.0	0.0	0.0
Facility RVU	**Work**	**PE**	**MP**	**Total**
80055	0.0	0.0	0.0	0.0
80081	0.0	0.0	0.0	0.0

80414

80414   Chorionic gonadotropin stimulation panel; testosterone response This panel must include the following: Testosterone (84403 x 2 on 3 pooled blood samples)

Explanation

This test may be ordered as a HCG "Stim" or human chorionic gonadotropin panel. Blood specimens may be drawn on two separate mornings before HCG is administered, usually by intramuscular injection. Injections may be repeated on two following days. Blood collection times may vary following HCG administration. The test is useful in diagnosis of certain cases of hypogonadotrophism as well as certain steroid deficiencies.

Relative Value Units/Medicare Edits

Non-Facility RVU	Work	PE	MP	Total
80414	0.0	0.0	0.0	0.0
Facility RVU	**Work**	**PE**	**MP**	**Total**
80414	0.0	0.0	0.0	0.0

80415

▲   80415   Chorionic gonadotropin stimulation panel; estradiol response This panel must include the following: Estradiol, total (82670 x 2 on 3 pooled blood samples)

Explanation

This test may be ordered as a HCG "Stim" or human chorionic gonadotropin panel. Blood specimens may be drawn on two separate mornings before HCG is administered, usually by intramuscular injection and sometimes in several sessions. Timing of blood draws may vary, but just prior to the first administration of HCG and four hours after is common for women. Estradiol is among the more active endogenous estrogens. The panel is useful in the diagnosis of certain menstrual disorders, fertility problems, and estrogen-producing tumors.

Relative Value Units/Medicare Edits

Non-Facility RVU	Work	PE	MP	Total
80415	0.0	0.0	0.0	0.0
Facility RVU	Work	PE	MP	Total
80415	0.0	0.0	0.0	0.0

81000

81000   Urinalysis, by dip stick or tablet reagent for bilirubin, glucose, hemoglobin, ketones, leukocytes, nitrite, pH, protein, specific gravity, urobilinogen, any number of these constituents; non-automated, with microscopy

Explanation

This type of test may be ordered by the brand name product and the analytes tested. Although screens are considered to show the presence of an analyte (qualitative), some newer products are semi-quantitative. Many are plastic strips that contain sites impregnated with chemicals that react with urine when the strip is dipped into a specimen. The result is a color change that is compared against a standardized chart. Most strips will test for numerous analytes, as well as for pH and specific gravity. Tablets work in a similar fashion. A drop of urine is placed on the tablet and a chemical reaction causes a color change that is compared to a standard chart. Usually only a single analyte is under consideration, per tablet. Code 81000 involves a manual (nonautomated) test and includes a microscopic examination. Microscopy involves examination of the urine sediments or solids. The urine is first centrifuged in a graduated tube to concentrate the sediments. Samples (either wet or dry) are examined, usually under both high and low power, and abnormal constituents are noted. These may include a wide range of biological abnormalities, such as blood cells, casts, and bacteria, as well as chemical anomalies, such as crystals.

Relative Value Units/Medicare Edits

Non-Facility RVU	Work	PE	MP	Total
81000	0.0	0.0	0.0	0.0
Facility RVU	Work	PE	MP	Total
81000	0.0	0.0	0.0	0.0

81001

81001   Urinalysis, by dip stick or tablet reagent for bilirubin, glucose, hemoglobin, ketones, leukocytes, nitrite, pH, protein, specific gravity, urobilinogen, any number of these constituents; automated, with microscopy

Explanation

This type of test may be ordered by the type of processor used and the analytes tested. The testing methodology is similar to the manual strips, except that the color change caused by the chemical reaction with urine is processed and read mechanically. The strip is exposed to the urine sample and is mechanically fed through a processor that reads the colors emitted by the reaction. The unit will be calibrated according to international standards and readings have a high degree of accuracy. The result may be displayed on a monitor, but is always printed or recorded in some form. Code 81001 also includes a microscopy.

Microscopy involves examination of the urine sediments or solids. The urine is first centrifuged in a graduated tube to concentrate the sediments. Samples (either wet or dry) are examined, usually under both high and low power, and abnormal constituents are noted. These may include a wide range of biological abnormalities, such as blood cells, casts, and bacteria, as well as chemical anomalies, such as crystals.

Relative Value Units/Medicare Edits

Non-Facility RVU	Work	PE	MP	Total
81001	0.0	0.0	0.0	0.0
Facility RVU	Work	PE	MP	Total
81001	0.0	0.0	0.0	0.0

81002

81002   Urinalysis, by dip stick or tablet reagent for bilirubin, glucose, hemoglobin, ketones, leukocytes, nitrite, pH, protein, specific gravity, urobilinogen, any number of these constituents; non-automated, without microscopy

Explanation

This type of test may be ordered by the brand name product and the analytes tested. Although usually considered screens to show the presence of an analyte (qualitative), some newer products are semi-quantitative. Many are plastic strips that contain sites impregnated with chemicals that react with urine when the strip is dipped into a specimen. The result is a color change that is compared against a standardized chart. Most strips will test for numerous analytes, as well as for pH and specific gravity. Tablets work in a similar fashion. A drop of urine is placed on the tablet and a chemical reaction causes a color change that is compared to a standard chart. Usually only a single analyte is under consideration per tablet, however. Code 81002 does not include a microscopic examination of the urine sample or its components.

Relative Value Units/Medicare Edits

Non-Facility RVU	Work	PE	MP	Total
81002	0.0	0.0	0.0	0.0
Facility RVU	Work	PE	MP	Total
81002	0.0	0.0	0.0	0.0

81003

81003   Urinalysis, by dip stick or tablet reagent for bilirubin, glucose, hemoglobin, ketones, leukocytes, nitrite, pH, protein, specific gravity, urobilinogen, any number of these constituents; automated, without microscopy

Explanation

This type of test may be ordered by the type of processor used and the analytes tested. The testing methodology is similar to the manual strips, except that the color change caused by the chemical reaction with urine is processed and read mechanically. The strip is exposed to the urine sample and is mechanically fed through a processor that reads the colors emitted by the reaction. The unit will be calibrated according to international standards and readings have a high degree of accuracy. The result may be displayed on a monitor, but is always printed or recorded in some form. Code 81003 does not include a microscopic examination of the urine sample or its components.

Non-Facility RVU	Work	PE	MP	Total
81003	0.0	0.0	0.0	0.0
Facility RVU	Work	PE	MP	Total
81003	0.0	0.0	0.0	0.0

81005

81005   Urinalysis; qualitative or semiquantitative, except immunoassays

Explanation

This test may be ordered by the type of processor used and the analytes under examination. The method will be any type of automated analyzer, usually colorimetry. The results of a semi-quantitative test indicate the presence or absence of an analyte and may be expressed as simply positive or negative. A qualitative result may be indicated as trace, 1+, 2+, etc.

Relative Value Units/Medicare Edits

Non-Facility RVU	Work	PE	MP	Total
81005	0.0	0.0	0.0	0.0
Facility RVU	Work	PE	MP	Total
81005	0.0	0.0	0.0	0.0

81007

81007   Urinalysis; bacteriuria screen, except by culture or dipstick

Explanation

This type of test may be ordered by the brand name of the commercial kit used and the bacteria that the kit screens for. Human urine is normally free of bacteria. However, bacteria can easily be introduced upon voiding. In addition, specimens containing any amount of pathological bacteria can have the organisms rapidly multiply after collection. For this reason, specimens are often examined shortly after collection. Method includes any method except culture or dipstick. The test is often performed by commercial kit. The type of kit used should be specified in the report.

Relative Value Units/Medicare Edits

Non-Facility RVU	Work	PE	MP	Total
81007	0.0	0.0	0.0	0.0
Facility RVU	Work	PE	MP	Total
81007	0.0	0.0	0.0	0.0

81015

81015   Urinalysis; microscopic only

Explanation

This test may be ordered as a microscopic analysis. Human urine is normally free of bacteria. However, bacteria can easily be introduced upon voiding. In addition, specimens containing any amount of pathological bacteria can have the organisms rapidly multiply after collection. For this reason, specimens are often examined shortly after collection. The sample may first be centrifuged into a graduated tube to concentrate the sediments, or solid matter, held in suspension. The concentration of bacteria as well as cell types, crystals, and other elements seen is reported.

Relative Value Units/Medicare Edits

Non-Facility RVU	Work	PE	MP	Total
81015	0.0	0.0	0.0	0.0
Facility RVU	Work	PE	MP	Total
81015	0.0	0.0	0.0	0.0

81020

81020   Urinalysis; 2 or 3 glass test

Explanation

This test may be ordered as a two-glass or three-glass test, a MacConkey-blood agar test, an MC-blood agar test, or any of the previous with a gram-positive plate. This is a culture for bacteria and will typically involve a culture plate of 5 percent sheep's blood agar and a MacConkey plate (a medium containing differentiate for lactose and nonlactose fermenters). A third plate of gram-positive media may offer further discrimination of bacteria cultured. The test is useful in determining the types and prevalence of bacteria in the urine.

Relative Value Units/Medicare Edits

Non-Facility RVU	Work	PE	MP	Total
81020	0.0	0.0	0.0	0.0
Facility RVU	Work	PE	MP	Total
81020	0.0	0.0	0.0	0.0

81025

81025   Urine pregnancy test, by visual color comparison methods

Explanation

This test may be ordered by any of the brand name kits available. The tests typically involve a dipstick impregnated with reagents that chemically react upon contact with urine. A change in color indicates positive or negative for the presence of hormones found in the urine of women in early pregnancy.

Relative Value Units/Medicare Edits

Non-Facility RVU	Work	PE	MP	Total
81025	0.0	0.0	0.0	0.0
Facility RVU	Work	PE	MP	Total
81025	0.0	0.0	0.0	0.0

82948

82948   Glucose; blood, reagent strip

Explanation

This test is used to monitor disorders of carbohydrate metabolism. Blood specimen is obtained by finger stick. A drop of blood is placed on the reagent strip for a specified amount of time. When the prescribed amount of time has elapsed, the strip is blotted and the reagent strip is compared to a color chart. Method is reagent strip with visual comparison.

Relative Value Units/Medicare Edits

Non-Facility RVU	Work	PE	MP	Total
82948	0.0	0.0	0.0	0.0
Facility RVU	Work	PE	MP	Total
82948	0.0	0.0	0.0	0.0

82950

82950   Glucose; post glucose dose (includes glucose)

Explanation

This test may also be requested as glucose, postprandial (PP). This test is used to monitor disorders of carbohydrate metabolism. The patient consumes a high carbohydrate meal or an oral glucose solution. Blood glucose levels are checked two hours after the meal or glucose solution. A one-hour postprandial screen may be used to evaluate pregnant women for gestational diabetes mellitus. Method of testing varies.

Relative Value Units/Medicare Edits

Non-Facility RVU	Work	PE	MP	Total
82950	0.0	0.0	0.0	0.0
Facility RVU	Work	PE	MP	Total
82950	0.0	0.0	0.0	0.0

82951-82952

82951   Glucose; tolerance test (GTT), 3 specimens (includes glucose)
+   82952   tolerance test, each additional beyond 3 specimens (List separately in addition to code for primary procedure)

Explanation

These tests may be requested as GTT, oral GTT, OGTT, intravenous GTT, or IVGTT. They monitor disorders of carbohydrate metabolism. These tests are normally performed using an oral dose of glucose, but may also be performed using intravenous glucose. A blood specimen is obtained prior to glucose administration and at intervals following glucose administration. Report 82951 for up to three specimens and 82952 for each additional specimen. Testing method varies.

Relative Value Units/Medicare Edits

Non-Facility RVU	Work	PE	MP	Total
82951	0.0	0.0	0.0	0.0
82952	0.0	0.0	0.0	0.0
Facility RVU	Work	PE	MP	Total
82951	0.0	0.0	0.0	0.0
82952	0.0	0.0	0.0	0.0

84112

84112   Evaluation of cervicovaginal fluid for specific amniotic fluid protein(s) (eg, placental alpha microglobulin-1 [PAMG-1], placental protein 12 [PP12], alpha-fetoprotein), qualitative, each specimen

Explanation

This is a noninvasive test to evaluate possible rupture of membranes (ROM) in a pregnant patient. During pregnancy, large quantities of placental alpha microglobulin-1 (PAMG-1) are secreted into the amniotic fluid. If the fetal membranes are intact, a low background level of PAMG-1 is measured in cervicovaginal secretions. High levels may be indicative of ROM. A swab is inserted two to three inches into the vagina and is withdrawn after one minute. The swab tip is placed into a vial and rinsed with solvent. A test strip is then placed into the vial with the solvent. Depending on the size of the amniotic fluid leak, results may be visible within five to 10 minutes.

Relative Value Units/Medicare Edits

Non-Facility RVU	Work	PE	MP	Total
84112	0.0	0.0	0.0	0.0
Facility RVU	Work	PE	MP	Total
84112	0.0	0.0	0.0	0.0

84702

84702   Gonadotropin, chorionic (hCG); quantitative

Explanation

This test may be ordered as hCG or as a serum pregnancy test. The specimen is serum. Method may be radioimmunoassay (RIA), two-site immunoradiometric assay (IRMA), two-site enzyme-linked immunosorbent assay (ELISA), and radioreceptor assay (RRA). This test is quantitative and measures the amount of hCG present, a determinate of pregnancy and certain tumors.

Relative Value Units/Medicare Edits

Non-Facility RVU	Work	PE	MP	Total
84702	0.0	0.0	0.0	0.0
Facility RVU	Work	PE	MP	Total
84702	0.0	0.0	0.0	0.0

84703

84703   Gonadotropin, chorionic (hCG); qualitative

Explanation

This test is also known as a beta-subunit human chorionic gonadotropin. The specimen is serum or random urine sample. Methods may include radioimmunoassay (RIA), immunoradiometric (IRMA), and enzyme immunoassay. The test may be ordered to determine pregnancy, ectopic pregnancy, and hCG tumors, and as a screening prior to select medical care (e.g., sterilization).

Relative Value Units/Medicare Edits

Non-Facility RVU	Work	PE	MP	Total
84703	0.0	0.0	0.0	0.0
Facility RVU	Work	PE	MP	Total
84703	0.0	0.0	0.0	0.0

84830

84830   Ovulation tests, by visual color comparison methods for human luteinizing hormone

Explanation

This test is used for the qualitative detection of the luteinizing hormone (LH) in urine. The specimen is urine. Method is rapid chromatographic immunoassay. LH is always present in the blood and urine, though its levels are higher in urine during ovulation. The LH surge and actual release of the egg is considered as the most fertile time of the cycle, and the most likely time for becoming pregnant.

Relative Value Units/Medicare Edits

Non-Facility RVU	Work	PE	MP	Total
84830	0.0	0.0	0.0	0.0
Facility RVU	Work	PE	MP	Total
84830	0.0	0.0	0.0	0.0

85004

85004   Blood count; automated differential WBC count

Explanation

This test may be ordered as a blood count with automated differential. The specimen is whole blood. Method is automated cell counter. The blood count typically includes a measurement of normal cell constituents including white blood cells or leukocytes, red blood cells, and platelets. In addition, this test includes a differential count of the white blood cells or "diff" in which the following leukocytes are differentiated and counted automatically: neutrophils or granulocytes, lymphocytes, monocytes, eosinophils, and basophils.

Relative Value Units/Medicare Edits

Non-Facility RVU	Work	PE	MP	Total
85004	0.0	0.0	0.0	0.0
Facility RVU	Work	PE	MP	Total
85004	0.0	0.0	0.0	0.0

85007-85008

85007   Blood count; blood smear, microscopic examination with manual differential WBC count

85008   blood smear, microscopic examination without manual differential WBC count

Explanation

These tests may be ordered as a manual blood smear examination, RBC smear, peripheral blood smear, or RBC morphology without differential parameters in 85008 and with manual WBC differential in 85007. The specimen is whole blood. The method is manual testing. A blood smear is prepared and microscopically examined for the presence of normal cell constituents, including white blood cells, red blood cells, and platelets. In 85008, the white blood cell and platelet or thrombocyte counts are estimated and red cell morphology is commented on if abnormal. In 85007, a manual differential of white blood cells is included in which the following leukocytes are differentiated: neutrophils or granulocytes, lymphocytes, monocytes, eosinophils, and basophils.

Relative Value Units/Medicare Edits

Non-Facility RVU	Work	PE	MP	Total
85007	0.0	0.0	0.0	0.0
85008	0.0	0.0	0.0	0.0
Facility RVU	Work	PE	MP	Total
85007	0.0	0.0	0.0	0.0
85008	0.0	0.0	0.0	0.0

85009

85009   Blood count; manual differential WBC count, buffy coat

Explanation

This test may be ordered as a buffy coat differential or as a differential WBC count, buffy coat. Specimen is whole blood. Other collection types (e.g., finger stick or heel stick) do not yield the volume of blood required for this test. Method is manual testing. The whole blood is centrifuged to concentrate the white blood cells, and a manual WBC differential is performed in which the following leukocytes are differentiated: neutrophils or granulocytes, lymphocytes, monocytes, eosinophils, and basophils. This test is usually performed when the number of WBCs or leukocytes is abnormally low and the presence of abnormal white cells (e.g., blasts or cancer cells) is suspected clinically.

Relative Value Units/Medicare Edits

Non-Facility RVU	Work	PE	MP	Total
85009	0.0	0.0	0.0	0.0
Facility RVU	Work	PE	MP	Total
85009	0.0	0.0	0.0	0.0

85013

85013   Blood count; spun microhematocrit

Explanation

This test may be ordered as a microhematocrit, a spun microhematocrit, or a "spun crit." The specimen (whole blood) is by finger stick or heel stick in infants. The sample is placed in a tube and into a microcentrifuge device. The vials can be read manually against a chart for the volume of packed red cells or a digital reader in the centrifuge device. A spun microhematocrit only reports the volume of packed red cells. It is typically performed at sites where limited testing is available, the patient is a very difficult blood draw, or on infants.

Relative Value Units/Medicare Edits

Non-Facility RVU	Work	PE	MP	Total
85013	0.0	0.0	0.0	0.0
Facility RVU	Work	PE	MP	Total
85013	0.0	0.0	0.0	0.0

85014

85014   Blood count; hematocrit (Hct)

Explanation

This test may be ordered as a hematocrit, Hmt, or Hct. The specimen is whole blood. Method is automated cell counter. The hematocrit or volume of packed red cells (VPRC) in the blood sample is calculated by multiplying the red blood cell count or RBC times the mean corpuscular volume or MCV.

Relative Value Units/Medicare Edits

Non-Facility RVU	Work	PE	MP	Total
85014	0.0	0.0	0.0	0.0
Facility RVU	Work	PE	MP	Total
85014	0.0	0.0	0.0	0.0

85018

85018   Blood count; hemoglobin (Hgb)

Explanation

This test may be ordered as hemoglobin, Hgb, or hemoglobin concentration. The specimen is whole blood. Method is usually automated cell counter but a manual method is seen in labs with a limited test menu and blood bank drawing stations. Hemoglobin is an index of the oxygen-carrying capacity of the blood.

Relative Value Units/Medicare Edits

Non-Facility RVU	Work	PE	MP	Total
85018	0.0	0.0	0.0	0.0
Facility RVU	Work	PE	MP	Total
85018	0.0	0.0	0.0	0.0

Coding Companion for Ob/Gyn

85025-85027

85025 Blood count; complete (CBC), automated (Hgb, Hct, RBC, WBC and platelet count) and automated differential WBC count

85027 complete (CBC), automated (Hgb, Hct, RBC, WBC and platelet count)

Explanation

These tests may be ordered as a complete automated blood count (CBC). The specimen is whole blood. Method is automated cell counter. These codes include the measurement of erythrocytes (red blood cells or RBC), leukocytes (white blood cells or WBC), hemoglobin, hematocrit (volume of packed red blood cells or VPRC), platelet or thrombocyte count, and indices (mean corpuscular hemoglobin or MCH, mean corpuscular hemoglobin concentration or MCHC, mean corpuscular volume or MCV, and red cell distribution width or RDW). Code 85025 includes an automated differential of the white blood cells or "diff" in which the following leukocytes are differentiated: neutrophils or granulocytes, lymphocytes, monocytes, eosinophils, and basophils. Report 85027 if the complete CBC, or automated blood count, is done without the differential WBC count.

Relative Value Units/Medicare Edits

Non-Facility RVU	Work	PE	MP	Total
85025	0.0	0.0	0.0	0.0
85027	0.0	0.0	0.0	0.0
Facility RVU	**Work**	**PE**	**MP**	**Total**
85025	0.0	0.0	0.0	0.0
85027	0.0	0.0	0.0	0.0

85041

85041 Blood count; red blood cell (RBC), automated

Explanation

This test may be ordered as red blood cell count or RBC. The specimen is by whole blood. Method is automated cell counter.

Relative Value Units/Medicare Edits

Non-Facility RVU	Work	PE	MP	Total
85041	0.0	0.0	0.0	0.0
Facility RVU	**Work**	**PE**	**MP**	**Total**
85041	0.0	0.0	0.0	0.0

85045

85045 Blood count; reticulocyte, automated

Explanation

This test may be ordered as an automated reticulocyte count, an "auto retic," or a reticulocyte by flow cytometry. The specimen is whole blood. Method is automated cell counter or flow cytometer. Reticulocytes are immature red blood cells that still contain mitochondria and ribosomes. The reticulocytes are reported as a percentage of total red blood cells.

Relative Value Units/Medicare Edits

Non-Facility RVU	Work	PE	MP	Total
85045	0.0	0.0	0.0	0.0
Facility RVU	**Work**	**PE**	**MP**	**Total**
85045	0.0	0.0	0.0	0.0

85046

85046 Blood count; reticulocytes, automated, including 1 or more cellular parameters (eg, reticulocyte hemoglobin content [CHr], immature reticulocyte fraction [IRF], reticulocyte volume [MRV], RNA content), direct measurement

Explanation

This test may be ordered as a reticulocyte count and hemoglobin concentration, "retics" and Hgb, or as an "auto retic" and hemoglobin. The specimen is whole blood. Method is automated cell counter. The blood is stained with a dye that marks the reticulum in immature red blood cells, or reticulocytes. The reticulocytes are reported as a percentage of total red blood cells. The automated reticulocyte blood count also includes one or more cellular parameters, such as the hemoglobin content of the reticulocytes (CHr), the fraction of immature reticulocytes (IRF), the RNA content, or the volume of reticulocytes.

Relative Value Units/Medicare Edits

Non-Facility RVU	Work	PE	MP	Total
85046	0.0	0.0	0.0	0.0
Facility RVU	**Work**	**PE**	**MP**	**Total**
85046	0.0	0.0	0.0	0.0

85048-85049

85048 Blood count; leukocyte (WBC), automated

85049 platelet, automated

Explanation

These tests may be ordered as an automated white blood cell or WBC count, white cell count, or leukocyte count for 85048 and as an automated platelet count in 85049. The specimen is whole blood. Method is automated cell counter. In 85048, the population of white blood cells, or WBCs in the blood sample, is counted by machine. Only the number of white blood cells or leukocytes is reported. In 85049, the population of platelets or thrombocytes in the blood sample is counted by machine. Only the number of platelets is reported.

Relative Value Units/Medicare Edits

Non-Facility RVU	Work	PE	MP	Total
85048	0.0	0.0	0.0	0.0
85049	0.0	0.0	0.0	0.0
Facility RVU	**Work**	**PE**	**MP**	**Total**
85048	0.0	0.0	0.0	0.0
85049	0.0	0.0	0.0	0.0

[86328]

● **86328** Immunoassay for infectious agent antibody(ies); qualitative or semiquantitative, single step method (eg, reagent strip); severe acute respiratory syndrome coronavirus 2 (SARS-CoV-2) (Coronavirus disease [COVID-19])

Explanation

This code reports immunoassay antibody testing for severe acute respiratory syndrome coronavirus 2 using a single-step method such as a reagent strip. The test may be requested as single-step qualitative or semi-quantitative; infectious agent specificity may also include terminology such as SARS-CoV-2, coronavirus disease, or COVID-19. In one method, a reagent strip, pre-coated with appropriate IgM and IgG antibodies, is taken from its sealed container following collection of blood or serum from the patient. The sample is placed in the specimen well and diluent is added. Once the specimen and reagents react with the strip's test area, the specimen is read and results are interpreted and reported.

● New   ▲ Revised   + Add On   ★ Telemedicine   [Resequenced]   © 2020 Optum360, LLC

Appendix

Relative Value Units/Medicare Edits

Non-Facility RVU	Work	PE	MP	Total
86328	0.0	0.0	0.0	0.0
Facility RVU	**Work**	**PE**	**MP**	**Total**
86328	0.0	0.0	0.0	0.0

[86413]

- **86413** Severe acute respiratory syndrome coronavirus 2 (SARS-CoV-2) (Coronavirus disease [COVID-19]) antibody, quantitative

Explanation

This antibody assay provides quantitative measurements of SARS-CoV-2 antibodies in order to examine the patient's adaptive immune response to the virus. Provision of precise measurement of the antibodies may help assess treatment effectiveness. Patient serum and diluent added to a SARS-CoV-2 spike protein receptor binding domain (RBD)-complexed solid-phase surface is incubated and washed. Antihuman-signal antibodies are then added to detect bound anti-RBD antibodies. The relative amount of the signal that is measured is directly proportionate to the specimen's anti-RBD antibody concentration. Interpretation is made using a standards-generated calibration curve. Results are reported in quantitative units.

Relative Value Units/Medicare Edits

Non-Facility RVU	Work	PE	MP	Total
86413				
Facility RVU	**Work**	**PE**	**MP**	**Total**
86413				

86592

86592 Syphilis test, non-treponemal antibody; qualitative (eg, VDRL, RPR, ART)

Explanation

This nontreponemal (screening) antibody test is commonly ordered as RPR (rapid plasma reagin), STS (serologic test for syphilis), VDRL (venereal disease research laboratory), or ART (automated reagin test). It may also be ordered as standard test for syphilis. The specimen is serum. The test is commonly used to provide a diagnosis (screening test) for syphilis. The method is by nontreponemal rapid plasma reagin (RPR)-particle agglutination test. More recently, it is being performed by automated methodology, such as enzyme-linked immunosorbent assay (ELISA).

Relative Value Units/Medicare Edits

Non-Facility RVU	Work	PE	MP	Total
86592	0.0	0.0	0.0	0.0
Facility RVU	**Work**	**PE**	**MP**	**Total**
86592	0.0	0.0	0.0	0.0

86593

86593 Syphilis test, non-treponemal antibody; quantitative

Explanation

This nontreponemal (screening) test is commonly ordered as quantitative RPR (rapid plasma reagin), STS (serologic test for syphilis), VDRL (venereal disease research laboratory), or ART (automated reagin test). This test may also be ordered as a standard test for syphilis. The specimen is serum. It is most commonly used to provide a monitor for treatment, or to establish a diagnosis of reinfection with syphilis. The method is nontreponemal rapid plasma reagin-particle agglutination test or anticardiolipin antibodies. More recently, it is being performed by automated methodology, such as by enzyme-linked immunosorbent assay (ELISA).

Relative Value Units/Medicare Edits

Non-Facility RVU	Work	PE	MP	Total
86593	0.0	0.0	0.0	0.0
Facility RVU	**Work**	**PE**	**MP**	**Total**
86593	0.0	0.0	0.0	0.0

86632

86632 Antibody; Chlamydia, IgM

Explanation

This test may be ordered as chlamydia IgM titer. The specimen is serum or finger stick in adults, or heel stick in infants. Complement fixation (CF), enzyme-linked immunosorbent assay (ELISA), and immunofluorescent antibody (IFA) are methods commonly used to determine previous exposure to chlamydia or a current infection. Chlamydomonas is a genus of algae that can cause nongonococcal urethritis, among other infections.

Relative Value Units/Medicare Edits

Non-Facility RVU	Work	PE	MP	Total
86632	0.0	0.0	0.0	0.0
Facility RVU	**Work**	**PE**	**MP**	**Total**
86632	0.0	0.0	0.0	0.0

86694-86696

86694 Antibody; herpes simplex, non-specific type test
86695 herpes simplex, type 1
86696 herpes simplex, type 2

Explanation

These tests may be ordered as HSV antibody titer, HSV titer, herpes simplex antibody titer, or HSV IgG/IGM. The specimen is serum or finger stick in adults, or heel stick in infants. A number of methodologies have been employed, such as complement fixation (CF), enzyme-linked immunosorbent assay (ELISA), indirect fluorescent antibody (IFA), enzyme immunoassay, and latex agglutination. This test has been used as a serologic method to detect previous or recent exposure to herpes simplex. To report non-specific type testing, see 86694; testing for type 1, see 86695; testing for type 2, see 86696.

Relative Value Units/Medicare Edits

Non-Facility RVU	Work	PE	MP	Total
86694	0.0	0.0	0.0	0.0
86695	0.0	0.0	0.0	0.0
86696	0.0	0.0	0.0	0.0
Facility RVU	**Work**	**PE**	**MP**	**Total**
86694	0.0	0.0	0.0	0.0
86695	0.0	0.0	0.0	0.0
86696	0.0	0.0	0.0	0.0

86701

86701 Antibody; HIV-1

Explanation

This test may be ordered as an HIV-1 serological test, an HIV-1 antibody, or by an internal code. HIV is a retrovirus and the causative agent of acquired immunodeficiency syndrome (AIDS). Specimen is serum. Numerous kits are now available that use a variety of viral proteins and serumsynthetic peptides as antigens. Methodology is enzyme immunoassay (EIA), enzyme-linked immunosorbent assay (ELISA), radioimmunoprecipitation assay (RIPA), or indirect fluorescent antibody (IFA). A negative test does not guarantee negative status and the test is often repeated several times.

Relative Value Units/Medicare Edits

Non-Facility RVU	Work	PE	MP	Total
86701	0.0	0.0	0.0	0.0
Facility RVU	Work	PE	MP	Total
86701	0.0	0.0	0.0	0.0

86702

86702 Antibody; HIV-2

Explanation

This test may be ordered as an HIV-2 serological antibody. This is an antibody test for HIV-2, a retrovirus closely related to simian AIDS and found initially in West African nations and Portugal, but with cases also being reported in the United States since 1987. Blood specimen is serum. Specific kits are now available that use a variety of viral proteins and synthetic peptides as antigens to test for HIV-2. Methodology is enzyme immunoassay (EIA), enzyme-linked immunosorbent assay (ELISA), radioimmunoprecipitation assay (RIPA), or indirect fluorescent antibody (IFA). A negative test does not guarantee negative status and the test is often repeated several times.

Relative Value Units/Medicare Edits

Non-Facility RVU	Work	PE	MP	Total
86702	0.0	0.0	0.0	0.0
Facility RVU	Work	PE	MP	Total
86702	0.0	0.0	0.0	0.0

86703

86703 Antibody; HIV-1 and HIV-2, single result

Explanation

This test may be ordered as a combined HIV-1 and -2 serological or a combined HIV-1 and -2 antibody. This is an antibody test that tests for both HIV-1 and HIV-2 with a single result. Both are retroviruses. HIV-1 is the causative agent of acquired immunodeficiency syndrome (AIDS), while HIV-2 is closely related to simian AIDS. Blood specimen is serum. Specific kits are now available that use a variety of viral proteins and synthetic peptides as antigens to test for both HIV-1 and HIV-2. Methodology is enzyme immunoassay (EIA), enzyme-linked immunosorbent assay (ELISA), radioimmunoprecipitation assay (RIPA), or indirect fluorescent antibody (IFA). A negative test does not guarantee negative status and the test is often repeated several times.

Relative Value Units/Medicare Edits

Non-Facility RVU	Work	PE	MP	Total
86703	0.0	0.0	0.0	0.0
Facility RVU	Work	PE	MP	Total
86703	0.0	0.0	0.0	0.0

86769

- **86769** Antibody; severe acute respiratory syndrome coronavirus 2 (SARS-CoV-2) (Coronavirus disease [COVID-19])

Explanation

This code reports testing to identify the presence of antibodies to the SARS-CoV-2 virus. Infectious agent specificity may also include terminology such as severe acute respiratory syndrome coronavirus 2, coronavirus disease, or COVID-19. In one method, following dilution in buffer of the plasma or serum sample, a measured portion of the diluted sample and controls are added to a sample plate. After incubation and washing, appropriate IgG and IgM antibodies are added and incubated. It is combined with a substrate, incubated, and read immediately.

Relative Value Units/Medicare Edits

Non-Facility RVU	Work	PE	MP	Total
86769	0.0	0.0	0.0	0.0
Facility RVU	Work	PE	MP	Total
86769	0.0	0.0	0.0	0.0

87081-87084

87081 Culture, presumptive, pathogenic organisms, screening only;
87084 with colony estimation from density chart

Explanation

These codes describe presumptive screening cultures for one or more pathogenic organisms. The methodology is by culture and the culture should be identified by type (e.g., anaerobic, aerobic) and specimen source (e.g., pleural, peritoneal, bronchial aspirates). If a specific organism is suspected, the person ordering the test typically uses common names, such as strep screen, staph screen, etc., to specify the organism for screening. Presumptive identification includes gram staining as well as up to three tests, such as a catalase, oxidase, or urease test. Screenings included in this code are nonmotile, catalase-positive, gram-positive rod bacteria. Report 87084 when an estimation of the number of organisms is also made, based on a density chart.

Relative Value Units/Medicare Edits

Non-Facility RVU	Work	PE	MP	Total
87081	0.0	0.0	0.0	0.0
87084	0.0	0.0	0.0	0.0
Facility RVU	Work	PE	MP	Total
87081	0.0	0.0	0.0	0.0
87084	0.0	0.0	0.0	0.0

87086-87088

87086 Culture, bacterial; quantitative colony count, urine
87088 with isolation and presumptive identification of each isolate, urine

Explanation

These codes report the performance of a urine bacterial culture with a calibrated inoculating device so that a colony count accurately correlates with the number of organisms in the urine. In 87088, isolation and presumptive identification of bacteria recovered from the sample is done by means of identifying colony morphology, subculturing organisms to selective media and the performance of a gram stain or other simple test to identify bacteria to the genus level. There are several automated systems that detect the presence of bacteria using colorimetric, radiometric, or spectrophotometric means. In 87086, quantified colony count numbers within the urine sample are measured.

Relative Value Units/Medicare Edits

Non-Facility RVU	Work	PE	MP	Total
87086	0.0	0.0	0.0	0.0
87088	0.0	0.0	0.0	0.0
Facility RVU	**Work**	**PE**	**MP**	**Total**
87086	0.0	0.0	0.0	0.0
87088	0.0	0.0	0.0	0.0

87110

87110   Culture, chlamydia, any source

Explanation

This test is commonly known as a Chlamydia culture. A swab of the infected site is placed in a vial of sucrose transport media containing antibiotics and glass beads. The specimen is generally kept refrigerated. The test method is by cell culture, fluorescent stain. The cell culture technique is to isolate for Chlamydia.

Relative Value Units/Medicare Edits

Non-Facility RVU	Work	PE	MP	Total
87110	0.0	0.0	0.0	0.0
Facility RVU	**Work**	**PE**	**MP**	**Total**
87110	0.0	0.0	0.0	0.0

87118

87118   Culture, mycobacterial, definitive identification, each isolate

Explanation

This procedure is a definitive identification of mycobacterial organisms isolated by procedure 87116. This procedure may be performed by a reference laboratory after isolation by a primary lab. Methodology is traditional biochemical tests for identification of mycobacterium.

Relative Value Units/Medicare Edits

Non-Facility RVU	Work	PE	MP	Total
87118	0.0	0.0	0.0	0.0
Facility RVU	**Work**	**PE**	**MP**	**Total**
87118	0.0	0.0	0.0	0.0

87186

87186   Susceptibility studies, antimicrobial agent; microdilution or agar dilution (minimum inhibitory concentration [MIC] or breakpoint), each multi-antimicrobial, per plate

Explanation

This procedure may be called an MIC, or a sensitivity test. It is a sensitivity test to determine the susceptibility of a bacterium to an antibiotic. The methodology is microtiter dilution (several commercial panels use this method). Results are given as a minimum inhibitory concentration (MIC) with an interpretation of sensitive, intermediate, or resistant. The antibiotics on commercial plates are numerous, but predetermined. The procedure is charged by plate not by antibiotic.

Relative Value Units/Medicare Edits

Non-Facility RVU	Work	PE	MP	Total
87186	0.0	0.0	0.0	0.0
Facility RVU	**Work**	**PE**	**MP**	**Total**
87186	0.0	0.0	0.0	0.0

87205

87205   Smear, primary source with interpretation; Gram or Giemsa stain for bacteria, fungi, or cell types

Explanation

Any smear done on a primary source (e.g., sputum, CSF, etc.) to identify bacteria, fungi, and cell types. An interpretation of findings is provided. Bacteria, fungi, WBCs, and epithelial cells may be estimated in quantity with an interpretation as to the possibility of contamination by normal flora. A gram stain may be the most commonly performed smear of this type.

Relative Value Units/Medicare Edits

Non-Facility RVU	Work	PE	MP	Total
87205	0.0	0.0	0.0	0.0
Facility RVU	**Work**	**PE**	**MP**	**Total**
87205	0.0	0.0	0.0	0.0

87206

87206   Smear, primary source with interpretation; fluorescent and/or acid fast stain for bacteria, fungi, parasites, viruses or cell types

Explanation

A fluorescent or acid-fast stain for bacteria, fungi, parasites, viruses, or cell types. These are stains usually for specific groups of organisms (e.g., mycobacterium and Nocardia). Identification of Cryptosporidium and related parasites are examples of parasites that can be identified by fluorescent or acid fast stain. An interpretation is included.

Relative Value Units/Medicare Edits

Non-Facility RVU	Work	PE	MP	Total
87206	0.0	0.0	0.0	0.0
Facility RVU	**Work**	**PE**	**MP**	**Total**
87206	0.0	0.0	0.0	0.0

87210

87210   Smear, primary source with interpretation; wet mount for infectious agents (eg, saline, India ink, KOH preps)

Explanation

This test may be requested as a KOH prep. A wet mount is prepared from a primary source to detect bacteria, fungi, or ova and parasites. Motility of organisms is visible on wet mounts and the addition of a simple stain, such as iodine, India ink, or simple dyes, may aid detection of bacteria, fungi, and parasites. An interpretation of findings is included.

Relative Value Units/Medicare Edits

Non-Facility RVU	Work	PE	MP	Total
87210	0.0	0.0	0.0	0.0
Facility RVU	**Work**	**PE**	**MP**	**Total**
87210	0.0	0.0	0.0	0.0

87220

87220 Tissue examination by KOH slide of samples from skin, hair, or nails for fungi or ectoparasite ova or mites (eg, scabies)

Explanation

Potassium hydroxide (KOH) prep and calcofluor stains are the most common methods of looking for hyphal elements and/ or yeast in tissue. The KOH causes a clearing of the specimen to make fungus more visible. The preparation is enhanced for microscopic observation by adding a drop of calcofluor, a type of fluorescent dye, to the slide and reading the preparation with a fluorescent microscope.

Relative Value Units/Medicare Edits

Non-Facility RVU	Work	PE	MP	Total
87220	0.0	0.0	0.0	0.0
Facility RVU	**Work**	**PE**	**MP**	**Total**
87220	0.0	0.0	0.0	0.0

87270

87270 Infectious agent antigen detection by immunofluorescent technique; Chlamydia trachomatis

Explanation

This test may be requested as Chlamydia trachomatis or C. trachomatis by DFA or by immunofluorescence. C. trachomatis is a frequently occurring sexually transmitted disease. It may cause nonspecific urethritis or pelvic inflammatory disease (PID), although it is frequently asymptomatic in women. Another serotype also causes conjunctivitis. Infectious agent antigen detection by immunofluorescence includes direct and indirect fluorescent antibody technique and involves using monoclonal antibodies and immunofluorescence microscopy. Cellular material must be obtained from the site for immunofluorescence to be an effective diagnostic technique.

Relative Value Units/Medicare Edits

Non-Facility RVU	Work	PE	MP	Total
87270	0.0	0.0	0.0	0.0
Facility RVU	**Work**	**PE**	**MP**	**Total**
87270	0.0	0.0	0.0	0.0

87390

▲ **87390** Infectious agent antigen detection by immunoassay technique, (eg, enzyme immunoassay [EIA], enzyme-linked immunosorbent assay [ELISA], fluorescence immunoassay [FIA], immunochemiluminometric assay [IMCA]) qualitative or semiquantitative; HIV-1

Explanation

This test may be requested as human immunodeficiency virus Type 1 (HIV-1) by immunoassay techniques such as enzyme immunoassay (EIA), enzyme-linked immunosorbent assay (ELISA), fluorescence immunoassay (FIA), or immunochemiluminometric assay (IMCA). HIV-1 is the causative agent of acquired immunodeficiency syndrome (AIDS). Blood specimen is obtained by venipuncture. If the specific immunoassay technique is positive, it is repeated. Two out of three tests must be positive before the test is reported as positive. All positive tests are confirmed with an additional test using a different technique, usually Western blot, which is reported separately.

Relative Value Units/Medicare Edits

Non-Facility RVU	Work	PE	MP	Total
87390	0.0	0.0	0.0	0.0
Facility RVU	**Work**	**PE**	**MP**	**Total**
87390	0.0	0.0	0.0	0.0

87391

▲ **87391** Infectious agent antigen detection by immunoassay technique, (eg, enzyme immunoassay [EIA], enzyme-linked immunosorbent assay [ELISA], fluorescence immunoassay [FIA], immunochemiluminometric assay [IMCA]) qualitative or semiquantitative; HIV-2

Explanation

This test may be requested as human immunodeficiency virus Type 2 (HIV-2) by immunoassay techniques such as enzyme immunoassay (EIA), enzyme-linked immunosorbent assay (ELISA), fluorescence immunoassay (FIA), or immunochemiluminometric assay (IMCA). HIV-2 is a retrovirus closely related to simian AIDS and found initially in West African nations and Portugal, but with cases also being reported in the United States since 1987. Blood specimen is serum. If the test is positive, it is repeated. Two out of three tests must be positive before the test is reported as positive. All positive tests are confirmed with an additional test using a different technique, usually Western blot, which is reported separately.

Relative Value Units/Medicare Edits

Non-Facility RVU	Work	PE	MP	Total
87391	0.0	0.0	0.0	0.0
Facility RVU	**Work**	**PE**	**MP**	**Total**
87391	0.0	0.0	0.0	0.0

87426

● **87426** Infectious agent antigen detection by immunoassay technique, (eg, enzyme immunoassay [EIA], enzyme-linked immunosorbent assay [ELISA], fluorescence immunoassay [FIA], immunochemiluminometric assay [IMCA]) qualitative or semiquantitative; severe acute respiratory syndrome coronavirus (eg, SARS-CoV, SARS-CoV-2 [COVID-19])

Explanation

This test may be requested as severe acute respiratory syndrome coronavirus (SARS-CoV or SARS-CoV-2 [COVID-19]) antigen detection. Methods include immunoassay techniques such as enzyme immunoassay (EIA), enzyme-linked immunosorbent assay (ELISA), fluorescence immunoassay (FIA), or immunochemiluminometric assay (IMCA). Assays currently available are incapable of differentiating between SARS-CoV and SARS-CoV-2; this immunoassay detects antigenic proteins for either. A nasopharyngeal swab is collected and placed into a reagent tube, where it is swirled to release viral nucleoprotein antigen. A portion of the sample is transferred to the test cassette sample well, which is placed into the analyzer along with quality control cassettes. A qualitative result is obtained and reported to the ordering health care professional.

Relative Value Units/Medicare Edits

Non-Facility RVU	Work	PE	MP	Total
87426	0.0	0.0	0.0	0.0
Facility RVU	**Work**	**PE**	**MP**	**Total**
87426	0.0	0.0	0.0	0.0

87482

87482   Infectious agent detection by nucleic acid (DNA or RNA); Candida species, quantification

Explanation

This test is used to diagnosis an infection by any species of Candida, but usually C. albicans. This test would normally be performed to diagnosis systemic (invasive) candidiasis. Blood is serum. The specimen is treated to isolate the nucleic acid (DNA, RNA). This code reports quantification only and is used primarily to assess extent of disease or disease progression.

Relative Value Units/Medicare Edits

Non-Facility RVU	Work	PE	MP	Total
87482	0.0	0.0	0.0	0.0
Facility RVU	Work	PE	MP	Total
87482	0.0	0.0	0.0	0.0

87490

87490   Infectious agent detection by nucleic acid (DNA or RNA); Chlamydia trachomatis, direct probe technique

Explanation

This test may be requested as Chlamydia trachomatis or C. trachomatis by direct DNA probe. C. trachomatis is a frequently occurring sexually transmitted disease. It may cause nonspecific urethritis or pelvic inflammatory disease (PID), although it is frequently asymptomatic in women. Another serotype also causes conjunctivitis. The specimen is treated to isolate the DNA using direct probe.

Relative Value Units/Medicare Edits

Non-Facility RVU	Work	PE	MP	Total
87490	0.0	0.0	0.0	0.0
Facility RVU	Work	PE	MP	Total
87490	0.0	0.0	0.0	0.0

87491

87491   Infectious agent detection by nucleic acid (DNA or RNA); Chlamydia trachomatis, amplified probe technique

Explanation

This test may be requested as Chlamydia trachomatis or C. trachomatis by polymerase chain reaction. C. trachomatis is a frequently occurring sexually transmitted disease. It may cause nonspecific urethritis or pelvic inflammatory disease (PID), although it is frequently asymptomatic in women. Another serotype also causes conjunctivitis. The DNA is amplified using a technique such as polymerase chain reaction (PCR).

Relative Value Units/Medicare Edits

Non-Facility RVU	Work	PE	MP	Total
87491	0.0	0.0	0.0	0.0
Facility RVU	Work	PE	MP	Total
87491	0.0	0.0	0.0	0.0

87492

87492   Infectious agent detection by nucleic acid (DNA or RNA); Chlamydia trachomatis, quantification

Explanation

This test may be requested as Chlamydia trachomatis or C. trachomatis DNA quantification. C. trachomatis is a frequently occurring sexually transmitted disease. It may cause nonspecific urethritis or pelvic inflammatory disease (PID), although it is frequently asymptomatic in women. Another serotype also causes conjunctivitis. This code reports quantification only.

Relative Value Units/Medicare Edits

Non-Facility RVU	Work	PE	MP	Total
87492	0.0	0.0	0.0	0.0
Facility RVU	Work	PE	MP	Total
87492	0.0	0.0	0.0	0.0

87528

87528   Infectious agent detection by nucleic acid (DNA or RNA); Herpes simplex virus, direct probe technique

Explanation

This test may be requested as HSV by direct DNA probe. Herpes simplex may be classified as HSV type 1 (HSV 1) or HSV type 2 (HSV 2). HSV 1 is primarily responsible for oral lesions frequently referred to as fever blisters or cold sores. HSV 2 is a sexually transmitted disease with lesions occurring primarily in the genitourinary tract. Lesion swab/scrapings are obtained. CSF is obtained by spinal puncture. Blood specimen is serum. The specimen is treated to isolate the DNA using direct probe. Detection and typing (HSV1, HSV2) by direct DNA probe is superior to culture methods.

Relative Value Units/Medicare Edits

Non-Facility RVU	Work	PE	MP	Total
87528	0.0	0.0	0.0	0.0
Facility RVU	Work	PE	MP	Total
87528	0.0	0.0	0.0	0.0

87529

87529   Infectious agent detection by nucleic acid (DNA or RNA); Herpes simplex virus, amplified probe technique

Explanation

This test may be requested as HSV by amplified DNA probe. Herpes simplex may be classified is HSV type 1 (HSV 1) or HSV type 2 (HSV 2). HSV 1 is primarily responsible for oral lesions frequently referred to as fever blisters or cold sores. HSV 2 is a sexually transmitted disease with lesions occurring primarily in the genitourinary tract. Lesion swab/scrapings are obtained. CSF is obtained by spinal puncture. Blood specimen is serum. The DNA is amplified using a technique such as polymerase chain reaction (PCR). Detection and typing (HSV 1, HSV 2) by amplified DNA probe is superior to culture methods.

Relative Value Units/Medicare Edits

Non-Facility RVU	Work	PE	MP	Total
87529	0.0	0.0	0.0	0.0
Facility RVU	Work	PE	MP	Total
87529	0.0	0.0	0.0	0.0

87530

87530   Infectious agent detection by nucleic acid (DNA or RNA); Herpes simplex virus, quantification

Explanation

This test may be requested as HSV quantification by molecular technique. Herpes simplex may be classified as HSV type 1 (HSV 1) or HSV type 2 (HSV 2). HSV 1 is primarily responsible for oral lesions frequently referred to as fever blisters or cold sores. HSV 2 is a sexually transmitted disease with lesions occurring primarily in the genitourinary tract. Lesion swab/scrapings are obtained. CSF is obtained by spinal puncture. Blood specimen is serum. This code reports quantification only.

Relative Value Units/Medicare Edits

Non-Facility RVU	Work	PE	MP	Total
87530	0.0	0.0	0.0	0.0
Facility RVU	Work	PE	MP	Total
87530	0.0	0.0	0.0	0.0

87534-87535, 87537-87538

87534 Infectious agent detection by nucleic acid (DNA or RNA); HIV-1, direct probe technique
87535 HIV-1, amplified probe technique, includes reverse transcription when performed
87537 HIV-2, direct probe technique
87538 HIV-2, amplified probe technique, includes reverse transcription when performed

Explanation

HIV is the causative agent of acquired immunodeficiency syndrome (AIDS). In 87534, the test may be requested as human immunodeficiency virus Type 1 (HIV-1) by direct nucleic acid (DNA, RNA) probe. A random urine sample is obtained. Tissue is obtained by separately reportable biopsy procedure. The specimen is treated to isolate the DNA using direct probe. In 87535, the testing includes an amplified probe technique or reverse transcription polymerase chain reaction (RT-PCR) in which the reversely transcribed DNA is repeatedly duplicated (amplified) and detected using various methods. In 87537 and 87538, the tests may be requested as human immunodeficiency virus Type 2 (HIV-2) by EIA. HIV-2 is a retrovirus closely related to simian AIDS and found initially in West African nations and Portugal, but with cases also being reported in the United States since 1987. In 87537, the specimen is treated to isolate the DNA using direct probe. In 87538, the test is used to detect infectious agents using the organism's DNA/RNA. In reverse transcription, the RNA from the organism is mapped to a single strand DNA allowing it to replicate. Report 87538 when the testing includes an amplified probe technique or reverse transcription polymerase chain reaction (RT-PCR) in which the reversely transcribed DNA is repeatedly duplicated (amplified) and detected using various methods. Blood specimen for these tests is serum. These tests are used primarily by research facilities.

Relative Value Units/Medicare Edits

Non-Facility RVU	Work	PE	MP	Total
87534	0.0	0.0	0.0	0.0
87535	0.0	0.0	0.0	0.0
87537	0.0	0.0	0.0	0.0
87538	0.0	0.0	0.0	0.0
Facility RVU	Work	PE	MP	Total
87534	0.0	0.0	0.0	0.0
87535	0.0	0.0	0.0	0.0
87537	0.0	0.0	0.0	0.0
87538	0.0	0.0	0.0	0.0

87536, 87539

87536 Infectious agent detection by nucleic acid (DNA or RNA); HIV-1, quantification, includes reverse transcription when performed
87539 HIV-2, quantification, includes reverse transcription when performed

Explanation

HIV is the causative agent of acquired immunodeficiency syndrome (AIDS). These codes may be may be requested as human immunodeficiency virus Type 1 (HIV-1) (87536) or human immunodeficiency virus Type 2 (HIV-2) (87539). HIV-2 is a retrovirus closely related to simian AIDS and found initially in West African nations and Portugal, but with cases also being reported in the United States since 1987. The tests are used to detect infectious agents using the organism's DNA/RNA. In reverse transcription, the RNA from the organism is mapped to a single strand DNA allowing it to replicate. Report these codes if quantification of the RNA/DNA is all that is performed to monitor the effects of treatment. Blood specimen is serum for both tests. These tests are used primarily by research facilities.

Relative Value Units/Medicare Edits

Non-Facility RVU	Work	PE	MP	Total
87536	0.0	0.0	0.0	0.0
87539	0.0	0.0	0.0	0.0
Facility RVU	Work	PE	MP	Total
87536	0.0	0.0	0.0	0.0
87539	0.0	0.0	0.0	0.0

[87623, 87624, 87625]

87623 Infectious agent detection by nucleic acid (DNA or RNA); Human Papillomavirus (HPV), low-risk types (eg, 6, 11, 42, 43, 44)
87624 Infectious agent detection by nucleic acid (DNA or RNA); Human Papillomavirus (HPV), high-risk types (eg, 16, 18, 31, 33, 35, 39, 45, 51, 52, 56, 58, 59, 68)
87625 Infectious agent detection by nucleic acid (DNA or RNA); Human Papillomavirus (HPV), types 16 and 18 only, includes type 45, if performed

Explanation

These tests may be requested as human papillomavirus (HPV) according to low-risk types (6, 11, 42, 43, and 44) (87623), high-risk types (16, 18, 31, 33, 35, 39, 45, 51, 52, 56, 58, 59, and 68) (87624), or by specified types 16 and 18 only with type 45 included, when performed (87625). Human papillomaviruses are a genus of viruses that cause warts (benign neoplasms of skin and mucous membranes). There are at least 58 known types. HPV is commonly associated with plantar and genital warts. HPV infection of the cervix is of particular concern as it may be associated with cervical cancer. Methodology is in situ hybridization (ISH) by chromogenic or fluorescence techniques, which are based on the complementary pairing of a labeled probe to HPV antigens or nucleic acids (DNA or mRNA) within paraffin-embedded tissue biopsies or cervical smears.

Relative Value Units/Medicare Edits

Non-Facility RVU	Work	PE	MP	Total
87623	0.0	0.0	0.0	0.0
87624	0.0	0.0	0.0	0.0
87625	0.0	0.0	0.0	0.0
Facility RVU	Work	PE	MP	Total
87623	0.0	0.0	0.0	0.0
87624	0.0	0.0	0.0	0.0
87625	0.0	0.0	0.0	0.0

● New   ▲ Revised   + Add On   ★ Telemedicine   [Resequenced]   © 2020 Optum360, LLC

87590

87590   Infectious agent detection by nucleic acid (DNA or RNA); Neisseria gonorrhoeae, direct probe technique

Explanation

This test may be requested as gonorrhea direct DNA probe, gonorrhea molecular probe assay, or DNA detection of gonorrhea. Neisseria gonorrhea is one of the most common sexually transmitted infections. Molecular (nucleic acid probe) techniques offer rapid, accurate identification of Neisseria gonorrhea. While a cervical or urethral swab is preferred, molecular techniques are sensitive enough to detect the organism in urine also. Neisseria gonorrhea can be detected by DNA, RNA, or rRNA probes.

Relative Value Units/Medicare Edits

Non-Facility RVU	Work	PE	MP	Total
87590	0.0	0.0	0.0	0.0
Facility RVU	**Work**	**PE**	**MP**	**Total**
87590	0.0	0.0	0.0	0.0

87591

87591   Infectious agent detection by nucleic acid (DNA or RNA); Neisseria gonorrhoeae, amplified probe technique

Explanation

This test may be requested as gonorrhea amplified DNA probe, gonorrhea molecular probe assay, or DNA detection of gonorrhea. Neisseria gonorrhea is one of the most common sexually transmitted infections. Molecular (nucleic acid probe) techniques offer rapid, accurate identification of Neisseria gonorrhea. While a cervical or urethral swab is preferred, molecular techniques are sensitive enough to detect the organism in urine also. Neisseria gonorrhea can be detected by DNA or rRNA probes. Amplification can be performed using a number of techniques. Polymerase chain reaction (PCR) and ligase chain reaction (LCR) detect gonorrhea DNA. An assay is also available which detects gonorrhea ribosomal RNA (rRNA)

Relative Value Units/Medicare Edits

Non-Facility RVU	Work	PE	MP	Total
87591	0.0	0.0	0.0	0.0
Facility RVU	**Work**	**PE**	**MP**	**Total**
87591	0.0	0.0	0.0	0.0

87592

87592   Infectious agent detection by nucleic acid (DNA or RNA); Neisseria gonorrhoeae, quantification

Explanation

This test may be requested as gonorrhea nucleic acid quantification. Neisseria gonorrhea is one of the most common sexually transmitted infections. Molecular (nucleic acid probe) techniques offer rapid, accurate identification of Neisseria gonorrhea. While a cervical or urethral swab is preferred, molecular techniques are sensitive enough to detect the organism in urine also. Neisseria gonorrhea can be detected by DNA or rRNA probes. This code reports quantification only.

Relative Value Units/Medicare Edits

Non-Facility RVU	Work	PE	MP	Total
87592	0.0	0.0	0.0	0.0
Facility RVU	**Work**	**PE**	**MP**	**Total**
87592	0.0	0.0	0.0	0.0

87635-87637

- 87635   Infectious agent detection by nucleic acid (DNA or RNA); severe acute respiratory syndrome coronavirus 2 (SARS-CoV-2) (Coronavirus disease [COVID-19]), amplified probe technique
- 87636   severe acute respiratory syndrome coronavirus 2 (SARS-CoV-2) (Coronavirus disease [COVID-19]) and influenza virus types A and B, multiplex amplified probe technique
- 87637   severe acute respiratory syndrome coronavirus 2 (SARS-CoV-2) (Coronavirus disease [COVID-19]), influenza virus types A and B, and respiratory syncytial virus, multiplex amplified probe technique

Explanation

This test is for the detection of SARS-CoV-2 and any pan-coronavirus types or subtypes. Specimens have been collected using one or more methods (bronchoalveolar lavage, lower respiratory tract or nasal/nasopharyngeal aspirate/wash, nasopharyngeal/oropharyngeal swab, or sputum induction), placed into appropriate containers, and transported to the laboratory. The test uses specific primers and amplified probe assay to detect DNA or RNA sequences specific for the SARS-CoV-2 virus. Infectious agent specificity may also include terminology such as severe acute respiratory syndrome coronavirus 2, coronavirus disease, or COVID-19. Report 87635 for severe acute respiratory syndrome coronavirus 2 (SARS-CoV-2) (coronavirus disease [COVID-19]), amplified probe technique; report 87636 for severe acute respiratory syndrome coronavirus 2 (SARS-CoV-2) (coronavirus disease [COVID-19]) and influenza virus types A and B, multiplex amplified probe technique; report 87637 for severe acute respiratory syndrome coronavirus 2 (SARS-CoV-2) (coronavirus disease [COVID-19]), influenza virus types A and B, and respiratory syncytial virus, multiplex amplified probe technique.

Relative Value Units/Medicare Edits

Non-Facility RVU	Work	PE	MP	Total
87635	0.0	0.0	0.0	0.0
87636				
87637				
Facility RVU	**Work**	**PE**	**MP**	**Total**
87635	0.0	0.0	0.0	0.0
87636				
87637				

87808

▲ 87808   Infectious agent antigen detection by immunoassay with direct optical (ie, visual) observation; Trichomonas vaginalis

Explanation

This test may be requested as a rapid antigen test for trichomonas. Sample is vaginal swab; detection is by immunoassay with direct optical observation. When referring to primary source infectious disease codes, direct optical observation is a testing platform that produces a signal, such as a colored band, on the reaction chamber that can be interpreted visually. In one proprietary method, a swab is collected from the vaginal cavity and mixed in sample buffer to make the trichomonas proteins more soluble. The test stick is placed into the sample mixture, which migrates along the membrane surface. Within approximately 10 minutes, the results are available. Positivity is indicated by the appearance of a visible blue test line along with the red control line.

Relative Value Units/Medicare Edits

Non-Facility RVU	Work	PE	MP	Total
87808	0.0	0.0	0.0	0.0
Facility RVU	Work	PE	MP	Total
87808	0.0	0.0	0.0	0.0

87850

▲ **87850** Infectious agent antigen detection by immunoassay with direct optical (ie, visual) observation; Neisseria gonorrhoeae

Explanation

This test may be requested as a rapid antigen test for Neisseria gonorrhea, one of the most common sexually transmitted infections. Specimen may include urethral or endocervical swab; detection is by immunoassay with direct optical observation. When referring to primary source infectious disease codes, direct optical observation is a testing platform that produces a signal, such as a colored band, on the reaction chamber that can be interpreted visually. In one proprietary method, a swab specimen is collected from the patient's urethra. The swab is placed into an extraction tube to which a specified amount of extraction buffer has been added. The swab is rotated against the tube to express the liquid; after two minutes, another extraction buffer is added. Extraction is performed for another minute in the same way. A specified amount of extracted specimen is added to the specimen well of the test cassette. A positive result is indicated by two colored bands appearing on the membrane and may be interpreted visually in approximately 15 minutes.

Relative Value Units/Medicare Edits

Non-Facility RVU	Work	PE	MP	Total
87850	0.0	0.0	0.0	0.0
Facility RVU	Work	PE	MP	Total
87850	0.0	0.0	0.0	0.0

87880

▲ **87880** Infectious agent antigen detection by immunoassay with direct optical (ie, visual) observation; Streptococcus, group A

Explanation

This test may be requested as a rapid antigen test for Strep A. Streptococcus A is a form of beta hemolytic Streptococcus, which causes pharyngitis. Untreated infection can cause rheumatic fever or glomerulonephritis. Sample is throat swab; detection is by immunoassay with direct optical observation. When referring to primary source infectious disease codes, direct optical observation is a testing platform that produces a signal, such as a colored band, on the reaction chamber that can be interpreted visually. In one test method, a throat swab specimen is collected, and antigen is extracted from the specimen with reagents. A dipstick is added to the extracted sample. If the sample contains Strep A antigen, a positive result is indicated by the appearance of a pink to red test line along with a blue control line on the dipstick.

Relative Value Units/Medicare Edits

Non-Facility RVU	Work	PE	MP	Total
87880	0.0	0.0	0.0	0.0
Facility RVU	Work	PE	MP	Total
87880	0.0	0.0	0.0	0.0

88141

88141 Cytopathology, cervical or vaginal (any reporting system), requiring interpretation by physician

Explanation

This test is for the interpretation by a physician of a Papanicolaou (Pap) smear. This code is used in addition to the code for the technical service.

Relative Value Units/Medicare Edits

Non-Facility RVU	Work	PE	MP	Total
88141	0.26	0.46	0.01	0.73
Facility RVU	Work	PE	MP	Total
88141	0.26	0.46	0.01	0.73

88142-88143

88142 Cytopathology, cervical or vaginal (any reporting system), collected in preservative fluid, automated thin layer preparation; manual screening under physician supervision

88143 with manual screening and rescreening under physician supervision

Explanation

These tests may be identified by the name "thin prep." Specimen collection is by cervical or endocervical scraping or aspiration of vaginal fluid. The physician obtaining the specimen places the specimen in a preservative suspension. At the laboratory, special instruments take the cells in the preservative suspension and "plate-out" a monolayer for screening-the careful review of the specimen for abnormal cells. Report 88142 for manual screening done under physician supervision and 88143 for manual screening followed by manual rescreening, done under physician supervision. System of reporting may be Bethesda or non-Bethesda.

Relative Value Units/Medicare Edits

Non-Facility RVU	Work	PE	MP	Total
88142	0.0	0.0	0.0	0.0
88143	0.0	0.0	0.0	0.0
Facility RVU	Work	PE	MP	Total
88142	0.0	0.0	0.0	0.0
88143	0.0	0.0	0.0	0.0

88147-88148

88147 Cytopathology smears, cervical or vaginal; screening by automated system under physician supervision

88148 screening by automated system with manual rescreening under physician supervision

Explanation

These tests may be identified as a cervical smear, Pap smear, or vaginal cytology. Specimen collection is by cervical or endocervical scraping or aspiration of vaginal fluid. Method is microscopy examination of a spray or liquid fixated smear. Code 88147 should be used to report smears screened by automated system under physician supervision, while 88148 reports automated screening with manual rescreening under physician supervision. System of reporting may be Bethesda or non-Bethesda.

Relative Value Units/Medicare Edits

Non-Facility RVU	Work	PE	MP	Total
88147	0.0	0.0	0.0	0.0
88148	0.0	0.0	0.0	0.0
Facility RVU	Work	PE	MP	Total
88147	0.0	0.0	0.0	0.0
88148	0.0	0.0	0.0	0.0

88150-88153

88150 Cytopathology, slides, cervical or vaginal; manual screening under physician supervision

88152 with manual screening and computer-assisted rescreening under physician supervision

88153 with manual screening and rescreening under physician supervision

Explanation

These tests may also be identified as a cervical smear, Pap smear, or vaginal cytology. The specimen cells are collected by scraping or brushing the cervix or endocervix or aspiration of vaginal fluid. The specimen is smeared onto a slide and chemically treated with a preservative. These codes should be reported when any system other than the Bethesda System of evaluating and describing cervical/vaginal cytopathology slides is used. Code selection is based on the screening process used, with manual screening under physician supervision being reported with 88150, manual screening and computer-assisted rescreening under physician supervision with 88152, and manual screening and rescreening under physician supervision with 88153.

Relative Value Units/Medicare Edits

Non-Facility RVU	Work	PE	MP	Total
88150	0.0	0.0	0.0	0.0
88152	0.0	0.0	0.0	0.0
88153	0.0	0.0	0.0	0.0
Facility RVU	Work	PE	MP	Total
88150	0.0	0.0	0.0	0.0
88152	0.0	0.0	0.0	0.0
88153	0.0	0.0	0.0	0.0

88155

+ 88155 Cytopathology, slides, cervical or vaginal, definitive hormonal evaluation (eg, maturation index, karyopyknotic index, estrogenic index) (List separately in addition to code[s] for other technical and interpretation services)

Explanation

This test may also be identified as the maturation index, cytologic estrogen effect, karyopyknotic index, or estrogenic index. Specimen collection is by tongue depressor or wooden spatula of the lateral vaginal wall. Method is microscopy examination of a spray or liquid fixated smear. The test may be used to determine the balance of estrogen and progesterone of the vaginal squamous epithelium.

Relative Value Units/Medicare Edits

Non-Facility RVU	Work	PE	MP	Total
88155	0.0	0.0	0.0	0.0
Facility RVU	Work	PE	MP	Total
88155	0.0	0.0	0.0	0.0

88164-88167

88164 Cytopathology, slides, cervical or vaginal (the Bethesda System); manual screening under physician supervision

88165 with manual screening and rescreening under physician supervision

88166 with manual screening and computer-assisted rescreening under physician supervision

88167 with manual screening and computer-assisted rescreening using cell selection and review under physician supervision

Explanation

These tests may be identified as a cervical smear, Pap smear, or vaginal cytology. Specimen collection is by scraping or brushing the cervix or endocervix, or aspiration of vaginal fluid. Method is microscopy examination of a spray or liquid coated smear. These codes should be reported when the Bethesda System of evaluating and describing cervical/vaginal cytopathology slides is used. Code selection is based on the screening process used, with manual screening under physician supervision being reported with 88164, manual screening and rescreening under physician supervision with 88165, manual screening and computer-assisted rescreening under physician supervision with 88166, manual screening and computer-assisted rescreening using cell selection and review under physician supervision with 88167.

Relative Value Units/Medicare Edits

Non-Facility RVU	Work	PE	MP	Total
88164	0.0	0.0	0.0	0.0
88165	0.0	0.0	0.0	0.0
88166	0.0	0.0	0.0	0.0
88167	0.0	0.0	0.0	0.0
Facility RVU	Work	PE	MP	Total
88164	0.0	0.0	0.0	0.0
88165	0.0	0.0	0.0	0.0
88166	0.0	0.0	0.0	0.0
88167	0.0	0.0	0.0	0.0

88174-88175

88174 Cytopathology, cervical or vaginal (any reporting system), collected in preservative fluid, automated thin layer preparation; screening by automated system, under physician supervision

88175 with screening by automated system and manual rescreening or review, under physician supervision

Explanation

These tests may be identified by the brand name ThinPrep. Specimen collection is by cervical or endocervical scraping or aspiration of vaginal fluid. Report 88174 for automated screening done under physician supervision and 88175 when automated screening is followed by manual rescreening or review under physician supervision.

Relative Value Units/Medicare Edits

Non-Facility RVU	Work	PE	MP	Total
88174	0.0	0.0	0.0	0.0
88175	0.0	0.0	0.0	0.0
Facility RVU	Work	PE	MP	Total
88174	0.0	0.0	0.0	0.0
88175	0.0	0.0	0.0	0.0

89253

89253 Assisted embryo hatching, microtechniques (any method)

Explanation

Assisted embryo hatching is performed in selected cases on the day of embryo transfer. A pipette is placed on one side of the embryo to keep it from moving. A very delicate, hollow needle called a hatching needle is placed on the other side of the embryo. An acidic solution is expelled from the needle against the outer shell (zona pellucida) of the embryo. The acidic solution digests a small area of the outer shell. The embryo is washed and replaced in the culture solution in the incubator.

Relative Value Units/Medicare Edits

Non-Facility RVU	Work	PE	MP	Total
89253	0.0	0.0	0.0	0.0
Facility RVU	**Work**	**PE**	**MP**	**Total**
89253	0.0	0.0	0.0	0.0

89254

89254   Oocyte identification from follicular fluid

Explanation

Because the egg (oocyte) is microscopic, only the follicle (fluid filled structure surrounding the egg) can be seen during the ultrasound-guided retrieval. Upon aspiration of the follicle, specially trained personnel use a microscope to search for the oocyte-cumulus complex, which includes the egg and surrounding cumulus cells from the ovary. This is accomplished by pouring the collected fluid into flat dishes and using a microscope to search for eggs.

Relative Value Units/Medicare Edits

Non-Facility RVU	Work	PE	MP	Total
89254	0.0	0.0	0.0	0.0
Facility RVU	**Work**	**PE**	**MP**	**Total**
89254	0.0	0.0	0.0	0.0

89255

89255   Preparation of embryo for transfer (any method)

Explanation

After the embryos have been cultured for two to six days, three to four healthy embryos are selected for transfer. Selected embryos are loaded into a transfer catheter. In a separately reportable procedure, the catheter is placed in the cervical canal and the embryos are transferred into the uterine cavity.

Relative Value Units/Medicare Edits

Non-Facility RVU	Work	PE	MP	Total
89255	0.0	0.0	0.0	0.0
Facility RVU	**Work**	**PE**	**MP**	**Total**
89255	0.0	0.0	0.0	0.0

89257

89257   Sperm identification from aspiration (other than seminal fluid)

Explanation

A separately reportable testicular biopsy with aspiration is performed to obtain sperm. This may be required in cases where azoospermia is due to suspected obstruction to the spermatic ducts or in instances where the patient has had a failed reversal of a vasectomy. This procedure reports microscopic examination of aspirated fluid for the presence of sperm. If sperm are identified, further evaluation services may be performed and would be reported separately.

Relative Value Units/Medicare Edits

Non-Facility RVU	Work	PE	MP	Total
89257	0.0	0.0	0.0	0.0
Facility RVU	**Work**	**PE**	**MP**	**Total**
89257	0.0	0.0	0.0	0.0

89258

89258   Cryopreservation; embryo(s)

Explanation

Embryos not required for current uterine transfer are frozen using a process referred to as cryopreservation. Pre-implantation embryo preservation is a relatively new procedure as compared to sperm preservation (see 89259), but more than two-thirds of the embryos survive the cryopreservation process and can be preserved for an indefinite period of time.

Relative Value Units/Medicare Edits

Non-Facility RVU	Work	PE	MP	Total
89258	0.0	0.0	0.0	0.0
Facility RVU	**Work**	**PE**	**MP**	**Total**
89258	0.0	0.0	0.0	0.0

89259

89259   Cryopreservation; sperm

Explanation

A cryoprotectant, usually glycerol or Dimethyl Sulfoxide (DMSO), is mixed with the semen to reduce damage to sperm during the freezing process. The semen specimen is placed in a vial and frozen in liquid nitrogen at -196 C. This halts all biologic and metabolic processes allowing the sperm to be preserved for many years.

Relative Value Units/Medicare Edits

Non-Facility RVU	Work	PE	MP	Total
89259	0.0	0.0	0.0	0.0
Facility RVU	**Work**	**PE**	**MP**	**Total**
89259	0.0	0.0	0.0	0.0

89260

89260   Sperm isolation; simple prep (eg, sperm wash and swim-up) for insemination or diagnosis with semen analysis

Explanation

Prior to insemination or further diagnostic studies, the sperm go through a spinning and washing process in a series of solutions. The purpose of this is to separate sperm from seminal fluids, allowing the sperm to go through a process referred to as capacitation. Capacitation is an invisible change mature spermatozoa must undergo to acquire accelerated movement, allowing them to navigate through the uterus and fallopian tube. In addition, this procedure checks the ability of the sperm to swim in a forward progressive fashion. This procedure includes a semen analysis (count, motility, volume and differential).

Relative Value Units/Medicare Edits

Non-Facility RVU	Work	PE	MP	Total
89260	0.0	0.0	0.0	0.0
Facility RVU	**Work**	**PE**	**MP**	**Total**
89260	0.0	0.0	0.0	0.0

89261

89261   Sperm isolation; complex prep (eg, Percoll gradient, albumin gradient) for insemination or diagnosis with semen analysis

Explanation

Prior to insemination or further diagnostic studies, the sperm go through a spinning and washing process in a series of solutions. The purpose of this is to separate sperm from seminal fluids, allowing the sperm to go through a process referred to as capacitation. Capacitation is an invisible change mature spermatozoa must undergo to acquire accelerated movement, allowing them to navigate through the uterus and fallopian tube. This complex prep includes a Percoll gradient and albumin gradient. This procedure includes a semen analysis (count, motility, volume and differential).

Relative Value Units/Medicare Edits

Non-Facility RVU	Work	PE	MP	Total
89261	0.0	0.0	0.0	0.0
Facility RVU	Work	PE	MP	Total
89261	0.0	0.0	0.0	0.0

89268

89268 Insemination of oocytes

Explanation

Insemination requires a sperm cell to be introduced to an egg (oocyte) for fertilization procedures. The sperm is prepared through a washing method, which separates the sperm cells from the seminal fluid. The washing filters out white blood cells, prostaglandins, and other debris, as well as cells with less motility, to provide the highest concentration of viable sperm. Once the concentrated spermatozoa have been prepared, they are placed in a culture medium with the eggs. If injection is required for fertilization, the protective coating of cells is removed from the egg and the sperm cell is directly injected.

Relative Value Units/Medicare Edits

Non-Facility RVU	Work	PE	MP	Total
89268	0.0	0.0	0.0	0.0
Facility RVU	Work	PE	MP	Total
89268	0.0	0.0	0.0	0.0

89272

89272 Extended culture of oocyte(s)/embryo(s), 4-7 days

Explanation

Culture of eggs (oocytes) or embryos usually occurs for 48 to 72 hours. This code describes an extended period of time for the cells to incubate in a culture medium, which will improve the identification of the most viable embryos. It is sometimes necessary to wait up to five days for the embryo to become a blastocyte before implantation due to high risk of multiple gestation or repeated IVF failures.

Relative Value Units/Medicare Edits

Non-Facility RVU	Work	PE	MP	Total
89272	0.0	0.0	0.0	0.0
Facility RVU	Work	PE	MP	Total
89272	0.0	0.0	0.0	0.0

89280-89281

89280 Assisted oocyte fertilization, microtechnique; less than or equal to 10 oocytes

89281 greater than 10 oocytes

Explanation

Assisted oocyte fertilization is done with microtechnique. A single sperm is injected into the egg (oocyte) to enable fertilization when sperm counts are very low or when sperm are non-motile. It requires micromanipulation of the sperm, which is also referred to as microtechnique. The usual method involves intracytoplasmic sperm injection (ICSI). Using ICSI technique, the mature egg is held in place with a holding pipette. A very delicate, sharp, hollow needle is used to immobilize and pick up a single sperm. This needle is inserted through the egg's outer shell (zona pellucida) into the cytoplasm of the egg. The sperm is injected into the cytoplasm and the needle removed. The eggs are checked the next day for evidence of fertilization. Report 89280 for 10 oocytes or less and 89281 for more than 10 oocytes.

Relative Value Units/Medicare Edits

Non-Facility RVU	Work	PE	MP	Total
89280	0.0	0.0	0.0	0.0
89281	0.0	0.0	0.0	0.0
Facility RVU	Work	PE	MP	Total
89280	0.0	0.0	0.0	0.0
89281	0.0	0.0	0.0	0.0

89290-89291

89290 Biopsy, oocyte polar body or embryo blastomere, microtechnique (for pre-implantation genetic diagnosis); less than or equal to 5 embryos

89291 greater than 5 embryos

Explanation

Biopsy of an egg (oocyte) polar body or embryo blastomere (an embryo with six to eight cells) is indicated for patients who carry genetic disorders such as Sickle cell anemia, hemophilia, Fragile X syndrome, and others, and for those experiencing difficulty with a successful IVF or ICSI. The process of a biopsy includes inserting a microneedle into a fertilized egg to extract polar bodies of the oocyte, or to extract a single cell from a six to eight cell embryo. Screenings are performed through the process of FISH (fluorescent in-situ hybridization) and PCR (polymerase chain reaction). During FISH, a small amount of DNA is analyzed through staining of fluorochromes. PCR is able to detect gene-sequences or single genes, which may have abnormal mutations. Report 89290 for a biopsy of five or less embryos and 89291 for six or more embryos.

Relative Value Units/Medicare Edits

Non-Facility RVU	Work	PE	MP	Total
89290	0.0	0.0	0.0	0.0
89291	0.0	0.0	0.0	0.0
Facility RVU	Work	PE	MP	Total
89290	0.0	0.0	0.0	0.0
89291	0.0	0.0	0.0	0.0

89300-89322

89300 Semen analysis; presence and/or motility of sperm including Huhner test (post coital)

89310 motility and count (not including Huhner test)

89320 volume, count, motility, and differential

89321 sperm presence and motility of sperm, if performed

89322 volume, count, motility, and differential using strict morphologic criteria (eg, Kruger)

Explanation

Semen analysis is generally performed in specialized infertility/andrology laboratories. Sexual activity culminating in ejaculation should be avoided for a minimum of 48 hours prior to testing. In 89300, a post coital specimen is obtained using a cervical swab. The test is timed to coincide with ovulation. Semen is tested for the presence (quantity) and/or motility of sperm. In 89310-89322, semen is collected using a condom-like seminal fluid collection device or by masturbation into a sterile container. In 89310, only sperm movement (motility) and number (concentration or count that measures how many million sperm are in each milliliter of fluid) are performed. Code 89320 reports a semen analysis that includes measurement of the ejaculate's volume, number, structure (shape) of sperm, sperm movement (motility), and direction of movement (forward motility). In addition, fluid thickness, acidity, and sugar content may be evaluated. Code 89321 tests only for the presence (quantity) and/or motility of sperm. In 89322, a detailed evaluation of the shape (morphology) is performed utilizing specially stained slides and microscopic examination of the sperm under high power magnification. In order to be considered normal, the sperm must meet a strict set of criteria regarding the shape and size of the head, mid-piece, and tail. A Kruger test is helpful in determining which reproductive techniques and methodologies may be most appropriate and successful. Tests reported with 89300-89322 may be accomplished using a variety of methods including semen function tests and computer-assisted sperm morphology/motility studies.

Relative Value Units/Medicare Edits

Non-Facility RVU	Work	PE	MP	Total
89300	0.0	0.0	0.0	0.0
89310	0.0	0.0	0.0	0.0
89320	0.0	0.0	0.0	0.0
89321	0.0	0.0	0.0	0.0
89322	0.0	0.0	0.0	0.0
Facility RVU	Work	PE	MP	Total
89300	0.0	0.0	0.0	0.0
89310	0.0	0.0	0.0	0.0
89320	0.0	0.0	0.0	0.0
89321	0.0	0.0	0.0	0.0
89322	0.0	0.0	0.0	0.0

89325

89325   Sperm antibodies

Explanation

This procedure tests for antisperm antibodies. A semen sample is placed with immunobeads; alternately, the semen sample may be placed with human or bovine cervical mucus together in a laboratory medium. The sperm antibody may be present in vaginal fluids or the male's blood or semen. Antisperm antibodies bind with the sperm inhibiting movement and their ability to fertilize an egg. The sperm appears clumped together on microscopic examination. Although the sample is sperm, some payers may cover as part of a fertility work-up for either partner.

Relative Value Units/Medicare Edits

Non-Facility RVU	Work	PE	MP	Total
89325	0.0	0.0	0.0	0.0
Facility RVU	Work	PE	MP	Total
89325	0.0	0.0	0.0	0.0

89329

89329   Sperm evaluation; hamster penetration test

Explanation

This test is also called sperm penetration assay (SPA) or hamster zona free ovum (HZFO) and tests the ability of the sperm to penetrate a hamster egg, which has been stripped of the zona pellucida (outer membrane). The patient should abstain from sexual activity culminating in ejaculation for a minimum of 48 hours. Semen is collected postcoitus using a condom-like seminal fluid collection device or by masturbation into a sterile container. Upon receiving the specimen in the laboratory, the sperm is washed and placed in a culture medium along with a single hamster egg. It is examined periodically using phase contrast microscopy. The test measures the ability of sperm to capacitate (invisible change which allows sperm to navigate rapidly forward), acrosome react (structural change fusing the outer membrane of the acrosome with the plasma membrane of the sperm head freeing enzymes in the acrosome which facilitate entry into the ovum), and fuse with the ovum.

Relative Value Units/Medicare Edits

Non-Facility RVU	Work	PE	MP	Total
89329	0.0	0.0	0.0	0.0
Facility RVU	Work	PE	MP	Total
89329	0.0	0.0	0.0	0.0

89330

89330   Sperm evaluation; cervical mucus penetration test, with or without spinnbarkeit test

Explanation

Sperm mucus interaction is assessed in vitro. Human or bovine ovulatory mucus is placed in a capillary tube. Sperm penetration is measured over a period of 90 minutes. Sperm progression measures which sperm have progressed the farthest down the tube. Patient sperm penetration can be compared with fertile sperm specimens using in vitro methods.

Relative Value Units/Medicare Edits

Non-Facility RVU	Work	PE	MP	Total
89330	0.0	0.0	0.0	0.0
Facility RVU	Work	PE	MP	Total
89330	0.0	0.0	0.0	0.0

89337

89337   Cryopreservation, mature oocyte(s)

Explanation

Cryopreservation is a technique of freezing and maintaining cells at extremely low temperatures to preserve the genetic and metabolic properties of the cell. The mature (M-II) oocyte specimens are first preserved in a cryoprotectant solution to reduce cellular damage and the tissue is placed in storage vials. The sample is gradually frozen in liquid nitrogen. Cryopreserved samples are stored at temperatures of -80 to -196 degrees centigrade. The amount of cells being frozen, the source and amount of protective solution used, and the cooling technique may vary. Oocyte cryopreservation (OC) enables patients who may be susceptible to losing ovarian function to preserve reproductive potential through the use of long-term storage of oocytes.

Relative Value Units/Medicare Edits

Non-Facility RVU	Work	PE	MP	Total
89337	0.0	0.0	0.0	0.0
Facility RVU	Work	PE	MP	Total
89337	0.0	0.0	0.0	0.0

89342-89346

89342 Storage (per year); embryo(s)
89343 sperm/semen
89344 reproductive tissue, testicular/ovarian
89346 oocyte(s)

Explanation

These codes report the long-term maintenance of preserved reproductive tissue samples and fertilized embryos in an appropriate storage facility per year. Report 89342 for embryo(s), 89343 for sperm/semen, 89344 for testicular or ovarian tissue, and 89346 for oocyte(s).

Relative Value Units/Medicare Edits

Non-Facility RVU	Work	PE	MP	Total
89342	0.0	0.0	0.0	0.0
89343	0.0	0.0	0.0	0.0
89344	0.0	0.0	0.0	0.0
89346	0.0	0.0	0.0	0.0
Facility RVU	**Work**	**PE**	**MP**	**Total**
89342	0.0	0.0	0.0	0.0
89343	0.0	0.0	0.0	0.0
89344	0.0	0.0	0.0	0.0
89346	0.0	0.0	0.0	0.0

90460-90461

90460 Immunization administration through 18 years of age via any route of administration, with counseling by physician or other qualified health care professional; first or only component of each vaccine or toxoid administered
+ 90461 each additional vaccine or toxoid component administered (List separately in addition to code for primary procedure)

Explanation

The physician or other qualified health care professional instructs the patient or family on the benefits and risks related to the vaccine or toxoid. The physician counsels the patient or family regarding signs and symptoms of adverse effects and when to seek medical attention for any adverse effects. A physician, nurse, or medical assistant administers an immunization by any route to the patient. It may be a single vaccine or a combination vaccine/toxoid in one immunization administration (e.g., diphtheria, pertussis, and tetanus toxoids are in a single DPT immunization). Report 90460 for the first or only vaccine/toxoid component. Report 90461 for each additional component. These codes report immunization administration to patients 18 years of age or younger.

Relative Value Units/Medicare Edits

Non-Facility RVU	Work	PE	MP	Total
90460	0.17	0.22	0.01	0.4
90461	0.15	0.2	0.01	0.36
Facility RVU	**Work**	**PE**	**MP**	**Total**
90460	0.17	0.22	0.01	0.4
90461	0.15	0.2	0.01	0.36

90471-90472

90471 Immunization administration (includes percutaneous, intradermal, subcutaneous, or intramuscular injections); 1 vaccine (single or combination vaccine/toxoid)
+ 90472 each additional vaccine (single or combination vaccine/toxoid) (List separately in addition to code for primary procedure)

Explanation

A physician, nurse, or medical assistant administers an injectable (percutaneous, intradermal, subcutaneous, or intramuscular) immunization to the patient. It may be a single vaccine or a combination vaccine/toxoid in one immunization administration (e.g., diphtheria, pertussis, and tetanus toxoids are in a single DPT immunization). Report 90471 for one vaccine and 90472 for each additional vaccine (single or combination vaccine/toxoid).

Relative Value Units/Medicare Edits

Non-Facility RVU	Work	PE	MP	Total
90471	0.17	0.22	0.01	0.4
90472	0.15	0.2	0.01	0.36
Facility RVU	**Work**	**PE**	**MP**	**Total**
90471	0.17	0.22	0.01	0.4
90472	0.15	0.2	0.01	0.36

90473-90474

90473 Immunization administration by intranasal or oral route; 1 vaccine (single or combination vaccine/toxoid)
+ 90474 each additional vaccine (single or combination vaccine/toxoid) (List separately in addition to code for primary procedure)

Explanation

A physician, nurse, or medical assistant administers an immunization to a patient via an intranasal (e.g., nasal spray) or an oral route (e.g., a liquid that is swallowed). It may be a single vaccine or a combination vaccine/toxoid in one immunization administration (e.g., adenovirus, Rotavirus, typhoid, poliovirus). Report 90473 for one vaccine and 90474 for each additional vaccine (single or combination vaccine/toxoid).

Relative Value Units/Medicare Edits

Non-Facility RVU	Work	PE	MP	Total
90473	0.17	0.22	0.01	0.4
90474	0.15	0.2	0.01	0.36
Facility RVU	**Work**	**PE**	**MP**	**Total**
90473	0.17	0.22	0.01	0.4
90474	0.15	0.2	0.01	0.36

[91300, 91301]

● **91300** Severe acute respiratory syndrome coronavirus 2 (SARS-CoV-2) (Coronavirus disease [COVID-19]) vaccine, mRNA-LNP, spike protein, preservative free, 30 mcg/0.3mL dosage, diluent reconstituted, for intramuscular use
● **91301** Severe acute respiratory syndrome coronavirus 2 (SARS-CoV2) (Coronavirus disease [COVID-19]) vaccine, mRNA-LNP, spike protein, preservative free, 100 mcg/0.5mL dosage, for intramuscular use

Explanation

A vaccine produces active immunization by inducing the immune system to build its own antibodies against specific microorganisms/viruses. The body retains memory of the antibody production pattern for long-term protection. These codes report a preservative-free spike protein vaccine against severe acute respiratory syndrome coronavirus 2, also known as SARS-CoV-2, Coronavirus disease, or COVID-19. Based on messenger RNA (mRNA) that utilizes a lipid nanoparticle (LNP) as a delivery platform, it is intended for intramuscular use. Report 91300 for a 30 mcg/0.3mL dosage (diluent reconstituted) and 91301 for a 100 mcg/0.5mL dosage. Report with the appropriate administration code for the first or second dose. These vaccines are currently pending FDA approval.

Relative Value Units/Medicare Edits

Non-Facility RVU	Work	PE	MP	Total
91300				
91301				
Facility RVU	**Work**	**PE**	**MP**	**Total**
91300				
91301				

90649-90651

90649 Human Papillomavirus vaccine, types 6, 11, 16, 18, quadrivalent (4vHPV), 3 dose schedule, for intramuscular use

90650 Human Papillomavirus vaccine, types 16, 18, bivalent (2vHPV), 3 dose schedule, for intramuscular use

90651 Human Papillomavirus vaccine types 6, 11, 16, 18, 31, 33, 45, 52, 58, nonavalent (9vHPV), 2 or 3 dose schedule, for intramuscular use

Explanation

A vaccine produces active immunization by inducing the immune system to manufacture its own antibodies against specific microorganisms/viruses. The body retains memory of the antibody production pattern for long-term protection. In 90649 and 90650, a human papilloma vaccine is prepared in a three-dose schedule for intramuscular use. The second dose is administered at least one to two months after the first dose and the third dose at least six months after the first dose. In 90651, the dose may be prepared in a two or three-dose schedule. The vaccine may be bivalent (2vHPV), types 16 and 18; quadrivalent (4vHPV), types 6, 11, 16, and 18; or nonavalent (9vHPV), types 6, 11, 16, 18, 31, 33, 45, 52, and 58. The vaccine immunizes a patient against HPV or assists in producing an immune reaction to the E6 and E7 viral proteins to prevent or destroy the growth of abnormal or cancerous cells. Report 90649 for the quadrivalent vaccine (4vHPV), 90650 for the bivalent vaccine (2bHPV), and 90651 for the nonavalent vaccine (9vHPV). Report these codes with the appropriate administration code.

Relative Value Units/Medicare Edits

Non-Facility RVU	Work	PE	MP	Total
90649	0.0	0.0	0.0	0.0
90650	0.0	0.0	0.0	0.0
90651	0.0	0.0	0.0	0.0
Facility RVU	**Work**	**PE**	**MP**	**Total**
90649	0.0	0.0	0.0	0.0
90650	0.0	0.0	0.0	0.0
90651	0.0	0.0	0.0	0.0

90653

90653 Influenza vaccine, inactivated (IIV), subunit, adjuvanted, for intramuscular use

Explanation

A vaccine produces active immunization by inducing the immune system to build its own antibodies against specific microorganisms/viruses. The body retains memory of the antibody production pattern for long-term protection. An inactive virus suspension of the prevalent strains of influenza (IIV), with added adjuvant, is prepared for intramuscular injection. Report this code in addition to the appropriate administration code.

Relative Value Units/Medicare Edits

Non-Facility RVU	Work	PE	MP	Total
90653	0.0	0.0	0.0	0.0
Facility RVU	**Work**	**PE**	**MP**	**Total**
90653	0.0	0.0	0.0	0.0

90654 [90630]

90654 Influenza virus vaccine, trivalent (IIV3), split virus, preservative-free, for intradermal use

90630 Influenza virus vaccine, quadrivalent (IIV4), split virus, preservative free, for intradermal use

Explanation

A vaccine produces active immunization by inducing the immune system to build its own antibodies against specific microorganisms/viruses. The body retains memory of the antibody production pattern for long-term protection. A trivalent (IIV3) or quadrivalent (IIV4), split virus suspension, preservative free vaccine of the prevalent strains of influenza is prepared for intradermal injection. Report 90654 for the trivalent vaccine and 90630 for the quadrivalent vaccine. Report these codes in addition to the appropriate administration code.

Relative Value Units/Medicare Edits

Non-Facility RVU	Work	PE	MP	Total
90630	0.0	0.0	0.0	0.0
90654	0.0	0.0	0.0	0.0
Facility RVU	**Work**	**PE**	**MP**	**Total**
90630	0.0	0.0	0.0	0.0
90654	0.0	0.0	0.0	0.0

90655-90656

90655 Influenza virus vaccine, trivalent (IIV3), split virus, preservative free, 0.25 mL dosage, for intramuscular use

90656 Influenza virus vaccine, trivalent (IIV3), split virus, preservative free, 0.5 mL dosage, for intramuscular use

Explanation

These codes report the supply of the vaccine only. A vaccine produces active immunization by inducing the immune system to build its own antibodies against specific microorganisms/viruses. The body retains memory of the antibody production pattern for long-term protection. A split virus suspension of three (two influenza A and one influenza B) (IIV3) of the most prevalent strains of influenza is prepared for intramuscular injection. Report 90655 for a 0.25 mL dose of preservative free, split virus influenza vaccine and 90656 for a 0.50 mL dose. Report these codes with the appropriate administration code.

Relative Value Units/Medicare Edits

Non-Facility RVU	Work	PE	MP	Total
90655	0.0	0.0	0.0	0.0
90656	0.0	0.0	0.0	0.0
Facility RVU	**Work**	**PE**	**MP**	**Total**
90655	0.0	0.0	0.0	0.0
90656	0.0	0.0	0.0	0.0

90657-90658

90657 Influenza virus vaccine, trivalent (IIV3), split virus, 0.25 mL dosage, for intramuscular use

90658 Influenza virus vaccine, trivalent (IIV3), split virus, 0.5 mL dosage, for intramuscular use

Explanation

These codes report the supply of the vaccine only. A vaccine produces active immunization by inducing the immune system to build its own antibodies against specific microorganisms/viruses. The body retains memory of the antibody production pattern for long-term protection. A split virus suspension of three (two influenza A and one influenza B) (IIV3) of the most prevalent strains of influenza is prepared for intramuscular use. Report 90657 for a 0.25 mL dose and 90658 for a 0.5 mL dose. The vaccine induces active immunity to the highly contagious infection of the respiratory tract caused by a myxovirus and transmitted by airborne droplet infection. Report these codes with the appropriate administration code.

Relative Value Units/Medicare Edits

Non-Facility RVU	Work	PE	MP	Total
90657	0.0	0.0	0.0	0.0
90658	0.0	0.0	0.0	0.0
Facility RVU	**Work**	**PE**	**MP**	**Total**
90657	0.0	0.0	0.0	0.0
90658	0.0	0.0	0.0	0.0

90660 [90672]

90660 Influenza virus vaccine, trivalent, live (LAIV3), for intranasal use

90672 Influenza virus vaccine, quadrivalent, live (LAIV4), for intranasal use

Explanation

A vaccine produces active immunization by inducing the immune system to build its own antibodies against specific microorganisms/viruses. The body retains memory of the antibody production pattern for long-term protection. A suspension of the prevalent strains of influenza virus is prepared for intranasal use. This live vaccination (LAIV3, LAIV4) contains the actual pathogen that has been weakened. Report these codes with the appropriate administration code. Report 90660 when the vaccine contains three strains. Report 90672 if the vaccine is comprised of four strains.

Relative Value Units/Medicare Edits

Non-Facility RVU	Work	PE	MP	Total
90660	0.0	0.0	0.0	0.0
90672	0.0	0.0	0.0	0.0
Facility RVU	**Work**	**PE**	**MP**	**Total**
90660	0.0	0.0	0.0	0.0
90672	0.0	0.0	0.0	0.0

[90673]

90673 Influenza virus vaccine, trivalent (RIV3), derived from recombinant DNA, hemagglutinin (HA) protein only, preservative and antibiotic free, for intramuscular use

Explanation

A vaccine produces active immunization by inducing the immune system to build its own antibodies against specific microorganisms/viruses. The body retains memory of the antibody production pattern for long-term protection. A suspension of recombinant hemagglutinin (HA) protein is prepared for intramuscular use. This is the only influenza vaccination that is manufactured

without the use of the influenza virus. Report this code with the appropriate administration code.

Relative Value Units/Medicare Edits

Non-Facility RVU	Work	PE	MP	Total
90673	0.0	0.0	0.0	0.0
Facility RVU	**Work**	**PE**	**MP**	**Total**
90673	0.0	0.0	0.0	0.0

90664-90668

90664 Influenza virus vaccine, live (LAIV), pandemic formulation, for intranasal use

90666 Influenza virus vaccine (IIV), pandemic formulation, split virus, preservative free, for intramuscular use

90667 Influenza virus vaccine (IIV), pandemic formulation, split virus, adjuvanted, for intramuscular use

90668 Influenza virus vaccine (IIV), pandemic formulation, split virus, for intramuscular use

Explanation

These codes report pandemic formulations of the influenza virus vaccine. An influenza pandemic is a large-scale eruption of disease that takes place when a new influenza virus emerges in the human population, spreading easily between individuals and resulting in serious illness. A pandemic can rapidly travel across a whole region, a continent, or the world. Unlike seasonal influenza, individuals have little immunity to this virus. A suspension of the live prevalent strain of pandemic influenza virus (LAIV) is prepared for intranasal use in 90664; this live vaccination contains the actual pathogen. Subvirion (split virus) vaccines do not contain the entire virus; rather, they contain purified portions. Split virus vaccines are believed to cause fewer adverse effects in children and young adults, while maintaining its ability to stimulate an immune response (immunogenicity) comparable to that of whole virus preparations. Due to their decreased rates of side effects, only split virus preparations are recommended for children younger than 13 years of age. A suspension of the prevalent strain of pandemic influenza virus (IIV) is prepared for intramuscular use; 90668 reports the split virus vaccine, 90666 reports the preservative-free split-virus version, and 90667 reports the adjuvanted version. These codes identify the vaccine products only and must be reported in addition to the appropriate immunization administration codes.

Relative Value Units/Medicare Edits

Non-Facility RVU	Work	PE	MP	Total
90664	0.0	0.0	0.0	0.0
90666	0.0	0.0	0.0	0.0
90667	0.0	0.0	0.0	0.0
90668	0.0	0.0	0.0	0.0
Facility RVU	**Work**	**PE**	**MP**	**Total**
90664	0.0	0.0	0.0	0.0
90666	0.0	0.0	0.0	0.0
90667	0.0	0.0	0.0	0.0
90668	0.0	0.0	0.0	0.0

90682-90689 [90756]

90756 Influenza virus vaccine, quadrivalent (ccIIV4), derived from cell cultures, subunit, antibiotic free, 0.5mL dosage, for intramuscular use

90682 Influenza virus vaccine, quadrivalent (RIV4), derived from recombinant DNA, hemagglutinin (HA) protein only, preservative and antibiotic free, for intramuscular use

90685 Influenza virus vaccine, quadrivalent (IIV4), split virus, preservative free, 0.25 mL, for intramuscular use

90686 Influenza virus vaccine, quadrivalent (IIV4), split virus, preservative free, 0.5 mL dosage, for intramuscular use

90687 Influenza virus vaccine, quadrivalent (IIV4), split virus, 0.25 mL dosage, for intramuscular use

90688 Influenza virus vaccine, quadrivalent (IIV4), split virus, 0.5 mL dosage, for intramuscular use

90689 Influenza virus vaccine quadrivalent (IIV4), inactivated, adjuvanted, preservative free, 0.25 mL dosage, for intramuscular use

Explanation

These codes report the supply of the vaccine only. A vaccine produces active immunization by inducing the immune system to build its own antibodies against specific microorganisms/viruses. The body retains memory of the antibody production pattern for long-term protection. A split virus suspension of four (two influenza A and two influenza B) (IIV4) of the most prevalent strains of influenza is prepared for intramuscular injection. Report 90682 for an antibiotic and preservative free, quadrivalent (RIV4) influenza vaccine derived from recombinant DNA, hemagglutinin (HA) protein only. Report 90685 for a preservative free, split virus influenza vaccine dose of 0.25 mL and 90686 for a 0.5 mL dose. Report 90689 for a preservative free, inactivated, and adjuvanted quadrivalent (IIV4) influenza vaccine dose of 0.25 mL. Report 90687 for a split virus influenza vaccine dose of 0.25 mL that is not preservative free and 90688 for a 0.5 mL dose. Report 90756 for an antibiotic, quadrivalent (ccIIV4) influenza vaccine derived from cell cultures. Report these codes with the appropriate administration code.

Relative Value Units/Medicare Edits

Non-Facility RVU	Work	PE	MP	Total
90682	0.0	0.0	0.0	0.0
90685	0.0	0.0	0.0	0.0
90686	0.0	0.0	0.0	0.0
90687	0.0	0.0	0.0	0.0
90688	0.0	0.0	0.0	0.0
90689	0.0	0.0	0.0	0.0
90756	0.0	0.0	0.0	0.0
Facility RVU	**Work**	**PE**	**MP**	**Total**
90682	0.0	0.0	0.0	0.0
90685	0.0	0.0	0.0	0.0
90686	0.0	0.0	0.0	0.0
90687	0.0	0.0	0.0	0.0
90688	0.0	0.0	0.0	0.0
90689	0.0	0.0	0.0	0.0
90756	0.0	0.0	0.0	0.0

90736 [90750]

90736 Zoster (shingles) vaccine (HZV), live, for subcutaneous injection

90750 Zoster (shingles) vaccine (HZV), recombinant, subunit, adjuvanted, for intramuscular use

Explanation

A vaccine produces active immunization by inducing the immune system to manufacture its own antibodies against specific microorganisms/viruses. The body retains memory of these antibody production patterns for long-term protection. In 90736, a live herpes zoster (HZV) or shingles vaccine for subcutaneous injection is administered. In 90750, a recombinant, subunit, adjuvanted vaccine is administered intramuscularly. Shingles is a reactivation of the herpes zoster virus that causes chickenpox. The virus persists in a dormant state and may reactivate with certain conditions or advancing age that cause or is associated with immune system compromise. This vaccine prevents herpes zoster and postherpetic neuralgia as a result of the dormant virus in sensory nerve cells. Report these codes with the appropriate administration code.

Relative Value Units/Medicare Edits

Non-Facility RVU	Work	PE	MP	Total
90736	0.0	0.0	0.0	0.0
90750	0.0	0.0	0.0	0.0
Facility RVU	**Work**	**PE**	**MP**	**Total**
90736	0.0	0.0	0.0	0.0
90750	0.0	0.0	0.0	0.0

90739-90747

90739 Hepatitis B vaccine (HepB), adult dosage, 2 dose schedule, for intramuscular use

90740 Hepatitis B vaccine (HepB), dialysis or immunosuppressed patient dosage, 3 dose schedule, for intramuscular use

90743 Hepatitis B vaccine (HepB), adolescent, 2 dose schedule, for intramuscular use

90744 Hepatitis B vaccine (HepB), pediatric/adolescent dosage, 3 dose schedule, for intramuscular use

90746 Hepatitis B vaccine (HepB), adult dosage, 3 dose schedule, for intramuscular use

90747 Hepatitis B vaccine (HepB), dialysis or immunosuppressed patient dosage, 4 dose schedule, for intramuscular use

Explanation

A vaccine produces active immunization by inducing the immune system to build its own antibodies against specific microorganisms/viruses. The body retains memory of these antibody production patterns for long-term protection. These codes are used to report the supply of a hepatitis B (HepB) vaccine for intramuscular use, prepared in various dosages. Report 90739 for an adult two-dose schedule; 90740 for a three-dose schedule for a dialysis or immunosuppressed patient; 90743 for an adolescent two-dose schedule; 90744 for a pediatric/adolescent three-dose schedule; 90746 for an adult three-dose schedule; and 90747 for a four-dose schedule for a dialysis or immunosuppressed patient. Report these codes with the appropriate administration code.

Relative Value Units/Medicare Edits

Non-Facility RVU	Work	PE	MP	Total
90739	0.0	0.0	0.0	0.0
90740	0.0	0.0	0.0	0.0
90743	0.0	0.0	0.0	0.0
90744	0.0	0.0	0.0	0.0
90746	0.0	0.0	0.0	0.0
90747	0.0	0.0	0.0	0.0
Facility RVU	**Work**	**PE**	**MP**	**Total**
90739	0.0	0.0	0.0	0.0
90740	0.0	0.0	0.0	0.0
90743	0.0	0.0	0.0	0.0
90744	0.0	0.0	0.0	0.0
90746	0.0	0.0	0.0	0.0
90747	0.0	0.0	0.0	0.0

90748

90748   Hepatitis B and Haemophilus influenzae type b vaccine (Hib-HepB), for intramuscular use

Explanation

A vaccine produces active immunization by inducing the immune system to build its own antibodies against specific microorganisms/viruses. The body retains memory of these antibody production patterns for long-term protection. This code describes a combined hepatitis B and Haemophilus influenzae type B (Hib-HepB) vaccine for intramuscular use. Report this code with the appropriate administration code.

Relative Value Units/Medicare Edits

Non-Facility RVU	Work	PE	MP	Total
90748	0.0	0.0	0.0	0.0
Facility RVU	**Work**	**PE**	**MP**	**Total**
90748	0.0	0.0	0.0	0.0

92950

92950   Cardiopulmonary resuscitation (eg, in cardiac arrest)

Explanation

Cardiopulmonary arrest occurs when the patient's heart and lungs suddenly stop. In a clinical setting, cardiopulmonary resuscitation, the attempt at restarting the heart and lungs, is usually directed by a physician or another health care provider who is certified in Advanced Cardiac Life Support (ACLS). The patient's lungs are ventilated by mouth-to-mouth breathing or by a bag and mask. The patient's circulation is assisted using external chest compression. An electronic defibrillator may be used to shock the heart into restarting. Medications used to restart the heart include epinephrine and lidocaine.

Relative Value Units/Medicare Edits

Non-Facility RVU	Work	PE	MP	Total
92950	4.0	4.77	0.39	9.16
Facility RVU	**Work**	**PE**	**MP**	**Total**
92950	4.0	0.97	0.39	5.36

93975

93975   Duplex scan of arterial inflow and venous outflow of abdominal, pelvic, scrotal contents and/or retroperitoneal organs; complete study

Explanation

The physician or assistant performs a Duplex ultrasound scan, which is a combination of real-time and Doppler studies, of the arteries and veins in the abdominal, pelvic, or genitorectal areas to evaluate vascular blood flow in relation to blockage. This code applies to a complete bilateral evaluation.

Relative Value Units/Medicare Edits

Non-Facility RVU	Work	PE	MP	Total
93975	1.16	6.55	0.12	7.83
Facility RVU	**Work**	**PE**	**MP**	**Total**
93975	1.16	6.55	0.12	7.83

93976

93976   Duplex scan of arterial inflow and venous outflow of abdominal, pelvic, scrotal contents and/or retroperitoneal organs; limited study

Explanation

The physician or assistant performs a Duplex ultrasound scan, which is a combination of real-time and Doppler studies, of the arteries and veins in the abdominal, pelvic, or genitorectal areas to evaluate vascular blood flow in relation to blockage. This code applies to a limited evaluation.

Relative Value Units/Medicare Edits

Non-Facility RVU	Work	PE	MP	Total
93976	0.8	3.77	0.07	4.64
Facility RVU	**Work**	**PE**	**MP**	**Total**
93976	0.8	3.77	0.07	4.64

96040

★96040   Medical genetics and genetic counseling services, each 30 minutes face-to-face with patient/family

Explanation

The trained genetic counselor meets with an individual, couple, or family to investigate family genetic history and assess the risks associated with genetic defects in offspring. This code covers 30 minutes of face-to-face counseling, review of medical data, or data collection (interviews).

Relative Value Units/Medicare Edits

Non-Facility RVU	Work	PE	MP	Total
96040	0.0	1.24	0.05	1.29
Facility RVU	**Work**	**PE**	**MP**	**Total**
96040	0.0	1.24	0.05	1.29

96160-96161

96160   Administration of patient-focused health risk assessment instrument (eg, health hazard appraisal) with scoring and documentation, per standardized instrument

96161   Administration of caregiver-focused health risk assessment instrument (eg, depression inventory) for the benefit of the patient, with scoring and documentation, per standardized instrument

Explanation

A provision in the Patient Protection and Affordable Care Act of 2010 (ACA) established a Medicare Wellness Visit, which included a Health Risk Assessment (HRA) and customized wellness or prevention plan. HRAs are typically completed by a patient or caregiver prior to the encounter with a physician or other qualified health care professional, but can involve the assistance of the clinician and/or staff members. The HRA tool is purposely designed to be brief, straightforward, and easy to comprehend with questions such as patient demographic information, personal and/or family history, a self-assessment of how the patient interprets his/her health to be, risk factors, biometric measurements, and compliance. Completion of the HRA tool takes approximately 20 minutes and may be done via the internet or on a paper-based document. Assessments that emphasize a patient or caregiver focus may be referred to as HRA plus assessments and as such should be person centered and culturally appropriate in all areas, including, but not limited to, the assessment instrument, the administration process of the assessment, clinician communication with the patient regarding findings, as well as followup and monitoring. Additionally, the patient-focused HRA takes into consideration the importance of care support services over and above the health care system; for example, by family members, community support services, or even in the workplace setting where the individual receiving care is not deemed to be a "patient." An emphasis is also placed on cultural competency as means of limited health disparities through respect of the patient's beliefs and understanding the mental and physical ways a patient can experience illness and health and working together to establish a health plan. Another area of patient-focused care involves areas of importance to patients as consumers, such as convenience as well as increasing outcomes that matter to patients; for example, improved quality of life and function. Similarly, caregiver-focused assessment tools serve to identify areas of concern such as stress levels, depression, and the burdens placed on the caregiver. HRAs contribute to the goals of the government to drive health improvements, quality of life, and value for the health care delivery system in the United States. Report 96160 for administration of a patient-focused health risk assessment tool and 96161 for administration of a caregiver-focused assessment tool. Both codes include scoring and documentation of the assessment tool.

Relative Value Units/Medicare Edits

Non-Facility RVU	Work	PE	MP	Total
96160	0.0	0.07	0.0	0.07
96161	0.0	0.07	0.0	0.07
Facility RVU	Work	PE	MP	Total
96160	0.0	0.07	0.0	0.07
96161	0.0	0.07	0.0	0.07

96360-96361

| | 96360 | Intravenous infusion, hydration; initial, 31 minutes to 1 hour |
| + | 96361 | each additional hour (List separately in addition to code for primary procedure) |

Explanation

A physician or an assistant under direct physician supervision infuses a hydration solution (prepackaged fluid and electrolytes) for 31 minutes to one hour through an intravenous catheter inserted by needle into a patient's vein or by infusion through an existing indwelling intravascular access catheter or port. Report 96361 for each additional hour beyond the first hour. Intravenous infusion for hydration lasting 30 minutes or less is not reported.

Relative Value Units/Medicare Edits

Non-Facility RVU	Work	PE	MP	Total
96360	0.17	0.77	0.02	0.96
96361	0.09	0.28	0.01	0.38
Facility RVU	Work	PE	MP	Total
96360	0.17	0.77	0.02	0.96
96361	0.09	0.28	0.01	0.38

96365-96368

	96365	Intravenous infusion, for therapy, prophylaxis, or diagnosis (specify substance or drug); initial, up to 1 hour
+	96366	each additional hour (List separately in addition to code for primary procedure)
+	96367	additional sequential infusion of a new drug/substance, up to 1 hour (List separately in addition to code for primary procedure)
+	96368	concurrent infusion (List separately in addition to code for primary procedure)

Explanation

A physician or an assistant under direct physician supervision injects or infuses a therapeutic, prophylactic (preventive), or diagnostic medication other than chemotherapy or other highly complex drugs or biologic agents via intravenous route. Infusions are administered through an intravenous catheter inserted by needle into a patient's vein or by injection or infusion through an existing indwelling intravascular access catheter or port. Report 96365 for the initial hour and 96366 for each additional hour. Report 96367 for each additional sequential infusion of a different substance or drug, up to one hour, and 96368 for each concurrent infusion of substances other than chemotherapy or other highly complex drugs or biologic agents.

Relative Value Units/Medicare Edits

Non-Facility RVU	Work	PE	MP	Total
96365	0.21	1.74	0.05	2.0
96366	0.18	0.42	0.01	0.61
96367	0.19	0.66	0.02	0.87
96368	0.17	0.41	0.01	0.59
Facility RVU	Work	PE	MP	Total
96365	0.21	1.74	0.05	2.0
96366	0.18	0.42	0.01	0.61
96367	0.19	0.66	0.02	0.87
96368	0.17	0.41	0.01	0.59

98966-98968

98966	Telephone assessment and management service provided by a qualified nonphysician health care professional to an established patient, parent, or guardian not originating from a related assessment and management service provided within the previous 7 days nor leading to an assessment and management service or procedure within the next 24 hours or soonest available appointment; 5-10 minutes of medical discussion
98967	11-20 minutes of medical discussion
98968	21-30 minutes of medical discussion

Explanation

A qualified health care professional (nonphysician) provides telephone assessment and management services to a patient in a non-face-to-face encounter. These episodes of care may be initiated by an established patient or by the patient's guardian. These codes are not reported if the telephone service results in a decision to see the patient within 24 hours or at the next available urgent visit appointment; instead, the phone encounter is regarded as part of the pre-service work of the subsequent face-to-face encounter. These codes are also not reported if the telephone call is in reference to a service performed and reported by the qualified health care professional that occurred within the past seven days or within the postoperative period of a previously completed procedure. This applies both to unsolicited patient follow-up or that requested by the health care professional. Report 98966 for telephone services requiring five to 10 minutes of medical discussion, 98967 for telephone services requiring 11 to 20 minutes of medical discussion, and 98968 for telephone services requiring 21 to 30 minutes of medical discussion.

Relative Value Units/Medicare Edits

Non-Facility RVU	Work	PE	MP	Total
98966	0.25	0.13	0.02	0.4
98967	0.5	0.23	0.05	0.78
98968	0.75	0.33	0.06	1.14
Facility RVU	Work	PE	MP	Total
98966	0.25	0.1	0.02	0.37
98967	0.5	0.19	0.05	0.74
98968	0.75	0.29	0.06	1.1

98970-98972

98970 Qualified nonphysician health care professional online digital assessment and management, for an established patient, for up to 7 days, cumulative time during the 7 days; 5-10 minutes

98971 11-20 minutes

98972 21 or more minutes

Explanation

Online digital evaluation and management services are non-face-to-face encounters originating from the established patient to a qualified nonphysician health care professional for evaluation or management of a problem utilizing internet resources. The service includes all communication, prescription, and laboratory orders with permanent storage in the patient's medical record. The service may include more than one provider responding to the same patient and is only reportable once during seven days for the same encounter. Do not report this code if the online patient request is related to an E/M service that occurred within the previous seven days or within the global period following a procedure. Report 98970 if the cumulative time during the seven-day period is five to 10 minutes; 98971 for 11 to 20 minutes; and 98972 for 21 or more minutes.

Relative Value Units/Medicare Edits

Non-Facility RVU	Work	PE	MP	Total
98970	0.0	0.0	0.0	0.0
98971	0.0	0.0	0.0	0.0
98972	0.0	0.0	0.0	0.0
Facility RVU	Work	PE	MP	Total
98970	0.0	0.0	0.0	0.0
98971	0.0	0.0	0.0	0.0
98972	0.0	0.0	0.0	0.0

99000

99000 Handling and/or conveyance of specimen for transfer from the office to a laboratory

Explanation

This code is adjunct to basic services rendered. This code is reported for the handling and/or conveyance of a specimen from the provider's office to a laboratory.

Relative Value Units/Medicare Edits

Non-Facility RVU	Work	PE	MP	Total
99000	0.0	0.0	0.0	0.0
Facility RVU	Work	PE	MP	Total
99000	0.0	0.0	0.0	0.0

99001

99001 Handling and/or conveyance of specimen for transfer from the patient in other than an office to a laboratory (distance may be indicated)

Explanation

This code is adjunct to basic services rendered. This code is reported for the handling and/or conveyance of a specimen from the patient in a location other than the provider's office to the laboratory.

Relative Value Units/Medicare Edits

Non-Facility RVU	Work	PE	MP	Total
99001	0.0	0.0	0.0	0.0
Facility RVU	Work	PE	MP	Total
99001	0.0	0.0	0.0	0.0

99026-99027

99026 Hospital mandated on call service; in-hospital, each hour

99027 out-of-hospital, each hour

Explanation

The code reports the time for hospital mandated on call service provided by the physician. This code does not include prolonged physician attendance time for standby services or the time spent performing other reportable procedures or services. Report 99026 for each hour of hospital mandated on call service spent in the hospital and 99027 for each hour of hospital mandated on call service spent outside the hospital.

Relative Value Units/Medicare Edits

Non-Facility RVU	Work	PE	MP	Total
99026	0.0	0.0	0.0	0.0
99027	0.0	0.0	0.0	0.0
Facility RVU	Work	PE	MP	Total
99026	0.0	0.0	0.0	0.0
99027	0.0	0.0	0.0	0.0

99050

99050 Services provided in the office at times other than regularly scheduled office hours, or days when the office is normally closed (eg, holidays, Saturday or Sunday), in addition to basic service

Explanation

This code is adjunct to basic services rendered. The physician reports this code to indicate services after posted office hours in addition to basic services.

Relative Value Units/Medicare Edits

Non-Facility RVU	Work	PE	MP	Total
99050	0.0	0.0	0.0	0.0
Facility RVU	Work	PE	MP	Total
99050	0.0	0.0	0.0	0.0

99051

99051   Service(s) provided in the office during regularly scheduled evening, weekend, or holiday office hours, in addition to basic service

Explanation

This code is adjunct to basic services rendered. The physician reports this code to indicate services provided during posted evening, weekend, or holiday office hours in addition to basic services.

Relative Value Units/Medicare Edits

Non-Facility RVU	Work	PE	MP	Total
99051	0.0	0.0	0.0	0.0
Facility RVU	Work	PE	MP	Total
99051	0.0	0.0	0.0	0.0

99053

99053   Service(s) provided between 10:00 PM and 8:00 AM at 24-hour facility, in addition to basic service

Explanation

This code is adjunct to basic services rendered. The physician reports this code to indicate services provided between 10 p.m. and 8 a.m. at a 24-hour facility in addition to basic services.

Relative Value Units/Medicare Edits

Non-Facility RVU	Work	PE	MP	Total
99053	0.0	0.0	0.0	0.0
Facility RVU	Work	PE	MP	Total
99053	0.0	0.0	0.0	0.0

99056

99056   Service(s) typically provided in the office, provided out of the office at request of patient, in addition to basic service

Explanation

This code is adjunct to basic services rendered. The physician reports this code to indicate services typically provided in the office that are provided in a different location at the request of a patient.

Relative Value Units/Medicare Edits

Non-Facility RVU	Work	PE	MP	Total
99056	0.0	0.0	0.0	0.0
Facility RVU	Work	PE	MP	Total
99056	0.0	0.0	0.0	0.0

99058

99058   Service(s) provided on an emergency basis in the office, which disrupts other scheduled office services, in addition to basic service

Explanation

This code is adjunct to basic services rendered. The physician reports this code to indicate services provided in the office on an emergency basis that disrupt other scheduled office services.

Relative Value Units/Medicare Edits

Non-Facility RVU	Work	PE	MP	Total
99058	0.0	0.0	0.0	0.0
Facility RVU	Work	PE	MP	Total
99058	0.0	0.0	0.0	0.0

99060

99060   Service(s) provided on an emergency basis, out of the office, which disrupts other scheduled office services, in addition to basic service

Explanation

This code is adjunct to basic services rendered. The physician reports this code to indicate services provided on an emergency basis in a location other than the physician's office that disrupt other scheduled office services.

Relative Value Units/Medicare Edits

Non-Facility RVU	Work	PE	MP	Total
99060	0.0	0.0	0.0	0.0
Facility RVU	Work	PE	MP	Total
99060	0.0	0.0	0.0	0.0

99601-99602

99601   Home infusion/specialty drug administration, per visit (up to 2 hours);

+   99602   each additional hour (List separately in addition to code for primary procedure)

Explanation

A home health professional visits the patient at home to perform the infusion of a specialty drug per a physician's order. The home health provider brings the supplies and medication required and administers and oversees the infusion. Each infusion takes up to two hours per visit for 99601. Report 99602 for each additional hour.

Relative Value Units/Medicare Edits

Non-Facility RVU	Work	PE	MP	Total
99601	0.0	0.0	0.0	0.0
99602	0.0	0.0	0.0	0.0
Facility RVU	Work	PE	MP	Total
99601	0.0	0.0	0.0	0.0
99602	0.0	0.0	0.0	0.0

0071T-0072T

0071T   Focused ultrasound ablation of uterine leiomyomata, including MR guidance; total leiomyomata volume less than 200 cc of tissue

0072T   total leiomyomata volume greater or equal to 200 cc of tissue

Explanation

Focused ultrasound ablation is a noninvasive surgical technique that uses thermal ablation to destroy uterine leiomyomata. In focused ultrasound ablation the ultrasound beam penetrates through soft tissues causing localized high temperatures for a few seconds at the targeted site, in this case the uterine leiomyomata. This produces thermocoagulation and necrosis of the uterine leiomyomata without damage to overlaying and surrounding tissues. Magnetic resonance (MR) guidance is used in conjunction with focused ultrasound ablation to provide more precise target definition. Since certain MR parameters are also temperature sensitive, MR guidance also allows estimation of optimal thermal doses to the uterine leiomyomata and detection of relatively small temperature elevations in surrounding tissues thereby preventing any irreversible damage to surrounding tissues. Report 0071T for total leiomyomata tissue volume less than 200 cc. Report 0072T for leiomyomata tissue volume equal to or greater than 200 cc.

0404T

0404T Transcervical uterine fibroid(s) ablation with ultrasound guidance, radiofrequency

Explanation

The physician performs transcervical uterine fibroid ablation. The physician utilizes a single system device comprised of a reusable intrauterine ultrasound (IUUS) probe and a single use, disposable articulating radiofrequency handpiece, along with integrated components that may include a radiofrequency generator and an ultrasound system with custom graphical user interface. The process enables the transcervical destruction of fibroids without incisions or general anesthesia. The patient is administered anesthesia (typically regional or conscious sedation with or without paracervical blockade). An electrode pad is placed on each front thigh area. Transvaginal ultrasound is used to identify the location and size of each fibroid. The cervix is dilated to approximately 8 mm and the handpiece is inserted transcervically into the uterus, along with a small amount of sterile water or 1.5% glycine for acoustic coupling. Once the size, angle, and location of the ablation is established, the physician advances the trocar-tipped introducer into the fibroid under intrauterine ultrasound imaging. Once properly positioned, the physician deploys the electrodes. Each fibroid receives one or more ablations at the discretion of the physician. One ablation usually destroys a 5 cm myoma. This technique permits the physician to plan exactly what will be ablated and avoid heating up the serosa and other tissues outside the uterus.

0475T-0478T

0475T Recording of fetal magnetic cardiac signal using at least 3 channels; patient recording and storage, data scanning with signal extraction, technical analysis and result, as well as supervision, review, and interpretation of report by a physician or other qualified health care professional

0476T patient recording, data scanning, with raw electronic signal transfer of data and storage

0477T signal extraction, technical analysis, and result

0478T review, interpretation, report by physician or other qualified health care professional

Explanation

The magnetic field created from electrical activity in the fetal heart is measured in a noninvasive technique that uses microfabricated optically pumped magnetometer (OPM) technology that works to fit the patient's abdomen at any stage of pregnancy. Individual sensors are inserted into a flexible belt-shaped holder, which is connected to light sources and electronics that are placed outside of a magnetically shielded room via optical and electrical cabling as fetal cardiac signals have only a very small magnitude. Two sensor belts are placed over a pregnant patient's abdomen and one over her chest. Recordings from the fetal magnetocardiogram placed over the patient's abdomen contains the mother's cardiac signal, which often dominates the fetal heart signals; to address this, orthogonal projection and independent component analysis signal processing methods are applied in order to obtain only fetal signals. In addition, the fetal heartrate is also removed from the fetal magnetocardiogram. These tests offer a lower cost means of evaluating certain kinds of fetal silent heart arrhythmias that may not be detected using standard echocardiography. Report 0475T for a complete test recording the fetal magnetic cardiac signal using a minimum of three channels with patient recording and storage, data scanning with signal extraction, analysis, and results including review, supervision, and interpretation from a physician or other qualified health care professional. Report 0476T for recording, data scanning, and raw electronic signal transfer of data

and storage. Report 0477T for signal extraction, technical analysis, and result only. Report 0478T for review and interpretation by the clinician.

0487T

0487T Biomechanical mapping, transvaginal, with report

Explanation

Biomechanical mapping is a diagnostic test used to assess vaginal conditions, muscles, and connective tissues in the female patient's pelvic floor that may contribute in analyzing various treatment options and identify the optimal treatment for women with prolapse, incontinence, atrophy, and some forms of pelvic pain. Vaginal tactile imaging (VTI) allows biomechanical characterization of soft tissue across the entire length of the front, back, and side vaginal walls, at rest as well as with manually induced pressure, muscle relaxation and contraction, and Valsalva maneuver. The VTI system is comprised of a vaginal probe and a movable computer display cart. The probe is equipped with 96 pressure or tactile sensors that are positioned every 2.5 mm along both sides of the probe, an orientation sensor, and temperature sensors with micro-heaters. The patient is placed in the dorsal lithotomy position with an empty bladder and rectum. The VTI probe is inserted into the patient's vagina using a lubricating jelly for both the patient's comfort and to provide reproducible boundary/contact conditions with deformed vaginal tissue. Data are sampled from the probe sensors and displayed on the VTI computer display in real time. The probe surfaces that contact the vaginal walls are preheated to human body temperature. The VTI software provides visualization, analysis, information, and reporting tools. The acquired data and information from the subsequent analysis can be used for quantitative assessment of the vaginal and pelvic floor conditions. A full VTI scan is performed and takes approximately five minutes to complete.

0500T

0500T Infectious agent detection by nucleic acid (DNA or RNA), human papillomavirus (HPV) for five or more separately reported high-risk HPV types (eg, 16, 18, 31, 33, 35, 39, 45, 51, 52, 56, 58, 59, 68) (ie, genotyping)

Explanation

This test may be requested as human papillomavirus (HPV) according to high-risk types (16, 18, 31, 33, 35, 39, 45, 51, 52, 56, 58, 59, and 68). Human papillomaviruses are a genus of viruses that cause warts (benign neoplasms of skin and mucous membranes). There are at least 58 known types. HPV is commonly associated with plantar and genital warts. HPV infection of the cervix is of particular concern as it may be associated with cervical cancer. Methodology is a diagnostic rapid batch, signal amplification, and cost-effective qualitative detection assay of 14 high-risk HPV genotypes, for the detection of cytological cervical squamous intraepithelial lesions (SIL), such as the careHPV Test. Specimen is cervical and vaginal specimens. This type of test is often used in resource-limited environments.

0548T-0551T

0548T Transperineal periurethral balloon continence device; bilateral placement, including cystoscopy and fluoroscopy

0549T unilateral placement, including cystoscopy and fluoroscopy

0550T removal, each balloon

0551T adjustment of balloon(s) fluid volume

Explanation

These procedures describe minimally invasive, long-term, and adjustable continence therapy for stress urinary incontinence (SUI) utilizing a proprietary balloon device. Indications often include post-prostatectomy incontinence in males and intrinsic sphincter deficiency or a previously failed surgery in females. Following appropriate anesthesia (general, spinal, or local), the patient is placed in a lithotomy position that enables access to the perineum. A cystourethroscopy is performed, leaving the cystoscope sheath in place during the procedure for visualization and palpation of the ureter. Via transverse perineal incisions and under fluoroscopic guidance, implantation instruments are advanced to the area of the bladder neck and the tissue is dilated to create a space for the balloon device. The balloon is inserted to the level of the bladder neck under fluoroscopic guidance and inflated using a needle to inject an isotonic filling solution into the port. The procedure is repeated on the contralateral side. Titanium ports are placed under the skin of the scrotum in males and under the skin of the labia majora in females. Incisions are closed with resorbable sutures and a dressing is applied. The fluid-filled balloons provide support and pressure to stop urine leakages during sneezing, coughing, exercising, or other physical exertion. Once implanted, the clinician can adjust the device at any time as required to meet the patient's needs. Report 0548T for bilateral placement and 0549T for unilateral placement. For removal, report 0550T for each balloon removed. Report 0551T for balloon fluid volume adjustments.

0567T-0568T

0567T Permanent fallopian tube occlusion with degradable biopolymer implant, transcervical approach, including transvaginal ultrasound

0568T Introduction of mixture of saline and air for sonosalpingography to confirm occlusion of fallopian tubes, transcervical approach, including transvaginal ultrasound and pelvic ultrasound

Explanation

This nonsurgical female contraception procedure consists of the implantation of a temporary biopolymer that triggers a natural healing response, causing scar tissue to form a permanent closure of the fallopian over time. The physician inserts a thin plastic tube into the uterus. Transvaginal ultrasound may be utilized. A small amount of degradable biopolymer material is delivered near the fallopian tubes. The tube is removed and the biopolymer begins a wound-healing response that results in scar tissue. The biopolymer is naturally excreted from the uterine cavity over time. Approximately three months following this procedure, the physician confirms the fallopian tube occlusion by introducing a mixture of saline and air for a sonosalpingogram. Report 0567T for the occlusion procedure and 0568T for the sonosalpingography to confirm occlusion. Transvaginal and pelvic ultrasound are included in 0568T.

0596T-0597T

● **0596T** Temporary female intraurethral valve-pump (ie, voiding prosthesis); initial insertion, including urethral measurement

● **0597T** replacement

Explanation

The physician treats permanent urinary retention due to impaired detrusor contractility (IDC) with a replaceable urinary prosthesis that mimics normal urination. This two-component system consists of a urethral insert with an internal valve-pump mechanism and a hand-held rechargeable activator that operates the valve-pump. Approximately one week prior to the insertion procedure, the correct device size is determined using a proprietary sizing tool. On the day of the procedure, the patient is placed in the lithotomy position and the meatus area is cleansed. Analgesic medical lubricant is applied to the external body of the device, after which it is inserted into the urethra using an introducer until the outer flange touches the edge of the meatus. The introducer's plunger is depressed, the device is released, and the introducer is removed. Following insertion, the physician performs a check for leakage and for proper device functioning using the activator. Holding the activator against the lower pubic area just above the urethral opening, the button is depressed to initiate urination. Upon completion of urination, the button is released and the activator is held in place for an additional three seconds until the valve has closed, completing the urination process. Report 0596T for the initial insertion and 0597T for a replacement procedure.

● New   ▲ Revised   + Add On   ★ Telemedicine   [Resequenced]

Correct Coding Initiative Update 26.3

❖Indicates Mutually Exclusive Edit

0071T 0213T, 0216T, 36000, 36410, 36591-36592, 51701-51702, 57180, 57400-57410, 57452, 57500, 57530, 57800, 58100, 61650, 62324-62327, 64415-64417, 64435, 64450, 64454, 64486-64490, 64493, 69990, 72195-72197, 74712, 76376-76380, 76940, 76970, 76998, 77013, 77021-77022, 96360, 96365, 96372, 96374-96377, 96523, 99446-99449, 99451-99452, G0471

0072T 0071T, 0213T, 0216T, 36000, 36410, 36591-36592, 51701-51702, 57180, 57400-57410, 57452, 57500, 57530, 57800, 58100, 61650, 62324-62327, 64415-64417, 64435, 64450, 64454, 64486-64490, 64493, 69990, 72195-72197, 74712, 76376-76380, 76940, 76970, 76998, 77013, 77021-77022, 96360, 96365, 96372, 96374-96377, 96523, 99446-99449, 99451-99452, G0471

0404T 0213T, 0216T, 0228T, 0230T, 0567T, 12001-12007, 12011-12057, 13100-13133, 13151-13153, 36000, 36400-36410, 36420-36430, 36440, 36600, 36640, 43752, 51701-51703, 57100, 57410, 57800, 58100, 62320-62327, 64400, 64405-64408, 64415-64435, 64445-64454, 64461, 64463, 64479, 64483, 64486-64490, 64493, 64505, 64510-64530, 69990, 76830-76831, 76856-76857, 76940, 76942, 76970, 76998, 92012-92014, 93000-93010, 93040-93042, 93318, 94002, 94200, 94250, 94680-94690, 94770, 95812-95816, 95819, 95822, 95829, 95955, 96360, 96365, 96372, 96374-96377, 96523, 99155, 99156, 99157, 99211-99223, 99231-99255, 99291-99292, 99304-99310, 99315-99316, 99334-99337, 99347-99350, 99374-99375, 99377-99378

0475T 0476T-0478T, 36591-36592, 76970, 96523, 99453-99454, 99473

0476T 36591-36592, 76970, 96523, 99453-99454, 99473

0477T 36591-36592, 96523, 99453-99454, 99473

0478T 36591-36592, 96523, 99453-99454, 99473

0487T 36591-36592, 51701-51702, 96523

0500T 80500-80502, 81400-81408, 87624-87625, 96523

0548T 0213T, 0216T, 0228T, 0230T, 0549T, 0551T, 11000-11006, 11042-11047, 12001-12007, 12011-12056, 36591-36592, 51990-51992, 52301, 53000-53025, 53080, 53444, 64450, 93318, 93355, 96365-96368, 96372, 96374-96377, 96523, 97597-97598, 97602, 99155, 99156, 99157, 99211-99223, 99231-99255, 99291-99292, 99304-99310, 99315-99316, 99334-99337, 99347-99350, 99374-99375, 99377-99378, 99446-99449, 99451-99452, 99495-99496, G0463, G0471

0549T 0213T, 0216T, 0228T, 0230T, 0551T, 11000-11006, 11042-11047, 12001-12007, 12011-12057, 13100-13133, 13151-13153, 36000, 36400-36410, 36420-36430, 36440, 36591-36592, 36600, 36640, 43752, 51701-51703, 51990-51992, 52000;52301, 53000-53025, 53080, 53444, 62320-62327, 64400, 64405-64408, 64415-64435, 64445-64450, 64461-64463, 64479-64505, 64510-64530, 69990, 76000, 77002, 92012-92014, 93000-93010, 93040-93042, 93318, 93355, 94002, 94200, 94250, 94680-94690, 94770, 95812-95816, 95819, 95822, 95829, 95955, 96360-96368, 96372, 96374-96377, 96523, 97597-97598, 97602, 99155, 99156, 99157, 99211-99223, 99231-99255, 99291-99292, 99304-99310, 99315-99316, 99334-99337, 99347-99350, 99374-99375, 99377-99378, 99446-99449, 99451-99452, 99495-99496, G0463, G0471

0550T 0213T, 0216T, 0228T, 0230T, 0551T, 11000-11006, 11042-11047, 12001-12007, 12011-12057, 13100-13133, 13151-13153, 36000, 36400-36410, 36420-36430, 36440, 36591-36592, 36600, 36640, 43752, 51701-51703, 52000, 53000-53025, 53080, 53445, 62320-62327, 64400, 64405-64408, 64415-64435, 64445-64450, 64461-64463, 64479-64505, 64510-64530, 69990, 92012-92014, 93000-93010, 93040-93042, 93318,

93355, 94002, 94200, 94250, 94680-94690, 94770, 95812-95816, 95819, 95822, 95829, 95955, 96360-96368, 96372, 96374-96377, 96523, 97597-97598, 97602, 99155, 99156, 99157, 99211-99223, 99231-99255, 99291-99292, 99304-99310, 99315-99316, 99334-99337, 99347-99350, 99374-99375, 99377-99378, 99446-99449, 99451-99452, 99495-99496, G0463, G0471

0551T No CCI edits apply to this code.

0567T 00952, 0213T, 0216T, 0228T, 0230T, 36591-36592, 57400-57410, 57800, 58100, 58555, 64450, 74742, 76000, 76816❖, 76998, 77001-77002, 93318, 93355, 96376, 96523, 99446-99449, 99451-99452, 99495-99496, G0463, G0471, J0670, J2001

0568T 00952, 0213T, 0216T, 0228T, 0230T, 36591-36592, 57410, 64450, 74742, 76000, 76998, 77001-77002, 93318, 93355, 96376, 96523, 99446-99449, 99451-99452, 99495-99496, G0463, G0471, J0670, J1642-J1644, J2001

0596T No CCI edits apply to this code.

0597T No CCI edits apply to this code.

10060 0213T, 0216T, 0228T, 0230T, 11055-11057, 11401-11406❖, 11421-11426❖, 11441-11471❖, 11600-11606❖, 11620-11646❖, 11719-11730, 11740, 11765, 12001-12007, 12011-12057, 13100-13133, 13151-13153, 20500, 29580-29581, 30000❖, 36000, 36400-36410, 36420-36430, 36440, 36591-36592, 36600, 36640, 43752, 51701-51703, 62320-62327, 64400, 64405-64408, 64415-64435, 64445-64454, 64461-64463, 64479-64505, 64510-64530, 69990, 92012-92014, 93000-93010, 93040-93042, 93318, 93355, 94002, 94200, 94250, 94680-94690, 94770, 95812-95816, 95819, 95822, 95829, 95955, 96360-96368, 96372, 96374-96377, 96523, 97597-97598, 97602-97608, 99155, 99156, 99157, 99211-99223, 99231-99255, 99291-99292, 99304-99310, 99315-99316, 99334-99337, 99347-99350, 99374-99375, 99377-99378, 99446-99449, 99451-99452, 99495-99496, G0127, G0463, G0471, J0670, J2001

10061 0213T, 0216T, 0228T, 0230T, 10060, 11055-11057, 11406❖, 11424-11440❖, 11444-11451❖, 11463-11471❖, 11604-11606❖, 11623-11626❖, 11643-11646❖, 11719-11730, 11740-11750, 11760, 11765, 12001-12007, 12011-12057, 13100-13133, 13151-13153, 20500, 29580-29581, 36000, 36400-36410, 36420-36430, 36440, 36591-36592, 36600, 36640, 43752, 51701-51703, 62320-62327, 64400, 64405-64408, 64415-64435, 64445-64454, 64461-64463, 64479-64505, 64510-64530, 69990, 92012-92014, 93000-93010, 93040-93042, 93318, 93355, 94002, 94200, 94250, 94680-94690, 94770, 95812-95816, 95819, 95822, 95829, 95955, 96360-96368, 96372, 96374-96377, 96523, 97597-97598, 97602-97608, 99155, 99156, 99157, 99211-99223, 99231-99255, 99291-99292, 99304-99310, 99315-99316, 99334-99337, 99347-99350, 99374-99375, 99377-99378, 99446-99449, 99451-99452, 99495-99496, G0127, G0463, G0471, J0670, J2001

10080 0213T, 0216T, 0228T, 0230T, 12001-12007, 12011-12057, 13100-13133, 13151-13153, 20500, 36000, 36400-36410, 36420-36430, 36440, 36591-36592, 36600, 36640, 43752, 51701-51703, 62320-62327, 64400, 64405-64408, 64415-64435, 64445-64454, 64461-64463, 64479-64505, 64510-64530, 69990, 92012-92014, 93000-93010, 93040-93042, 93318, 93355, 94002, 94200, 94250, 94680-94690, 94770, 95812-95816, 95819, 95822, 95829, 95955, 96360-96368, 96372, 96374-96377, 96523, 99155, 99156, 99157, 99211-99223, 99231-99255, 99291-99292, 99304-99310, 99315-99316, 99334-99337, 99347-99350, 99374-99375, 99377-99378, 99446-99449, 99451-99452, 99495-99496, G0463, G0471, J0670, J2001

10081 0213T, 0216T, 0228T, 0230T, 10080, 12001-12007, 12011-12057, 13100-13133, 13151-13153, 20500, 36000, 36400-36410, 36420-36430, 36440, 36591-36592, 36600, 36640, 43752, 51701-51703, 62320-62327, 64400, 64405-64408, 64415-64435, 64445-64454, 64461-64463, 64479-64505, 64510-64530, 69990, 92012-92014, 93000-93010, 93040-93042, 93318, 93355, 94002, 94200, 94250, 94680-94690, 94770, 95812-95816, 95819, 95822, 95829, 95955, 96360-96368, 96372, 96374-96377, 96523, 99155, 99156, 99157, 99211-99223, 99231-99255, 99291-99292, 99304-99310, 99315-99316, 99334-99337, 99347-99350, 99374-99375, 99377-99378, 99446-99449, 99451-99452, 99495-99496, G0463, G0471, J0670, J2001

10120 0213T, 0216T, 0228T, 0230T, 11000-11006, 11042-11047, 11055-11057, 11719-11721, 12001-12007, 12011-12057, 13100-13133, 13151-13153, 36000, 36400-36410, 36420-36430, 36440, 36591-36592, 36600, 36640, 43752, 51701-51703, 62320-62327, 64400, 64405-64408, 64415-64435, 64445-64454, 64461-64463, 64479-64505, 64510-64530, 69990, 92012-92014, 93000-93010, 93040-93042, 93318, 93355, 94002, 94200, 94250, 94680-94690, 94770, 95812-95816, 95819, 95822, 95829, 95955, 96360-96368, 96372, 96374-96377, 96523, 97597-97598, 97602, 99155, 99156, 99157, 99211-99223, 99231-99255, 99291-99292, 99304-99310, 99315-99316, 99334-99337, 99347-99350, 99374-99375, 99377-99378, 99446-99449, 99451-99452, 99495-99496, G0127, G0463, G0471, J0670, J2001

10121 0213T, 0216T, 0228T, 0230T, 10120, 11000-11006, 11042-11047, 11720-11721, 12001-12007, 12011-12057, 13100-13133, 13151-13153, 36000, 36400-36410, 36420-36430, 36440, 36591-36592, 36600, 36640, 43752, 51701-51703, 62320-62327, 64400, 64405-64408, 64415-64435, 64445-64454, 64461-64463, 64479-64505, 64510-64530, 69990, 92012-92014, 93000-93010, 93040-93042, 93318, 93355, 94002, 94200, 94250, 94680-94690, 94770, 95812-95816, 95819, 95822, 95829, 95955, 96360-96368, 96372, 96374-96377, 96523, 97597-97598, 97602, 99155, 99156, 99157, 99211-99223, 99231-99255, 99291-99292, 99304-99310, 99315-99316, 99334-99337, 99347-99350, 99374-99375, 99377-99378, 99446-99449, 99451-99452, 99495-99496, G0463, G0471, J0670, J2001

10140 0213T, 0216T, 0228T, 0230T, 11055-11057, 11719-11721, 12001-12007, 12011-12057, 13100-13133, 13151-13153, 29580-29581, 36000, 36400-36410, 36420-36430, 36440, 36591-36592, 36600, 36640, 43752, 51701-51703, 62320-62327, 64400, 64405-64408, 64415-64435, 64445-64454, 64461-64463, 64479-64505, 64510-64530, 69990, 76000, 76942, 76998, 77002, 77012, 77021, 92012-92014, 93000-93010, 93040-93042, 93318, 93355, 94002, 94200, 94250, 94680-94690, 94770, 95812-95816, 95819, 95822, 95829, 95955, 96360-96368, 96372, 96374-96377, 96523, 99155, 99156, 99157, 99211-99223, 99231-99255, 99291-99292, 99304-99310, 99315-99316, 99334-99337, 99347-99350, 99374-99375, 99377-99378, 99446-99449, 99451-99452, 99495-99496, G0127, G0463, G0471, J0670, J2001

10160 0213T, 0216T, 0228T, 0230T, 10061✧, 10140✧, 11055-11057, 11719-11721, 12001-12007, 12011-12057, 13100-13133, 13151-13153, 29580-29581, 36000, 36400-36410, 36420-36430, 36440, 36591-36592, 36600, 36640, 43752, 51701-51703, 62320-62327, 64400, 64405-64408, 64415-64435, 64445-64454, 64461-64463, 64479-64505, 64510-64530, 69990, 92012-92014, 93000-93010, 93040-93042, 93318, 93355, 94002, 94200, 94250, 94680-94690, 94770, 95812-95816, 95819, 95822, 95829, 95955, 96360-96368, 96372, 96374-96377, 96523, 99155, 99156, 99157, 99211-99223, 99231-99255, 99291-99292, 99304-99310, 99315-99316, 99334-99337, 99347-99350, 99374-99375, 99377-99378, 99446-99449, 99451-99452, 99495-99496, G0127, G0463, G0471, J0670, J2001

10180 0213T, 0216T, 0228T, 0230T, 11720-11721, 12001-12007, 12011-12057, 13100-13133, 13151-13153, 20500, 36000, 36400-36410, 36420-36430, 36440, 36591-36592, 36600, 36640, 43752, 51701-51703, 62320-62327, 64400, 64405-64408, 64415-64435, 64445-64454, 64461-64463, 64479-64505, 64510-64530, 69990, 92012-92014, 93000-93010, 93040-93042, 93318, 93355, 94002, 94200, 94250, 94680-94690, 94770, 95812-95816, 95819, 95822, 95829, 95955, 96360-96368, 96372, 96374-96377, 96523, 99155, 99156, 99157, 99211-99223, 99231-99255, 99291-99292, 99304-99310, 99315-99316, 99334-99337, 99347-99350, 99374-99375, 99377-99378, 99446-99449, 99451-99452, 99495-99496, G0463, G0471, J0670, J2001

11004 0213T, 0216T, 0228T, 0230T, 0437T, 0552T, 10030, 10060-10061, 11000, 11010-11012, 11042-11044, 11102-11107, 12001-12007, 12011-12018, 12021-12057, 13100-13133, 13151-13153, 15769, 15777, 20552-20553, 20560-20561, 20700-20701, 36000, 36400-36410, 36420-36430, 36440, 36591-36592, 36600, 36640, 43752, 57267, 62320-62327, 64400, 64405-64408, 64415-64435, 64445-64454, 64461-64463, 64479-64505, 64510-64530, 66987-66988, 69990, 92012-92014, 93000-93010, 93040-93042, 93318, 93355, 94002, 94200, 94250, 94680-94690, 94770, 95812-95816, 95819, 95822, 95829, 95955, 96360-96368, 96372, 96374-96377, 96523, 97597-97598, 97610, 99155, 99156, 99157, 99211-99223, 99231-99255, 99291-99292, 99304-99310, 99315-99316, 99334-99337, 99347-99350, 99374-99375, 99377-99378, 99446-99449, 99451-99452, 99495-99496, G0463, G0471

11005 0213T, 0216T, 0228T, 0230T, 0437T, 0552T, 10030, 10060-10061, 11000, 11004, 11010-11012, 11042-11044, 11102-11107, 12001-12007, 12011-12018, 12021-12057, 13100-13133, 13151-13153, 15769, 15777, 20552-20553, 20560-20561, 20700-20701, 36000, 36400-36410, 36420-36430, 36440, 36591-36592, 36600, 36640, 43752, 57267, 62320-62327, 64400, 64405-64408, 64415-64435, 64445-64454, 64461-64463, 64479-64505, 64510-64530, 66987-66988, 69990, 92012-92014, 93000-93010, 93040-93042, 93318, 93355, 94002, 94200, 94250, 94680-94690, 94770, 95812-95816, 95819, 95822, 95829, 95955, 96360-96368, 96372, 96374-96377, 96523, 97597-97598, 97610, 99155, 99156, 99157, 99211-99223, 99231-99255, 99291-99292, 99304-99310, 99315-99316, 99334-99337, 99347-99350, 99374-99375, 99377-99378, 99446-99449, 99451-99452, 99495-99496, G0463, G0471

11006 0213T, 0216T, 0228T, 0230T, 0437T, 0552T, 10030, 10060-10061, 11000, 11004-11005, 11010-11012, 11042-11044, 11102-11107, 12001-12007, 12011-12018, 12021-12057, 13100-13133, 13151-13153, 15769, 15777, 20552-20553, 20560-20561, 20700-20701, 36000, 36400-36410, 36420-36430, 36440, 36591-36592, 36600, 36640, 43752, 57267, 62320-62327, 64400, 64405-64408, 64415-64435, 64445-64454, 64461-64463, 64479-64505, 64510-64530, 66987-66988, 69990, 92012-92014, 93000-93010, 93040-93042, 93318, 93355, 94002, 94200, 94250, 94680-94690, 94770, 95812-95816, 95819, 95822, 95829, 95955, 96360-96368, 96372, 96374-96377, 96523, 97597-97598, 97610, 99155, 99156, 99157, 99211-99223, 99231-99255, 99291-99292, 99304-99310, 99315-99316, 99334-99337, 99347-99350, 99374-99375, 99377-99378, 99446-99449, 99451-99452, 99495-99496, G0463, G0471

11008 36591-36592, 96523

11420 00400, 0213T, 0216T, 0228T, 0230T, 0470T-0471T, 10030✧, 10060-10061✧, 11000-11006, 11042-11047, 11102, 11104, 11106, 11719, 11900-11901, 12001-12007, 12011-12057, 13100-13133, 13151-13153, 17000✧, 17250, 36000, 36400-36410, 36420-36430, 36440, 36591-36592, 36600, 36640, 43752, 51701-51703, 62320-62327, 64400, 64405-64408, 64415-64435, 64445-64454, 64461-64463, 64479-64505, 64510-64530, 69990, 92012-92014, 93000-93010, 93040-93042, 93318, 93355, 94002, 94200, 94250, 94680-94690,

94770, 95812-95816, 95819, 95822, 95829, 95955, 96360-96368, 96372, 96374-96377, 96405-96406, 96523, 96931-96936, 97597-97598, 97602, 99155, 99156, 99157, 99211-99223, 99231-99255, 99291-99292, 99304-99310, 99315-99316, 99334-99337, 99347-99350, 99374-99375, 99377-99378, 99446-99449, 99451-99452, 99495-99496, G0168, G0463, G0471, J0670, J2001

11421 00400, 0213T, 0216T, 0228T, 0230T, 0470T-0471T, 10061❖, 11000-11006, 11042-11047, 11102, 11104, 11106, 11719, 11900-11901, 12001-12007, 12011-12018, 17000❖, 17004❖, 17250, 36000, 36400-36410, 36420-36430, 36440, 36591-36592, 36600, 36640, 43752, 51701-51703, 62320-62327, 64400, 64405-64408, 64415-64435, 64445-64454, 64461-64463, 64479-64505, 64510-64530, 69990, 92012-92014, 93000-93010, 93040-93042, 93318, 93355, 94002, 94200, 94250, 94680-94690, 94770, 95812-95816, 95819, 95822, 95829, 95955, 96360-96368, 96372, 96374-96377, 96405-96406, 96523, 96931-96936, 97597-97598, 97602, 99155, 99156, 99157, 99211-99223, 99231-99255, 99291-99292, 99304-99310, 99315-99316, 99334-99337, 99347-99350, 99374-99375, 99377-99378, 99446-99449, 99451-99452, 99495-99496, G0168, G0463, G0471, J0670, J2001

11422 00400, 0213T, 0216T, 0228T, 0230T, 0470T-0471T, 10061❖, 11000-11006, 11042-11047, 11102, 11104, 11106, 11900-11901, 12001-12007, 12011-12018, 17000❖, 17004❖, 17250, 36000, 36400-36410, 36420-36430, 36440, 36591-36592, 36600, 36640, 43752, 51701-51703, 62320-62327, 64400, 64405-64408, 64415-64435, 64445-64454, 64461-64463, 64479-64505, 64510-64530, 69990, 92012-92014, 93000-93010, 93040-93042, 93318, 93355, 94002, 94200, 94250, 94680-94690, 94770, 95812-95816, 95819, 95822, 95829, 95955, 96360-96368, 96372, 96374-96377, 96405-96406, 96523, 96931-96936, 97597-97598, 97602, 99155, 99156, 99157, 99211-99223, 99231-99255, 99291-99292, 99304-99310, 99315-99316, 99334-99337, 99347-99350, 99374-99375, 99377-99378, 99446-99449, 99451-99452, 99495-99496, G0168, G0463, G0471, J0670, J2001

11423 00400, 0213T, 0216T, 0228T, 0230T, 0470T-0471T, 10061❖, 11000-11006, 11042-11047, 11102, 11104, 11106, 11900-11901, 12001-12007, 12011-12018, 17000❖, 17004❖, 17250, 36000, 36400-36410, 36420-36430, 36440, 36591-36592, 36600, 36640, 43752, 51701-51703, 62320-62327, 64400, 64405-64408, 64415-64435, 64445-64454, 64461-64463, 64479-64505, 64510-64530, 69990, 92012-92014, 93000-93010, 93040-93042, 93318, 93355, 94002, 94200, 94250, 94680-94690, 94770, 95812-95816, 95819, 95822, 95829, 95955, 96360-96368, 96372, 96374-96377, 96405-96406, 96523, 96931-96936, 97597-97598, 97602, 99155, 99156, 99157, 99211-99223, 99231-99255, 99291-99292, 99304-99310, 99315-99316, 99334-99337, 99347-99350, 99374-99375, 99377-99378, 99446-99449, 99451-99452, 99495-99496, G0168, G0463, G0471, J0670, J2001

11424 00400, 0213T, 0216T, 0228T, 0230T, 0470T-0471T, 11000-11006, 11042-11047, 11102, 11104, 11106, 11900-11901, 12001-12007, 12011-12018, 17000❖, 17004❖, 17250, 36000, 36400-36410, 36420-36430, 36440, 36591-36592, 36600, 36640, 43752, 51701-51703, 62320-62327, 64400, 64405-64408, 64415-64435, 64445-64454, 64461-64463, 64479-64505, 64510-64530, 69990, 92012-92014, 93000-93010, 93040-93042, 93318, 93355, 94002, 94200, 94250, 94680-94690, 94770, 95812-95816, 95819, 95822, 95829, 95955, 96360-96368, 96372, 96374-96377, 96405-96406, 96523, 96931-96936, 97597-97598, 97602, 99155, 99156, 99157, 99211-99223, 99231-99255, 99291-99292, 99304-99310, 99315-99316, 99334-99337, 99347-99350, 99374-99375, 99377-99378, 99446-99449, 99451-99452, 99495-99496, G0168, G0463, G0471, J0670, J2001

11426 00400, 0213T, 0216T, 0228T, 0230T, 0470T-0471T, 11000-11006, 11042-11047, 11102, 11104, 11106, 11900-11901, 12001-12007, 12011-12018, 17000❖, 17004❖, 17250, 36000, 36400-36410, 36420-36430, 36440, 36591-36592, 36600, 36640, 43752, 51701-51703, 62320-62327, 64400, 64405-64408, 64415-64435, 64445-64454, 64461-64463, 64479-64505, 64510-64530, 69990, 92012-92014, 93000-93010, 93040-93042, 93318, 93355, 94002, 94200, 94250, 94680-94690, 94770, 95812-95816, 95819, 95822, 95829, 95955, 96360-96368, 96372, 96374-96377, 96405-96406, 96523, 96931-96936, 97597-97598, 97602, 99155, 99156, 99157, 99211-99223, 99231-99255, 99291-99292, 99304-99310, 99315-99316, 99334-99337, 99347-99350, 99374-99375, 99377-99378, 99446-99449, 99451-99452, 99495-99496, G0168, G0463, G0471, J0670, J2001

11620 00400, 0213T, 0216T, 0228T, 0230T, 10061❖, 11000-11006, 11042-11047, 11102, 11104, 11106, 11900-11901, 12001-12007, 12011-12018, 17000❖, 17004❖, 17250, 17262-17266❖, 17271-17276❖, 17281-17286❖, 36000, 36400-36410, 36420-36430, 36440, 36591-36592, 36600, 36640, 43752, 51701-51703, 62320-62327, 64400, 64405-64408, 64415-64435, 64445-64454, 64461-64463, 64479-64505, 64510-64530, 69990, 92012-92014, 93000-93010, 93040-93042, 93318, 93355, 94002, 94200, 94250, 94680-94690, 94770, 95812-95816, 95819, 95822, 95829, 95955, 96360-96368, 96372, 96374-96377, 96523, 97597-97598, 97602, 99155, 99156, 99157, 99211-99223, 99231-99255, 99291-99292, 99304-99310, 99315-99316, 99334-99337, 99347-99350, 99374-99375, 99377-99378, 99446-99449, 99451-99452, 99495-99496, G0168, G0463, G0471, J0670, J2001

11621 00400, 0213T, 0216T, 0228T, 0230T, 10061❖, 11000-11006, 11042-11047, 11102, 11104, 11106, 11900-11901, 12001-12007, 12011-12018, 17000❖, 17004❖, 17250, 17266❖, 17273-17276❖, 17282-17286❖, 36000, 36400-36410, 36420-36430, 36440, 36591-36592, 36600, 36640, 43752, 51701-51703, 62320-62327, 64400, 64405-64408, 64415-64435, 64445-64454, 64461-64463, 64479-64505, 64510-64530, 69990, 92012-92014, 93000-93010, 93040-93042, 93318, 93355, 94002, 94200, 94250, 94680-94690, 94770, 95812-95816, 95819, 95822, 95829, 95955, 96360-96368, 96372, 96374-96377, 96523, 97597-97598, 97602, 99155, 99156, 99157, 99211-99223, 99231-99255, 99291-99292, 99304-99310, 99315-99316, 99334-99337, 99347-99350, 99374-99375, 99377-99378, 99446-99449, 99451-99452, 99495-99496, G0168, G0463, G0471, J0670, J2001

11622 00400, 0213T, 0216T, 0228T, 0230T, 10061❖, 11000-11006, 11042-11047, 11102, 11104, 11106, 11900-11901, 12001-12007, 12011-12018, 17000❖, 17004❖, 17250, 17274-17276❖, 17283-17286❖, 36000, 36400-36410, 36420-36430, 36440, 36591-36592, 36600, 36640, 43752, 51701-51703, 62320-62327, 64400, 64405-64408, 64415-64435, 64445-64454, 64461-64463, 64479-64505, 64510-64530, 69990, 92012-92014, 93000-93010, 93040-93042, 93318, 93355, 94002, 94200, 94250, 94680-94690, 94770, 95812-95816, 95819, 95822, 95829, 95955, 96360-96368, 96372, 96374-96377, 96523, 97597-97598, 97602, 99155, 99156, 99157, 99211-99223, 99231-99255, 99291-99292, 99304-99310, 99315-99316, 99334-99337, 99347-99350, 99374-99375, 99377-99378, 99446-99449, 99451-99452, 99495-99496, G0168, G0463, G0471, J0670, J2001

11623 00400, 0213T, 0216T, 0228T, 0230T, 11000-11006, 11042-11047, 11102, 11104, 11106, 11900-11901, 12001-12007, 12011-12018, 17000❖, 17004❖, 17250, 17276❖, 17284-17286❖, 36000, 36400-36410, 36420-36430, 36440, 36591-36592, 36600, 36640, 43752, 51701-51703, 62320-62327, 64400, 64405-64408, 64415-64435, 64445-64454, 64461-64463, 64479-64505, 64510-64530, 69990, 92012-92014, 93000-93010, 93040-93042, 93318, 93355, 94002, 94200, 94250, 94680-94690, 94770, 95812-95816, 95819, 95822, 95829, 95955,

96360-96368, 96372, 96374-96377, 96523, 97597-97598, 97602, 99155, 99156, 99157, 99211-99223, 99231-99255, 99291-99292, 99304-99310, 99315-99316, 99334-99337, 99347-99350, 99374-99375, 99377-99378, 99446-99449, 99451-99452, 99495-99496, G0168, G0463, G0471, J0670, J2001

11624 00400, 0213T, 0216T, 0228T, 0230T, 11000-11006, 11042-11047, 11102, 11104, 11106, 11900-11901, 12001-12007, 12011-12018, 17000✦, 17004✦, 17250, 17286✦, 36000, 36400-36410, 36420-36430, 36440, 36591-36592, 36600, 36640, 43752, 51701-51703, 62320-62327, 64400, 64405-64408, 64415-64435, 64445-64454, 64461-64463, 64479-64505, 64510-64530, 69990, 92012-92014, 93000-93010, 93040-93042, 93318, 93355, 94002, 94200, 94250, 94680-94690, 94770, 95812-95816, 95819, 95822, 95829, 95955, 96360-96368, 96372, 96374-96377, 96523, 97597-97598, 97602, 99155, 99156, 99157, 99211-99223, 99231-99255, 99291-99292, 99304-99310, 99315-99316, 99334-99337, 99347-99350, 99374-99375, 99377-99378, 99446-99449, 99451-99452, 99495-99496, G0168, G0463, G0471, J0670, J2001

11626 00400, 0213T, 0216T, 0228T, 0230T, 11000-11006, 11042-11047, 11102, 11104, 11106, 11900-11901, 12001-12007, 12011-12018, 15002✦, 17000✦, 17004✦, 17250, 17286✦, 36000, 36400-36410, 36420-36430, 36440, 36591-36592, 36600, 36640, 43752, 51701-51703, 62320-62327, 64400, 64405-64408, 64415-64435, 64445-64454, 64461-64463, 64479-64505, 64510-64530, 69990, 92012-92014, 93000-93010, 93040-93042, 93318, 93355, 94002, 94200, 94250, 94680-94690, 94770, 95812-95816, 95819, 95822, 95829, 95955, 96360-96368, 96372, 96374-96377, 96523, 97597-97598, 97602, 99155, 99156, 99157, 99211-99223, 99231-99255, 99291-99292, 99304-99310, 99315-99316, 99334-99337, 99347-99350, 99374-99375, 99377-99378, 99446-99449, 99451-99452, 99495-99496, G0168, G0463, G0471, J0670, J2001

11770 0213T, 0216T, 0228T, 0230T, 10080-10081, 11000-11006, 11042-11047, 11900-11901, 12001-12007, 12011-12057, 13100-13133, 13151-13153, 17250, 20500, 36000, 36400-36410, 36420-36430, 36440, 36591-36592, 36600, 36640, 43752, 51701-51703, 62320-62327, 64400, 64405-64408, 64415-64435, 64445-64454, 64461-64463, 64479-64505, 64510-64530, 69990, 92012-92014, 93000-93010, 93040-93042, 93318, 93355, 94002, 94200, 94250, 94680-94690, 94770, 95812-95816, 95819, 95822, 95829, 95955, 96360-96368, 96372, 96374-96377, 96405-96406, 96523, 97597-97598, 97602, 99155, 99156, 99157, 99211-99223, 99231-99255, 99291-99292, 99304-99310, 99315-99316, 99334-99337, 99347-99350, 99374-99375, 99377-99378, 99446-99449, 99451-99452, 99495-99496, G0463, G0471, J0670, J2001

11771 0213T, 0216T, 0228T, 0230T, 10080-10081, 11000-11006, 11042-11047, 11770, 11900-11901, 12001-12007, 12011-12057, 13100-13133, 13151-13153, 17250, 20500, 36000, 36400-36410, 36420-36430, 36440, 36591-36592, 36600, 36640, 43752, 51701-51703, 62320-62327, 64400, 64405-64408, 64415-64435, 64445-64454, 64461-64463, 64479-64505, 64510-64530, 69990, 92012-92014, 93000-93010, 93040-93042, 93318, 93355, 94002, 94200, 94250, 94680-94690, 94770, 95812-95816, 95819, 95822, 95829, 95955, 96360-96368, 96372, 96374-96377, 96405-96406, 96523, 97597-97598, 97602, 99155, 99156, 99157, 99211-99223, 99231-99255, 99291-99292, 99304-99310, 99315-99316, 99334-99337, 99347-99350, 99374-99375, 99377-99378, 99446-99449, 99451-99452, 99495-99496, G0463, G0471, J0670, J2001

11772 0213T, 0216T, 0228T, 0230T, 10080-10081, 11000-11006, 11042-11047, 11770-11771, 11900-11901, 12001-12007, 12011-12057, 13100-13133, 13151-13153, 17250, 17313✦, 36000, 36400-36410, 36420-36430, 36440, 36591-36592, 36600, 36640, 43752, 51701-51703, 62320-62327, 64400, 64405-64408, 64415-64435, 64445-64454, 64461-64463,

64479-64505, 64510-64530, 69990, 92012-92014, 93000-93010, 93040-93042, 93318, 93355, 94002, 94200, 94250, 94680-94690, 94770, 95812-95816, 95819, 95822, 95829, 95955, 96360-96368, 96372, 96374-96377, 96405-96406, 96523, 97597-97598, 97602, 99155, 99156, 99157, 99211-99223, 99231-99255, 99291-99292, 99304-99310, 99315-99316, 99334-99337, 99347-99350, 99374-99375, 99377-99378, 99446-99449, 99451-99452, 99495-99496, G0463, G0471, J0670, J2001

11976 0213T, 0216T, 0228T, 0230T, 11000-11006, 11042-11047, 12001-12007, 12011-12057, 13100-13133, 13151-13153, 36000, 36400-36410, 36420-36430, 36440, 36591-36592, 36600, 36640, 43752, 51701-51703, 62320-62327, 64400, 64405-64408, 64415-64435, 64445-64454, 64461-64463, 64479-64505, 64510-64530, 92012-92014, 93000-93010, 93040-93042, 93318, 93355, 94002, 94200, 94250, 94680-94690, 94770, 95812-95816, 95819, 95822, 95829, 95955, 96360-96368, 96372, 96374-96377, 96523, 97597-97598, 97602, 99155, 99156, 99157, 99211-99223, 99231-99255, 99291-99292, 99304-99310, 99315-99316, 99334-99337, 99347-99350, 99374-99375, 99377-99378, 99446-99449, 99451-99452, 99495-99496, G0463, G0471, J2001

11980 0213T, 0216T, 0228T, 0230T, 11900, 12001-12007, 12011-12057, 13100-13133, 13151-13153, 36000, 36400-36410, 36420-36430, 36440, 36591-36592, 36600, 36640, 43752, 51701-51703, 62320-62327, 64400, 64405-64408, 64415-64435, 64445-64454, 64461-64463, 64479-64505, 64510-64530, 92012-92014, 93000-93010, 93040-93042, 93318, 93355, 94002, 94200, 94250, 94680-94690, 94770, 95812-95816, 95819, 95822, 95829, 95955, 96360-96368, 96372, 96374-96377, 96523, 99155, 99156, 99157, 99211-99223, 99231-99255, 99291-99292, 99304-99310, 99315-99316, 99334-99337, 99347-99350, 99374-99375, 99377-99378, 99446-99449, 99451-99452, 99495-99496, G0463, G0471, J0670, J2001

11981 0213T, 0216T, 11000-11006, 11042-11047, 11982✦, 36000, 36410, 36591-36592, 61650, 62324-62327, 64415-64417, 64450, 64454, 64486-64490, 64493, 96360, 96365, 96372, 96374-96377, 96523, 97597-97598, 97602, G0516-G0517✦, J0670, J2001

11982 0213T, 0216T, 11000-11006, 11042-11047, 11976✦, 20701, 36000, 36410, 36591-36592, 61650, 62324-62327, 64415-64417, 64450, 64454, 64486-64490, 64493, 96360, 96365, 96372, 96374-96377, 96523, 97597-97598, 97602, G0517✦, J0670, J2001

11983 0213T, 0216T, 11000-11006, 11042-11047, 11976, 11981-11982, 36000, 36410, 36591-36592, 61650, 62324-62327, 64415-64417, 64450, 64454, 64486-64490, 64493, 96360, 96365, 96372, 96374-96377, 96523, 97597-97598, 97602, G0516-G0518✦, J0670, J2001

12001 0213T, 0216T, 0228T, 0230T, 0543T-0544T, 0545T, 0567T-0574T, 0580T, 0581T, 0582T, 11042, 11055-11056, 11719, 11740-11750, 11900-11901, 20560-20561, 36000, 36400-36410, 36420-36430, 36440, 36591-36592, 36600, 36640, 43752, 51701-51703, 64400, 64405-64408, 64415-64435, 64445-64450, 64479-64484, 64490-64505, 64510-64530, 66987-66988, 69990, 92012-92014, 93000-93010, 93040-93042, 93318, 93355, 94002, 94200, 94250, 94680-94690, 94770, 95812-95816, 95819, 95822, 95829, 95955, 96360-96368, 96372, 96374-96377, 96523, 97597-97598, 97602-97608, 99155, 99156, 99157, 99211-99223, 99231-99255, 99291-99292, 99304-99310, 99315-99316, 99334-99337, 99347-99350, 99374-99375, 99377-99378, 99446-99449, 99451-99452, 99495-99496, G0168, G0463, G0471, J0670, J2001

12002 0213T, 0216T, 0228T, 0230T, 0543T-0544T, 0545T, 0567T-0574T, 0580T, 0581T, 0582T, 11042, 11740, 11900-11901, 12001, 12013-12014✦, 20560-20561, 20701, 36000, 36400-36410, 36420-36430, 36440, 36591-36592, 36600, 36640, 43752, 51701-51703, 64400, 64405-64408, 64415-64435, 64445-64450, 64479-64484, 64490-64505, 64510-64530, 66987-66988, 69990, 92012-92014, 93000-93010, 93040-93042, 93318,

93355, 94002, 94200, 94250, 94680-94690, 94770, 95812-95816,
95819, 95822, 95829, 95955, 96360-96368, 96372, 96374-96377,
96523, 97597-97598, 97602-97608, 99155, 99156, 99157, 99211-99223,
99231-99255, 99291-99292, 99304-99310, 99315-99316, 99334-99337,
99347-99350, 99374-99375, 99377-99378, 99446-99449, 99451-99452,
99495-99496, G0168, G0463, G0471, J0670, J2001

12004 0213T, 0216T, 0228T, 0230T, 0543T-0544T, 0545T, 0567T-0574T, 0580T,
0581T, 0582T, 11042, 11900-11901, 12001-12002, 12015✦,
20560-20561, 20701, 36000, 36400-36410, 36420-36430, 36440,
36591-36592, 36600, 36640, 43752, 51701-51703, 64400, 64405-64408,
64415-64435, 64445-64450, 64479-64484, 64490-64505, 64510-64530,
66987-66988, 69990, 92012-92014, 93000-93010, 93040-93042, 93318,
93355, 94002, 94200, 94250, 94680-94690, 94770, 95812-95816,
95819, 95822, 95829, 95955, 96360-96368, 96372, 96374-96377,
96523, 97597-97598, 97602-97608, 99155, 99156, 99157, 99211-99223,
99231-99255, 99291-99292, 99304-99310, 99315-99316, 99334-99337,
99347-99350, 99374-99375, 99377-99378, 99446-99449, 99451-99452,
99495-99496, G0168, G0463, G0471, J0670, J2001

12005 0213T, 0216T, 0228T, 0230T, 0543T-0544T, 0545T, 0567T-0574T, 0580T,
0581T, 0582T, 11042-11043, 11900-11901, 12001-12004, 12016✦,
20560-20561, 20700-20701, 36000, 36400-36410, 36420-36430, 36440,
36591-36592, 36600, 36640, 43752, 51701-51703, 64400, 64405-64408,
64415-64435, 64445-64451, 64479-64484, 64490-64505, 64510-64530,
66987-66988, 69990, 92012-92014, 93000-93010, 93040-93042, 93318,
93355, 94002, 94200, 94250, 94680-94690, 94770, 95812-95816,
95819, 95822, 95829, 95955, 96360-96368, 96372, 96374-96377,
96523, 97597-97598, 97602-97608, 99155, 99156, 99157, 99211-99223,
99231-99255, 99291-99292, 99304-99310, 99315-99316, 99334-99337,
99347-99350, 99374-99375, 99377-99378, 99446-99449, 99451-99452,
99495-99496, G0168, G0463, G0471, J0670, J2001

12006 0213T, 0216T, 0228T, 0230T, 0543T-0544T, 0545T, 0567T-0574T, 0580T,
0581T, 0582T, 11042-11043, 11900-11901, 12001-12005, 12017✦,
20560-20561, 20700-20701, 36000, 36400-36410, 36420-36430, 36440,
36591-36592, 36600, 36640, 43752, 51701-51703, 64400, 64405-64408,
64415-64435, 64445-64451, 64479-64484, 64490-64505, 64510-64530,
66987-66988, 69990, 92012-92014, 93000-93010, 93040-93042, 93318,
93355, 94002, 94200, 94250, 94680-94690, 94770, 95812-95816,
95819, 95822, 95829, 95955, 96360-96368, 96372, 96374-96377,
96523, 97597-97598, 97602-97608, 99155, 99156, 99157, 99211-99223,
99231-99255, 99291-99292, 99304-99310, 99315-99316, 99334-99337,
99347-99350, 99374-99375, 99377-99378, 99446-99449, 99451-99452,
99495-99496, G0168, G0463, G0471, J0670, J2001

12007 0213T, 0216T, 0228T, 0230T, 0543T-0544T, 0545T, 0567T-0574T, 0580T,
0581T, 0582T, 11900-11901, 12001-12006, 12018✦, 15772, 15774,
20560-20561, 20700-20701, 36000, 36400-36410, 36420-36430, 36440,
36591-36592, 36600, 36640, 43752, 51701-51703, 64400, 64405-64408,
64415-64435, 64445-64451, 64479-64484, 64490-64505, 64510-64530,
66987-66988, 69990, 92012-92014, 93000-93010, 93040-93042, 93318,
93355, 94002, 94200, 94250, 94680-94690, 94770, 95812-95816,
95819, 95822, 95829, 95955, 96360-96368, 96372, 96374-96377,
96523, 97597-97598, 97602-97608, 99155, 99156, 99157, 99211-99223,
99231-99255, 99291-99292, 99304-99310, 99315-99316, 99334-99337,
99347-99350, 99374-99375, 99377-99378, 99446-99449, 99451-99452,
99495-99496, G0168, G0463, G0471, J0670, J2001

12020 0213T, 0216T, 0228T, 0230T, 0543T-0544T, 0545T, 0567T-0574T, 0580T,
0581T, 0582T, 11000-11006, 11042-11047, 11900-11901, 12021, 15772,
15774, 20560-20561, 20700-20701, 36000, 36400-36410, 36420-36430,
36440, 36591-36592, 36600, 36640, 43752, 51701-51703, 64400,
64405-64408, 64415-64435, 64445-64451, 64479-64484, 64490-64505,

64510-64530, 66987-66988, 69990, 92012-92014, 93000-93010,
93040-93042, 93318, 93355, 94002, 94200, 94250, 94680-94690,
94770, 95812-95816, 95819, 95822, 95829, 95955, 96360-96368,
96372, 96374-96377, 96523, 97597-97598, 97602-97608, 99155, 99156,
99157, 99211-99223, 99231-99255, 99291-99292, 99304-99310,
99315-99316, 99334-99337, 99347-99350, 99374-99375, 99377-99378,
99446-99449, 99451-99452, 99495-99496, G0168, G0463, G0471,
J0670, J2001

12021 0213T, 0216T, 0228T, 0230T, 0543T-0544T, 0567T-0574T, 0580T, 0581T,
0582T, 11042, 11900-11901, 20560-20561, 20700-20701, 36000,
36400-36410, 36420-36430, 36440, 36591-36592, 36600, 36640, 43752,
51701-51703, 64400, 64405-64408, 64415-64435, 64445-64451,
64479-64484, 64490-64505, 64510-64530, 66987-66988, 69990,
92012-92014, 93000-93010, 93040-93042, 93318, 93355, 94002, 94200,
94250, 94680-94690, 94770, 95812-95816, 95819, 95822, 95829,
95955, 96360-96368, 96372, 96374-96377, 96523, 97597-97598,
97602-97608, 99155, 99156, 99157, 99211-99223, 99231-99255,
99291-99292, 99304-99310, 99315-99316, 99334-99337, 99347-99350,
99374-99375, 99377-99378, 99446-99449, 99451-99452, 99495-99496,
G0168, G0463, G0471, J2001

12031 0213T, 0216T, 0228T, 0230T, 0543T-0544T, 0567T-0574T, 0580T, 0581T,
0582T, 11042, 11055-11056, 11900-11901, 12051✦, 20560-20561,
20700-20701, 36000, 36400-36410, 36420-36430, 36440, 36591-36592,
36600, 36640, 43752, 51701-51703, 64400, 64405-64408, 64415-64435,
64445-64451, 64479-64484, 64490-64505, 64510-64530, 66987-66988,
69990, 92012-92014, 93000-93010, 93040-93042, 93318, 93355, 94002,
94200, 94250, 94680-94690, 94770, 95812-95816, 95819, 95822,
95829, 95955, 96360-96368, 96372, 96374-96377, 96523, 97597-97598,
97602-97608, 99155, 99156, 99157, 99211-99223, 99231-99255,
99291-99292, 99304-99310, 99315-99316, 99334-99337, 99347-99350,
99374-99375, 99377-99378, 99446-99449, 99451-99452, 99495-99496,
G0168, G0463, G0471, J0670, J2001

12032 0213T, 0216T, 0228T, 0230T, 0543T-0544T, 0567T-0574T, 0580T, 0581T,
0582T, 11042-11043, 11900-11901, 12031, 12042✦, 12052-12053✦,
15772, 15774, 20560-20561, 20700-20701, 36000, 36400-36410,
36420-36430, 36440, 36591-36592, 36600, 36640, 43752, 51701-51703,
64400, 64405-64408, 64415-64435, 64445-64451, 64479-64484,
64490-64505, 64510-64530, 66987-66988, 69990, 92012-92014,
93000-93010, 93040-93042, 93318, 93355, 94002, 94200, 94250,
94680-94690, 94770, 95812-95816, 95819, 95822, 95829, 95955,
96360-96368, 96372, 96374-96377, 96523, 97597-97598, 97602-97608,
99155, 99156, 99157, 99211-99223, 99231-99255, 99291-99292,
99304-99310, 99315-99316, 99334-99337, 99347-99350, 99374-99375,
99377-99378, 99446-99449, 99451-99452, 99495-99496, G0168,
G0463, G0471, J0670, J2001

12034 0213T, 0216T, 0228T, 0230T, 0543T-0544T, 0567T-0574T, 0580T, 0581T,
0582T, 11042-11043, 11900-11901, 12031-12032, 12044✦, 12054✦,
15772, 15774, 20560-20561, 20700-20701, 36000, 36400-36410,
36420-36430, 36440, 36591-36592, 36600, 36640, 43752, 51701-51703,
64400, 64405-64408, 64415-64435, 64445-64451, 64479-64484,
64490-64505, 64510-64530, 66987-66988, 69990, 92012-92014,
93000-93010, 93040-93042, 93318, 93355, 94002, 94200, 94250,
94680-94690, 94770, 95812-95816, 95819, 95822, 95829, 95955,
96360-96368, 96372, 96374-96377, 96523, 97597-97598, 97602-97608,
99155, 99156, 99157, 99211-99223, 99231-99255, 99291-99292,
99304-99310, 99315-99316, 99334-99337, 99347-99350, 99374-99375,
99377-99378, 99446-99449, 99451-99452, 99495-99496, G0168,
G0463, G0471, J0670, J2001

12035 0213T, 0216T, 0228T, 0230T, 0543T-0544T, 0567T-0574T, 0580T, 0581T, 0582T, 11042-11044, 11900-11901, 12031-12034, 12045✦, 12055✦, 15772, 15774, 20560-20561, 20700-20701, 36000, 36400-36410, 36420-36430, 36440, 36591-36592, 36600, 36640, 43752, 51701-51703, 64400, 64405-64408, 64415-64435, 64445-64451, 64479-64484, 64490-64505, 64510-64530, 64625, 66987-66988, 69990, 92012-92014, 93000-93010, 93040-93042, 93318, 93355, 94002, 94200, 94250, 94680-94690, 94770, 95812-95816, 95819, 95822, 95829, 95955, 96360-96368, 96372, 96374-96377, 96523, 97597-97598, 97602-97608, 99155, 99156, 99157, 99211-99223, 99231-99255, 99291-99292, 99304-99310, 99315-99316, 99334-99337, 99347-99350, 99374-99375, 99377-99378, 99446-99449, 99451-99452, 99495-99496, G0168, G0463, G0471, J0670, J2001

12036 0213T, 0216T, 0228T, 0230T, 0543T-0544T, 0567T-0574T, 0580T, 0581T, 0582T, 11043, 11900-11901, 12031-12035, 12046✦, 12056✦, 15772, 15774, 20560-20561, 20700-20701, 36000, 36400-36410, 36420-36430, 36440, 36591-36592, 36600, 36640, 43752, 51701-51703, 64400, 64405-64408, 64415-64435, 64445-64451, 64479-64484, 64490-64505, 64510-64530, 64625, 66987-66988, 69990, 92012-92014, 93000-93010, 93040-93042, 93318, 93355, 94002, 94200, 94250, 94680-94690, 94770, 95812-95816, 95819, 95822, 95829, 95955, 96360-96368, 96372, 96374-96377, 96523, 97597-97598, 97602-97608, 99155, 99156, 99157, 99211-99223, 99231-99255, 99291-99292, 99304-99310, 99315-99316, 99334-99337, 99347-99350, 99374-99375, 99377-99378, 99446-99449, 99451-99452, 99495-99496, G0168, G0463, G0471, J0670, J2001

12037 0213T, 0216T, 0228T, 0230T, 0543T-0544T, 0567T-0574T, 0580T, 0581T, 0582T, 11043-11044, 11900-11901, 12031-12036, 12057✦, 15772, 15774, 20560-20561, 20700-20701, 36000, 36400-36410, 36420-36430, 36440, 36591-36592, 36600, 36640, 43752, 51701-51703, 64400, 64405-64408, 64415-64435, 64445-64451, 64479-64484, 64490-64505, 64510-64530, 64625, 66987-66988, 69990, 92012-92014, 93000-93010, 93040-93042, 93318, 93355, 94002, 94200, 94250, 94680-94690, 94770, 95812-95816, 95819, 95822, 95829, 95955, 96360-96368, 96372, 96374-96377, 96523, 97597-97598, 97602-97608, 99155, 99156, 99157, 99211-99223, 99231-99255, 99291-99292, 99304-99310, 99315-99316, 99334-99337, 99347-99350, 99374-99375, 99377-99378, 99446-99449, 99451-99452, 99495-99496, G0168, G0463, G0471, J0670, J2001

12041 0213T, 0216T, 0228T, 0230T, 0543T-0544T, 0567T-0574T, 0580T, 0581T, 0582T, 11055-11056, 11740, 11900-11901, 12031, 20560-20561, 20700-20701, 36000, 36400-36410, 36420-36430, 36440, 36591-36592, 36600, 36640, 43752, 51701-51703, 64400, 64405-64408, 64415-64435, 64445-64451, 64479-64484, 64490-64505, 64510-64530, 66987-66988, 69990, 92012-92014, 93000-93010, 93040-93042, 93318, 93355, 94002, 94200, 94250, 94680-94690, 94770, 95812-95816, 95819, 95822, 95829, 95955, 96360-96368, 96372, 96374-96377, 96523, 97597-97598, 97602-97608, 99155, 99156, 99157, 99211-99223, 99231-99255, 99291-99292, 99304-99310, 99315-99316, 99334-99337, 99347-99350, 99374-99375, 99377-99378, 99446-99449, 99451-99452, 99495-99496, G0168, G0463, G0471, J0670, J2001

12042 0213T, 0216T, 0228T, 0230T, 0567T-0574T, 0580T, 0581T, 0582T, 11042, 11740, 11900-11901, 12041, 15772, 15774, 20560-20561, 20700-20701, 36000, 36400-36410, 36420-36430, 36440, 36591-36592, 36600, 36640, 43752, 51701-51703, 64400, 64405-64408, 64415-64435, 64445-64451, 64479-64484, 64490-64505, 64510-64530, 66987-66988, 69990, 92012-92014, 93000-93010, 93040-93042, 93318, 93355, 94002, 94200, 94250, 94680-94690, 94770, 95812-95816, 95819, 95822, 95829, 95955, 96360-96368, 96372, 96374-96377, 96523, 97597-97598, 97602-97608, 99155, 99156, 99157, 99211-99223, 99231-99255,

99291-99292, 99304-99310, 99315-99316, 99334-99337, 99347-99350, 99374-99375, 99377-99378, 99446-99449, 99451-99452, 99495-99496, G0168, G0463, G0471, J0670, J2001

12044 0213T, 0216T, 0228T, 0230T, 0567T-0574T, 0580T, 0581T, 0582T, 11043-11044, 11900-11901, 12041-12042, 12054✦, 15772, 15774, 20560-20561, 20700-20701, 36000, 36400-36410, 36420-36430, 36440, 36591-36592, 36600, 36640, 43752, 51701-51703, 64400, 64405-64408, 64415-64435, 64445-64451, 64479-64484, 64490-64505, 64510-64530, 66987-66988, 69990, 92012-92014, 93000-93010, 93040-93042, 93318, 93355, 94002, 94200, 94250, 94680-94690, 94770, 95812-95816, 95819, 95822, 95829, 95955, 96360-96368, 96372, 96374-96377, 96523, 97597-97598, 97602-97608, 99155, 99156, 99157, 99211-99223, 99231-99255, 99291-99292, 99304-99310, 99315-99316, 99334-99337, 99347-99350, 99374-99375, 99377-99378, 99446-99449, 99451-99452, 99495-99496, G0168, G0463, G0471, J0670, J2001

12045 0213T, 0216T, 0228T, 0230T, 0567T-0574T, 0580T, 0581T, 0582T, 11042, 11900-11901, 12041-12044, 12055✦, 15772, 15774, 20560-20561, 20700-20701, 36000, 36400-36410, 36420-36430, 36440, 36591-36592, 36600, 36640, 43752, 51701-51703, 64400, 64405-64408, 64415-64435, 64445-64451, 64479-64484, 64490-64505, 64510-64530, 64625, 66987-66988, 69990, 92012-92014, 93000-93010, 93040-93042, 93318, 93355, 94002, 94200, 94250, 94680-94690, 94770, 95812-95816, 95819, 95822, 95829, 95955, 96360-96368, 96372, 96374-96377, 96523, 97597-97598, 97602-97608, 99155, 99156, 99157, 99211-99223, 99231-99255, 99291-99292, 99304-99310, 99315-99316, 99334-99337, 99347-99350, 99374-99375, 99377-99378, 99446-99449, 99451-99452, 99495-99496, G0168, G0463, G0471, J0670, J2001

12046 0213T, 0216T, 0228T, 0230T, 0567T-0574T, 0580T, 0581T, 0582T, 11043-11044, 11900-11901, 12041-12045, 12056✦, 15772, 15774, 20560-20561, 20700-20701, 36000, 36400-36410, 36420-36430, 36440, 36591-36592, 36600, 36640, 43752, 51701-51703, 64400, 64405-64408, 64415-64435, 64445-64451, 64479-64484, 64490-64505, 64510-64530, 64625, 66987-66988, 69990, 92012-92014, 93000-93010, 93040-93042, 93318, 93355, 94002, 94200, 94250, 94680-94690, 94770, 95812-95816, 95819, 95822, 95829, 95955, 96360-96368, 96372, 96374-96377, 96523, 97597-97598, 97602-97608, 99155, 99156, 99157, 99211-99223, 99231-99255, 99291-99292, 99304-99310, 99315-99316, 99334-99337, 99347-99350, 99374-99375, 99377-99378, 99446-99449, 99451-99452, 99495-99496, G0168, G0463, G0471, J0670, J2001

12047 0213T, 0216T, 0228T, 0230T, 0567T-0574T, 0580T, 0581T, 0582T, 11900-11901, 12037-12046, 12057✦, 15772, 15774, 20560-20561, 20700-20701, 36000, 36400-36410, 36420-36430, 36440, 36591-36592, 36600, 36640, 43752, 51701-51703, 64400, 64405-64408, 64415-64435, 64445-64451, 64479-64484, 64490-64505, 64510-64530, 64625, 66987-66988, 69990, 92012-92014, 93000-93010, 93040-93042, 93318, 93355, 94002, 94200, 94250, 94680-94690, 94770, 95812-95816, 95819, 95822, 95829, 95955, 96360-96368, 96372, 96374-96377, 96523, 97597-97598, 97602-97608, 99155, 99156, 99157, 99211-99223, 99231-99255, 99291-99292, 99304-99310, 99315-99316, 99334-99337, 99347-99350, 99374-99375, 99377-99378, 99446-99449, 99451-99452, 99495-99496, G0168, G0463, G0471, J0670, J2001

13100 0213T, 0216T, 0228T, 0230T, 0543T-0544T, 0548T, 0567T-0574T, 0580T, 0581T, 0582T, 11000, 11010-11012, 11042-11044, 11900-11901, 13102, 13160✦, 15772, 15774, 20560-20561, 20700-20701, 36000, 36400-36410, 36420-36430, 36440, 36591-36592, 36600, 36640, 43752, 51701-51703, 64400, 64405-64408, 64415-64435, 64445-64451, 64479-64484, 64490-64505, 64510-64530, 66987-66988, 69990, 92012-92014, 93000-93010, 93040-93042, 93318, 93355, 94002, 94200, 94250, 94680-94690, 94770, 95812-95816, 95819, 95822, 95829,

95955, 96360-96368, 96372, 96374-96377, 96523, 97597-97598, 97602-97608, 99155, 99156, 99157, 99211-99223, 99231-99255, 99291-99292, 99304-99310, 99315-99316, 99334-99337, 99347-99350, 99374-99375, 99377-99378, 99446-99449, 99451-99452, 99495-99496, G0168, G0463, G0471, J0670, J2001

13101 0213T, 0216T, 0228T, 0230T, 0543T-0544T, 0548T, 0567T-0574T, 0580T, 0581T, 0582T, 11000, 11010-11012, 11042-11044, 11900-11901, 13100, 13160✧, 15772, 15774, 20560-20561, 20700-20701, 36000, 36400-36410, 36420-36430, 36440, 36591-36592, 36600, 36640, 43752, 51701-51703, 64400, 64405-64408, 64415-64435, 64445-64451, 64479-64484, 64490-64505, 64510-64530, 64625, 66987-66988, 69990, 92012-92014, 93000-93010, 93040-93042, 93318, 93355, 94002, 94200, 94250, 94680-94690, 94770, 95812-95816, 95819, 95822, 95829, 95955, 96360-96368, 96372, 96374-96377, 96523, 97597-97598, 97602-97608, 99155, 99156, 99157, 99211-99223, 99231-99255, 99291-99292, 99304-99310, 99315-99316, 99334-99337, 99347-99350, 99374-99375, 99377-99378, 99446-99449, 99451-99452, 99495-99496, G0168, G0463, G0471, J0670, J2001

13102 0543T-0544T, 0548T, 0567T-0574T, 0580T, 0581T, 0582T, 11900-11901, 13160✧, 20560-20561, 20701, 36591-36592, 66987-66988, 69990, 96523, J0670, J2001

13131 0213T, 0216T, 0228T, 0230T, 0548T, 0567T-0574T, 0580T, 0581T, 0582T, 11000, 11010-11012, 11042-11044, 11900-11901, 13133, 13160✧, 15772, 15774, 20560-20561, 20700-20701, 36000, 36400-36410, 36420-36430, 36440, 36591-36592, 36600, 36640, 43752, 51701-51703, 64400, 64405-64408, 64415-64435, 64445-64451, 64479-64484, 64490-64505, 64510-64530, 64625, 66987-66988, 69990, 92012-92014, 93000-93010, 93040-93042, 93318, 93355, 94002, 94200, 94250, 94680-94690, 94770, 95812-95816, 95819, 95822, 95829, 95955, 96360-96368, 96372, 96374-96377, 96523, 97597-97598, 97602-97608, 99155, 99156, 99157, 99211-99223, 99231-99255, 99291-99292, 99304-99310, 99315-99316, 99334-99337, 99347-99350, 99374-99375, 99377-99378, 99446-99449, 99451-99452, 99495-99496, G0168, G0463, G0471, J0670, J2001

13132 0213T, 0216T, 0228T, 0230T, 0548T, 0567T-0574T, 0580T, 0581T, 0582T, 11000, 11010-11012, 11042-11044, 11056, 11900-11901, 13131, 13160✧, 15772, 15774, 20560-20561, 20700-20701, 36000, 36400-36410, 36420-36430, 36440, 36591-36592, 36600, 36640, 43752, 51701-51703, 64400, 64405-64408, 64415-64435, 64445-64451, 64479-64484, 64490-64505, 64510-64530, 64625, 66987-66988, 69990, 92012-92014, 93000-93010, 93040-93042, 93318, 93355, 94002, 94200, 94250, 94680-94690, 94770, 95812-95816, 95819, 95822, 95829, 95955, 96360-96368, 96372, 96374-96377, 96523, 97597-97598, 97602-97608, 99155, 99156, 99157, 99211-99223, 99231-99255, 99291-99292, 99304-99310, 99315-99316, 99334-99337, 99347-99350, 99374-99375, 99377-99378, 99446-99449, 99451-99452, 99495-99496, G0168, G0463, G0471, J0670, J2001

13133 0548T, 0567T-0574T, 0580T, 0581T, 0582T, 11900-11901, 13160✧, 20560-20561, 20700-20701, 36591-36592, 64451, 66987-66988, 69990, 96523, J0670, J2001

13160 0213T, 0216T, 0228T, 0230T, 10180, 11000-11006, 11010-11012, 11042-11047, 11102, 11104, 11106, 11900-11901, 12001-12007, 12011-12057, 36000, 36400-36410, 36420-36430, 36440, 36591-36592, 36600, 36640, 43752, 51701-51703, 62320-62327, 64400, 64405-64408, 64415-64435, 64445-64454, 64461-64463, 64479-64505, 64510-64530, 69990, 92012-92014, 93000-93010, 93040-93042, 93318, 93355, 94002, 94200, 94250, 94680-94690, 94770, 95812-95816, 95819, 95822, 95829, 95955, 96360-96368, 96372, 96374-96377, 96523, 97597-97598, 97602-97608, 99155, 99156, 99157, 99211-99223, 99231-99255,

99291-99292, 99304-99310, 99315-99316, 99334-99337, 99347-99350, 99374-99375, 99377-99378, 99446-99449, 99451-99452, 99495-99496, G0168, G0463, G0471

14040 0213T, 0216T, 0228T, 0230T, 0490T, 11000-11006, 11042-11047, 11055-11056, 11102, 11104, 11106, 11400-11471, 11600-11606, 11620-11646, 12001-12007, 12011-12057, 13100-13133, 13151-13153, 15852, 20526-20553, 20560-20561, 25259, 26340, 29086, 36000, 36400-36410, 36420-36430, 36440, 36591-36592, 36600, 36640, 43752, 51701-51703, 62320-62327, 64400, 64405-64408, 64415-64435, 64445-64454, 64461-64463, 64479-64505, 64510-64530, 69990, 92012-92014, 93000-93010, 93040-93042, 93318, 93355, 94002, 94200, 94250, 94680-94690, 94770, 95812-95816, 95819, 95822, 95829, 95955, 96360-96368, 96372, 96374-96377, 96523, 97597-97598, 97602-97608, 99155, 99156, 99157, 99211-99223, 99231-99255, 99291-99292, 99304-99310, 99315-99316, 99334-99337, 99347-99350, 99374-99375, 99377-99378, 99446-99449, 99451-99452, 99495-99496, G0168, G0463, G0471, J0670, J2001

14041 0213T, 0216T, 0228T, 0230T, 11000-11006, 11042-11047, 11102, 11104, 11106, 11400-11471, 11600-11606, 11620-11646, 12001-12007, 12011-12057, 13100-13133, 13151-13153, 14040, 20526, 20551-20553, 20560-20561, 25259, 26340, 29086, 36000, 36400-36410, 36420-36430, 36440, 36591-36592, 36600, 36640, 43752, 51701-51703, 62320-62327, 64400, 64405-64408, 64415-64435, 64445-64454, 64461-64463, 64479-64505, 64510-64530, 69990, 92012-92014, 93000-93010, 93040-93042, 93318, 93355, 94002, 94200, 94250, 94680-94690, 94770, 95812-95816, 95819, 95822, 95829, 95955, 96360-96368, 96372, 96374-96377, 96523, 97597-97598, 97602-97608, 99155, 99156, 99157, 99211-99223, 99231-99255, 99291-99292, 99304-99310, 99315-99316, 99334-99337, 99347-99350, 99374-99375, 99377-99378, 99446-99449, 99451-99452, 99495-99496, G0168, G0463, G0471, J0670, J2001

17270 0213T, 0216T, 0228T, 0230T, 0419T-0420T✧, 11102, 11104, 11106, 11600-11606✧, 11620-11646✧, 11900-11901, 12001-12007, 12011-12057, 13100-13133, 13151-13153, 17000✧, 17004✧, 17110-17111✧, 17340, 36000, 36400-36410, 36420-36430, 36440, 36591-36592, 36600, 36640, 43752, 51701-51703, 62320-62327, 64400, 64405-64408, 64415-64435, 64445-64454, 64461-64463, 64479-64505, 64510-64530, 69990, 92012-92014, 93000-93010, 93040-93042, 93318, 93355, 94002, 94200, 94250, 94680-94690, 94770, 95812-95816, 95819, 95822, 95829, 95955, 96360-96368, 96372, 96374-96377, 96523, 99155, 99156, 99157, 99211-99223, 99231-99255, 99291-99292, 99304-99310, 99315-99316, 99334-99337, 99347-99350, 99374-99375, 99377-99378, 99446-99449, 99451-99452, 99495-99496, G0463, G0471, J0670, J2001

17271 0213T, 0216T, 0228T, 0230T, 11102, 11104, 11106, 11601-11606✧, 11621-11646✧, 11900-11901, 12001-12007, 12011-12057, 13100-13133, 13151-13153, 17000✧, 17004✧, 17110-17111✧, 17340, 36000, 36400-36410, 36420-36430, 36440, 36591-36592, 36600, 36640, 43752, 51701-51703, 62320-62327, 64400, 64405-64408, 64415-64435, 64445-64454, 64461-64463, 64479-64505, 64510-64530, 69990, 92012-92014, 93000-93010, 93040-93042, 93318, 93355, 94002, 94200, 94250, 94680-94690, 94770, 95812-95816, 95819, 95822, 95829, 95955, 96360-96368, 96372, 96374-96377, 96523, 99155, 99156, 99157, 99211-99223, 99231-99255, 99291-99292, 99304-99310, 99315-99316, 99334-99337, 99347-99350, 99374-99375, 99377-99378, 99446-99449, 99451-99452, 99495-99496, G0463, G0471, J0670, J2001

17272 0213T, 0216T, 0228T, 0230T, 11102, 11104, 11106, 11601-11606✧, 11621-11626✧, 11641-11646✧, 11900-11901, 12001-12007, 12011-12057, 13100-13133, 13151-13153, 17000✧, 17004✧,

17110-17111❖, 17340, 36000, 36400-36410, 36420-36430, 36440, 36591-36592, 36600, 36640, 43752, 51701-51703, 62320-62327, 64400, 64405-64408, 64415-64435, 64445-64454, 64461-64463, 64479-64505, 64510-64530, 69990, 92012-92014, 93000-93010, 93040-93042, 93318, 93355, 94002, 94200, 94250, 94680-94690, 94770, 95812-95816, 95819, 95822, 95829, 95955, 96360-96368, 96372, 96374-96377, 96523, 99155, 99156, 99157, 99211-99223, 99231-99255, 99291-99292, 99304-99310, 99315-99316, 99334-99337, 99347-99350, 99374-99375, 99377-99378, 99446-99449, 99451-99452, 99495-99496, G0463, G0471, J0670, J2001

17273 0213T, 0216T, 0228T, 0230T, 11102, 11104, 11106, 11602-11606❖, 11622-11626❖, 11641-11646❖, 11900-11901, 12001-12007, 12011-12057, 13100-13133, 13151-13153, 17000❖, 17004❖, 17110-17111❖, 17340, 36000, 36400-36410, 36420-36430, 36440, 36591-36592, 36600, 36640, 43752, 51701-51703, 62320-62327, 64400, 64405-64408, 64415-64435, 64445-64454, 64461-64463, 64479-64505, 64510-64530, 69990, 92012-92014, 93000-93010, 93040-93042, 93318, 93355, 94002, 94200, 94250, 94680-94690, 94770, 95812-95816, 95819, 95822, 95829, 95955, 96360-96368, 96372, 96374-96377, 96523, 99155, 99156, 99157, 99211-99223, 99231-99255, 99291-99292, 99304-99310, 99315-99316, 99334-99337, 99347-99350, 99374-99375, 99377-99378, 99446-99449, 99451-99452, 99495-99496, G0463, G0471, J0670, J2001

17274 0213T, 0216T, 0228T, 0230T, 11102, 11104, 11106, 11606❖, 11623-11626❖, 11642-11646❖, 11900-11901, 12001-12007, 12011-12057, 13100-13133, 13151-13153, 17000❖, 17004❖, 17110-17111❖, 17340, 36000, 36400-36410, 36420-36430, 36440, 36591-36592, 36600, 36640, 43752, 51701-51703, 62320-62327, 64400, 64405-64408, 64415-64435, 64445-64454, 64461-64463, 64479-64505, 64510-64530, 69990, 92012-92014, 93000-93010, 93040-93042, 93318, 93355, 94002, 94200, 94250, 94680-94690, 94770, 95812-95816, 95819, 95822, 95829, 95955, 96360-96368, 96372, 96374-96377, 96523, 99155, 99156, 99157, 99211-99223, 99231-99255, 99291-99292, 99304-99310, 99315-99316, 99334-99337, 99347-99350, 99374-99375, 99377-99378, 99446-99449, 99451-99452, 99495-99496, G0463, G0471, J0670, J2001

17276 0213T, 0216T, 0228T, 0230T, 11102, 11104, 11106, 11606❖, 11624-11626❖, 11643-11646❖, 11900-11901, 12001-12007, 12011-12057, 13100-13133, 13151-13153, 17000❖, 17004❖, 17110-17111❖, 17340, 36000, 36400-36410, 36420-36430, 36440, 36591-36592, 36600, 36640, 43752, 51701-51703, 62320-62327, 64400, 64405-64408, 64415-64435, 64445-64454, 64461-64463, 64479-64505, 64510-64530, 69990, 92012-92014, 93000-93010, 93040-93042, 93318, 93355, 94002, 94200, 94250, 94680-94690, 94770, 95812-95816, 95819, 95822, 95829, 95955, 96360-96368, 96372, 96374-96377, 96523, 99155, 99156, 99157, 99211-99223, 99231-99255, 99291-99292, 99304-99310, 99315-99316, 99334-99337, 99347-99350, 99374-99375, 99377-99378, 99446-99449, 99451-99452, 99495-99496, G0463, G0471, J0670, J2001

35840 0213T, 0216T, 0228T, 0230T, 12001-12007, 12011-12057, 13100-13133, 13151-13153, 36000, 36002, 36400-36410, 36420-36430, 36440, 36591-36592, 36595-36596❖, 36600, 36640, 43752, 49000-49002, 51701-51703, 62320-62327, 64400, 64405-64408, 64415-64435, 64445-64454, 64461-64463, 64479-64505, 64510-64530, 69990, 75625, 75630, 75635, 75726, 75731, 75733, 75810, 75825, 75831, 75833, 75840, 75842, 75885, 75887, 75889, 75891, 92012-92014, 93000-93010, 93040-93042, 93318, 93355, 94002, 94200, 94250, 94680-94690, 94770, 95812-95816, 95819, 95822, 95829, 95955, 96360-96368, 96372, 96374-96377, 96523, 99155, 99156, 99157, 99211-99223, 99231-99255, 99291-99292, 99304-99310, 99315-99316,

99334-99337, 99347-99350, 99374-99375, 99377-99378, 99446-99449, 99451-99452, 99495-99496, G0463, G0471

36415 36591-36592, 96523, 99211

36416 36591-36592, 96523

36460 36591-36592, 69990, 96523

38562 0213T, 0216T, 0228T, 0230T, 11000-11006, 11042-11047, 12001-12007, 12011-12057, 13100-13133, 13151-13153, 36000, 36400-36410, 36420-36430, 36440, 36591-36592, 36600, 36640, 43752, 44005, 44180, 44602-44605, 44820-44850, 44950, 44970, 49000-49010, 49255, 49320-49321, 49570, 51701-51703, 52000, 62320-62327, 64400, 64405-64408, 64415-64435, 64445-64454, 64461-64463, 64479-64505, 64510-64530, 69990, 92012-92014, 93000-93010, 93040-93042, 93318, 93355, 94002, 94200, 94250, 94680-94690, 94770, 95812-95816, 95819, 95822, 95829, 95955, 96360-96368, 96372, 96374-96377, 96523, 97597-97598, 97602, 99155, 99156, 99157, 99211-99223, 99231-99255, 99291-99292, 99304-99310, 99315-99316, 99334-99337, 99347-99350, 99374-99375, 99377-99378, 99446-99449, 99451-99452, 99495-99496, G0463, G0471

38747 11000-11006, 11042-11047, 36591-36592, 38500, 38531, 38570, 44950, 44970, 49000-49002, 49320-49321, 96523, 97597-97598, 97602

38760 0213T, 0216T, 0228T, 0230T, 11000-11006, 11042-11047, 12001-12007, 12011-12057, 13100-13133, 13151-13153, 36000, 36400-36410, 36420-36430, 36440, 36591-36592, 36600, 36640, 38500, 38531❖, 43752, 51701-51703, 62320-62327, 64400, 64405-64408, 64415-64435, 64445-64454, 64461-64463, 64479-64505, 64510-64530, 69990, 92012-92014, 93000-93010, 93040-93042, 93318, 93355, 94002, 94200, 94250, 94680-94690, 94770, 95812-95816, 95819, 95822, 95829, 95955, 96360-96368, 96372, 96374-96377, 96523, 97597-97598, 97602, 99155, 99156, 99157, 99211-99223, 99231-99255, 99291-99292, 99304-99310, 99315-99316, 99334-99337, 99347-99350, 99374-99375, 99377-99378, 99446-99449, 99451-99452, 99495-99496, G0463, G0471

38765 0213T, 0216T, 0228T, 0230T, 11000-11006, 11042-11047, 12001-12007, 12011-12057, 13100-13133, 13151-13153, 36000, 36400-36410, 36420-36430, 36440, 36591-36592, 36600, 36640, 38500, 38531❖, 38562, 38571, 38760, 38770, 43752, 51701-51703, 52000, 62320-62327, 64400, 64405-64408, 64415-64435, 64445-64454, 64461-64463, 64479-64505, 64510-64530, 69990, 92012-92014, 93000-93010, 93040-93042, 93318, 93355, 94002, 94200, 94250, 94680-94690, 94770, 95812-95816, 95819, 95822, 95829, 95955, 96360-96368, 96372, 96374-96377, 96523, 97597-97598, 97602, 99155, 99156, 99157, 99211-99223, 99231-99255, 99291-99292, 99304-99310, 99315-99316, 99334-99337, 99347-99350, 99374-99375, 99377-99378, 99446-99449, 99451-99452, 99495-99496, G0463, G0471, J0670, J2001

38770 0213T, 0216T, 0228T, 0230T, 11000-11006, 11042-11047, 12001-12007, 12011-12057, 13100-13133, 13151-13153, 36000, 36400-36410, 36420-36430, 36440, 36591-36592, 36600, 36640, 38500, 38531, 38562-38564, 38571, 38760, 43752, 44005, 44180, 44602-44605, 44820-44850, 44950, 44970, 49000-49010, 49320-49321, 49570, 51701-51703, 52000, 62320-62327, 64400, 64405-64408, 64415-64435, 64445-64454, 64461-64463, 64479-64505, 64510-64530, 69990, 92012-92014, 93000-93010, 93040-93042, 93318, 93355, 94002, 94200, 94250, 94680-94690, 94770, 95812-95816, 95819, 95822, 95829, 95955, 96360-96368, 96372, 96374-96377, 96523, 97597-97598, 97602, 99155, 99156, 99157, 99211-99223, 99231-99255, 99291-99292, 99304-99310, 99315-99316, 99334-99337, 99347-99350, 99374-99375, 99377-99378, 99446-99449, 99451-99452, 99495-99496, G0463, G0471

38780 0213T, 0216T, 0228T, 0230T, 11000-11006, 11042-11047, 12001-12007, 12011-12057, 13100-13133, 13151-13153, 36000, 36400-36410,

36420-36430, 36440, 36591-36592, 36600, 36640, 38500, 38531,
38562-38572, 38765, 38770, 43752, 44005, 44180, 44602-44605,
44820-44850, 44950, 44970, 49000-49010, 49320-49321, 49570,
51701-51703, 52000, 62320-62327, 64400, 64405-64408, 64415-64435,
64445-64454, 64461-64463, 64479-64505, 64510-64530, 69990,
92012-92014, 93000-93010, 93040-93042, 93318, 93355, 94002, 94200,
94250, 94680-94690, 94770, 95812-95816, 95819, 95822, 95829,
95955, 96360-96368, 96372, 96374-96377, 96523, 97597-97598, 97602,
99155, 99156, 99157, 99211-99223, 99231-99255, 99291-99292,
99304-99310, 99315-99316, 99334-99337, 99347-99350, 99374-99375,
99377-99378, 99446-99449, 99451-99452, 99495-99496, G0463, G0471

44180 0213T, 0216T, 0228T, 0230T, 12001-12007, 12011-12057, 13100-13133,
13151-13153, 36000, 36400-36410, 36420-36430, 36440, 36591-36592,
36600, 36640, 43752, 44701, 49082-49084, 49320, 49400,
51701-51703, 62320-62327, 64400, 64405-64408, 64415-64435,
64445-64454, 64461-64463, 64479-64505, 64510-64530, 69990, 76000,
77001-77002, 92012-92014, 93000-93010, 93040-93042, 93318, 93355,
94002, 94200, 94250, 94680-94690, 94770, 95812-95816, 95819,
95822, 95829, 95955, 96360-96368, 96372, 96374-96377, 96523,
99155, 99156, 99157, 99211-99223, 99231-99255, 99291-99292,
99304-99310, 99315-99316, 99334-99337, 99347-99350, 99374-99375,
99377-99378, 99446-99449, 99451-99452, 99495-99496, G0463, G0471

45560 0213T, 0216T, 0228T, 0230T, 0437T, 12001-12007, 12011-12057,
13100-13133, 13151-13153, 15777, 36000, 36400-36410, 36420-36430,
36440, 36591-36592, 36600, 36640, 43752, 44602-44605, 44701,
45900-45990, 46040, 46080, 46220, 46600-46601, 46940-46942,
49000-49002, 49320, 49568, 51701-51703, 52000, 62320-62327, 64400,
64405-64408, 64415-64435, 64445-64454, 64461-64463, 64479-64505,
64510-64530, 69990, 92012-92014, 93000-93010, 93040-93042, 93318,
93355, 94002, 94200, 94250, 94680-94690, 94770, 95812-95816,
95819, 95822, 95829, 95955, 96360-96368, 96372, 96374-96377,
96523, 99155, 99156, 99157, 99211-99223, 99231-99255, 99291-99292,
99304-99310, 99315-99316, 99334-99337, 99347-99350, 99374-99375,
99377-99378, 99446-99449, 99451-99452, 99495-99496, G0463, G0471

46900 00902, 0213T, 0216T, 0228T, 0230T, 12001-12007, 12011-12057,
13100-13133, 13151-13153, 36000, 36400-36410, 36420-36430, 36440,
36591-36592, 36600, 36640, 43752, 45900-45990, 46040, 46080,
46220, 46600-46601, 46940-46942, 51701-51703, 62320-62327, 64400,
64405-64408, 64415-64435, 64445-64454, 64461-64463, 64479-64505,
64510-64530, 69990, 92012-92014, 93000-93010, 93040-93042, 93318,
93355, 94002, 94200, 94250, 94680-94690, 94770, 95812-95816,
95819, 95822, 95829, 95955, 96360-96368, 96372, 96374-96377,
96523, 99155, 99156, 99157, 99211-99223, 99231-99255, 99291-99292,
99304-99310, 99315-99316, 99334-99337, 99347-99350, 99374-99375,
99377-99378, 99446-99449, 99451-99452, 99495-99496, G0463,
G0471, J0670, J2001

46910 00902, 0213T, 0216T, 0228T, 0230T, 12001-12007, 12011-12057,
13100-13133, 13151-13153, 36000, 36400-36410, 36420-36430, 36440,
36591-36592, 36600, 36640, 43752, 45900-45990, 46040, 46080,
46220, 46600-46601, 46940-46942, 51701-51703, 62320-62327, 64400,
64405-64408, 64415-64435, 64445-64454, 64461-64463, 64479-64505,
64510-64530, 69990, 92012-92014, 93000-93010, 93040-93042, 93318,
93355, 94002, 94200, 94250, 94680-94690, 94770, 95812-95816,
95819, 95822, 95829, 95955, 96360-96368, 96372, 96374-96377,
96523, 99155, 99156, 99157, 99211-99223, 99231-99255, 99291-99292,
99304-99310, 99315-99316, 99334-99337, 99347-99350, 99374-99375,
99377-99378, 99446-99449, 99451-99452, 99495-99496, G0463,
G0471, J0670, J2001

46916 00902, 0213T, 0216T, 0228T, 0230T, 12001-12007, 12011-12057,
13100-13133, 13151-13153, 36000, 36400-36410, 36420-36430, 36440,
36591-36592, 36600, 36640, 43752, 45900-45990, 46040, 46080,
46220, 46600-46601, 46940-46942, 51701-51703, 62320-62327, 64400,
64405-64408, 64415-64435, 64445-64454, 64461-64463, 64479-64505,
64510-64530, 69990, 92012-92014, 93000-93010, 93040-93042, 93318,
93355, 94002, 94200, 94250, 94680-94690, 94770, 95812-95816,
95819, 95822, 95829, 95955, 96360-96368, 96372, 96374-96377,
96523, 99155, 99156, 99157, 99211-99223, 99231-99255, 99291-99292,
99304-99310, 99315-99316, 99334-99337, 99347-99350, 99374-99375,
99377-99378, 99446-99449, 99451-99452, 99495-99496, G0463,
G0471, J0670, J2001

46917 00902, 0213T, 0216T, 0228T, 0230T, 12001-12007, 12011-12057,
13100-13133, 13151-13153, 36000, 36400-36410, 36420-36430, 36440,
36591-36592, 36600, 36640, 43752, 45900-45990, 46040, 46080,
46220, 46600-46601, 46940-46942, 51701-51703, 62320-62327, 64400,
64405-64408, 64415-64435, 64445-64454, 64461-64463, 64479-64505,
64510-64530, 69990, 92012-92014, 93000-93010, 93040-93042, 93318,
93355, 94002, 94200, 94250, 94680-94690, 94770, 95812-95816,
95819, 95822, 95829, 95955, 96360-96368, 96372, 96374-96377,
96523, 99155, 99156, 99157, 99211-99223, 99231-99255, 99291-99292,
99304-99310, 99315-99316, 99334-99337, 99347-99350, 99374-99375,
99377-99378, 99446-99449, 99451-99452, 99495-99496, G0463,
G0471, J0670, J2001

46922 00902, 0213T, 0216T, 0228T, 0230T, 11000-11006, 11042-11047,
12001-12007, 12011-12057, 13100-13133, 13151-13153, 36000,
36400-36410, 36420-36430, 36440, 36591-36592, 36600, 36640, 43752,
45900-45990, 46040, 46080, 46220, 46600-46601, 46940-46942,
51701-51703, 62320-62327, 64400, 64405-64408, 64415-64435,
64445-64454, 64461-64463, 64479-64505, 64510-64530, 69990,
92012-92014, 93000-93010, 93040-93042, 93318, 93355, 94002, 94200,
94250, 94680-94690, 94770, 95812-95816, 95819, 95822, 95829,
95955, 96360-96368, 96372, 96374-96377, 96523, 97597-97598, 97602,
99155, 99156, 99157, 99211-99223, 99231-99255, 99291-99292,
99304-99310, 99315-99316, 99334-99337, 99347-99350, 99374-99375,
99377-99378, 99446-99449, 99451-99452, 99495-99496, G0463,
G0471, J0670, J2001

49000 0213T, 0216T, 0228T, 0230T, 10005, 10007, 10009, 10011, 10021,
11000-11006, 11042-11047, 12001-12007, 12011-12057, 13100-13133,
13151-13153, 20102, 36000, 36400-36410, 36420-36430, 36440,
36591-36592, 36600, 36640, 43752, 44015, 44180, 44950, 44970,
49013-49014, 49255, 51701-51703, 57410, 62320-62327, 64400,
64405-64408, 64415-64435, 64445-64454, 64461-64463, 64479-64505,
64510-64530, 69990, 92012-92014, 93000-93010, 93040-93042, 93318,
93355, 94002, 94200, 94250, 94680-94690, 94770, 95812-95816,
95819, 95822, 95829, 95955, 96360-96368, 96372, 96374-96377,
96523, 97597-97598, 97602, 99155, 99156, 99157, 99211-99223,
99231-99255, 99291-99292, 99304-99310, 99315-99316, 99334-99337,
99347-99350, 99374-99375, 99377-99378, 99446-99449, 99451-99452,
99495-99496, G0463, G0471

49002 0213T, 0216T, 0228T, 0230T, 11000-11006, 11042-11047, 12001-12007,
12011-12057, 13100-13133, 13151-13153, 20102, 36000, 36400-36410,
36420-36430, 36440, 36591-36592, 36600, 36640, 43752, 44005,
44180, 44820-44850, 44950, 44970, 49000, 49010-49014, 49255,
49570, 51701-51703, 62320-62327, 64400, 64405-64408, 64415-64435,
64445-64454, 64461-64463, 64479-64505, 64510-64530, 69990,
92012-92014, 93000-93010, 93040-93042, 93318, 93355, 94002, 94200,
94250, 94680-94690, 94770, 95812-95816, 95819, 95822, 95829,
95955, 96360-96368, 96372, 96374-96377, 96523, 97597-97598, 97602,
99155, 99156, 99157, 99211-99223, 99231-99255, 99291-99292,

99304-99310, 99315-99316, 99334-99337, 99347-99350, 99374-99375, 99377-99378, 99446-99449, 99451-99452, 99495-99496, G0463, G0471

49020 0213T, 0216T, 0228T, 0230T, 12001-12007, 12011-12057, 13100-13133, 13151-13153, 20102, 36000, 36400-36410, 36420-36430, 36440, 36591-36592, 36600, 36640, 43752, 44005, 44180, 44602-44605, 44820-44850, 44950, 44970, 49000-49014, 49185, 49203-49204, 49255, 49320, 49402, 49406-49407, 49424, 49570, 51701-51703, 62320-62327, 64400, 64405-64408, 64415-64435, 64445-64454, 64461-64463, 64479-64505, 64510-64530, 69990, 76000, 77001-77002, 92012-92014, 93000-93010, 93040-93042, 93318, 93355, 94002, 94200, 94250, 94680-94690, 94770, 95812-95816, 95819, 95822, 95829, 95955, 96360-96368, 96372, 96374-96377, 96523, 99155, 99156, 99157, 99211-99223, 99231-99255, 99291-99292, 99304-99310, 99315-99316, 99334-99337, 99347-99350, 99374-99375, 99377-99378, 99446-99449, 99451-99452, 99495-99496, G0463, G0471

49082 0213T, 0216T, 0228T, 0230T, 12001-12007, 12011-12057, 13100-13133, 13151-13153, 20102, 36000, 36400-36410, 36420-36430, 36440, 36591-36592, 36600, 36640, 43752, 49013-49014, 51701-51703, 62320-62327, 64400, 64405-64408, 64415-64435, 64445-64454, 64461-64463, 64479-64505, 64510-64530, 69990, 76000, 76380, 76942, 76970, 76998, 77001-77002, 77012, 77021, 92012-92014, 93000-93010, 93040-93042, 93318, 93355, 94002, 94200, 94250, 94680-94690, 94770, 95812-95816, 95819, 95822, 95829, 95955, 96360-96368, 96372, 96374-96377, 96523, 99155, 99156, 99157, 99211-99223, 99231-99255, 99291-99292, 99304-99310, 99315-99316, 99334-99337, 99347-99350, 99374-99375, 99377-99378, 99446-99449, 99451-99452, 99495-99496, G0463, G0471

49083 0213T, 0216T, 0228T, 0230T, 12001-12007, 12011-12057, 13100-13133, 13151-13153, 20102, 36000, 36400-36410, 36420-36430, 36440, 36591-36592, 36600, 36640, 43752, 49013-49014, 49082, 51701-51703, 62320-62327, 64400, 64405-64408, 64415-64435, 64445-64454, 64461-64463, 64479-64505, 64510-64530, 69990, 76000, 76380, 76942, 76970, 76998, 77001-77002, 77012, 77021, 92012-92014, 93000-93010, 93040-93042, 93318, 93355, 94002, 94200, 94250, 94680-94690, 94770, 95812-95816, 95819, 95822, 95829, 95955, 96360-96368, 96372, 96374-96377, 96523, 99155, 99156, 99157, 99211-99223, 99231-99255, 99291-99292, 99304-99310, 99315-99316, 99334-99337, 99347-99350, 99374-99375, 99377-99378, 99446-99449, 99451-99452, 99495-99496, G0463, G0471

49084 0213T, 0216T, 0228T, 0230T, 12001-12007, 12011-12057, 13100-13133, 13151-13153, 20102, 36000, 36400-36410, 36420-36430, 36440, 36591-36592, 36600, 36640, 43752, 49013-49014, 49082-49083, 51701-51703, 62320-62327, 64400, 64405-64408, 64415-64435, 64445-64454, 64461-64463, 64479-64505, 64510-64530, 69990, 76000, 76380, 76942, 76970, 76998, 77001-77002, 77012, 77021, 92012-92014, 93000-93010, 93040-93042, 93318, 93355, 94002, 94200, 94250, 94680-94690, 94770, 95812-95816, 95819, 95822, 95829, 95955, 96360-96368, 96372, 96374-96377, 96523, 99155, 99156, 99157, 99211-99223, 99231-99255, 99291-99292, 99304-99310, 99315-99316, 99334-99337, 99347-99350, 99374-99375, 99377-99378, 99446-99449, 99451-99452, 99495-99496, G0463, G0471

49180 0213T, 0216T, 0228T, 0230T, 10005, 10007, 10009, 10011, 10021, 12001-12007, 12011-12057, 13100-13133, 13151-13153, 36000, 36400-36410, 36420-36430, 36440, 36591-36592, 36600, 36640, 43752, 44950, 44970, 51701-51703, 62320-62327, 64400, 64405-64408, 64415-64435, 64445-64454, 64461-64463, 64479-64505, 64510-64530, 69990, 92012-92014, 93000-93010, 93040-93042, 93318, 93355, 94002, 94200, 94250, 94680-94690, 94770, 95812-95816, 95819, 95822, 95829, 95955, 96360-96368, 96372, 96374-96377, 96523, 99155,

99156, 99157, 99211-99223, 99231-99255, 99291-99292, 99304-99310, 99315-99316, 99334-99337, 99347-99350, 99374-99375, 99377-99378, 99446-99449, 99451-99452, 99495-99496, G0463, G0471, J0670, J1642-J1644, J2001

49203 0213T, 0216T, 0228T, 0230T, 11000-11006, 11042-11047, 12001-12007, 12011-12057, 13100-13133, 13151-13153, 36000, 36400-36410, 36420-36430, 36440, 36591-36592, 36600, 36640, 38500, 38531, 38770, 38780, 43752, 43832, 44005, 44180, 44602-44605, 44820-44850, 44950, 44970, 47382-47383✧, 49000-49010, 49040, 49255, 49320, 49322-49323, 49406, 49560-49566, 49570-49572, 49580, 49582-49587, 50010, 50205, 50220, 50280-50290, 50592-50593, 50722-50725, 57410, 58700-58720, 58805, 58900-58940, 58943, 58950, 58960, 60540-60545, 62320-62327, 64400, 64405-64408, 64415-64435, 64445-64454, 64461-64463, 64479-64505, 64510-64530, 69990, 92012-92014, 93000-93010, 93040-93042, 93318, 93355, 94002, 94200, 94250, 94680-94690, 94770, 95812-95816, 95819, 95822, 95829, 95955, 96360-96368, 96372, 96374-96377, 96523, 97597-97598, 97602, 99155, 99156, 99157, 99211-99223, 99231-99255, 99291-99292, 99304-99310, 99315-99316, 99334-99337, 99347-99350, 99374-99375, 99377-99378, 99446-99449, 99451-99452, 99495-99496, G0463

49204 0213T, 0216T, 0228T, 0230T, 11000-11006, 11042-11047, 12001-12007, 12011-12057, 13100-13133, 13151-13153, 36000, 36400-36410, 36420-36430, 36440, 36591-36592, 36600, 36640, 38500, 38531, 38770, 38780, 43752, 43832, 44005, 44160-44180, 44602-44605, 44820-44850, 44950, 44970, 47370-47371✧, 47380-47383✧, 49000-49010, 49040, 49203, 49255, 49320, 49322-49323, 49406, 49560-49566, 49570-49572, 49580, 49582-49587, 50010, 50205, 50220-50234, 50250-50290, 50542, 50592-50593, 50715, 50722-50725, 57410, 58200, 58700-58720, 58805, 58900-58940, 58943, 58950-58951, 58956, 58960, 60540-60545, 62320-62327, 64400, 64405-64408, 64415-64435, 64445-64454, 64461-64463, 64479-64505, 64510-64530, 69990, 92012-92014, 93000-93010, 93040-93042, 93318, 93355, 94002, 94200, 94250, 94680-94690, 94770, 95812-95816, 95819, 95822, 95829, 95955, 96360-96368, 96372, 96374-96377, 96523, 97597-97598, 97602, 99155, 99156, 99157, 99211-99223, 99231-99255, 99291-99292, 99304-99310, 99315-99316, 99334-99337, 99347-99350, 99374-99375, 99377-99378, 99446-99449, 99451-99452, 99495-99496, G0463

49205 0213T, 0216T, 0228T, 0230T, 11000-11006, 11042-11047, 12001-12007, 12011-12057, 13100-13133, 13151-13153, 36000, 36400-36410, 36420-36430, 36440, 36591-36592, 36600, 36640, 38500, 38531, 38770, 38780, 43752, 43832, 44005, 44160-44180, 44602-44605, 44820-44850, 44950, 44970, 47370-47371✧, 47380-47383✧, 49000-49010, 49020, 49040, 49203-49204, 49255, 49320, 49322-49323, 49406, 49560-49566, 49570-49572, 49580, 49582-49587, 50010, 50205, 50220-50236, 50250-50290, 50542, 50592-50593, 50715, 50722-50725, 57410, 58200, 58700-58720, 58805, 58900-58940, 58943, 58950-58952, 58956-58960, 60540-60545, 62320-62327, 64400, 64405-64408, 64415-64435, 64445-64454, 64461-64463, 64479-64505, 64510-64530, 69990, 92012-92014, 93000-93010, 93040-93042, 93318, 93355, 94002, 94200, 94250, 94680-94690, 94770, 95812-95816, 95819, 95822, 95829, 95955, 96360-96368, 96372, 96374-96377, 96523, 97597-97598, 97602, 99155, 99156, 99157, 99211-99223, 99231-99255, 99291-99292, 99304-99310, 99315-99316, 99334-99337, 99347-99350, 99374-99375, 99377-99378, 99446-99449, 99451-99452, 99495-99496, G0463

49320 0213T, 0216T, 0228T, 0230T, 12001-12007, 12011-12057, 13100-13133, 13151-13153, 36000, 36400-36410, 36420-36430, 36440, 36591-36592, 36600, 36640, 43752, 44005, 47001, 49082-49084, 49400, 50715, 51701-51703, 57410, 62320-62327, 64400, 64405-64408, 64415-64435, 64445-64454, 64461-64463, 64479-64505, 64510-64530, 69990, 76000, 77001-77002, 92012-92014, 93000-93010, 93040-93042, 93318, 93355,

94002, 94200, 94250, 94680-94690, 94770, 95812-95816, 95819, 95822, 95829, 95955, 96360-96368, 96372, 96374-96377, 96523, 99155, 99156, 99157, 99211-99223, 99231-99255, 99291-99292, 99304-99310, 99315-99316, 99334-99337, 99347-99350, 99374-99375, 99377-99378, 99446-99449, 99451-99452, 99495-99496, G0463, G0471

49321 0213T, 0216T, 0228T, 0230T, 10005, 10007, 10009, 10011, 10021, 12001-12007, 12011-12057, 13100-13133, 13151-13153, 36000, 36400-36410, 36420-36430, 36440, 36591-36592, 36600, 36640, 43653, 43752, 44005, 44180, 44602-44605, 44950, 47001, 49082-49084, 49320, 49400, 50715, 51701-51703, 57410, 62320-62327, 64400, 64405-64408, 64415-64435, 64445-64454, 64461-64463, 64479-64505, 64510-64530, 69990, 76000, 77001-77002, 92012-92014, 93000-93010, 93040-93042, 93318, 93355, 94002, 94200, 94250, 94680-94690, 94770, 95812-95816, 95819, 95822, 95829, 95955, 96360-96368, 96372, 96374-96377, 96523, 99155, 99156, 99157, 99211-99223, 99231-99255, 99291-99292, 99304-99310, 99315-99316, 99334-99337, 99347-99350, 99374-99375, 99377-99378, 99446-99449, 99451-99452, 99495-99496, G0463, G0471

49322 0213T, 0216T, 0228T, 0230T, 12001-12007, 12011-12057, 13100-13133, 13151-13153, 36000, 36400-36410, 36420-36430, 36440, 36591-36592, 36600, 36640, 43653, 43752, 44005, 44180, 44602-44605, 44950, 44970, 49082-49084, 49320, 49400, 50715, 51701-51703, 57410, 62320-62327, 64400, 64405-64408, 64415-64435, 64445-64454, 64461-64463, 64479-64505, 64510-64530, 69990, 76000, 77001-77002, 92012-92014, 93000-93010, 93040-93042, 93318, 93355, 94002, 94200, 94250, 94680-94690, 94770, 95812-95816, 95819, 95822, 95829, 95955, 96360-96368, 96372, 96374-96377, 96523, 99155, 99156, 99157, 99211-99223, 99231-99255, 99291-99292, 99304-99310, 99315-99316, 99334-99337, 99347-99350, 99374-99375, 99377-99378, 99446-99449, 99451-99452, 99495-99496, G0463, G0471

49324 0213T, 0216T, 0228T, 0230T, 11000-11006, 11042-11047, 12001-12007, 12011-12057, 13100-13133, 13151-13153, 36000, 36400-36410, 36420-36430, 36440, 36591-36592, 36600, 36640, 43653, 43752, 44005, 44180, 44602-44605, 44950, 44970, 49000, 49082-49084, 49320, 49400, 49421-49422❖, 49436, 50715, 51701-51703, 58660, 62320-62327, 64400, 64405-64408, 64415-64435, 64445-64454, 64461-64463, 64479-64505, 64510-64530, 69990, 76000, 77001-77002, 92012-92014, 93000-93010, 93040-93042, 93318, 93355, 94002, 94200, 94250, 94680-94690, 94770, 95812-95816, 95819, 95822, 95829, 95955, 96360-96368, 96372, 96374-96377, 96523, 97597-97598, 97602, 99155, 99156, 99157, 99211-99223, 99231-99255, 99291-99292, 99304-99310, 99315-99316, 99334-99337, 99347-99350, 99374-99375, 99377-99378, 99446-99449, 99451-99452, 99495-99496, G0463, G0471

49325 0213T, 0216T, 0228T, 0230T, 11000-11006, 11042-11047, 12001-12007, 12011-12057, 13100-13133, 13151-13153, 36000, 36400-36410, 36420-36430, 36440, 36591-36592, 36600, 36640, 43653, 43752, 44005, 44180, 44602-44605, 44950, 44970, 49000, 49082-49084, 49320, 49324❖, 49400, 49421-49422❖, 50715, 51701-51703, 58660, 62320-62327, 64400, 64405-64408, 64415-64435, 64445-64454, 64461-64463, 64479-64505, 64510-64530, 69990, 76000, 77001-77002, 92012-92014, 93000-93010, 93040-93042, 93318, 93355, 94002, 94200, 94250, 94680-94690, 94770, 95812-95816, 95819, 95822, 95829, 95955, 96360-96368, 96372, 96374-96377, 96523, 97597-97598, 97602, 99155, 99156, 99157, 99211-99223, 99231-99255, 99291-99292, 99304-99310, 99315-99316, 99334-99337, 99347-99350, 99374-99375, 99377-99378, 99446-99449, 99451-99452, 99495-99496, G0463, G0471

49326 36591-36592, 49082-49084, 49400, 96523

49327 36591-36592, 43653, 44005, 44180, 44970, 49082-49084, 49320, 49400, 50715, 57410, 58660, 76000, 76380, 76942, 76970, 76998, 77002, 77012, 77021, 96523

49402 0213T, 0216T, 11000-11006, 11042-11047, 12001-12007, 12011-12057, 13100-13133, 13151-13153, 20102, 36000, 36400-36410, 36420-36430, 36440, 36591-36592, 36600, 36640, 43752, 44005, 44180, 44602-44605, 44820-44850, 44950, 44970, 49000-49014, 49255, 49320, 49429, 49560-49566, 49570-49572, 49580, 49582-49587, 51701-51703, 62320-62327, 64400, 64405-64408, 64415-64435, 64445-64454, 64461-64463, 64479-64505, 64510-64530, 69990, 92012-92014, 93000-93010, 93040-93042, 93318, 93355, 94002, 94200, 94250, 94680-94690, 94770, 95812-95816, 95819, 95822, 95829, 95955, 96360-96368, 96372, 96374-96377, 96523, 97597-97598, 97602, 99155, 99156, 99157, 99211-99223, 99231-99255, 99291-99292, 99304-99310, 99315-99316, 99334-99337, 99347-99350, 99374-99375, 99377-99378, 99446-99449, 99451-99452, 99495-99496, G0463, G0471

49406 00910, 0213T, 0216T, 0228T, 0230T, 12001-12007, 12011-12057, 13100-13133, 13151-13153, 36000, 36400-36410, 36420-36430, 36440, 36591-36592, 36600, 36640, 43752, 44005, 44180, 44602-44605, 44701, 44820-44850, 44950, 44970, 49000-49010, 49082-49084❖, 49180-49185, 49255, 49320, 49322, 49400, 49402, 49423-49424, 49570, 50010, 50205, 50715, 51045, 51570, 51701-51703, 57410, 58660, 58700, 58800, 58900, 62320-62327, 64400, 64405-64408, 64415-64435, 64445-64454, 64461-64463, 64479-64505, 64510-64530, 69990, 75989, 76000, 76380, 76942, 76970, 76998, 77001-77003, 77012, 77021, 92012-92014, 93000-93010, 93040-93042, 93318, 93355, 94002, 94200, 94250, 94680-94690, 94770, 95812-95816, 95819, 95822, 95829, 95955, 96360-96368, 96372, 96374-96377, 96523, 99155, 99156, 99157, 99211-99223, 99231-99255, 99291-99292, 99304-99310, 99315-99316, 99334-99337, 99347-99350, 99374-99375, 99377-99378, 99446-99449, 99451-99452, G0463, G0471, J0670, J2001

49407 0213T, 0216T, 0228T, 0230T, 12001-12007, 12011-12057, 13100-13133, 13151-13153, 36000, 36400-36410, 36420-36430, 36440, 36591-36592, 36600, 36640, 43752, 44701, 45005, 45900-45990, 46040, 46080, 46220, 46600-46601, 46940-46942, 49082-49084❖, 49185, 49322, 49406, 49423-49424, 50715, 51701-51703, 57410, 58660, 58805, 58900, 62320-62327, 64400, 64405-64408, 64415-64435, 64445-64454, 64461-64463, 64479-64505, 64510-64530, 69990, 75989, 76000, 76380, 76942, 76970, 76998, 77001-77003, 77012, 77021, 92012-92014, 93000-93010, 93040-93042, 93318, 93355, 94002, 94200, 94250, 94680-94690, 94770, 95812-95816, 95819, 95822, 95829, 95955, 96360-96368, 96372, 96374-96377, 96523, 99155, 99156, 99157, 99211-99223, 99231-99255, 99291-99292, 99304-99310, 99315-99316, 99334-99337, 99347-99350, 99374-99375, 99377-99378, 99446-99449, 99451-99452, G0463, G0471, J0670, J2001

50722 00910, 0213T, 0216T, 0228T, 0230T, 12001-12007, 12011-12057, 13100-13133, 13151-13153, 36000, 36400-36410, 36420-36430, 36440, 36591-36592, 36600, 36640, 43752, 44602-44605, 44850, 44950, 44970, 49000-49010, 50600-50605, 50715, 50900, 51701-51703, 62320-62327, 64400, 64405-64408, 64415-64435, 64445-64454, 64461-64463, 64479-64505, 64510-64530, 69990, 92012-92014, 93000-93010, 93040-93042, 93318, 93355, 94002, 94200, 94250, 94680-94690, 94770, 95812-95816, 95819, 95822, 95829, 95955, 96360-96368, 96372, 96374-96377, 96523, 99155, 99156, 99157, 99211-99223, 99231-99255, 99291-99292, 99304-99310, 99315-99316, 99334-99337, 99347-99350, 99374-99375, 99377-99378, 99446-99449, 99451-99452, 99495-99496, G0463, G0471

51020 00910, 0213T, 0216T, 0228T, 0230T, 11000-11006, 11042-11047, 12001-12007, 12011-12057, 13100-13133, 13151-13153, 36000,

36400-36410, 36420-36430, 36440, 36591-36592, 36600, 36640, 43752,
44602-44605, 44950, 44970, 49000-49002, 49320, 50715, 51045,
51100-51102, 51520-51525, 51701-51703, 52000, 62320-62327, 64400,
64405-64408, 64415-64435, 64445-64454, 64461-64463, 64479-64505,
64510-64530, 69990, 92012-92014, 93000-93010, 93040-93042, 93318,
93355, 94002, 94200, 94250, 94680-94690, 94770, 95812-95816,
95819, 95822, 95829, 95955, 96360-96368, 96372, 96374-96377,
96523, 97597-97598, 97602, 99155, 99156, 99157, 99211-99223,
99231-99255, 99291-99292, 99304-99310, 99315-99316, 99334-99337,
99347-99350, 99374-99375, 99377-99378, 99446-99449, 99451-99452,
99495-99496, G0463, G0471

51030 00910, 0213T, 0216T, 0228T, 0230T, 11000-11006, 11042-11047,
12001-12007, 12011-12057, 13100-13133, 13151-13153, 36000,
36400-36410, 36420-36430, 36440, 36591-36592, 36600, 36640, 43752,
44602-44605, 44950, 44970, 49000-49002, 49320, 50715, 51045,
51100-51102, 51520-51525, 51701-51703, 52000, 62320-62327, 64400,
64405-64408, 64415-64435, 64445-64454, 64461-64463, 64479-64505,
64510-64530, 69990, 92012-92014, 93000-93010, 93040-93042, 93318,
93355, 94002, 94200, 94250, 94680-94690, 94770, 95812-95816,
95819, 95822, 95829, 95955, 96360-96368, 96372, 96374-96377,
96523, 97597-97598, 97602, 99155, 99156, 99157, 99211-99223,
99231-99255, 99291-99292, 99304-99310, 99315-99316, 99334-99337,
99347-99350, 99374-99375, 99377-99378, 99446-99449, 99451-99452,
99495-99496, G0463, G0471

51045 00910, 0213T, 0216T, 0228T, 0230T, 11000-11006, 11042-11047,
12001-12007, 12011-12057, 13100-13133, 13151-13153, 36000,
36400-36410, 36420-36430, 36440, 36591-36592, 36600, 36640, 43752,
44602-44605, 44950, 44970, 49000-49002, 49320, 50715, 51701-51703,
52000, 62320-62327, 64400, 64405-64408, 64415-64435, 64445-64454,
64461-64463, 64479-64505, 64510-64530, 69990, 92012-92014,
93000-93010, 93040-93042, 93318, 93355, 94002, 94200, 94250,
94680-94690, 94770, 95812-95816, 95819, 95822, 95829, 95955,
96360-96368, 96372, 96374-96377, 96523, 97597-97598, 97602, 99155,
99156, 99157, 99211-99223, 99231-99255, 99291-99292, 99304-99310,
99315-99316, 99334-99337, 99347-99350, 99374-99375, 99377-99378,
99446-99449, 99451-99452, 99495-99496, G0463, G0471

51100 00910, 0213T, 0216T, 0228T, 0230T, 12001-12007, 12011-12057,
13100-13133, 13151-13153, 36000, 36400-36410, 36420-36430, 36440,
36591-36592, 36600, 36640, 43752, 44970, 51701, 52000,
62320-62327, 64400, 64405-64408, 64415-64435, 64445-64454,
64461-64463, 64479-64505, 64510-64530, 69990, 92012-92014,
93000-93010, 93040-93042, 93318, 93355, 94002, 94200, 94250,
94680-94690, 94770, 95812-95816, 95819, 95822, 95829, 95955,
96360-96368, 96372, 96374-96377, 96523, 99155, 99156, 99157,
99211-99223, 99231-99255, 99291-99292, 99304-99310, 99315-99316,
99334-99337, 99347-99350, 99374-99375, 99377-99378, 99446-99449,
99451-99452, 99495-99496, G0463, J0670, J2001

51101 00910, 0213T, 0216T, 0228T, 0230T, 12001-12007, 12011-12057,
13100-13133, 13151-13153, 36000, 36400-36410, 36420-36430, 36440,
36591-36592, 36600, 36640, 43752, 44970, 51100, 51701, 52000,
62320-62327, 64400, 64405-64408, 64415-64435, 64445-64454,
64461-64463, 64479-64505, 64510-64530, 69990, 76000, 77001,
92012-92014, 93000-93010, 93040-93042, 93318, 93355, 94002, 94200,
94250, 94680-94690, 94770, 95812-95816, 95819, 95822, 95829,
95955, 96360-96368, 96372, 96374-96377, 96523, 99155, 99156,
99157, 99211-99223, 99231-99255, 99291-99292, 99304-99310,
99315-99316, 99334-99337, 99347-99350, 99374-99375, 99377-99378,
99446-99449, 99451-99452, 99495-99496, G0463, J0670, J2001

51102 00910, 0213T, 0216T, 0228T, 0230T, 11000-11006, 11042-11047,
12001-12007, 12011-12057, 13100-13133, 13151-13153, 36000,
36400-36410, 36420-36430, 36440, 36591-36592, 36600, 36640, 43752,
44970, 51100-51101✦, 51701-51702, 52000, 52281, 62320-62327,
64400, 64405-64408, 64415-64435, 64445-64454, 64461-64463,
64479-64505, 64510-64530, 69990, 76000, 77001, 92012-92014,
93000-93010, 93040-93042, 93318, 93355, 94002, 94200, 94250,
94680-94690, 94770, 95812-95816, 95819, 95822, 95829, 95955,
96360-96368, 96372, 96374-96377, 96523, 97597-97598, 97602, 99155,
99156, 99157, 99211-99223, 99231-99255, 99291-99292, 99304-99310,
99315-99316, 99334-99337, 99347-99350, 99374-99375, 99377-99378,
99446-99449, 99451-99452, 99495-99496, G0463, G0471, J0670, J2001

51597 00910, 0213T, 0216T, 0228T, 0230T, 11000-11006, 11042-11047,
12001-12007, 12011-12057, 13100-13133, 13151-13153, 36000,
36400-36410, 36420-36430, 36440, 36591-36592, 36600, 36640,
38562-38564, 38571-38573, 38770, 38780, 43752, 44005, 44140-44151,
44155-44158, 44180, 44188, 44320-44346, 44602-44605, 44620-44625,
44820-44850, 44950-44970, 45110-45135, 45160, 45171-45172, 45190,
45395-45397, 45505, 45540, 46080-46200, 46220-46280, 46285,
46600-46601, 46940-46942, 46947-46948, 49000-49010, 49020, 49040,
49082-49084, 49203-49205, 49255, 49320-49321, 49560-49566, 49570,
49580, 49582-49587, 50650, 50715, 50800, 50810, 50860,
51040-51045, 51520-51525, 51550-51596, 51701-51703, 52000, 52204,
55821-55845, 55866, 57106, 57410, 57530-57556, 58100, 58120-58200,
58210-58263, 58267-58280, 58290-58294, 58541-58544, 58548, 58558,
58570-58575, 58660, 58662, 58950-58958, 62320-62327, 64400,
64405-64408, 64415-64435, 64445-64454, 64461-64463, 64479-64505,
64510-64530, 69990, 92012-92014, 93000-93010, 93040-93042, 93318,
93355, 94002, 94200, 94250, 94680-94690, 94770, 95812-95816,
95819, 95822, 95829, 95955, 96360-96368, 96372, 96374-96377,
96523, 97597-97598, 97602, 99155, 99156, 99157, 99211-99223,
99231-99255, 99291-99292, 99304-99310, 99315-99316, 99334-99337,
99347-99350, 99374-99375, 99377-99378, 99446-99449, 99451-99452,
99495-99496, G0463, G0471, P9612

51701 0543T-0544T, 0548T, 0567T-0574T, 0580T, 0581T, 0582T, 11000-11006,
11042-11047, 13102, 13122, 13133, 13153, 20560-20561, 36400-36406,
36420-36430, 36440, 36591-36592, 36600, 64480, 64484, 66987-66988,
69990, 92012-92014, 93000-93010, 93040-93042, 93318, 93355, 94002,
94200, 94250, 94680-94690, 94770, 95812-95816, 95819, 95822,
95829, 95955, 96360-96368, 96372, 96374-96377, 96523, 97597-97598,
97602, 99155, 99156, 99157, 99211-99223, 99231-99255, 99291-99292,
99304-99310, 99315-99316, 99334-99337, 99347-99350, 99374-99375,
99377-99378, 99446-99449, 99451-99452, 99495-99496, G0463, J0670,
J2001, P9612-P9615✦

51702 0543T-0544T, 0548T, 0567T-0574T, 0580T, 0581T, 0582T, 11000-11006,
11042-11047, 13102, 13122, 13133, 13153, 20560-20561, 36400-36406,
36420-36430, 36440, 36591-36592, 36600, 51701, 64480, 64484,
66987-66988, 69990, 92012-92014, 93000-93010, 93040-93042, 93318,
93355, 94002, 94200, 94250, 94680-94690, 94770, 95812-95816,
95819, 95822, 95829, 95955, 96360-96368, 96372, 96374-96377,
96523, 97597-97598, 97602, 99155, 99156, 99157, 99211-99223,
99231-99255, 99291-99292, 99304-99310, 99315-99316, 99334-99337,
99347-99350, 99374-99375, 99377-99378, 99446-99449, 99451-99452,
99495-99496, G0463, J0670, J2001, P9612

51703 0543T-0544T, 0548T, 0567T-0574T, 0580T, 0581T, 0582T, 11000-11006,
11042-11047, 13102, 13122, 13133, 13153, 20560-20561, 20701,
36400-36406, 36420-36430, 36440, 36591-36592, 36600, 51700-51702,
53080, 64415, 64417, 64450, 64480, 64484-64489, 66987-66988,
69990, 92012-92014, 93000-93010, 93040-93042, 93318, 93355, 94002,
94200, 94250, 94680-94690, 94770, 95812-95816, 95819, 95822,

95829, 95955, 96360-96368, 96372, 96374-96377, 96523, 97597-97598, 97602, 99155, 99156, 99157, 99211-99223, 99231-99255, 99291-99292, 99304-99310, 99315-99316, 99334-99337, 99347-99350, 99374-99375, 99377-99378, 99446-99449, 99451-99452, 99495-99496, G0463, G0471, J0670, J2001, P9612

51725 00910, 0213T, 0216T, 0228T, 0230T, 12001-12007, 12011-12057, 13100-13133, 13151-13153, 36000, 36400-36410, 36420-36430, 36440, 36591-36592, 36600, 36640, 43752, 50715, 51701-51703, 62320-62327, 64400, 64405-64408, 64415-64435, 64445-64454, 64461-64463, 64479-64505, 64510-64530, 69990, 92012-92014, 93000-93010, 93040-93042, 93318, 93355, 94002, 94200, 94250, 94680-94690, 94770, 95812-95816, 95819, 95822, 95829, 95955, 96360-96368, 96372, 96374-96377, 96523, 99155, 99156, 99157, 99211-99223, 99231-99255, 99291-99292, 99304-99310, 99315-99316, 99334-99337, 99347-99350, 99374-99375, 99377-99378, 99446-99449, 99451-99452, 99495-99496, G0463, G0471, P9612

51726 00910, 0228T, 0230T, 12001-12007, 12011-12057, 13100-13133, 13151-13153, 36000, 36400-36410, 36420-36430, 36440, 36591-36592, 36600, 36640, 43752, 50715, 51701-51703, 51725, 62320-62327, 64400, 64405-64408, 64415-64435, 64445-64454, 64461-64463, 64479-64505, 64510-64530, 69990, 92012-92014, 93000-93010, 93040-93042, 93318, 93355, 94002, 94200, 94250, 94680-94690, 94770, 95812-95816, 95819, 95822, 95829, 95955, 96360-96368, 96372, 96374-96377, 96523, 99155, 99156, 99157, 99211-99223, 99231-99255, 99291-99292, 99304-99310, 99315-99316, 99334-99337, 99347-99350, 99374-99375, 99377-99378, 99446-99449, 99451-99452, 99495-99496, G0463, G0471, P9612

51727 00910, 0213T, 0216T, 0228T, 0230T, 11000-11006, 11042-11047, 12001-12007, 12011-12057, 13100-13133, 13151-13153, 36000, 36400-36410, 36420-36430, 36440, 36591-36592, 36600, 36640, 43752, 50715, 51701-51703, 51725-51726, 62320-62327, 64400, 64405-64408, 64415-64435, 64445-64454, 64461-64463, 64479-64505, 64510-64530, 69990, 92012-92014, 93000-93010, 93040-93042, 93318, 93355, 94002, 94200, 94250, 94680-94690, 94770, 95812-95816, 95819, 95822, 95829, 95955, 96360-96368, 96372, 96374-96377, 96523, 97597-97598, 97602, 99155, 99156, 99157, 99211-99223, 99231-99255, 99291-99292, 99304-99310, 99315-99316, 99334-99337, 99347-99350, 99374-99375, 99377-99378, 99446-99449, 99451-99452, 99495-99496, G0463, G0471, J0670, J2001, P9612

51728 00910, 0213T, 0216T, 0228T, 0230T, 12001-12007, 12011-12057, 13100-13133, 13151-13153, 36000, 36400-36410, 36420-36430, 36440, 36591-36592, 36600, 36640, 43752, 50715, 51701-51703, 51725-51727, 62320-62327, 64400, 64405-64408, 64415-64435, 64445-64454, 64461-64463, 64479-64505, 64510-64530, 69990, 90901, 92012-92014, 93000-93010, 93040-93042, 93318, 93355, 94002, 94200, 94250, 94680-94690, 94770, 95812-95816, 95819, 95822, 95829, 95955, 96360-96368, 96372, 96374-96377, 96523, 99155, 99156, 99157, 99211-99223, 99231-99255, 99291-99292, 99304-99310, 99315-99316, 99334-99337, 99347-99350, 99374-99375, 99377-99378, 99446-99449, 99451-99452, 99495-99496, G0463, G0471, J0670, J2001, P9612

51729 00910, 0213T, 0216T, 0228T, 0230T, 11000-11006, 11042-11047, 12001-12007, 12011-12057, 13100-13133, 13151-13153, 36000, 36400-36410, 36420-36430, 36440, 36591-36592, 36600, 36640, 43752, 50715, 51701-51703, 51725-51728, 62320-62327, 64400, 64405-64408, 64415-64435, 64445-64454, 64461-64463, 64479-64505, 64510-64530, 69990, 90901, 92012-92014, 93000-93010, 93040-93042, 93318, 93355, 94002, 94200, 94250, 94680-94690, 94770, 95812-95816, 95819, 95822, 95829, 95955, 96360-96368, 96372, 96374-96377, 96523, 97597-97598, 97602, 99155, 99156, 99157, 99211-99223, 99231-99255,

99291-99292, 99304-99310, 99315-99316, 99334-99337, 99347-99350, 99374-99375, 99377-99378, 99446-99449, 99451-99452, 99495-99496, G0463, G0471, J0670, J2001, P9612

51736 00910, 0213T, 0216T, 0228T, 0230T, 36000, 36400-36410, 36420-36430, 36440, 36591-36592, 36600, 36640, 43752, 50715, 51701-51703, 61650, 62320-62327, 64400, 64405-64408, 64415-64435, 64445-64454, 64461, 64463, 64479, 64483, 64486-64490, 64493, 64505, 64510-64530, 69990, 93000-93010, 93040-93042, 93318, 93355, 94002, 94200, 94250, 94680-94690, 94770, 95812-95816, 95819, 95822, 95829, 95955, 96360, 96365, 96372, 96374-96377, 96523, 99155, 99156, 99157, G0471, P9612

51741 00910, 0213T, 0216T, 0228T, 0230T, 36000, 36400-36410, 36420-36430, 36440, 36591-36592, 36600, 36640, 43752, 50715, 51701-51703, 51736, 61650, 62320-62327, 64400, 64405-64408, 64415-64435, 64445-64454, 64461, 64463, 64479, 64483, 64486-64490, 64493, 64505, 64510-64530, 69990, 93000-93010, 93040-93042, 93318, 93355, 94002, 94200, 94250, 94680-94690, 94770, 95812-95816, 95819, 95822, 95829, 95955, 96360, 96365, 96372, 96374-96377, 96523, 99155, 99156, 99157, G0471, P9612

51840 00910, 0213T, 0216T, 0228T, 0230T, 12001-12007, 12011-12057, 13100-13133, 13151-13153, 36000, 36400-36410, 36420-36430, 36440, 36591-36592, 36600, 36640, 43752, 44602-44605, 44950, 44970, 49000-49002, 49320, 50715, 51040, 51595❖, 51701-51703, 52000-52005, 53000-53025, 53660-53661, 62320-62327, 64400, 64405-64408, 64415-64435, 64445-64454, 64461-64463, 64479-64505, 64510-64530, 69990, 92012-92014, 93000-93010, 93040-93042, 93318, 93355, 94002, 94200, 94250, 94680-94690, 94770, 95812-95816, 95819, 95822, 95829, 95955, 96360-96368, 96372, 96374-96377, 96523, 99155, 99156, 99157, 99211-99223, 99231-99255, 99291-99292, 99304-99310, 99315-99316, 99334-99337, 99347-99350, 99374-99375, 99377-99378, 99446-99449, 99451-99452, 99495-99496, G0463, G0471

51841 00910, 0213T, 0216T, 0228T, 0230T, 12001-12007, 12011-12057, 13100-13133, 13151-13153, 36000, 36400-36410, 36420-36430, 36440, 36591-36592, 36600, 36640, 43752, 44602-44605, 44950, 44970, 49000-49002, 49320, 50715, 51595❖, 51701-51703, 51840, 52000-52001, 53000-53025, 57285❖, 62320-62327, 64400, 64405-64408, 64415-64435, 64445-64454, 64461-64463, 64479-64505, 64510-64530, 69990, 92012-92014, 93000-93010, 93040-93042, 93318, 93355, 94002, 94200, 94250, 94680-94690, 94770, 95812-95816, 95819, 95822, 95829, 95955, 96360-96368, 96372, 96374-96377, 96523, 99155, 99156, 99157, 99211-99223, 99231-99255, 99291-99292, 99304-99310, 99315-99316, 99334-99337, 99347-99350, 99374-99375, 99377-99378, 99446-99449, 99451-99452, 99495-99496, G0463, G0471

51845 00910, 0213T, 0216T, 0228T, 0230T, 12001-12007, 12011-12057, 13100-13133, 13151-13153, 36000, 36400-36410, 36420-36430, 36440, 36591-36592, 36600, 36640, 43752, 44602-44605, 44820-44850, 44950, 44970, 49000-49010, 49255, 49320, 50715, 51040, 51701-51703, 51840-51841❖, 52000-52005, 52281, 52332, 52356, 53660-53661, 57250, 57265, 57289, 62320-62327, 64400, 64405-64408, 64415-64435, 64445-64454, 64461-64463, 64479-64505, 64510-64530, 69990, 92012-92014, 93000-93010, 93040-93042, 93318, 93355, 94002, 94200, 94250, 94680-94690, 94770, 95812-95816, 95819, 95822, 95829, 95955, 96360-96368, 96372, 96374-96377, 96523, 99155, 99156, 99157, 99211-99223, 99231-99255, 99291-99292, 99304-99310, 99315-99316, 99334-99337, 99347-99350, 99374-99375, 99377-99378, 99446-99449, 99451-99452, 99495-99496, G0463, G0471

51900 00910, 0213T, 0216T, 0228T, 0230T, 11000-11006, 11042-11047, 12001-12007, 12011-12057, 13100-13133, 13151-13153, 36000, 36400-36410, 36420-36430, 36440, 36591-36592, 36600, 36640, 43752,

44602-44605, 44850, 44950, 44970, 49000-49010, 49255, 49320,
50715, 51701-51703, 51860-51880, 52000, 62320-62327, 64400,
64405-64408, 64415-64435, 64445-64454, 64461-64463, 64479-64505,
64510-64530, 69990, 92012-92014, 93000-93010, 93040-93042, 93318,
93355, 94002, 94200, 94250, 94680-94690, 94770, 95812-95816,
95819, 95822, 95829, 95955, 96360-96368, 96372, 96374-96377,
96523, 97597-97598, 97602, 99155, 99156, 99157, 99211-99223,
99231-99255, 99291-99292, 99304-99310, 99315-99316, 99334-99337,
99347-99350, 99374-99375, 99377-99378, 99446-99449, 99451-99452,
99495-99496, G0463, G0471

51920 00910, 0213T, 0216T, 0228T, 0230T, 11000-11006, 11042-11047,
12001-12007, 12011-12057, 13100-13133, 13151-13153, 36000,
36400-36410, 36420-36430, 36440, 36591-36592, 36600, 36640, 43752,
44602-44605, 44850, 44950, 44970, 49000-49010, 49255, 49320,
50715, 51701-51703, 51860-51880, 52000, 62320-62327, 64400,
64405-64408, 64415-64435, 64445-64454, 64461-64463, 64479-64505,
64510-64530, 69990, 92012-92014, 93000-93010, 93040-93042, 93318,
93355, 94002, 94200, 94250, 94680-94690, 94770, 95812-95816,
95819, 95822, 95829, 95955, 96360-96368, 96372, 96374-96377,
96523, 97597-97598, 97602, 99155, 99156, 99157, 99211-99223,
99231-99255, 99291-99292, 99304-99310, 99315-99316, 99334-99337,
99347-99350, 99374-99375, 99377-99378, 99446-99449, 99451-99452,
99495-99496, G0463, G0471

51925 00910, 0213T, 0216T, 0228T, 0230T, 11000-11006, 11042-11047,
12001-12007, 12011-12057, 13100-13133, 13151-13153, 36000,
36400-36410, 36420-36430, 36440, 36591-36592, 36600, 36640, 43752,
44005, 44180, 44602-44605, 44850, 44950, 44970, 49000-49010,
49255, 49320-49321, 50715, 51701-51703, 51860-51880, 51920, 52000,
57505, 57530, 57550-57555❖, 57558, 58120-58140, 58146-58180,
58260-58263, 58267-58280, 58290-58294, 58545-58546, 58561,
62320-62327, 64400, 64405-64408, 64415-64435, 64445-64454,
64461-64463, 64479-64505, 64510-64530, 69990, 92012-92014,
93000-93010, 93040-93042, 93318, 93355, 94002, 94200, 94250,
94680-94690, 94770, 95812-95816, 95819, 95822, 95829, 95955,
96360-96368, 96372, 96374-96377, 96523, 97597-97598, 97602, 99155,
99156, 99157, 99211-99223, 99231-99255, 99291-99292, 99304-99310,
99315-99316, 99334-99337, 99347-99350, 99374-99375, 99377-99378,
99446-99449, 99451-99452, 99495-99496, G0463, G0471

51990 00910, 0213T, 0216T, 0228T, 0230T, 12001-12007, 12011-12057,
13100-13133, 13151-13153, 36000, 36400-36410, 36420-36430, 36440,
36591-36592, 36600, 36640, 43653, 43752, 44005, 44180,
44602-44605, 44950, 44970, 49082-49084, 49320, 49400, 50715,
51701-51703, 51992❖, 52000, 57285, 58660, 62320-62327, 64400,
64405-64408, 64415-64435, 64445-64454, 64461-64463, 64479-64505,
64510-64530, 69990, 76000, 77001-77002, 92012-92014, 93000-93010,
93040-93042, 93318, 93355, 94002, 94200, 94250, 94680-94690,
94770, 95812-95816, 95819, 95822, 95829, 95955, 96360-96368,
96372, 96374-96377, 96523, 99155, 99156, 99157, 99211-99223,
99231-99255, 99291-99292, 99304-99310, 99315-99316, 99334-99337,
99347-99350, 99374-99375, 99377-99378, 99446-99449, 99451-99452,
99495-99496, G0463, G0471

51992 00910, 0213T, 0216T, 0228T, 0230T, 12001-12007, 12011-12057,
13100-13133, 13151-13153, 36000, 36400-36410, 36420-36430, 36440,
36591-36592, 36600, 36640, 43653, 43752, 44005, 44180,
44602-44605, 44950, 44970, 49082-49084, 49320, 49400, 50715,
51701-51703, 52000, 53000-53025, 58660, 62320-62327, 64400,
64405-64408, 64415-64435, 64445-64454, 64461-64463, 64479-64505,
64510-64530, 69990, 76000, 77001-77002, 92012-92014, 93000-93010,
93040-93042, 93318, 93355, 94002, 94200, 94250, 94680-94690,
94770, 95812-95816, 95819, 95822, 95829, 95955, 96360-96368,

96372, 96374-96377, 96523, 99155, 99156, 99157, 99211-99223,
99231-99255, 99291-99292, 99304-99310, 99315-99316, 99334-99337,
99347-99350, 99374-99375, 99377-99378, 99446-99449, 99451-99452,
99495-99496, G0463, G0471

52000 00910, 00916, 0213T, 0216T, 0228T, 0230T, 0548T, 0582T,
12001-12007, 12011-12057, 13100-13133, 13151-13153, 36000,
36400-36410, 36420-36430, 36440, 36591-36592, 36600, 36640, 43752,
51700-51703, 53000-53025, 53600-53621, 53660-53665, 57410,
62320-62327, 64400, 64405-64408, 64415-64435, 64445-64454,
64461-64463, 64479-64505, 64510-64530, 69990, 76000, 77001-77002,
92012-92014, 93000-93010, 93040-93042, 93318, 93355, 94002, 94200,
94250, 94680-94690, 94770, 95812-95816, 95819, 95822, 95829,
95955, 96360-96368, 96372, 96374-96377, 96523, 99155, 99156,
99157, 99211-99223, 99231-99255, 99291-99292, 99304-99310,
99315-99316, 99334-99337, 99347-99350, 99374-99375, 99377-99378,
99446-99449, 99451-99452, 99495-99496, C9738, G0463, G0471,
J2001, P9612

53060 0213T, 0216T, 0228T, 0230T, 12001-12007, 12011-12057, 13100-13133,
13151-13153, 36000, 36400-36410, 36420-36430, 36440, 36591-36592,
36600, 36640, 43752, 51701-51703, 53000-53025, 53080, 53270❖,
62320-62327, 64400, 64405-64408, 64415-64435, 64445-64454,
64461-64463, 64479-64505, 64510-64530, 69990, 92012-92014,
93000-93010, 93040-93042, 93318, 93355, 94002, 94200, 94250,
94680-94690, 94770, 95812-95816, 95819, 95822, 95829, 95955,
96360-96368, 96372, 96374-96377, 96523, 99155, 99156, 99157,
99211-99223, 99231-99255, 99291-99292, 99304-99310, 99315-99316,
99334-99337, 99347-99350, 99374-99375, 99377-99378, 99446-99449,
99451-99452, 99495-99496, G0463, G0471, J2001

53230 0213T, 0216T, 0228T, 0230T, 11000-11006, 11042-11047, 12001-12007,
12011-12057, 13100-13133, 13151-13153, 36000, 36400-36410,
36420-36430, 36440, 36591-36592, 36600, 36640, 43752, 51701-51703,
52000, 52301, 53000-53025, 62320-62327, 64400, 64405-64408,
64415-64435, 64445-64454, 64461-64463, 64479-64505, 64510-64530,
69990, 92012-92014, 93000-93010, 93040-93042, 93318, 93355, 94002,
94200, 94250, 94680-94690, 94770, 95812-95816, 95819, 95822,
95829, 95955, 96360-96368, 96372, 96374-96377, 96523, 97597-97598,
97602, 99155, 99156, 99157, 99211-99223, 99231-99255, 99291-99292,
99304-99310, 99315-99316, 99334-99337, 99347-99350, 99374-99375,
99377-99378, 99446-99449, 99451-99452, 99495-99496, G0463, G0471

53240 0213T, 0216T, 0228T, 0230T, 12001-12007, 12011-12057, 13100-13133,
13151-13153, 36000, 36400-36410, 36420-36430, 36440, 36591-36592,
36600, 36640, 43752, 51701-51703, 52000, 52301, 53000-53025,
53230, 62320-62327, 64400, 64405-64408, 64415-64435, 64445-64454,
64461-64463, 64479-64505, 64510-64530, 69990, 92012-92014,
93000-93010, 93040-93042, 93318, 93355, 94002, 94200, 94250,
94680-94690, 94770, 95812-95816, 95819, 95822, 95829, 95955,
96360-96368, 96372, 96374-96377, 96523, 99155, 99156, 99157,
99211-99223, 99231-99255, 99291-99292, 99304-99310, 99315-99316,
99334-99337, 99347-99350, 99374-99375, 99377-99378, 99446-99449,
99451-99452, 99495-99496, G0463, G0471

53260 0213T, 0216T, 0228T, 0230T, 11000-11006, 11042-11047, 12001-12007,
12011-12057, 13100-13133, 13151-13153, 36000, 36400-36410,
36420-36430, 36440, 36591-36592, 36600, 36640, 43752, 51701-51703,
52000, 53000-53025, 53080, 53230, 62320-62327, 64400, 64405-64408,
64415-64435, 64445-64454, 64461-64463, 64479-64505, 64510-64530,
69990, 92012-92014, 93000-93010, 93040-93042, 93318, 93355, 94002,
94200, 94250, 94680-94690, 94770, 95812-95816, 95819, 95822,
95829, 95955, 96360-96368, 96372, 96374-96377, 96523, 97597-97598,
97602, 99155, 99156, 99157, 99211-99223, 99231-99255, 99291-99292,

99304-99310, 99315-99316, 99334-99337, 99347-99350, 99374-99375, 99377-99378, 99446-99449, 99451-99452, 99495-99496, G0463, G0471, J2001

53265 0213T, 0216T, 0228T, 0230T, 11000-11006, 11042-11047, 12001-12007, 12011-12057, 13100-13133, 13151-13153, 36000, 36400-36410, 36420-36430, 36440, 36591-36592, 36600, 36640, 43752, 51701-51703, 52000, 53000-53025, 53080, 53230, 62320-62327, 64400, 64405-64408, 64415-64435, 64445-64454, 64461-64463, 64479-64505, 64510-64530, 69990, 92012-92014, 93000-93010, 93040-93042, 93318, 93355, 94002, 94200, 94250, 94680-94690, 94770, 95812-95816, 95819, 95822, 95829, 95955, 96360-96368, 96372, 96374-96377, 96523, 97597-97598, 97602, 99155, 99156, 99157, 99211-99223, 99231-99255, 99291-99292, 99304-99310, 99315-99316, 99334-99337, 99347-99350, 99374-99375, 99377-99378, 99446-99449, 99451-99452, 99495-99496, G0463, G0471, J0670, J2001

53270 0213T, 0216T, 0228T, 0230T, 11000-11006, 11042-11047, 12001-12007, 12011-12057, 13100-13133, 13151-13153, 36000, 36400-36410, 36420-36430, 36440, 36591-36592, 36600, 36640, 43752, 51701-51703, 52000, 53000-53025, 53080, 53230, 62320-62327, 64400, 64405-64408, 64415-64435, 64445-64454, 64461-64463, 64479-64505, 64510-64530, 69990, 92012-92014, 93000-93010, 93040-93042, 93318, 93355, 94002, 94200, 94250, 94680-94690, 94770, 95812-95816, 95819, 95822, 95829, 95955, 96360-96368, 96372, 96374-96377, 96523, 97597-97598, 97602, 99155, 99156, 99157, 99211-99223, 99231-99255, 99291-99292, 99304-99310, 99315-99316, 99334-99337, 99347-99350, 99374-99375, 99377-99378, 99446-99449, 99451-99452, 99495-99496, G0463, G0471, J2001

53275 0213T, 0216T, 0228T, 0230T, 11000-11006, 11042-11047, 12001-12007, 12011-12057, 13100-13133, 13151-13153, 36000, 36400-36410, 36420-36430, 36440, 36591-36592, 36600, 36640, 43752, 51701-51703, 52000, 53000-53025, 53080, 53230, 62320-62327, 64400, 64405-64408, 64415-64435, 64445-64454, 64461-64463, 64479-64505, 64510-64530, 69990, 92012-92014, 93000-93010, 93040-93042, 93318, 93355, 94002, 94200, 94250, 94680-94690, 94770, 95812-95816, 95819, 95822, 95829, 95955, 96360-96368, 96372, 96374-96377, 96523, 97597-97598, 97602, 99155, 99156, 99157, 99211-99223, 99231-99255, 99291-99292, 99304-99310, 99315-99316, 99334-99337, 99347-99350, 99374-99375, 99377-99378, 99446-99449, 99451-99452, 99495-99496, G0463, G0471

53430 0213T, 0216T, 0228T, 0230T, 11000-11006, 11042-11047, 12001-12007, 12011-12057, 13100-13133, 13151-13153, 36000, 36400-36410, 36420-36430, 36440, 36591-36592, 36600, 36640, 43752, 51701-51703, 51990-51992, 52000, 52301, 53000-53025, 53080, 53502-53520, 53860✦, 62320-62327, 64400, 64405-64408, 64415-64435, 64445-64454, 64461-64463, 64479-64505, 64510-64530, 69990, 92012-92014, 93000-93010, 93040-93042, 93318, 93355, 94002, 94200, 94250, 94680-94690, 94770, 95812-95816, 95819, 95822, 95829, 95955, 96360-96368, 96372, 96374-96377, 96523, 97597-97598, 97602, 99155, 99156, 99157, 99211-99223, 99231-99255, 99291-99292, 99304-99310, 99315-99316, 99334-99337, 99347-99350, 99374-99375, 99377-99378, 99446-99449, 99451-99452, 99495-99496, G0463, G0471

53500 00910, 0213T, 0216T, 0228T, 0230T, 12001-12007, 12011-12057, 13100-13133, 13151-13153, 36000, 36400-36410, 36420-36430, 36440, 36591-36592, 36600, 36640, 43752, 51700-51703, 52000, 52310-52315, 53000-53025, 53080, 53502-53510, 53520-53621, 53660-53665, 62320-62327, 64400, 64405-64408, 64415-64435, 64445-64454, 64461-64463, 64479-64505, 64510-64530, 69990, 92012-92014, 93000-93010, 93040-93042, 93318, 93355, 94002, 94200, 94250, 94680-94690, 94770, 95812-95816, 95819, 95822, 95829, 95955, 96360-96368, 96372, 96374-96377, 96523, 99155, 99156, 99157,

99211-99223, 99231-99255, 99291-99292, 99304-99310, 99315-99316, 99334-99337, 99347-99350, 99374-99375, 99377-99378, 99446-99449, 99451-99452, 99495-99496, G0463, G0471

53502 0213T, 0216T, 0228T, 0230T, 12001-12007, 12011-12057, 13100-13133, 13151-13153, 36000, 36400-36410, 36420-36430, 36440, 36591-36592, 36600, 36640, 43752, 51701-51703, 52000, 52301, 53000-53025, 53080, 62320-62327, 64400, 64405-64408, 64415-64435, 64445-64454, 64461-64463, 64479-64505, 64510-64530, 69990, 92012-92014, 93000-93010, 93040-93042, 93318, 93355, 94002, 94200, 94250, 94680-94690, 94770, 95812-95816, 95819, 95822, 95829, 95955, 96360-96368, 96372, 96374-96377, 96523, 99155, 99156, 99157, 99211-99223, 99231-99255, 99291-99292, 99304-99310, 99315-99316, 99334-99337, 99347-99350, 99374-99375, 99377-99378, 99446-99449, 99451-99452, 99495-99496, G0463, G0471

53660 0213T, 0216T, 0228T, 0230T, 0421T, 12001-12007, 12011-12057, 13100-13133, 13151-13153, 36000, 36400-36410, 36420-36430, 36440, 36591-36592, 36600, 36640, 43752, 51701-51703, 53000-53025, 53080, 53661✦, 62320-62327, 64400, 64405-64408, 64415-64435, 64445-64454, 64461-64463, 64479-64505, 64510-64530, 69990, 92012-92014, 93000-93010, 93040-93042, 93318, 93355, 94002, 94200, 94250, 94680-94690, 94770, 95812-95816, 95819, 95822, 95829, 95955, 96360-96368, 96372, 96374-96377, 96523, 99155, 99156, 99157, 99211-99223, 99231-99255, 99291-99292, 99304-99310, 99315-99316, 99334-99337, 99347-99350, 99374-99375, 99377-99378, 99446-99449, 99451-99452, 99495-99496, G0463, G0471, J0670, J2001, P9612

53661 0213T, 0216T, 0228T, 0230T, 0421T, 12001-12007, 12011-12057, 13100-13133, 13151-13153, 36000, 36400-36410, 36420-36430, 36440, 36591-36592, 36600, 36640, 43752, 51700-51703, 53000-53025, 53080, 62320-62327, 64400, 64405-64408, 64415-64435, 64445-64454, 64461-64463, 64479-64505, 64510-64530, 69990, 92012-92014, 93000-93010, 93040-93042, 93318, 93355, 94002, 94200, 94250, 94680-94690, 94770, 95812-95816, 95819, 95822, 95829, 95955, 96360-96368, 96372, 96374-96377, 96523, 99155, 99156, 99157, 99211-99223, 99231-99255, 99291-99292, 99304-99310, 99315-99316, 99334-99337, 99347-99350, 99374-99375, 99377-99378, 99446-99449, 99451-99452, 99495-99496, G0463, G0471, J0670, J2001, P9612

53665 0213T, 0216T, 0228T, 0230T, 0421T, 12001-12007, 12011-12057, 13100-13133, 13151-13153, 36000, 36400-36410, 36420-36430, 36440, 36591-36592, 36600, 36640, 43752, 51701-51703, 53000-53025, 53080, 53660-53661✦, 62320-62327, 64400, 64405-64408, 64415-64435, 64445-64454, 64461-64463, 64479-64505, 64510-64530, 69990, 92012-92014, 93000-93010, 93040-93042, 93318, 93355, 94002, 94200, 94250, 94680-94690, 94770, 95812-95816, 95819, 95822, 95829, 95955, 96360-96368, 96372, 96374-96377, 96523, 99151✦, 99152✦, 99153✦, 99155, 99156, 99157, 99211-99223, 99231-99255, 99291-99292, 99304-99310, 99315-99316, 99334-99337, 99347-99350, 99374-99375, 99377-99378, 99446-99449, 99451-99452, 99495-99496, G0463, G0471

53860 12001-12007, 12011-12057, 13100-13133, 13151-13153, 36000, 36400-36410, 36420-36430, 36440, 36591-36592, 36600, 36640, 43752, 51102, 51700-51703, 52000-52001, 52281, 52285✦, 52310-52315, 52500, 53000-53025, 53080, 53660-53665, 62320-62327, 64400, 64405-64408, 64415-64435, 64445-64454, 64461-64463, 64479-64505, 64510-64530, 69990, 92012-92014, 93000-93010, 93040-93042, 93318, 93355, 94002, 94200, 94250, 94680-94690, 94770, 95812-95816, 95819, 95822, 95829, 95955, 96360-96368, 96372, 96374-96377, 96523, 99155, 99156, 99157, 99211-99223, 99231-99255, 99291-99292, 99304-99310, 99315-99316, 99334-99337, 99347-99350, 99374-99375,

99377-99378, 99446-99449, 99451-99452, 99495-99496, G0463,
G0471, J0670, J2001, P9612

55920 0213T, 0216T, 0228T, 0230T, 0347T✦, 10035-10036✦, 12001-12007,
12011-12057, 13100-13133, 13151-13153, 20555✦, 36000,
36400-36410, 36420-36430, 36440, 36591-36592, 36600, 36640, 43752,
57155-57156, 58346, 62320-62327, 64400, 64405-64408, 64415-64435,
64445-64454, 64461-64463, 64479-64505, 64510-64530, 69990,
92012-92014, 93000-93010, 93040-93042, 93318, 93355, 94002, 94200,
94250, 94680-94690, 94770, 95812-95816, 95819, 95822, 95829,
95955, 96360-96368, 96372, 96374-96377, 96523, 99155, 99156,
99157, 99211-99223, 99231-99255, 99291-99292, 99304-99310,
99315-99316, 99334-99337, 99347-99350, 99374-99375, 99377-99378,
99446-99449, 99451-99452, 99495-99496, G0463

56405 00940, 0213T, 0216T, 0228T, 0230T, 12001-12007, 12011-12057,
13100-13133, 13151-13153, 36000, 36400-36410, 36420-36430, 36440,
36591-36592, 36600, 36640, 43752, 51701-51703, 56440, 56605,
56810-56820, 57100, 57180, 57500, 62320-62327, 64400, 64405-64408,
64415-64435, 64445-64454, 64461-64463, 64479-64505, 64510-64530,
69990, 92012-92014, 93000-93010, 93040-93042, 93318, 93355, 94002,
94200, 94250, 94680-94690, 94770, 95812-95816, 95819, 95822,
95829, 95955, 96360-96368, 96372, 96374-96377, 96523, 99155,
99156, 99157, 99211-99223, 99231-99255, 99291-99292, 99304-99310,
99315-99316, 99334-99337, 99347-99350, 99374-99375, 99377-99378,
99446-99449, 99451-99452, 99495-99496, G0463, G0471, J0670, J2001

56420 00940, 0213T, 0216T, 0228T, 0230T, 12001-12007, 12011-12057,
13100-13133, 13151-13153, 36000, 36400-36410, 36420-36430, 36440,
36591-36592, 36600, 36640, 43752, 51701-51703, 56405, 56440,
56605, 56820, 57100, 57180, 57500, 62320-62327, 64400,
64405-64408, 64415-64435, 64445-64454, 64461-64463, 64479-64505,
64510-64530, 69990, 92012-92014, 93000-93010, 93040-93042, 93318,
93355, 94002, 94200, 94250, 94680-94690, 94770, 95812-95816,
95819, 95822, 95829, 95955, 96360-96368, 96372, 96374-96377,
96523, 99155, 99156, 99157, 99211-99223, 99231-99255, 99291-99292,
99304-99310, 99315-99316, 99334-99337, 99347-99350, 99374-99375,
99377-99378, 99446-99449, 99451-99452, 99495-99496, G0463,
G0471, J0670, J2001

56440 00940, 0213T, 0216T, 0228T, 0230T, 12001-12007, 12011-12057,
13100-13133, 13151-13153, 36000, 36400-36410, 36420-36430, 36440,
36591-36592, 36600, 36640, 43752, 51701-51703, 56605, 56820,
57100, 57180, 57500, 62320-62327, 64400, 64405-64408, 64415-64435,
64445-64454, 64461-64463, 64479-64505, 64510-64530, 69990,
92012-92014, 93000-93010, 93040-93042, 93318, 93355, 94002, 94200,
94250, 94680-94690, 94770, 95812-95816, 95819, 95822, 95829,
95955, 96360-96368, 96372, 96374-96377, 96523, 99155, 99156,
99157, 99211-99223, 99231-99255, 99291-99292, 99304-99310,
99315-99316, 99334-99337, 99347-99350, 99374-99375, 99377-99378,
99446-99449, 99451-99452, 99495-99496, G0463, G0471, J2001

56441 00940, 0213T, 0216T, 0228T, 0230T, 12001-12007, 12011-12057,
13100-13133, 13151-13153, 36000, 36400-36410, 36420-36430, 36440,
36591-36592, 36600, 36640, 43752, 51701-51703, 56820, 57100,
57180, 57500, 62320-62327, 64400, 64405-64408, 64415-64435,
64445-64454, 64461-64463, 64479-64505, 64510-64530, 69990,
92012-92014, 93000-93010, 93040-93042, 93318, 93355, 94002, 94200,
94250, 94680-94690, 94770, 95812-95816, 95819, 95822, 95829,
95955, 96360-96368, 96372, 96374-96377, 96523, 99155, 99156,
99157, 99211-99223, 99231-99255, 99291-99292, 99304-99310,
99315-99316, 99334-99337, 99347-99350, 99374-99375, 99377-99378,
99446-99449, 99451-99452, 99495-99496, G0463, G0471, J0670, J2001

56442 00940, 0213T, 0216T, 0228T, 0230T, 11000-11006, 11042-11047,
12001-12007, 12011-12057, 13100-13133, 13151-13153, 36000,
36400-36410, 36420-36430, 36440, 36591-36592, 36600, 36640, 43752,
51701-51703, 56605, 56820, 57100, 57180, 57410, 57500, 57800,
58100, 62320-62327, 64400, 64405-64408, 64415-64435, 64445-64454,
64461-64463, 64479-64505, 64510-64530, 69990, 92012-92014,
93000-93010, 93040-93042, 93318, 93355, 94002, 94200, 94250,
94680-94690, 94770, 95812-95816, 95819, 95822, 95829, 95955,
96360-96368, 96372, 96374-96377, 96523, 97597-97598, 97602, 99155,
99156, 99157, 99211-99223, 99231-99255, 99291-99292, 99304-99310,
99315-99316, 99334-99337, 99347-99350, 99374-99375, 99377-99378,
99446-99449, 99451-99452, 99495-99496, G0463, G0471

56501 00940, 0213T, 0216T, 0228T, 0230T, 12001-12007, 12011-12057,
13100-13133, 13151-13153, 36000, 36400-36410, 36420-36430, 36440,
36591-36592, 36600, 36640, 43752, 51701-51703, 55815✦, 56441✦,
56810-56820, 57100, 57180, 57410, 57500, 57800, 58100,
62320-62327, 64400, 64405-64408, 64415-64435, 64445-64454,
64461-64463, 64479-64505, 64510-64530, 69990, 92012-92014,
93000-93010, 93040-93042, 93318, 93355, 94002, 94200, 94250,
94680-94690, 94770, 95812-95816, 95819, 95822, 95829, 95955,
96360-96368, 96372, 96374-96377, 96523, 99155, 99156, 99157,
99211-99223, 99231-99255, 99291-99292, 99304-99310, 99315-99316,
99334-99337, 99347-99350, 99374-99375, 99377-99378, 99446-99449,
99451-99452, 99495-99496, G0463, G0471, J0670, J2001

56515 00940, 0213T, 0216T, 0228T, 0230T, 12001-12007, 12011-12057,
13100-13133, 13151-13153, 36000, 36400-36410, 36420-36430, 36440,
36591-36592, 36600, 36640, 43752, 51701-51703, 53270, 56441,
56501, 56605, 56810-56820, 57100, 57180, 57410, 57500, 57800,
58100, 62320-62327, 64400, 64405-64408, 64415-64435, 64445-64454,
64461-64463, 64479-64505, 64510-64530, 69990, 92012-92014,
93000-93010, 93040-93042, 93318, 93355, 94002, 94200, 94250,
94680-94690, 94770, 95812-95816, 95819, 95822, 95829, 95955,
96360-96368, 96372, 96374-96377, 96523, 99155, 99156, 99157,
99211-99223, 99231-99255, 99291-99292, 99304-99310, 99315-99316,
99334-99337, 99347-99350, 99374-99375, 99377-99378, 99446-99449,
99451-99452, 99495-99496, G0463, G0471, J0670, J2001

56605 00940, 0213T, 0216T, 0228T, 0230T, 10005, 10007, 10009, 10011,
10021, 11102-11107✦, 12001-12007, 12011-12057, 13100-13133,
13151-13153, 36000, 36400-36410, 36420-36430, 36440, 36591-36592,
36600, 36640, 43752, 51701-51703, 56820, 57100, 57180, 57410,
57500, 57800, 62320-62327, 64400, 64405-64408, 64415-64435,
64445-64454, 64461-64463, 64479-64505, 64510-64530, 69990,
92012-92014, 93000-93010, 93040-93042, 93318, 93355, 94002, 94200,
94250, 94680-94690, 94770, 95812-95816, 95819, 95822, 95829,
95955, 96360-96368, 96372, 96374-96377, 96523, 99155, 99156,
99157, 99211-99223, 99231-99255, 99291-99292, 99304-99310,
99315-99316, 99334-99337, 99347-99350, 99374-99375, 99377-99378,
99446-99449, 99451-99452, 99495-99496, G0463, G0471

56606 10005, 10007, 10009, 10011, 10021, 11102-11107✦, 36591-36592,
64430-64435, 96523

56620 00940, 0213T, 0216T, 0228T, 0230T, 11000-11006, 11042-11047,
12001-12007, 12011-12057, 13100-13133, 13151-13153, 36000,
36400-36410, 36420-36430, 36440, 36591-36592, 36600, 36640, 43752,
51701-51703, 56605-56606, 56810-56821, 57100, 57180, 57410, 57500,
58100, 62320-62327, 64400, 64405-64408, 64415-64435, 64445-64454,
64461-64463, 64479-64505, 64510-64530, 69990, 92012-92014,
93000-93010, 93040-93042, 93318, 93355, 94002, 94200, 94250,
94680-94690, 94770, 95812-95816, 95819, 95822, 95829, 95955,
96360-96368, 96372, 96374-96377, 96523, 97597-97598, 97602, 99155,

99156, 99157, 99211-99223, 99231-99255, 99291-99292, 99304-99310, 99315-99316, 99334-99337, 99347-99350, 99374-99375, 99377-99378, 99446-99449, 99451-99452, 99495-99496, G0463, G0471

56625 00940, 0213T, 0216T, 0228T, 0230T, 11000-11006, 11042-11047, 12001-12007, 12011-12057, 13100-13133, 13151-13153, 36000, 36400-36410, 36420-36430, 36440, 36591-36592, 36600, 36640, 43752, 51701-51703, 56605-56620, 56810-56821, 57100, 57180, 57410, 57500, 57800, 58100, 62320-62327, 64400, 64405-64408, 64415-64435, 64445-64454, 64461-64463, 64479-64505, 64510-64530, 69990, 92012-92014, 93000-93010, 93040-93042, 93318, 93355, 94002, 94200, 94250, 94680-94690, 94770, 95812-95816, 95819, 95822, 95829, 95955, 96360-96368, 96372, 96374-96377, 96523, 97597-97598, 97602, 99155, 99156, 99157, 99211-99223, 99231-99255, 99291-99292, 99304-99310, 99315-99316, 99334-99337, 99347-99350, 99374-99375, 99377-99378, 99446-99449, 99451-99452, 99495-99496, G0463, G0471

56630 00940, 0213T, 0216T, 0228T, 0230T, 11000-11006, 11042-11047, 12001-12007, 12011-12057, 13100-13133, 13151-13153, 36000, 36400-36410, 36420-36430, 36440, 36591-36592, 36600, 36640, 43752, 51701-51703, 56605-56625❖, 56810-56821, 57100, 57180, 57410, 57500, 57800, 58100, 62320-62327, 64400, 64405-64408, 64415-64435, 64445-64454, 64461-64463, 64479-64505, 64510-64530, 69990, 92012-92014, 93000-93010, 93040-93042, 93318, 93355, 94002, 94200, 94250, 94680-94690, 94770, 95812-95816, 95819, 95822, 95829, 95955, 96360-96368, 96372, 96374-96377, 96523, 97597-97598, 97602, 99155, 99156, 99157, 99211-99223, 99231-99255, 99291-99292, 99304-99310, 99315-99316, 99334-99337, 99347-99350, 99374-99375, 99377-99378, 99446-99449, 99451-99452, 99495-99496, G0463, G0471

56631 00940, 0213T, 0216T, 0228T, 0230T, 11000-11006, 11042-11047, 12001-12007, 12011-12057, 13100-13133, 13151-13153, 36000, 36400-36410, 36420-36430, 36440, 36591-36592, 36600, 36640, 38505, 38531, 38760, 43752, 51701-51703, 56605-56630, 56810-56821, 57100, 57180, 57410, 57500, 57800, 58100, 62320-62327, 64400, 64405-64408, 64415-64435, 64445-64454, 64461-64463, 64479-64505, 64510-64530, 69990, 92012-92014, 93000-93010, 93040-93042, 93318, 93355, 94002, 94200, 94250, 94680-94690, 94770, 95812-95816, 95819, 95822, 95829, 95955, 96360-96368, 96372, 96374-96377, 96523, 97597-97598, 97602, 99155, 99156, 99157, 99211-99223, 99231-99255, 99291-99292, 99304-99310, 99315-99316, 99334-99337, 99347-99350, 99374-99375, 99377-99378, 99446-99449, 99451-99452, 99495-99496, G0463, G0471

56632 00940, 0213T, 0216T, 0228T, 0230T, 11000-11006, 11042-11047, 12001-12007, 12011-12057, 13100-13133, 13151-13153, 36000, 36400-36410, 36420-36430, 36440, 36591-36592, 36600, 36640, 38505, 38531, 38760, 38765, 43752, 51701-51703, 56605-56631❖, 56633-56634❖, 56810-56821, 57100, 57180, 57410, 57500, 57800, 58100, 62320-62327, 64400, 64405-64408, 64415-64435, 64445-64454, 64461-64463, 64479-64505, 64510-64530, 69990, 92012-92014, 93000-93010, 93040-93042, 93318, 93355, 94002, 94200, 94250, 94680-94690, 94770, 95812-95816, 95819, 95822, 95829, 95955, 96360-96368, 96372, 96374-96377, 96523, 97597-97598, 97602, 99155, 99156, 99157, 99211-99223, 99231-99255, 99291-99292, 99304-99310, 99315-99316, 99334-99337, 99347-99350, 99374-99375, 99377-99378, 99446-99449, 99451-99452, 99495-99496, G0463, G0471

56633 00940, 0213T, 0216T, 0228T, 0230T, 11000-11006, 11042-11047, 12001-12007, 12011-12057, 13100-13133, 13151-13153, 36000, 36400-36410, 36420-36430, 36440, 36591-36592, 36600, 36640, 43752, 51701-51703, 56605-56631❖, 56810-56821, 57100, 57180, 57410, 57500, 57800, 58100, 62320-62327, 64400, 64405-64408, 64415-64435, 64445-64454, 64461-64463, 64479-64505, 64510-64530, 69990,

92012-92014, 93000-93010, 93040-93042, 93318, 93355, 94002, 94200, 94250, 94680-94690, 94770, 95812-95816, 95819, 95822, 95829, 95955, 96360-96368, 96372, 96374-96377, 96523, 97597-97598, 97602, 99155, 99156, 99157, 99211-99223, 99231-99255, 99291-99292, 99304-99310, 99315-99316, 99334-99337, 99347-99350, 99374-99375, 99377-99378, 99446-99449, 99451-99452, 99495-99496, G0463, G0471

56634 00940, 0213T, 0216T, 0228T, 0230T, 11000-11006, 11042-11047, 12001-12007, 12011-12057, 13100-13133, 13151-13153, 36000, 36400-36410, 36420-36430, 36440, 36591-36592, 36600, 36640, 38505, 38531, 38760, 43752, 51701-51703, 56605-56631❖, 56633, 56810-56821, 57100, 57180, 57410, 57500, 57800, 58100, 62320-62327, 64400, 64405-64408, 64415-64435, 64445-64454, 64461-64463, 64479-64505, 64510-64530, 69990, 92012-92014, 93000-93010, 93040-93042, 93318, 93355, 94002, 94200, 94250, 94680-94690, 94770, 95812-95816, 95819, 95822, 95829, 95955, 96360-96368, 96372, 96374-96377, 96523, 97597-97598, 97602, 99155, 99156, 99157, 99211-99223, 99231-99255, 99291-99292, 99304-99310, 99315-99316, 99334-99337, 99347-99350, 99374-99375, 99377-99378, 99446-99449, 99451-99452, 99495-99496, G0463, G0471

56637 00940, 0213T, 0216T, 0228T, 0230T, 11000-11006, 11042-11047, 12001-12007, 12011-12057, 13100-13133, 13151-13153, 36000, 36400-36410, 36420-36430, 36440, 36591-36592, 36600, 36640, 38505, 38531, 38760, 38765, 43752, 51701-51703, 56605-56634❖, 56640❖, 56810-56821, 57100, 57180, 57410, 57500, 57800, 58100, 62320-62327, 64400, 64405-64408, 64415-64435, 64445-64454, 64461-64463, 64479-64505, 64510-64530, 69990, 92012-92014, 93000-93010, 93040-93042, 93318, 93355, 94002, 94200, 94250, 94680-94690, 94770, 95812-95816, 95819, 95822, 95829, 95955, 96360-96368, 96372, 96374-96377, 96523, 97597-97598, 97602, 99155, 99156, 99157, 99211-99223, 99231-99255, 99291-99292, 99304-99310, 99315-99316, 99334-99337, 99347-99350, 99374-99375, 99377-99378, 99446-99449, 99451-99452, 99495-99496, G0463, G0471

56640 00940, 0213T, 0216T, 0228T, 0230T, 11000-11006, 11042-11047, 12001-12007, 12011-12057, 13100-13133, 13151-13153, 36000, 36400-36410, 36420-36430, 36440, 36591-36592, 36600, 36640, 38500-38505, 38531, 38562-38573, 38760, 38765, 38770, 38780, 43752, 49010, 51701-51703, 52000, 56605-56634❖, 56810-56821, 57100, 57180, 57410, 57500, 57800, 58100, 62320-62327, 64400, 64405-64408, 64415-64435, 64445-64454, 64461-64463, 64479-64505, 64510-64530, 69990, 92012-92014, 93000-93010, 93040-93042, 93318, 93355, 94002, 94200, 94250, 94680-94690, 94770, 95812-95816, 95819, 95822, 95829, 95955, 96360-96368, 96372, 96374-96377, 96523, 97597-97598, 97602, 99155, 99156, 99157, 99211-99223, 99231-99255, 99291-99292, 99304-99310, 99315-99316, 99334-99337, 99347-99350, 99374-99375, 99377-99378, 99446-99449, 99451-99452, 99495-99496, G0463, G0471

56700 00940, 0213T, 0216T, 0228T, 0230T, 11000-11006, 11042-11047, 12001-12007, 12011-12057, 13100-13133, 13151-13153, 36000, 36400-36410, 36420-36430, 36440, 36591-36592, 36600, 36640, 43752, 51701-51703, 56442, 56605-56606, 56820, 57100, 57180, 57410, 57500, 57800, 58100, 62320-62327, 64400, 64405-64408, 64415-64435, 64445-64454, 64461-64463, 64479-64505, 64510-64530, 69990, 92012-92014, 93000-93010, 93040-93042, 93318, 93355, 94002, 94200, 94250, 94680-94690, 94770, 95812-95816, 95819, 95822, 95829, 95955, 96360-96368, 96372, 96374-96377, 96523, 97597-97598, 97602, 99155, 99156, 99157, 99211-99223, 99231-99255, 99291-99292, 99304-99310, 99315-99316, 99334-99337, 99347-99350, 99374-99375, 99377-99378, 99446-99449, 99451-99452, 99495-99496, G0463, G0471, J2001

56740 00940, 0213T, 0216T, 0228T, 0230T, 11000-11006, 11042-11047, 12001-12007, 12011-12057, 13100-13133, 13151-13153, 36000, 36400-36410, 36420-36430, 36440, 36591-36592, 36600, 36640, 43752, 51701-51703, 56420-56440, 56605-56606, 56820, 57100, 57180, 57410, 57500, 57800, 58100, 62320-62327, 64400, 64405-64408, 64415-64435, 64445-64454, 64461-64463, 64479-64505, 64510-64530, 69990, 92012-92014, 93000-93010, 93040-93042, 93318, 93355, 94002, 94200, 94250, 94680-94690, 94770, 95812-95816, 95819, 95822, 95829, 95955, 96360-96368, 96372, 96374-96377, 96523, 97597-97598, 97602, 99155, 99156, 99157, 99211-99223, 99231-99255, 99291-99292, 99304-99310, 99315-99316, 99334-99337, 99347-99350, 99374-99375, 99377-99378, 99446-99449, 99451-99452, 99495-99496, G0463, G0471, J2001

56800 00940, 0213T, 0216T, 0228T, 0230T, 12001-12007, 12011-12057, 13100-13133, 13151-13153, 36000, 36400-36410, 36420-36430, 36440, 36591-36592, 36600, 36640, 43752, 51701-51703, 56605-56606, 56810-56820, 57100, 57180, 57410, 57500, 57800, 58100, 62320-62327, 64400, 64405-64408, 64415-64435, 64445-64454, 64461-64463, 64479-64505, 64510-64530, 69990, 92012-92014, 93000-93010, 93040-93042, 93318, 93355, 94002, 94200, 94250, 94680-94690, 94770, 95812-95816, 95819, 95822, 95829, 95955, 96360-96368, 96372, 96374-96377, 96523, 99155, 99156, 99157, 99211-99223, 99231-99255, 99291-99292, 99304-99310, 99315-99316, 99334-99337, 99347-99350, 99374-99375, 99377-99378, 99446-99449, 99451-99452, 99495-99496, G0463, G0471

56805 00940, 0213T, 0216T, 0228T, 0230T, 11000-11006, 11042-11047, 12001-12007, 12011-12057, 13100-13133, 13151-13153, 36000, 36400-36410, 36420-36430, 36440, 36591-36592, 36600, 36640, 43752, 51701-51703, 56605-56606, 56820, 57100, 57180, 57410, 57500, 58100, 62320-62327, 64400, 64405-64408, 64415-64435, 64445-64454, 64461-64463, 64479-64505, 64510-64530, 69990, 92012-92014, 93000-93010, 93040-93042, 93318, 93355, 94002, 94200, 94250, 94680-94690, 94770, 95812-95816, 95819, 95822, 95829, 95955, 96360-96368, 96372, 96374-96377, 96523, 97597-97598, 97602, 99155, 99156, 99157, 99211-99223, 99231-99255, 99291-99292, 99304-99310, 99315-99316, 99334-99337, 99347-99350, 99374-99375, 99377-99378, 99446-99449, 99451-99452, 99495-99496, G0463, G0471

56810 00940, 0213T, 0216T, 0228T, 0230T, 11000-11006, 11042-11047, 12001-12007, 12011-12057, 13100-13133, 13151-13153, 36000, 36400-36410, 36420-36430, 36440, 36591-36592, 36600, 36640, 43752, 51701-51703, 56605-56606, 56820, 57100, 57180, 57410, 57500, 57800, 58100, 62320-62327, 64400, 64405-64408, 64415-64435, 64445-64454, 64461-64463, 64479-64505, 64510-64530, 69990, 92012-92014, 93000-93010, 93040-93042, 93318, 93355, 94002, 94200, 94250, 94680-94690, 94770, 95812-95816, 95819, 95822, 95829, 95955, 96360-96368, 96372, 96374-96377, 96523, 97597-97598, 97602, 99155, 99156, 99157, 99211-99223, 99231-99255, 99291-99292, 99304-99310, 99315-99316, 99334-99337, 99347-99350, 99374-99375, 99377-99378, 99446-99449, 99451-99452, 99495-99496, G0463, G0471

56820 00940, 0213T, 0216T, 0228T, 0230T, 12001-12007, 12011-12057, 13100-13133, 13151-13153, 36000, 36400-36410, 36420-36430, 36440, 36591-36592, 36600, 36640, 43752, 51701-51703, 57410, 62320-62327, 64400, 64405-64408, 64415-64435, 64445-64454, 64461-64463, 64479-64505, 64510-64530, 69990, 76000, 77001-77002, 92012-92014, 93000-93010, 93040-93042, 93318, 93355, 94002, 94200, 94250, 94680-94690, 94770, 95812-95816, 95819, 95822, 95829, 95955, 96360-96368, 96372, 96374-96377, 96523, 99155, 99156, 99157, 99211-99223, 99231-99255, 99291-99292, 99304-99310, 99315-99316, 99334-99337, 99347-99350, 99374-99375, 99377-99378, 99446-99449, 99451-99452, 99495-99496, G0463, G0471

56821 00940, 0213T, 0216T, 0228T, 0230T, 10005, 10007, 10009, 10011, 10021, 12001-12007, 12011-12057, 13100-13133, 13151-13153, 36000, 36400-36410, 36420-36430, 36440, 36591-36592, 36600, 36640, 43752, 51701-51703, 56605, 56820, 57410, 62320-62327, 64400, 64405-64408, 64415-64435, 64445-64454, 64461-64463, 64479-64505, 64510-64530, 69990, 76000, 77001-77002, 92012-92014, 93000-93010, 93040-93042, 93318, 93355, 94002, 94200, 94250, 94680-94690, 94770, 95812-95816, 95819, 95822, 95829, 95955, 96360-96368, 96372, 96374-96377, 96523, 99155, 99156, 99157, 99211-99223, 99231-99255, 99291-99292, 99304-99310, 99315-99316, 99334-99337, 99347-99350, 99374-99375, 99377-99378, 99446-99449, 99451-99452, 99495-99496, G0463, G0471, J0670, J2001

57000 00940, 0213T, 0216T, 0228T, 0230T, 11000-11006, 11042-11047, 12001-12007, 12011-12057, 13100-13133, 13151-13153, 36000, 36400-36410, 36420-36430, 36440, 36591-36592, 36600, 36640, 43752, 49407, 51701-51703, 56810, 57020, 57100, 57150, 57180, 57410-57420, 57452, 57500, 57800, 58100, 58800, 62320-62327, 64400, 64405-64408, 64415-64435, 64445-64454, 64461-64463, 64479-64505, 64510-64530, 69990, 92012-92014, 93000-93010, 93040-93042, 93318, 93355, 94002, 94200, 94250, 94680-94690, 94770, 95812-95816, 95819, 95822, 95829, 95955, 96360-96368, 96372, 96374-96377, 96523, 97597-97598, 97602, 99155, 99156, 99157, 99211-99223, 99231-99255, 99291-99292, 99304-99310, 99315-99316, 99334-99337, 99347-99350, 99374-99375, 99377-99378, 99446-99449, 99451-99452, 99495-99496, G0463, G0471, P9612

57010 00940, 0213T, 0216T, 0228T, 0230T, 11000-11006, 11042-11047, 12001-12007, 12011-12057, 13100-13133, 13151-13153, 36000, 36400-36410, 36420-36430, 36440, 36591-36592, 36600, 36640, 43752, 49407, 51701-51703, 56810, 57000, 57020, 57100, 57150, 57180, 57410-57420, 57452, 57500, 57800, 58100, 58800, 58820, 62320-62327, 64400, 64405-64408, 64415-64435, 64445-64454, 64461-64463, 64479-64505, 64510-64530, 69990, 92012-92014, 93000-93010, 93040-93042, 93318, 93355, 94002, 94200, 94250, 94680-94690, 94770, 95812-95816, 95819, 95822, 95829, 95955, 96360-96368, 96372, 96374-96377, 96523, 97597-97598, 97602, 99155, 99156, 99157, 99211-99223, 99231-99255, 99291-99292, 99304-99310, 99315-99316, 99334-99337, 99347-99350, 99374-99375, 99377-99378, 99446-99449, 99451-99452, 99495-99496, G0463, G0471, P9612

57020 00940, 0213T, 0216T, 0228T, 0230T, 12001-12007, 12011-12057, 13100-13133, 13151-13153, 36000, 36400-36410, 36420-36430, 36440, 36591-36592, 36600, 36640, 43752, 49407, 51701-51703, 57100, 57150, 57180, 57410-57420, 57452, 57500, 57800, 58100, 58800, 62320-62327, 64400, 64405-64408, 64415-64435, 64445-64454, 64461-64463, 64479-64505, 64510-64530, 69990, 92012-92014, 93000-93010, 93040-93042, 93318, 93355, 94002, 94200, 94250, 94680-94690, 94770, 95812-95816, 95819, 95822, 95829, 95955, 96360-96368, 96372, 96374-96377, 96523, 99155, 99156, 99157, 99211-99223, 99231-99255, 99291-99292, 99304-99310, 99315-99316, 99334-99337, 99347-99350, 99374-99375, 99377-99378, 99446-99449, 99451-99452, 99495-99496, G0463, G0471

57022 00940, 0213T, 0216T, 0228T, 0230T, 12001-12007, 12011-12057, 13100-13133, 13151-13153, 36000, 36400-36410, 36420-36430, 36440, 36591-36592, 36600, 36640, 43752, 49407, 51701-51703, 57000-57020, 57100, 57150, 57180, 57400-57420, 57452, 57500, 57800, 58100, 58800, 62320-62327, 64400, 64405-64408, 64415-64435, 64445-64454, 64461-64463, 64479-64505, 64510-64530, 69990, 92012-92014, 93000-93010, 93040-93042, 93318, 93355, 94002, 94200, 94250, 94680-94690, 94770, 95812-95816, 95819, 95822, 95829, 95955, 96360-96368, 96372, 96374-96377, 96523, 99155, 99156, 99157, 99211-99223, 99231-99255, 99291-99292, 99304-99310, 99315-99316,

99334-99337, 99347-99350, 99374-99375, 99377-99378, 99446-99449, 99451-99452, 99495-99496, G0463, G0471, P9612

57023 00940, 0213T, 0216T, 0228T, 0230T, 12001-12007, 12011-12057, 13100-13133, 13151-13153, 36000, 36400-36410, 36420-36430, 36440, 36591-36592, 36600, 36640, 43752, 49407, 51701-51703, 56810, 57000-57020, 57100, 57150, 57180, 57400-57420, 57452, 57500, 57800, 58100, 58800, 62320-62327, 64400, 64405-64408, 64415-64435, 64445-64454, 64461-64463, 64479-64505, 64510-64530, 69990, 92012-92014, 93000-93010, 93040-93042, 93318, 93355, 94002, 94200, 94250, 94680-94690, 94770, 95812-95816, 95819, 95822, 95829, 95955, 96360-96368, 96372, 96374-96377, 96523, 99155, 99156, 99157, 99211-99223, 99231-99255, 99291-99292, 99304-99310, 99315-99316, 99334-99337, 99347-99350, 99374-99375, 99377-99378, 99446-99449, 99451-99452, 99495-99496, G0463, G0471, P9612

57061 00940, 0213T, 0216T, 0228T, 0230T, 12001-12007, 12011-12057, 13100-13133, 13151-13153, 36000, 36400-36410, 36420-36430, 36440, 36591-36592, 36600, 36640, 43752, 51701-51703, 57100, 57150, 57180, 57410-57415, 57452, 57500, 57800, 58100, 62320-62327, 64400, 64405-64408, 64415-64435, 64445-64454, 64461-64463, 64479-64505, 64510-64530, 69990, 92012-92014, 93000-93010, 93040-93042, 93318, 93355, 94002, 94200, 94250, 94680-94690, 94770, 95812-95816, 95819, 95822, 95829, 95955, 96360-96368, 96372, 96374-96377, 96523, 99155, 99156, 99157, 99211-99223, 99231-99255, 99291-99292, 99304-99310, 99315-99316, 99334-99337, 99347-99350, 99374-99375, 99377-99378, 99446-99449, 99451-99452, 99495-99496, G0463, G0471, J0670, J2001

57065 00940, 0213T, 0216T, 0228T, 0230T, 12001-12007, 12011-12057, 13100-13133, 13151-13153, 36000, 36400-36410, 36420-36430, 36440, 36591-36592, 36600, 36640, 43752, 51701-51703, 57061, 57100, 57150, 57180, 57410-57420, 57452, 57500, 57800, 58100, 62320-62327, 64400, 64405-64408, 64415-64435, 64445-64454, 64461-64463, 64479-64505, 64510-64530, 92012-92014, 93000-93010, 93040-93042, 93318, 93355, 94002, 94200, 94250, 94680-94690, 94770, 95812-95816, 95819, 95822, 95829, 95955, 96360-96368, 96372, 96374-96377, 96523, 99155, 99156, 99157, 99211-99223, 99231-99255, 99291-99292, 99304-99310, 99315-99316, 99334-99337, 99347-99350, 99374-99375, 99377-99378, 99446-99449, 99451-99452, 99495-99496, G0463, G0471, J0670, J2001, P9612

57100 00940, 0213T, 0216T, 0228T, 0230T, 10005, 10007, 10009, 10011, 10021, 12001-12007, 12011-12057, 13100-13133, 13151-13153, 36000, 36400-36410, 36420-36430, 36440, 36591-36592, 36600, 36640, 43752, 51701-51703, 57415, 62320-62327, 64400, 64405-64408, 64415-64435, 64445-64454, 64461-64463, 64479-64505, 64510-64530, 69990, 92012-92014, 93000-93010, 93040-93042, 93318, 93355, 94002, 94200, 94250, 94680-94690, 94770, 95812-95816, 95819, 95822, 95829, 95955, 96360-96368, 96372, 96374-96377, 96523, 99155, 99156, 99157, 99211-99223, 99231-99255, 99291-99292, 99304-99310, 99315-99316, 99334-99337, 99347-99350, 99374-99375, 99377-99378, 99446-99449, 99451-99452, 99495-99496, G0463, G0471, J2001

57105 00940, 0213T, 0216T, 0228T, 0230T, 10005, 10007, 10009, 10011, 10021, 12001-12007, 12011-12057, 13100-13133, 13151-13153, 36000, 36400-36410, 36420-36430, 36440, 36591-36592, 36600, 36640, 43752, 51701-51703, 57061, 57100, 57150, 57180, 57410-57420, 57452, 57500, 57800, 58100, 62320-62327, 64400, 64405-64408, 64415-64435, 64445-64454, 64461-64463, 64479-64505, 64510-64530, 69990, 92012-92014, 93000-93010, 93040-93042, 93318, 93355, 94002, 94200, 94250, 94680-94690, 94770, 95812-95816, 95819, 95822, 95829, 95955, 96360-96368, 96372, 96374-96377, 96523, 99155, 99156, 99157, 99211-99223, 99231-99255, 99291-99292, 99304-99310,

99315-99316, 99334-99337, 99347-99350, 99374-99375, 99377-99378, 99446-99449, 99451-99452, 99495-99496, G0463, G0471, J2001

57106 00940, 0213T, 0216T, 0228T, 0230T, 11000-11006, 11042-11047, 12001-12007, 12011-12057, 13100-13133, 13151-13153, 35840, 36000, 36400-36410, 36420-36430, 36440, 36591-36592, 36600, 36640, 43752, 44950, 44970, 50715, 51701-51703, 52000, 56810, 57000, 57061, 57065-57105, 57120-57150, 57180, 57268-57270, 57410-57421, 57452, 57500, 57800, 58100, 62320-62327, 64400, 64405-64408, 64415-64435, 64445-64454, 64461-64463, 64479-64505, 64510-64530, 69990, 92012-92014, 93000-93010, 93040-93042, 93318, 93355, 94002, 94200, 94250, 94680-94690, 94770, 95812-95816, 95819, 95822, 95829, 95955, 96360-96368, 96372, 96374-96377, 96523, 97597-97598, 97602, 99155, 99156, 99157, 99211-99223, 99231-99255, 99291-99292, 99304-99310, 99315-99316, 99334-99337, 99347-99350, 99374-99375, 99377-99378, 99446-99449, 99451-99452, 99495-99496, G0463, G0471, P9612

57107 00940, 0213T, 0216T, 0228T, 0230T, 11000-11006, 11042-11047, 12001-12007, 12011-12057, 13100-13133, 13151-13153, 35840, 36000, 36400-36410, 36420-36430, 36440, 36591-36592, 36600, 36640, 43752, 44950, 44970, 50715, 51701-51703, 52000, 56810, 57000, 57061, 57065-57106, 57111❖, 57120-57150, 57180, 57268-57270, 57410-57421, 57452, 57555, 57800, 58100, 62320-62327, 64400, 64405-64408, 64415-64435, 64445-64454, 64461-64463, 64479-64505, 64510-64530, 69990, 92012-92014, 93000-93010, 93040-93042, 93318, 93355, 94002, 94200, 94250, 94680-94690, 94770, 95812-95816, 95819, 95822, 95829, 95955, 96360-96368, 96372, 96374-96377, 96523, 97597-97598, 97602, 99155, 99156, 99157, 99211-99223, 99231-99255, 99291-99292, 99304-99310, 99315-99316, 99334-99337, 99347-99350, 99374-99375, 99377-99378, 99446-99449, 99451-99452, 99495-99496, G0463, G0471, P9612

57109 00940, 0213T, 0216T, 0228T, 0230T, 10005, 10007, 10009, 10011, 10021, 11000-11006, 11042-11047, 12001-12007, 12011-12057, 13100-13133, 13151-13153, 35840, 36000, 36400-36410, 36420-36430, 36440, 36591-36592, 36600, 36640, 38570-38573, 38770, 38780, 43752, 44950, 44970, 50715, 51701-51703, 52000, 56810, 57000, 57061, 57065-57107, 57120-57150, 57180, 57268-57270, 57410-57421, 57452, 57555, 57800, 58100, 62320-62327, 64400, 64405-64408, 64415-64435, 64445-64454, 64461-64463, 64479-64505, 64510-64530, 69990, 92012-92014, 93000-93010, 93040-93042, 93318, 93355, 94002, 94200, 94250, 94680-94690, 94770, 95812-95816, 95819, 95822, 95829, 95955, 96360-96368, 96372, 96374-96377, 96523, 97597-97598, 97602, 99155, 99156, 99157, 99211-99223, 99231-99255, 99291-99292, 99304-99310, 99315-99316, 99334-99337, 99347-99350, 99374-99375, 99377-99378, 99446-99449, 99451-99452, 99495-99496, G0463, G0471, P9612

57110 00940, 0213T, 0216T, 0228T, 0230T, 11000-11006, 11042-11047, 12001-12007, 12011-12057, 13100-13133, 13151-13153, 36000, 36400-36410, 36420-36430, 36440, 36591-36592, 36600, 36640, 43752, 44950, 44970, 50715, 51701-51703, 52000, 56810, 57061, 57065-57107, 57109, 57120-57150, 57180, 57268-57270, 57410-57421, 57452, 57500, 57800, 58100, 62320-62327, 64400, 64405-64408, 64415-64435, 64445-64454, 64461-64463, 64479-64505, 64510-64530, 69990, 92012-92014, 93000-93010, 93040-93042, 93318, 93355, 94002, 94200, 94250, 94680-94690, 94770, 95812-95816, 95819, 95822, 95829, 95955, 96360-96368, 96372, 96374-96377, 96523, 97597-97598, 97602, 99155, 99156, 99157, 99211-99223, 99231-99255, 99291-99292, 99304-99310, 99315-99316, 99334-99337, 99347-99350, 99374-99375, 99377-99378, 99446-99449, 99451-99452, 99495-99496, G0463, G0471, P9612

57111 00940, 0213T, 0216T, 0228T, 0230T, 11000-11006, 11042-11047, 12001-12007, 12011-12057, 13100-13133, 13151-13153, 35840, 36000, 36400-36410, 36420-36430, 36440, 36591-36592, 36600, 36640, 43752, 44950, 44970, 50715, 51701-51703, 52000, 56810, 57061, 57065-57106, 57109-57110, 57120-57150, 57180, 57268-57270, 57410-57421, 57452, 57500, 57800, 58100, 62320-62327, 64400, 64405-64408, 64415-64435, 64445-64454, 64461-64463, 64479-64505, 64510-64530, 69990, 92012-92014, 93000-93010, 93040-93042, 93318, 93355, 94002, 94200, 94250, 94680-94690, 94770, 95812-95816, 95819, 95822, 95829, 95955, 96360-96368, 96372, 96374-96377, 96523, 97597-97598, 97602, 99155, 99156, 99157, 99211-99223, 99231-99255, 99291-99292, 99304-99310, 99315-99316, 99334-99337, 99347-99350, 99374-99375, 99377-99378, 99446-99449, 99451-99452, 99495-99496, G0463, G0471, P9612

57120 00940, 0213T, 0216T, 0228T, 0230T, 12001-12007, 12011-12057, 13100-13133, 13151-13153, 36000, 36400-36410, 36420-36430, 36440, 36591-36592, 36600, 36640, 43752, 50715, 51701-51703, 52000, 56810, 57000, 57061, 57065-57105, 57130-57150, 57180, 57268-57270, 57410-57420, 57452, 57500, 57800, 58100, 62320-62327, 64400, 64405-64408, 64415-64435, 64445-64454, 64461-64463, 64479-64505, 64510-64530, 69990, 92012-92014, 93000-93010, 93040-93042, 93318, 93355, 94002, 94200, 94250, 94680-94690, 94770, 95812-95816, 95819, 95822, 95829, 95955, 96360-96368, 96372, 96374-96377, 96523, 99155, 99156, 99157, 99211-99223, 99231-99255, 99291-99292, 99304-99310, 99315-99316, 99334-99337, 99347-99350, 99374-99375, 99377-99378, 99446-99449, 99451-99452, 99495-99496, G0463, G0471, P9612

57130 00940, 0213T, 0216T, 0228T, 0230T, 11000-11006, 11042-11047, 12001-12007, 12011-12057, 13100-13133, 13151-13153, 36000, 36400-36410, 36420-36430, 36440, 36591-36592, 36600, 36640, 43752, 50715, 51701-51703, 56810, 57000, 57022, 57100-57105, 57150, 57180, 57410-57420, 57452, 57500, 57800, 58100, 62320-62327, 64400, 64405-64408, 64415-64435, 64445-64454, 64461-64463, 64479-64505, 64510-64530, 69990, 92012-92014, 93000-93010, 93040-93042, 93318, 93355, 94002, 94200, 94250, 94680-94690, 94770, 95812-95816, 95819, 95822, 95829, 95955, 96360-96368, 96372, 96374-96377, 96523, 97597-97598, 97602, 99155, 99156, 99157, 99211-99223, 99231-99255, 99291-99292, 99304-99310, 99315-99316, 99334-99337, 99347-99350, 99374-99375, 99377-99378, 99446-99449, 99451-99452, 99495-99496, G0463, G0471, J0670, J2001

57135 00940, 0213T, 0216T, 0228T, 0230T, 11000-11006, 11042-11047, 12001-12007, 12011-12057, 13100-13133, 13151-13153, 36000, 36400-36410, 36420-36430, 36440, 36591-36592, 36600, 36640, 43752, 50715, 51701-51703, 56810, 57000, 57061, 57065-57105, 57150, 57180, 57410-57421, 57452, 57500, 57800, 58100, 62320-62327, 64400, 64405-64408, 64415-64435, 64445-64454, 64461-64463, 64479-64505, 64510-64530, 69990, 92012-92014, 93000-93010, 93040-93042, 93318, 93355, 94002, 94200, 94250, 94680-94690, 94770, 95812-95816, 95819, 95822, 95829, 95955, 96360-96368, 96372, 96374-96377, 96523, 97597-97598, 97602, 99155, 99156, 99157, 99211-99223, 99231-99255, 99291-99292, 99304-99310, 99315-99316, 99334-99337, 99347-99350, 99374-99375, 99377-99378, 99446-99449, 99451-99452, 99495-99496, G0463, G0471, J0670, J2001, P9612

57150 00940, 0213T, 0216T, 0228T, 0230T, 12001-12007, 12011-12057, 13100-13133, 13151-13153, 36000, 36400-36410, 36420-36430, 36440, 36591-36592, 36600, 36640, 43752, 50715, 51701-51703, 57100, 57410, 57420, 57452, 57500, 57800, 58100, 62320-62327, 64400, 64405-64408, 64415-64435, 64445-64454, 64461-64463, 64479-64505, 64510-64530, 69990, 92012-92014, 93000-93010, 93040-93042, 93318,

93355, 94002, 94200, 94250, 94680-94690, 94770, 95812-95816, 95819, 95822, 95829, 95955, 96360-96368, 96372, 96374-96377, 96523, 99155, 99156, 99157, 99211-99223, 99231-99255, 99291-99292, 99304-99310, 99315-99316, 99334-99337, 99347-99350, 99374-99375, 99377-99378, 99446-99449, 99451-99452, 99495-99496, G0463, G0471

57155 00940, 0213T, 0216T, 0228T, 0230T, 11000-11006, 11042-11047, 12001-12007, 12011-12057, 13100-13133, 13151-13153, 36000, 36400-36410, 36420-36430, 36440, 36591-36592, 36600, 36640, 43752, 50715, 51701-51703, 57100, 57150, 57156♦, 57180, 57400-57420, 57452, 57530, 57800, 58100, 62320-62327, 64400, 64405-64408, 64415-64435, 64445-64454, 64461-64463, 64479-64505, 64510-64530, 69990, 92012-92014, 93000-93010, 93040-93042, 93318, 93355, 94002, 94200, 94250, 94680-94690, 94770, 95812-95816, 95819, 95822, 95829, 95955, 96360-96368, 96372, 96374-96377, 96523, 97597-97598, 97602, 99155, 99156, 99157, 99211-99223, 99231-99255, 99291-99292, 99304-99310, 99315-99316, 99334-99337, 99347-99350, 99374-99375, 99377-99378, 99446-99449, 99451-99452, 99495-99496, G0463, G0471, P9612

57156 00940, 0213T, 0216T, 11000-11006, 11042-11047, 12001-12007, 12011-12057, 13100-13133, 13151-13153, 36000, 36400-36410, 36420-36430, 36440, 36591-36592, 36600, 36640, 43752, 50715, 51701-51703, 57100, 57150, 57180, 57400-57420, 57452, 57530, 57800, 58100, 62320-62327, 64400, 64405-64408, 64415-64435, 64445-64454, 64461-64463, 64479-64505, 64510-64530, 69990, 92012-92014, 93000-93010, 93040-93042, 93318, 93355, 94002, 94200, 94250, 94680-94690, 94770, 95812-95816, 95819, 95822, 95829, 95955, 96360-96368, 96372, 96374-96377, 96523, 97597-97598, 97602, 99155, 99156, 99157, 99211-99223, 99231-99255, 99291-99292, 99304-99310, 99315-99316, 99334-99337, 99347-99350, 99374-99375, 99377-99378, 99446-99449, 99451-99452, 99495-99496, G0463, G0471, P9612

57160 00940, 0213T, 0216T, 0228T, 0230T, 11000-11006, 11042-11047, 12001-12007, 12011-12057, 13100-13133, 13151-13153, 36000, 36400-36410, 36420-36430, 36440, 36591-36592, 36600, 36640, 43752, 50715, 51701-51703, 57100, 57150, 57180, 57410, 57420, 57452, 57500, 57800, 62320-62327, 64400, 64405-64408, 64415-64435, 64445-64454, 64461-64463, 64479-64505, 64510-64530, 69990, 92012-92014, 93000-93010, 93040-93042, 93318, 93355, 94002, 94200, 94250, 94680-94690, 94770, 95812-95816, 95819, 95822, 95829, 95955, 96360-96368, 96372, 96374-96377, 96523, 97597-97598, 97602, 99155, 99156, 99157, 99211-99223, 99231-99255, 99291-99292, 99304-99310, 99315-99316, 99334-99337, 99347-99350, 99374-99375, 99377-99378, 99446-99449, 99451-99452, 99495-99496, G0463, G0471

57170 00940, 0213T, 0216T, 0228T, 0230T, 12001-12007, 12011-12057, 13100-13133, 13151-13153, 36000, 36400-36410, 36420-36430, 36440, 36591-36592, 36600, 36640, 43752, 50715, 51701-51703, 57100, 57150, 57410, 57420, 57452, 57500, 57800, 58100, 62320-62327, 64400, 64405-64408, 64415-64435, 64445-64454, 64461-64463, 64479-64505, 64510-64530, 69990, 92012-92014, 93000-93010, 93040-93042, 93318, 93355, 94002, 94200, 94250, 94680-94690, 94770, 95812-95816, 95819, 95822, 95829, 95955, 96360-96368, 96372, 96374-96377, 96523, 99155, 99156, 99157, 99211-99223, 99231-99255, 99291-99292, 99304-99310, 99315-99316, 99334-99337, 99347-99350, 99374-99375, 99377-99378, 99446-99449, 99451-99452, 99495-99496, G0463, G0471, J2001

57180 00940, 0213T, 0216T, 0228T, 0230T, 12001-12007, 12011-12057, 13100-13133, 13151-13153, 36000, 36400-36410, 36420-36430, 36440, 36591-36592, 36600, 36640, 43752, 50715, 51701-51703, 57100, 57800, 62320-62327, 64400, 64405-64408, 64415-64435, 64445-64454,

64461-64463, 64479-64505, 64510-64530, 69990, 92012-92014, 93000-93010, 93040-93042, 93318, 93355, 94002, 94200, 94250, 94680-94690, 94770, 95812-95816, 95819, 95822, 95829, 95955, 96360-96368, 96372, 96374-96377, 96523, 99155, 99156, 99157, 99211-99223, 99231-99255, 99291-99292, 99304-99310, 99315-99316, 99334-99337, 99347-99350, 99374-99375, 99377-99378, 99446-99449, 99451-99452, 99495-99496, G0463, G0471, J0670, J2001

57200 00940, 0213T, 0216T, 0228T, 0230T, 12001-12007, 12011-12057, 13100-13133, 13151-13153, 36000, 36400-36410, 36420-36430, 36440, 36591-36592, 36600, 36640, 43752, 44950, 44970, 50715, 51701-51703, 52000, 56810, 57100-57105, 57150, 57180, 57410, 57420, 57452, 57500, 57800, 58100, 62320-62327, 64400, 64405-64408, 64415-64435, 64445-64454, 64461-64463, 64479-64505, 64510-64530, 69990, 92012-92014, 93000-93010, 93040-93042, 93318, 93355, 94002, 94200, 94250, 94680-94690, 94770, 95812-95816, 95819, 95822, 95829, 95955, 96360-96368, 96372, 96374-96377, 96523, 99155, 99156, 99157, 99211-99223, 99231-99255, 99291-99292, 99304-99310, 99315-99316, 99334-99337, 99347-99350, 99374-99375, 99377-99378, 99446-99449, 99451-99452, 99495-99496, G0463, G0471, P9612

57210 00940, 0213T, 0216T, 0228T, 0230T, 12001-12007, 12011-12057, 13100-13133, 13151-13153, 36000, 36400-36410, 36420-36430, 36440, 36591-36592, 36600, 36640, 43752, 44950, 44970, 45560, 50715, 51701-51703, 52000, 56605-56606, 56800, 56810, 57100-57105, 57150, 57180-57200, 57410, 57420, 57452, 57500, 57800, 58100, 59300, 62320-62327, 64400, 64405-64408, 64415-64435, 64445-64454, 64461-64463, 64479-64505, 64510-64530, 69990, 92012-92014, 93000-93010, 93040-93042, 93318, 93355, 94002, 94200, 94250, 94680-94690, 94770, 95812-95816, 95819, 95822, 95829, 95955, 96360-96368, 96372, 96374-96377, 96523, 99155, 99156, 99157, 99211-99223, 99231-99255, 99291-99292, 99304-99310, 99315-99316, 99334-99337, 99347-99350, 99374-99375, 99377-99378, 99446-99449, 99451-99452, 99495-99496, G0463, G0471, P9612

57220 00940, 0213T, 0216T, 0228T, 0230T, 12001-12007, 12011-12057, 13100-13133, 13151-13153, 36000, 36400-36410, 36420-36430, 36440, 36591-36592, 36600, 36640, 43752, 44950, 44970, 45560, 50715, 51701-51703, 52000, 53000-53025, 53200, 56810, 57000, 57061, 57065-57105, 57150, 57180, 57210, 57268, 57410, 57420, 57452, 57500, 57800, 58100, 62320-62327, 64400, 64405-64408, 64415-64435, 64445-64454, 64461-64463, 64479-64505, 64510-64530, 69990, 92012-92014, 93000-93010, 93040-93042, 93318, 93355, 94002, 94200, 94250, 94680-94690, 94770, 95812-95816, 95819, 95822, 95829, 95955, 96360-96368, 96372, 96374-96377, 96523, 99155, 99156, 99157, 99211-99223, 99231-99255, 99291-99292, 99304-99310, 99315-99316, 99334-99337, 99347-99350, 99374-99375, 99377-99378, 99446-99449, 99451-99452, 99495-99496, G0463, G0471, P9612

57230 00940, 0213T, 0216T, 0228T, 0230T, 12001-12007, 12011-12057, 13100-13133, 13151-13153, 36000, 36400-36410, 36420-36430, 36440, 36591-36592, 36600, 36640, 43752, 44950, 44970, 45560, 50715, 51701-51703, 52000, 53000-53025, 53200, 53275, 53450-53460, 56810, 57100-57105, 57150, 57180, 57220, 57268, 57410, 57420, 57452, 57500, 57800, 58100, 62320-62327, 64400, 64405-64408, 64415-64435, 64445-64454, 64461-64463, 64479-64505, 64510-64530, 69990, 92012-92014, 93000-93010, 93040-93042, 93318, 93355, 94002, 94200, 94250, 94680-94690, 94770, 95812-95816, 95819, 95822, 95829, 95955, 96360-96368, 96372, 96374-96377, 96523, 99155, 99156, 99157, 99211-99223, 99231-99255, 99291-99292, 99304-99310, 99315-99316, 99334-99337, 99347-99350, 99374-99375, 99377-99378, 99446-99449, 99451-99452, 99495-99496, G0463, G0471, P9612

57240 00940, 0213T, 0216T, 0228T, 0230T, 0437T, 12001-12007, 12011-12057, 13100-13133, 13151-13153, 15777, 36000, 36400-36410, 36420-36430, 36440, 36591-36592, 36600, 36640, 43752, 44950, 44970, 49568, 50715, 51701-51703, 52000, 53000-53025, 56810, 57000, 57065-57106, 57150, 57180-57200, 57220-57230, 57250, 57285, 57410, 57420, 57452, 57500, 57800, 58100, 62320-62327, 64400, 64405-64408, 64415-64435, 64445-64454, 64461-64463, 64479-64505, 64510-64530, 69990, 92012-92014, 93000-93010, 93040-93042, 93318, 93355, 94002, 94200, 94250, 94680-94690, 94770, 95812-95816, 95819, 95822, 95829, 95955, 96360-96368, 96372, 96374-96377, 96523, 99155, 99156, 99157, 99211-99223, 99231-99255, 99291-99292, 99304-99310, 99315-99316, 99334-99337, 99347-99350, 99374-99375, 99377-99378, 99446-99449, 99451-99452, 99495-99496, G0463, G0471, P9612

57250 00940, 0213T, 0216T, 0228T, 0230T, 0437T, 12001-12007, 12011-12057, 13100-13133, 13151-13153, 15777, 36000, 36400-36410, 36420-36430, 36440, 36591-36592, 36600, 36640, 43752, 44950, 44970, 45560, 49568, 50715, 51701-51703, 52000, 56810, 57000, 57061, 57100-57106, 57135-57150, 57180, 57210, 57289✣, 57410, 57420, 57452, 57500, 57800, 58100, 62320-62327, 64400, 64405-64408, 64415-64435, 64445-64454, 64461-64463, 64479-64505, 64510-64530, 69990, 92012-92014, 93000-93010, 93040-93042, 93318, 93355, 94002, 94200, 94250, 94680-94690, 94770, 95812-95816, 95819, 95822, 95829, 95955, 96360-96368, 96372, 96374-96377, 96523, 99155, 99156, 99157, 99211-99223, 99231-99255, 99291-99292, 99304-99310, 99315-99316, 99334-99337, 99347-99350, 99374-99375, 99377-99378, 99446-99449, 99451-99452, 99495-99496, G0463, G0471, P9612

57260 00940, 0213T, 0216T, 0228T, 0230T, 0437T, 12001-12007, 12011-12057, 13100-13133, 13151-13153, 15777, 36000, 36400-36410, 36420-36430, 36440, 36591-36592, 36600, 36640, 43752, 44950, 44970, 45560, 49568, 50715, 51701-51703, 52000, 53620, 53660, 56800, 56810, 57000, 57061, 57100-57106, 57120, 57150, 57180, 57210-57250, 57268-57270, 57285, 57410, 57420, 57452, 57500, 57800, 58100, 62320-62327, 64400, 64405-64408, 64415-64435, 64445-64454, 64461-64463, 64479-64505, 64510-64530, 69990, 92012-92014, 93000-93010, 93040-93042, 93318, 93355, 94002, 94200, 94250, 94680-94690, 94770, 95812-95816, 95819, 95822, 95829, 95955, 96360-96368, 96372, 96374-96377, 96523, 99155, 99156, 99157, 99211-99223, 99231-99255, 99291-99292, 99304-99310, 99315-99316, 99334-99337, 99347-99350, 99374-99375, 99377-99378, 99446-99449, 99451-99452, 99495-99496, G0463, G0471, P9612

57265 00940, 0213T, 0216T, 0228T, 0230T, 0437T, 12001-12007, 12011-12057, 13100-13133, 13151-13153, 15777, 36000, 36400-36410, 36420-36430, 36440, 36591-36592, 36600, 36640, 43752, 44950, 44970, 45560, 49407, 49568, 50715, 51701-51703, 52000, 56800, 56810, 57000, 57061, 57100-57106, 57150, 57180, 57210-57260, 57268-57270, 57284-57285, 57410, 57420, 57452, 57500, 57800, 58100, 58800, 62320-62327, 64400, 64405-64408, 64415-64435, 64445-64454, 64461-64463, 64479-64505, 64510-64530, 69990, 92012-92014, 93000-93010, 93040-93042, 93318, 93355, 94002, 94200, 94250, 94680-94690, 94770, 95812-95816, 95819, 95822, 95829, 95955, 96360-96368, 96372, 96374-96377, 96523, 99155, 99156, 99157, 99211-99223, 99231-99255, 99291-99292, 99304-99310, 99315-99316, 99334-99337, 99347-99350, 99374-99375, 99377-99378, 99446-99449, 99451-99452, 99495-99496, G0463, G0471, P9612

57267 0437T✣, 11000-11001, 11042-11047, 15777✣, 36591-36592, 56810, 57000, 57100-57105, 57150, 57180, 57210, 96523, 97597-97598, 97602

57268 00940, 0213T, 0216T, 0228T, 0230T, 12001-12007, 12011-12057, 13100-13133, 13151-13153, 36000, 36400-36410, 36420-36430, 36440, 36591-36592, 36600, 36640, 43752, 44950, 44970, 45560, 49407,

50715, 51701-51703, 52000, 56810, 57000, 57061, 57100-57105, 57135-57150, 57180, 57210, 57267, 57270, 57410, 57420, 57452, 57500, 57800, 58100, 58800, 62320-62327, 64400, 64405-64408, 64415-64435, 64445-64454, 64461-64463, 64479-64505, 64510-64530, 69990, 92012-92014, 93000-93010, 93040-93042, 93318, 93355, 94002, 94200, 94250, 94680-94690, 94770, 95812-95816, 95819, 95822, 95829, 95955, 96360-96368, 96372, 96374-96377, 96523, 99155, 99156, 99157, 99211-99223, 99231-99255, 99291-99292, 99304-99310, 99315-99316, 99334-99337, 99347-99350, 99374-99375, 99377-99378, 99446-99449, 99451-99452, 99495-99496, G0463, G0471, P9612

57270 00940, 0213T, 0216T, 0228T, 0230T, 12001-12007, 12011-12057, 13100-13133, 13151-13153, 36000, 36400-36410, 36420-36430, 36440, 36591-36592, 36600, 36640, 43752, 44005, 44180, 44602-44605, 44850, 44950, 44970, 49000-49010, 49255, 49320, 50715, 51701-51703, 52000, 56810, 57100, 57180, 57267, 57410, 57420, 57452, 57500, 57800, 58100, 62320-62327, 64400, 64405-64408, 64415-64435, 64445-64454, 64461-64463, 64479-64505, 64510-64530, 92012-92014, 93000-93010, 93040-93042, 93318, 93355, 94002, 94200, 94250, 94680-94690, 94770, 95812-95816, 95819, 95822, 95829, 95955, 96360-96368, 96372, 96374-96377, 96523, 99155, 99156, 99157, 99211-99223, 99231-99255, 99291-99292, 99304-99310, 99315-99316, 99334-99337, 99347-99350, 99374-99375, 99377-99378, 99446-99449, 99451-99452, 99495-99496, G0463, G0471, P9612

57280 00940, 0213T, 0216T, 0228T, 0230T, 12001-12007, 12011-12057, 13100-13133, 13151-13153, 36000, 36400-36410, 36420-36430, 36440, 36591-36592, 36600, 36640, 43752, 44005, 44180, 44602-44605, 44850, 44950, 44970, 49000-49010, 49255, 49320, 49570, 50715, 51701-51703, 52000, 57100, 57180, 57267-57270, 57282-57283♦, 57410, 57420, 57425, 57452, 57500, 57800, 62320-62327, 64400, 64405-64408, 64415-64435, 64445-64454, 64461-64463, 64479-64505, 64510-64530, 69990, 92012-92014, 93000-93010, 93040-93042, 93318, 93355, 94002, 94200, 94250, 94680-94690, 94770, 95812-95816, 95819, 95822, 95829, 95955, 96360-96368, 96372, 96374-96377, 96523, 99155, 99156, 99157, 99211-99223, 99231-99255, 99291-99292, 99304-99310, 99315-99316, 99334-99337, 99347-99350, 99374-99375, 99377-99378, 99446-99449, 99451-99452, 99495-99496, G0463, G0471, P9612

57282 00940, 0213T, 0216T, 0228T, 0230T, 12001-12007, 12011-12057, 13100-13133, 13151-13153, 36000, 36400-36410, 36420-36430, 36440, 36591-36592, 36600, 36640, 43752, 44005, 44180, 44602-44605, 44850, 44950, 44970, 49000-49010, 50715, 51701-51703, 52000, 56810, 57000, 57100, 57150, 57180, 57268-57270, 57410, 57420, 57452, 57500, 57800, 58100, 62320-62327, 64400, 64405-64408, 64415-64435, 64445-64454, 64461-64463, 64479-64505, 64510-64530, 69990, 92012-92014, 93000-93010, 93040-93042, 93318, 93355, 94002, 94200, 94250, 94680-94690, 94770, 95812-95816, 95819, 95822, 95829, 95955, 96360-96368, 96372, 96374-96377, 96523, 99155, 99156, 99157, 99211-99223, 99231-99255, 99291-99292, 99304-99310, 99315-99316, 99334-99337, 99347-99350, 99374-99375, 99377-99378, 99446-99449, 99451-99452, 99495-99496, G0463, G0471

57283 00940, 0213T, 0216T, 0228T, 0230T, 12001-12007, 12011-12057, 13100-13133, 13151-13153, 36000, 36400-36410, 36420-36430, 36440, 36591-36592, 36600, 36640, 43752, 44005, 44180, 44950, 44970, 50715, 51701-51703, 52000, 56810, 57000, 57100, 57150, 57180, 57268-57270, 57282♦, 57410, 57420, 57452, 57500, 57800, 58100, 62320-62327, 64400, 64405-64408, 64415-64435, 64445-64454, 64461-64463, 64479-64505, 64510-64530, 69990, 92012-92014, 93000-93010, 93040-93042, 93318, 93355, 94002, 94200, 94250, 94680-94690, 94770, 95812-95816, 95819, 95822, 95829, 95955, 96360-96368, 96372, 96374-96377, 96523, 99155, 99156, 99157,

99211-99223, 99231-99255, 99291-99292, 99304-99310, 99315-99316, 99334-99337, 99347-99350, 99374-99375, 99377-99378, 99446-99449, 99451-99452, 99495-99496, G0463, G0471

57284 00940, 0213T, 0216T, 0228T, 0230T, 12001-12007, 12011-12057, 13100-13133, 13151-13153, 36000, 36400-36410, 36420-36430, 36440, 36591-36592, 36600, 36640, 43653, 43752, 44005, 44180, 44602-44605, 44820-44850, 44950, 44970, 49000-49010, 49255, 49320, 49570, 50715, 51701-51703, 51715, 51840-51841, 51990, 52000, 57100, 57240, 57260, 57268-57270, 57285♦, 57410, 57420, 57423, 57452, 57500, 57800, 58100, 58660, 62320-62327, 64400, 64405-64408, 64415-64435, 64445-64454, 64461-64463, 64479-64505, 64510-64530, 69990, 92012-92014, 93000-93010, 93040-93042, 93318, 93355, 94002, 94200, 94250, 94680-94690, 94770, 95812-95816, 95819, 95822, 95829, 95955, 96360-96368, 96372, 96374-96377, 96523, 99155, 99156, 99157, 99211-99223, 99231-99255, 99291-99292, 99304-99310, 99315-99316, 99334-99337, 99347-99350, 99374-99375, 99377-99378, 99446-99449, 99451-99452, 99495-99496, G0463, G0471, P9612

57285 00940, 0213T, 0216T, 0228T, 0230T, 0437T, 12001-12007, 12011-12057, 13100-13133, 13151-13153, 15777, 36000, 36400-36410, 36420-36430, 36440, 36591-36592, 36600, 36640, 43752, 49568, 51701-51703, 51840♦, 52000, 56810, 57020, 57100, 57150, 57180, 57268, 57400-57420, 57423, 57452, 57500, 57530, 57800, 58100, 62320-62327, 64400, 64405-64408, 64415-64435, 64445-64454, 64461-64463, 64479-64505, 64510-64530, 69990, 92012-92014, 93000-93010, 93040-93042, 93318, 93355, 94002, 94200, 94250, 94680-94690, 94770, 95812-95816, 95819, 95822, 95829, 95955, 96360-96368, 96372, 96374-96377, 96523, 99155, 99156, 99157, 99211-99223, 99231-99255, 99291-99292, 99304-99310, 99315-99316, 99334-99337, 99347-99350, 99374-99375, 99377-99378, 99446-99449, 99451-99452, 99495-99496, G0463, G0471, P9612

57287 00940, 0213T, 0216T, 0228T, 0230T, 11000-11006, 11042-11047, 12001-12007, 12011-12057, 13100-13133, 13151-13153, 36000, 36400-36410, 36420-36430, 36440, 36591-36592, 36600, 36640, 43752, 44950, 44970, 50715, 51701-51703, 51992♦, 52000, 53000-53025, 57000, 57020, 57100, 57150, 57180, 57220, 57268, 57288-57289, 57410, 57420, 57452, 57500, 57800, 58100, 58267♦, 58293♦, 62320-62327, 64400, 64405-64408, 64415-64435, 64445-64454, 64461-64463, 64479-64505, 64510-64530, 69990, 92012-92014, 93000-93010, 93040-93042, 93318, 93355, 94002, 94200, 94250, 94680-94690, 94770, 95812-95816, 95819, 95822, 95829, 95955, 96360-96368, 96372, 96374-96377, 96523, 97597-97598, 97602, 99155, 99156, 99157, 99211-99223, 99231-99255, 99291-99292, 99304-99310, 99315-99316, 99334-99337, 99347-99350, 99374-99375, 99377-99378, 99446-99449, 99451-99452, 99495-99496, G0463, G0471, P9612

57288 00940, 0213T, 0216T, 0228T, 0230T, 12001-12007, 12011-12057, 13100-13133, 13151-13153, 36000, 36400-36410, 36420-36430, 36440, 36591-36592, 36600, 36640, 43752, 44950, 44970, 50715, 51701-51703, 51992, 52000, 53000-53025, 56810, 57000, 57100, 57150, 57180, 57220, 57267-57268, 57289, 57410, 57420, 57452, 57500, 57800, 58100, 58267♦, 58293♦, 62320-62327, 64400, 64405-64408, 64415-64435, 64445-64454, 64461-64463, 64479-64505, 64510-64530, 92012-92014, 93000-93010, 93040-93042, 93318, 93355, 94002, 94200, 94250, 94680-94690, 94770, 95812-95816, 95819, 95822, 95829, 95955, 96360-96368, 96372, 96374-96377, 96523, 99155, 99156, 99157, 99211-99223, 99231-99255, 99291-99292, 99304-99310, 99315-99316, 99334-99337, 99347-99350, 99374-99375, 99377-99378, 99446-99449, 99451-99452, 99495-99496, G0463, G0471, P9612

57289 00940, 0213T, 0216T, 0228T, 0230T, 12001-12007, 12011-12057, 13100-13133, 13151-13153, 36000, 36400-36410, 36420-36430, 36440, 36591-36592, 36600, 36640, 43752, 44950, 44970, 50715, 51701-51703, 51840❖, 52000, 56810, 57000, 57100, 57150, 57180-57200, 57230-57240, 57260, 57268, 57410, 57420, 57452, 57500, 57800, 58100, 62320-62327, 64400, 64405-64408, 64415-64435, 64445-64454, 64461-64463, 64479-64505, 64510-64530, 69990, 92012-92014, 93000-93010, 93040-93042, 93318, 93355, 94002, 94200, 94250, 94680-94690, 94770, 95812-95816, 95819, 95822, 95829, 95955, 96360-96368, 96372, 96374-96377, 96523, 99155, 99156, 99157, 99211-99223, 99231-99255, 99291-99292, 99304-99310, 99315-99316, 99334-99337, 99347-99350, 99374-99375, 99377-99378, 99446-99449, 99451-99452, 99495-99496, G0463, G0471, P9612

57291 00940, 0213T, 0216T, 0228T, 0230T, 12001-12007, 12011-12057, 13100-13133, 13151-13153, 36000, 36400-36410, 36420-36430, 36440, 36591-36592, 36600, 36640, 43752, 44950, 44970, 50715, 51701-51703, 52000, 56810, 57100, 57150, 57180, 57295❖, 57410, 57420, 57452, 57500, 57800, 58100, 62320-62327, 64400, 64405-64408, 64415-64435, 64445-64454, 64461-64463, 64479-64505, 64510-64530, 69990, 92012-92014, 93000-93010, 93040-93042, 93318, 93355, 94002, 94200, 94250, 94680-94690, 94770, 95812-95816, 95819, 95822, 95829, 95955, 96360-96368, 96372, 96374-96377, 96523, 99155, 99156, 99157, 99211-99223, 99231-99255, 99291-99292, 99304-99310, 99315-99316, 99334-99337, 99347-99350, 99374-99375, 99377-99378, 99446-99449, 99451-99452, 99495-99496, G0463, G0471

57292 00940, 0213T, 0216T, 0228T, 0230T, 12001-12007, 12011-12057, 13100-13133, 13151-13153, 36000, 36400-36410, 36420-36430, 36440, 36591-36592, 36600, 36640, 43752, 44950, 44970, 50715, 51701-51703, 52000, 56810, 57100, 57150, 57180, 57291, 57295❖, 57410, 57420, 57452, 57500, 57800, 58100, 62320-62327, 64400, 64405-64408, 64415-64435, 64445-64454, 64461-64463, 64479-64505, 64510-64530, 69990, 92012-92014, 93000-93010, 93040-93042, 93318, 93355, 94002, 94200, 94250, 94680-94690, 94770, 95812-95816, 95819, 95822, 95829, 95955, 96360-96368, 96372, 96374-96377, 96523, 99155, 99156, 99157, 99211-99223, 99231-99255, 99291-99292, 99304-99310, 99315-99316, 99334-99337, 99347-99350, 99374-99375, 99377-99378, 99446-99449, 99451-99452, 99495-99496, G0463, G0471

57295 00940, 0213T, 0216T, 0228T, 0230T, 11000-11006, 11042-11047, 12001-12007, 12011-12057, 13100-13133, 13151-13153, 36000, 36400-36410, 36420-36430, 36440, 36591-36592, 36600, 36640, 43752, 51701-51703, 52000, 56810, 57000, 57100-57105, 57150, 57180, 57210-57230, 57400-57420, 57452, 57500, 57800, 58100, 62320-62327, 64400, 64405-64408, 64415-64435, 64445-64454, 64461-64463, 64479-64505, 64510-64530, 69990, 92012-92014, 93000-93010, 93040-93042, 93318, 93355, 94002, 94200, 94250, 94680-94690, 94770, 95812-95816, 95819, 95822, 95829, 95955, 96360-96368, 96372, 96374-96377, 96523, 97597-97598, 97602, 99155, 99156, 99157, 99211-99223, 99231-99255, 99291-99292, 99304-99310, 99315-99316, 99334-99337, 99347-99350, 99374-99375, 99377-99378, 99446-99449, 99451-99452, 99495-99496, G0463, G0471

57296 00940, 0213T, 0216T, 0228T, 0230T, 11000-11006, 11042-11047, 12001-12007, 12011-12057, 13100-13133, 13151-13153, 36000, 36400-36410, 36420-36430, 36440, 36591-36592, 36600, 36640, 43752, 44005, 44180, 44602-44605, 44820-44850, 44950, 44970, 49000-49010, 49255, 49320, 49570, 51701-51703, 52000, 56810, 57100, 57150, 57180, 57291-57295❖, 57400-57420, 57426, 57452, 57500, 62320-62327, 64400, 64405-64408, 64415-64435, 64445-64454, 64461-64463, 64479-64505, 64510-64530, 69990, 92012-92014, 93000-93010, 93040-93042, 93318, 93355, 94002, 94200, 94250, 94680-94690, 94770, 95812-95816, 95819, 95822, 95829, 95955,

96360-96368, 96372, 96374-96377, 96523, 97597-97598, 97602, 99155, 99156, 99157, 99211-99223, 99231-99255, 99291-99292, 99304-99310, 99315-99316, 99334-99337, 99347-99350, 99374-99375, 99377-99378, 99446-99449, 99451-99452, 99495-99496, G0463, G0471

57300 00940, 0213T, 0216T, 0228T, 0230T, 11000-11006, 11042-11047, 12001-12007, 12011-12057, 13100-13133, 13151-13153, 36000, 36400-36410, 36420-36430, 36440, 36591-36592, 36600, 36640, 43752, 44950, 44970, 45560, 50715, 51701-51703, 56810, 57000, 57100-57105, 57150, 57180-57210, 57250, 57305❖, 57410, 57420, 57452, 57500, 57800, 58100, 62320-62327, 64400, 64405-64408, 64415-64435, 64445-64454, 64461-64463, 64479-64505, 64510-64530, 69990, 92012-92014, 93000-93010, 93040-93042, 93318, 93355, 94002, 94200, 94250, 94680-94690, 94770, 95812-95816, 95819, 95822, 95829, 95955, 96360-96368, 96372, 96374-96377, 96523, 97597-97598, 97602, 99155, 99156, 99157, 99211-99223, 99231-99255, 99291-99292, 99304-99310, 99315-99316, 99334-99337, 99347-99350, 99374-99375, 99377-99378, 99446-99449, 99451-99452, 99495-99496, G0463, G0471, P9612

57305 00940, 0213T, 0216T, 0228T, 0230T, 11000-11006, 11042-11047, 12001-12007, 12011-12057, 13100-13133, 13151-13153, 36000, 36400-36410, 36420-36430, 36440, 36591-36592, 36600, 36640, 43752, 44005, 44180, 44602-44605, 44850, 44950, 44970, 49000-49010, 49255, 49320, 49570, 50715, 51701-51703, 56810, 57100, 57180, 57410, 57500, 57800, 58100, 62320-62327, 64400, 64405-64408, 64415-64435, 64445-64454, 64461-64463, 64479-64505, 64510-64530, 69990, 92012-92014, 93000-93010, 93040-93042, 93318, 93355, 94002, 94200, 94250, 94680-94690, 94770, 95812-95816, 95819, 95822, 95829, 95955, 96360-96368, 96372, 96374-96377, 96523, 97597-97598, 97602, 99155, 99156, 99157, 99211-99223, 99231-99255, 99291-99292, 99304-99310, 99315-99316, 99334-99337, 99347-99350, 99374-99375, 99377-99378, 99446-99449, 99451-99452, 99495-99496, G0463, G0471, P9612

57307 00940, 0213T, 0216T, 0228T, 0230T, 11000-11006, 11042-11047, 12001-12007, 12011-12057, 13100-13133, 13151-13153, 36000, 36400-36410, 36420-36430, 36440, 36591-36592, 36600, 36640, 43752, 44005, 44180, 44320, 44602-44605, 44820-44850, 44950, 44970, 49000-49010, 49255, 49320, 49570, 50715, 51701-51703, 56810, 57100, 57180, 57305, 57410, 57420, 57452, 57500, 57800, 58100, 62320-62327, 64400, 64405-64408, 64415-64435, 64445-64454, 64461-64463, 64479-64505, 64510-64530, 69990, 92012-92014, 93000-93010, 93040-93042, 93318, 93355, 94002, 94200, 94250, 94680-94690, 94770, 95812-95816, 95819, 95822, 95829, 95955, 96360-96368, 96372, 96374-96377, 96523, 97597-97598, 97602, 99155, 99156, 99157, 99211-99223, 99231-99255, 99291-99292, 99304-99310, 99315-99316, 99334-99337, 99347-99350, 99374-99375, 99377-99378, 99446-99449, 99451-99452, 99495-99496, G0463, G0471, P9612

57308 00940, 0213T, 0216T, 0228T, 0230T, 11000-11006, 11042-11047, 12001-12007, 12011-12057, 13100-13133, 13151-13153, 36000, 36400-36410, 36420-36430, 36440, 36591-36592, 36600, 36640, 43752, 44950, 44970, 50715, 51701-51703, 56810, 57410, 57420, 57452, 62320-62327, 64400, 64405-64408, 64415-64435, 64445-64454, 64461-64463, 64479-64505, 64510-64530, 69990, 92012-92014, 93000-93010, 93040-93042, 93318, 93355, 94002, 94200, 94250, 94680-94690, 94770, 95812-95816, 95819, 95822, 95829, 95955, 96360-96368, 96372, 96374-96377, 96523, 97597-97598, 97602, 99155, 99156, 99157, 99211-99223, 99231-99255, 99291-99292, 99304-99310, 99315-99316, 99334-99337, 99347-99350, 99374-99375, 99377-99378, 99446-99449, 99451-99452, 99495-99496, G0463, G0471

57310 00940, 0213T, 0216T, 0228T, 0230T, 11000-11006, 11042-11047, 12001-12007, 12011-12057, 13100-13133, 13151-13153, 36000, 36400-36410, 36420-36430, 36440, 36591-36592, 36600, 36640, 43752, 44950, 44970, 50715, 51701-51703, 52000, 53200, 53275, 53502, 53520, 56810, 57100, 57150, 57180-57200, 57220-57230, 57410, 57420, 57452, 57500, 57800, 58100, 62320-62327, 64400, 64405-64408, 64415-64435, 64445-64454, 64461-64463, 64479-64505, 64510-64530, 69990, 92012-92014, 93000-93010, 93040-93042, 93318, 93355, 94002, 94200, 94250, 94680-94690, 94770, 95812-95816, 95819, 95822, 95829, 95955, 96360-96368, 96372, 96374-96377, 96523, 97597-97598, 97602, 99155, 99156, 99157, 99211-99223, 99231-99255, 99291-99292, 99304-99310, 99315-99316, 99334-99337, 99347-99350, 99374-99375, 99377-99378, 99446-99449, 99451-99452, 99495-99496, G0463, G0471, P9612

57311 00940, 0213T, 0216T, 0228T, 0230T, 11000-11006, 11042-11047, 12001-12007, 12011-12057, 13100-13133, 13151-13153, 36000, 36400-36410, 36420-36430, 36440, 36591-36592, 36600, 36640, 43752, 44950, 44970, 50715, 51701-51703, 52000, 56810, 57100, 57150, 57180, 57310, 57410, 57420, 57452, 57500, 57800, 58100, 62320-62327, 64400, 64405-64408, 64415-64435, 64445-64454, 64461-64463, 64479-64505, 64510-64530, 69990, 92012-92014, 93000-93010, 93040-93042, 93318, 93355, 94002, 94200, 94250, 94680-94690, 94770, 95812-95816, 95819, 95822, 95829, 95955, 96360-96368, 96372, 96374-96377, 96523, 97597-97598, 97602, 99155, 99156, 99157, 99211-99223, 99231-99255, 99291-99292, 99304-99310, 99315-99316, 99334-99337, 99347-99350, 99374-99375, 99377-99378, 99446-99449, 99451-99452, 99495-99496, G0463, G0471

57320 00940, 0213T, 0216T, 0228T, 0230T, 11000-11006, 11042-11047, 12001-12007, 12011-12057, 13100-13133, 13151-13153, 36000, 36400-36410, 36420-36430, 36440, 36591-36592, 36600, 36640, 43752, 44950, 44970, 50715, 51701-51703, 52000, 56810, 57000, 57100-57105, 57150, 57180, 57210, 57410, 57420, 57452, 57500, 57800, 58100, 62320-62327, 64400, 64405-64408, 64415-64435, 64445-64454, 64461-64463, 64479-64505, 64510-64530, 69990, 92012-92014, 93000-93010, 93040-93042, 93318, 93355, 94002, 94200, 94250, 94680-94690, 94770, 95812-95816, 95819, 95822, 95829, 95955, 96360-96368, 96372, 96374-96377, 96523, 97597-97598, 97602, 99155, 99156, 99157, 99211-99223, 99231-99255, 99291-99292, 99304-99310, 99315-99316, 99334-99337, 99347-99350, 99374-99375, 99377-99378, 99446-99449, 99451-99452, 99495-99496, G0463, G0471

57330 00940, 0213T, 0216T, 0228T, 0230T, 11000-11006, 11042-11047, 12001-12007, 12011-12057, 13100-13133, 13151-13153, 36000, 36400-36410, 36420-36430, 36440, 36591-36592, 36600, 36640, 43752, 44950, 44970, 50715, 51701-51703, 52000, 56810, 57000, 57100, 57150, 57180, 57320, 57410, 57420, 57452, 57500, 57800, 58100, 62320-62327, 64400, 64405-64408, 64415-64435, 64445-64454, 64461-64463, 64479-64505, 64510-64530, 69990, 92012-92014, 93000-93010, 93040-93042, 93318, 93355, 94002, 94200, 94250, 94680-94690, 94770, 95812-95816, 95819, 95822, 95829, 95955, 96360-96368, 96372, 96374-96377, 96523, 97597-97598, 97602, 99155, 99156, 99157, 99211-99223, 99231-99255, 99291-99292, 99304-99310, 99315-99316, 99334-99337, 99347-99350, 99374-99375, 99377-99378, 99446-99449, 99451-99452, 99495-99496, G0463, G0471

57335 00940, 0213T, 0216T, 0228T, 0230T, 11000-11006, 11042-11047, 12001-12007, 12011-12057, 13100-13133, 13151-13153, 36000, 36400-36410, 36420-36430, 36440, 36591-36592, 36600, 36640, 43752, 44950, 44970, 50715, 51701-51703, 56810, 57100, 57150, 57180, 57410, 57420, 57452, 57500, 57800, 58100, 62320-62327, 64400, 64405-64408, 64415-64435, 64445-64454, 64461-64463, 64479-64505, 64510-64530, 69990, 92012-92014, 93000-93010, 93040-93042, 93318, 93355, 94002, 94200, 94250, 94680-94690, 94770, 95812-95816, 95819, 95822, 95829, 95955, 96360-96368, 96372, 96374-96377, 96523, 97597-97598, 97602, 99155, 99156, 99157, 99211-99223, 99231-99255, 99291-99292, 99304-99310, 99315-99316, 99334-99337, 99347-99350, 99374-99375, 99377-99378, 99446-99449, 99451-99452, 99495-99496, G0463, G0471

57400 00940, 0213T, 0216T, 0228T, 0230T, 12001-12007, 12011-12057, 13100-13133, 13151-13153, 36000, 36400-36410, 36420-36430, 36440, 36591-36592, 36600, 36640, 43752, 51701-51703, 57100, 57180, 57410-57421, 57452-57461, 57500, 57530, 57800, 58100, 62320-62327, 64400, 64405-64408, 64415-64435, 64445-64454, 64461-64463, 64479-64505, 64510-64530, 69990, 92012-92014, 93000-93010, 93040-93042, 93318, 93355, 94002, 94200, 94250, 94680-94690, 94770, 95812-95816, 95819, 95822, 95829, 95955, 96360-96368, 96372, 96374-96377, 96523, 99155, 99156, 99157, 99211-99223, 99231-99255, 99291-99292, 99304-99310, 99315-99316, 99334-99337, 99347-99350, 99374-99375, 99377-99378, 99446-99449, 99451-99452, 99495-99496, G0463, G0471

57410 00940, 0213T, 0216T, 0228T, 0230T, 12001-12007, 12011-12057, 13100-13133, 13151-13153, 36000, 36400-36410, 36420-36430, 36440, 36591-36592, 36600, 36640, 43752, 51701-51703, 57100, 57180, 57500, 57800, 58100, 62320-62327, 64400, 64405-64408, 64415-64435, 64445-64454, 64461-64463, 64479-64505, 64510-64530, 69990, 92012-92014, 93000-93010, 93040-93042, 93318, 93355, 94002, 94200, 94250, 94680-94690, 94770, 95812-95816, 95819, 95822, 95829, 95955, 96360-96368, 96372, 96374-96377, 96523, 99155, 99156, 99157, 99211-99223, 99231-99255, 99291-99292, 99304-99310, 99315-99316, 99334-99337, 99347-99350, 99374-99375, 99377-99378, 99446-99449, 99451-99452, 99495-99496, G0463, G0471

57415 00940, 0213T, 0216T, 0228T, 0230T, 11000-11006, 11042-11047, 12001-12007, 12011-12057, 13100-13133, 13151-13153, 36000, 36400-36410, 36420-36430, 36440, 36591-36592, 36600, 36640, 43752, 51701-51703, 57150, 57180, 57410, 57420, 57452, 57500, 57800, 58100, 62320-62327, 64400, 64405-64408, 64415-64435, 64445-64454, 64461-64463, 64479-64505, 64510-64530, 69990, 92012-92014, 93000-93010, 93040-93042, 93318, 93355, 94002, 94200, 94250, 94680-94690, 94770, 95812-95816, 95819, 95822, 95829, 95955, 96360-96368, 96372, 96374-96377, 96523, 97597-97598, 97602, 99155, 99156, 99157, 99211-99223, 99231-99255, 99291-99292, 99304-99310, 99315-99316, 99334-99337, 99347-99350, 99374-99375, 99377-99378, 99446-99449, 99451-99452, 99495-99496, G0463, G0471

57420 00940, 0213T, 0216T, 0228T, 0230T, 12001-12007, 12011-12057, 13100-13133, 13151-13153, 36000, 36400-36410, 36420-36430, 36440, 36591-36592, 36600, 36640, 43752, 51701-51703, 57061, 57100, 57180, 57410, 57452, 62320-62327, 64400, 64405-64408, 64415-64435, 64445-64454, 64461-64463, 64479-64505, 64510-64530, 69990, 76000, 77001-77002, 92012-92014, 93000-93010, 93040-93042, 93318, 93355, 94002, 94200, 94250, 94680-94690, 94770, 95812-95816, 95819, 95822, 95829, 95955, 96360-96368, 96372, 96374-96377, 96523, 99155, 99156, 99157, 99211-99223, 99231-99255, 99291-99292, 99304-99310, 99315-99316, 99334-99337, 99347-99350, 99374-99375, 99377-99378, 99446-99449, 99451-99452, 99495-99496, G0463, G0471

57421 00940, 0213T, 0216T, 0228T, 0230T, 10005, 10007, 10009, 10011, 10021, 12001-12007, 12011-12057, 13100-13133, 13151-13153, 36000, 36400-36410, 36420-36430, 36440, 36591-36592, 36600, 36640, 43752, 51701-51703, 57061, 57100, 57150, 57180, 57410, 57420, 57452, 57455-57456, 57500-57505, 57800, 58100, 62320-62327, 64400, 64405-64408, 64415-64435, 64445-64454, 64461-64463, 64479-64505, 64510-64530, 69990, 76000, 77001-77002, 92012-92014, 93000-93010,

93040-93042, 93318, 93355, 94002, 94200, 94250, 94680-94690, 94770, 95812-95816, 95819, 95822, 95829, 95955, 96360-96368, 96372, 96374-96377, 96523, 99155, 99156, 99157, 99211-99223, 99231-99255, 99291-99292, 99304-99310, 99315-99316, 99334-99337, 99347-99350, 99374-99375, 99377-99378, 99446-99449, 99451-99452, 99495-99496, G0463, G0471, J0670, J2001

57423 0213T, 0216T, 0228T, 0230T, 12001-12007, 12011-12057, 13100-13133, 13151-13153, 36000, 36400-36410, 36420-36430, 36440, 36591-36592, 36600, 36640, 43752, 44180, 44602-44605, 49082-49084, 49320, 49400, 51701-51703, 51840-51841, 51990, 52000, 57180, 57240, 57260-57265, 57410, 58660, 62320-62327, 64400, 64405-64408, 64415-64435, 64445-64454, 64461-64463, 64479-64505, 64510-64530, 69990, 76000, 77001-77002, 92012-92014, 93000-93010, 93040-93042, 93318, 93355, 94002, 94200, 94250, 94680-94690, 94770, 95812-95816, 95819, 95822, 95829, 95955, 96360-96368, 96372, 96374-96377, 96523, 99155, 99156, 99157, 99211-99223, 99231-99255, 99291-99292, 99304-99310, 99315-99316, 99334-99337, 99347-99350, 99374-99375, 99377-99378, 99446-99449, 99451-99452, 99495-99496, G0463, G0471

57425 0213T, 0216T, 0228T, 0230T, 12001-12007, 12011-12057, 13100-13133, 13151-13153, 36000, 36400-36410, 36420-36430, 36440, 36591-36592, 36600, 36640, 43752, 44180, 44602-44605, 44950, 44970, 49082-49084, 49320, 49400, 50715, 51701-51703, 52000, 57267-57268, 57282, 57410, 58660, 62320-62327, 64400, 64405-64408, 64415-64435, 64445-64454, 64461-64463, 64479-64505, 64510-64530, 69990, 76000, 77001-77002, 92012-92014, 93000-93010, 93040-93042, 93318, 93355, 94002, 94200, 94250, 94680-94690, 94770, 95812-95816, 95819, 95822, 95829, 95955, 96360-96368, 96372, 96374-96377, 96523, 99155, 99156, 99157, 99211-99223, 99231-99255, 99291-99292, 99304-99310, 99315-99316, 99334-99337, 99347-99350, 99374-99375, 99377-99378, 99446-99449, 99451-99452, 99495-99496, G0463, G0471

57426 0213T, 0216T, 0228T, 0230T, 11000-11006, 11042-11047, 12001-12007, 12011-12057, 13100-13133, 13151-13153, 36000, 36400-36410, 36420-36430, 36440, 36591-36592, 36600, 36640, 43752, 44005, 44180, 44602-44605, 49082-49084, 49320, 49400, 50715, 51701-51703, 52000, 57100, 57150, 57180, 57295, 57400-57415, 57500, 57800, 58100, 58660, 62320-62327, 64400, 64405-64408, 64415-64435, 64445-64454, 64461-64463, 64479-64505, 64510-64530, 69990, 92012-92014, 93000-93010, 93040-93042, 93318, 93355, 94002, 94200, 94250, 94680-94690, 94770, 95812-95816, 95819, 95822, 95829, 95955, 96360-96368, 96372, 96374-96377, 96523, 97597-97598, 97602, 99155, 99156, 99157, 99211-99223, 99231-99255, 99291-99292, 99304-99310, 99315-99316, 99334-99337, 99347-99350, 99374-99375, 99377-99378, 99446-99449, 99451-99452, 99495-99496, G0463, G0471

57452 00940, 0213T, 0216T, 0228T, 0230T, 12001-12007, 12011-12057, 13100-13133, 13151-13153, 36000, 36400-36410, 36420-36430, 36440, 36591-36592, 36600, 36640, 43752, 51701-51703, 57100, 57180, 57410, 62320-62327, 64400, 64405-64408, 64415-64435, 64445-64454, 64461-64463, 64479-64505, 64510-64530, 69990, 76000, 77001-77002, 92012-92014, 93000-93010, 93040-93042, 93318, 93355, 94002, 94200, 94250, 94680-94690, 94770, 95812-95816, 95819, 95822, 95829, 95955, 96360-96368, 96372, 96374-96377, 96523, 99155, 99156, 99157, 99211-99223, 99231-99255, 99291-99292, 99304-99310, 99315-99316, 99334-99337, 99347-99350, 99374-99375, 99377-99378, 99446-99449, 99451-99452, 99495-99496, G0463, G0471

57454 00940, 0213T, 0216T, 0228T, 0230T, 10005, 10007, 10009, 10011, 10021, 12001-12007, 12011-12057, 13100-13133, 13151-13153, 36000, 36400-36410, 36420-36430, 36440, 36591-36592, 36600, 36640, 43752, 51701-51703, 57100, 57180, 57410, 57420-57421, 57452, 57455-57456,

57500-57505, 57800, 58100, 62320-62327, 64400, 64405-64408, 64415-64435, 64445-64454, 64461-64463, 64479-64505, 64510-64530, 69990, 76000, 77001-77002, 92012-92014, 93000-93010, 93040-93042, 93318, 93355, 94002, 94200, 94250, 94680-94690, 94770, 95812-95816, 95819, 95822, 95829, 95955, 96360-96368, 96372, 96374-96377, 96523, 99155, 99156, 99157, 99211-99223, 99231-99255, 99291-99292, 99304-99310, 99315-99316, 99334-99337, 99347-99350, 99374-99375, 99377-99378, 99446-99449, 99451-99452, 99495-99496, G0463, G0471

57455 00940, 0213T, 0216T, 0228T, 0230T, 10005, 10007, 10009, 10011, 10021, 12001-12007, 12011-12057, 13100-13133, 13151-13153, 36000, 36400-36410, 36420-36430, 36440, 36591-36592, 36600, 36640, 43752, 51701-51703, 57100, 57180, 57410, 57420, 57452, 57500-57505, 57800, 58100, 62320-62327, 64400, 64405-64408, 64415-64435, 64445-64454, 64461-64463, 64479-64505, 64510-64530, 69990, 76000, 77001-77002, 92012-92014, 93000-93010, 93040-93042, 93318, 93355, 94002, 94200, 94250, 94680-94690, 94770, 95812-95816, 95819, 95822, 95829, 95955, 96360-96368, 96372, 96374-96377, 96523, 99155, 99156, 99157, 99211-99223, 99231-99255, 99291-99292, 99304-99310, 99315-99316, 99334-99337, 99347-99350, 99374-99375, 99377-99378, 99446-99449, 99451-99452, 99495-99496, G0463, G0471

57456 00940, 0213T, 0216T, 0228T, 0230T, 12001-12007, 12011-12057, 13100-13133, 13151-13153, 36000, 36400-36410, 36420-36430, 36440, 36591-36592, 36600, 36640, 43752, 51701-51703, 57100, 57180, 57410, 57420, 57452, 57500-57505, 57800, 58100, 62320-62327, 64400, 64405-64408, 64415-64435, 64445-64454, 64461-64463, 64479-64505, 64510-64530, 69990, 76000, 77001-77002, 92012-92014, 93000-93010, 93040-93042, 93318, 93355, 94002, 94200, 94250, 94680-94690, 94770, 95812-95816, 95819, 95822, 95829, 95955, 96360-96368, 96372, 96374-96377, 96523, 99155, 99156, 99157, 99211-99223, 99231-99255, 99291-99292, 99304-99310, 99315-99316, 99334-99337, 99347-99350, 99374-99375, 99377-99378, 99446-99449, 99451-99452, 99495-99496, G0463, G0471

57460 00940, 0213T, 0216T, 0228T, 0230T, 10005, 10007, 10009, 10011, 10021, 12001-12007, 12011-12057, 13100-13133, 13151-13153, 36000, 36400-36410, 36420-36430, 36440, 36591-36592, 36600, 36640, 43752, 51701-51703, 57100, 57180, 57410, 57420-57421, 57452-57455, 57500, 57800, 58100, 62320-62327, 64400, 64405-64408, 64415-64435, 64445-64454, 64461-64463, 64479-64505, 64510-64530, 69990, 76000, 77001-77002, 92012-92014, 93000-93010, 93040-93042, 93318, 93355, 94002, 94200, 94250, 94680-94690, 94770, 95812-95816, 95819, 95822, 95829, 95955, 96360-96368, 96372, 96374-96377, 96523, 99155, 99156, 99157, 99211-99223, 99231-99255, 99291-99292, 99304-99310, 99315-99316, 99334-99337, 99347-99350, 99374-99375, 99377-99378, 99446-99449, 99451-99452, 99495-99496, G0463, G0471, J0670, J2001

57461 00940, 0213T, 0216T, 0228T, 0230T, 12001-12007, 12011-12057, 13100-13133, 13151-13153, 36000, 36400-36410, 36420-36430, 36440, 36591-36592, 36600, 36640, 43752, 51701-51703, 57100, 57180, 57410, 57420-57421, 57452-57460, 57500, 57800, 58100, 62320-62327, 64400, 64405-64408, 64415-64435, 64445-64454, 64461-64463, 64479-64505, 64510-64530, 69990, 76000, 77001-77002, 92012-92014, 93000-93010, 93040-93042, 93318, 93355, 94002, 94200, 94250, 94680-94690, 94770, 95812-95816, 95819, 95822, 95829, 95955, 96360-96368, 96372, 96374-96377, 96523, 99155, 99156, 99157, 99211-99223, 99231-99255, 99291-99292, 99304-99310, 99315-99316, 99334-99337, 99347-99350, 99374-99375, 99377-99378, 99446-99449, 99451-99452, 99495-99496, G0463, G0471, J0670, J2001

57465 No CCI edits apply to this code.

57500 0213T, 0216T, 0228T, 0230T, 10005, 10007, 10009, 10011, 10021, 11000-11006, 11042-11047, 12001-12007, 12011-12057, 13100-13133, 13151-13153, 36000, 36400-36410, 36420-36430, 36440, 36591-36592, 36600, 36640, 43752, 51701-51703, 57100, 57180, 57420, 57452, 62320-62327, 64400, 64405-64408, 64415-64435, 64445-64454, 64461-64463, 64479-64505, 64510-64530, 69990, 92012-92014, 93000-93010, 93040-93042, 93318, 93355, 94002, 94200, 94250, 94680-94690, 94770, 95812-95816, 95819, 95822, 95829, 95955, 96360-96368, 96372, 96374-96377, 96523, 97597-97598, 97602, 99155, 99156, 99157, 99211-99223, 99231-99255, 99291-99292, 99304-99310, 99315-99316, 99334-99337, 99347-99350, 99374-99375, 99377-99378, 99446-99449, 99451-99452, 99495-99496, G0463, G0471, J0670, J2001

57505 0213T, 0216T, 0228T, 0230T, 12001-12007, 12011-12057, 13100-13133, 13151-13153, 36000, 36400-36410, 36420-36430, 36440, 36591-36592, 36600, 36640, 43752, 51701-51703, 57100, 57180, 57410, 57420, 57452, 57520✤, 57530, 57800, 58100, 58120✤, 62320-62327, 64400, 64405-64408, 64415-64435, 64445-64454, 64461-64463, 64479-64505, 64510-64530, 69990, 92012-92014, 93000-93010, 93040-93042, 93318, 93355, 94002, 94200, 94250, 94680-94690, 94770, 95812-95816, 95819, 95822, 95829, 95955, 96360-96368, 96372, 96374-96377, 96523, 99155, 99156, 99157, 99211-99223, 99231-99255, 99291-99292, 99304-99310, 99315-99316, 99334-99337, 99347-99350, 99374-99375, 99377-99378, 99446-99449, 99451-99452, 99495-99496, G0463, G0471, J0670, J2001

57510 0213T, 0216T, 0228T, 0230T, 12001-12007, 12011-12057, 13100-13133, 13151-13153, 36000, 36400-36410, 36420-36430, 36440, 36591-36592, 36600, 36640, 43752, 51701-51703, 57100, 57180, 57410, 57420, 57452, 57500, 57530, 57800, 58100, 62320-62327, 64400, 64405-64408, 64415-64435, 64445-64454, 64461-64463, 64479-64505, 64510-64530, 69990, 92012-92014, 93000-93010, 93040-93042, 93318, 93355, 94002, 94200, 94250, 94680-94690, 94770, 95812-95816, 95819, 95822, 95829, 95955, 96360-96368, 96372, 96374-96377, 96523, 99155, 99156, 99157, 99211-99223, 99231-99255, 99291-99292, 99304-99310, 99315-99316, 99334-99337, 99347-99350, 99374-99375, 99377-99378, 99446-99449, 99451-99452, 99495-99496, G0463, G0471, J0670, J2001

57511 0213T, 0216T, 0228T, 0230T, 12001-12007, 12011-12057, 13100-13133, 13151-13153, 36000, 36400-36410, 36420-36430, 36440, 36591-36592, 36600, 36640, 43752, 51701-51703, 57100, 57180, 57410, 57420, 57452, 57500, 57510✤, 57522-57530, 57800, 58100, 62320-62327, 64400, 64405-64408, 64415-64435, 64445-64454, 64461-64463, 64479-64505, 64510-64530, 69990, 92012-92014, 93000-93010, 93040-93042, 93318, 93355, 94002, 94200, 94250, 94680-94690, 94770, 95812-95816, 95819, 95822, 95829, 95955, 96360-96368, 96372, 96374-96377, 96523, 99155, 99156, 99157, 99211-99223, 99231-99255, 99291-99292, 99304-99310, 99315-99316, 99334-99337, 99347-99350, 99374-99375, 99377-99378, 99446-99449, 99451-99452, 99495-99496, G0463, G0471, J0670, J2001

57513 0213T, 0216T, 0228T, 0230T, 12001-12007, 12011-12057, 13100-13133, 13151-13153, 36000, 36400-36410, 36420-36430, 36440, 36591-36592, 36600, 36640, 43752, 51701-51703, 57100, 57180, 57410, 57420, 57452, 57500, 57510-57511✤, 57522-57530, 57800, 58100, 62320-62327, 64400, 64405-64408, 64415-64435, 64445-64454, 64461-64463, 64479-64505, 64510-64530, 69990, 92012-92014, 93000-93010, 93040-93042, 93318, 93355, 94002, 94200, 94250, 94680-94690, 94770, 95812-95816, 95819, 95822, 95829, 95955, 96360-96368, 96372, 96374-96377, 96523, 99155, 99156, 99157, 99211-99223, 99231-99255, 99291-99292, 99304-99310, 99315-99316, 99334-99337, 99347-99350, 99374-99375, 99377-99378, 99446-99449, 99451-99452, 99495-99496, G0463, G0471, J0670, J2001

57520 0213T, 0216T, 0228T, 0230T, 12001-12007, 12011-12057, 13100-13133, 13151-13153, 36000, 36400-36410, 36420-36430, 36440, 36591-36592, 36600, 36640, 43752, 51701-51703, 57100, 57180, 57410, 57420, 57452-57455, 57460-57461, 57500, 57510-57513, 57522-57530, 57720-57800, 58100, 58120, 62320-62327, 64400, 64405-64408, 64415-64435, 64445-64454, 64461-64463, 64479-64505, 64510-64530, 69990, 92012-92014, 93000-93010, 93040-93042, 93318, 93355, 94002, 94200, 94250, 94680-94690, 94770, 95812-95816, 95819, 95822, 95829, 95955, 96360-96368, 96372, 96374-96377, 96523, 99155, 99156, 99157, 99211-99223, 99231-99255, 99291-99292, 99304-99310, 99315-99316, 99334-99337, 99347-99350, 99374-99375, 99377-99378, 99446-99449, 99451-99452, 99495-99496, G0463, G0471, J0670, J2001, P9612

57522 0213T, 0216T, 0228T, 0230T, 11000-11006, 11042-11047, 12001-12007, 12011-12057, 13100-13133, 13151-13153, 36000, 36400-36410, 36420-36430, 36440, 36591-36592, 36600, 36640, 43752, 51701-51703, 57100, 57180, 57410, 57420-57421, 57452-57455, 57460-57461, 57500, 57510✤, 57530, 57800, 58100, 58120, 62320-62327, 64400, 64405-64408, 64415-64435, 64445-64454, 64461-64463, 64479-64505, 64510-64530, 69990, 92012-92014, 93000-93010, 93040-93042, 93318, 93355, 94002, 94200, 94250, 94680-94690, 94770, 95812-95816, 95819, 95822, 95829, 95955, 96360-96368, 96372, 96374-96377, 96523, 97597-97598, 97602, 99155, 99156, 99157, 99211-99223, 99231-99255, 99291-99292, 99304-99310, 99315-99316, 99334-99337, 99347-99350, 99374-99375, 99377-99378, 99446-99449, 99451-99452, 99495-99496, G0463, G0471, J0670, J2001, P9612

57530 0213T, 0216T, 0228T, 0230T, 11000-11006, 11042-11047, 12001-12007, 12011-12057, 13100-13133, 13151-13153, 36000, 36400-36410, 36420-36430, 36440, 36591-36592, 36600, 36640, 43752, 44950, 44970, 50715, 51701-51703, 52000, 57100, 57160-57180, 57410, 57420-57421, 57452-57461, 57500, 58100, 62320-62327, 64400, 64405-64408, 64415-64435, 64445-64454, 64461-64463, 64479-64505, 64510-64530, 69990, 92012-92014, 93000-93010, 93040-93042, 93318, 93355, 94002, 94200, 94250, 94680-94690, 94770, 95812-95816, 95819, 95822, 95829, 95955, 96360-96368, 96372, 96374-96377, 96523, 97597-97598, 97602, 99155, 99156, 99157, 99211-99223, 99231-99255, 99291-99292, 99304-99310, 99315-99316, 99334-99337, 99347-99350, 99374-99375, 99377-99378, 99446-99449, 99451-99452, 99495-99496, G0463, G0471, P9612

57531 0213T, 0216T, 0228T, 0230T, 10005, 10007, 10009, 10011, 10021, 11000-11006, 11042-11047, 12001-12007, 12011-12057, 13100-13133, 13151-13153, 36000, 36400-36410, 36420-36430, 36440, 36591-36592, 36600, 36640, 38562-38573, 38765, 38770, 38780, 43752, 44950, 44970, 49000-49010, 50715, 51701-51703, 52000, 57000, 57410, 57420-57421, 57452, 57530, 58150, 58700-58720, 58940, 58960, 62320-62327, 64400, 64405-64408, 64415-64435, 64445-64454, 64461-64463, 64479-64505, 64510-64530, 69990, 92012-92014, 93000-93010, 93040-93042, 93318, 93355, 94002, 94200, 94250, 94680-94690, 94770, 95812-95816, 95819, 95822, 95829, 95955, 96360-96368, 96372, 96374-96377, 96523, 97597-97598, 97602, 99155, 99156, 99157, 99211-99223, 99231-99255, 99291-99292, 99304-99310, 99315-99316, 99334-99337, 99347-99350, 99374-99375, 99377-99378, 99446-99449, 99451-99452, 99495-99496, G0463, G0471

57540 0213T, 0216T, 0228T, 0230T, 11000-11006, 11042-11047, 12001-12007, 12011-12057, 13100-13133, 13151-13153, 36000, 36400-36410, 36420-36430, 36440, 36591-36592, 36600, 36640, 43752, 44005, 44180, 44602-44605, 44850, 44950, 44970, 49000-49010, 49255, 49320, 49570, 50715, 51701-51703, 52000, 57100, 57180, 57410, 57420-57421, 57452-57455, 57460, 57500, 57522-57530, 57800, 58100✤, 62320-62327, 64400, 64405-64408, 64415-64435,

Coding Companion for Ob/Gyn

64445-64454, 64461-64463, 64479-64505, 64510-64530, 69990, 92012-92014, 93000-93010, 93040-93042, 93318, 93355, 94002, 94200, 94250, 94680-94690, 94770, 95812-95816, 95819, 95822, 95829, 95955, 96360-96368, 96372, 96374-96377, 96523, 97597-97598, 97602, 99155, 99156, 99157, 99211-99223, 99231-99255, 99291-99292, 99304-99310, 99315-99316, 99334-99337, 99347-99350, 99374-99375, 99377-99378, 99446-99449, 99451-99452, 99495-99496, G0463, G0471, P9612

57545 0213T, 0216T, 0228T, 0230T, 11000-11006, 11042-11047, 12001-12007, 12011-12057, 13100-13133, 13151-13153, 36000, 36400-36410, 36420-36430, 36440, 36591-36592, 36600, 36640, 43752, 44005, 44180, 44602-44605, 44850, 44950, 44970, 49000-49010, 49255, 49320, 49570, 50715, 51701-51703, 52000, 57100, 57180-57200, 57260, 57280, 57284, 57410, 57420-57421, 57452-57455, 57460, 57500, 57522-57530, 57540, 57800, 58100❖, 62320-62327, 64400, 64405-64408, 64415-64435, 64445-64454, 64461-64463, 64479-64505, 64510-64530, 69990, 92012-92014, 93000-93010, 93040-93042, 93318, 93355, 94002, 94200, 94250, 94680-94690, 94770, 95812-95816, 95819, 95822, 95829, 95955, 96360-96368, 96372, 96374-96377, 96523, 97597-97598, 97602, 99155, 99156, 99157, 99211-99223, 99231-99255, 99291-99292, 99304-99310, 99315-99316, 99334-99337, 99347-99350, 99374-99375, 99377-99378, 99446-99449, 99451-99452, 99495-99496, G0463, G0471, P9612

57550 0213T, 0216T, 0228T, 0230T, 11000-11006, 11042-11047, 12001-12007, 12011-12057, 13100-13133, 13151-13153, 36000, 36400-36410, 36420-36430, 36440, 36591-36592, 36600, 36640, 43752, 50715, 51701-51703, 52000, 57000, 57100-57105, 57150, 57180-57210, 57410, 57420-57421, 57452-57455, 57460, 57500, 57522-57530, 57545❖, 57800, 58100❖, 62320-62327, 64400, 64405-64408, 64415-64435, 64445-64454, 64461-64463, 64479-64505, 64510-64530, 69990, 92012-92014, 93000-93010, 93040-93042, 93318, 93355, 94002, 94200, 94250, 94680-94690, 94770, 95812-95816, 95819, 95822, 95829, 95955, 96360-96368, 96372, 96374-96377, 96523, 97597-97598, 97602, 99155, 99156, 99157, 99211-99223, 99231-99255, 99291-99292, 99304-99310, 99315-99316, 99334-99337, 99347-99350, 99374-99375, 99377-99378, 99446-99449, 99451-99452, 99495-99496, G0463, G0471, P9612

57555 0213T, 0216T, 0228T, 0230T, 11000-11006, 11042-11047, 12001-12007, 12011-12057, 13100-13133, 13151-13153, 36000, 36400-36410, 36420-36430, 36440, 36591-36592, 36600, 36640, 43752, 50715, 51701-51703, 52000, 57000, 57100-57106, 57180-57200, 57240-57260, 57400-57410, 57420-57421, 57452-57455, 57460, 57500, 57522-57530, 57550, 57556, 57800, 58100❖, 62320-62327, 64400, 64405-64408, 64415-64435, 64445-64454, 64461-64463, 64479-64505, 64510-64530, 69990, 92012-92014, 93000-93010, 93040-93042, 93318, 93355, 94002, 94200, 94250, 94680-94690, 94770, 95812-95816, 95819, 95822, 95829, 95955, 96360-96368, 96372, 96374-96377, 96523, 97597-97598, 97602, 99155, 99156, 99157, 99211-99223, 99231-99255, 99291-99292, 99304-99310, 99315-99316, 99334-99337, 99347-99350, 99374-99375, 99377-99378, 99446-99449, 99451-99452, 99495-99496, G0463, G0471, P9612

57556 0213T, 0216T, 0228T, 0230T, 11000-11006, 11042-11047, 12001-12007, 12011-12057, 13100-13133, 13151-13153, 36000, 36400-36410, 36420-36430, 36440, 36591-36592, 36600, 36640, 43752, 50715, 51701-51703, 52000, 57000, 57100, 57180-57200, 57260-57265, 57268, 57283, 57400-57410, 57420-57421, 57452-57455, 57460, 57500, 57522-57530, 57550, 57800, 58100❖, 62320-62327, 64400, 64405-64408, 64415-64435, 64445-64454, 64461-64463, 64479-64505, 64510-64530, 69990, 92012-92014, 93000-93010, 93040-93042, 93318, 93355, 94002, 94200, 94250, 94680-94690, 94770, 95812-95816,

95819, 95822, 95829, 95955, 96360-96368, 96372, 96374-96377, 96523, 97597-97598, 97602, 99155, 99156, 99157, 99211-99223, 99231-99255, 99291-99292, 99304-99310, 99315-99316, 99334-99337, 99347-99350, 99374-99375, 99377-99378, 99446-99449, 99451-99452, 99495-99496, G0463, G0471, P9612

57558 0213T, 0216T, 0228T, 0230T, 12001-12007, 12011-12057, 13100-13133, 13151-13153, 36000, 36400-36410, 36420-36430, 36440, 36591-36592, 36600, 36640, 43752, 51701-51703, 57100, 57180, 57400-57410, 57420, 57452, 57500, 57530, 57800, 58100, 62320-62327, 64400, 64405-64408, 64415-64435, 64445-64454, 64461-64463, 64479-64505, 64510-64530, 69990, 92012-92014, 93000-93010, 93040-93042, 93318, 93355, 94002, 94200, 94250, 94680-94690, 94770, 95812-95816, 95819, 95822, 95829, 95955, 96360-96368, 96372, 96374-96377, 96523, 99155, 99156, 99157, 99211-99223, 99231-99255, 99291-99292, 99304-99310, 99315-99316, 99334-99337, 99347-99350, 99374-99375, 99377-99378, 99446-99449, 99451-99452, 99495-99496, G0463, G0471, J2001

57700 0213T, 0216T, 0228T, 0230T, 12001-12007, 12011-12057, 13100-13133, 13151-13153, 36000, 36400-36410, 36420-36430, 36440, 36591-36592, 36600, 36640, 43752, 51701-51703, 57100, 57180, 57400-57410, 57420, 57452, 57500, 57530, 57800, 58100, 62320-62327, 64400, 64405-64408, 64415-64435, 64445-64454, 64461-64463, 64479-64505, 64510-64530, 69990, 92012-92014, 93000-93010, 93040-93042, 93318, 93355, 94002, 94200, 94250, 94680-94690, 94770, 95812-95816, 95819, 95822, 95829, 95955, 96360-96368, 96372, 96374-96377, 96523, 99155, 99156, 99157, 99211-99223, 99231-99255, 99291-99292, 99304-99310, 99315-99316, 99334-99337, 99347-99350, 99374-99375, 99377-99378, 99446-99449, 99451-99452, 99495-99496, G0463, G0471, P9612

57720 0213T, 0216T, 0228T, 0230T, 12001-12007, 12011-12057, 13100-13133, 13151-13153, 36000, 36400-36410, 36420-36430, 36440, 36591-36592, 36600, 36640, 43752, 51701-51703, 52000, 57000, 57100-57105, 57150, 57180, 57210, 57400-57410, 57420, 57452, 57500, 57530, 57800, 58100, 62320-62327, 64400, 64405-64408, 64415-64435, 64445-64454, 64461-64463, 64479-64505, 64510-64530, 69990, 92012-92014, 93000-93010, 93040-93042, 93318, 93355, 94002, 94200, 94250, 94680-94690, 94770, 95812-95816, 95819, 95822, 95829, 95955, 96360-96368, 96372, 96374-96377, 96523, 99155, 99156, 99157, 99211-99223, 99231-99255, 99291-99292, 99304-99310, 99315-99316, 99334-99337, 99347-99350, 99374-99375, 99377-99378, 99446-99449, 99451-99452, 99495-99496, G0463, G0471, J2001, P9612

57800 0213T, 0216T, 0228T, 0230T, 12001-12007, 12011-12057, 13100-13133, 13151-13153, 36000, 36400-36410, 36420-36430, 36440, 36591-36592, 36600, 36640, 43752, 51701-51703, 57100, 57420, 57452, 57500, 57530, 62320-62327, 64400, 64405-64408, 64415-64435, 64445-64454, 64461-64463, 64479-64505, 64510-64530, 69990, 92012-92014, 93000-93010, 93040-93042, 93318, 93355, 94002, 94200, 94250, 94680-94690, 94770, 95812-95816, 95819, 95822, 95829, 95955, 96360-96368, 96372, 96374-96377, 96523, 99155, 99156, 99157, 99211-99223, 99231-99255, 99291-99292, 99304-99310, 99315-99316, 99334-99337, 99347-99350, 99374-99375, 99377-99378, 99446-99449, 99451-99452, 99495-99496, G0463, G0471, J2001

58100 0213T, 0216T, 0228T, 0230T, 10005, 10007, 10009, 10011, 10021, 12001-12007, 12011-12057, 13100-13133, 13151-13153, 36000, 36400-36410, 36420-36430, 36440, 36591-36592, 36600, 36640, 43752, 51701-51703, 57100, 57180, 57452, 57500, 57800, 62320-62327, 64400, 64405-64408, 64415-64435, 64445-64454, 64461-64463, 64479-64505, 64510-64530, 69990, 92012-92014, 93000-93010, 93040-93042, 93318, 93355, 94002, 94200, 94250, 94680-94690,

94770, 95812-95816, 95819, 95822, 95829, 95955, 96360-96368, 96372, 96374-96377, 96523, 99155, 99156, 99157, 99211-99223, 99231-99255, 99291-99292, 99304-99310, 99315-99316, 99334-99337, 99347-99350, 99374-99375, 99377-99378, 99446-99449, 99451-99452, 99495-99496, G0463, G0471

58110 0213T, 0216T, 10005, 10007, 10009, 10011, 10021, 36000, 36410, 36591-36592, 43752, 61650, 62324-62327, 64415-64417, 64450, 64454, 64486-64490, 64493, 69990, 96360, 96365, 96372, 96374-96377, 96523

58120 0213T, 0216T, 0228T, 0230T, 12001-12007, 12011-12057, 13100-13133, 13151-13153, 36000, 36400-36410, 36420-36430, 36440, 36591-36592, 36600, 36640, 43752, 51701-51703, 57100, 57180, 57400-57410, 57452, 57500, 57530, 57800, 58100, 62320-62327, 64400, 64405-64408, 64415-64435, 64445-64454, 64461-64463, 64479-64505, 64510-64530, 69990, 92012-92014, 93000-93010, 93040-93042, 93318, 93355, 94002, 94200, 94250, 94680-94690, 94770, 95812-95816, 95819, 95822, 95829, 95955, 96360-96368, 96372, 96374-96377, 96523, 99155, 99156, 99157, 99211-99223, 99231-99255, 99291-99292, 99304-99310, 99315-99316, 99334-99337, 99347-99350, 99374-99375, 99377-99378, 99446-99449, 99451-99452, 99495-99496, G0463, G0471, J0670, J2001, P9612

58140 0071T, 0072T, 0213T, 0216T, 0228T, 0230T, 0404T✤, 11000-11006, 11042-11047, 12001-12007, 12011-12057, 13100-13133, 13151-13153, 36000, 36400-36410, 36420-36430, 36440, 36591-36592, 36600, 36640, 43752, 44005, 44180, 44602-44605, 44850, 44950, 44970, 49000-49010, 49255, 49320-49321, 49570, 50715, 51701-51703, 57410, 58100, 58545-58546, 58550, 58561, 58605, 58662, 58674✤, 58700, 58740, 58900, 62320-62327, 64400, 64405-64408, 64415-64435, 64445-64454, 64461-64463, 64479-64505, 64510-64530, 69990, 92012-92014, 93000-93010, 93040-93042, 93318, 93355, 94002, 94200, 94250, 94680-94690, 94770, 95812-95816, 95819, 95822, 95829, 95955, 96360-96368, 96372, 96374-96377, 96523, 97597-97598, 97602, 99155, 99156, 99157, 99211-99223, 99231-99255, 99291-99292, 99304-99310, 99315-99316, 99334-99337, 99347-99350, 99374-99375, 99377-99378, 99446-99449, 99451-99452, 99495-99496, G0463, G0471

58145 0071T, 0072T, 0213T, 0216T, 0228T, 0230T, 0404T✤, 11000-11006, 11042-11047, 12001-12007, 12011-12057, 13100-13133, 13151-13153, 36000, 36400-36410, 36420-36430, 36440, 36591-36592, 36600, 36640, 43752, 50715, 51701-51703, 57210, 57410, 57420, 57452, 57500, 57800, 58100, 58120-58140, 58545-58546, 58561✤, 58605, 58662, 58700, 58900, 62320-62327, 64400, 64405-64408, 64415-64435, 64445-64454, 64461-64463, 64479-64505, 64510-64530, 69990, 92012-92014, 93000-93010, 93040-93042, 93318, 93355, 94002, 94200, 94250, 94680-94690, 94770, 95812-95816, 95819, 95822, 95829, 95955, 96360-96368, 96372, 96374-96377, 96523, 97597-97598, 97602, 99155, 99156, 99157, 99211-99223, 99231-99255, 99291-99292, 99304-99310, 99315-99316, 99334-99337, 99347-99350, 99374-99375, 99377-99378, 99446-99449, 99451-99452, 99495-99496, G0463, G0471, P9612

58146 0071T, 0072T, 0213T, 0216T, 0228T, 0230T, 0404T✤, 11000-11006, 11042-11047, 12001-12007, 12011-12057, 13100-13133, 13151-13153, 36000, 36400-36410, 36420-36430, 36440, 36591-36592, 36600, 36640, 43752, 44005, 44180, 44602-44605, 44850, 44950, 44970, 49000-49010, 49255, 49320-49321, 49570, 50715, 57410, 58100, 58140-58145, 58550, 58552-58553, 58561, 58570-58572, 58605, 58662, 58674✤, 58700, 58740, 58900, 62320-62327, 64400, 64405-64408, 64415-64435, 64445-64454, 64461-64463, 64479-64505, 64510-64530, 69990, 92012-92014, 93000-93010, 93040-93042, 93318, 93355, 94002, 94200, 94250, 94680-94690, 94770, 95812-95816, 95819, 95822, 95829, 95955, 96360-96368, 96372, 96374-96377, 96523, 97597-97598,

97602, 99155, 99156, 99157, 99211-99223, 99231-99255, 99291-99292, 99304-99310, 99315-99316, 99334-99337, 99347-99350, 99374-99375, 99377-99378, 99446-99449, 99451-99452, 99495-99496, G0463

58150 0071T, 0072T, 01962-01963, 01969, 0213T, 0216T, 0228T, 0230T, 11000-11006, 11042-11047, 12001-12007, 12011-12057, 13100-13133, 13151-13153, 36000, 36400-36410, 36420-36430, 36440, 36591-36592, 36600, 36640, 43752, 44005, 44180, 44602-44605, 44850, 44950, 44970, 49000-49010, 49082-49084, 49180, 49255, 49320-49322, 49406, 49560-49566, 49570, 50715, 51701-51703, 51840, 52000, 57410, 57454-57455, 57460, 57505, 57522-57530, 57540-57555✤, 57558, 58100, 58110-58146, 58180, 58353-58356, 58541-58543, 58545-58546, 58550, 58552-58554, 58558, 58561, 58570, 58575, 58660-58674✤, 58700-58740, 58805, 58822, 58900-58940, 62320-62327, 64400, 64405-64408, 64415-64435, 64445-64454, 64461-64463, 64479-64505, 64510-64530, 69990, 92012-92014, 93000-93010, 93040-93042, 93318, 93355, 94002, 94200, 94250, 94680-94690, 94770, 95812-95816, 95819, 95822, 95829, 95955, 96360-96368, 96372, 96374-96377, 96523, 97597-97598, 97602, 99155, 99156, 99157, 99211-99223, 99231-99255, 99291-99292, 99304-99310, 99315-99316, 99334-99337, 99347-99350, 99374-99375, 99377-99378, 99446-99449, 99451-99452, 99495-99496, G0463, G0471, P9612

58152 0071T, 0072T, 01962-01963, 01969, 0213T, 0216T, 0228T, 0230T, 11000-11006, 11042-11047, 12001-12007, 12011-12057, 13100-13133, 13151-13153, 36000, 36400-36410, 36420-36430, 36440, 36591-36592, 36600, 36640, 38573, 43752, 44005, 44180, 44602-44605, 44850, 44950, 44970, 49000-49010, 49082-49084, 49255, 49320-49322, 49406, 49560-49566, 49570, 50715, 51701-51703, 51840-51841, 52000, 57284, 57410, 57423, 57454-57455, 57460, 57500-57505, 57522-57530, 57540-57555✤, 57558, 58100, 58110-58150, 58180, 58353-58356, 58541-58546, 58550, 58552-58554, 58558, 58561, 58570-58572✤, 58660, 58662, 58674✤, 58700-58740, 58805, 58900, 58925-58940, 62320-62327, 64400, 64405-64408, 64415-64435, 64445-64454, 64461-64463, 64479-64505, 64510-64530, 69990, 92012-92014, 93000-93010, 93040-93042, 93318, 93355, 94002, 94200, 94250, 94680-94690, 94770, 95812-95816, 95819, 95822, 95829, 95955, 96360-96368, 96372, 96374-96377, 96523, 97597-97598, 97602, 99155, 99156, 99157, 99211-99223, 99231-99255, 99291-99292, 99304-99310, 99315-99316, 99334-99337, 99347-99350, 99374-99375, 99377-99378, 99446-99449, 99451-99452, 99495-99496, G0463, G0471, P9612

58180 0071T, 0072T, 01962-01963, 01969, 0213T, 0216T, 0228T, 0230T, 11000-11006, 11042-11047, 12001-12007, 12011-12057, 13100-13133, 13151-13153, 36000, 36400-36410, 36420-36430, 36440, 36591-36592, 36600, 36640, 43752, 44005, 44180, 44602-44605, 44850, 44950, 44970, 49000-49010, 49082-49084, 49255, 49320-49322, 49406, 49560-49566, 49570, 50715, 51701-51703, 52000, 57410, 57505, 57522-57530, 57540-57555✤, 57558, 58100, 58110-58146, 58353-58356, 58541✤, 58545-58546, 58550, 58552-58554, 58558, 58561, 58570✤, 58575, 58660-58674✤, 58700-58740, 58805, 58900-58940, 62320-62327, 64400, 64405-64408, 64415-64435, 64445-64454, 64461-64463, 64479-64505, 64510-64530, 69990, 92012-92014, 93000-93010, 93040-93042, 93318, 93355, 94002, 94200, 94250, 94680-94690, 94770, 95812-95816, 95819, 95822, 95829, 95955, 96360-96368, 96372, 96374-96377, 96523, 97597-97598, 97602, 99155, 99156, 99157, 99211-99223, 99231-99255, 99291-99292, 99304-99310, 99315-99316, 99334-99337, 99347-99350, 99374-99375, 99377-99378, 99446-99449, 99451-99452, 99495-99496, G0463, G0471, P9612

58200 0071T, 0072T, 01962-01963, 01969, 0213T, 0216T, 0228T, 0230T, 11000-11006, 11042-11047, 12001-12007, 12011-12057, 13100-13133, 13151-13153, 36000, 36400-36410, 36420-36430, 36440, 36591-36592,

36600, 36640, 38562, 38573, 43752, 44005, 44180, 44602-44605, 44820-44850, 44950, 44970, 49000-49010, 49082-49084, 49203, 49255, 49320-49322, 49406, 49560-49566, 49570, 50715, 51701-51703, 51840, 52000, 57105-57107, 57109-57112, 57410, 57454-57455, 57460, 57505, 57522-57530, 57540-57555✦, 57558, 58100, 58110-58180, 58260-58263, 58267-58280, 58290-58294, 58353-58356, 58541-58546, 58550, 58552-58554, 58558, 58561, 58570-58575, 58660-58674✦, 58700-58740, 58805, 58822, 58900-58940, 58943, 62320-62327, 64400, 64405-64408, 64415-64435, 64445-64454, 64461-64463, 64479-64505, 64510-64530, 69990, 92012-92014, 93000-93010, 93040-93042, 93318, 93355, 94002, 94200, 94250, 94680-94690, 94770, 95812-95816, 95819, 95822, 95829, 95955, 96360-96368, 96372, 96374-96377, 96523, 97597-97598, 97602, 99155, 99156, 99157, 99211-99223, 99231-99255, 99291-99292, 99304-99310, 99315-99316, 99334-99337, 99347-99350, 99374-99375, 99377-99378, 99446-99449, 99451-99452, 99495-99496, G0463, G0471, P9612

58210 0071T, 0072T, 01962-01963, 01969, 0213T, 0216T, 0228T, 0230T, 10005, 10007, 10009, 10011, 10021, 11000-11006, 11042-11047, 12001-12007, 12011-12057, 13100-13133, 13151-13153, 36000, 36400-36410, 36420-36430, 36440, 36591-36592, 36600, 36640, 38562, 38570-38573, 38770, 38780, 43752, 44005, 44180, 44602-44605, 44820-44850, 44950, 44970, 49000-49010, 49082-49084, 49180, 49203-49205, 49255, 49320-49322, 49406, 49560-49566, 49570, 50715, 51040, 51701-51703, 52000, 57106-57107, 57109-57112, 57410, 57454-57455, 57460, 57505, 57522-57555✦, 57558, 58100, 58110-58150, 58353-58356, 58541-58550, 58552-58554, 58558, 58561, 58570-58575, 58660-58674✦, 58700-58740, 58805, 58822, 58900-58940, 58943, 62320-62327, 64400, 64405-64408, 64415-64435, 64445-64454, 64461-64463, 64479-64505, 64510-64530, 69990, 92012-92014, 93000-93010, 93040-93042, 93318, 93355, 94002, 94200, 94250, 94680-94690, 94770, 95812-95816, 95819, 95822, 95829, 95955, 96360-96368, 96372, 96374-96377, 96523, 97597-97598, 97602, 99155, 99156, 99157, 99211-99223, 99231-99255, 99291-99292, 99304-99310, 99315-99316, 99334-99337, 99347-99350, 99374-99375, 99377-99378, 99446-99449, 99451-99452, 99495-99496, G0463, G0471, P9612

58240 0071T, 0072T, 0213T, 0216T, 0228T, 0230T, 11000-11006, 11042-11047, 12001-12007, 12011-12057, 13100-13133, 13151-13153, 36000, 36400-36410, 36420-36430, 36440, 36591-36592, 36600, 36640, 38562-38564, 38571-38573, 38770, 38780, 43752, 44005, 44140-44151, 44155-44158, 44180, 44188, 44320-44346, 44602-44605, 44620-44625, 44820-44850, 44950-44970, 45110-45123, 45130-45135, 45160, 45171-45172, 45190, 45395-45397, 45505, 45540, 46080-46200, 46220-46280, 46285, 46600-46601, 46940-46942, 46947-46948, 49000-49010, 49020, 49040, 49082-49084, 49203-49205, 49255, 49320-49322, 49406, 49560-49566, 49570, 49580, 49582-49587, 50650, 50715, 50800, 50810-50815, 50820, 50860, 51040-51045, 51520-51525, 51550-51596, 51701-51703, 52000, 55821-55845, 55866, 57106-57107, 57109-57112, 57410, 57454-57455, 57460, 57505, 57522-57556, 58100, 58110-58200, 58210, 58260-58263, 58267-58280, 58290-58294, 58353-58356, 58541-58546, 58550, 58552-58554, 58558, 58561, 58570-58575, 58660-58674✦, 58700-58740, 58805, 58822, 58900-58940, 58943, 58950-58958, 62320-62327, 64400, 64405-64408, 64415-64435, 64445-64454, 64461-64463, 64479-64505, 64510-64530, 69990, 92012-92014, 93000-93010, 93040-93042, 93318, 93355, 94002, 94200, 94250, 94680-94690, 94770, 95812-95816, 95819, 95822, 95829, 95955, 96360-96368, 96372, 96374-96377, 96523, 97597-97598, 97602, 99155, 99156, 99157, 99211-99223, 99231-99255, 99291-99292, 99304-99310, 99315-99316, 99334-99337, 99347-99350, 99374-99375,

58260 0071T, 0072T, 01962-01963, 01969, 0213T, 0216T, 0228T, 0230T, 11000-11006, 11042-11047, 12001-12007, 12011-12057, 13100-13133, 13151-13153, 36000, 36400-36410, 36420-36430, 36440, 36591-36592, 36600, 36640, 43752, 50715, 51040, 51701-51703, 52000, 57000, 57100-57106, 57150, 57180, 57210, 57268, 57280-57284, 57410, 57420, 57452-57455, 57460, 57500-57505, 57522-57530, 57550-57555✦, 57558, 57800, 58100, 58110-58146, 58280✦, 58353-58356, 58545-58546, 58550, 58552, 58554, 58558, 58660, 58662, 58674✦, 58720, 62320-62327, 64400, 64405-64408, 64415-64435, 64445-64454, 64461-64463, 64479-64505, 64510-64530, 69990, 92012-92014, 93000-93010, 93040-93042, 93318, 93355, 94002, 94200, 94250, 94680-94690, 94770, 95812-95816, 95819, 95822, 95829, 95955, 96360-96368, 96372, 96374-96377, 96523, 97597-97598, 97602, 99155, 99156, 99157, 99211-99223, 99231-99255, 99291-99292, 99304-99310, 99315-99316, 99334-99337, 99347-99350, 99374-99375, 99377-99378, 99446-99449, 99451-99452, 99495-99496, G0463, G0471, P9612

58262 0071T, 0072T, 01962-01963, 01969, 0213T, 0216T, 0228T, 0230T, 11000-11006, 11042-11047, 12001-12007, 12011-12057, 13100-13133, 13151-13153, 36000, 36400-36410, 36420-36430, 36440, 36591-36592, 36600, 36640, 43752, 49322, 49407, 50715, 51040, 51701-51703, 52000, 57000, 57100-57106, 57150, 57180, 57210, 57280-57284, 57410, 57420, 57452-57455, 57460, 57500-57505, 57522-57530, 57550-57555✦, 57558, 57800, 58100, 58110-58146, 58260, 58290, 58353-58356, 58541✦, 58545-58546, 58550, 58552-58554, 58558, 58570✦, 58575, 58660-58674✦, 58700-58740, 58800, 58820, 58900, 58925-58940, 62320-62327, 64400, 64405-64408, 64415-64435, 64445-64454, 64461-64463, 64479-64505, 64510-64530, 69990, 92012-92014, 93000-93010, 93040-93042, 93318, 93355, 94002, 94200, 94250, 94680-94690, 94770, 95812-95816, 95819, 95822, 95829, 95955, 96360-96368, 96372, 96374-96377, 96523, 97597-97598, 97602, 99155, 99156, 99157, 99211-99223, 99231-99255, 99291-99292, 99304-99310, 99315-99316, 99334-99337, 99347-99350, 99374-99375, 99377-99378, 99446-99449, 99451-99452, 99495-99496, G0463, G0471, P9612

58263 0071T, 0072T, 01962-01963, 01969, 0213T, 0216T, 0228T, 0230T, 11000-11006, 11042-11047, 12001-12007, 12011-12057, 13100-13133, 13151-13153, 36000, 36400-36410, 36420-36430, 36440, 36591-36592, 36600, 36640, 43752, 45560, 49322, 49407, 50715, 51040, 51701-51703, 52000, 57000, 57100-57106, 57150, 57180, 57210, 57250-57260, 57268, 57280-57284, 57410, 57420, 57452-57455, 57460, 57500-57505, 57522-57530, 57550-57555✦, 57558, 57800, 58100, 58110-58146, 58260-58262, 58270, 58290-58291, 58353-58356, 58541-58543✦, 58545-58546, 58550, 58552, 58554, 58558, 58570✦, 58575, 58660-58674✦, 58700-58740, 58800, 58820, 58900, 58925-58940, 62320-62327, 64400, 64405-64408, 64415-64435, 64445-64454, 64461-64463, 64479-64505, 64510-64530, 69990, 92012-92014, 93000-93010, 93040-93042, 93318, 93355, 94002, 94200, 94250, 94680-94690, 94770, 95812-95816, 95819, 95822, 95829, 95955, 96360-96368, 96372, 96374-96377, 96523, 97597-97598, 97602, 99155, 99156, 99157, 99211-99223, 99231-99255, 99291-99292, 99304-99310, 99315-99316, 99334-99337, 99347-99350, 99374-99375, 99377-99378, 99446-99449, 99451-99452, 99495-99496, G0463, G0471, P9612

58267 0071T, 0072T, 01962-01963, 01969, 0213T, 0216T, 0228T, 0230T, 11000-11006, 11042-11047, 12001-12007, 12011-12057, 13100-13133, 13151-13153, 36000, 36400-36410, 36420-36430, 36440, 36591-36592, 36600, 36640, 43752, 50715, 51040, 51701-51703, 51840-51845,

52000, 52204, 57000, 57100-57106, 57150, 57180, 57210-57220, 57240, 57260, 57280-57285, 57289, 57410, 57420, 57423, 57452-57455, 57460, 57500-57505, 57522-57530, 57550-57555❖, 57558, 57800, 58100, 58110-58146, 58260-58263, 58270, 58290, 58353-58356, 58541-58546, 58550, 58552, 58554, 58558, 58570-58571❖, 58660, 58662, 58674❖, 58720, 62320-62327, 64400, 64405-64408, 64415-64435, 64445-64454, 64461-64463, 64479-64505, 64510-64530, 69990, 92012-92014, 93000-93010, 93040-93042, 93318, 93355, 94002, 94200, 94250, 94680-94690, 94770, 95812-95816, 95819, 95822, 95829, 95955, 96360-96368, 96372, 96374-96377, 96523, 97597-97598, 97602, 99155, 99156, 99157, 99211-99223, 99231-99255, 99291-99292, 99304-99310, 99315-99316, 99334-99337, 99347-99350, 99374-99375, 99377-99378, 99446-99449, 99451-99452, 99495-99496, G0463, G0471, P9612

58270 0071T, 0072T, 01962-01963, 01969, 0213T, 0216T, 0228T, 0230T, 11000-11006, 11042-11047, 12001-12007, 12011-12057, 13100-13133, 13151-13153, 36000, 36400-36410, 36420-36430, 36440, 36591-36592, 36600, 36640, 43752, 45560, 50715, 51040, 51701-51703, 52000, 57000, 57100-57106, 57150, 57180, 57210, 57250-57260, 57268-57284, 57410, 57420, 57452-57455, 57460, 57500-57505, 57522-57530, 57550-57555❖, 57558, 57800, 58100, 58110-58150❖, 58260-58262, 58290, 58353-58356, 58541❖, 58545-58546, 58550, 58552, 58554, 58558, 58660, 58662, 58674❖, 58720, 62320-62327, 64400, 64405-64408, 64415-64435, 64445-64454, 64461-64463, 64479-64505, 64510-64530, 69990, 92012-92014, 93000-93010, 93040-93042, 93318, 93355, 94002, 94200, 94250, 94680-94690, 94770, 95812-95816, 95819, 95822, 95829, 95955, 96360-96368, 96372, 96374-96377, 96523, 97597-97598, 97602, 99155, 99156, 99157, 99211-99223, 99231-99255, 99291-99292, 99304-99310, 99315-99316, 99334-99337, 99347-99350, 99374-99375, 99377-99378, 99446-99449, 99451-99452, 99495-99496, G0463, G0471, P9612

58275 0071T, 0072T, 01962-01963, 01969, 0213T, 0216T, 0228T, 0230T, 11000-11006, 11042-11047, 12001-12007, 12011-12057, 13100-13133, 13151-13153, 36000, 36400-36410, 36420-36430, 36440, 36591-36592, 36600, 36640, 43752, 49407, 50715, 51040, 51701-51703, 52000, 57000, 57100-57107, 57109-57112, 57150, 57180, 57210, 57280-57284, 57410, 57420, 57452-57455, 57460, 57500-57505, 57522-57530, 57550-57555❖, 57558, 57800, 58100, 58110-58146, 58353-58356, 58541-58543❖, 58545-58546, 58550, 58552, 58554, 58558, 58570❖, 58660, 58662, 58674❖, 58700-58720, 58800, 58820, 58900-58940, 62320-62327, 64400, 64405-64408, 64415-64435, 64445-64454, 64461-64463, 64479-64505, 64510-64530, 69990, 92012-92014, 93000-93010, 93040-93042, 93318, 93355, 94002, 94200, 94250, 94680-94690, 94770, 95812-95816, 95819, 95822, 95829, 95955, 96360-96368, 96372, 96374-96377, 96523, 97597-97598, 97602, 99155, 99156, 99157, 99211-99223, 99231-99255, 99291-99292, 99304-99310, 99315-99316, 99334-99337, 99347-99350, 99374-99375, 99377-99378, 99446-99449, 99451-99452, 99495-99496, G0463, G0471, P9612

58280 0071T, 0072T, 01962-01963, 01969, 0213T, 0216T, 0228T, 0230T, 11000-11006, 11042-11047, 12001-12007, 12011-12057, 13100-13133, 13151-13153, 36000, 36400-36410, 36420-36430, 36440, 36591-36592, 36600, 36640, 43752, 45560, 49407, 50715, 51040, 51701-51703, 52000, 57000, 57100-57107, 57109-57112, 57150, 57180, 57210, 57260-57265, 57268-57284, 57410, 57420, 57452-57455, 57460, 57500-57505, 57522-57530, 57550-57555❖, 57558, 57800, 58100, 58110-58146, 58263❖, 58270-58275, 58353-58356, 58541-58546, 58550, 58552, 58554, 58558, 58570-58571❖, 58660, 58662, 58674❖, 58700-58720, 58800, 58900-58940, 62320-62327, 64400, 64405-64408, 64415-64435, 64445-64454, 64461-64463, 64479-64505, 64510-64530, 69990, 92012-92014, 93000-93010, 93040-93042, 93318, 93355, 94002,

94200, 94250, 94680-94690, 94770, 95812-95816, 95819, 95822, 95829, 95955, 96360-96368, 96372, 96374-96377, 96523, 97597-97598, 97602, 99155, 99156, 99157, 99211-99223, 99231-99255, 99291-99292, 99304-99310, 99315-99316, 99334-99337, 99347-99350, 99374-99375, 99377-99378, 99446-99449, 99451-99452, 99495-99496, G0463, G0471, P9612

58285 0071T, 0072T, 01962-01963, 01969, 0213T, 0216T, 0228T, 0230T, 11000-11006, 11042-11047, 12001-12007, 12011-12057, 13100-13133, 13151-13153, 36000, 36400-36410, 36420-36430, 36440, 36591-36592, 36600, 36640, 43752, 45560, 49407, 50715, 51040, 51701-51703, 52000, 57000, 57100-57107, 57109-57112, 57150, 57180, 57210, 57280-57284, 57410, 57420, 57452-57455, 57460, 57500-57505, 57522-57530, 57550-57555❖, 57558, 57800, 58100, 58110-58146, 58353-58356, 58541-58546, 58550, 58552, 58554, 58558, 58570-58573❖, 58660, 58662, 58674❖, 58700-58720, 58800, 58900-58925, 62320-62327, 64400, 64405-64408, 64415-64435, 64445-64454, 64461-64463, 64479-64505, 64510-64530, 69990, 92012-92014, 93000-93010, 93040-93042, 93318, 93355, 94002, 94200, 94250, 94680-94690, 94770, 95812-95816, 95819, 95822, 95829, 95955, 96360-96368, 96372, 96374-96377, 96523, 97597-97598, 97602, 99155, 99156, 99157, 99211-99223, 99231-99255, 99291-99292, 99304-99310, 99315-99316, 99334-99337, 99347-99350, 99374-99375, 99377-99378, 99446-99449, 99451-99452, 99495-99496, G0463, G0471, P9612

58290 0071T, 0072T, 01962-01963, 01969, 0213T, 0216T, 0228T, 0230T, 11000-11006, 11042-11047, 12001-12007, 12011-12057, 13100-13133, 13151-13153, 36000, 36400-36410, 36420-36430, 36440, 36591-36592, 36600, 36640, 43752, 50715, 51040, 51701-51703, 52000, 57000, 57100-57106, 57150, 57180, 57210, 57268, 57280-57284, 57410, 57420, 57452-57455, 57460, 57500-57505, 57522-57530, 57550-57555❖, 57558, 57800, 58100, 58110-58145, 58260, 58280❖, 58353-58356, 58541-58544❖, 58550, 58552-58554, 58558, 58570-58572❖, 58660, 58662, 58674❖, 58720, 62320-62327, 64400, 64405-64408, 64415-64435, 64445-64454, 64461-64463, 64479-64505, 64510-64530, 69990, 92012-92014, 93000-93010, 93040-93042, 93318, 93355, 94002, 94200, 94250, 94680-94690, 94770, 95812-95816, 95819, 95822, 95829, 95955, 96360-96368, 96372, 96374-96377, 96523, 97597-97598, 97602, 99155, 99156, 99157, 99211-99223, 99231-99255, 99291-99292, 99304-99310, 99315-99316, 99334-99337, 99347-99350, 99374-99375, 99377-99378, 99446-99449, 99451-99452, 99495-99496, G0463, G0471, P9612

58291 0071T, 0072T, 01962-01963, 01969, 0213T, 0216T, 0228T, 0230T, 11000-11006, 11042-11047, 12001-12007, 12011-12057, 13100-13133, 13151-13153, 36000, 36400-36410, 36420-36430, 36440, 36591-36592, 36600, 36640, 43752, 49322, 49407, 50715, 51040, 51701-51703, 52000, 57000, 57100-57106, 57150, 57180, 57210, 57280-57284, 57410, 57420, 57452-57455, 57460, 57500-57505, 57522-57530, 57550-57555❖, 57558, 57800, 58100, 58110-58145, 58260-58262, 58267-58270, 58353-58356, 58541-58544❖, 58550, 58552-58554, 58558, 58570-58572❖, 58575, 58660-58674❖, 58700-58740, 58800, 58820, 58900, 58925-58940, 62320-62327, 64400, 64405-64408, 64415-64435, 64445-64454, 64461-64463, 64479-64505, 64510-64530, 69990, 92012-92014, 93000-93010, 93040-93042, 93318, 93355, 94002, 94200, 94250, 94680-94690, 94770, 95812-95816, 95819, 95822, 95829, 95955, 96360-96368, 96372, 96374-96377, 96523, 97597-97598, 97602, 99155, 99156, 99157, 99211-99223, 99231-99255, 99291-99292, 99304-99310, 99315-99316, 99334-99337, 99347-99350, 99374-99375, 99377-99378, 99446-99449, 99451-99452, 99495-99496, G0463, G0471, P9612

58292 0071T, 0072T, 01962-01963, 01969, 0213T, 0216T, 0228T, 0230T, 11000-11006, 11042-11047, 12001-12007, 12011-12057, 13100-13133, 13151-13153, 36000, 36400-36410, 36420-36430, 36440, 36591-36592, 36600, 36640, 43752, 45560, 49322, 49407, 50715, 51040, 51701-51703, 52000, 57000, 57100-57106, 57150, 57180, 57210, 57250-57260, 57268-57284, 57410, 57420, 57452-57455, 57460, 57500-57505, 57522-57530, 57550-57555❖, 57558, 57800, 58100, 58110-58145, 58260-58263, 58267-58270, 58280❖, 58291, 58294, 58353-58356, 58541-58544❖, 58550, 58552-58554, 58558, 58570-58575, 58660-58674❖, 58700-58740, 58800, 58820, 58900, 58925-58940, 62320-62327, 64400, 64405-64408, 64415-64435, 64445-64454, 64461-64463, 64479-64505, 64510-64530, 69990, 92012-92014, 93000-93010, 93040-93042, 93318, 93355, 94002, 94200, 94250, 94680-94690, 94770, 95812-95816, 95819, 95822, 95829, 95955, 96360-96368, 96372, 96374-96377, 96523, 97597-97598, 97602, 99155, 99156, 99157, 99211-99223, 99231-99255, 99291-99292, 99304-99310, 99315-99316, 99334-99337, 99347-99350, 99374-99375, 99377-99378, 99446-99449, 99451-99452, 99495-99496, G0463, G0471, P9612

58294 0071T, 0072T, 01962-01963, 01969, 0213T, 0216T, 0228T, 0230T, 11000-11006, 11042-11047, 12001-12007, 12011-12057, 13100-13133, 13151-13153, 36000, 36400-36410, 36420-36430, 36440, 36591-36592, 36600, 36640, 43752, 45560, 50715, 51040, 51701-51703, 52000, 57000, 57100-57106, 57150, 57180, 57210, 57250-57260, 57268-57284, 57410, 57420, 57452-57455, 57460, 57500-57505, 57522-57530, 57550-57555❖, 57558, 57800, 58100, 58110-58145, 58150❖, 58260-58263, 58267-58270, 58280❖, 58291, 58293, 58353-58356, 58541-58544❖, 58550, 58552-58554, 58558, 58570-58572❖, 58660, 58662, 58674❖, 58720, 62320-62327, 64400, 64405-64408, 64415-64435, 64445-64454, 64461-64463, 64479-64505, 64510-64530, 69990, 92012-92014, 93000-93010, 93040-93042, 93318, 93355, 94002, 94200, 94250, 94680-94690, 94770, 95812-95816, 95819, 95822, 95829, 95955, 96360-96368, 96372, 96374-96377, 96523, 97597-97598, 97602, 99155, 99156, 99157, 99211-99223, 99231-99255, 99291-99292, 99304-99310, 99315-99316, 99334-99337, 99347-99350, 99374-99375, 99377-99378, 99446-99449, 99451-99452, 99495-99496, G0463, G0471, P9612

58300 11000-11006, 11042-11047, 36591-36592, 96523, 97597-97598, 97602

58301 0213T, 0216T, 0228T, 0230T, 11000-11006, 11042-11047, 12001-12007, 12011-12057, 13100-13133, 13151-13153, 36000, 36400-36410, 36420-36430, 36440, 36591-36592, 36600, 36640, 43752, 51701-51703, 57410, 57500, 57800, 62320-62327, 64400, 64405-64408, 64415-64435, 64445-64454, 64461-64463, 64479-64505, 64510-64530, 69990, 92012-92014, 93000-93010, 93040-93042, 93318, 93355, 94002, 94200, 94250, 94680-94690, 94770, 95812-95816, 95819, 95822, 95829, 95955, 96360-96368, 96372, 96374-96377, 96523, 97597-97598, 97602, 99155, 99156, 99157, 99211-99223, 99231-99255, 99291-99292, 99304-99310, 99315-99316, 99334-99337, 99347-99350, 99374-99375, 99377-99378, 99446-99449, 99451-99452, 99495-99496, G0463, G0471, J0670, J2001

58321 0213T, 0216T, 0228T, 0230T, 12001-12007, 12011-12057, 13100-13133, 13151-13153, 36000, 36400-36410, 36420-36430, 36440, 36591-36592, 36600, 36640, 43752, 51701-51703, 57410, 62320-62327, 64400, 64405-64408, 64415-64435, 64445-64454, 64461-64463, 64479-64505, 64510-64530, 69990, 92012-92014, 93000-93010, 93040-93042, 93318, 93355, 94002, 94200, 94250, 94680-94690, 94770, 95812-95816, 95819, 95822, 95829, 95955, 96360-96368, 96372, 96374-96377, 96523, 99155, 99156, 99157, 99211-99223, 99231-99255, 99291-99292, 99304-99310, 99315-99316, 99334-99337, 99347-99350, 99374-99375, 99377-99378, 99446-99449, 99451-99452, 99495-99496, G0463, G0471, J0670, J2001

58322 0213T, 0216T, 0228T, 0230T, 12001-12007, 12011-12057, 13100-13133, 13151-13153, 36000, 36400-36410, 36420-36430, 36440, 36591-36592, 36600, 36640, 43752, 51701-51703, 57410, 62320-62327, 64400, 64405-64408, 64415-64435, 64445-64454, 64461-64463, 64479-64505, 64510-64530, 69990, 92012-92014, 93000-93010, 93040-93042, 93318, 93355, 94002, 94200, 94250, 94680-94690, 94770, 95812-95816, 95819, 95822, 95829, 95955, 96360-96368, 96372, 96374-96377, 96523, 99155, 99156, 99157, 99211-99223, 99231-99255, 99291-99292, 99304-99310, 99315-99316, 99334-99337, 99347-99350, 99374-99375, 99377-99378, 99446-99449, 99451-99452, 99495-99496, G0463, G0471, J0670, J2001

58323 0213T, 0216T, 0228T, 0230T, 12001-12007, 12011-12057, 13100-13133, 13151-13153, 36000, 36400-36410, 36420-36430, 36440, 36591-36592, 36600, 36640, 43752, 51701-51703, 57410, 62320-62327, 64400, 64405-64408, 64415-64435, 64445-64454, 64461-64463, 64479-64505, 64510-64530, 69990, 92012-92014, 93000-93010, 93040-93042, 93318, 93355, 94002, 94200, 94250, 94680-94690, 94770, 95812-95816, 95819, 95822, 95829, 95955, 96360-96368, 96372, 96374-96377, 96523, 99155, 99156, 99157, 99211-99223, 99231-99255, 99291-99292, 99304-99310, 99315-99316, 99334-99337, 99347-99350, 99374-99375, 99377-99378, 99446-99449, 99451-99452, 99495-99496, G0463, G0471

58340 00952, 0213T, 0216T, 0228T, 0230T, 0567T-0568T, 12001-12007, 12011-12057, 13100-13133, 13151-13153, 36000, 36400-36410, 36420-36430, 36440, 36591-36592, 36600, 36640, 43752, 51701-51703, 57410, 62320-62327, 64400, 64405-64408, 64415-64435, 64445-64454, 64461-64463, 64479-64505, 64510-64530, 69990, 76000, 76942, 76970, 76998, 77001-77002, 92012-92014, 93000-93010, 93040-93042, 93318, 93355, 94002, 94200, 94250, 94680-94690, 94770, 95812-95816, 95819, 95822, 95829, 95955, 96360-96368, 96372, 96374-96377, 96523, 99155, 99156, 99157, 99211-99223, 99231-99255, 99291-99292, 99304-99310, 99315-99316, 99334-99337, 99347-99350, 99374-99375, 99377-99378, 99446-99449, 99451-99452, 99495-99496, G0463, G0471, J0670, J1642-J1644, J2001

58345 00952, 0213T, 0216T, 0228T, 0230T, 0568T, 12001-12007, 12011-12057, 13100-13133, 13151-13153, 36000, 36400-36410, 36420-36430, 36440, 36591-36592, 36600, 36640, 43752, 51701-51703, 57410, 58340, 62320-62327, 64400, 64405-64408, 64415-64435, 64445-64454, 64461-64463, 64479-64505, 64510-64530, 69990, 76000, 76942, 76970, 76998, 77001-77002, 92012-92014, 93000-93010, 93040-93042, 93318, 93355, 94002, 94200, 94250, 94680-94690, 94770, 95812-95816, 95819, 95822, 95829, 95955, 96360-96368, 96372, 96374-96377, 96523, 99155, 99156, 99157, 99211-99223, 99231-99255, 99291-99292, 99304-99310, 99315-99316, 99334-99337, 99347-99350, 99374-99375, 99377-99378, 99446-99449, 99451-99452, 99495-99496, G0463, G0471

58346 0213T, 0216T, 0228T, 0230T, 11000-11006, 11042-11047, 12001-12007, 12011-12057, 13100-13133, 13151-13153, 36000, 36400-36410, 36420-36430, 36440, 36591-36592, 36600, 36640, 43752, 51701-51703, 57180, 57400-57410, 57558, 57800, 58100, 62320-62327, 64400, 64405-64408, 64415-64435, 64445-64454, 64461-64463, 64479-64505, 64510-64530, 69990, 92012-92014, 93000-93010, 93040-93042, 93318, 93355, 94002, 94200, 94250, 94680-94690, 94770, 95812-95816, 95819, 95822, 95829, 95955, 96360-96368, 96372, 96374-96377, 96523, 97597-97598, 97602, 99155, 99156, 99157, 99211-99223, 99231-99255, 99291-99292, 99304-99310, 99315-99316, 99334-99337, 99347-99350, 99374-99375, 99377-99378, 99446-99449, 99451-99452, 99495-99496, G0463, G0471

58350 0213T, 0216T, 0228T, 0230T, 12001-12007, 12011-12057, 13100-13133, 13151-13153, 36000, 36400-36410, 36420-36430, 36440, 36591-36592, 36600, 36640, 43752, 51701-51703, 57410, 62320-62327, 64400, 64405-64408, 64415-64435, 64445-64454, 64461-64463, 64479-64505, 64510-64530, 69990, 92012-92014, 93000-93010, 93040-93042, 93318, 93355, 94002, 94200, 94250, 94680-94690, 94770, 95812-95816, 95819, 95822, 95829, 95955, 96360-96368, 96372, 96374-96377, 96523, 99155, 99156, 99157, 99211-99223, 99231-99255, 99291-99292, 99304-99310, 99315-99316, 99334-99337, 99347-99350, 99374-99375, 99377-99378, 99446-99449, 99451-99452, 99495-99496, G0463, G0471, J0670, J2001

58353 0213T, 0216T, 0228T, 0230T, 12001-12007, 12011-12057, 13100-13133, 13151-13153, 36000, 36400-36410, 36420-36430, 36440, 36591-36592, 36600, 36640, 43752, 51701-51703, 57100, 57400-57410, 57800, 58100, 58120, 58555-58560, 58562-58563, 62320-62327, 64400, 64405-64408, 64415-64435, 64445-64454, 64461-64463, 64479-64505, 64510-64530, 69990, 92012-92014, 93000-93010, 93040-93042, 93318, 93355, 94002, 94200, 94250, 94680-94690, 94770, 95812-95816, 95819, 95822, 95829, 95955, 96360-96368, 96372, 96374-96377, 96523, 99155, 99156, 99157, 99211-99223, 99231-99255, 99291-99292, 99304-99310, 99315-99316, 99334-99337, 99347-99350, 99374-99375, 99377-99378, 99446-99449, 99451-99452, 99495-99496, G0463, G0471, J0670, J2001

58356 00940, 0213T, 0216T, 0228T, 0230T, 0567T-0568T, 12001-12007, 12011-12057, 13100-13133, 13151-13153, 36000, 36400-36410, 36420-36430, 36440, 36591-36592, 36600, 36640, 43752, 51701-51703, 57180, 57400-57410, 57452, 57500, 57800, 58100, 58120, 58340, 58353❖, 58558, 58563❖, 62320-62327, 64400, 64405-64408, 64415-64435, 64445-64454, 64461-64463, 64479-64505, 64510-64530, 69990, 76380, 76700, 76830, 76856-76857, 76940, 76942, 76970, 76998, 77013, 77022, 92012-92014, 93000-93010, 93040-93042, 93318, 93355, 94002, 94200, 94250, 94680-94690, 94770, 95812-95816, 95819, 95822, 95829, 95955, 96360-96368, 96372, 96374-96377, 96523, 99155, 99156, 99157, 99211-99223, 99231-99255, 99291-99292, 99304-99310, 99315-99316, 99334-99337, 99347-99350, 99374-99375, 99377-99378, 99446-99449, 99451-99452, 99495-99496, G0463, G0471, J0670, J2001

58400 0213T, 0216T, 0228T, 0230T, 12001-12007, 12011-12057, 13100-13133, 13151-13153, 36000, 36400-36410, 36420-36430, 36440, 36591-36592, 36600, 36640, 43752, 44005, 44180, 44602-44605, 44820-44850, 44950, 44970, 49000-49010, 49255, 49320, 49570, 50715, 51701-51703, 52000, 57410, 62320-62327, 64400, 64405-64408, 64415-64435, 64445-64454, 64461-64463, 64479-64505, 64510-64530, 69990, 92012-92014, 93000-93010, 93040-93042, 93318, 93355, 94002, 94200, 94250, 94680-94690, 94770, 95812-95816, 95819, 95822, 95829, 95955, 96360-96368, 96372, 96374-96377, 96523, 99155, 99156, 99157, 99211-99223, 99231-99255, 99291-99292, 99304-99310, 99315-99316, 99334-99337, 99347-99350, 99374-99375, 99377-99378, 99446-99449, 99451-99452, 99495-99496, G0463, G0471

58410 0213T, 0216T, 0228T, 0230T, 11000-11006, 11042-11047, 12001-12007, 12011-12057, 13100-13133, 13151-13153, 36000, 36400-36410, 36420-36430, 36440, 36591-36592, 36600, 36640, 43752, 44005, 44180, 44602-44605, 44820-44850, 44950, 44970, 49000-49010, 49255, 49320, 49570, 50715, 51701-51703, 52000, 57410, 58400, 62320-62327, 64400, 64405-64408, 64415-64435, 64445-64454, 64461-64463, 64479-64505, 64510-64530, 69990, 92012-92014, 93000-93010, 93040-93042, 93318, 93355, 94002, 94200, 94250, 94680-94690, 94770, 95812-95816, 95819, 95822, 95829, 95955, 96360-96368, 96372, 96374-96377, 96523, 97597-97598, 97602, 99155, 99156, 99157, 99211-99223, 99231-99255, 99291-99292, 99304-99310,

99315-99316, 99334-99337, 99347-99350, 99374-99375, 99377-99378, 99446-99449, 99451-99452, 99495-99496, G0463, G0471

58520 0213T, 0216T, 0228T, 0230T, 12001-12007, 12011-12057, 13100-13133, 13151-13153, 36000, 36400-36410, 36420-36430, 36440, 36591-36592, 36600, 36640, 43752, 44005, 44180, 44602-44605, 44820-44850, 44950, 44970, 49000-49010, 49255, 49320, 49570, 50715, 51701-51703, 52000, 57410, 58140-58146, 62320-62327, 64400, 64405-64408, 64415-64435, 64445-64454, 64461-64463, 64479-64505, 64510-64530, 69990, 92012-92014, 93000-93010, 93040-93042, 93318, 93355, 94002, 94200, 94250, 94680-94690, 94770, 95812-95816, 95819, 95822, 95829, 95955, 96360-96368, 96372, 96374-96377, 96523, 99155, 99156, 99157, 99211-99223, 99231-99255, 99291-99292, 99304-99310, 99315-99316, 99334-99337, 99347-99350, 99374-99375, 99377-99378, 99446-99449, 99451-99452, 99495-99496, G0463, G0471

58540 0213T, 0216T, 0228T, 0230T, 11000-11006, 11042-11047, 12001-12007, 12011-12057, 13100-13133, 13151-13153, 36000, 36400-36410, 36420-36430, 36440, 36591-36592, 36600, 36640, 43752, 44005, 44180, 44602-44605, 44820-44850, 44950, 44970, 49000-49010, 49255, 49320, 49570, 50715, 51701-51703, 52000, 57410, 58140-58146, 58520, 62320-62327, 64400, 64405-64408, 64415-64435, 64445-64454, 64461-64463, 64479-64505, 64510-64530, 69990, 92012-92014, 93000-93010, 93040-93042, 93318, 93355, 94002, 94200, 94250, 94680-94690, 94770, 95812-95816, 95819, 95822, 95829, 95955, 96360-96368, 96372, 96374-96377, 96523, 97597-97598, 97602, 99155, 99156, 99157, 99211-99223, 99231-99255, 99291-99292, 99304-99310, 99315-99316, 99334-99337, 99347-99350, 99374-99375, 99377-99378, 99446-99449, 99451-99452, 99495-99496, G0463, G0471

58541 0213T, 0216T, 0228T, 0230T, 11000-11006, 11042-11047, 12001-12007, 12011-12057, 13100-13133, 13151-13153, 36000, 36400-36410, 36420-36430, 36440, 36591-36592, 36600, 36640, 43752, 44005, 44180, 44602-44605, 44950, 44970, 49082-49084, 49320-49321, 49400, 50715, 51701-51703, 52000, 57000, 57020, 57100, 57180, 57400-57420, 57452, 57500-57505, 57530, 57550-57555❖, 57558, 57800, 58100, 58110-58146, 58260❖, 58545-58546, 58558, 58561, 58575, 58660-58661, 58670-58673, 58700-58720, 58940, 62320-62327, 64400, 64405-64408, 64415-64435, 64445-64454, 64461-64463, 64479-64505, 64510-64530, 69990, 76000, 77001-77002, 92012-92014, 93000-93010, 93040-93042, 93318, 93355, 94002, 94200, 94250, 94680-94690, 94770, 95812-95816, 95819, 95822, 95829, 95955, 96360-96368, 96372, 96374-96377, 96523, 97597-97598, 97602, 99155, 99156, 99157, 99211-99223, 99231-99255, 99291-99292, 99304-99310, 99315-99316, 99334-99337, 99347-99350, 99374-99375, 99377-99378, 99446-99449, 99451-99452, 99495-99496, G0463, G0471, P9612

58542 0213T, 0216T, 0228T, 0230T, 11000-11006, 11042-11047, 12001-12007, 12011-12057, 13100-13133, 13151-13153, 36000, 36400-36410, 36420-36430, 36440, 36591-36592, 36600, 36640, 43752, 44005, 44180, 44602-44605, 44950, 44970, 49082-49084, 49320-49321, 49400, 50715, 51701-51703, 52000, 57000, 57020, 57100, 57180, 57400-57420, 57452, 57500-57505, 57530, 57550-57555❖, 57558, 57800, 58100, 58110-58146, 58180❖, 58260-58262❖, 58270❖, 58541, 58545-58546, 58550❖, 58558, 58561, 58570❖, 58575, 58660-58661, 58670-58674, 58700-58720, 58940, 62320-62327, 64400, 64405-64408, 64415-64435, 64445-64454, 64461-64463, 64479-64505, 64510-64530, 69990, 76000, 77001-77002, 92012-92014, 93000-93010, 93040-93042, 93318, 93355, 94002, 94200, 94250, 94680-94690, 94770, 95812-95816, 95819, 95822, 95829, 95955, 96360-96368, 96372, 96374-96377, 96523, 97597-97598, 97602, 99155, 99156, 99157, 99211-99223, 99231-99255, 99291-99292, 99304-99310, 99315-99316, 99334-99337, 99347-99350, 99374-99375, 99377-99378, 99446-99449, 99451-99452, 99495-99496, G0463, G0471, P9612

Coding Companion for Ob/Gyn

58543 0213T, 0216T, 0228T, 0230T, 11000-11006, 11042-11047, 12001-12007, 12011-12057, 13100-13133, 13151-13153, 36000, 36400-36410, 36420-36430, 36440, 36591-36592, 36600, 36640, 43752, 44005, 44180, 44602-44605, 44950, 44970, 49082-49084, 49320-49321, 49400, 50715, 51701-51703, 52000, 57000, 57020, 57100, 57180, 57400-57420, 57452, 57500-57505, 57530, 57550-57555✦, 57558, 57800, 58100, 58110-58146, 58180✦, 58260-58262✦, 58270✦, 58541-58542✦, 58545-58546, 58550✦, 58552✦, 58558, 58561, 58570✦, 58575, 58660-58661, 58670-58674, 58700-58720, 58940, 62320-62327, 64400, 64405-64408, 64415-64435, 64445-64454, 64461-64463, 64479-64505, 64510-64530, 69990, 76000, 77001-77002, 92012-92014, 93000-93010, 93040-93042, 93318, 93355, 94002, 94200, 94250, 94680-94690, 94770, 95812-95816, 95819, 95822, 95829, 95955, 96360-96368, 96372, 96374-96377, 96523, 97597-97598, 97602, 99155, 99156, 99157, 99211-99223, 99231-99255, 99291-99292, 99304-99310, 99315-99316, 99334-99337, 99347-99350, 99374-99375, 99377-99378, 99446-99449, 99451-99452, 99495-99496, G0463, G0471, P9612

58544 0213T, 0216T, 0228T, 0230T, 11000-11006, 11042-11047, 12001-12007, 12011-12057, 13100-13133, 13151-13153, 36000, 36400-36410, 36420-36430, 36440, 36591-36592, 36600, 36640, 43752, 44005, 44180, 44602-44605, 44950, 44970, 49082-49084, 49320-49321, 49400, 50715, 51701-51703, 52000, 57000, 57020, 57100, 57180, 57400-57420, 57452, 57500-57505, 57530, 57550-57555✦, 57558, 57800, 58100, 58110-58150, 58180✦, 58260-58263✦, 58270-58275✦, 58541-58543, 58545-58546, 58550✦, 58552✦, 58558, 58561, 58570-58571✦, 58575, 58660-58661, 58670-58674, 58700-58720, 58940, 62320-62327, 64400, 64405-64408, 64415-64435, 64445-64454, 64461-64463, 64479-64505, 64510-64530, 69990, 76000, 77001-77002, 92012-92014, 93000-93010, 93040-93042, 93318, 93355, 94002, 94200, 94250, 94680-94690, 94770, 95812-95816, 95819, 95822, 95829, 95955, 96360-96368, 96372, 96374-96377, 96523, 97597-97598, 97602, 99155, 99156, 99157, 99211-99223, 99231-99255, 99291-99292, 99304-99310, 99315-99316, 99334-99337, 99347-99350, 99374-99375, 99377-99378, 99446-99449, 99451-99452, 99495-99496, G0463, G0471, P9612

58545 0213T, 0216T, 0228T, 0230T, 0404T✦, 11000-11006, 11042-11047, 12001-12007, 12011-12057, 13100-13133, 13151-13153, 36000, 36400-36410, 36420-36430, 36440, 36591-36592, 36600, 36640, 43653, 43752, 44005, 44180, 44602-44605, 44950, 44970, 49082-49084, 49320-49321, 49400, 50715, 51701-51703, 57410, 58550, 58660, 58674, 62320-62327, 64400, 64405-64408, 64415-64435, 64445-64454, 64461-64463, 64479-64505, 64510-64530, 69990, 76000, 77001-77002, 92012-92014, 93000-93010, 93040-93042, 93318, 93355, 94002, 94200, 94250, 94680-94690, 94770, 95812-95816, 95819, 95822, 95829, 95955, 96360-96368, 96372, 96374-96377, 96523, 97597-97598, 97602, 99155, 99156, 99157, 99211-99223, 99231-99255, 99291-99292, 99304-99310, 99315-99316, 99334-99337, 99347-99350, 99374-99375, 99377-99378, 99446-99449, 99451-99452, 99495-99496, G0463, G0471

58546 0213T, 0216T, 0228T, 0230T, 0404T✦, 11000-11006, 11042-11047, 12001-12007, 12011-12057, 13100-13133, 13151-13153, 36000, 36400-36410, 36420-36430, 36440, 36591-36592, 36600, 36640, 43653, 43752, 44005, 44180, 44602-44605, 44950, 44970, 49082-49084, 49320-49321, 49400, 50715, 51701-51703, 57410, 58545, 58550, 58552, 58570-58571, 58660, 58674, 62320-62327, 64400, 64405-64408, 64415-64435, 64445-64454, 64461-64463, 64479-64505, 64510-64530, 69990, 76000, 77001-77002, 92012-92014, 93000-93010, 93040-93042, 93318, 93355, 94002, 94200, 94250, 94680-94690, 94770, 95812-95816, 95819, 95822, 95829, 95955, 96360-96368, 96372, 96374-96377, 96523, 97597-97598, 97602, 99155, 99156, 99157, 99211-99223, 99231-99255, 99291-99292, 99304-99310, 99315-99316,

99334-99337, 99347-99350, 99374-99375, 99377-99378, 99446-99449, 99451-99452, 99495-99496, G0463, G0471

58548 0213T, 0216T, 0228T, 0230T, 10005, 10007, 10009, 10011, 10021, 11000-11006, 11042-11047, 12001-12007, 12011-12057, 13100-13133, 13151-13153, 36000, 36400-36410, 36420-36430, 36440, 36591-36592, 36600, 36640, 38562-38573, 38765, 38770, 38780, 43653, 43752, 44005, 44180, 44602-44605, 44950, 44970, 49082-49084, 49320-49321, 49400, 50715, 51701-51703, 52000, 57000, 57020, 57100, 57180, 57400-57420, 57452-57455, 57460, 57500-57505, 57530, 57550-57555✦, 57558, 57800, 58100, 58110-58200✦, 58260-58263✦, 58267-58294✦, 58541-58546, 58550, 58552-58554, 58558, 58561, 58570-58575, 58660-58674, 58700-58720, 58940, 62320-62327, 64400, 64405-64408, 64415-64435, 64445-64454, 64461-64463, 64479-64505, 64510-64530, 69990, 76000, 77001-77002, 92012-92014, 93000-93010, 93040-93042, 93318, 93355, 94002, 94200, 94250, 94680-94690, 94770, 95812-95816, 95819, 95822, 95829, 95955, 96360-96368, 96372, 96374-96377, 96523, 97597-97598, 97602, 99155, 99156, 99157, 99211-99223, 99231-99255, 99291-99292, 99304-99310, 99315-99316, 99334-99337, 99347-99350, 99374-99375, 99377-99378, 99446-99449, 99451-99452, 99495-99496, G0463, G0471, P9612

58550 0213T, 0216T, 0228T, 0230T, 11000-11006, 11042-11047, 12001-12007, 12011-12057, 13100-13133, 13151-13153, 36000, 36400-36410, 36420-36430, 36440, 36591-36592, 36600, 36640, 43653, 43752, 44005, 44180, 44602-44605, 44950, 44970, 49082-49084, 49320-49322, 49400, 50715, 51701-51703, 52000, 57000, 57020, 57100-57106, 57150, 57180, 57210, 57280-57284, 57400-57420, 57452-57455, 57460, 57500-57505, 57530, 57550-57555✦, 57558, 57800, 58100, 58110-58120, 58145, 58541✦, 58558, 58561, 58575, 58660-58661, 58670-58674, 58700-58720, 58940, 62320-62327, 64400, 64405-64408, 64415-64435, 64445-64454, 64461-64463, 64479-64505, 64510-64530, 69990, 76000, 77001-77002, 92012-92014, 93000-93010, 93040-93042, 93318, 93355, 94002, 94200, 94250, 94680-94690, 94770, 95812-95816, 95819, 95822, 95829, 95955, 96360-96368, 96372, 96374-96377, 96523, 97597-97598, 97602, 99155, 99156, 99157, 99211-99223, 99231-99255, 99291-99292, 99304-99310, 99315-99316, 99334-99337, 99347-99350, 99374-99375, 99377-99378, 99446-99449, 99451-99452, 99495-99496, G0463, G0471, P9612

58552 0213T, 0216T, 0228T, 0230T, 11000-11006, 11042-11047, 12001-12007, 12011-12057, 13100-13133, 13151-13153, 36000, 36400-36410, 36420-36430, 36440, 36591-36592, 36600, 36640, 43653, 43752, 44005, 44180, 44602-44605, 44950, 44970, 49082-49084, 49320-49322, 49400, 50715, 51701-51703, 52000, 57000, 57020, 57100-57106, 57150, 57180, 57210, 57280-57284, 57400-57420, 57452-57455, 57460, 57500-57505, 57530, 57550-57555✦, 57558, 57800, 58100, 58110-58145, 58541-58542✦, 58545, 58550, 58558, 58561, 58570✦, 58575, 58660-58661, 58670-58674, 58700-58720, 58900, 58940, 62320-62327, 64400, 64405-64408, 64415-64435, 64445-64454, 64461-64463, 64479-64505, 64510-64530, 69990, 76000, 77001-77002, 92012-92014, 93000-93010, 93040-93042, 93318, 93355, 94002, 94200, 94250, 94680-94690, 94770, 95812-95816, 95819, 95822, 95829, 95955, 96360-96368, 96372, 96374-96377, 96523, 97597-97598, 97602, 99155, 99156, 99157, 99211-99223, 99231-99255, 99291-99292, 99304-99310, 99315-99316, 99334-99337, 99347-99350, 99374-99375, 99377-99378, 99446-99449, 99451-99452, 99495-99496, G0463, G0471, P9612

58553 0213T, 0216T, 0228T, 0230T, 11000-11006, 11042-11047, 12001-12007, 12011-12057, 13100-13133, 13151-13153, 36000, 36400-36410, 36420-36430, 36440, 36591-36592, 36600, 36640, 43653, 43752, 44005, 44180, 44602-44605, 44950, 44970, 49082-49084, 49320-49321, 49400, 50715, 51701-51703, 52000, 57000, 57020, 57100-57106,

Coding Companion for Ob/Gyn

57150, 57180, 57210, 57280-57284, 57400-57420, 57452-57455, 57460, 57500-57505, 57530, 57550-57555✢, 57558, 57800, 58100, 58110-58145, 58541-58546, 58550, 58552, 58558, 58561, 58570-58571✢, 58575, 58661, 58670-58674, 58700-58720, 62320-62327, 64400, 64405-64408, 64415-64435, 64445-64454, 64461-64463, 64479-64505, 64510-64530, 69990, 76000, 77001-77002, 92012-92014, 93000-93010, 93040-93042, 93318, 93355, 94002, 94200, 94250, 94680-94690, 94770, 95812-95816, 95819, 95822, 95829, 95955, 96360-96368, 96372, 96374-96377, 96523, 97597-97598, 97602, 99155, 99156, 99157, 99211-99223, 99231-99255, 99291-99292, 99304-99310, 99315-99316, 99334-99337, 99347-99350, 99374-99375, 99377-99378, 99446-99449, 99451-99452, 99495-99496, G0463, G0471, P9612

58554 0213T, 0216T, 0228T, 0230T, 11000-11006, 11042-11047, 12001-12007, 12011-12057, 13100-13133, 13151-13153, 36000, 36400-36410, 36420-36430, 36440, 36591-36592, 36600, 36640, 38573, 43653, 43752, 44005, 44180, 44602-44605, 44950, 44970, 49082-49084, 49320-49322, 49400, 50715, 51701-51703, 52000, 57000, 57020, 57100-57106, 57150, 57180, 57210, 57280-57284, 57400-57420, 57452-57455, 57460, 57500-57505, 57530, 57550-57555✢, 57558, 57800, 58100, 58110-58146, 58541-58546, 58550, 58552-58553, 58558, 58561, 58570-58572✢, 58575, 58660-58661, 58670-58674, 58700-58720, 58900, 58940, 62320-62327, 64400, 64405-64408, 64415-64435, 64445-64454, 64461-64463, 64479-64505, 64510-64530, 69990, 76000, 77001-77002, 92012-92014, 93000-93010, 93040-93042, 93318, 93355, 94002, 94200, 94250, 94680-94690, 94770, 95812-95816, 95819, 95822, 95829, 95955, 96360-96368, 96372, 96374-96377, 96523, 97597-97598, 97602, 99155, 99156, 99157, 99211-99223, 99231-99255, 99291-99292, 99304-99310, 99315-99316, 99334-99337, 99347-99350, 99374-99375, 99377-99378, 99446-99449, 99451-99452, 99495-99496, G0463, G0471, P9612

58555 00952, 0213T, 0216T, 0228T, 0230T, 12001-12007, 12011-12057, 13100-13133, 13151-13153, 36000, 36400-36410, 36420-36430, 36440, 36591-36592, 36600, 36640, 43752, 50715, 51701-51703, 57100, 57410, 57800, 58100, 62320-62327, 64400, 64405-64408, 64415-64435, 64445-64454, 64461-64463, 64479-64505, 64510-64530, 69990, 76000, 77001-77002, 92012-92014, 93000-93010, 93040-93042, 93318, 93355, 94002, 94200, 94250, 94680-94690, 94770, 95812-95816, 95819, 95822, 95829, 95955, 96360-96368, 96372, 96374-96377, 96523, 99155, 99156, 99157, 99211-99223, 99231-99255, 99291-99292, 99304-99310, 99315-99316, 99334-99337, 99347-99350, 99374-99375, 99377-99378, 99446-99449, 99451-99452, 99495-99496, G0463, G0471, J0670, J2001

58558 00952, 0213T, 0216T, 0228T, 0230T, 10005, 10007, 10009, 10011, 10021, 11000-11006, 11042-11047, 12001-12007, 12011-12057, 13100-13133, 13151-13153, 36000, 36400-36410, 36420-36430, 36440, 36591-36592, 36600, 36640, 43752, 50715, 51701-51703, 57100, 57410, 57800, 58100, 58120, 58555, 62320-62327, 64400, 64405-64408, 64415-64435, 64445-64454, 64461-64463, 64479-64505, 64510-64530, 69990, 76000, 77001-77002, 92012-92014, 93000-93010, 93040-93042, 93318, 93355, 94002, 94200, 94250, 94680-94690, 94770, 95812-95816, 95819, 95822, 95829, 95955, 96360-96368, 96372, 96374-96377, 96523, 97597-97598, 97602, 99155, 99156, 99157, 99211-99223, 99231-99255, 99291-99292, 99304-99310, 99315-99316, 99334-99337, 99347-99350, 99374-99375, 99377-99378, 99446-99449, 99451-99452, 99495-99496, G0463, G0471, J0670, J2001

58559 00952, 0213T, 0216T, 0228T, 0230T, 12001-12007, 12011-12057, 13100-13133, 13151-13153, 36000, 36400-36410, 36420-36430, 36440, 36591-36592, 36600, 36640, 43752, 50715, 51701-51703, 57100, 57410, 57800, 58100, 58555, 62320-62327, 64400, 64405-64408,

64415-64435, 64445-64454, 64461-64463, 64479-64505, 64510-64530, 69990, 76000, 77001-77002, 92012-92014, 93000-93010, 93040-93042, 93318, 93355, 94002, 94200, 94250, 94680-94690, 94770, 95812-95816, 95819, 95822, 95829, 95955, 96360-96368, 96372, 96374-96377, 96523, 99155, 99156, 99157, 99211-99223, 99231-99255, 99291-99292, 99304-99310, 99315-99316, 99334-99337, 99347-99350, 99374-99375, 99377-99378, 99446-99449, 99451-99452, 99495-99496, G0463, G0471

58560 00952, 0213T, 0216T, 0228T, 0230T, 11000-11006, 11042-11047, 12001-12007, 12011-12057, 13100-13133, 13151-13153, 36000, 36400-36410, 36420-36430, 36440, 36591-36592, 36600, 36640, 43752, 50715, 51701-51703, 57100, 57410, 57800, 58100, 58555, 62320-62327, 64400, 64405-64408, 64415-64435, 64445-64454, 64461-64463, 64479-64505, 64510-64530, 69990, 76000, 77001-77002, 92012-92014, 93000-93010, 93040-93042, 93318, 93355, 94002, 94200, 94250, 94680-94690, 94770, 95812-95816, 95819, 95822, 95829, 95955, 96360-96368, 96372, 96374-96377, 96523, 97597-97598, 97602, 99155, 99156, 99157, 99211-99223, 99231-99255, 99291-99292, 99304-99310, 99315-99316, 99334-99337, 99347-99350, 99374-99375, 99377-99378, 99446-99449, 99451-99452, 99495-99496, G0463, G0471

58561 00952, 0213T, 0216T, 0228T, 0230T, 0404T✢, 11000-11006, 11042-11047, 12001-12007, 12011-12057, 13100-13133, 13151-13153, 36000, 36400-36410, 36420-36430, 36440, 36591-36592, 36600, 36640, 43752, 50715, 51701-51703, 57100, 57410, 57800, 58100, 58353, 58555-58558, 62320-62327, 64400, 64405-64408, 64415-64435, 64445-64454, 64461-64463, 64479-64505, 64510-64530, 69990, 76000, 77001-77002, 92012-92014, 93000-93010, 93040-93042, 93318, 93355, 94002, 94200, 94250, 94680-94690, 94770, 95812-95816, 95819, 95822, 95829, 95955, 96360-96368, 96372, 96374-96377, 96523, 97597-97598, 97602, 99155, 99156, 99157, 99211-99223, 99231-99255, 99291-99292, 99304-99310, 99315-99316, 99334-99337, 99347-99350, 99374-99375, 99377-99378, 99446-99449, 99451-99452, 99495-99496, G0463, G0471

58562 00952, 0213T, 0216T, 0228T, 0230T, 11000-11006, 11042-11047, 12001-12007, 12011-12057, 13100-13133, 13151-13153, 36000, 36400-36410, 36420-36430, 36440, 36591-36592, 36600, 36640, 43752, 50715, 51701-51703, 57100, 57410, 57800, 58100, 58301, 58555-58558, 62320-62327, 64400, 64405-64408, 64415-64435, 64445-64454, 64461-64463, 64479-64505, 64510-64530, 69990, 76000, 77001-77002, 92012-92014, 93000-93010, 93040-93042, 93318, 93355, 94002, 94200, 94250, 94680-94690, 94770, 95812-95816, 95819, 95822, 95829, 95955, 96360-96368, 96372, 96374-96377, 96523, 97597-97598, 97602, 99155, 99156, 99157, 99211-99223, 99231-99255, 99291-99292, 99304-99310, 99315-99316, 99334-99337, 99347-99350, 99374-99375, 99377-99378, 99446-99449, 99451-99452, 99495-99496, G0463, G0471, J0670, J2001

58563 00952, 0213T, 0216T, 0228T, 0230T, 11000-11006, 11042-11047, 12001-12007, 12011-12057, 13100-13133, 13151-13153, 36000, 36400-36410, 36420-36430, 36440, 36591-36592, 36600, 36640, 43752, 50715, 51701-51703, 57100, 57410, 57800, 58100, 58120, 58555-58558, 62320-62327, 64400, 64405-64408, 64415-64435, 64445-64454, 64461-64463, 64479-64505, 64510-64530, 69990, 76000, 77001-77002, 92012-92014, 93000-93010, 93040-93042, 93318, 93355, 94002, 94200, 94250, 94680-94690, 94770, 95812-95816, 95819, 95822, 95829, 95955, 96360-96368, 96372, 96374-96377, 96523, 97597-97598, 97602, 99155, 99156, 99157, 99211-99223, 99231-99255, 99291-99292, 99304-99310, 99315-99316, 99334-99337, 99347-99350, 99374-99375, 99377-99378, 99446-99449, 99451-99452, 99495-99496, G0463, G0471, J0670, J2001

58565 00952, 0213T, 0216T, 0228T, 0230T, 0567T, 12001-12007, 12011-12057, 13100-13133, 13151-13153, 36000, 36400-36410, 36420-36430, 36440, 36591-36592, 36600, 36640, 43752, 51701-51703, 57400-57410, 57800, 58100, 58555, 58615✦, 58671✦, 62320-62327, 64400, 64405-64408, 64415-64435, 64445-64454, 64461-64463, 64479-64505, 64510-64530, 69990, 76000, 77001-77002, 92012-92014, 93000-93010, 93040-93042, 93318, 93355, 94002, 94200, 94250, 94680-94690, 94770, 95812-95816, 95819, 95822, 95829, 95955, 96360-96368, 96372, 96374-96377, 96523, 99155, 99156, 99157, 99211-99223, 99231-99255, 99291-99292, 99304-99310, 99315-99316, 99334-99337, 99347-99350, 99374-99375, 99377-99378, 99446-99449, 99451-99452, 99495-99496, G0463, G0471, J0670, J2001

58570 0213T, 0216T, 0228T, 0230T, 11000-11006, 11042-11047, 12001-12007, 12011-12057, 13100-13133, 13151-13153, 36000, 36400-36410, 36420-36430, 36440, 36591-36592, 36600, 36640, 43752, 44180, 44602-44605, 44950, 44970, 49082-49084, 49320-49321, 49400, 51701-51703, 52000, 57000, 57020, 57100, 57180, 57400-57420, 57452-57455, 57460, 57500-57505, 57530, 57550-57555✦, 57558, 57800, 58100, 58110-58145, 58260✦, 58270✦, 58541✦, 58545, 58550✦, 58558, 58561, 58660-58661, 58670-58673, 58700-58720, 58940, 62320-62327, 64400, 64405-64408, 64415-64435, 64445-64454, 64461-64463, 64479-64505, 64510-64530, 69990, 76000, 77001-77002, 92012-92014, 93000-93010, 93040-93042, 93318, 93355, 94002, 94200, 94250, 94680-94690, 94770, 95812-95816, 95819, 95822, 95829, 95955, 96360-96368, 96372, 96374-96377, 96523, 97597-97598, 97602, 99155, 99156, 99157, 99211-99223, 99231-99255, 99291-99292, 99304-99310, 99315-99316, 99334-99337, 99347-99350, 99374-99375, 99377-99378, 99446-99449, 99451-99452, 99495-99496, G0463, G0471, P9612

58571 0213T, 0216T, 0228T, 0230T, 11000-11006, 11042-11047, 12001-12007, 12011-12057, 13100-13133, 13151-13153, 36000, 36400-36410, 36420-36430, 36440, 36591-36592, 36600, 36640, 43752, 44180, 44602-44605, 44950, 44970, 49082-49084, 49320-49321, 49400, 51701-51703, 52000, 57000, 57020, 57100, 57180, 57400-57420, 57452-57455, 57460, 57500-57505, 57530, 57550-57555✦, 57558, 57800, 58100, 58110-58145, 58150, 58180✦, 58260-58263✦, 58270-58275✦, 58541-58543✦, 58545, 58550✦, 58552✦, 58558, 58561, 58570, 58660-58661, 58670-58674, 58700-58720, 58940, 62320-62327, 64400, 64405-64408, 64415-64435, 64445-64454, 64461-64463, 64479-64505, 64510-64530, 69990, 76000, 77001-77002, 92012-92014, 93000-93010, 93040-93042, 93318, 93355, 94002, 94200, 94250, 94680-94690, 94770, 95812-95816, 95819, 95822, 95829, 95955, 96360-96368, 96372, 96374-96377, 96523, 97597-97598, 97602, 99155, 99156, 99157, 99211-99223, 99231-99255, 99291-99292, 99304-99310, 99315-99316, 99334-99337, 99347-99350, 99374-99375, 99377-99378, 99446-99449, 99451-99452, 99495-99496, G0463, G0471, P9612

58572 0213T, 0216T, 0228T, 0230T, 11000-11006, 11042-11047, 12001-12007, 12011-12057, 13100-13133, 13151-13153, 36000, 36400-36410, 36420-36430, 36440, 36591-36592, 36600, 36640, 43752, 44005, 44180, 44602-44605, 44950, 44970, 49082-49084, 49320-49321, 49400, 50715, 51701-51703, 52000, 57000, 57020, 57100, 57180, 57400-57420, 57452-57455, 57460, 57500-57505, 57530, 57550-57555✦, 57558, 57800, 58100, 58110-58145, 58150, 58180✦, 58260-58263✦, 58267-58280✦, 58541-58546, 58550✦, 58552-58553✦, 58558, 58561, 58570-58571✦, 58660-58661, 58670-58674, 58700-58720, 58940, 58943, 58950, 62320-62327, 64400, 64405-64408, 64415-64435, 64445-64454, 64461-64463, 64479-64505, 64510-64530, 69990, 76000, 77001-77002, 92012-92014, 93000-93010, 93040-93042, 93318, 93355, 94002, 94200, 94250, 94680-94690, 94770, 95812-95816, 95819, 95822, 95829, 95955, 96360-96368, 96372,

58573 0213T, 0216T, 0228T, 0230T, 11000-11006, 11042-11047, 12001-12007, 12011-12057, 13100-13133, 13151-13153, 36000, 36400-36410, 36420-36430, 36440, 36591-36592, 36600, 36640, 43752, 44005, 44180, 44602-44605, 44950, 44970, 49082-49084, 49320-49321, 49400, 50715, 51701-51703, 52000, 57000, 57020, 57100, 57180, 57400-57420, 57452-57455, 57460, 57500-57505, 57530, 57550-57555✦, 57558, 57800, 58100, 58110-58180✦, 58260-58263✦, 58267-58280✦, 58290-58291✦, 58294✦, 58541-58546, 58550✦, 58552-58554✦, 58558, 58561, 58570-58572, 58660-58661, 58670-58674, 58700-58720, 58940, 58943, 58950, 58956, 62320-62327, 64400, 64405-64408, 64415-64435, 64445-64454, 64461-64463, 64479-64505, 64510-64530, 69990, 76000, 77001-77002, 92012-92014, 93000-93010, 93040-93042, 93318, 93355, 94002, 94200, 94250, 94680-94690, 94770, 95812-95816, 95819, 95822, 95829, 95955, 96360-96368, 96372, 96374-96377, 96523, 97597-97598, 97602, 99155, 99156, 99157, 99211-99223, 99231-99255, 99291-99292, 99304-99310, 99315-99316, 99334-99337, 99347-99350, 99374-99375, 99377-99378, 99446-99449, 99451-99452, 99495-99496, G0463, G0471, P9612

58575 0213T, 0216T, 0228T, 0230T, 11000-11006, 11042-11047, 12001-12007, 12011-12057, 13100-13133, 13151-13153, 36000, 36400-36410, 36420-36430, 36440, 36591-36592, 36600, 36640, 43653, 43752, 44005, 44180, 44602-44605, 44950, 44970, 49082-49084, 49255, 49320-49322, 49400, 50715, 51701-51703, 52000, 57000, 57020, 57100, 57180, 57400-57420, 57452-57455, 57460, 57500-57505, 57530, 57550-57555✦, 57558, 57800, 58100, 58110-58146, 58152✦, 58260✦, 58267-58290✦, 58293-58294✦, 58545-58546, 58558, 58561, 58570-58573, 58660-58661, 58670-58674, 58740, 58940, 62320-62327, 64400, 64405-64408, 64415-64435, 64445-64454, 64461-64463, 64479-64505, 64510-64530, 69990, 76000, 77001-77002, 92012-92014, 93000-93010, 93040-93042, 93318, 93355, 94002, 94200, 94250, 94680-94690, 94770, 95812-95816, 95819, 95822, 95829, 95955, 96360-96368, 96372, 96374-96377, 96523, 97597-97598, 97602, 99155, 99156, 99157, 99211-99223, 99231-99255, 99291-99292, 99304-99310, 99315-99316, 99334-99337, 99347-99350, 99374-99375, 99377-99378, 99446-99449, 99451-99452, 99495-99496, G0463, G0471, P9612

58600 00851, 0213T, 0216T, 0228T, 0230T, 12001-12007, 12011-12057, 13100-13133, 13151-13153, 36000, 36400-36410, 36420-36430, 36440, 36591-36592, 36600, 36640, 43752, 44005, 44180, 44602-44605, 44820-44850, 44950, 44970, 49000-49010, 49255, 49320, 49406, 49570, 50715, 51701-51703, 57000-57010, 57100-57105, 57150, 57180, 57210, 57410, 58350, 58605, 58670-58671, 58700, 58805, 58900, 62320-62327, 64400, 64405-64408, 64415-64435, 64445-64454, 64461-64463, 64479-64505, 64510-64530, 69990, 92012-92014, 93000-93010, 93040-93042, 93318, 93355, 94002, 94200, 94250, 94680-94690, 94770, 95812-95816, 95819, 95822, 95829, 95955, 96360-96368, 96372, 96374-96377, 96523, 99155, 99156, 99157, 99211-99223, 99231-99255, 99291-99292, 99304-99310, 99315-99316, 99334-99337, 99347-99350, 99374-99375, 99377-99378, 99446-99449, 99451-99452, 99495-99496, G0463, G0471

58605 00851, 0213T, 0216T, 0228T, 0230T, 12001-12007, 12011-12057, 13100-13133, 13151-13153, 36000, 36400-36410, 36420-36430, 36440, 36591-36592, 36600, 36640, 43752, 44005, 44180, 44602-44605, 44820-44850, 44950, 44970, 49000-49010, 49255, 49320, 49406, 49570, 50715, 51701-51703, 57000-57010, 57100-57105, 57150, 57180, 57210, 57410, 58350, 58670-58671, 58805, 58900, 62320-62327, 64400, 64405-64408, 64415-64435, 64445-64454, 64461-64463,

64479-64505, 64510-64530, 69990, 92012-92014, 93000-93010, 93040-93042, 93318, 93355, 94002, 94200, 94250, 94680-94690, 94770, 95812-95816, 95819, 95822, 95829, 95955, 96360-96368, 96372, 96374-96377, 96523, 99155, 99156, 99157, 99211-99223, 99231-99255, 99291-99292, 99304-99310, 99315-99316, 99334-99337, 99347-99350, 99374-99375, 99377-99378, 99446-99449, 99451-99452, 99495-99496, G0463, G0471

58611 00851, 36591-36592, 44180, 50715, 57410, 58350, 58670-58671, 96523

58615 00851, 0213T, 0216T, 0228T, 0230T, 0567T✣, 12001-12007, 12011-12057, 13100-13133, 13151-13153, 36000, 36400-36410, 36420-36430, 36440, 36591-36592, 36600, 36640, 43752, 44005, 44180, 44602-44605, 44820-44850, 44950, 44970, 49000-49010, 49255, 49406, 49570, 50715, 51701-51703, 57000-57010, 57100-57105, 57150, 57180, 57210, 57410, 58350, 58605, 58700-58720, 58805, 58900, 62320-62327, 64400, 64405-64408, 64415-64435, 64445-64454, 64461-64463, 64479-64505, 64510-64530, 69990, 92012-92014, 93000-93010, 93040-93042, 93318, 93355, 94002, 94200, 94250, 94680-94690, 94770, 95812-95816, 95819, 95822, 95829, 95955, 96360-96368, 96372, 96374-96377, 96523, 99155, 99156, 99157, 99211-99223, 99231-99255, 99291-99292, 99304-99310, 99315-99316, 99334-99337, 99347-99350, 99374-99375, 99377-99378, 99446-99449, 99451-99452, 99495-99496, G0463, G0471

58660 0213T, 0216T, 0228T, 0230T, 12001-12007, 12011-12057, 13100-13133, 13151-13153, 36000, 36400-36410, 36420-36430, 36440, 36591-36592, 36600, 36640, 43653, 43752, 44005, 44180, 44602-44605, 49082-49084, 49320, 49400, 50715, 51701-51703, 57410, 58350, 58740, 62320-62327, 64400, 64405-64408, 64415-64435, 64445-64454, 64461-64463, 64479-64505, 64510-64530, 69990, 76000, 77001-77002, 92012-92014, 93000-93010, 93040-93042, 93318, 93355, 94002, 94200, 94250, 94680-94690, 94770, 95812-95816, 95819, 95822, 95829, 95955, 96360-96368, 96372, 96374-96377, 96523, 99155, 99156, 99157, 99211-99223, 99231-99255, 99291-99292, 99304-99310, 99315-99316, 99334-99337, 99347-99350, 99374-99375, 99377-99378, 99446-99449, 99451-99452, 99495-99496, G0463, G0471

58661 0213T, 0216T, 0228T, 0230T, 11000-11006, 11042-11047, 12001-12007, 12011-12057, 13100-13133, 13151-13153, 36000, 36400-36410, 36420-36430, 36440, 36591-36592, 36600, 36640, 43653, 43752, 44005, 44180, 44602-44605, 44950, 44970, 49082-49084, 49320-49322, 49400, 50715, 51701-51703, 52000, 57410, 58660, 58670, 58672-58673, 58740, 58900, 62320-62327, 64400, 64405-64408, 64415-64435, 64445-64454, 64461-64463, 64479-64505, 64510-64530, 69990, 76000, 77001-77002, 92012-92014, 93000-93010, 93040-93042, 93318, 93355, 94002, 94200, 94250, 94680-94690, 94770, 95812-95816, 95819, 95822, 95829, 95955, 96360-96368, 96372, 96374-96377, 96523, 97597-97598, 97602, 99155, 99156, 99157, 99211-99223, 99231-99255, 99291-99292, 99304-99310, 99315-99316, 99334-99337, 99347-99350, 99374-99375, 99377-99378, 99446-99449, 99451-99452, 99495-99496, G0463, G0471

58662 0213T, 0216T, 0228T, 0230T, 11000-11006, 11042-11047, 12001-12007, 12011-12057, 13100-13133, 13151-13153, 36000, 36400-36410, 36420-36430, 36440, 36591-36592, 36600, 36640, 43653, 43752, 44005, 44180, 44602-44605, 44950, 44970, 49082-49084, 49320, 49400, 50715, 51701-51703, 52000, 57410, 58350, 58660, 62320-62327, 64400, 64405-64408, 64415-64435, 64445-64454, 64461-64463, 64479-64505, 64510-64530, 69990, 76000, 77001-77002, 92012-92014, 93000-93010, 93040-93042, 93318, 93355, 94002, 94200, 94250, 94680-94690, 94770, 95812-95816, 95819, 95822, 95829, 95955, 96360-96368, 96372, 96374-96377, 96523, 97597-97598, 97602, 99155, 99156, 99157, 99211-99223, 99231-99255, 99291-99292,

99304-99310, 99315-99316, 99334-99337, 99347-99350, 99374-99375, 99377-99378, 99446-99449, 99451-99452, 99495-99496, G0463, G0471

58670 00851, 0213T, 0216T, 0228T, 0230T, 12001-12007, 12011-12057, 13100-13133, 13151-13153, 36000, 36400-36410, 36420-36430, 36440, 36591-36592, 36600, 36640, 43653, 43752, 44005, 44180, 44602-44605, 44950, 44970, 49082-49084, 49320, 49400, 50715, 51701-51703, 57410, 58350, 58660, 58671✣, 62320-62327, 64400, 64405-64408, 64415-64435, 64445-64454, 64461-64463, 64479-64505, 64510-64530, 69990, 76000, 77001-77002, 92012-92014, 93000-93010, 93040-93042, 93318, 93355, 94002, 94200, 94250, 94680-94690, 94770, 95812-95816, 95819, 95822, 95829, 95955, 96360-96368, 96372, 96374-96377, 96523, 99155, 99156, 99157, 99211-99223, 99231-99255, 99291-99292, 99304-99310, 99315-99316, 99334-99337, 99347-99350, 99374-99375, 99377-99378, 99446-99449, 99451-99452, 99495-99496, G0463, G0471

58671 00851, 0213T, 0216T, 0228T, 0230T, 0567T✣, 12001-12007, 12011-12057, 13100-13133, 13151-13153, 36000, 36400-36410, 36420-36430, 36440, 36591-36592, 36600, 36640, 43653, 43752, 44005, 44180, 44602-44605, 44950, 44970, 49082-49084, 49320, 49400, 50715, 51701-51703, 57410, 58350, 58660, 62320-62327, 64400, 64405-64408, 64415-64435, 64445-64454, 64461-64463, 64479-64505, 64510-64530, 69990, 76000, 77001-77002, 92012-92014, 93000-93010, 93040-93042, 93318, 93355, 94002, 94200, 94250, 94680-94690, 94770, 95812-95816, 95819, 95822, 95829, 95955, 96360-96368, 96372, 96374-96377, 96523, 99155, 99156, 99157, 99211-99223, 99231-99255, 99291-99292, 99304-99310, 99315-99316, 99334-99337, 99347-99350, 99374-99375, 99377-99378, 99446-99449, 99451-99452, 99495-99496, G0463, G0471

58672 0213T, 0216T, 0228T, 0230T, 11000-11006, 11042-11047, 12001-12007, 12011-12057, 13100-13133, 13151-13153, 36000, 36400-36410, 36420-36430, 36440, 36591-36592, 36600, 36640, 43653, 43752, 44005, 44180, 44602-44605, 44950, 44970, 49082-49084, 49320, 49400, 50715, 51701-51703, 57410, 58350, 58660, 62320-62327, 64400, 64405-64408, 64415-64435, 64445-64454, 64461-64463, 64479-64505, 64510-64530, 69990, 76000, 77001-77002, 92012-92014, 93000-93010, 93040-93042, 93318, 93355, 94002, 94200, 94250, 94680-94690, 94770, 95812-95816, 95819, 95822, 95829, 95955, 96360-96368, 96372, 96374-96377, 96523, 97597-97598, 97602, 99155, 99156, 99157, 99211-99223, 99231-99255, 99291-99292, 99304-99310, 99315-99316, 99334-99337, 99347-99350, 99374-99375, 99377-99378, 99446-99449, 99451-99452, 99495-99496, G0463, G0471

58673 0213T, 0216T, 0228T, 0230T, 12001-12007, 12011-12057, 13100-13133, 13151-13153, 36000, 36400-36410, 36420-36430, 36440, 36591-36592, 36600, 36640, 43653, 43752, 44005, 44180, 44602-44605, 44950, 44970, 49082-49084, 49320, 49400, 50715, 51701-51703, 57410, 58350, 58660, 62320-62327, 64400, 64405-64408, 64415-64435, 64445-64454, 64461-64463, 64479-64505, 64510-64530, 69990, 76000, 77001-77002, 92012-92014, 93000-93010, 93040-93042, 93318, 93355, 94002, 94200, 94250, 94680-94690, 94770, 95812-95816, 95819, 95822, 95829, 95955, 96360-96368, 96372, 96374-96377, 96523, 99155, 99156, 99157, 99211-99223, 99231-99255, 99291-99292, 99304-99310, 99315-99316, 99334-99337, 99347-99350, 99374-99375, 99377-99378, 99446-99449, 99451-99452, 99495-99496, G0463, G0471

58674 0071T, 0072T, 0213T, 0216T, 0228T, 0230T, 12001-12007, 12011-12057, 13100-13133, 13151-13153, 36000, 36400-36410, 36420-36430, 36440, 36591-36592, 36600, 36640, 37243✣, 43752, 44005, 44180, 49320, 50715, 51701-51703, 52000, 57410, 58145✣, 58541, 58561✣, 58570, 58660, 61650, 62320-62327, 64400, 64405-64408, 64415-64435, 64445-64454, 64461-64463, 64479-64505, 64510-64530, 69990, 76940,

76942, 76970, 76998, 92012-92014, 93000-93010, 93040-93042, 93318, 93355, 94002, 94200, 94250, 94680-94690, 94770, 95812-95816, 95819, 95822, 95829, 95955, 96360-96368, 96372, 96374-96377, 96523, 99155, 99156, 99157, 99211-99223, 99231-99255, 99291-99292, 99304-99310, 99315-99316, 99334-99337, 99347-99350, 99374-99375, 99377-99378, 99446-99449, 99451-99452, G0463, G0471

58700 0213T, 0216T, 0228T, 0230T, 11000-11006, 11042-11047, 12001-12007, 12011-12057, 13100-13133, 13151-13153, 36000, 36400-36410, 36420-36430, 36440, 36591-36592, 36600, 36640, 43752, 44005, 44180, 44602-44605, 44820-44850, 44950, 44970, 49000-49010, 49255, 49320-49321, 49570, 50715, 51701-51703, 52000, 57410, 58575, 58605, 58661-58673, 58740, 58900, 62320-62327, 64400, 64405-64408, 64415-64435, 64445-64454, 64461-64463, 64479-64505, 64510-64530, 69990, 92012-92014, 93000-93010, 93040-93042, 93318, 93355, 94002, 94200, 94250, 94680-94690, 94770, 95812-95816, 95819, 95822, 95829, 95955, 96360-96368, 96372, 96374-96377, 96523, 97597-97598, 97602, 99155, 99156, 99157, 99211-99223, 99231-99255, 99291-99292, 99304-99310, 99315-99316, 99334-99337, 99347-99350, 99374-99375, 99377-99378, 99446-99449, 99451-99452, 99495-99496, G0463, G0471

58720 0213T, 0216T, 0228T, 0230T, 11000-11006, 11042-11047, 12001-12007, 12011-12057, 13100-13133, 13151-13153, 36000, 36400-36410, 36420-36430, 36440, 36591-36592, 36600, 36640, 43752, 44005, 44180, 44602-44605, 44820-44850, 44950, 44970, 49000-49010, 49255, 49320-49321, 49406, 49570, 50715, 51701-51703, 52000, 57410, 58575, 58605, 58661-58673, 58700, 58740, 58805, 58900, 62320-62327, 64400, 64405-64408, 64415-64435, 64445-64454, 64461-64463, 64479-64505, 64510-64530, 69990, 92012-92014, 93000-93010, 93040-93042, 93318, 93355, 94002, 94200, 94250, 94680-94690, 94770, 95812-95816, 95819, 95822, 95829, 95955, 96360-96368, 96372, 96374-96377, 96523, 97597-97598, 97602, 99155, 99156, 99157, 99211-99223, 99231-99255, 99291-99292, 99304-99310, 99315-99316, 99334-99337, 99347-99350, 99374-99375, 99377-99378, 99446-99449, 99451-99452, 99495-99496, G0463, G0471

58740 0213T, 0216T, 0228T, 0230T, 12001-12007, 12011-12057, 13100-13133, 13151-13153, 36000, 36400-36410, 36420-36430, 36440, 36591-36592, 36600, 36640, 43752, 44005, 44180, 44602-44605, 44820-44850, 44950, 44970, 49000-49010, 49255, 49320, 49406, 49570, 50715, 51701-51703, 57410, 58350, 58805, 58900, 62320-62327, 64400, 64405-64408, 64415-64435, 64445-64454, 64461-64463, 64479-64505, 64510-64530, 69990, 92012-92014, 93000-93010, 93040-93042, 93318, 93355, 94002, 94200, 94250, 94680-94690, 94770, 95812-95816, 95819, 95822, 95829, 95955, 96360-96368, 96372, 96374-96377, 96523, 99155, 99156, 99157, 99211-99223, 99231-99255, 99291-99292, 99304-99310, 99315-99316, 99334-99337, 99347-99350, 99374-99375, 99377-99378, 99446-99449, 99451-99452, 99495-99496, G0463, G0471

58750 0213T, 0216T, 0228T, 0230T, 12001-12007, 12011-12057, 13100-13133, 13151-13153, 36000, 36400-36410, 36420-36430, 36440, 36591-36592, 36600, 36640, 43752, 44005, 44180, 44602-44605, 44820-44850, 44950, 44970, 49000-49010, 49255, 49320, 49406, 49570, 50715, 51701-51703, 57410, 58350, 58660, 58805, 58900, 62320-62327, 64400, 64405-64408, 64415-64435, 64445-64454, 64461-64463, 64479-64505, 64510-64530, 69990, 92012-92014, 93000-93010, 93040-93042, 93318, 93355, 94002, 94200, 94250, 94680-94690, 94770, 95812-95816, 95819, 95822, 95829, 95955, 96360-96368, 96372, 96374-96377, 96523, 99155, 99156, 99157, 99211-99223, 99231-99255, 99291-99292, 99304-99310, 99315-99316, 99334-99337, 99347-99350, 99374-99375, 99377-99378, 99446-99449, 99451-99452, 99495-99496, G0463, G0471

58752 0213T, 0216T, 0228T, 0230T, 12001-12007, 12011-12057, 13100-13133, 13151-13153, 36000, 36400-36410, 36420-36430, 36440, 36591-36592, 36600, 36640, 43752, 44005, 44180, 44602-44605, 44820-44850, 44950, 44970, 49000-49010, 49255, 49320, 49406, 49570, 50715, 51701-51703, 57410, 58350, 58660, 58805, 58900, 62320-62327, 64400, 64405-64408, 64415-64435, 64445-64454, 64461-64463, 64479-64505, 64510-64530, 69990, 92012-92014, 93000-93010, 93040-93042, 93318, 93355, 94002, 94200, 94250, 94680-94690, 94770, 95812-95816, 95819, 95822, 95829, 95955, 96360-96368, 96372, 96374-96377, 96523, 99155, 99156, 99157, 99211-99223, 99231-99255, 99291-99292, 99304-99310, 99315-99316, 99334-99337, 99347-99350, 99374-99375, 99377-99378, 99446-99449, 99451-99452, 99495-99496, G0463, G0471

58760 0213T, 0216T, 0228T, 0230T, 11000-11006, 11042-11047, 12001-12007, 12011-12057, 13100-13133, 13151-13153, 36000, 36400-36410, 36420-36430, 36440, 36591-36592, 36600, 36640, 43752, 44005, 44180, 44602-44605, 44820-44850, 44950, 44970, 49000-49010, 49255, 49320, 49406, 49570, 50715, 51701-51703, 57410, 58350, 58660, 58672, 58805, 58900, 62320-62327, 64400, 64405-64408, 64415-64435, 64445-64454, 64461-64463, 64479-64505, 64510-64530, 69990, 92012-92014, 93000-93010, 93040-93042, 93318, 93355, 94002, 94200, 94250, 94680-94690, 94770, 95812-95816, 95819, 95822, 95829, 95955, 96360-96368, 96372, 96374-96377, 96523, 97597-97598, 97602, 99155, 99156, 99157, 99211-99223, 99231-99255, 99291-99292, 99304-99310, 99315-99316, 99334-99337, 99347-99350, 99374-99375, 99377-99378, 99446-99449, 99451-99452, 99495-99496, G0463, G0471

58770 0213T, 0216T, 0228T, 0230T, 12001-12007, 12011-12057, 13100-13133, 13151-13153, 36000, 36400-36410, 36420-36430, 36440, 36591-36592, 36600, 36640, 43752, 44005, 44180, 44602-44605, 44820-44850, 44950, 44970, 49000-49010, 49255, 49320, 49406, 49570, 50715, 51701-51703, 57410, 58350, 58660, 58673, 58805, 58900, 62320-62327, 64400, 64405-64408, 64415-64435, 64445-64454, 64461-64463, 64479-64505, 64510-64530, 69990, 92012-92014, 93000-93010, 93040-93042, 93318, 93355, 94002, 94200, 94250, 94680-94690, 94770, 95812-95816, 95819, 95822, 95829, 95955, 96360-96368, 96372, 96374-96377, 96523, 99155, 99156, 99157, 99211-99223, 99231-99255, 99291-99292, 99304-99310, 99315-99316, 99334-99337, 99347-99350, 99374-99375, 99377-99378, 99446-99449, 99451-99452, 99495-99496, G0463, G0471

58800 0213T, 0216T, 0228T, 0230T, 12001-12007, 12011-12057, 13100-13133, 13151-13153, 36000, 36400-36410, 36420-36430, 36440, 36591-36592, 36600, 36640, 43752, 49322, 49407, 50715, 51701-51703, 57410, 58660, 58900, 62320-62327, 64400, 64405-64408, 64415-64435, 64445-64454, 64461-64463, 64479-64505, 64510-64530, 69990, 92012-92014, 93000-93010, 93040-93042, 93318, 93355, 94002, 94200, 94250, 94680-94690, 94770, 95812-95816, 95819, 95822, 95829, 95955, 96360-96368, 96372, 96374-96377, 96523, 99155, 99156, 99157, 99211-99223, 99231-99255, 99291-99292, 99304-99310, 99315-99316, 99334-99337, 99347-99350, 99374-99375, 99377-99378, 99446-99449, 99451-99452, 99495-99496, G0463, G0471, J0670, J2001

58805 0213T, 0216T, 0228T, 0230T, 12001-12007, 12011-12057, 13100-13133, 13151-13153, 36000, 36400-36410, 36420-36430, 36440, 36591-36592, 36600, 36640, 43752, 44005, 44180, 44602-44605, 44820-44850, 44950, 44970, 49000-49010, 49255, 49320, 49322, 49406, 49570, 50715, 51701-51703, 57410, 58660, 58700, 58800✦, 62320-62327, 64400, 64405-64408, 64415-64435, 64445-64454, 64461-64463, 64479-64505, 64510-64530, 69990, 92012-92014, 93000-93010, 93040-93042, 93318, 93355, 94002, 94200, 94250, 94680-94690, 94770, 95812-95816, 95819, 95822, 95829, 95955, 96360-96368, 96372, 96374-96377, 96523, 99155, 99156, 99157, 99211-99223,

99231-99255, 99291-99292, 99304-99310, 99315-99316, 99334-99337, 99347-99350, 99374-99375, 99377-99378, 99446-99449, 99451-99452, 99495-99496, G0463, G0471

58820 0213T, 0216T, 0228T, 0230T, 12001-12007, 12011-12057, 13100-13133, 13151-13153, 36000, 36400-36410, 36420-36430, 36440, 36591-36592, 36600, 36640, 43752, 49406-49407, 50715, 51701-51703, 57000, 57100-57105, 57150, 57180, 57210, 57410, 58660, 58800-58805, 58822❖, 58900, 62320-62327, 64400, 64405-64408, 64415-64435, 64445-64454, 64461-64463, 64479-64505, 64510-64530, 69990, 92012-92014, 93000-93010, 93040-93042, 93318, 93355, 94002, 94200, 94250, 94680-94690, 94770, 95812-95816, 95819, 95822, 95829, 95955, 96360-96368, 96372, 96374-96377, 96523, 99155, 99156, 99157, 99211-99223, 99231-99255, 99291-99292, 99304-99310, 99315-99316, 99334-99337, 99347-99350, 99374-99375, 99377-99378, 99446-99449, 99451-99452, 99495-99496, G0463, G0471

58822 0213T, 0216T, 0228T, 0230T, 12001-12007, 12011-12057, 13100-13133, 13151-13153, 36000, 36400-36410, 36420-36430, 36440, 36591-36592, 36600, 36640, 43752, 44005, 44180, 44602-44605, 44850, 44950, 44970, 49000-49010, 49255, 49320, 49406-49407❖, 49570, 50715, 51701-51703, 57410, 58660, 58700, 58800, 58900, 62320-62327, 64400, 64405-64408, 64415-64435, 64445-64454, 64461-64463, 64479-64505, 64510-64530, 92012-92014, 93000-93010, 93040-93042, 93318, 93355, 94002, 94200, 94250, 94680-94690, 94770, 95812-95816, 95819, 95822, 95829, 95955, 96360-96368, 96372, 96374-96377, 96523, 99155, 99156, 99157, 99211-99223, 99231-99255, 99291-99292, 99304-99310, 99315-99316, 99334-99337, 99347-99350, 99374-99375, 99377-99378, 99446-99449, 99451-99452, 99495-99496, G0463, G0471

58825 0213T, 0216T, 0228T, 0230T, 12001-12007, 12011-12057, 13100-13133, 13151-13153, 36000, 36400-36410, 36420-36430, 36440, 36591-36592, 36600, 36640, 43752, 44005, 44180, 44602-44605, 44820-44850, 44950, 44970, 49000-49010, 49255, 49320, 49406, 49570, 50715, 51701-51703, 57410, 58660, 58805, 58900, 62320-62327, 64400, 64405-64408, 64415-64435, 64445-64454, 64461-64463, 64479-64505, 64510-64530, 69990, 92012-92014, 93000-93010, 93040-93042, 93318, 93355, 94002, 94200, 94250, 94680-94690, 94770, 95812-95816, 95819, 95822, 95829, 95955, 96360-96368, 96372, 96374-96377, 96523, 99155, 99156, 99157, 99211-99223, 99231-99255, 99291-99292, 99304-99310, 99315-99316, 99334-99337, 99347-99350, 99374-99375, 99377-99378, 99446-99449, 99451-99452, 99495-99496, G0463, G0471

58900 0213T, 0216T, 0228T, 0230T, 10005, 10007, 10009, 10011, 10021, 12001-12007, 12011-12057, 13100-13133, 13151-13153, 36000, 36400-36410, 36420-36430, 36440, 36591-36592, 36600, 36640, 43752, 44005, 44180, 44602-44605, 44820-44850, 44950, 44970, 49000-49010, 49255, 49320, 49570, 50715, 51701-51703, 57410, 58660, 58805, 62320-62327, 64400, 64405-64408, 64415-64435, 64445-64454, 64461-64463, 64479-64505, 64510-64530, 69990, 92012-92014, 93000-93010, 93040-93042, 93318, 93355, 94002, 94200, 94250, 94680-94690, 94770, 95812-95816, 95819, 95822, 95829, 95955, 96360-96368, 96372, 96374-96377, 96523, 99155, 99156, 99157, 99211-99223, 99231-99255, 99291-99292, 99304-99310, 99315-99316, 99334-99337, 99347-99350, 99374-99375, 99377-99378, 99446-99449, 99451-99452, 99495-99496, G0463, G0471

58920 0213T, 0216T, 0228T, 0230T, 11000-11006, 11042-11047, 12001-12007, 12011-12057, 13100-13133, 13151-13153, 36000, 36400-36410, 36420-36430, 36440, 36591-36592, 36600, 36640, 43752, 44005, 44180, 44602-44605, 44820-44850, 44950, 44970, 49000-49010, 49255, 49320, 49322, 49406, 49570, 50715, 51701-51703, 57410, 58575, 58660-58662, 58805, 58900, 62320-62327, 64400, 64405-64408,

64415-64435, 64445-64454, 64461-64463, 64479-64505, 64510-64530, 69990, 92012-92014, 93000-93010, 93040-93042, 93318, 93355, 94002, 94200, 94250, 94680-94690, 94770, 95812-95816, 95819, 95822, 95829, 95955, 96360-96368, 96372, 96374-96377, 96523, 97597-97598, 97602, 99155, 99156, 99157, 99211-99223, 99231-99255, 99291-99292, 99304-99310, 99315-99316, 99334-99337, 99347-99350, 99374-99375, 99377-99378, 99446-99449, 99451-99452, 99495-99496, G0463, G0471

58925 0213T, 0216T, 0228T, 0230T, 11000-11006, 11042-11047, 12001-12007, 12011-12057, 13100-13133, 13151-13153, 36000, 36400-36410, 36420-36430, 36440, 36591-36592, 36600, 36640, 43752, 44005, 44180, 44602-44605, 44820-44850, 44950, 44970, 49000-49010, 49255, 49320-49322, 49406, 49570, 50715, 51701-51703, 57410, 58575, 58660-58662, 58740, 58805, 58900, 62320-62327, 64400, 64405-64408, 64415-64435, 64445-64454, 64461-64463, 64479-64505, 64510-64530, 69990, 92012-92014, 93000-93010, 93040-93042, 93318, 93355, 94002, 94200, 94250, 94680-94690, 94770, 95812-95816, 95819, 95822, 95829, 95955, 96360-96368, 96372, 96374-96377, 96523, 97597-97598, 97602, 99155, 99156, 99157, 99211-99223, 99231-99255, 99291-99292, 99304-99310, 99315-99316, 99334-99337, 99347-99350, 99374-99375, 99377-99378, 99446-99449, 99451-99452, 99495-99496, G0463, G0471

58940 0213T, 0216T, 0228T, 0230T, 11000-11006, 11042-11047, 12001-12007, 12011-12057, 13100-13133, 13151-13153, 36000, 36400-36410, 36420-36430, 36440, 36591-36592, 36600, 36640, 43752, 44005, 44180, 44602-44605, 44820-44850, 44950, 44970, 49000-49010, 49255, 49320-49322, 49406, 49570, 50715, 51701-51703, 52000, 57410, 58660-58662, 58740, 58805, 58900, 62320-62327, 64400, 64405-64408, 64415-64435, 64445-64454, 64461-64463, 64479-64505, 64510-64530, 69990, 92012-92014, 93000-93010, 93040-93042, 93318, 93355, 94002, 94200, 94250, 94680-94690, 94770, 95812-95816, 95819, 95822, 95829, 95955, 96360-96368, 96372, 96374-96377, 96523, 97597-97598, 97602, 99155, 99156, 99157, 99211-99223, 99231-99255, 99291-99292, 99304-99310, 99315-99316, 99334-99337, 99347-99350, 99374-99375, 99377-99378, 99446-99449, 99451-99452, 99495-99496, G0463, G0471

58943 0213T, 0216T, 0228T, 0230T, 10005, 10007, 10009, 10011, 10021, 11000-11006, 11042-11047, 12001-12007, 12011-12057, 13100-13133, 13151-13153, 36000, 36400-36410, 36420-36430, 36440, 36591-36592, 36600, 36640, 38562, 38573, 43752, 44005, 44180, 44602-44605, 44820-44850, 44950, 44970, 49000-49010, 49255, 49320-49322, 49406, 49570, 50715, 51701-51703, 52000, 57410, 58541-58544, 58548-58550, 58552, 58554, 58570-58571, 58575, 58660-58673, 58740, 58805, 58900, 58940, 62320-62327, 64400, 64405-64408, 64415-64435, 64445-64454, 64461-64463, 64479-64505, 64510-64530, 69990, 92012-92014, 93000-93010, 93040-93042, 93318, 93355, 94002, 94200, 94250, 94680-94690, 94770, 95812-95816, 95819, 95822, 95829, 95955, 96360-96368, 96372, 96374-96377, 96523, 97597-97598, 97602, 99155, 99156, 99157, 99211-99223, 99231-99255, 99291-99292, 99304-99310, 99315-99316, 99334-99337, 99347-99350, 99374-99375, 99377-99378, 99446-99449, 99451-99452, 99495-99496, G0463, G0471

58950 0213T, 0216T, 0228T, 0230T, 11000-11006, 11042-11047, 12001-12007, 12011-12057, 13100-13133, 13151-13153, 36000, 36400-36410, 36420-36430, 36440, 36591-36592, 36600, 36640, 43752, 44005, 44180, 44602-44605, 44820-44850, 44950, 44970, 49000-49010, 49082-49084, 49180, 49255, 49320-49322, 49406, 49570, 50715, 51701-51703, 52000, 57410, 57530-57545, 58140-58200, 58210, 58260-58263, 58267-58285, 58541-58544, 58548-58550, 58552, 58554, 58570-58571, 58575, 58660-58673, 58700-58740, 58805, 58900-58925, 58943, 58960, 62320-62327, 64400, 64405-64408, 64415-64435, 64445-64454, 64461-64463, 64479-64505, 64510-64530, 69990, 92012-92014, 93000-93010, 93040-93042, 93318, 93355, 94002, 94200, 94250, 94680-94690, 94770, 95812-95816, 95819, 95822, 95829,

95955, 96360-96368, 96372, 96374-96377, 96523, 97597-97598, 97602, 99155, 99156, 99157, 99211-99223, 99231-99255, 99291-99292, 99304-99310, 99315-99316, 99334-99337, 99347-99350, 99374-99375, 99377-99378, 99446-99449, 99451-99452, 99495-99496, G0463, G0471

58951 0213T, 0216T, 0228T, 0230T, 11000-11006, 11042-11047, 12001-12007, 12011-12057, 13100-13133, 13151-13153, 36000, 36400-36410, 36420-36430, 36440, 36591-36592, 36600, 36640, 38562, 38570-38573, 38770, 38780, 43752, 44005, 44180, 44602-44605, 44820-44850, 44950, 44970, 49000-49010, 49082-49084, 49180, 49203, 49255, 49320-49322, 49406, 49570, 50715, 51701-51703, 52000, 57410, 57454-57455, 57460, 57505, 57530-57555❖, 57558, 58100, 58110-58200, 58210, 58541-58550, 58552, 58554, 58558, 58561, 58570-58575, 58660-58673, 58700-58740, 58805, 58900-58925, 58943, 58950, 58960, 62320-62327, 64400, 64405-64408, 64415-64435, 64445-64454, 64461-64463, 64479-64505, 64510-64530, 69990, 92012-92014, 93000-93010, 93040-93042, 93318, 93355, 94002, 94200, 94250, 94680-94690, 94770, 95812-95816, 95819, 95822, 95829, 95955, 96360-96368, 96372, 96374-96377, 96523, 97597-97598, 97602, 99155, 99156, 99157, 99211-99223, 99231-99255, 99291-99292, 99304-99310, 99315-99316, 99334-99337, 99347-99350, 99374-99375, 99377-99378, 99446-99449, 99451-99452, 99495-99496, G0463, G0471

58952 0213T, 0216T, 0228T, 0230T, 11000-11006, 11042-11047, 12001-12007, 12011-12057, 13100-13133, 13151-13153, 36000, 36400-36410, 36420-36430, 36440, 36591-36592, 36600, 36640, 38562, 38573, 38770, 38780, 43752, 44005, 44180, 44602-44605, 44820-44850, 44950, 44970, 49000-49010, 49082-49084, 49180, 49203-49204, 49215, 49255, 49320-49322, 49406, 49570, 50715, 51701-51703, 52000, 57410, 57530-57545, 58110, 58140-58200, 58210, 58260-58263, 58267-58285, 58541-58544, 58548-58550, 58552, 58554, 58570-58575, 58660-58673, 58700-58740, 58805, 58900-58940, 58943, 58950-58951, 58957, 58960, 62320-62327, 64400, 64405-64408, 64415-64435, 64445-64454, 64461-64463, 64479-64505, 64510-64530, 69990, 92012-92014, 93000-93010, 93040-93042, 93318, 93355, 94002, 94200, 94250, 94680-94690, 94770, 95812-95816, 95819, 95822, 95829, 95955, 96360-96368, 96372, 96374-96377, 96523, 97597-97598, 97602, 99155, 99156, 99157, 99211-99223, 99231-99255, 99291-99292, 99304-99310, 99315-99316, 99334-99337, 99347-99350, 99374-99375, 99377-99378, 99446-99449, 99451-99452, 99495-99496, G0463, G0471

58953 0213T, 0216T, 0228T, 0230T, 11000-11006, 11042-11047, 12001-12007, 12011-12057, 13100-13133, 13151-13153, 36000, 36400-36410, 36420-36430, 36440, 36591-36592, 36600, 36640, 38562, 38573, 38770, 38780, 43752, 44005, 44180, 44602-44605, 44820-44850, 44950, 44970, 49000-49010, 49082-49084, 49180, 49203-49215, 49255, 49320-49322, 49406, 49570, 50715, 51701-51703, 52000, 57410, 57454-57455, 57460, 57505, 57530-57555❖, 58100, 58110-58200, 58210, 58260-58263, 58267-58285, 58541-58550, 58558, 58561, 58570-58575, 58660-58673, 58700-58740, 58805, 58822, 58900-58940, 58943, 58950-58952, 58956-58960, 62320-62327, 64400, 64405-64408, 64415-64435, 64445-64454, 64461-64463, 64479-64505, 64510-64530, 69990, 92012-92014, 93000-93010, 93040-93042, 93318, 93355, 94002, 94200, 94250, 94680-94690, 94770, 95812-95816, 95819, 95822, 95829, 95955, 96360-96368, 96372, 96374-96377, 96523, 97597-97598, 97602, 99155, 99156, 99157, 99211-99223, 99231-99255, 99291-99292, 99304-99310, 99315-99316, 99334-99337, 99347-99350, 99374-99375, 99377-99378, 99446-99449, 99451-99452, 99495-99496, G0463, G0471, P9612

58954 0213T, 0216T, 0228T, 0230T, 11000-11006, 11042-11047, 12001-12007, 12011-12057, 13100-13133, 13151-13153, 36000, 36400-36410, 36420-36430, 36440, 36591-36592, 36600, 36640, 38562, 38570-38573, 38770, 38780, 43752, 44005, 44180, 44602-44605, 44820-44850,

44950, 44970, 49000-49010, 49082-49084, 49180, 49203-49215, 49255, 49320-49322, 49406, 49570, 50715, 51701-51703, 52000, 57410, 57454-57455, 57460, 57505, 57530-57555❖, 58100, 58110-58200, 58210, 58260-58263, 58267-58285, 58541-58550, 58558, 58561, 58570-58575, 58660-58673, 58700-58740, 58805, 58822, 58900-58940, 58943, 58950-58953, 58956-58960, 62320-62327, 64400, 64405-64408, 64415-64435, 64445-64454, 64461-64463, 64479-64505, 64510-64530, 69990, 92012-92014, 93000-93010, 93040-93042, 93318, 93355, 94002, 94200, 94250, 94680-94690, 94770, 95812-95816, 95819, 95822, 95829, 95955, 96360-96368, 96372, 96374-96377, 96523, 97597-97598, 97602, 99155, 99156, 99157, 99211-99223, 99231-99255, 99291-99292, 99304-99310, 99315-99316, 99334-99337, 99347-99350, 99374-99375, 99377-99378, 99446-99449, 99451-99452, 99495-99496, G0463, G0471, P9612

58956 0213T, 0216T, 0228T, 0230T, 11000-11006, 11042-11047, 12001-12007, 12011-12057, 13100-13133, 13151-13153, 36000, 36400-36410, 36420-36430, 36440, 36591-36592, 36600, 36640, 38562, 38573, 38770, 38780, 43752, 44005, 44180, 44602-44605, 44820-44850, 44950, 44970, 49000-49010, 49082-49084, 49180, 49203, 49255, 49320-49322, 49406, 49570, 50715, 51701-51703, 52000, 57410, 57454-57455, 57460, 57505, 57530-57555❖, 57558, 58100, 58110-58200, 58210, 58260-58263, 58267-58294, 58541-58550, 58552-58554, 58558, 58561, 58570-58572, 58575, 58660-58673, 58700-58740, 58805, 58822, 58900-58940, 58943, 58950-58952, 58960, 62320-62327, 64400, 64405-64408, 64415-64435, 64445-64454, 64461-64463, 64479-64505, 64510-64530, 69990, 92012-92014, 93000-93010, 93040-93042, 93318, 93355, 94002, 94200, 94250, 94680-94690, 94770, 95812-95816, 95819, 95822, 95829, 95955, 96360-96368, 96372, 96374-96377, 96523, 97597-97598, 97602, 99155, 99156, 99157, 99211-99223, 99231-99255, 99291-99292, 99304-99310, 99315-99316, 99334-99337, 99347-99350, 99374-99375, 99377-99378, 99446-99449, 99451-99452, 99495-99496, G0463, G0471, P9612

58957 0213T, 0216T, 0228T, 0230T, 11000-11006, 11042-11047, 12001-12007, 12011-12057, 13100-13133, 13151-13153, 36000, 36400-36410, 36420-36430, 36440, 36591-36592, 36600, 36640, 38570-38573, 38770, 38780, 43752, 44005, 44180, 44602-44605, 44820-44850, 44950, 44970, 49000-49010, 49082-49084, 49180, 49203-49204, 49215, 49255, 49320-49321, 49570, 50715, 51701-51703, 52000, 57410, 58541-58544, 58548, 58570-58575, 58660-58673, 58700-58740, 58900-58940, 58943, 58950-58951, 58956, 58960, 62320-62327, 64400, 64405-64408, 64415-64435, 64445-64454, 64461-64463, 64479-64505, 64510-64530, 69990, 92012-92014, 93000-93010, 93040-93042, 93318, 93355, 94002, 94200, 94250, 94680-94690, 94770, 95812-95816, 95819, 95822, 95829, 95955, 96360-96368, 96372, 96374-96377, 96523, 97597-97598, 97602, 99155, 99156, 99157, 99211-99223, 99231-99255, 99291-99292, 99304-99310, 99315-99316, 99334-99337, 99347-99350, 99374-99375, 99377-99378, 99446-99449, 99451-99452, 99495-99496, G0463, G0471

58958 0213T, 0216T, 0228T, 0230T, 11000-11006, 11042-11047, 12001-12007, 12011-12057, 13100-13133, 13151-13153, 36000, 36400-36410, 36420-36430, 36440, 36591-36592, 36600, 36640, 38570-38573, 38770, 38780, 43752, 44005, 44180, 44602-44605, 44820-44850, 44950, 44970, 49000-49010, 49082-49084, 49180, 49203-49204, 49215, 49255, 49320-49321, 49570, 50715, 51701-51703, 52000, 57410, 58541-58544, 58548, 58570-58575, 58660-58673, 58700-58740, 58900-58940, 58943, 58950-58952, 58956-58957, 58960, 62320-62327, 64400, 64405-64408, 64415-64435, 64445-64454, 64461-64463, 64479-64505, 64510-64530, 69990, 92012-92014, 93000-93010, 93040-93042, 93318, 93355, 94002, 94200, 94250, 94680-94690, 94770, 95812-95816, 95819, 95822, 95829, 95955, 96360-96368, 96372, 96374-96377, 96523, 97597-97598, 97602, 99155, 99156, 99157, 99211-99223, 99231-99255, 99291-99292,

99304-99310, 99315-99316, 99334-99337, 99347-99350, 99374-99375, 99377-99378, 99446-99449, 99451-99452, 99495-99496, G0463, G0471

58960 0213T, 0216T, 0228T, 0230T, 10005, 10007, 10009, 10011, 10021, 11000-11006, 11042-11047, 12001-12007, 12011-12057, 13100-13133, 13151-13153, 36000, 36400-36410, 36420-36430, 36440, 36591-36592, 36600, 36640, 38562, 38571-38572, 38770, 38780, 43752, 44005, 44180, 44602-44605, 44820-44850, 44950, 44970, 49000-49010, 49255, 49320-49321, 49406, 49570, 50715, 51701-51703, 52000, 57410, 58548, 58660, 58720, 58805, 58900, 62320-62327, 64400, 64405-64408, 64415-64435, 64445-64454, 64461-64463, 64479-64505, 64510-64530, 69990, 92012-92014, 93000-93010, 93040-93042, 93318, 93355, 94002, 94200, 94250, 94680-94690, 94770, 95812-95816, 95819, 95822, 95829, 95955, 96360-96368, 96372, 96374-96377, 96523, 97597-97598, 97602, 99155, 99156, 99157, 99211-99223, 99231-99255, 99291-99292, 99304-99310, 99315-99316, 99334-99337, 99347-99350, 99374-99375, 99377-99378, 99446-99449, 99451-99452, 99495-99496, G0463, G0471

58970 0213T, 0216T, 0228T, 0230T, 12001-12007, 12011-12057, 13100-13133, 13151-13153, 36000, 36400-36410, 36420-36430, 36440, 36591-36592, 36600, 36640, 43752, 49320, 51701-51703, 57410, 62320-62327, 64400, 64405-64408, 64415-64435, 64445-64454, 64461-64463, 64479-64505, 64510-64530, 69990, 76000, 76942, 76970, 76998, 77001-77002, 92012-92014, 93000-93010, 93040-93042, 93318, 93355, 94002, 94200, 94250, 94680-94690, 94770, 95812-95816, 95819, 95822, 95829, 95955, 96360-96368, 96372, 96374-96377, 96523, 99155, 99156, 99157, 99211-99223, 99231-99255, 99291-99292, 99304-99310, 99315-99316, 99334-99337, 99347-99350, 99374-99375, 99377-99378, 99446-99449, 99451-99452, 99495-99496, G0463, G0471

58974 0213T, 0216T, 0228T, 0230T, 12001-12007, 12011-12057, 13100-13133, 13151-13153, 36000, 36400-36410, 36420-36430, 36440, 36591-36592, 36600, 36640, 43752, 51701-51703, 57410, 62320-62327, 64400, 64405-64408, 64415-64435, 64445-64454, 64461-64463, 64479-64505, 64510-64530, 69990, 92012-92014, 93000-93010, 93040-93042, 93318, 93355, 94002, 94200, 94250, 94680-94690, 94770, 95812-95816, 95819, 95822, 95829, 95955, 96360-96368, 96372, 96374-96377, 96523, 99155, 99156, 99157, 99211-99223, 99231-99255, 99291-99292, 99304-99310, 99315-99316, 99334-99337, 99347-99350, 99374-99375, 99377-99378, 99446-99449, 99451-99452, 99495-99496, G0463, G0471

58976 0213T, 0216T, 0228T, 0230T, 12001-12007, 12011-12057, 13100-13133, 13151-13153, 36000, 36400-36410, 36420-36430, 36440, 36591-36592, 36600, 36640, 43752, 51701-51703, 57410, 62320-62327, 64400, 64405-64408, 64415-64435, 64445-64454, 64461-64463, 64479-64505, 64510-64530, 69990, 92012-92014, 93000-93010, 93040-93042, 93318, 93355, 94002, 94200, 94250, 94680-94690, 94770, 95812-95816, 95819, 95822, 95829, 95955, 96360-96368, 96372, 96374-96377, 96523, 99155, 99156, 99157, 99211-99223, 99231-99255, 99291-99292, 99304-99310, 99315-99316, 99334-99337, 99347-99350, 99374-99375, 99377-99378, 99446-99449, 99451-99452, 99495-99496, G0463, G0471

59000 0213T, 0216T, 0228T, 0230T, 12001-12007, 12011-12057, 13100-13133, 13151-13153, 36000, 36400-36410, 36420-36430, 36440, 36591-36592, 36600, 36640, 43752, 51701-51703, 57410, 62320-62327, 64400, 64405-64408, 64415-64435, 64445-64454, 64461-64463, 64479-64505, 64510-64530, 69990, 76000, 76942, 76970, 76998, 77001-77002, 92012-92014, 93000-93010, 93040-93042, 93318, 93355, 94002, 94200, 94250, 94680-94690, 94770, 95812-95816, 95819, 95822, 95829, 95955, 96360-96368, 96372, 96374-96377, 96523, 99155, 99156, 99157, 99211-99223, 99231-99255, 99291-99292, 99304-99310, 99315-99316, 99334-99337, 99347-99350, 99374-99375, 99377-99378, 99446-99449, 99451-99452, 99495-99496, G0463, G0471

59001 0213T, 0216T, 0228T, 0230T, 12001-12007, 12011-12057, 13100-13133, 13151-13153, 36000, 36400-36410, 36420-36430, 36440, 36591-36592, 36600, 36640, 43752, 51701-51703, 57410, 59000, 62320-62327, 64400, 64405-64408, 64415-64435, 64445-64454, 64461-64463, 64479-64505, 64510-64530, 69990, 76941-76942, 76945-76946, 76970, 76998, 92012-92014, 93000-93010, 93040-93042, 93318, 93355, 94002, 94200, 94250, 94680-94690, 94770, 95812-95816, 95819, 95822, 95829, 95955, 96360-96368, 96372, 96374-96377, 96523, 99155, 99156, 99157, 99211-99223, 99231-99255, 99291-99292, 99304-99310, 99315-99316, 99334-99337, 99347-99350, 99374-99375, 99377-99378, 99446-99449, 99451-99452, 99495-99496, G0463, G0471

59012 0213T, 0216T, 0228T, 0230T, 12001-12007, 12011-12057, 13100-13133, 13151-13153, 36000, 36400-36410, 36420-36430, 36440, 36591-36592, 36600, 36640, 43752, 51701-51703, 57410, 62320-62327, 64400, 64405-64408, 64415-64435, 64445-64454, 64461-64463, 64479-64505, 64510-64530, 69990, 76000, 76942, 76970, 76998, 77001-77002, 92012-92014, 93000-93010, 93040-93042, 93318, 93355, 94002, 94200, 94250, 94680-94690, 94770, 95812-95816, 95819, 95822, 95829, 95955, 96360-96368, 96372, 96374-96377, 96523, 99155, 99156, 99157, 99211-99223, 99231-99255, 99291-99292, 99304-99310, 99315-99316, 99334-99337, 99347-99350, 99374-99375, 99377-99378, 99446-99449, 99451-99452, 99495-99496, G0463, G0471

59015 0213T, 0216T, 0228T, 0230T, 12001-12007, 12011-12057, 13100-13133, 13151-13153, 36000, 36400-36410, 36420-36430, 36440, 36591-36592, 36600, 36640, 43752, 51701-51703, 57410, 62320-62327, 64400, 64405-64408, 64415-64435, 64445-64454, 64461-64463, 64479-64505, 64510-64530, 69990, 76000, 76942, 76970, 76998, 77001-77002, 92012-92014, 93000-93010, 93040-93042, 93318, 93355, 94002, 94200, 94250, 94680-94690, 94770, 95812-95816, 95819, 95822, 95829, 95955, 96360-96368, 96372, 96374-96377, 96523, 99155, 99156, 99157, 99211-99223, 99231-99255, 99291-99292, 99304-99310, 99315-99316, 99334-99337, 99347-99350, 99374-99375, 99377-99378, 99446-99449, 99451-99452, 99495-99496, G0463, G0471

59020 0213T, 0216T, 0228T, 0230T, 12001-12007, 12011-12057, 13100-13133, 13151-13153, 36000, 36400-36410, 36420-36430, 36440, 36591-36592, 36600, 36640, 43752, 51701-51703, 57410, 62320-62327, 64400, 64405-64408, 64415-64435, 64445-64454, 64461-64463, 64479-64505, 64510-64530, 69990, 92012-92014, 93000-93010, 93040-93042, 93318, 93355, 94002, 94200, 94250, 94680-94690, 94770, 95812-95816, 95819, 95822, 95829, 95955, 96360-96368, 96372, 96374-96377, 96523, 99155, 99156, 99157, 99211-99223, 99231-99255, 99291-99292, 99304-99310, 99315-99316, 99334-99337, 99347-99350, 99374-99375, 99377-99378, 99446-99449, 99451-99452, 99495-99496, G0463, G0471

59025 0213T, 0216T, 0228T, 0230T, 12001-12007, 12011-12057, 13100-13133, 13151-13153, 36000, 36400-36410, 36420-36430, 36440, 36591-36592, 36600, 36640, 43752, 51701-51703, 57410, 62320-62327, 64400, 64405-64408, 64415-64435, 64445-64454, 64461-64463, 64479-64505, 64510-64530, 69990, 92012-92014, 93000-93010, 93040-93042, 93318, 93355, 94002, 94200, 94250, 94680-94690, 94770, 95812-95816, 95819, 95822, 95829, 95955, 96361, 96366-96368, 96523, 99155, 99156, 99157, 99211-99223, 99231-99255, 99291-99292, 99304-99310, 99315-99316, 99334-99337, 99347-99350, 99374-99375, 99377-99378, 99446-99449, 99451-99452, 99495-99496, G0463, G0471

59030 0213T, 0216T, 0228T, 0230T, 12001-12007, 12011-12057, 13100-13133, 13151-13153, 36000, 36400-36410, 36420-36430, 36440, 36591-36592, 36600, 36640, 43752, 51701-51702, 57410, 62320-62327, 64400, 64405-64408, 64415-64435, 64445-64454, 64461-64463, 64479-64505, 64510-64530, 69990, 92012-92014, 93000-93010, 93040-93042, 93318, 93355, 94002, 94200, 94250, 94680-94690, 94770, 95812-95816,

95819, 95822, 95829, 95955, 96360-96368, 96372, 96374-96377, 96523, 99155, 99156, 99157, 99211-99223, 99231-99255, 99291-99292, 99304-99310, 99315-99316, 99334-99337, 99347-99350, 99374-99375, 99377-99378, 99446-99449, 99451-99452, 99495-99496, G0463, G0471

59050 0213T, 0216T, 36000, 36410, 36591-36592, 51701-51702, 57410, 59051, 61650, 62324-62327, 64415-64417, 64450, 64454, 64486-64490, 64493, 69990, 96360, 96365, 96523, G0471

59051 0213T, 0216T, 36000, 36410, 36591-36592, 51701-51703, 57410, 61650, 62324-62327, 64415-64417, 64450, 64454, 64486-64490, 64493, 69990, 96360, 96365, 96523, G0471

59070 0213T, 0216T, 0228T, 0230T, 12001-12007, 12011-12057, 13100-13133, 13151-13153, 36000, 36400-36410, 36420-36430, 36440, 36591-36592, 36600, 36640, 43752, 51701-51703, 57410, 62320-62327, 64400, 64405-64408, 64415-64435, 64445-64454, 64461-64463, 64479-64505, 64510-64530, 69990, 76941-76942, 76945-76946, 76970, 76998, 92012-92014, 93000-93010, 93040-93042, 93318, 93355, 94002, 94200, 94250, 94680-94690, 94770, 95812-95816, 95819, 95822, 95829, 95955, 96360-96368, 96372, 96374-96377, 96523, 99155, 99156, 99157, 99211-99223, 99231-99255, 99291-99292, 99304-99310, 99315-99316, 99334-99337, 99347-99350, 99374-99375, 99377-99378, 99446-99449, 99451-99452, 99495-99496, G0463, G0471, J0670, J2001

59072 0213T, 0216T, 0228T, 0230T, 12001-12007, 12011-12057, 13100-13133, 13151-13153, 36000, 36400-36410, 36420-36430, 36440, 36591-36592, 36600, 36640, 43752, 51701-51703, 57410, 62320-62327, 64400, 64405-64408, 64415-64435, 64445-64454, 64461-64463, 64479-64505, 64510-64530, 69990, 76941-76942, 76945-76946, 76970, 76998, 92012-92014, 93000-93010, 93040-93042, 93318, 93355, 94002, 94200, 94250, 94680-94690, 94770, 95812-95816, 95819, 95822, 95829, 95955, 96360-96368, 96372, 96374-96377, 96523, 99155, 99156, 99157, 99211-99223, 99231-99255, 99291-99292, 99304-99310, 99315-99316, 99334-99337, 99347-99350, 99374-99375, 99377-99378, 99446-99449, 99451-99452, 99495-99496, G0463, G0471

59074 0213T, 0216T, 0228T, 0230T, 12001-12007, 12011-12057, 13100-13133, 13151-13153, 36000, 36400-36410, 36420-36430, 36440, 36591-36592, 36600, 36640, 43752, 51701-51703, 57410, 62320-62327, 64400, 64405-64408, 64415-64435, 64445-64454, 64461-64463, 64479-64505, 64510-64530, 69990, 76941-76942, 76945-76946, 76970, 76998, 92012-92014, 93000-93010, 93040-93042, 93318, 93355, 94002, 94200, 94250, 94680-94690, 94770, 95812-95816, 95819, 95822, 95829, 95955, 96360-96368, 96372, 96374-96377, 96523, 99155, 99156, 99157, 99211-99223, 99231-99255, 99291-99292, 99304-99310, 99315-99316, 99334-99337, 99347-99350, 99374-99375, 99377-99378, 99446-99449, 99451-99452, 99495-99496, G0463, G0471, J0670, J2001

59076 0213T, 0216T, 0228T, 0230T, 12001-12007, 12011-12057, 13100-13133, 13151-13153, 36000, 36400-36410, 36420-36430, 36440, 36591-36592, 36600, 36640, 43752, 51701-51703, 57410, 62320-62327, 64400, 64405-64408, 64415-64435, 64445-64454, 64461-64463, 64479-64505, 64510-64530, 69990, 76941-76942, 76945-76946, 76970, 76998, 92012-92014, 93000-93010, 93040-93042, 93318, 93355, 94002, 94200, 94250, 94680-94690, 94770, 95812-95816, 95819, 95822, 95829, 95955, 96360-96368, 96372, 96374-96377, 96523, 99155, 99156, 99157, 99211-99223, 99231-99255, 99291-99292, 99304-99310, 99315-99316, 99334-99337, 99347-99350, 99374-99375, 99377-99378, 99446-99449, 99451-99452, 99495-99496, G0463, G0471

59100 0213T, 0216T, 0228T, 0230T, 11000-11006, 11042-11047, 12001-12007, 12011-12057, 13100-13133, 13151-13153, 36000, 36400-36410, 36420-36430, 36440, 36591-36592, 36600, 36640, 43752, 44005, 44180, 44602-44605, 44850, 49000-49010, 49255, 49320, 49570, 51701-51703, 57410, 59856-59857✣, 62320-62327, 64400,

64405-64408, 64415-64435, 64445-64454, 64461-64463, 64479-64505, 64510-64530, 69990, 92012-92014, 93000-93010, 93040-93042, 93318, 93355, 94002, 94200, 94250, 94680-94690, 94770, 95812-95816, 95819, 95822, 95829, 95955, 96360-96368, 96372, 96374-96377, 96523, 97597-97598, 97602, 99155, 99156, 99157, 99211-99223, 99231-99255, 99291-99292, 99304-99310, 99315-99316, 99334-99337, 99347-99350, 99374-99375, 99377-99378, 99446-99449, 99451-99452, 99495-99496, G0463, G0471

59120 0213T, 0216T, 0228T, 0230T, 11000-11006, 11042-11047, 12001-12007, 12011-12057, 13100-13133, 13151-13153, 36000, 36400-36410, 36420-36430, 36440, 36591-36592, 36600, 36640, 43752, 44005, 44180, 44602-44605, 44850, 49000-49010, 49255, 49320-49321, 49570, 51701-51703, 57410, 58700-58720, 59856-59866, 62320-62327, 64400, 64405-64408, 64415-64435, 64445-64454, 64461-64463, 64479-64505, 64510-64530, 69990, 92012-92014, 93000-93010, 93040-93042, 93318, 93355, 94002, 94200, 94250, 94680-94690, 94770, 95812-95816, 95819, 95822, 95829, 95955, 96360-96368, 96372, 96374-96377, 96523, 97597-97598, 97602, 99155, 99156, 99157, 99211-99223, 99231-99255, 99291-99292, 99304-99310, 99315-99316, 99334-99337, 99347-99350, 99374-99375, 99377-99378, 99446-99449, 99451-99452, 99495-99496, G0463, G0471

59121 0213T, 0216T, 0228T, 0230T, 11000-11006, 11042-11047, 12001-12007, 12011-12057, 13100-13133, 13151-13153, 36000, 36400-36410, 36420-36430, 36440, 36591-36592, 36600, 36640, 43752, 44005, 44180, 44602-44605, 44850, 49000-49010, 49255, 49320, 49570, 51701-51703, 57410, 58700-58720, 59856-59866, 62320-62327, 64400, 64405-64408, 64415-64435, 64445-64454, 64461-64463, 64479-64505, 64510-64530, 69990, 92012-92014, 93000-93010, 93040-93042, 93318, 93355, 94002, 94200, 94250, 94680-94690, 94770, 95812-95816, 95819, 95822, 95829, 95955, 96360-96368, 96372, 96374-96377, 96523, 97597-97598, 97602, 99155, 99156, 99157, 99211-99223, 99231-99255, 99291-99292, 99304-99310, 99315-99316, 99334-99337, 99347-99350, 99374-99375, 99377-99378, 99446-99449, 99451-99452, 99495-99496, G0463, G0471

59130 0213T, 0216T, 0228T, 0230T, 12001-12007, 12011-12057, 13100-13133, 13151-13153, 36000, 36400-36410, 36420-36430, 36440, 36591-36592, 36600, 36640, 43752, 44005, 44180, 44602-44605, 44820-44850, 49000-49002, 49255, 49320, 49570, 51701-51703, 57410, 59857-59866, 62320-62327, 64400, 64405-64408, 64415-64435, 64445-64454, 64461-64463, 64479-64505, 64510-64530, 69990, 92012-92014, 93000-93010, 93040-93042, 93318, 93355, 94002, 94200, 94250, 94680-94690, 94770, 95812-95816, 95819, 95822, 95829, 95955, 96360-96368, 96372, 96374-96377, 96523, 99155, 99156, 99157, 99211-99223, 99231-99255, 99291-99292, 99304-99310, 99315-99316, 99334-99337, 99347-99350, 99374-99375, 99377-99378, 99446-99449, 99451-99452, 99495-99496, G0463, G0471

59135 0213T, 0216T, 0228T, 0230T, 11000-11006, 11042-11047, 12001-12007, 12011-12057, 13100-13133, 13151-13153, 36000, 36400-36410, 36420-36430, 36440, 36591-36592, 36600, 36640, 43752, 44005, 44180, 44602-44605, 44820-44850, 49000-49010, 49255, 49320-49321, 49570, 51701-51703, 57410, 58140, 58146, 59866, 62320-62327, 64400, 64405-64408, 64415-64435, 64445-64454, 64461-64463, 64479-64505, 64510-64530, 69990, 92012-92014, 93000-93010, 93040-93042, 93318, 93355, 94002, 94200, 94250, 94680-94690, 94770, 95812-95816, 95819, 95822, 95829, 95955, 96360-96368, 96372, 96374-96377, 96523, 97597-97598, 97602, 99155, 99156, 99157, 99211-99223, 99231-99255, 99291-99292, 99304-99310, 99315-99316, 99334-99337, 99347-99350, 99374-99375, 99377-99378, 99446-99449, 99451-99452, 99495-99496, G0463, G0471

59136 0213T, 0216T, 0228T, 0230T, 11000-11006, 11042-11047, 12001-12007, 12011-12057, 13100-13133, 13151-13153, 36000, 36400-36410, 36420-36430, 36440, 36591-36592, 36600, 36640, 43752, 44005, 44180, 44602-44605, 44820-44850, 49000-49010, 49255, 49320, 49570, 51701-51703, 57410, 59857-59866, 62320-62327, 64400, 64405-64408, 64415-64435, 64445-64454, 64461-64463, 64479-64505, 64510-64530, 69990, 92012-92014, 93000-93010, 93040-93042, 93318, 93355, 94002, 94200, 94250, 94680-94690, 94770, 95812-95816, 95819, 95822, 95829, 95955, 96360-96368, 96372, 96374-96377, 96523, 97597-97598, 97602, 99155, 99156, 99157, 99211-99223, 99231-99255, 99291-99292, 99304-99310, 99315-99316, 99334-99337, 99347-99350, 99374-99375, 99377-99378, 99446-99449, 99451-99452, 99495-99496, G0463, G0471

59140 0213T, 0216T, 0228T, 0230T, 12001-12007, 12011-12057, 13100-13133, 13151-13153, 36000, 36400-36410, 36420-36430, 36440, 36591-36592, 36600, 36640, 43752, 44005, 44180, 44602-44605, 44850, 49000-49010, 49255, 49320, 49570, 51701-51703, 57410, 59856-59866, 62320-62327, 64400, 64405-64408, 64415-64435, 64445-64454, 64461-64463, 64479-64505, 64510-64530, 69990, 92012-92014, 93000-93010, 93040-93042, 93318, 93355, 94002, 94200, 94250, 94680-94690, 94770, 95812-95816, 95819, 95822, 95829, 95955, 96360-96368, 96372, 96374-96377, 96523, 99155, 99156, 99157, 99211-99223, 99231-99255, 99291-99292, 99304-99310, 99315-99316, 99334-99337, 99347-99350, 99374-99375, 99377-99378, 99446-99449, 99451-99452, 99495-99496, G0463, G0471, J2001

59150 0213T, 0216T, 0228T, 0230T, 11000-11006, 11042-11047, 12001-12007, 12011-12057, 13100-13133, 13151-13153, 36000, 36400-36410, 36420-36430, 36440, 36591-36592, 36600, 36640, 43752, 49320, 49400, 51701-51703, 57410, 58700-58720, 59856-59866, 62320-62327, 64400, 64405-64408, 64415-64435, 64445-64454, 64461-64463, 64479-64505, 64510-64530, 69990, 92012-92014, 93000-93010, 93040-93042, 93318, 93355, 94002, 94200, 94250, 94680-94690, 94770, 95812-95816, 95819, 95822, 95829, 95955, 96360-96368, 96372, 96374-96377, 96523, 97597-97598, 97602, 99155, 99156, 99157, 99211-99223, 99231-99255, 99291-99292, 99304-99310, 99315-99316, 99334-99337, 99347-99350, 99374-99375, 99377-99378, 99446-99449, 99451-99452, 99495-99496, G0463, G0471

59151 0213T, 0216T, 0228T, 0230T, 11000-11006, 11042-11047, 12001-12007, 12011-12057, 13100-13133, 13151-13153, 36000, 36400-36410, 36420-36430, 36440, 36591-36592, 36600, 36640, 43752, 49320-49321, 49400, 51701-51703, 57410, 58700-58720, 59150, 59866, 62320-62327, 64400, 64405-64408, 64415-64435, 64445-64454, 64461-64463, 64479-64505, 64510-64530, 69990, 92012-92014, 93000-93010, 93040-93042, 93318, 93355, 94002, 94200, 94250, 94680-94690, 94770, 95812-95816, 95819, 95822, 95829, 95955, 96360-96368, 96372, 96374-96377, 96523, 97597-97598, 97602, 99155, 99156, 99157, 99211-99223, 99231-99255, 99291-99292, 99304-99310, 99315-99316, 99334-99337, 99347-99350, 99374-99375, 99377-99378, 99446-99449, 99451-99452, 99495-99496, G0463, G0471

59160 0213T, 0216T, 0228T, 0230T, 12001-12007, 12011-12057, 13100-13133, 13151-13153, 36000, 36400-36410, 36420-36430, 36440, 36591-36592, 36600, 36640, 43752, 51701-51703, 57410, 57505, 57800, 58120, 59856-59857✢, 62320-62327, 64400, 64405-64408, 64415-64435, 64445-64454, 64461-64463, 64479-64505, 64510-64530, 69990, 92012-92014, 93000-93010, 93040-93042, 93318, 93355, 94002, 94200, 94250, 94680-94690, 94770, 95812-95816, 95819, 95822, 95829, 95955, 96360-96368, 96372, 96374-96377, 96523, 99155, 99156, 99157, 99211-99223, 99231-99255, 99291-99292, 99304-99310, 99315-99316, 99334-99337, 99347-99350, 99374-99375, 99377-99378, 99446-99449, 99451-99452, 99495-99496, G0463, G0471, J2001

59200 0213T, 0216T, 0228T, 0230T, 11000-11006, 11042-11047, 12001-12007, 12011-12057, 13100-13133, 13151-13153, 36000, 36400-36410, 36420-36430, 36440, 36591-36592, 36600, 36640, 43752, 51701-51703, 57410, 62320-62327, 64400, 64405-64408, 64415-64435, 64445-64454, 64461-64463, 64479-64505, 64510-64530, 69990, 92012-92014, 93000-93010, 93040-93042, 93318, 93355, 94002, 94200, 94250, 94680-94690, 94770, 95812-95816, 95819, 95822, 95829, 95955, 96360-96368, 96372, 96374-96377, 96523, 97597-97598, 97602, 99155, 99156, 99157, 99211-99223, 99231-99255, 99291-99292, 99304-99310, 99315-99316, 99334-99337, 99347-99350, 99374-99375, 99377-99378, 99446-99449, 99451-99452, 99495-99496, G0463, G0471, J2001

59300 0213T, 0216T, 0228T, 0230T, 11000-11006, 11042-11047, 12001-12007, 12011-12057, 13100-13133, 13151-13153, 36000, 36400-36410, 36420-36430, 36440, 36591-36592, 36600, 36640, 43752, 51701-51703, 57410, 62320-62327, 64400, 64405-64408, 64415-64435, 64445-64454, 64461-64463, 64479-64505, 64510-64530, 69990, 92012-92014, 93000-93010, 93040-93042, 93318, 93355, 94002, 94200, 94250, 94680-94690, 94770, 95812-95816, 95819, 95822, 95829, 95955, 96360-96368, 96372, 96374-96377, 96523, 97597-97598, 97602, 99155, 99156, 99157, 99211-99223, 99231-99255, 99291-99292, 99304-99310, 99315-99316, 99334-99337, 99347-99350, 99374-99375, 99377-99378, 99446-99449, 99451-99452, 99495-99496, G0463, G0471, J0670, J2001

59320 0213T, 0216T, 0228T, 0230T, 12001-12007, 12011-12057, 13100-13133, 13151-13153, 36000, 36400-36410, 36420-36430, 36440, 36591-36592, 36600, 36640, 43752, 51701-51703, 57410, 62320-62327, 64400, 64405-64408, 64415-64435, 64445-64454, 64461-64463, 64479-64505, 64510-64530, 69990, 92012-92014, 93000-93010, 93040-93042, 93318, 93355, 94002, 94200, 94250, 94680-94690, 94770, 95812-95816, 95819, 95822, 95829, 95955, 96360-96368, 96372, 96374-96377, 96523, 99155, 99156, 99157, 99211-99223, 99231-99255, 99291-99292, 99304-99310, 99315-99316, 99334-99337, 99347-99350, 99374-99375, 99377-99378, 99446-99449, 99451-99452, 99495-99496, G0463, G0471

59325 0213T, 0216T, 0228T, 0230T, 12001-12007, 12011-12057, 13100-13133, 13151-13153, 36000, 36400-36410, 36420-36430, 36440, 36591-36592, 36600, 36640, 43752, 44005, 44180, 44602-44605, 44820-44850, 49000-49010, 49255, 49320, 49570, 51701-51703, 57410, 62320-62327, 64400, 64405-64408, 64415-64435, 64445-64454, 64461-64463, 64479-64505, 64510-64530, 69990, 92012-92014, 93000-93010, 93040-93042, 93318, 93355, 94002, 94200, 94250, 94680-94690, 94770, 95812-95816, 95819, 95822, 95829, 95955, 96360-96368, 96372, 96374-96377, 96523, 99155, 99156, 99157, 99211-99223, 99231-99255, 99291-99292, 99304-99310, 99315-99316, 99334-99337, 99347-99350, 99374-99375, 99377-99378, 99446-99449, 99451-99452, 99495-99496, G0463, G0471

59350 0213T, 0216T, 0228T, 0230T, 12001-12007, 12011-12057, 13100-13133, 13151-13153, 36000, 36400-36410, 36420-36430, 36440, 36591-36592, 36600, 36640, 43752, 44005, 44180, 44602-44605, 44820-44850, 49000-49010, 49255, 49320, 49570, 51701-51703, 57410, 59866, 62320-62327, 64400, 64405-64408, 64415-64435, 64445-64454, 64461-64463, 64479-64505, 64510-64530, 69990, 92012-92014, 93000-93010, 93040-93042, 93318, 93355, 94002, 94200, 94250, 94680-94690, 94770, 95812-95816, 95819, 95822, 95829, 95955, 96360-96368, 96372, 96374-96377, 96523, 99155, 99156, 99157, 99211-99223, 99231-99255, 99291-99292, 99304-99310, 99315-99316, 99334-99337, 99347-99350, 99374-99375, 99377-99378, 99446-99449, 99451-99452, 99495-99496, G0463, G0471

59400 01958, 01960, 01967, 0213T, 0216T, 0230T, 11000-11006, 11042-11047, 12001-12007, 12011-12057, 13100-13133, 13151-13153, 36000, 36410, 36591-36592, 49407, 51701-51702, 57720, 58800, 59050-59051,

Coding Companion for Ob/Gyn

59200-59300, 59414, 59610❖, 61650, 62322-62327, 64415-64417, 64430-64435, 64450, 64454, 64483, 64486-64490, 64493, 69990, 81000, 81002, 96360, 96365, 96372, 96374-96377, 96523, 97597-97598, 97602, 99201-99239, 99304-99310, 99315-99318, 99324-99328, 99334-99337, 99341-99350, 99483, 99497, G0463, G0471

59409 01958, 01960, 01967, 0213T, 0216T, 0230T, 11000-11006, 11042-11047, 12001-12007, 12011-12057, 13100-13133, 13151-13153, 36000, 36410, 36591-36592, 51701-51702, 59050-59051, 59200-59300, 59414, 59430, 59610❖, 61650, 62322-62327, 64415-64417, 64430-64435, 64450, 64454, 64483, 64486-64490, 64493, 69990, 96360, 96365, 96372, 96374-96377, 96523, 97597-97598, 97602, G0471

59410 01958, 01960, 01967, 0213T, 0216T, 0230T, 11000-11006, 11042-11047, 12001-12007, 12011-12057, 13100-13133, 13151-13153, 36000, 36410, 36591-36592, 51701-51702, 57720, 59050-59051, 59200-59300, 59409, 59414, 59430, 59610❖, 61650, 62322-62327, 64415-64417, 64430-64435, 64450, 64454, 64483, 64486-64490, 64493, 69990, 96360, 96365, 96372, 96374-96377, 96523, 97597-97598, 97602, 99201-99239, 99304-99310, 99315-99318, 99324-99328, 99334-99337, 99341-99350, 99483, 99497, G0463, G0471

59412 01958, 01960, 01967, 0213T, 0216T, 0230T, 36000, 36410, 36591-36592, 51701-51702, 61650, 62322-62327, 64415-64417, 64430-64435, 64450, 64454, 64483, 64486-64490, 64493, 69990, 96360, 96365, 96372, 96374-96377, 96523, G0471

59414 01960, 01967, 0213T, 0216T, 0230T, 36000, 36410, 36591-36592, 51701-51702, 59430, 61650, 62322-62327, 64415-64417, 64430-64435, 64450, 64454, 64483, 64486-64490, 64493, 69990, 96360, 96365, 96372, 96374-96377, 96523, G0471

59425 0213T, 0216T, 36000, 36410, 36591-36592, 59426❖, 59610❖, 61650, 62324-62327, 64415-64417, 64450, 64454, 64486-64490, 64493, 69990, 81000, 81002, 96360, 96365, 96372, 96374-96377, 96523, 99201-99215, 99483, 99497, G0463

59426 0213T, 0216T, 36000, 36410, 36591-36592, 59610❖, 61650, 62324-62327, 64415-64417, 64450, 64454, 64486-64490, 64493, 69990, 81000, 81002, 96360, 96365, 96372, 96374-96377, 96523, 99201-99215, 99483, 99497, G0463

59430 0213T, 0216T, 36000, 36410, 36591-36592, 49010, 61650, 62324-62327, 64415-64417, 64450, 64454, 64486-64490, 64493, 69990, 96360, 96365, 96372, 96374-96377, 96523, 99201-99215, 99483, 99497, G0463

59510 01958, 01961, 01968, 0213T, 0216T, 0230T, 12001-12007, 12011-12057, 13100-13133, 13151-13153, 36000, 36410, 36591-36592, 44005, 44180, 44602-44605, 44820-44850, 49000-49010, 49255, 49570, 51701-51702, 59050-59051, 59300, 59414, 59430, 61650, 62322-62327, 64415-64417, 64430-64435, 64450, 64454, 64483, 64486-64490, 64493, 69990, 81000, 81002, 96360, 96365, 96372, 96374-96377, 96523, 99201-99239, 99304-99310, 99315-99318, 99324-99328, 99334-99337, 99341-99350, 99483, 99497, G0463, G0471

59514 01958, 01961, 01968, 0213T, 0216T, 0230T, 12001-12007, 12011-12057, 13100-13133, 13151-13153, 36000, 36410, 36591-36592, 44005, 44180, 44602-44605, 44820-44850, 49000-49010, 49255, 49570, 51701-51702, 59050-59051, 59300, 59414, 61650, 62322-62327, 64415-64417, 64430-64435, 64450, 64454, 64483, 64486-64490, 64493, 69990, 96360, 96365, 96372, 96374-96377, 96523, G0471

59515 01961, 01968, 0213T, 0216T, 0230T, 12001-12007, 12011-12057, 13100-13133, 13151-13153, 36000, 36410, 36591-36592, 44005, 44180, 44602-44605, 44820-44850, 49000-49010, 49255, 49570, 51701-51702, 59050-59051, 59300, 59414, 59430, 59514, 61650, 62322-62327,

64415-64417, 64430-64435, 64450, 64454, 64483, 64486-64490, 64493, 69990, 96360, 96365, 96372, 96374-96377, 96523, 99201-99239, 99304-99310, 99315-99318, 99324-99328, 99334-99337, 99341-99350, 99483, 99497, G0463, G0471

59525 01962-01963, 01969, 0230T, 11000-11006, 11042-11047, 44602-44605, 44820-44850, 49000-49010, 49255, 49570, 59430, 59857❖, 62322-62323, 64430-64435, 64483, 96523, 97597-97598, 97602

59610 01958, 01960, 01967, 0213T, 0216T, 0230T, 11000-11006, 11042-11047, 12001-12007, 12011-12057, 13100-13133, 13151-13153, 36000, 36410, 36591-36592, 51701-51702, 59050-59051, 59300, 59414, 59430, 59510-59515, 59525, 59612-59618❖, 61650, 62322-62327, 64415-64417, 64430-64435, 64450, 64454, 64483, 64486-64490, 64493, 69990, 81000, 81002, 96360, 96365, 96372, 96374-96377, 96523, 97597-97598, 97602, 99201-99239, 99304-99310, 99315-99318, 99324-99328, 99334-99337, 99341-99350, 99483, 99497, G0463, G0471

59612 01958, 01960, 01967, 0213T, 0216T, 0230T, 11000-11006, 11042-11047, 12001-12007, 12011-12057, 13100-13133, 13151-13153, 36000, 36410, 36591-36592, 51701-51702, 59050-59051, 59300, 59400-59410, 59414, 59515, 59525, 59618-59622❖, 61650, 62322-62327, 64415-64417, 64430-64435, 64450, 64454, 64483, 64486-64490, 64493, 69990, 96360, 96365, 96372, 96374-96377, 96523, 97597-97598, 97602, G0471

59614 01958, 01960, 01967, 0213T, 0216T, 0230T, 11000-11006, 11042-11047, 12001-12007, 12011-12057, 13100-13133, 13151-13153, 36000, 36410, 36591-36592, 51701-51702, 59050-59051, 59300, 59400-59410, 59414, 59430, 59510-59515, 59525, 59612, 59618-59622❖, 61650, 62322-62327, 64415-64417, 64430-64435, 64450, 64454, 64483, 64486-64490, 64493, 69990, 96360, 96365, 96372, 96374-96377, 96523, 97597-97598, 97602, 99201-99239, 99304-99310, 99315-99318, 99324-99328, 99334-99337, 99341-99350, 99483, 99497, G0463, G0471

59618 01958, 01961, 01968, 0213T, 0216T, 0230T, 12001-12007, 12011-12057, 13100-13133, 13151-13153, 36000, 36410, 36591-36592, 44602-44605, 44820-44850, 49000-49010, 49255, 49570, 51701-51702, 59050-59051, 59300, 59400-59410, 59414, 59425-59430, 59510-59515, 59620-59622, 61650, 62322-62327, 64415-64417, 64430-64435, 64450, 64454, 64483, 64486-64490, 64493, 69990, 81000, 81002, 96360, 96365, 96372, 96374-96377, 96523, 99201-99239, 99304-99310, 99315-99318, 99324-99328, 99334-99337, 99341-99350, 99483, 99497, G0463, G0471

59620 01958, 01961, 01968, 0213T, 0216T, 0230T, 12001-12007, 12011-12057, 13100-13133, 13151-13153, 36000, 36410, 36591-36592, 44005, 44180, 44602-44605, 44820-44850, 49000-49002, 49255, 49570, 51701-51702, 59050-59051, 59300, 59400-59410, 59414, 59510-59515, 59610❖, 61650, 62322-62327, 64415-64417, 64430-64435, 64450, 64454, 64483, 64486-64490, 64493, 69990, 96360, 96365, 96372, 96374-96377, 96523, G0471

59622 01958, 01961, 01968, 0213T, 0216T, 0230T, 12001-12007, 12011-12057, 13100-13133, 13151-13153, 36000, 36410, 36591-36592, 44005, 44180, 44602-44605, 44820-44850, 49000-49010, 49255, 49570, 51701-51702, 59050-59051, 59300, 59400-59410, 59414, 59430, 59510-59515, 59610❖, 59620, 61650, 62322-62327, 64415-64417, 64430-64435, 64450, 64454, 64483, 64486-64490, 64493, 69990, 96360, 96365, 96372, 96374-96377, 96523, 99201-99239, 99304-99310, 99315-99318, 99324-99328, 99334-99337, 99341-99350, 99483, 99497, G0463, G0471

59812 01965-01966, 0213T, 0216T, 0228T, 0230T, 12001-12007, 12011-12057, 13100-13133, 13151-13153, 36000, 36400-36410, 36420-36430, 36440, 36591-36592, 36600, 36640, 43752, 51701-51703, 57410, 57505, 58120, 59855-59866✦, 62320-62327, 64400, 64405-64408, 64415-64435, 64445-64454, 64461-64463, 64479-64505, 64510-64530, 69990, 92012-92014, 93000-93010, 93040-93042, 93318, 93355, 94002, 94200, 94250, 94680-94690, 94770, 95812-95816, 95819, 95822, 95829, 95955, 96360-96368, 96372, 96374-96377, 96523, 99155, 99156, 99157, 99211-99223, 99231-99255, 99291-99292, 99304-99310, 99315-99316, 99334-99337, 99347-99350, 99374-99375, 99377-99378, 99446-99449, 99451-99452, 99495-99496, G0463, G0471, J0670, J2001

59820 01965-01966, 0213T, 0216T, 0228T, 0230T, 12001-12007, 12011-12057, 13100-13133, 13151-13153, 36000, 36400-36410, 36420-36430, 36440, 36591-36592, 36600, 36640, 43752, 51701-51703, 57410, 57505, 58120, 59821✦, 59855-59866✦, 62320-62327, 64400, 64405-64408, 64415-64435, 64445-64454, 64461-64463, 64479-64505, 64510-64530, 69990, 92012-92014, 93000-93010, 93040-93042, 93318, 93355, 94002, 94200, 94250, 94680-94690, 94770, 95812-95816, 95819, 95822, 95829, 95955, 96360-96368, 96372, 96374-96377, 96523, 99155, 99156, 99157, 99211-99223, 99231-99255, 99291-99292, 99304-99310, 99315-99316, 99334-99337, 99347-99350, 99374-99375, 99377-99378, 99446-99449, 99451-99452, 99495-99496, G0463, G0471, J0670, J2001

59821 01965-01966, 0213T, 0216T, 0228T, 0230T, 12001-12007, 12011-12057, 13100-13133, 13151-13153, 36000, 36400-36410, 36420-36430, 36440, 36591-36592, 36600, 36640, 43752, 51701-51703, 57410, 57505, 58120, 59855-59857✦, 62320-62327, 64400, 64405-64408, 64415-64435, 64445-64454, 64461-64463, 64479-64505, 64510-64530, 69990, 92012-92014, 93000-93010, 93040-93042, 93318, 93355, 94002, 94200, 94250, 94680-94690, 94770, 95812-95816, 95819, 95822, 95829, 95955, 96360-96368, 96372, 96374-96377, 96523, 99155, 99156, 99157, 99211-99223, 99231-99255, 99291-99292, 99304-99310, 99315-99316, 99334-99337, 99347-99350, 99374-99375, 99377-99378, 99446-99449, 99451-99452, 99495-99496, G0463, G0471, J0670, J2001

59830 01965-01966, 0213T, 0216T, 0228T, 0230T, 12001-12007, 12011-12057, 13100-13133, 13151-13153, 36000, 36400-36410, 36420-36430, 36440, 36591-36592, 36600, 36640, 43752, 51701-51703, 57410, 57505, 58120, 59856-59857✦, 62320-62327, 64400, 64405-64408, 64415-64435, 64445-64454, 64461-64463, 64479-64505, 64510-64530, 69990, 92012-92014, 93000-93010, 93040-93042, 93318, 93355, 94002, 94200, 94250, 94680-94690, 94770, 95812-95816, 95819, 95822, 95829, 95955, 96360-96368, 96372, 96374-96377, 96523, 99155, 99156, 99157, 99211-99223, 99231-99255, 99291-99292, 99304-99310, 99315-99316, 99334-99337, 99347-99350, 99374-99375, 99377-99378, 99446-99449, 99451-99452, 99495-99496, G0463, G0471

59840 01965-01966, 0213T, 0216T, 0228T, 0230T, 12001-12007, 12011-12057, 13100-13133, 13151-13153, 36000, 36400-36410, 36420-36430, 36440, 36591-36592, 36600, 36640, 43752, 51701-51703, 57410, 57505, 58120, 59855-59866✦, 62320-62327, 64400, 64405-64408, 64415-64435, 64445-64454, 64461-64463, 64479-64505, 64510-64530, 69990, 92012-92014, 93000-93010, 93040-93042, 93318, 93355, 94002, 94200, 94250, 94680-94690, 94770, 95812-95816, 95819, 95822, 95829, 95955, 96360-96368, 96372, 96374-96377, 96523, 99155, 99156, 99157, 99211-99223, 99231-99255, 99291-99292, 99304-99310, 99315-99316, 99334-99337, 99347-99350, 99374-99375, 99377-99378, 99446-99449, 99451-99452, 99495-99496, G0463, G0471

59841 01965-01966, 0213T, 0216T, 0228T, 0230T, 12001-12007, 12011-12057, 13100-13133, 13151-13153, 36000, 36400-36410, 36420-36430, 36440, 36591-36592, 36600, 36640, 43752, 51701-51703, 57410, 57505, 58120, 59855-59857✦, 62320-62327, 64400, 64405-64408,

59850 *(continued)*
64415-64435, 64445-64454, 64461-64463, 64479-64505, 64510-64530, 69990, 92012-92014, 93000-93010, 93040-93042, 93318, 93355, 94002, 94200, 94250, 94680-94690, 94770, 95812-95816, 95819, 95822, 95829, 95955, 96360-96368, 96372, 96374-96377, 96523, 99155, 99156, 99157, 99211-99223, 99231-99255, 99291-99292, 99304-99310, 99315-99316, 99334-99337, 99347-99350, 99374-99375, 99377-99378, 99446-99449, 99451-99452, 99495-99496, G0463, G0471, J0670, J2001

59850 01965-01966, 0213T, 0216T, 0228T, 0230T, 12001-12007, 12011-12057, 13100-13133, 13151-13153, 36000, 36400-36410, 36420-36430, 36440, 36591-36592, 36600, 36640, 43752, 51701-51703, 57410, 59200, 59856-59857✦, 62320-62327, 64400, 64405-64408, 64415-64435, 64445-64454, 64461-64463, 64479-64505, 64510-64530, 69990, 92012-92014, 93000-93010, 93040-93042, 93318, 93355, 94002, 94200, 94250, 94680-94690, 94770, 95812-95816, 95819, 95822, 95829, 95955, 96360-96368, 96372, 96374-96377, 96523, 99155, 99156, 99157, 99211-99223, 99231-99255, 99291-99292, 99304-99310, 99315-99316, 99334-99337, 99347-99350, 99374-99375, 99377-99378, 99446-99449, 99451-99452, 99495-99496, G0463, G0471

59851 01965-01966, 0213T, 0216T, 0228T, 0230T, 12001-12007, 12011-12057, 13100-13133, 13151-13153, 36000, 36400-36410, 36420-36430, 36440, 36591-36592, 36600, 36640, 43752, 51701-51703, 57410, 59200, 59850, 59856✦, 62320-62327, 64400, 64405-64408, 64415-64435, 64445-64454, 64461-64463, 64479-64505, 64510-64530, 69990, 92012-92014, 93000-93010, 93040-93042, 93318, 93355, 94002, 94200, 94250, 94680-94690, 94770, 95812-95816, 95819, 95822, 95829, 95955, 96360-96368, 96372, 96374-96377, 96523, 99155, 99156, 99157, 99211-99223, 99231-99255, 99291-99292, 99304-99310, 99315-99316, 99334-99337, 99347-99350, 99374-99375, 99377-99378, 99446-99449, 99451-99452, 99495-99496, G0463, G0471

59852 01965-01966, 0213T, 0216T, 0228T, 0230T, 11000-11006, 11042-11047, 12001-12007, 12011-12057, 13100-13133, 13151-13153, 36000, 36400-36410, 36420-36430, 36440, 36591-36592, 36600, 36640, 43752, 44602-44605, 49000-49002, 49320, 51701-51703, 57410, 59200, 59850, 59857✦, 62320-62327, 64400, 64405-64408, 64415-64435, 64445-64454, 64461-64463, 64479-64505, 64510-64530, 69990, 92012-92014, 93000-93010, 93040-93042, 93318, 93355, 94002, 94200, 94250, 94680-94690, 94770, 95812-95816, 95819, 95822, 95829, 95955, 96360-96368, 96372, 96374-96377, 96523, 97597-97598, 97602, 99155, 99156, 99157, 99211-99223, 99231-99255, 99291-99292, 99304-99310, 99315-99316, 99334-99337, 99347-99350, 99374-99375, 99377-99378, 99446-99449, 99451-99452, 99495-99496, G0463, G0471

59855 01965-01966, 0213T, 0216T, 0228T, 0230T, 12001-12007, 12011-12057, 13100-13133, 13151-13153, 36000, 36400-36410, 36420-36430, 36440, 36591-36592, 36600, 36640, 43752, 51701-51703, 57410, 59100✦, 59120-59121✦, 59130-59200, 59510-59515✦, 59525✦, 59610-59622✦, 59830✦, 59850-59852✦, 62320-62327, 64400, 64405-64408, 64415-64435, 64445-64454, 64461-64463, 64479-64505, 64510-64530, 69990, 92012-92014, 93000-93010, 93040-93042, 93318, 93355, 94002, 94200, 94250, 94680-94690, 94770, 95812-95816, 95819, 95822, 95829, 95955, 96360-96368, 96372, 96374-96377, 96523, 99155, 99156, 99157, 99211-99223, 99231-99255, 99291-99292, 99304-99310, 99315-99316, 99334-99337, 99347-99350, 99374-99375, 99377-99378, 99446-99449, 99451-99452, 99495-99496, G0463, G0471

59856 01965-01966, 0213T, 0216T, 0228T, 0230T, 12001-12007, 12011-12057, 13100-13133, 13151-13153, 36000, 36400-36410, 36420-36430, 36440, 36591-36592, 36600, 36640, 43752, 51701-51703, 57410, 59130-59136✦, 59151✦, 59200, 59510-59515✦, 59525✦, 59610-59622✦, 59852✦, 62320-62327, 64400, 64405-64408, 64415-64435, 64445-64454, 64461-64463, 64479-64505, 64510-64530, 69990,

Coding Companion for Ob/Gyn

92012-92014, 93000-93010, 93040-93042, 93318, 93355, 94002, 94200, 94250, 94680-94690, 94770, 95812-95816, 95819, 95822, 95829, 95955, 96360-96368, 96372, 96374-96377, 96523, 99155, 99156, 99157, 99211-99223, 99231-99255, 99291-99292, 99304-99310, 99315-99316, 99334-99337, 99347-99350, 99374-99375, 99377-99378, 99446-99449, 99451-99452, 99495-99496, G0463, G0471

59857 01965-01966, 0213T, 0216T, 0228T, 0230T, 11000-11006, 11042-11047, 12001-12007, 12011-12057, 13100-13133, 13151-13153, 36000, 36400-36410, 36420-36430, 36440, 36591-36592, 36600, 36640, 43752, 44005, 44180, 44602-44605, 44820-44850, 49000-49010, 49255, 49320, 51701-51703, 57410, 59135✦, 59200, 59510-59515✦, 59610-59622✦, 59851, 59855, 62320-62327, 64400, 64405-64408, 64415-64435, 64445-64454, 64461-64463, 64479-64505, 64510-64530, 69990, 92012-92014, 93000-93010, 93040-93042, 93318, 93355, 94002, 94200, 94250, 94680-94690, 94770, 95812-95816, 95819, 95822, 95829, 95955, 96360-96368, 96372, 96374-96377, 96523, 97597-97598, 97602, 99155, 99156, 99157, 99211-99223, 99231-99255, 99291-99292, 99304-99310, 99315-99316, 99334-99337, 99347-99350, 99374-99375, 99377-99378, 99446-99449, 99451-99452, 99495-99496, G0463, G0471

59866 01965-01966, 0213T, 0216T, 0228T, 0230T, 12001-12007, 12011-12057, 13100-13133, 13151-13153, 36000, 36400-36410, 36420-36430, 36440, 36591-36592, 36600, 36640, 43752, 51701-51703, 57410, 59160, 59821-59830✦, 59841-59857✦, 62320-62327, 64400, 64405-64408, 64415-64435, 64445-64454, 64461-64463, 64479-64505, 64510-64530, 69990, 92012-92014, 93000-93010, 93040-93042, 93318, 93355, 94002, 94200, 94250, 94680-94690, 94770, 95812-95816, 95819, 95822, 95829, 95955, 96360-96368, 96372, 96374-96377, 96523, 99155, 99156, 99157, 99211-99223, 99231-99255, 99291-99292, 99304-99310, 99315-99316, 99334-99337, 99347-99350, 99374-99375, 99377-99378, 99446-99449, 99451-99452, 99495-99496, G0463, G0471, J2001

59870 01965-01966, 0213T, 0216T, 0228T, 0230T, 12001-12007, 12011-12057, 13100-13133, 13151-13153, 36000, 36400-36410, 36420-36430, 36440, 36591-36592, 36600, 36640, 43752, 51701-51703, 57410, 57505, 58120, 59855-59866, 62320-62327, 64400, 64405-64408, 64415-64435, 64445-64454, 64461-64463, 64479-64505, 64510-64530, 69990, 92012-92014, 93000-93010, 93040-93042, 93318, 93355, 94002, 94200, 94250, 94680-94690, 94770, 95812-95816, 95819, 95822, 95829, 95955, 96360-96368, 96372, 96374-96377, 96523, 99155, 99156, 99157, 99211-99223, 99231-99255, 99291-99292, 99304-99310, 99315-99316, 99334-99337, 99347-99350, 99374-99375, 99377-99378, 99446-99449, 99451-99452, 99495-99496, G0463, G0471

59871 0213T, 0216T, 0228T, 0230T, 11000-11006, 11042-11047, 12001-12007, 12011-12057, 13100-13133, 13151-13153, 15851, 36000, 36400-36410, 36420-36430, 36440, 36591-36592, 36600, 36640, 43752, 51701-51703, 57410, 62320-62327, 64400, 64405-64408, 64415-64435, 64445-64454, 64461-64463, 64479-64505, 64510-64530, 69990, 92012-92014, 93000-93010, 93040-93042, 93318, 93355, 94002, 94200, 94250, 94680-94690, 94770, 95812-95816, 95819, 95822, 95829, 95955, 96360-96368, 96372, 96374-96377, 96523, 97597-97598, 97602, 99155, 99156, 99157, 99211-99223, 99231-99255, 99291-99292, 99304-99310, 99315-99316, 99334-99337, 99347-99350, 99374-99375, 99377-99378, 99446-99449, 99451-99452, 99495-99496, G0463, G0471, J0670, J2001

64430 01991-01992, 0333T, 0464T, 0543T-0544T, 0548T, 0567T-0574T, 0580T, 0581T, 0582T, 20550-20551, 20560-20561, 36000, 36400-36410, 36420-36430, 36440, 36591-36592, 36600, 51701-51703, 66987-66988, 69990, 76000, 76970, 76998, 77001, 92012-92014, 92585, 93000-93010, 93040-93042, 93318, 93355, 94002, 94200, 94250, 94680-94690, 94770, 95812-95816, 95819, 95822, 95829, 95860-95870, 95907-95913, 95925-95933, 95937-95940, 95955, 96360-96368, 96372,

96374-96377, 96523, 99155, 99156, 99157, 99211-99223, 99231-99255, 99291-99292, 99304-99310, 99315-99316, 99334-99337, 99347-99350, 99374-99375, 99377-99378, 99446-99449, 99451-99452, 99495-99496, G0453, G0459, G0463, G0471, J0670, J2001

64435 01991-01992, 0333T, 0464T, 0543T-0544T, 0548T, 0567T-0574T, 0580T, 0581T, 0582T, 20560-20561, 36000, 36400-36410, 36420-36430, 36440, 36591-36592, 36600, 51701-51703, 66987-66988, 69990, 76000, 76970, 76998, 77001, 92012-92014, 92585, 93000-93010, 93040-93042, 93318, 93355, 94002, 94200, 94250, 94680-94690, 94770, 95812-95816, 95819, 95822, 95829, 95860-95870, 95907-95913, 95925-95933, 95937-95940, 95955, 96360-96368, 96372, 96374-96377, 96523, 99155, 99156, 99157, 99211-99223, 99231-99255, 99291-99292, 99304-99310, 99315-99316, 99334-99337, 99347-99350, 99374-99375, 99377-99378, 99446-99449, 99451-99452, 99495-99496, G0453, G0459, G0463, G0471, J0670, J2001

64486 01991-01992, 0333T, 0464T, 0543T-0544T, 0548T, 0567T-0574T, 0580T, 0581T, 0582T, 12001-12007, 12011-12057, 13100-13133, 13151-13153, 20560-20561, 20701, 36000, 36400-36410, 36420-36430, 36440, 36591-36592, 36600, 51701-51702, 66987-66988, 69990, 76000, 76380, 76942, 76970, 76998, 77001-77002, 77012, 77021, 92012-92014, 92585, 93000-93010, 93040-93042, 93318, 93355, 94002, 94200, 94250, 94680-94690, 94770, 95812-95816, 95819, 95822, 95829, 95860-95870, 95907-95913, 95925-95933, 95937-95941, 95955, 96360-96368, 96372, 96374-96377, 96523, 99155, 99156, 99157, 99211-99223, 99231-99255, 99291-99292, 99304-99310, 99315-99316, 99334-99337, 99347-99350, 99374-99375, 99377-99378, 99446-99449, 99451-99452, 99495-99496, G0453, G0459, G0463, G0471, J0670, J2001

64487 01991-01992, 0333T, 0464T, 0543T-0544T, 0548T, 0567T-0574T, 0580T, 0581T, 0582T, 12001-12007, 12011-12057, 13100-13133, 13151-13153, 20560-20561, 20701, 36000, 36400-36410, 36420-36430, 36440, 36591-36592, 36600, 51701-51702, 64486✦, 66987-66988, 69990, 76000, 76380, 76942, 76970, 76998, 77001-77002, 77012, 77021, 92012-92014, 92585, 93000-93010, 93040-93042, 93318, 93355, 94002, 94200, 94250, 94680-94690, 94770, 95812-95816, 95819, 95822, 95829, 95860-95870, 95907-95913, 95925-95933, 95937-95941, 95955, 96360-96368, 96372, 96374-96377, 96523, 99155, 99156, 99157, 99211-99223, 99231-99255, 99291-99292, 99304-99310, 99315-99316, 99334-99337, 99347-99350, 99374-99375, 99377-99378, 99446-99449, 99451-99452, 99495-99496, G0453, G0459, G0463, G0471, J0670, J2001

64488 01991-01992, 0333T, 0464T, 0543T-0544T, 0548T, 0567T-0574T, 0580T, 0581T, 0582T, 12001-12007, 12011-12057, 13100-13133, 13151-13153, 20560-20561, 20700-20701, 36000, 36400-36410, 36420-36430, 36440, 36591-36592, 36600, 51701-51702, 64451, 64486-64487✦, 66987-66988, 69990, 76000, 76380, 76942, 76970, 76998, 77001-77002, 77012, 77021, 92012-92014, 92585, 93000-93010, 93040-93042, 93318, 93355, 94002, 94200, 94250, 94680-94690, 94770, 95812-95816, 95819, 95822, 95829, 95860-95870, 95907-95913, 95925-95933, 95937-95941, 95955, 96360-96368, 96372, 96374-96377, 96523, 99155, 99156, 99157, 99211-99223, 99231-99255, 99291-99292, 99304-99310, 99315-99316, 99334-99337, 99347-99350, 99374-99375, 99377-99378, 99446-99449, 99451-99452, 99495-99496, G0453, G0459, G0463, G0471, J0670, J2001

64489 01991-01992, 0333T, 0464T, 0543T-0544T, 0548T, 0567T-0574T, 0580T, 0581T, 0582T, 12001-12007, 12011-12057, 13100-13133, 13151-13153, 20560-20561, 20700-20701, 36000, 36400-36410, 36420-36430, 36440, 36591-36592, 36600, 51701-51702, 64451, 64486-64488✦, 66987-66988, 69990, 76000, 76380, 76942, 76970, 76998,

77001-77002, 77012, 77021, 92012-92014, 92585, 93000-93010, 93040-93042, 93318, 93355, 94002, 94200, 94250, 94680-94690, 94770, 95812-95816, 95819, 95822, 95829, 95860-95870, 95907-95913, 95925-95933, 95937-95941, 95955, 96360-96368, 96372, 96374-96377, 96523, 99155, 99156, 99157, 99211-99223, 99231-99255, 99291-99292, 99304-99310, 99315-99316, 99334-99337, 99347-99350, 99374-99375, 99377-99378, 99446-99449, 99451-99452, 99495-99496, G0453, G0459, G0463, G0471, J0670, J2001

64517 01991-01992, 0333T, 0464T, 0543T-0544T, 0548T, 0567T-0574T, 0580T, 0581T, 0582T, 20560-20561, 20700-20701, 36000, 36400-36410, 36420-36430, 36440, 36591-36592, 36600, 51701-51703, 62329, 64451, 66987-66988, 69990, 76000, 76800, 76970, 76998, 77001, 92012-92014, 92585, 93000-93010, 93040-93042, 93318, 93355, 94002, 94200, 94250, 94680-94690, 94770, 95812-95816, 95819, 95822, 95829, 95860-95870, 95907-95913, 95925-95933, 95937-95940, 95955, 96360-96368, 96372, 96374-96377, 96523, 99155, 99156, 99157, 99211-99223, 99231-99255, 99291-99292, 99304-99310, 99315-99316, 99334-99337, 99347-99350, 99374-99375, 99377-99378, 99446-99449, 99451-99452, 99495-99496, G0453, G0459, G0463, G0471, J0670, J2001

64681 0216T, 0228T, 0230T, 0333T, 0464T, 12001-12007, 12011-12057, 13100-13133, 13151-13153, 20550-20553, 20560-20561, 36000, 36400-36410, 36420-36430, 36440, 36591-36592, 36600, 36640, 43752, 51701-51703, 62320-62327, 64400, 64405-64408, 64415-64435, 64445-64454, 64461-64463, 64479-64489, 64493-64505, 64510-64530, 69990, 76000, 77001-77003, 92012-92014, 92585, 93000-93010, 93040-93042, 93318, 93355, 94002, 94200, 94250, 94680-94690, 94770, 95812-95816, 95819, 95822, 95829, 95860-95870, 95907-95913, 95925-95933, 95937-95940, 95955, 96360-96368, 96372, 96374-96377, 96523, 99155, 99156, 99157, 99211-99223, 99231-99255, 99291-99292, 99304-99310, 99315-99316, 99334-99337, 99347-99350, 99374-99375, 99377-99378, 99446-99449, 99451-99452, 99495-99496, G0453, G0463, G0471

69990 0543T-0544T, 0548T, 0567T-0574T, 0580T, 0581T, 0582T, 0583T, 15772, 15774, 20560-20561, 20700-20701, 36591-36592, 62329, 64451, 64625, 66987-66988, 96523

76641 0581T, 36591-36592, 76642, 76882, 76942, 76970, 76981-76983✧, 76998, 96523

76642 0581T, 36591-36592, 76882, 76942, 76970, 76983✧, 76998, 96523

76700 36591-36592, 51701-51702, 76705, 76942, 76970, 76981-76983✧, 76998, 96523, G0471

76705 36591-36592, 51701-51702, 76942, 76970, 76983✧, 76998, 96523, G0471

76801 0567T✧, 36591-36592, 76805-76810, 76812, 76815-76816, 76830✧, 76942, 76970, 76998, 96523, 99446-99449, 99451-99452

76802 36591-36592, 76942, 76970, 76998, 96523, 99446-99449, 99451-99452

76805 0567T✧, 36591-36592, 51701-51702, 76802, 76812, 76815-76816, 76830-76831✧, 76856-76857✧, 76942, 76970, 76998, 96523, 99446-99449, 99451-99452, G0471

76810 36591-36592, 51701-51702, 76815, 76942, 76970, 76998, 96523, 99446-99449, 99451-99452, G0471

76811 0567T✧, 36591-36592, 51701-51702, 76801, 76805, 76815-76816, 76830-76831✧, 76856-76857✧, 76941-76942, 76970, 76998, 96523, 99446-99449, 99451-99452, G0471

76812 36591-36592, 51701-51702, 76942, 76970, 76998, 96523, 99446-99449, 99451-99452, G0471

76813 0567T✧, 36591-36592, 51701-51702, 76815, 76830✧, 76857✧, 76942, 76970, 76998, 96523, 99446-99449, 99451-99452, G0471

76814 36591-36592, 76942, 76970, 76998, 96523, 99446-99449, 99451-99452

76815 0567T✧, 36591-36592, 51701-51702, 76827-76828, 76857✧, 76942, 76970, 76998, 96523, 99446-99449, 99451-99452, G0471

76816 36591-36592, 51701-51702, 76810✧, 76815✧, 76857✧, 76942, 76970, 76998, 96523, 99446-99449, 99451-99452, G0471

76817 0567T✧, 36591-36592, 51701-51702, 76830-76831✧, 76856-76857✧, 76941-76942, 76970, 76998, 96523, 99446-99449, 99451-99452, G0471

76818 36591-36592, 51701-51702, 59025, 76376-76377, 76819, 76970, 76998, 96523, 99446-99449, 99451-99452, G0471

76819 36591-36592, 51701-51702, 59020-59025, 76376-76377, 76970, 76998, 96523, 99446-99449, 99451-99452, G0471

76820 36591-36592, 93325, 96523, 99446-99449, 99451-99452

76821 36591-36592, 76376-76377, 76815, 93325, 96523, 99446-99449, 99451-99452

76825 36591-36592, 51701-51702, 76815, 76970, 76998, 96523, 99446-99449, 99451-99452, G0471

76826 36591-36592, 51701-51702, 76815, 76825, 76970, 76998, 96523, 99446-99449, 99451-99452, G0471

76827 36591-36592, 51701-51702, 76376-76377, 76970, 76998, 96523, 99446-99449, 99451-99452, G0471

76828 36591-36592, 51701-51702, 76376-76377, 76827✧, 76970, 76998, 96523, 99446-99449, 99451-99452, G0471

76830 0567T-0568T, 36591-36592, 51701-51702, 76815-76816✧, 76942, 76970, 76981-76983✧, 76998, 96523, 99446-99449, 99451-99452, G0471

76856 0567T-0568T, 36591-36592, 51701-51702, 51798, 76801✧, 76813✧, 76815-76816✧, 76857, 76941-76942, 76970, 76981-76983✧, 76998, 93976, 93980✧, 96523, G0471

76857 0567T-0568T, 36591-36592, 51701-51702, 51798, 76801✧, 76810✧, 76941-76942, 76970, 76998, 93975-93981✧, 96523, G0471

76945 36591-36592, 76000, 76942, 76946, 76970, 76998, 77001-77002, 77012, 77021, 96523, 99446-99449, 99451-99452

76946 36591-36592, 76000, 76942, 76970, 76998, 77001-77002, 77012, 77021, 96523, 99446-99449, 99451-99452

76948 36591-36592, 76000, 76942, 76945✧, 76970, 76998, 77001-77002, 77012, 77021, 96523, 99446-99449, 99451-99452

80050 96523

80051 82374, 82435, 84132, 84295, 96523

80055 96523

80081 0064U, 0065U, 85004, 85007-85009, 85013-85018, 85025-85027, 85032-85041, 85048-85049, 86592, 86762, 86780, 86850, 86900-86901, 87340, 87389, 96523, G0306-G0307

80414 80415✧, 80500-80502, 84403, 96523

80415 80500-80502, 82670, 96523

81000 81002, 81015, 96523

81001 81000✧, 81002-81003, 81007, 81015✧, 96523

81002 81007✧, 81015✧, 96523

81003 81000, 81002✧, 81007✧, 81015✧, 96523

81005 81000, 81002-81003✧, 81007✧, 81015✧, 96523

81007 81000✧, 81015✧, 87086, 87088, 96523

81015 96523

81020 81000, 96523

81025 96523

82948 82950✤, 82952✤, 96523

82950 82951✤, 96523

82951 80500-80502, 82948, 96523

82952 80500-80502, 82947✤, 96523

84112 82105-82107, 96523

84702 80500-80502, 96523

84703 96523

84830 96523

85004 85008, 96523

85007 85004, 96523

85008 85007✤, 96523

85009 85004, 96523

85013 88738✤, 96523

85014 85013✤, 88738✤, 96523

85018 85008✤, 88738✤, 96523

85025 85004, 85007-85009, 85013-85018, 85027, 85032-85041, 85048-85049, 88738, 96523, G0306-G0307

85027 85004, 85008, 85013-85018, 85032-85041, 85048-85049, 88738, 96523, G0307

85041 85032, 96523

85045 85044, 96523

85046 85044-85045, 96523

85048 85008, 85032, 96523

85049 85008, 85032, 96523

86328 No CCI edits apply to this code.

86413 No CCI edits apply to this code.

86592 96523

86593 96523

86632 96523

86694 96523

86695 96523

86696 96523

86701 96523

86702 96523

86703 96523

86769 No CCI edits apply to this code.

87081 87040-87045✤, 87075✤, 87084✤, 87088✤, 88387-88388, 96523

87084 87040-87045✤, 87070✤, 87075✤, 88387-88388, 96523

87086 87070-87071, 87073-87075, 87081, 87084✤, 88387-88388, 96523

87088 87070-87071, 87073-87075, 87084✤, 88387-88388, 96523

87110 88387-88388, 96523

87118 88387-88388, 96523

87186 87188-87190✤, 88387-88388, 96523

87205 80500-80502, 88387-88388, 96523

87206 80500-80502, 87177✤, 88387-88388, 96523

87210 80500-80502, 87177✤, 88387-88388, 96523

87220 80500-80502, 87177✤, 88387-88388, 96523

87270 80500-80502, 87320✤, 87490-87492✤, 88346, 96523

87390 87535✤, 96523

87391 96523

87426 No CCI edits apply to this code.

87482 80500-80502, 81400-81408, 96523

87490 80500-80502, 81400-81408, 87206, 87491-87492✤, 96523

87491 80500-80502, 81400-81408, 87492✤, 96523

87492 80500-80502, 81400-81408, 96523

87528 80500-80502, 81400-81408, 87529-87530✤, 96523

87529 80500-80502, 81400-81408, 87206, 87530✤, 96523

87530 80500-80502, 81400-81408, 96523

87534 80500-80502, 81400-81408, 87535-87536✤, 96523

87535 80500-80502, 81400-81408, 87536✤, 96523

87536 80500-80502, 81400-81408, 87389-87390✤, 96523

87537 80500-80502, 81400-81408, 87538-87539✤, 96523

87538 80500-80502, 81400-81408, 87539✤, 96523

87539 80500-80502, 81400-81408, 96523

87590 80500-80502, 81400-81408, 87206, 87449, 87591-87592✤, 96523

87591 80500-80502, 81400-81408, 87592✤, 96523

87592 80500-80502, 81400-81408, 96523

87623 0112U✤, 80500-80502, 81400-81408, 87149-87150✤, 87153✤, 96523

87624 0112U✤, 80500-80502, 81400-81408, 87149-87150✤, 87153✤, 87623, 87625, 96523, G0476✤

87625 0112U✤, 80500-80502, 81400-81408, 87149-87150✤, 87153✤, 96523

87635 No CCI edits apply to this code.

87636 No CCI edits apply to this code.

87637 No CCI edits apply to this code.

87808 80500-80502, 96523

87850 80500-80502, 87590-87592✤, 96523

87880 80500-80502, 87650-87652✤, 96523

88141 88387, 96523, G0123-G0124, G0141-G0148, P3000

88142 88108, 88147-88150, 88152-88153, 88164-88167, 88387, 96523, G0123, G0143-G0148, P3000

88143 88142, 88147-88150, 88152-88153, 88164-88167, 88387, 96523, G0123, G0143-G0148, P3000

88147 88150, 88164, 88387, 96523, G0123, G0143-G0148, P3000

88148 88147, 88150, 88153, 88164-88165, 88387, 96523, G0123, G0143-G0148, P3000

88150 88104-88106, 88108, 88160-88162, 88387, 96523, G0123, G0143-G0148, P3000

88152 88108, 88147-88150, 88153, 88164-88165, 88387, 96523, G0123, G0143-G0148, P3000

88153 88147, 88150, 88164, 88387, 96523, G0123, G0143-G0148, P3000

88155 88104-88106, 88108, 88387, 96523

88164 88104-88106, 88108, 88150, 88160-88162, 88387, 96523, G0123, G0143-G0148, P3000

88165 88147, 88150, 88153, 88164, 88387, 96523, G0123, G0143-G0148, P3000

Coding Companion for Ob/Gyn

88166 88108, 88147-88150, 88152-88153, 88164-88165, 88387, 96523, G0123, G0143-G0148, P3000

88167 88147-88150, 88152-88153, 88164-88166, 88387, 96523, G0123, G0143-G0148, P3000

88174 88108, 88142-88143, 88147-88150, 88152-88153, 88164-88167, 88387, 96523, G0123, G0143-G0148, P3000

88175 88108, 88142-88143, 88147-88150, 88152-88153, 88164-88167, 88174, 88387, 96523, G0123, G0143-G0148, P3000

89253 96523

89254 96523

89255 96523

89257 80500-80502, 96523

89258 96523

89259 96523

89260 80500-80502, 89300-89321, 96523, G0027

89261 80500-80502, 89300-89321, 96523, G0027

89268 96523

89272 96523

89280 96523

89281 96523

89290 96523

89291 96523

89300 80500-80502, 89310✦, 89321✦, 96523, G0027

89310 80500-80502, 89321, 96523, G0027

89320 80500-80502, 89300-89310, 89321, 96523, G0027

89321 89257✦, 89264✦, 96523

89322 89300-89321, 96523, G0027

89325 80500-80502, 96523

89329 80500-80502, 96523

89330 80500-80502, 89329✦, 96523

89337 0058T, 88240, 96523

89342 96523

89343 96523

89344 96523

89346 96523

90384 36591-36592, 96523

90385 36591-36592, 96523

90386 36591-36592, 96523

90460 0591T-0593T, 36591-36592, 90471, 90473, 96160-96161, 96372, 96377, 96523, 99201-99215, 99241-99245, 99281-99285, 99381-99412, 99483, 99497, G0008-G0010, G0442-G0445, G0463

90461 0591T-0593T, 36591-36592, 96160-96161, 96523, 99201-99215, 99241-99245, 99281-99285, 99381-99412, 99483, 99497, G0442-G0445, G0463

90471 0591T-0593T, 36591-36592, 90473, 96160-96161, 96523, 99201-99215, 99241-99245, 99281-99285, 99381-99412, 99483, 99497, G0008-G0010✦, G0442-G0445, G0463

90472 0591T-0593T, 36591-36592, 96160-96161, 96523, 99201-99215, 99241-99245, 99281-99285, 99381-99412, 99483, 99497, G0442-G0445, G0463

90473 0591T-0593T, 36591-36592, 96160-96161, 96523, 99201-99215, 99241-99245, 99281-99285, 99381-99412, 99483, 99497, G0008✦, G0442-G0445, G0463

90474 0591T-0593T, 36591-36592, 96160-96161, 96523, 99201-99215, 99241-99245, 99281-99285, 99381-99412, 99483, 99497, G0442-G0445, G0463

90630 36591-36592, 90653✦, 90654✦, 90655-90658✦, 90660-90662✦, 90664✦, 90666-90668✦, 90672-90674✦, 90682-90689✦, 90694✦, 90756✦, 96523, Q2034-Q2039✦

90649 36591-36592, 96523

90650 36591-36592, 90649✦, 96523

90651 36591-36592, 90649✦, 90650✦, 96523

90653 36591-36592, 90689✦, 90694✦, 96523, Q2035-Q2039✦

90654 36591-36592, 90653✦, 90655-90658✦, 90660-90662✦, 90664✦, 90666-90668✦, 90673-90674✦, 90682-90689✦, 90694✦, 90756✦, 96523, Q2034✦

90655 36591-36592, 90653✦, 90657-90658✦, 90660-90662✦, 90664✦, 90666-90668✦, 90689✦, 90694✦, 96523, Q2034✦

90656 36591-36592, 90653✦, 90655✦, 90657-90658✦, 90660-90662✦, 90664✦, 90666-90668✦, 90673-90674✦, 90682-90689✦, 90694✦, 90756✦, 96523, Q2034✦

90657 36591-36592, 90653✦, 90658✦, 90660-90662✦, 90664✦, 90666-90668✦, 90689✦, 90694✦, 96523

90658 36591-36592, 90653✦, 90660-90662✦, 90664✦, 90666-90668✦, 90689✦, 90694✦, 96523

90660 36591-36592, 90653✦, 90661-90662✦, 90664✦, 90666-90668✦, 90689✦, 90694✦, 96523

90664 36591-36592, 90653✦, 90666-90668✦, 90689✦, 90694✦, 96523

90666 36591-36592, 90653✦, 90667-90668✦, 90689✦, 90694✦, 96523

90667 36591-36592, 90653✦, 90668✦, 90689✦, 90694✦, 96523

90668 36591-36592, 90653✦, 90689✦, 90694✦, 96523

90672 36591-36592, 90653✦, 90654✦, 90655-90658✦, 90660-90662✦, 90664✦, 90666-90668✦, 90673-90674✦, 90682-90689✦, 90694✦, 90756✦, 96523, Q2034-Q2039✦

90673 36591-36592, 90389✦, 90653✦, 90655✦, 90657-90658✦, 90660-90662✦, 90664✦, 90666-90668✦, 90694✦, 96523, Q2034✦

90682 36591-36592, 90653✦, 90655✦, 90657-90658✦, 90660-90662✦, 90664✦, 90666-90668✦, 90673✦, 90685-90689✦, 90694✦, 90756✦, 96523, Q2034-Q2039✦

90685 36591-36592, 90653✦, 90655✦, 90657-90658✦, 90660-90662✦, 90664✦, 90666-90668✦, 90673✦, 90686-90689✦, 90756✦, 96523, Q2034✦

90686 36591-36592, 90653✦, 90655✦, 90657-90658✦, 90660-90662✦, 90664✦, 90666-90668✦, 90673✦, 90687-90689✦, 90694✦, 96523, Q2034✦

90687 36591-36592, 90653✦, 90655✦, 90657-90658✦, 90660-90662✦, 90664✦, 90666-90668✦, 90673✦, 90688-90689✦, 90694✦, 96523, Q2034✦

90688 36591-36592, 90653✦, 90655✦, 90657-90658✦, 90660-90662✦, 90664✦, 90666-90668✦, 90673✦, 90689✦, 90694✦, 96523, Q2034✦

90689 36591-36592, 90694✦, 96523

90736 36591-36592, 96523

90739 36591-36592, 96523

90740 36591-36592, 90739✦, 90747✦, 96523

90743 36591-36592, 90739-90740✦, 90744✦, 90746-90747✦, 96523

90744 36591-36592, 90739-90740✦, 90746-90747✦, 96523

Coding Companion for Ob/Gyn

90746 36591-36592, 90739-90740✦, 90747✦, 96523

90747 36591-36592, 90739✦, 96523

90748 36591-36592, 90739✦, 96523

90750 36591-36592, 90736✦, 96523

90756 36591-36592, 90653✦, 90655✦, 90657-90658✦, 90660-90662✦, 90664✦, 90666-90668✦, 90673✦, 90686-90689✦, 90694✦, 96523, Q2034-Q2039✦

91300 No CCI edits apply to this code.

91301 No CCI edits apply to this code.

92950 12001-12007, 12011-12057, 13100-13133, 13151-13153, 36000, 36400-36410, 36420-36430, 36440, 36591-36592, 36600, 36640, 43752, 51701-51703, 62320-62327, 64400, 64405-64408, 64415-64435, 64445-64454, 64461-64463, 64479-64505, 64510-64530, 92012-92014, 92961✦, 93000-93010, 93040-93042, 93318, 93355, 94002, 94200, 94250, 94680-94690, 94770, 95812-95816, 95819, 95822, 95829, 95955, 96360-96368, 96372, 96374-96377, 96523, 99155, 99156, 99157, 99211-99223, 99231-99255, 99291-99292, 99304-99310, 99315-99316, 99334-99337, 99347-99350, 99374-99375, 99377-99378, 99446-99449, 99451-99452, 99495-99496, G0463, G0471

93975 36591-36592, 76700-76776, 76856, 76970, 76998, 93976-93979, 96523

93976 36591-36592, 76700-76776, 76970, 76998, 93978-93979, 96523

96040 36591-36592, 96523

96160 0373T, 36591-36592, 94002-94004, 94660-94662, 96110, 96164-96171, 96523, 97153-97158, 99091, 99172-99173, 99474

96161 0373T, 36591-36592, 94002-94004, 94660-94662, 96110, 96164-96171, 96523, 97153-97158, 99091, 99172-99173, 99474

96360 0543T-0544T, 0548T, 0567T-0574T, 0580T, 0581T, 0582T, 36000, 36410, 36425, 36591-36592, 64450, 66987-66988, 96372, 96374, 96377, 96523, 99201-99215, 99354-99355, 99358-99359, 99455-99456, 99483, 99497, E0781, G0463

96361 0543T-0544T, 0548T, 0567T-0574T, 0580T, 0581T, 0582T, 36591-36592, 66987-66988, 96523, 99354-99355, 99358-99359, E0781

96365 0543T-0544T, 0567T-0574T, 0580T, 0581T, 0582T, 36000, 36410, 36425, 36591-36592, 64450, 66987-66988, 96360, 96372, 96374, 96377, 96523, 99201-99215, 99354-99355, 99358-99359, 99455-99456, 99483, 99497, E0781, G0463, J1642-J1644

96366 0543T-0544T, 0567T-0574T, 0580T, 0581T, 0582T, 36591-36592, 66987-66988, 96523, 99354-99355, 99358-99359, E0781

96367 0543T-0544T, 0567T-0574T, 0580T, 0581T, 0582T, 36591-36592, 66987-66988, 96523, 99354-99355, 99358-99359, E0781

96368 0543T-0544T, 0567T-0574T, 0580T, 0581T, 0582T, 36591-36592, 66987-66988, 96523, 99354-99355, 99358-99359

98966 36591-36592, 93792, 93793, 96523, G0250

98967 36591-36592, 93792, 93793, 96523, 99421, G0250

98968 36591-36592, 93792, 93793, 96523, 99421-99422, 99446-99447, G0250

98970 36591-36592, 96523, 99489, G0250, G2061-G2063

98971 36591-36592, 96523, 99489, G0250, G2061-G2063

98972 36591-36592, 96523, 99489, G0250, G2061-G2063

99000 36591-36592, 96523

99001 36591-36592, 96523

99026 36591-36592, 96523

99027 36591-36592, 96523

99050 36591-36592, 96523

99051 36591-36592, 96523

99053 36591-36592, 96523

99056 36591-36592, 96523

99058 36591-36592, 96523

99060 36591-36592, 96523

99202 0362T, 0373T, 0469T, 36591-36592, 43752, 80500-80502, 90863, 90940, 92002-92014, 92227-92228, 92531-92532, 93561-93562, 93792, 93793, 94002-94004, 94660-94662, 95851-95852, 96020, 96105, 96116, 96125, 96130, 96132, 96136, 96138, 96146, 96156-96159, 96164-96168, 96523, 97151, 97153-97158, 97169-97172, 97802-97804, 99091, 99172-99173, 99174, 99177, 99201, 99211-99215, 99408-99409, 99421-99423, 99446-99449, 99463✦, 99474, 99605-99606, G0102, G0117-G0118, G0245-G0246, G0248, G0250, G0270-G0271, G0396-G0397, G0406-G0408✦, G0425-G0427✦, G0442-G0447, G0459, G0473, G0508-G0509✦, G2011

99203 0362T, 0373T, 0469T, 36591-36592, 43752, 80500-80502, 90863, 90940, 92002-92014, 92227-92228, 92531-92532, 93561-93562, 93792, 93793, 94002-94004, 94660-94662, 95851-95852, 96020, 96105, 96116, 96125, 96130, 96132, 96136, 96138, 96146, 96156-96159, 96164-96168, 96523, 97151, 97153-97158, 97169-97172, 97802-97804, 99091, 99172-99173, 99174, 99177, 99201-99202, 99211-99215, 99408-99409, 99421-99423, 99446-99449, 99463✦, 99474, 99605-99606, G0102, G0117-G0118, G0245-G0246, G0248, G0250, G0270-G0271, G0396-G0397, G0406-G0408✦, G0425-G0427✦, G0442-G0447, G0459, G0473, G0508-G0509✦, G2011

99204 0362T, 0373T, 0469T, 36591-36592, 43752, 80500-80502, 90863, 90940, 92002-92014, 92227-92228, 92531-92532, 93561-93562, 93792, 93793, 94002-94004, 94660-94662, 95851-95852, 96020, 96105, 96116, 96125, 96130, 96132, 96136, 96138, 96146, 96156-96159, 96164-96168, 96523, 97151, 97153-97158, 97169-97172, 97802-97804, 99091, 99172-99173, 99174, 99177, 99201-99203, 99211-99215, 99408-99409, 99421-99423, 99446-99449, 99463✦, 99474, 99605-99606, G0102, G0117-G0118, G0245-G0246, G0248, G0250, G0270-G0271, G0396-G0397, G0406-G0408✦, G0425-G0427✦, G0442-G0447, G0459, G0473, G0508-G0509✦, G2011

99205 0362T, 0373T, 0469T, 36591-36592, 43752, 80500-80502, 90863, 90940, 92002-92014, 92227-92228, 92531-92532, 93561-93562, 93792, 93793, 94002-94004, 94660-94662, 95851-95852, 96020, 96105, 96116, 96125, 96130, 96132, 96136, 96138, 96146, 96156-96159, 96164-96168, 96523, 97151, 97153-97158, 97169-97172, 97802-97804, 99091, 99172-99173, 99174, 99177, 99201-99204, 99211-99215, 99408-99409, 99421-99423, 99446-99449, 99463✦, 99474, 99605-99606, G0102, G0117-G0118, G0245-G0246, G0248, G0250, G0270-G0271, G0396-G0397, G0406-G0408✦, G0425-G0427✦, G0442-G0447, G0459, G0473, G0508-G0509✦, G2011

99211 0362T, 0373T, 0469T, 0543T-0544T, 0567T-0574T, 0580T, 0581T, 0582T, 36591-36592, 43752, 80500-80502, 90863, 90940, 92002-92014, 92227-92228, 92531-92532, 93561-93562, 93792, 93793, 94002-94004, 94660-94662, 95851-95852, 96020, 96105, 96116, 96125, 96130, 96132, 96136, 96138, 96146, 96156-96159, 96164-96168, 96523, 97151, 97153-97158, 97169-97172, 97802-97804, 99091, 99172-99173, 99174, 99177, 99408-99409, 99446-99449, 99474, 99605-99606, G0102, G0117-G0118, G0245-G0246, G0248, G0250, G0270-G0271, G0396-G0397, G0406-G0408✦, G0425-G0427✦, G0442-G0447, G0459, G0473, G0508-G0509✦, G2011

99212 0362T, 0373T, 0469T, 0543T-0544T, 0567T-0574T, 0580T, 0581T, 0582T, 20560-20561, 36591-36592, 43752, 80500-80502, 90863, 90940, 92002-92014, 92227-92228, 92531-92532, 93561-93562, 93792, 93793, 94002-94004, 94660-94662, 95851-95852, 96020, 96105, 96116, 96125,

96130, 96132, 96136, 96138, 96146, 96156-96159, 96164-96168, 96523, 97151, 97153-97158, 97169-97172, 97802-97804, 99091, 99172-99173, 99174, 99177, 99211, 99408-99409, 99421, 99446-99449, 99474, 99605-99606, G0102, G0117-G0118, G0245-G0246, G0248, G0250, G0270-G0271, G0396-G0397, G0406-G0408♦, G0425-G0427♦, G0442-G0447, G0459, G0473, G0508-G0509♦, G2011

99213 0362T, 0373T, 0469T, 0543T-0544T, 0567T-0574T, 0580T, 0581T, 0582T, 20560-20561, 36591-36592, 43752, 80500-80502, 90863, 90940, 92002-92014, 92227-92228, 92531-92532, 93561-93562, 93792, 93793, 94002-94004, 94660-94662, 95851-95852, 96020, 96105, 96116, 96125, 96130, 96132, 96136, 96138, 96146, 96156-96159, 96164-96168, 96523, 97151, 97153-97158, 97169-97172, 97802-97804, 99091, 99172-99173, 99174, 99177, 99211-99212, 99408-99409, 99421-99423, 99446-99449, 99463♦, 99474, 99605-99606, G0102, G0117-G0118, G0245-G0246, G0248, G0250, G0270-G0271, G0396-G0397, G0406-G0408♦, G0425-G0427♦, G0442-G0447, G0459, G0473, G0508-G0509♦, G2011

99214 0362T, 0373T, 0469T, 0543T-0544T, 0567T-0574T, 0580T, 0581T, 0582T, 20560-20561, 20700-20701, 36591-36592, 43752, 80500-80502, 90863, 90940, 92002-92014, 92227-92228, 92531-92532, 93561-93562, 93792, 93793, 94002-94004, 94660-94662, 95851-95852, 96020, 96105, 96116, 96125, 96130, 96132, 96136, 96138, 96146, 96156-96159, 96164-96168, 96523, 97151, 97153-97158, 97169-97172, 97802-97804, 99091, 99172-99173, 99174, 99177, 99211-99213, 99408-99409, 99421-99423, 99446-99449, 99463♦, 99474, 99605-99606, G0102, G0117-G0118, G0245-G0246, G0248, G0250, G0270-G0271, G0396-G0397, G0406-G0408♦, G0425-G0427♦, G0442-G0447, G0459, G0473, G0508-G0509♦, G2011

99215 0362T, 0373T, 0469T, 0543T-0544T, 0567T-0574T, 0580T, 0581T, 0582T, 20560-20561, 20700-20701, 36591-36592, 43752, 62329, 80500-80502, 90863, 90940, 92002-92014, 92227-92228, 92531-92532, 93561-93562, 93792, 93793, 94002-94004, 94660-94662, 95851-95852, 96020, 96105, 96116, 96125, 96130, 96132, 96136, 96138, 96146, 96156-96159, 96164-96168, 96523, 97151, 97153-97158, 97169-97172, 97802-97804, 99091, 99172-99173, 99174, 99177, 99211-99214, 99408-99409, 99421-99423, 99446-99449, 99463♦, 99474, 99605-99606, G0102, G0117-G0118, G0245-G0246, G0248, G0250, G0270-G0271, G0396-G0397, G0406-G0408♦, G0425-G0427♦, G0442-G0447, G0459, G0473, G0508-G0509♦, G2011

99217 0362T, 0373T, 0469T, 0543T-0544T, 0567T-0574T, 0580T, 0581T, 0582T, 20560-20561, 20701, 36591-36592, 43752, 90863, 90940, 92002-92014, 92227-92228, 92531-92532, 93792, 93793, 94002-94004, 94644, 94660-94662, 95851-95852, 96020, 96105, 96116, 96125-96130, 96132, 96136, 96138, 96146, 96156-96159, 96164-96168, 96360, 96365, 96369, 96372-96374, 96377, 96401-96406, 96409, 96413, 96416, 96420-96422, 96425-96440, 96446-96450, 96523, 97151, 97153-97158, 97169-97172, 97802-97804, 99091, 99172-99173, 99174, 99177, 99281-99285, 99408-99409, 99446-99449, 99451-99452, 99474, 99605-99606, G0102, G0245-G0246, G0250, G0270-G0271, G0396-G0397, G0442-G0447, G0459, G0473, G0498, G2011

99218 0362T, 0373T, 0469T, 0543T-0544T, 0567T-0574T, 0580T, 0581T, 0582T, 0591T-0593T, 20560-20561, 20700-20701, 36591-36592, 43752, 90863, 90940, 92002-92014, 92227-92228, 92531-92532, 93792, 93793, 94002-94004, 94644, 94660-94662, 95851-95852, 96020, 96105, 96116, 96125-96130, 96132, 96136, 96138, 96146, 96156-96159, 96164-96168, 96360, 96365, 96369, 96372-96374, 96377, 96401-96406, 96409, 96413, 96416, 96420-96422, 96425-96440, 96446-96450, 96523, 97151, 97153-97158, 97169-97172, 97802-97804, 99091, 99172-99173, 99174, 99177, 99201-99217, 99224-99226, 99238-99239, 99281-99285,

99307-99310, 99315-99318, 99324-99328, 99334-99337, 99341-99350, 99381-99404, 99408-99412, 99446-99449, 99451-99452, 99474, 99483, 99497, 99605-99606, G0102, G0245-G0246, G0250, G0270-G0271, G0380-G0384, G0396-G0397, G0442-G0447, G0459, G0463, G0473, G0498, G2011

99219 0362T, 0373T, 0469T, 0543T-0544T, 0567T-0574T, 0580T, 0581T, 0582T, 0591T-0593T, 15772, 15774, 20560-20561, 20700-20701, 36591-36592, 43752, 90863, 90940, 92002-92014, 92227-92228, 92531-92532, 93792, 93793, 94002-94004, 94644, 94660-94662, 95851-95852, 96020, 96105, 96116, 96125-96130, 96132, 96136, 96138, 96146, 96156-96159, 96164-96168, 96360, 96365, 96369, 96372-96374, 96377, 96401-96406, 96409, 96413, 96416, 96420-96422, 96425-96440, 96446-96450, 96523, 97151, 97153-97158, 97169-97172, 97802-97804, 99091, 99172-99173, 99174, 99177, 99201-99218, 99224-99226, 99238-99239, 99281-99285, 99307-99310, 99315-99318, 99324-99328, 99334-99337, 99341-99350, 99381-99404, 99408-99412, 99446-99449, 99451-99452, 99463♦, 99474, 99483, 99497, 99605-99606, G0102, G0245-G0246, G0250, G0270-G0271, G0380-G0384, G0396-G0397, G0442-G0447, G0459, G0463, G0473, G0498, G2011

99220 0362T, 0373T, 0469T, 0543T-0544T, 0567T-0574T, 0580T, 0581T, 0582T, 0591T-0593T, 15772, 15774, 20560-20561, 20700-20701, 36591-36592, 43752, 62329, 90863, 90940, 92002-92014, 92227-92228, 92531-92532, 93792, 93793, 94002-94004, 94644, 94660-94662, 95851-95852, 96020, 96105, 96116, 96125-96130, 96132, 96136, 96138, 96146, 96156-96159, 96164-96168, 96360, 96365, 96369, 96372-96374, 96377, 96401-96406, 96409, 96413, 96416, 96420-96422, 96425-96440, 96446-96450, 96523, 97151, 97153-97158, 97169-97172, 97802-97804, 99091, 99172-99173, 99174, 99177, 99201-99219, 99224-99226, 99238-99239, 99281-99285, 99307-99310, 99315-99318, 99324-99328, 99334-99337, 99341-99350, 99381-99404, 99408-99412, 99446-99449, 99451-99452, 99463♦, 99474, 99483, 99497, 99605-99606, G0102, G0245-G0246, G0250, G0270-G0271, G0380-G0384, G0396-G0397, G0442-G0447, G0459, G0463, G0473, G0498, G2011

99221 0362T, 0373T, 0469T, 0543T-0544T, 0567T-0574T, 0580T, 0581T, 0582T, 0591T-0593T, 20560-20561, 20700-20701, 36591-36592, 43752, 80500-80502, 90863, 90940, 92002-92014, 92227-92228, 92531-92532, 93792, 93793, 94002-94004, 94644, 94660-94662, 95851-95852, 96020, 96105, 96116, 96125-96130, 96132, 96136, 96138, 96146, 96156-96159, 96164-96168, 96360, 96365, 96369, 96372-96374, 96377, 96401-96406, 96409, 96413, 96416, 96420-96422, 96425-96440, 96446-96450, 96523, 97151, 97153-97158, 97169-97172, 97802-97804, 99091, 99172-99173, 99174, 99177, 99184, 99201-99220, 99224-99233, 99238-99239, 99281-99285, 99304-99310, 99315-99318, 99324-99328, 99334-99337, 99341-99350, 99381-99404, 99408-99412, 99446-99449, 99451-99452, 99460, 99462-99463♦, 99474, 99483, 99497, 99605-99606, G0102, G0245-G0246, G0250, G0270-G0271, G0380-G0384, G0396-G0397, G0406-G0408, G0424-G0427, G0442-G0447, G0459, G0463, G0473, G0498, G0508-G0509, G2011

99222 0362T, 0373T, 0469T, 0543T-0544T, 0567T-0574T, 0580T, 0581T, 0582T, 0591T-0593T, 15774, 20560-20561, 20700-20701, 36591-36592, 43752, 62329, 80500-80502, 90863, 90940, 92002-92014, 92227-92228, 92531-92532, 93792, 93793, 94002-94004, 94644, 94660-94662, 95851-95852, 96020, 96105, 96116, 96125-96130, 96132, 96136, 96138, 96146, 96156-96159, 96164-96168, 96360, 96365, 96369, 96372-96374, 96377, 96401-96406, 96409, 96413, 96416, 96420-96422, 96425-96440, 96446-96450, 96523, 97151, 97153-97158, 97169-97172, 97802-97804, 99091, 99172-99173, 99174, 99177, 99184, 99201-99221, 99224-99233, 99238-99239, 99281-99285, 99304-99310, 99315-99318, 99324-99328, 99334-99337, 99341-99350, 99381-99404, 99408-99412, 99446-99449, 99451-99452, 99460, 99462-99463♦, 99474,

99479-99480, 99483, 99497, 99605-99606, G0102, G0245-G0246, G0250, G0270-G0271, G0380-G0384, G0396-G0397, G0406-G0408, G0424-G0427, G0442-G0447, G0459, G0463, G0473, G0498, G0508-G0509, G2011

99223 0362T, 0373T, 0469T, 0543T-0544T, 0567T-0574T, 0580T, 0581T, 0582T, 0591T-0593T, 15772, 15774, 20560-20561, 20700-20701, 36591-36592, 43752, 62329, 80500-80502, 90863, 90940, 92002-92014, 92227-92228, 92531-92532, 93792, 93793, 94002-94004, 94644, 94660-94662, 95851-95852, 96020, 96105, 96116, 96125-96130, 96132, 96136, 96138, 96146, 96156-96159, 96164-96168, 96360, 96365, 96369, 96372-96374, 96377, 96401-96406, 96409, 96413, 96416, 96420-96422, 96425-96440, 96446-96450, 96523, 97151, 97153-97158, 97169-97172, 97802-97804, 99091, 99172-99173, 99174, 99177, 99184, 99201-99222, 99224-99233, 99238-99239, 99281-99285, 99304-99310, 99315-99318, 99324-99328, 99334-99337, 99341-99350, 99381-99404, 99408-99412, 99446-99449, 99451-99452, 99460-99463✦, 99474, 99478-99480, 99483, 99497, 99605-99606, G0102, G0245-G0246, G0250, G0270-G0271, G0380-G0384, G0396-G0397, G0406-G0408, G0424-G0427, G0442-G0447, G0459, G0463, G0473, G0498, G0508-G0509, G2011

99224 0362T, 0373T, 0469T, 36591-36592, 43752, 90863, 90940, 92002-92014, 92227-92228, 92531-92532, 93792, 93793, 94002-94004, 94644, 94660-94662, 95851-95852, 96020, 96116, 96127, 96156-96159, 96164-96168, 96360, 96365, 96369, 96372-96374, 96377, 96401-96406, 96409, 96413, 96416, 96420-96422, 96425-96440, 96446-96450, 96523, 97151, 97153-97158, 97169-97172, 97802-97804, 99091, 99172-99173, 99174, 99177, 99201-99217, 99281-99285, 99307-99310, 99318, 99324-99328, 99334-99337, 99341-99350, 99408-99409, 99446-99449, 99451-99452, 99460-99462, 99474, 99483, 99497, 99605-99606, G0102, G0245-G0246, G0250, G0270-G0271, G0380-G0384, G0396-G0397, G0442-G0447, G0459, G0463, G0473, G0498, G2011

99225 0362T, 0373T, 0469T, 36591-36592, 43752, 90863, 90940, 92002-92014, 92227-92228, 92531-92532, 93792, 93793, 94002-94004, 94644, 94660-94662, 95851-95852, 96020, 96116, 96127, 96360, 96365, 96369, 96372-96374, 96377, 96401-96406, 96409, 96413, 96416, 96420-96422, 96425-96440, 96446-96450, 96523, 97151, 97153-97158, 97802-97804, 99091, 99172-99173, 99174, 99177, 99201-99217, 99224, 99281-99285, 99307-99310, 99318, 99324-99328, 99334-99337, 99341-99350, 99408-99409, 99446-99449, 99451-99452, 99460-99462, 99483, 99497, 99605-99606, G0102, G0245-G0246, G0250, G0270-G0271, G0380-G0384, G0396-G0397, G0442-G0447, G0459, G0463, G0473, G0498, G2011

99226 0362T, 0373T, 0469T, 36591-36592, 43752, 90863, 90940, 92002-92014, 92227-92228, 92531-92532, 93792, 93793, 94002-94004, 94644, 94660-94662, 95851-95852, 96020, 96116, 96127, 96360, 96365, 96369, 96372-96374, 96377, 96401-96406, 96409, 96413, 96416, 96420-96422, 96425-96440, 96446-96450, 96523, 97151, 97153-97158, 97802-97804, 99091, 99172-99173, 99174, 99177, 99201-99217, 99224-99225, 99281-99285, 99307-99310, 99318, 99324-99328, 99334-99337, 99341-99350, 99408-99409, 99446-99449, 99451-99452, 99460-99462, 99483, 99497, 99605-99606, G0102, G0245-G0246, G0250, G0270-G0271, G0380-G0384, G0396-G0397, G0442-G0447, G0459, G0463, G0473, G0498, G2011

99231 0362T, 0373T, 0469T, 0543T-0544T, 0567T-0574T, 0580T, 0581T, 0582T, 20560-20561, 36591-36592, 43752, 80500-80502, 90863, 90940, 92002-92014, 92227-92228, 92531-92532, 93792, 93793, 94002-94004, 94644, 94660-94662, 95851-95852, 96020, 96105, 96116, 96125-96130, 96132, 96136, 96138, 96146, 96156-96159, 96164-96168, 96360, 96365, 96369, 96372-96374, 96377, 96401-96406, 96409, 96413,

96416, 96420-96422, 96425-96440, 96446-96450, 96523, 97151, 97153-97158, 97169-97172, 97802-97804, 99091, 99172-99173, 99174, 99177, 99184, 99281-99285, 99408-99409, 99446-99449, 99451-99452, 99474, 99605-99606, G0102, G0245-G0246, G0250, G0270-G0271, G0380-G0384, G0396-G0397, G0406-G0408, G0425-G0427, G0442-G0447, G0459, G0473, G0498, G0508-G0509, G2011

99232 0362T, 0373T, 0469T, 0543T-0544T, 0567T-0574T, 0580T, 0581T, 0582T, 20560-20561, 20701, 36591-36592, 43752, 80500-80502, 90863, 90940, 92002-92014, 92227-92228, 92531-92532, 93792, 93793, 94002-94004, 94644, 94660-94662, 95851-95852, 96020, 96105, 96116, 96125-96130, 96132, 96136, 96138, 96146, 96156-96159, 96164-96168, 96360, 96365, 96369, 96372-96374, 96377, 96401-96406, 96409, 96413, 96416, 96420-96422, 96425-96440, 96446-96450, 96523, 97151, 97153-97158, 97169-97172, 97802-97804, 99091, 99172-99173, 99174, 99177, 99184, 99231, 99281-99285, 99408-99409, 99446-99449, 99451-99452, 99462, 99474, 99605-99606, G0102, G0245-G0246, G0250, G0270-G0271, G0380-G0384, G0396-G0397, G0406-G0408, G0425-G0427, G0442-G0447, G0459, G0473, G0498, G0508-G0509, G2011

99233 0362T, 0373T, 0469T, 0543T-0544T, 0567T-0574T, 0580T, 0581T, 0582T, 20560-20561, 20700-20701, 36591-36592, 43752, 80500-80502, 90863, 90940, 92002-92014, 92227-92228, 92531-92532, 93792, 93793, 94002-94004, 94644, 94660-94662, 95851-95852, 96020, 96105, 96116, 96125-96130, 96132, 96136, 96138, 96146, 96156-96159, 96164-96168, 96360, 96365, 96369, 96372-96374, 96377, 96401-96406, 96409, 96413, 96416, 96420-96422, 96425-96440, 96446-96450, 96523, 97151, 97153-97158, 97169-97172, 97802-97804, 99091, 99172-99173, 99174, 99177, 99184, 99231-99232, 99281-99285, 99408-99409, 99446-99449, 99451-99452, 99460, 99462-99463✦, 99474, 99605-99606, G0102, G0245-G0246, G0250, G0270-G0271, G0380-G0384, G0396-G0397, G0406-G0408, G0425-G0427, G0442-G0447, G0459, G0473, G0498, G0508-G0509, G2011

99234 0362T, 0373T, 0469T, 0543T-0544T, 0567T-0574T, 0580T, 0581T, 0582T, 15772, 15774, 20560-20561, 20700-20701, 36591-36592, 43752, 62329, 80500-80502, 90863, 90940, 92002-92014, 92227-92228, 92531-92532, 93792, 93793, 94002-94004, 94644, 94660-94662, 95851-95852, 96020, 96105, 96116, 96125-96130, 96132, 96136, 96138, 96146, 96156-96159, 96164-96168, 96360, 96365, 96369, 96372-96374, 96377, 96401-96406, 96409, 96413, 96416, 96420-96422, 96425-96440, 96446-96450, 96523, 97151, 97153-97158, 97169-97172, 97802-97804, 99091, 99172-99173, 99174, 99177, 99201-99233, 99238-99239, 99281-99285, 99307-99310, 99318, 99324-99328, 99334-99337, 99341-99350, 99408-99409, 99446-99449, 99451-99452, 99474, 99483, 99497, 99605-99606, G0102, G0245-G0246, G0250, G0270-G0271, G0380-G0384, G0396-G0397, G0406-G0408, G0425-G0427, G0442-G0447, G0459, G0463, G0473, G0498, G0508-G0509, G2011

99235 0362T, 0373T, 0469T, 0543T-0544T, 0567T-0574T, 0580T, 0581T, 0582T, 15772, 15774, 20560-20561, 20700-20701, 36591-36592, 43752, 62329, 80500-80502, 90863, 90940, 92002-92014, 92227-92228, 92531-92532, 93792, 93793, 94002-94004, 94644, 94660-94662, 95851-95852, 96020, 96105, 96116, 96125-96130, 96132, 96136, 96138, 96146, 96156-96159, 96164-96168, 96360, 96365, 96369, 96372-96374, 96377, 96401-96406, 96409, 96413, 96416, 96420-96422, 96425-96440, 96446-96450, 96523, 97151, 97153-97158, 97169-97172, 97802-97804, 99091, 99172-99173, 99174, 99177, 99201-99234, 99238-99239, 99281-99285, 99307-99310, 99318, 99324-99328, 99334-99337, 99341-99350, 99408-99409, 99446-99449, 99451-99452, 99474, 99483, 99497, 99605-99606, G0102, G0245-G0246, G0250, G0270-G0271, G0380-G0384, G0396-G0397, G0406-G0408, G0425-G0427, G0442-G0447, G0459, G0463, G0473, G0498, G0508-G0509, G2011

99236 0362T, 0373T, 0469T, 0543T-0544T, 0567T-0574T, 0580T, 0581T, 0582T, 15772, 15774, 20560-20561, 20700-20701, 36591-36592, 43752, 62329, 80500-80502, 90863, 90940, 92002-92014, 92227-92228, 92531-92532, 93792, 93793, 94002-94004, 94644, 94660-94662, 95851-95852, 96020, 96105, 96116, 96125-96130, 96132, 96136, 96138, 96146, 96156-96159, 96164-96168, 96360, 96365, 96369, 96372-96374, 96377, 96401-96406, 96409, 96413, 96416, 96420-96422, 96425-96440, 96446-96450, 96523, 97151, 97153-97158, 97169-97172, 97802-97804, 99091, 99172-99173, 99174, 99177, 99201-99235, 99238-99239, 99281-99285, 99307-99310, 99318, 99324-99328, 99334-99337, 99341-99350, 99408-99409, 99446-99449, 99451-99452, 99474, 99483, 99497, 99605-99606, G0102, G0245-G0246, G0250, G0270-G0271, G0380-G0384, G0396-G0397, G0406-G0408, G0425-G0427, G0442-G0447, G0459, G0463, G0473, G0498, G0508-G0509, G2011

99238 0362T, 0373T, 0469T, 0543T-0544T, 0567T-0574T, 0580T, 0581T, 0582T, 20560-20561, 20701, 36591-36592, 43752, 80500-80502, 90863, 90940, 92002-92014, 92227-92228, 92531-92532, 93792, 93793, 94002-94004, 94644, 94660-94662, 95851-95852, 96020, 96105, 96116, 96125-96130, 96132, 96136, 96138, 96146, 96156-96159, 96164-96168, 96360, 96365, 96369, 96372-96374, 96377, 96401-96406, 96409, 96413, 96416, 96420-96422, 96425-96440, 96446-96450, 96523, 97151, 97153-97158, 97169-97172, 97802-97804, 99091, 99172-99173, 99174, 99177, 99201-99217✦, 99231-99233, 99281-99285, 99408-99409, 99446-99449, 99451-99452, 99474, 99483, 99605-99606, G0102, G0245-G0246, G0250, G0270-G0271, G0380-G0384, G0396-G0397, G0442-G0447, G0459, G0463, G0473, G0498, G2011

99239 0362T, 0373T, 0469T, 0543T-0544T, 0567T-0574T, 0580T, 0581T, 0582T, 20560-20561, 20700-20701, 36591-36592, 43752, 80500-80502, 90863, 90940, 92002-92014, 92227-92228, 92531-92532, 93792, 93793, 94002-94004, 94644, 94660-94662, 95851-95852, 96020, 96105, 96116, 96125-96130, 96132, 96136, 96138, 96146, 96156-96159, 96164-96168, 96360, 96365, 96369, 96372-96374, 96377, 96401-96406, 96409, 96413, 96416, 96420-96422, 96425-96440, 96446-96450, 96523, 97151, 97153-97158, 97169-97172, 97802-97804, 99091, 99172-99173, 99174, 99177, 99201-99217✦, 99231-99233, 99238, 99281-99285, 99408-99409, 99446-99449, 99451-99452, 99474, 99483, 99605-99606, G0102, G0245-G0246, G0250, G0270-G0271, G0380-G0384, G0396-G0397, G0442-G0447, G0459, G0463, G0473, G0498, G2011

99241 0362T, 0373T, 0469T, 0543T-0544T, 0567T-0574T, 0580T, 0581T, 0582T, 20560-20561, 36591-36592, 90863, 93792, 93793, 94002-94004, 94660-94662, 96523, 97151, 97153-97158, 99091, 99172-99173, 99174, 99177, 99421-99422, 99446-99449, 99451-99452, 99474, G0406-G0408✦, G0425-G0427✦, G0459✦, G0473, G0508-G0509✦

99242 0362T, 0373T, 0469T, 0543T-0544T, 0567T-0574T, 0580T, 0581T, 0582T, 20560-20561, 20701, 36591-36592, 90863, 93792, 93793, 94002-94004, 94660-94662, 96523, 97151, 97153-97158, 99091, 99172-99173, 99174, 99177, 99421-99423, 99446-99449, 99451-99452, 99474, G0406-G0408✦, G0425-G0427✦, G0459✦, G0473, G0508-G0509✦

99243 0362T, 0373T, 0469T, 0543T-0544T, 0567T-0574T, 0580T, 0581T, 0582T, 20560-20561, 20700-20701, 36591-36592, 90863, 93792, 93793, 94002-94004, 94660-94662, 96523, 97151, 97153-97158, 99091, 99172-99173, 99174, 99177, 99421-99423, 99446-99449, 99451-99452, 99474, G0406-G0408✦, G0425-G0427✦, G0459✦, G0473, G0508-G0509✦

99244 0362T, 0373T, 0469T, 0543T-0544T, 0567T-0574T, 0580T, 0581T, 0582T, 15774, 20560-20561, 20700-20701, 36591-36592, 62329, 90863, 93792, 93793, 94002-94004, 94660-94662, 96523, 97151, 97153-97158, 99091, 99172-99173, 99174, 99177, 99421-99423, 99446-99449, 99451-99452, 99474, G0406-G0408✦, G0425-G0427✦, G0459✦, G0473, G0508-G0509✦

99245 0362T, 0373T, 0469T, 0543T-0544T, 0567T-0574T, 0580T, 0581T, 0582T, 15774, 20560-20561, 20700-20701, 36591-36592, 62329, 90863, 93792, 93793, 94002-94004, 94660-94662, 96523, 97151, 97153-97158, 99091, 99172-99173, 99174, 99177, 99421-99423, 99446-99449, 99451-99452, 99474, G0406-G0408✦, G0425-G0427✦, G0459✦, G0473, G0508-G0509✦

99251 0362T, 0373T, 0469T, 0543T-0544T, 0567T-0574T, 0580T, 0581T, 0582T, 20560-20561, 20701, 36591-36592, 90863, 93792, 93793, 94002-94004, 94660-94662, 96127, 96523, 97151, 97153-97158, 99091, 99172-99173, 99174, 99177, 99241-99245, 99446-99449, 99451-99452, 99474, G0406-G0408✦, G0425-G0427✦, G0459✦, G0473, G0508-G0509✦

99252 0362T, 0373T, 0469T, 0543T-0544T, 0567T-0574T, 0580T, 0581T, 0582T, 20560-20561, 20701, 36591-36592, 90863, 93792, 93793, 94002-94004, 94660-94662, 96127, 96523, 97151, 97153-97158, 99091, 99172-99173, 99174, 99177, 99241-99245, 99446-99449, 99451-99452, 99474, G0406-G0408✦, G0425-G0427✦, G0459✦, G0473, G0508-G0509✦

99253 0362T, 0373T, 0469T, 0543T-0544T, 0567T-0574T, 0580T, 0581T, 0582T, 20560-20561, 20700-20701, 36591-36592, 62329, 90863, 93792, 93793, 94002-94004, 94660-94662, 96127, 96523, 97151, 97153-97158, 99091, 99172-99173, 99174, 99177, 99241-99245, 99446-99449, 99451-99452, 99474, G0406-G0408✦, G0425-G0427✦, G0459✦, G0473, G0508-G0509✦

99254 0362T, 0373T, 0469T, 0543T-0544T, 0567T-0574T, 0580T, 0581T, 0582T, 20560-20561, 20700-20701, 36591-36592, 62329, 90863, 93792, 93793, 94002-94004, 94660-94662, 96127, 96523, 97151, 97153-97158, 99091, 99172-99173, 99174, 99177, 99241-99245, 99446-99449, 99451-99452, 99474, G0406-G0408✦, G0425-G0427✦, G0459✦, G0473, G0508-G0509✦

99255 0362T, 0373T, 0469T, 0543T-0544T, 0567T-0574T, 0580T, 0581T, 0582T, 20560-20561, 20700-20701, 36591-36592, 62329, 90863, 93792, 93793, 94002-94004, 94660-94662, 96127, 96523, 97151, 97153-97158, 99091, 99172-99173, 99174, 99177, 99241-99245, 99446-99449, 99451-99452, 99474, G0406-G0408✦, G0425-G0427✦, G0459✦, G0473, G0508-G0509✦

99281 0362T, 0373T, 0469T, 36591-36592, 43752, 90863, 90940, 92002-92014, 92227-92228, 92531-92532, 93792, 93793, 94002-94004, 94660-94662, 95851-95852, 96020, 96105, 96116, 96125-96130, 96132, 96136, 96138, 96146, 96156-96159, 96164-96168, 96360, 96365, 96369, 96372-96374, 96377, 96401-96406, 96409, 96413, 96416, 96420-96422, 96425-96440, 96446-96450, 96523, 97151, 97153-97172, 97802-97804, 99091, 99172-99173, 99174, 99177, 99408-99409, 99446-99449, 99451-99452, 99474, 99605-99606, G0102, G0245-G0246, G0270-G0271, G0380✦, G0382-G0384✦, G0396-G0397, G0406-G0408, G0425-G0427, G0442-G0447, G0459, G0473, G0498, G0508-G0509, G2011

99282 0362T, 0373T, 0469T, 36591-36592, 43752, 90863, 90940, 92002-92014, 92227-92228, 92531-92532, 93792, 93793, 94002-94004, 94660-94662, 95851-95852, 96020, 96105, 96116, 96125-96130, 96132, 96136, 96138, 96146, 96156-96159, 96164-96168, 96360, 96365, 96369, 96372-96374, 96377, 96401-96406, 96409, 96413, 96416, 96420-96422, 96425-96440, 96446-96450, 96523, 97151, 97153-97172, 97802-97804, 99091, 99172-99173, 99174, 99177, 99281, 99408-99409, 99446-99449, 99451-99452, 99474, 99605-99606, G0102, G0245-G0246, G0270-G0271, G0380-G0384✦, G0396-G0397, G0406-G0408, G0425-G0427, G0442-G0447, G0459, G0473, G0498, G0508-G0509, G2011

99283 0362T, 0373T, 0469T, 36591-36592, 43752, 90863, 90940, 92002-92014, 92227-92228, 92531-92532, 93792, 93793, 94002-94004, 94660-94662, 95851-95852, 96020, 96105, 96116, 96125-96130, 96132, 96136, 96138, 96146, 96156-96159, 96164-96168, 96360, 96365, 96369, 96372-96374, 96377, 96401-96406, 96409, 96413, 96416, 96420-96422, 96425-96440, 96446-96450, 96523, 97151, 97153-97172, 97802-97804,

99091, 99172-99173, 99174, 99177, 99281-99282, 99408-99409,
99446-99449, 99451-99452, 99474, 99605-99606, G0102,
G0245-G0246, G0270-G0271, G0380-G0384✦, G0396-G0397,
G0406-G0408, G0425-G0427, G0442-G0447, G0459, G0473, G0498,
G0508-G0509, G2011

99284 0362T, 0373T, 0469T, 36591-36592, 43752, 90863, 90940, 92002-92014,
92227-92228, 92531-92532, 93792, 93793, 94002-94004, 94660-94662,
95851-95852, 96020, 96105, 96116, 96125-96130, 96132, 96136,
96138, 96146, 96156-96159, 96164-96168, 96360, 96365, 96369,
96372-96374, 96377, 96401-96406, 96409, 96413, 96416, 96420-96422,
96425-96440, 96446-96450, 96523, 97151, 97153-97172, 97802-97804,
99091, 99172-99173, 99174, 99177, 99281-99283, 99408-99409,
99446-99449, 99451-99452, 99463✦, 99474, 99605-99606, G0102,
G0245-G0246, G0270-G0271, G0380-G0384✦, G0396-G0397,
G0406-G0408, G0425-G0427, G0442-G0447, G0459, G0473, G0498,
G0508-G0509, G2011

99285 0362T, 0373T, 0469T, 36591-36592, 43752, 90863, 90940, 92002-92014,
92227-92228, 92531-92532, 93792, 93793, 94002-94004, 94660-94662,
95851-95852, 96020, 96105, 96116, 96125-96130, 96132, 96136,
96138, 96146, 96156-96159, 96164-96168, 96360, 96365, 96369,
96372-96374, 96377, 96401-96406, 96409, 96413, 96416, 96420-96422,
96425-96440, 96446-96450, 96523, 97151, 97153-97172, 97802-97804,
99091, 99172-99173, 99174, 99177, 99281-99284, 99408-99409,
99446-99449, 99451-99452, 99463✦, 99474, 99605-99606, G0102,
G0245-G0246, G0270-G0271, G0380-G0384✦, G0396-G0397,
G0406-G0408, G0425-G0427, G0442-G0447, G0459, G0473, G0498,
G0508-G0509, G2011

99291 0362T, 0373T, 0469T, 0543T-0544T, 0567T-0574T, 0580T, 0581T, 0582T,
15772, 15774, 20560-20561, 20700-20701, 36000, 36410-36415,
36591-36592, 36600, 43752-43753, 62329, 71045-71047, 80500-80502,
90846-90849, 90940, 92002-92014, 92227-92228, 92531-92532,
92953-92960, 93040-93042, 93318, 93355, 93561-93562, 93701, 93792,
93793, 94002-94004, 94375-94450, 94610, 94644, 94660-94662,
94760-94762, 94780-94781, 95851-95852, 96020, 96105, 96116,
96125-96130, 96132, 96136, 96138, 96146, 96156-96159, 96164-96168,
96360, 96365, 96369, 96372-96374, 96377, 96401-96406, 96409,
96413, 96416, 96420-96422, 96425-96440, 96446-96450, 96523, 97151,
97153-97158, 97169-97172, 97802-97804, 99091, 99172-99173, 99174,
99177, 99281-99285, 99408-99409, 99446-99449, 99451-99452,
99460-99462, 99474, 99477-99480, 99497-99498, 99605-99606, G0102,
G0245-G0246, G0250, G0270-G0271, G0380-G0384, G0396-G0397,
G0442-G0447, G0459, G0471, G0473, G0498, G0508-G0509, G2011

99292 0362T, 0373T, 0469T, 0543T-0544T, 0567T-0574T, 0580T, 0581T, 0582T,
20560-20561, 20700-20701, 36000, 36410, 36591-36592, 36600,
43752-43753, 62329, 71045-71047, 80500-80502, 90846-90849, 90940,
92002-92014, 92953-92960, 93040-93042, 93318, 93355, 93561-93562,
93792, 93793, 94002-94004, 94375-94450, 94660-94662, 94760-94762,
94780-94781, 95851-95852, 96020, 96116, 96127, 96156-96159,
96164-96168, 96523, 97151, 97153-97158, 97169-97172, 97802-97804,
99091, 99172-99173, 99174, 99177, 99281-99285, 99408-99409,
99446-99449, 99451-99452, 99474, 99497-99498, G0102,
G0245-G0246, G0250, G0270-G0271, G0396-G0397, G0442-G0447,
G0459, G0473, G2011

99354 0362T, 0373T, 0469T, 36591-36592, 43752, 90940, 92531-92532,
93561-93562, 93792, 93793, 94002-94004, 94660-94662, 96020, 96105,
96116, 96125, 96130, 96132, 96136, 96138, 96146, 96156-96159,
96164-96168, 96523, 97151, 97153-97158, 99091, 99172-99173, 99174,
99177, 99408-99409, 99415-99416, 99446-99449, 99451-99452,

99463✦, 99474, G0102, G0396-G0397, G0406-G0408✦, G0425-G0427✦,
G0442-G0447, G0459✦, G0473, G0508-G0509✦, G2011

99355 0362T, 0373T, 0469T, 36591-36592, 43752, 92531-92532, 93561-93562,
93792, 93793, 94002-94004, 94660-94662, 96020, 96105, 96116,
96125, 96130, 96132, 96136, 96138, 96146, 96156-96159,
96164-96168, 96523, 97151, 97153-97158, 99091, 99172-99173, 99174,
99177, 99408-99409, 99415-99416, 99446-99449, 99451-99452,
99463✦, 99474, G0102, G0396-G0397, G0406-G0408✦, G0425-G0427✦,
G0442-G0447, G0459✦, G0473, G0508-G0509✦, G2011

99356 0362T, 0373T, 0469T, 36591-36592, 43752, 90940, 92531-92532, 93792,
93793, 94002-94004, 94660-94662, 96020, 96105, 96116, 96125-96130,
96132, 96136, 96138, 96146, 96156-96159, 96164-96168, 96523,
97151, 97153-97158, 99091, 99172-99173, 99174, 99177, 99408-99409,
99446-99449, 99451-99452, 99463✦, 99474, G0102, G0396-G0397,
G0442-G0447, G0473, G2011

99357 0362T, 0373T, 0469T, 36591-36592, 43752, 92531-92532, 93792, 93793,
94002-94004, 94660-94662, 96020, 96105, 96116, 96125-96130, 96132,
96136, 96138, 96146, 96156-96159, 96164-96168, 96523, 97151,
97153-97158, 99091, 99172-99173, 99174, 99177, 99408-99409,
99446-99449, 99451-99452, 99463✦, 99474, G0102, G0396-G0397,
G0442-G0447, G0473, G2011

99358 0362T, 0373T, 0469T, 36591-36592, 43752, 90940, 92531-92532,
93561-93562, 93792, 93793, 94002-94004, 94660-94662, 96020, 96105,
96116, 96125-96130, 96132, 96136, 96138, 96146, 96156-96159,
96164-96168, 97151, 97153-97158, 98970-98972, 99091, 99172-99173,
99174, 99177, 99339-99340, 99366-99368, 99374-99375, 99377-99380,
99415-99416, 99421-99423, 99446-99449, 99452, 99474, G0102,
G0396-G0397, G0406-G0408✦, G0425-G0427✦, G0442-G0447, G0459✦,
G0473, G2011, G2061-G2063

99359 0362T, 0373T, 0469T, 36591-36592, 43752, 92531-92532, 93561-93562,
93792, 93793, 94002-94004, 94660-94662, 96020, 96105, 96116,
96125-96130, 96132, 96136, 96138, 96146, 96156-96159, 96164-96168,
97151, 97153-97158, 98970-98972, 99091, 99172-99173, 99174, 99177,
99339-99340, 99366-99368, 99374-99375, 99377-99380, 99415-99416,
99421-99423, 99446-99449, 99452, 99474, G0102, G0396-G0397,
G0406-G0408✦, G0425-G0427✦, G0442-G0447, G0459✦, G0473, G2011,
G2061-G2063

99360 0362T, 0373T, 0469T, 36591-36592, 43752, 92531-92532, 93792, 93793,
94002-94004, 94660-94662, 96020, 96116, 96127, 96156-96159,
96164-96168, 96523, 97151, 97153-97158, 97802-97804, 99091,
99172-99173, 99174, 99177, 99408-99409, 99474, G0102,
G0270-G0271, G0396-G0397, G0442-G0443, G2011

99384 0362T, 0373T, 0469T, 36591-36592, 93792, 93793, 94002-94004,
94660-94662, 96523, 97151, 97153-97158, 99091, 99446-99449,
99451-99452, 99474, G0444

99385 0362T, 0373T, 0469T, 36591-36592, 93792, 93793, 94002-94004,
94660-94662, 96523, 97151, 97153-97158, 99091, 99446-99449,
99451-99452, 99474, G0444

99386 0362T, 0373T, 0469T, 36591-36592, 93792, 93793, 94002-94004,
94660-94662, 96523, 97151, 97153-97158, 99091, 99446-99449,
99451-99452, 99474, G0444

99387 0362T, 0373T, 0469T, 36591-36592, 93792, 93793, 94002-94004,
94660-94662, 96523, 97151, 97153-97158, 99091, 99446-99449,
99451-99452, 99474, G0444

99394 0362T, 0373T, 0469T, 36591-36592, 93792, 93793, 94002-94004,
94660-94662, 96523, 97151, 97153-97158, 99091, 99446-99449,
99451-99452, 99474, G0444

99395 0362T, 0373T, 0469T, 36591-36592, 93792, 93793, 94002-94004, 94660-94662, 96523, 97151, 97153-97158, 99091, 99446-99449, 99451-99452, 99474, G0444

99396 0362T, 0373T, 0469T, 36591-36592, 93792, 93793, 94002-94004, 94660-94662, 96523, 97151, 97153-97158, 99091, 99446-99449, 99451-99452, 99474, G0444

99397 0362T, 0373T, 0469T, 36591-36592, 93792, 93793, 94002-94004, 94660-94662, 96523, 97151, 97153-97158, 99091, 99446-99449, 99451-99452, 99474, G0444

99415 0362T, 0373T, 0469T, 36591-36592, 43752, 90940, 92531-92532, 93561-93562, 93792, 93793, 94002-94004, 94660-94662, 96020, 96105, 96116, 96125, 96130, 96132, 96136, 96138, 96146, 96156-96159, 96164-96168, 96523, 97151, 97153-97158, 99091, 99172-99173, 99174, 99177, 99408-99409, 99446-99449, 99451-99452, G0102, G0396-G0397, G0442-G0447, G0473, G2011

99416 0362T, 0373T, 0469T, 36591-36592, 43752, 92531-92532, 93561-93562, 93792, 93793, 94002-94004, 94660-94662, 96020, 96105, 96116, 96125, 96130, 96132, 96136, 96138, 96146, 96156-96159, 96164-96168, 96523, 97151, 97153-97158, 99091, 99172-99173, 99174, 99177, 99408-99409, 99446-99449, 99451-99452, G0102, G0396-G0397, G0442-G0447, G0473, G2011

99417 No CCI edits apply to this code.

99421 0362T, 0373T, 0469T, 36591-36592, 93792, 93793, 94002-94004, 94660-94662, 96127, 96523, 97151, 97153-97158, 98966, 98970-98972, 99172-99173, 99174, 99177, 99211, 99441, 99474, G0250, G0378-G0379, G2061-G2063, Q3014

99422 0362T, 0373T, 0469T, 36591-36592, 93792, 93793, 94002-94004, 94660-94662, 96127, 96523, 97151, 97153-97158, 98966-98967, 98970-98972, 99172-99173, 99174, 99177, 99201, 99211-99212, 99421, 99441-99442, 99446, 99474, G0250, G0378-G0379, G2061-G2063, Q3014

99423 0362T, 0373T, 0469T, 36591-36592, 93792, 93793, 94002-94004, 94660-94662, 96127, 96523, 97151, 97153-97158, 98966-98968, 98970-98972, 99172-99173, 99174, 99177, 99201, 99211-99212, 99241, 99421-99422, 99441-99443, 99446-99447, 99451-99452, 99474, 99490, G0250, G0378-G0379, G0406, G2061-G2063, Q3014

99441 0362T, 0373T, 0469T, 36591-36592, 93792, 93793, 94002-94004, 94660-94662, 96127, 96523, 97151, 97153-97158, 98970-98972, 99091, 99172-99173, 99174, 99177, 99474, G0250, G2061-G2063

99442 0362T, 0373T, 0469T, 36591-36592, 93792, 93793, 94002-94004, 94660-94662, 96127, 96523, 97151, 97153-97158, 98970-98972, 99091, 99172-99173, 99174, 99177, 99421, 99474, G0250, G2061-G2063

99443 0362T, 0373T, 0469T, 36591-36592, 93792, 93793, 94002-94004, 94660-94662, 96127, 96523, 97151, 97153-97158, 98970-98972, 99091, 99172-99173, 99174, 99177, 99421-99422, 99446-99447, 99474, G0250, G2061-G2063

99446 0362T, 0373T, 0469T, 36591-36592, 76140, 93792, 93793, 94002-94004, 94660-94662, 96127, 96523, 97151-97158, 98966-98967, 98970-98972, 99091, 99172-99173, 99174, 99177, 99421, 99441-99442, 99451-99452✦, 99474, G0250

99447 0362T, 0373T, 0469T, 36591-36592, 76140, 93792, 93793, 94002-94004, 94660-94662, 96127, 96523, 97151, 97153-97158, 98966-98967, 98970-98972, 99091, 99172-99173, 99174, 99177, 99421-99422, 99441-99442, 99446, 99451-99452✦, 99474, G0250

99448 0362T, 0373T, 0469T, 36591-36592, 76140, 93792, 93793, 94002-94004, 94660-94662, 96127, 96523, 97151, 97153-97158, 98966-98968,

98970-98972, 99091, 99172-99173, 99174, 99177, 99421-99423, 99441-99443, 99446-99447, 99451-99452✦, 99474, G0250

99449 0362T, 0373T, 0469T, 36591-36592, 76140, 93792, 93793, 94002-94004, 94660-94662, 96127, 96523, 97151, 97153-97158, 98966-98968, 98970-98972, 99091, 99172-99173, 99174, 99177, 99421-99423, 99441-99443, 99446-99448, 99451-99452✦, 99474, G0250

99451 0362T, 0373T, 0469T, 36591-36592, 76140, 93792, 93793, 94002-94004, 94660-94662, 96127, 96523, 97151-97154, 97156-97158, 99091, 99172-99173, 99174, 99177, 99358-99359, 99421-99422, 99452✦, 99474, G0250

99452 0362T, 0373T, 0469T, 36591-36592, 93792, 93793, 94002-94004, 94660-94662, 96127, 96523, 99091, 99172-99173, 99174, 99177, 99421-99422, 99474, G0250

99464 0362T, 0373T, 0469T, 36591-36592, 43752, 92531-92532, 93792, 93793, 94002-94004, 94660-94662, 95851-95852, 96020, 96105, 96116, 96125-96130, 96132, 96136, 96138, 96146, 96156-96159, 96164-96168, 96369, 96523, 97151, 97153-97172, 97802-97804, 99091, 99172-99173, 99174, 99177, 99360, 99408-99409, 99446-99449, 99451-99452, 99462, 99474, G0102, G0270-G0271, G0396-G0397, G0442-G0443, G2011

99465 0362T, 0373T, 0469T, 36591-36592, 43752, 92531-92532, 93792, 93793, 94002-94004, 94660-94662, 95851-95852, 96020, 96105, 96116, 96125-96130, 96132, 96136, 96138, 96146, 96156-96159, 96164-96168, 96360, 96365, 96369, 96372-96374, 96377, 96401-96406, 96409, 96413, 96416, 96420-96422, 96425-96440, 96446-96450, 96523, 97151, 97153-97158, 97169-97172, 97802-97804, 99091, 99172-99173, 99174, 99177, 99408-99409, 99446-99449, 99451-99452, 99464, 99474, 99605-99606, G0102, G0270-G0271, G0396-G0397, G0442-G0443, G0498, G2011

99500 36591-36592, 96523

99501 36591-36592, 96523

99601 36591-36592, 96523

99602 36591-36592, 96523

G0101 36591-36592, 57410✦, 96523, 99201-99239, 99281-99285, 99291-99292, 99304-99310, 99315-99318, 99324-99328, 99334-99337, 99341-99350, 99354-99360, 99415-99416, 99446-99449, 99451-99452, 99455-99456, 99460-99466, 99468-99472, 99475-99480, 99483, 99485, 99497, G0181-G0182, G0380-G0384, G0406-G0408, G0425-G0427, G0463, G0508-G0509

G0124 88142-88143, 88147-88150, 88152-88153, 88164-88167, 88174-88175, G0141, G0147-G0148, P3000-P3001

G0130 0508T✦, 36591-36592, 76977✦, 77080✦, 78445, 96523

G0141 88142-88143, 88147-88150, 88152-88153, 88164-88167, 88174-88175, G0123, G0143-G0144, P3000

G0168 0213T, 0216T, 0228T, 0230T, 11000-11006, 11042-11047, 11900-11901, 13102, 13122, 13133, 13153, 36000, 36400-36410, 36420-36430, 36440, 36591-36592, 36600, 36640, 43752, 51701-51703, 62320-62327, 64400, 64405-64408, 64415-64435, 64445-64454, 64461-64463, 64479-64505, 64510-64530, 92012-92014, 93000-93010, 93040-93042, 93318, 93355, 94002, 94200, 94250, 94680-94690, 94770, 95812-95816, 95819, 95822, 95829, 95955, 96360-96368, 96372, 96374-96377, 96523, 97597-97598, 97602, 99155, 99156, 99157, 99211-99223, 99231-99255, 99291-99292, 99304-99310, 99315-99316, 99334-99337, 99347-99350, 99374-99375, 99377-99378, 99446-99449, 99451-99452, 99495-99496, G0463, G0471, J0670, J2001

G0425 36591-36592, 43752, 80500-80502, 90832-90833✦, 90836✦, 90839-90840✦, 90940, 92002-92014, 92531-92532, 93793, 94002-94004, 94644, 94660-94662, 95851-95852, 96020, 96116, 96127,

96156-96159, 96164-96168, 96360, 96365, 96369, 96372-96374, 96377, 96401-96406, 96409, 96413, 96416, 96420-96422, 96425-96440, 96446-96450, 96523, 97169-97172, 97802-97804, 99421-99423, 99452✣, G0102, G0245-G0246, G0250, G0270-G0271, G0406-G0408, G0424, G0459, G0498

G0426 36591-36592, 43752, 80500-80502, 90832-90834✣, 90836✣, 90839-90840✣, 90940, 92002-92014, 92531-92532, 93793, 94002-94004, 94644, 94660-94662, 95851-95852, 96020, 96116, 96127, 96156-96159, 96164-96168, 96360, 96365, 96369, 96372-96374, 96377, 96401-96406, 96409, 96413, 96416, 96420-96422, 96425-96440, 96446-96450, 96523, 97169-97172, 97802-97804, 99421-99423, 99452✣, G0102, G0245-G0246, G0250, G0270-G0271, G0406-G0408, G0424-G0425, G0459, G0498, G0508-G0509

G0427 36591-36592, 43752, 80500-80502, 90832-90834✣, 90836-90840✣, 90940, 92002-92014, 92531-92532, 93793, 94002-94004, 94644, 94660-94662, 95851-95852, 96020, 96116, 96127, 96156-96159, 96164-96168, 96360, 96365, 96369, 96372-96374, 96377, 96401-96406, 96409, 96413, 96416, 96420-96422, 96425-96440, 96446-96450, 96523, 97169-97172, 97802-97804, 99421-99423, 99452✣, G0102, G0245-G0246, G0250, G0270-G0271, G0406-G0408, G0424-G0426, G0459, G0498, G0508-G0509

G0438 36591-36592, 90791-90792, 90832-90834, 90836-90839, 90845, 92002-92014, 93793, 95851-95852, 96116, 96127, 96156-96159, 96164-96168, 96523, 97161-97172, 97802-97804, 99201-99215✣, 99281-99285✣, 99304-99310✣, 99315-99318✣, 99324-99328✣, 99334-99337✣, 99341-99350✣, 99446-99449, 99451-99452, G0250, G0270-G0271, G0380-G0384✣, G0439, G0444, G0459, G0463✣

G0439 36591-36592, 90791-90792, 90832-90834, 90836-90839, 90845, 92002-92014, 93793, 95851-95852, 96116, 96127, 96156-96159, 96164-96168, 96523, 97161-97172, 97802-97804, 99201-99215✣, 99281-99285✣, 99304-99310✣, 99315-99318✣, 99324-99328✣, 99334-99337✣, 99341-99350✣, 99446-99449, 99451-99452, G0250, G0270-G0271, G0380-G0384✣, G0459, G0463✣

P3001 88141-88143, 88147-88150, 88152-88153, 88164-88167, 88174-88175, 99201-99239, 99281-99285, 99291-99292, 99304-99310, 99315-99318, 99324-99328, 99334-99337, 99341-99350, 99354-99360, 99415-99416, 99455-99456, 99460-99466, 99468-99472, 99475-99480, 99483, 99485, 99497, G0123, G0141-G0148, G0380-G0384, G0406-G0408, G0425-G0427, G0463, G0508-G0509

Q0091 99201-99239, 99281-99285, 99291-99292, 99304-99310, 99315-99318, 99324-99328, 99334-99337, 99341-99350, 99354-99360, 99415-99416, 99455-99456, 99460-99466, 99468-99472, 99475-99480, 99483, 99485, 99497, G0181-G0182, G0380-G0384, G0406-G0408, G0425-G0427, G0463, G0508-G0509

CPT Index

A

Abdomen, Abdominal
Abscess, 49020
  Incision and Drainage
    Skin and Subcutaneous Tissue,
      10060-10061
  Open
    Peritoneal, 49020
    Peritonitis, Localized, 49020
Biopsy
  Open, 49000
  Percutaneous, 49180
Celiotomy, 49000
Cyst
  Destruction/Excision, 49203-49205
Delivery
  After Attempted Vaginal Delivery
    Delivery Only, 59620
    Postpartum Care, 59622
    Routine Care, 59618
  Delivery Only, 59514
  Peritoneal Abscess
    Open, 49020
    Peritonitis, Localized, 49020
  Postpartum Care, 59515
  Routine Care, 59510
  Tubal Ligation at Time of, 58611
  with Hysterectomy, 59525
Drainage, 49020
  Fluid, 49082-49083
  Skin and Subcutaneous Tissue, 10060-10061
Ectopic Pregnancy, 59130
Endometrioma, 49203-49205
  Destruction/Excision, 49203-49205
Exploration, 49000-49002, 49020, 49082-49084
  Blood Vessel, 35840
  Staging, 58960
Incision, 49000-49002, 49020, 49082-49084
  Staging, 58960
Insertion
  Catheter, 49324
Intraperitoneal
  Catheter Insertion, 49324
  Catheter Revision, 49325
Laparoscopy, 49320-49322, 49324-49327
Laparotomy
  Exploration, 49000-49002, 58960
  Hemorrhage Control, 49002
  Reopening, 49002
  Second Look, 58960
  Staging, 58960
  with Biopsy, 49000
Needle Biopsy
  Mass, 49180
Paracentesis, 49082-49083
Peritoneal Abscess, 49020
Peritoneal Lavage, 49084
Radical Resection, 51597
Tumor
  Destruction/Excision, 49203-49205
Tumor Staging, 58960
Ultrasound, 76700-76705
Wall
  Debridement
    Infected, 11005-11006
  Removal
    Mesh, 11008
    Prosthesis, 11008
Abdominal Plane Block
Bilateral, 64488-64489
Unilateral, 64486-64487
Abdominohysterectomy
Radical, 58210
Resection of Ovarian Malignancy, 58951, 58953-58956
Supracervical, 58180
Total, 58150, 58200
  with Colpo-Urethrocystopexy, 58152
  with Omentectomy, 58956

Abdominohysterectomy — *continued*
Total — *continued*
  with Partial Vaginectomy, 58200
Ablation
Endometrial, 58353-58356, 58563
Endometrium
  Ultrasound Guidance, 58356
Ultrasound
  Ultrasound Focused, 0071T-0072T
  Uterine Tumor, 0071T-0072T
Uterus
  Fibroids, 0404T [58674]
  Leiomyomata, 0071T-0072T
  Tumor
    Ultrasound, Focused, 0071T-0072T
Abortion
Incomplete, 59812
Induced by
  Amniocentesis Injection, 59850-59852
  Dilation and Curettage, 59840
  Dilation and Evacuation, 59841
  Saline, 59850-59851
  Vaginal Suppositories, 59855-59856
  with Hysterotomy, 59100, 59852, 59857
Missed
  First Trimester, 59820
  Second Trimester, 59821
Septic, 59830
Spontaneous, 59812
Therapeutic, 59840-59852
  by Saline, 59850
    with Dilatation and Curettage, 59851
    with Hysterotomy, 59852
Abscess
Abdomen
  Drainage, 49020
    Peritoneal
      Open, 49020
      Peritonitis, Localized, 49020
    Skin and Subcutaneous Tissue
      Complicated, 10061
      Multiple, 10061
      Simple, 10060
      Single, 10060
Bartholin's Gland
  Incision and Drainage, 56420
Ovarian
  Incision and Drainage, 58820-58822
    Abdominal Approach, 58822
    Vaginal Approach, 58820
Ovary
  Incision and Drainage
    Abdominal Approach, 58822
    Vaginal Approach, 58820
Paraurethral Gland
  Incision and Drainage, 53060
Perineum
  Incision and Drainage, 56405
Peritoneum
  Incision and Drainage
    Open, 49020
Skene's Gland
  Incision and Drainage, 53060
Skin
  Incision and Drainage, 10060-10061
    Complicated, 10061
    Multiple, 10061
    Simple, 10060
    Single, 10060
  Puncture Aspiration, 10160
Vagina
  Incision and Drainage, 57010
Vulva
  Incision and Drainage, 56405
Absolute Neutrophil Count (ANC), 85048
Adenovirus
Antigen Detection
  Enzyme Immunoassay, 87390-87391, 87426

Adhesion, Adhesions
Intestinal
  Enterolysis
    Laparoscopic, 44180
Intrauterine
  Lysis, 58559
Labial
  Lysis, 56441
Pelvic
  Lysis, 58660, 58662, 58740
Urethral
  Lysis, 53500
Adjustment
Transperineal Periurethral Balloon, 0551T
Administration
Health Risk Assessment, 96160-96161
Immunization
  with Counseling, 90460-90461
  without Counseling, 90471-90474
Adrenogenital Syndrome, 56805, 57335
Advanced Life Support
Emergency Department Services, 99281-99285
Advancement Flap
Skin, Adjacent Tissue Transfer, 14040-14041
AFI, 76815
Afluria, 90655-90658
After Hours Medical Services, 99050-99060
AGTT, 82951-82952
AIDS
Antibodies, 86701-86703
Virus, 86701, 86703
Alexander's Operation, 58400-58410
Amniocentesis
Diagnostic, 59000
Induced Abortion, 59850
  with Dilation and Curettage, 59851
  with Dilation and Evacuation, 59851
  with Hysterotomy, 59852
Urine
  with Amniotic Fluid Reduction, 59001
with Amniotic Fluid Reduction, 59001
Amnioinfusion
Transabdominal, 59070
Amnion
Amniocentesis, 59000
  with Amniotic Fluid Reduction, 59001
Amnioinfusion
  Transabdominal, 59070
Amniotic Fluid
Index, 76815
Amputation
Cervix
  Total, 57530
Analysis
Semen, 89320-89322
  Sperm Isolation, 89260-89261
Anastomosis
Fallopian Tube, 58750
Oviduct, 58750
Tubotubal, 58750
ANC, 85048
Anesthesia
Emergency, 99058
Pelvis
  Examination, 57400
Vagina
  Dilation, 57400
  Removal
    Foreign Body, 57415
Antepartum Care
Antepartum Care Only, 59425-59426
Cesarean Delivery, 59510
  Previous, 59610-59618
Included with
  Cesarean Delivery, 59510
    Failed NSVD, Previous C–Section, 59618
  Vaginal Delivery, 59400
    Previous C–Section, 59610
Vaginal Delivery, 59425-59426
Anti D Immunoglobulin, 90384-90386

Antibiotic Sensitivity
Minimum Inhibitory Concentration, 87186
Antibody Identification
Immunoassay, 86769 [86328]
Antibody
Chlamydia, 86632
Coronavirus Disease (COVID-19), 86769 [86328, 86413]
Herpes Simplex, 86694-86696
HIV, 86701-86703
HIV–1, 86701, 86703
HIV–2, 86702-86703
Severe Acute Respiratory Syndrome Coronavirus 2 (SARS-CoV-2), 86769 [86328, 86413]
Sperm, 89325
Antigen Detection
Enzyme Immunoassay, 87390-87391, 87426
  HIV–1, 87390
  HIV–2, 87391
  Severe Acute Respiratory Syndrome Coronavirus (eg, SARS-CoV, SARS-CoV-2 [COVID-19]), 87426
Immunoassay
  Direct Optical (Visual), 87808, 87850-87880
    Neisseria Gonorrhoeae, 87850
    Streptococcus, Group A, 87880
    Trichomonas Vaginalis, 87808
Immunofluorescence, 87270
  Chlamydia Trachomatis, 87270
Anus
Lesion
  Destruction, 46900-46917
  Excision, 46922
ART, 86592-86593
Artery
Middle Cerebral Artery, Fetal Vascular Studies, 76821
Umbilical
  Vascular Study, 76820
Artificial Insemination, 58976
In Vitro Fertilization
  Culture Oocyte, 89272
  Fertilize Oocyte, 89280-89281
  Retrieve Oocyte, 58970
  Transfer Embryo, 58974-58976
  Transfer Gamete, 58976
Intracervical, 58321
Intrauterine, 58322
Sperm Washing, 58323
Aspiration
Amniotic Fluid
  Diagnostic, 59000
  Therapeutic, 59001
Bladder, 51100-51102
Cyst
  Ovarian, 49322
Fetal Fluid, 59074
Pelvis
  Endoscopy, 49322
Assessment
Health Risk
  Caregiver-Focused, 96161
  Patient-Focused, 96160
Online
  Consult Physician, 99446-99449 [99451]
  Nonphysician, 98970-98972
  Physician, [99421, 99422, 99423]
  Referral, [99452]
Telephone
  Consult Physician, 99446-99449 [99451]
  Nonphysician, 98966-98968
  Physician, 99441-99443
  Referral, [99452]
Assisted
Zonal Hatching (AZH), 89253
Attendance and Resuscitation Services
Newborn, 99464
AutoPap, 88152

CPT Index

Furuncle
Incision and Drainage, 10060-10061

G

Gamete Intrafallopian Transfer (GIFT), 58976
Gamete Transfer
In Vitro Fertilization, 58976
GARDASIL, 90649
Genitalia
Tissue Transfer, Adjacent, 14040-14041
GIFT, 58976
Globulin, Rh Immune, 90384-90386
Globulin
Immune, 90384-90386
Glucose
Blood Test, 82948-82950
Tolerance Test, 82951-82952
Gonadotropin
Chorionic, 84702-84703
GTT, 82951-82952

H

Hamster Penetration Test, 89329
Handling
Specimen, 99000-99001
Harvesting
Eggs for In Vitro Fertilization, 58970
HCG, 84702-84703
Hct, 85013-85014
Health Risk Assessment Instrument, 96160-96161
Heart
Resuscitation, 92950
Heel
Collection of Blood, 36415-36416
Hematoma
Incision and Drainage
Skin, 10140
Puncture Aspiration, 10160
Skin
Incision and Drainage, 10140
Puncture Aspiration, 10160
Vagina
Incision and Drainage, 57022-57023
Hemogram
Added Indices, 85025-85027
Automated, 85025-85027
Manual, 85014-85018
Hemophilus Influenza
B Vaccine, 90748
Hemorrhage
Abdomen, 49002
Uterus
Postpartum, 59160
Vagina, 57180
Hepatitis B and Hib, 90748
Hepatitis B Immunization, 90739-90748
Hepatitis B Vaccine
Dosage
Adolescent, 90743-90744
Adult, 90739, 90746
Dialysis Patient, 90747
Immunosuppressed, 90740, 90747
Pediatric, 90744
Adolescent, 90743-90744
with Hemophilus Influenza Vaccine, 90748
Herpes Simplex Virus
Antibody, 86696
Antigen Detection
Nucleic Acid, 87528-87530
Hgb, 85018
Hidradenitis
Suppurative
Incision and Drainage, 10060-10061
History and Physical
Pelvic Exam Under Anesthesia, 57410
Preventive
Established Patient, 99394-99397
New Patient, 99384-99387
HIV Antibody, 86701-86703
HIV Detection
Antibody, 86701-86703
Antigen, 87390-87391, 87534-87539

HIV-1
Antigen Detection
Enzyme Immunoassay, 87390
HIV-2
Antigen Detection
Enzyme Immunoassay, 87391
HIV, 86701-86703, 87390-87391, 87534-87539
Home Services
Home Infusion Procedures, 99601-99602
Postnatal Assessment, 99501
Prenatal Monitoring, 99500
Hormone Pellet Implantation, 11980
Hospital Services
Inpatient Services
Discharge Services, 99238-99239
Initial Care New or Established Patient, 99221-99223
Initial Hospital Care, 99221-99223
Newborn, 99464-99465
Prolonged Services, 99356-99357
Subsequent Hospital Care, 99231-99233
Observation
Discharge Services, 99234-99236
Initial Care, 99218-99220
New or Established Patient, 99218-99220
Same Day Admission
Discharge Services, 99234-99236
HSG, 58340
Huhner Test, 89300-89320
Human
Papillomavirus Detection, [87623, 87624, 87625]
Papillomavirus Vaccine, 90649-90651
Hydatidiform Mole
Evacuation and Curettage, 59870
Excision, 59100
Hydration, 96360-96361
Hydrotubation, 58350
Hymen
Excision, 56700
Incision, 56442
Hymenal Ring
Revision, 56700
Hymenectomy, 56700
Hymenotomy, 56442
Hypogastric Plexus
Destruction, 64681
Injection
Anesthetic, 64517
Neurolytic, 64681
Hysterectomy
Abdominal
Radical, 58210
Resection of Ovarian Malignancy, 58951, 58953-58956
Supracervical, 58180
Total, 58150, 58200
with Colpo-Urethrocystopexy, 58152
with Omentectomy, 58956
with Partial Vaginectomy, 58200
Cesarean
After Cesarean Section, 59525
with Closure of Vesicouterine Fistula, 51925
Laparoscopic, 58541-58544, 58548, 58570-58575
Vaginal, 58260-58270, 58290-58294, 58550-58554
Laparoscopic, 58550
Radical, 58285
Removal Tubes
Ovaries, 58262-58263, 58291-58292, 58552, 58554
Repair of Enterocele, 58263, 58292-58294
with Colpectomy, 58275-58280
with Colpo-Urethrocystopexy, 58267
Wertheim, 58210
Hysterolysis, 58559
Hysteroplasty, 58540
Hysterorrhaphy, 58520, 59350
Hysterosalpingography
Catheterization, 58345

Hysterosalpingography — continued
Catheterization — continued
Introduction of Contrast, 58340
Hysteroscopy
Ablation
Endometrial, 58563
Diagnostic, 58555
Lysis
Adhesions, 58559
Placement
Fallopian Tube Implants, 58565
Removal
Impacted Foreign Body, 58562
Leiomyomata, 58561
Resection
of Intrauterine Septum, 58560
Surgical with Biopsy, 58558
with Endometrial Ablation, 58563
with Lysis of Adhesions, 58559
Hysterotomy, 59100
Induced Abortion
with Amniotic Injections, 59852
with Vaginal Suppositories, 59857
Hysterotrachelectomy, 57530

I

Ichthyosis, Sex-Linked, 86592-86593
Identification
Oocyte from Follicular Fluid, 89254
Sperm
from Aspiration, 89257
Immune Globulin Administration, 96365-96368
Immune Globulins
Rho (D), 90384-90386
Immunization
Active
Hemophilus Influenza B, 90748
Hepatitis B, 90740-90748
Hepatitis B, Hemophilus Influenza B (HIB), 90748
Influenza, 90655-90660
Administration
with Counseling, 90460-90461
without Counseling, 90471-90474
Passive
Hyperimmune Serum Globulin, 90384-90386
Immunoassay
Infectious Agent, [86328]
Immunodeficiency Virus Type 1, Human, 87390
Immunodeficiency Virus Type 2, Human, 87391
Implant
Drug Delivery Device, 11981, 11983
Fallopian Tube, 58565
Hormone Pellet, 11980
Mesh
Vaginal Repair, 57267
Ovum, 58976
Tubouterine, 58752
In Vitro Fertilization
Biopsy Oocyte, 89290-89291
Culture Oocyte
Extended, 89272
Embryo Hatching, 89253
Fertilize Oocyte
Microtechnique, 89280-89281
Identify Oocyte, 89254
Insemination of Oocyte, 89268
Prepare Embryo, 89255
Retrieve Oocyte, 58970
Transfer Embryo, 58974-58976
Transfer Gamete, 58976
Incision and Drainage
Abdomen
Fluid, 49082-49083
Abscess
Abdomen, Abdominal
Peritoneal, 49020
Peritonitis, Localized, 49020
Skin and Subcutaneous Tissue
Complicated, 10061
Multiple, 10061
Simple, 10060
Single, 10060
Bartholin's Gland, 56420
Ovary, 58820-58822

Incision and Drainage — continued
Abscess — continued
Ovary — continued
Abdominal Approach, 58822
Vaginal Approach, 58820
Paraurethral Gland, 53060
Perineum, 56405
Peritoneum
Open, 49020
Skene's Gland, 53060
Skin, 10060-10061
Vagina, 57010-57020
Vulva, 56405
Bulla
Skin
Puncture Aspiration, 10160
Cyst
Ovarian, 58800-58805
Skin, 10060-10061
Pilonidal, 10080-10081
Puncture Aspiration, 10160
Fluid Collection
Skin, 10140
Foreign Body
Skin, 10120-10121
Furuncle, 10060-10061
Hematoma
Skin, 10140
Puncture Aspiration, 10160
Vagina, 57022-57023
Pilonidal Cyst, 10080-10081
Seroma
Skin, 10140
Vagina, 57020
Wound Infection
Skin, 10180
Incision
Abdomen, 49000
Exploration, 58960
Bladder
Catheterization, 51045
with Destruction, 51020-51030
with Radiotracer, 51020
Hymenotomy, 56442
Skin, 10060-10180
Uterus
Remove Lesion, 59100
Vagina
Exploration, 57000
Inclusion Bodies
Smear, 87210
Incomplete
Abortion, 59812
Induced
Abortion
by Dilation and Curettage, 59840
by Dilation and Evacuation, 59841
by Saline, 59850-59851
by Vaginal Suppositories, 59855-59856
with Hysterotomy, 59100, 59852, 59857
Infection
Drainage
Postoperative Wound, 10180
Immunoassay, [86328]
Infectious Agent Detection
Antigen Detection
Enzyme Immunoassay, 87390-87391, 87426
HIV-1, 87390
HIV-2, 87391
Severe Acute Respiratory Syndrome Coronavirus (eg, SARS-CoV, SARS-CoV-2 [COVID-19]), 87426
Immunoassay
Direct Optical (Visual), 87808, 87850-87880
Neisseria Gonorrhoeae, 87850
Streptococcus, Group A, 87880
Trichomonas Vaginalis, 87808
Immunofluorescence, 87270

CPT Index

© 2020 Optum360, LLC   ● **New**   ▲ **Revised**   ✛ **Add On**   **AMA: CPT Assist [Resequenced]**

Coding Companion for Ob/Gyn

CPT Index